Pharmacology and Therapeutics for Dentistry

7TH EDITION

PHARMACOLOGY AND THERAPEUTICS FOR DENTISTRY

FRANK J. DOWD, DDS, PhD
Professor Emeritus
Pharmacology
Creighton University, School of Medicine and School of Dentistry
Omaha, Nebraska

BARTON S. JOHNSON, DDS, MS
Director, General Practice Residency Program
Swedish Medical Center
Private Practice
Seattle Special Care Dentistry
Seattle, Washington

ANGELO J. MARIOTTI, DDS, PhD
Professor and Chair
Periodontology
The Ohio State University
Columbus, Ohio

ELSEVIER

ELSEVIER

3251 Riverport Lane
St. Louis, Missouri 63043

PHARMACOLOGY AND THERAPEUTICS FOR DENTISTRY,
SEVENTH EDITION ISBN: 978-0-323-39307-2

Notices

Knowledge and best practice in this field are constantly changing. As new research and experience broaden our understanding, changes in research methods, professional practices, or medical treatment may become necessary.

Practitioners and researchers must always rely on their own experience and knowledge in evaluating and using any information, methods, compounds, or experiments described herein. In using such information or methods they should be mindful of their own safety and the safety of others, including parties for whom they have a professional responsibility.

With respect to any drug or pharmaceutical products identified, readers are advised to check the most current information provided (i) on procedures featured or (ii) by the manufacturer of each product to be administered, to verify the recommended dose or formula, the method and duration of administration, and contraindications. It is the responsibility of practitioners, relying on their own experience and knowledge of their patients, to make diagnoses, to determine dosages and the best treatment for each individual patient, and to take all appropriate safety precautions.

To the fullest extent of the law, neither the Publisher nor the authors, contributors, or editors, assume any liability for any injury and/or damage to persons or property as a matter of products liability, negligence or otherwise, or from any use or operation of any methods, products, instructions, or ideas contained in the material herein.

Library of Congress Cataloging-in-Publication Data

Names: Dowd, Frank J., 1939- editor. | Johnson, Barton S., editor. | Mariotti, Angelo J., editor.
Title: Pharmacology and therapeutics for dentistry / [edited by] Frank J. Dowd, Barton S. Johnson, Angelo J. Mariotti.
Description: 7th edition. | St. Louis, Missouri : Elsevier, Inc., [2017] | Includes bibliographical references and index.
Identifiers: LCCN 2016020799| ISBN 9780323393072 (hardback : alk. paper) | ISBN 9780323445955 (e-book)
Subjects: | MESH: Pharmacological Phenomena | Dentistry | Pharmaceutical Preparations | Pharmaceutical Preparations, Dental | Drug-Related Side Effects and Adverse Reactions
Classification: LCC RM300 | NLM QV 50 | DDC 615.102/46176--dc23 LC record available at https://lccn.loc.gov/2016020799

Executive Content Strategist: Kathy Falk
Content Development Manager: Jolynn Gower
Associate Content Development Specialist: Laura Klein
Publishing Services Manager: Deepthi Unni
Project Manager: Kamatchi Madhavan
Book Designer: Brian Salisbury

Printed in United States of America.

Last digit is the print number: 9 8 7 6 5 4 3 2

REMEMBERING JOHN A. YAGIELA, DDS, PhD, AND ENID A. NEIDLE, PhD

Since the publishing of our last edition (6th) of this textbook, we have lost two of our former editors, dear friends, and true giants in the field of dental education: John A. Yagiela and Enid A. Neidle. Both had been editors through all of the previous editions of this textbook, and both were very instrumental in providing the initial focus and establishing its content. This is the first time since 1980 that the names of these two outstanding individuals will not appear on the book as editors. John and Enid have left a lasting legacy. We dedicate this edition to their memory as we carry on the tradition of providing a current and thorough treatment of pharmacology for dental students and the dental profession.

John Allen Yagiela was born in Washington, DC, but grew up in Los Angeles.

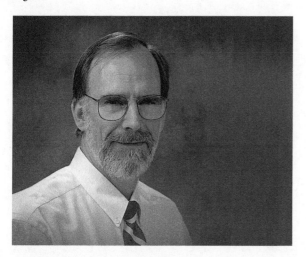

He received his dental degree from UCLA in 1971 and his PhD in pharmacology from the University of Utah in 1975 and completed a residency in anesthesiology from the UCLA School of Medicine in 1983. Dr. Yagiela used his expertise in pharmacology and anesthesiology to make this textbook the standard reference for all dental students. His contributions to critical chapters in principles of pharmacology and dental anesthesia were immensely important for the foundation of basic pharmacologic principles for dental students and professionals. Moreover, as the lead editor, he was tireless in his effort to make certain all chapters were accurate and current. John applied his vast knowledge and abundant energy to all the things that are required to insure a quality textbook. He was always helpful to contributors and often helped authors who needed assistance with certain aspects of their chapters. This included everything from providing expert advice on the text, to providing figures to authors, down to simply explaining when to correctly use a dash. We always found him supportive and willing to provide information and advice on many areas of pharmacology. The field of dental anesthesiology and dental education in general, as well as this text, will be forever in his debt. John was active as a clinician in the area of dental anesthesiology. Indeed, he was a key and devoted advocate for the field of dental anesthesiology and was largely responsible for spearheading the recognition of anesthesiology as a specialty of dentistry. John spent the majority of his academic carrier at UCLA School of Dentistry where he held several leadership positions, including professor (later Professor Emeritus) and Chair, Department of Diagnostic and Surgical Sciences. He was also in demand as a keynote speaker and has received many academic awards. On a personal note, he was a kind, fun, and an ever-inquisitive man who delighted in the wonders of the universe.

Enid Anne Neidle received her PhD from the Department of Physiology at Columbia University.

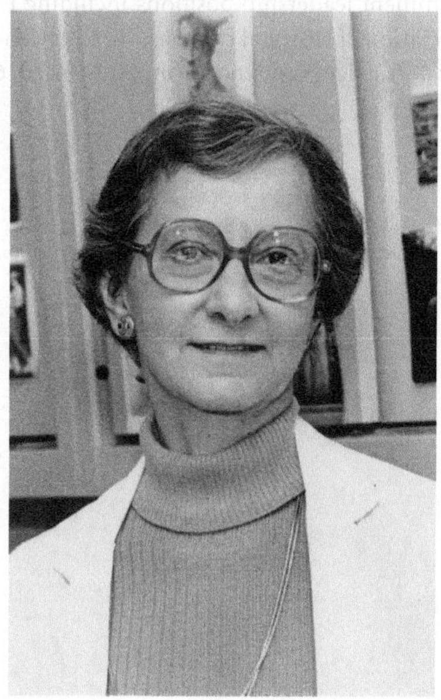

Her first faculty position was in the Department of Pharmacology at the Jefferson Medical College in 1950, but she moved to New York University in 1955 to become an Instructor in the Department of Physiology, which began a long career in the College of Dentistry. Dr. Neidle was the initial force behind this text and has had a key role in the previous editions. It was her insight that brought to fruition the first thorough textbook of pharmacology and therapeutics designed for the dental profession. As the textbook's first lead editor, she was dedicated to finding key people to contribute to the text and deciding on its focus to better serve the dental community. She was also a major contributor to dental education. Dr. Neidle was professor (later Professor Emeritus) and Chair, Department of Pharmacology, New York University School of Dentistry. Her initial research contributed to the field of cholinergic and anticholinergic drugs and later to dental education. She spent 33 years of her career at New York University, and she held several positions in organized dentistry, including Assistant Executive Director of Scientific Affairs for the America Dental Association for 6.5 years. One of her passions was to further the cause of women in dentistry. She received several honors for her work and dedication, including a national scholarship named in her honor. Enid was also in demand as a public speaker and was an early advocate of evidence-based dentistry. Those of us who knew her from the first edition of this textbook remember Enid for her abundant organizational skills and devotion to academic dentistry. (From those early years on, I found her most supportive and instructive. – FD)

HONORING BART JOHNSON, DDS, MS

We are deeply saddened by the recent passing of Bart Johnson, one of the three editors of this textbook. Bart was an editor not only of this edition but also the sixth edition as well as an author over the previous three editions. In 2015, Dr. Johnson was diagnosed with stage 4 colon cancer. Nonetheless, he remained an editor until this edition was finished.

Barton Johnson received his DDS degree in 1985 from UCLA. He continued on at UCLA in a general practice residency, and later earned an MS degree in Oral Biology. He was a faculty member at the University of Washington School of Dentistry from 1991 to 2007, and directed its General Practice Residency program during that time. Bart held many prominent leadership positions including President of the American Association of Hospital Dentists. He had been Director of the Swedish General Practice Residency from 2009 to 2016. Dr. Johnson specialized in special care dentistry, serving the needs of patients with significant underlying medical issues. He also contributed his knowledge and experience as editor and author. His expertise included pharmacology, internal medicine, medical emergencies, hospital dentistry, and basic and advanced cardiac life support.

We deeply appreciate all the wonderful work he did with the book, especially with the battle he had and with his extensive clinical responsibilities. He made several critical editorial contributions to the book. He was a trusted colleague who offered expert advice, and is the sole author of two chapters in the book. We are all grateful and proud of his many contributions to dental pharmacology. It has been a joy to work with Bart and to witness his courage and positive attitude while dealing with his disease. We appreciate his dedication to the book and his professionalism even when it was a special challenge.

It is with the utmost respect and gratitude that we honor Bart.

ABOUT THE EDITORS

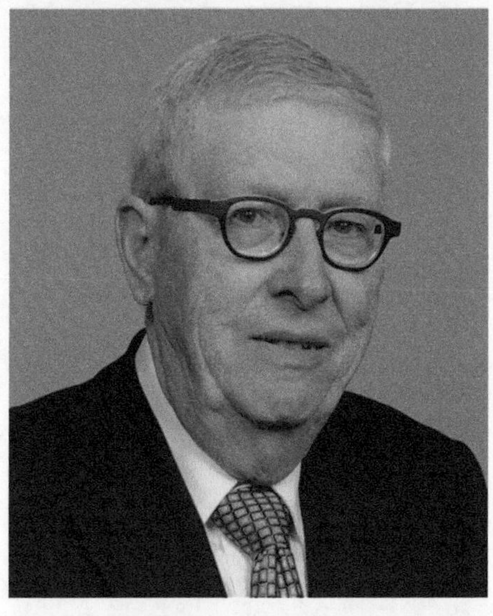

FRANK J. DOWD

Frank J. Dowd is Professor Emeritus, Creighton University School of Medicine and School of Dentistry. He received his DDS degree from Creighton University School of Dentistry and his PhD degree in pharmacology from Baylor College of Medicine. He spent his professional career at Creighton University, most of it as Chair, Department of Pharmacology, School of Medicine.

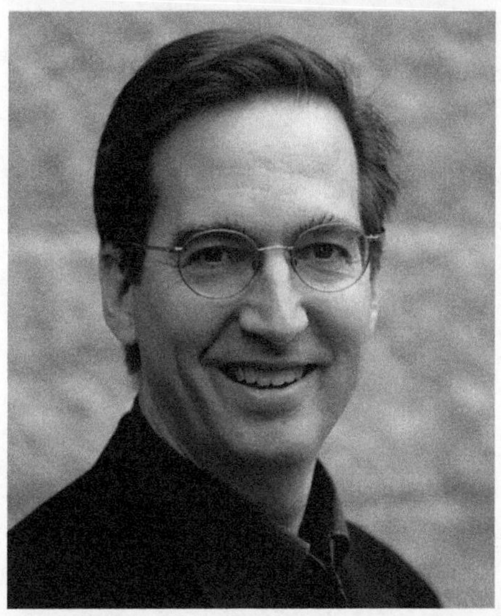

BARTON S. JOHNSON

Barton S. Johnson received his DDS, GPR Certificate, and MS in oral biology (with a molecular biology focus) from UCLA. His career has focused on the dental care of high-risk medically, mentally, emotionally, and physically challenged people. He was, until his passing, the Director of the Swedish Medical Center GPR program in Seattle.

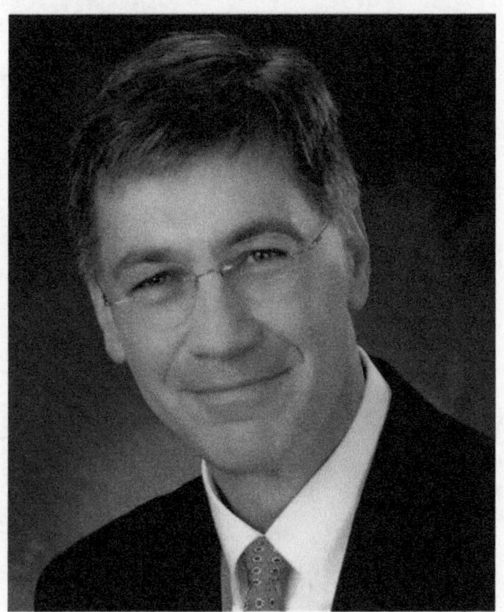

ANGELO J. MARIOTTI

Angelo J. Mariotti graduated from Grove City College with a BS in biology and education and received his PhD in pharmacology/toxicology and DDS from West Virginia University as well as specialty training in periodontology from Virginia Commonwealth University. He currently serves as Professor and Chair of Periodontology at The Ohio State University.

CONTRIBUTORS

Peter W. Abel, PhD
Professor
Department of Pharmacology
Creighton University School of Medicine
Omaha, Nebraska

Marc-Alain Babi, MD
Neurocritical Care Fellow
Department of Neurology
Duke University Hospital
Durham, North Carolina

Jeffrey D. Bennett, DMD
Professor and Chair
Department of Oral Surgery and Hospital Dentistry
School of Dentistry
Indiana University
Indianapolis, Indiana

Charles S. Bockman, PhD
Assistant Professor
Department of Pharmacology
Creighton University School of Medicine
Omaha, Nebraska

James T. Boyd, MD
Associate Professor
Department of Neurological Sciences
University of Vermont
Burlington, Vermont

George A. Cook, PhD
Professor
Department of Pharmacology
University of Tennessee
Health Science Center
Memphis, Tennessee

Matthew R. Cooke, DDS, MD, MPH
Assistant Professor
Department of Dental Anesthesiology
School of Dental Medicine
Pittsburgh University
Pittsburgh, Pennsylvania

Xi-Qin Ding, PhD
Associate Professor
Department of Cell Biology
College of Medicine
University of Oklahoma Health Sciences Center
Oklahoma City, Oklahoma

Raymond A. Dionne, DDS, PhD
Research Professor
Department of Pharmacology and Toxicology
Brody School of Medicine at East Carolina University
Greenville, North Carolina

Clayton English, PharmD
Associate Professor
Department of Pharmacology Practice
Albany College of Pharmacy and Health Sciences
Colchester, Vermont
Psychiatric Pharmacist
University of Vermont
Medical Center
Burlington, Vermont
Adjunct Assistant Professor
Department of Psychiatry
University of Vermont
Burlington, Vermont

Sean Flynn, PhD
Assistant Professor
Department of Neurological Sciences
University of Vermont
Burlington, Vermont

Gail T. Galasko, PhD
Professor and Pharmacology Course Director
Department of Biomedical Sciences
College of Medicine
Florida State University
Tallahassee, Florida

Steven I. Ganzberg, DMD, MS
Clinical Professor of Anesthesiology
UCLA School of Dentistry
Los Angeles, California
Editor-in-Chief, Anesthesia Progress

James N. Gibson, PharmD
Clinical Pharmacist-Hematology/Oncology
University of Washington Medical Center
Seattle Cancer Care Alliance
Seattle, Washington
Clinical Instructor
University of Washington
School of Pharmacy
Seattle, Washington

Joseph A. Giovannitti Jr., DMD
Professor and Chair
Department of Dental Anesthesiology
Director of Anesthesia
Center for Patients with Special Needs
University of Pittsburgh
School of Dental Medicine
Pittsburgh, Pennsylvania

Denis M. Grant, PhD
Professor
Department of Pharmacology and Toxicology
University of Toronto
Toronto, Ontario, Canada

Karen S. Gregson, PhD
Adjunct Professor
Pharmacology
Bradley University
Peoria, Illinois

David A. Haas, DDS, PhD
Dean and Professor
Faculty of Dentistry
University of Toronto
Toronto, Ontario, Canada

David W. Hein, PhD
Vice Provost for Academic Strategy
Peter K Knoefel Endowed Chair
Professor and Chair
Department of Pharmacology and Toxicology
University of Louisville
Louisville, Kentucky

Elliot V. Hersh, DMD, MS, PhD
Professor of Oral and Maxillofacial Surgery/Pharmacology
University of Pennsylvania, School of Dental Medicine
Philadelphia, Pennsylvania

Harrell E. Hurst, MS, PhD
Professor Emeritus
Pharmacology and Toxicology
University of Louisville
School of Medicine
Louisville, Kentucky

William B. Jeffries, PhD
Senior Associate Dean for Medical Education
Professor of Pharmacology
University of Vermont
College of Medicine
Burlington, Vermont

Anahid Jewett, PhD, MPH
Professor and Director of Tumor Immunology Laboratory
Division of Oral Biology and Medicine
The Jane and Jerry Weintraub Center for Reconstructive Biotechnology
Jonsson Comprehensive Cancer Center
UCLA School of Dentistry
Los Angeles, California

Mo Kwan Kang, MS, PhD
Professor and Chair
Section of Endodontics and Division of Constitutive & Regenerative Sciences
UCLA, School of Dentistry
Los Angeles, California

Purnima Kumar, BDS, MS, PhD
Associate Professor
Division of Periodontology
College of Dentistry
The Ohio State University
Columbus, Ohio

Karl Kwok, PharmD, RPh
Clinical Pharmacist-Hematology/Oncology
University of Washington Medical Center
Seattle Cancer Care Alliance
Seattle, Washington

Binnaz Leblebicioglu, DDS, MS, PhD
Professor
Division of Periodontology
College of Dentistry
The Ohio State University
Columbus, Ohio

Vahn A. Lewis, PharmD, MS, PhD
Associate Professor
Diagnostic and Biomedical Science
UTHealth, School of Dentistry
Houston, Texas

Karen M. Lounsbury, PhD
Professor
Department of Pharmacology
University of Vermont
Burlington, Vermont

Michael D. Martin, DMD, MSD, MPH, MA, PhD
Professor
Department of Oral Medicine
University of Washington
Seattle, Washington

Robert L. Merrill, DDS, MS
Clinical Professor
Oral Biology and Medicine
UCLA
Los Angeles, California

Michael Ossipov, PhD
Research Professor Emeritus
Department of Pharmacology
University of Arizona
College of Medicine
Tucson, Arizona

No-Hee Park, DMD, PhD
Distinguished Professor of Dentistry and Dean Emeritus
UCLA School of Dentistry
Distinguished Professor of Medicine
David Geffen School of Medicine at UCLA
Los Angeles, California

James C. Phero, D.M.D.
Professor Emeritus
Anesthesiology
University of Cincinnati
College of Medicine
Anesthesiology Affiliate Medical Staff
University of Cincinnati Medical Center (UCMC)
Director Advanced Cardiac Life Support (ACLS), AHA Training Center, UCMC
Department of Anesthesiology
University of Cincinnati Medical Center
Cincinnati, Ohio

Michael T. Piascik, PhD
Professor and Director of Education
Department of Pharmacology and Nutritional Sciences
University of Kentucky, College of Medicine
Lexington, Kentucky

Frank Porreca, PhD
Professor
Department of Pharmacology
College of Medicine
University of Arizona
Tucson, Arizona

Christine Quinn, DDS, MS
Clinical Professor
Dental Anesthesiology
UCLA School of Dentistry
Los Angeles, California

Robert B. Raffa, PhD
Professor Emeritus and Past Chair
Department of Pharmaceutical Sciences
Temple University
School of Pharmacy
Philadelphia, Pennsylvania
Adjunct Professor
University of Arizona College of Pharmacy
Tucson, Arizona

Morton B. Rosenberg, DMD
Professor Emeritus of Oral and Maxillofacial Surgery
Head, Division of Anesthesia and Pain Control
Tufts University School of Dental Medicine
Boston, Massachusetts
Professor of Anesthesiology
Tufts University School of Medicine
Boston, Massachusetts

David H. Shaw, PhD
Professor and Chairman
Oral Biology
University of Nebraska Medical Center
College of Dentistry
Lincoln, Nebraska

Ki-Hyuk Shin, PhD
Associate Professor
Oral Biology and Medicine
School of Dentistry
UCLA
Los Angeles, California

Han-Ching Tseng, PhD, MS
Quality Manager
Blood Bank Laboratory Manager
Grifols Pharmaceuticals
Los Angeles, California

Yaping Tu, PhD
Professor
Department of Pharmacology
Creighton University School of Medicine
Omaha, Nebraska

Erica C. Vincent, PharmD, BCOP, RPh
Clinical Pharmacist-Hematology/Oncology
University of Washington Medical Center
Seattle Cancer Care Alliance
Seattle, Washington
Clinical Instructor
University of Washington School of Pharmacy
Seattle, Washington

Dennis W. Wolff, PhD
Clinical Associate Professor of Pharmacology
Department of Biomedical Sciences
University of South Carolina School of Medicine
Greenville, South Carolina

PREFACE

HOW TO APPROACH PHARMACOLOGY

Although pharmacology can be considered a basic science, the ultimate purpose of pharmacology in the health science setting is to apply basic principles to clinical practice. This book, which is targeted to the dental student and dental practitioner, is designed to meet that need. Pharmacology is important to the dentist not only because of the drugs that he or she prescribes or uses in the dental office but also because of other drugs that the patient takes. Every drug can affect the entire body. Moreover, when more than one drug is given concurrently, there is a potential for drug interactions that could have adverse consequences.

This book is designed to make specific dental applications to each drug class. Included in this information are the benefits and risks associated with those drug classes.

In the study of pharmacology, it is important to learn drugs by their classes on the basis of similarity of mechanism of action rather than individual stand-alone medications. Thus armed with the knowledge of the properties of a class of drugs and examples of drugs within that class, one can streamline the learning process. Organization of drug information can then be arranged around the following subcategories (these will be useful in studying most drugs):

1. Name of drug class and examples
2. Mechanism of action
3. Pharmacokinetics
4. Indications
5. Adverse effects
6. Contraindications
7. Miscellaneous information, including drug interactions
8. Implications for dentistry

Some devices can help in the learning of drug names. The nonproprietary (generic) names for drugs within a given class often have similarities. Being familiar with a list of suffixes of generic drug names can be helpful in identifying an individual drug. Such a list is given next.

SUFFIXES AS CUES FOR REMEMBERING DRUG CLASSES

Suffix	Drug Class	Example
"azole"	Azole-type antifungal drug or antibacterial-antiparasitic drug	Fluconazole Metronidazole
"caine"	Local anesthetic	Lidocaine
"coxib"	Cyclooxygenase-2 (COX-2) inhibitor	Celecoxib
"dipine"	Dihydropyridine Ca^{++} channel blocker	Amlodipine
"ilol" or "alol"	β-Adrenergic receptor blocker that also blocks the α_1-adrenergic receptor	Carvedilol, labetalol
"mab"	Monoclonal antibody	Infliximab
"olol"	β-Adrenergic receptor blocker	Metoprolol
"onium" or "urium"	Quaternary ammonium compound, usually used as a peripheral competitive skeletal muscle relaxer	Pancuronium, atracurium
"osin"	α_1-Adrenergic receptor blocker	Prazosin
"pam" or "lam"	Benzodiazepine antianxiety agent or sedative hypnotic	Diazepam, triazolam
"pril" or "prilat"	Angiotensin-converting enzyme (ACE) inhibitor	Captopril
"sartan"	Angiotensin II receptor blocker	Losartan
"statin"	HMG CoA reductase inhibitor antilipid drug	Lovastatin
"triptan"	Serotonin 5-$HT_{1B/1D}$ agonist antimigraine drug	Sumatriptan
"vir"	Antiviral drug	Acyclovir

Application of information to clinical cases can increase retention and appreciation of pharmacology. The cases presented in this book help to make that application. The dentist will encounter drugs prescribed by a physician that have adverse effects on the oral cavity. Knowledge of a drug is essential in determining the likelihood of a drug causing adverse oral effects, and what strategies can be used to reduce these effects without compromising the intended therapy. On the other hand, a drug administered by the dentist could impact therapy by the physician. Here again, the dentist will need to have knowledge of that drug to determine whether or not it is advisable to use it in a given patient. These situations require knowledge of how drugs act, including the receptors involved, and what responses are linked to these receptors.

The landscape of pharmacology is ever expanding with the constant development of new drugs, new drug classes, and new information on older drugs. Furthermore, the growth in our knowledge in areas such as pharmacogenetics and pharmacogenomics promises to lead to the practice of tailoring drug therapy to the individual.

All in all, pharmacology is an exciting and dynamic discipline. This book covers the major areas of pharmacology and provides an intellectual framework on which to use drugs in a rational manner.

Frank J. Dowd
Barton S. Johnson
Angelo J. Mariotti

ACKNOWLEDGMENTS

The competing demands of academia in the modern health science setting make the writing of textbooks such as *Pharmacology and Therapeutics for Dentistry* a challenging task. In this effort, we have been aided greatly by our contributing authors, past and present, who have given their time and expertise to ensure that the information provided herein is both accurate and current. We wish to especially acknowledge Dr. John Yagiela and Dr. Enid Neidle, past chief editors of this textbook, for the foundations they set. (Separate tributes to each of them are given earlier.) We specifically acknowledge the contributors to this text who have devoted time and expertise to advancing dental pharmacology. We also must express gratitude to our families, Pat Dowd, Bridgette Mariotti, and Kim Franz, for their forbearance in dealing with our distractions and preoccupations on everything pharmacologic.

We wish to thank several individuals who made special contributions to this work. Ms. Laura Klein, Associate Content Development Specialist with Elsevier, has been our primary contact and associate. She has been most helpful, responsive, kind, and essential to this effort. We deeply appreciate our good times working with her. Ms. Jodie Bernard has been our expert in both her help and responsiveness in her artist role. We also appreciate the work of the following additional professionals at Elsevier: Kathy Falk, the Executive Content Specialist, has given wise direction in this project. Brandi Graham and Jolynn Gower, with their content help, have provided useful assistance in this endeavor. Deepthi Unni has insured that the production of this book has gone smoothly. Jennifer Bertucci has been timely in helping with online submission of documents. Kamatchi Madhavan has provided expert assistance in correcting proofs of the manuscript, and has been our adept project manager. We also recognize Brian Salisbury for his artistic help in the book design.

Frank J. Dowd
Barton S. Johnson
Angelo J. Mariotti

INTRODUCTION

*Pharmacology may be defined as the science of drugs and how they affect living systems. The term derives from *pharmakon,* the Greek word for drug or medicine, and *logia,* the Latin suffix traditionally used to designate a body of knowledge and its study. As an organized discipline, pharmacology is of recent origin, but the study of medicinal substances is as old as civilization itself.

HISTORY

Sir William Osler (1849 to 1919) once said, "The desire to take medicine is perhaps the greatest feature which distinguishes man from animals." This serves to illustrate the historical relationship between drugs and human beings. The use of natural products to cure disease and alter mentation dates back to the dawn of time. By the writing of the Ebers papyrus (c. 1550 BCE), more than 700 prescriptions for various ailments were known. Many of the ingredients incorporated in these preparations—lizard's blood, virgin's hair, fly excreta—are humorous by modern standards, but also included were many compounds recognized today as pharmacologically active. A summary of folk remedies and other medicinals that have withstood scientific scrutiny would list such substances as opium (morphine), belladonna (atropine), squill and foxglove (digitalis), cinchona bark (quinine and quinidine), coca leaves (cocaine), and ma huang (ephedrine). The empirical study of plant derivatives and animal products must have been extensive to be so fruitful.

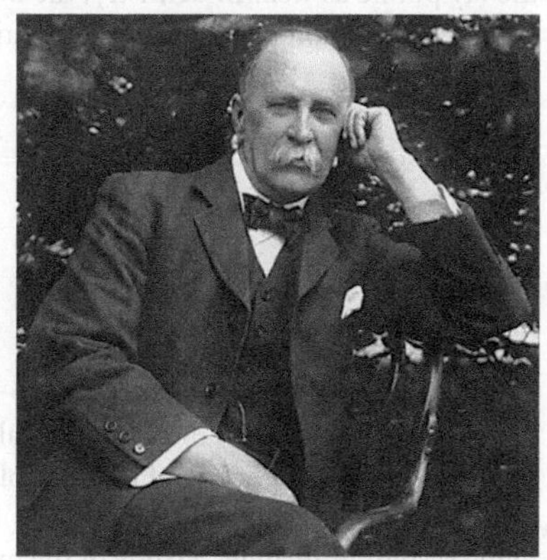

A major hindrance to the effective use of these drugs, however, was the large number of materials usually present in apothecary formulations. For example, the most popular drug of the 15th century, triaca, contained more than 100 separate components. Aureolus Paracelsus (1493 to 1541) was the first to recognize that the indiscriminate mixing of numerous substances did little but dilute whatever effective compounds may have been present initially. The focus of Paracelsus on single agents was refined by Felice Fontana (1720 to 1805), who deduced from his own experiments that each crude drug contains an "active principle" that, when administered, yields a characteristic effect on the body. One of the greatest scientific achievements of the 19th century was the isolation and objective evaluation of such "active principles."

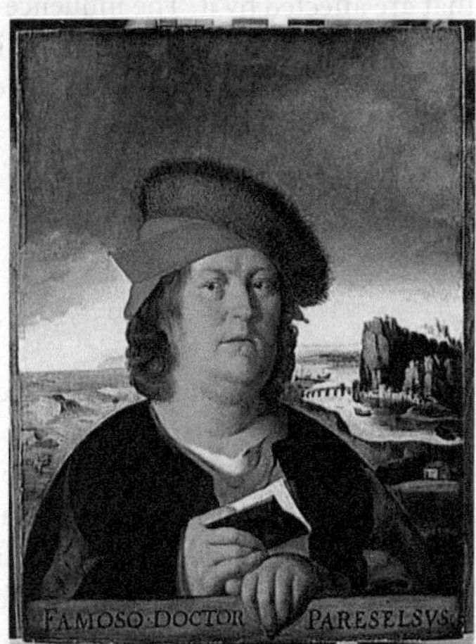

In 1803, a young German pharmacist, Frederick Sertürner (1780 to 1841), extracted the alkaloid morphine from opium. This singular achievement not only marked the beginning of pharmaceutical chemistry, but it also led to a revolution in experimental biology. The availability of newly purified drugs and the standardization of existing biologic preparations encouraged pioneers like Francois Magendie (1783 to 1855) and Claude Bernard (1813 to 1878) to use pharmacologic agents as probes in the study of physiologic processes. The use of curare by Bernard for the elucidation of the neuromuscular junction is but one example of the successes obtained with this approach. Perhaps because drugs became associated with several biologic sciences and were, of course, considered under the domain of the various medical specialties, the development of pharmacology as a separate discipline was delayed.

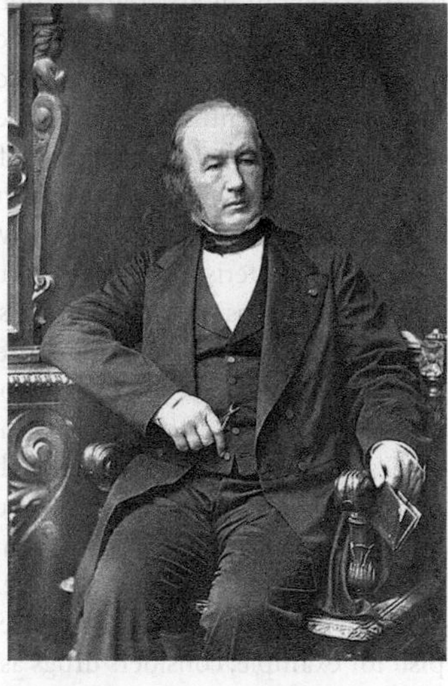

*(Photos in this introduction are as follows: From Wellcome Library, London L0074448, Sir William Osler (1849 to 1919), Canadian physician, aged 63. Copyrighted work available under Creative Commons Attribution only license CC BY 4.0 http://creativecommons.org/licenses/by/4.0/. *Paracelsus,* © Musée du Louvre, © Direction des Musées de France, 1999; *Claude Bernard,* public domain; *John Jacob Abel,* public domain; *Agonist concentration-response curve; Dioscorides' Material Medica,* public domain; *aspirin tablets,* photo © istock.com).

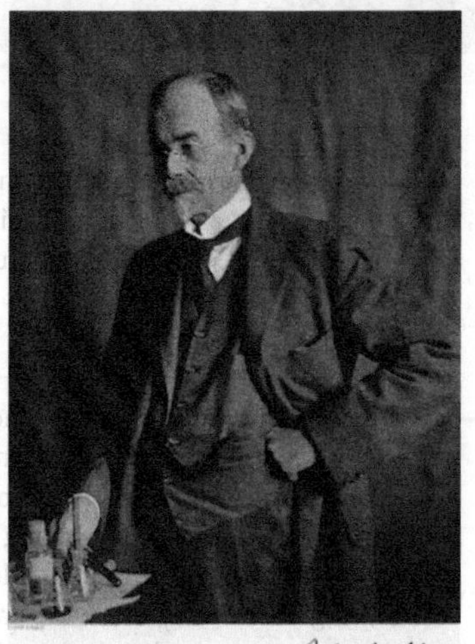

Rudolf Buchheim (1820 to 1879) and Oswald Schmiedeberg (1838 to 1921) were the two individuals most responsible for establishing pharmacology as a science in its own right. Buchheim organized the first laboratory exclusively devoted to pharmacology and became the first professor of his discipline. A student of Buchheim's, Schmiedeberg founded the first scientific journal of pharmacology. More importantly, through his tutelage Schmiedeberg helped spread acceptance of pharmacology throughout the world. One protégé of Schmiedeberg was John J. Abel (1857 to 1938), generally regarded as the father of American pharmacology.

Once an obscure experimental science, pharmacology has expanded its purview to such an extent that the subject has become an important area of study for all health professionals and holds certain interests for the lay public as well. In dentistry, the impact of pharmacology was formally recognized by the American Dental Association in 1934 with publication of the first edition of *Accepted Dental Remedies.*

SCOPE OF PHARMACOLOGY

Pharmacology is one of the few medical sciences that straddles the division between the basic and the clinical. The scope of pharmacology is so extensive that several subdivisions have come to be recognized. *Pharmacodynamics* is the study of the biologic activity that a drug has on a living system. It includes a study of the mechanisms of action of the drug and the exact processes that are affected by it. The influence of chemical structure on drug action (the structure–activity relationship) is also a concern of this branch of pharmacology. *Pharmacokinetics* deals with the magnitude and time course of drug effect, and it attempts to explain these aspects of drug action through a consideration of dosage and the absorption, distribution, and fate of chemicals in living systems.

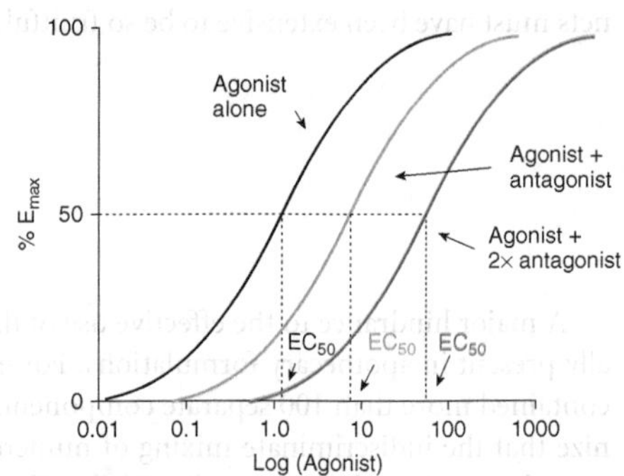

Pharmacotherapeutics is the proper selection of an agent whose biologic effect on a living organism is most appropriate to treat a particular disease state. It requires a consideration of, among many other things, dose, duration of therapy, and side effects of drug treatment. The practice of *pharmacy* involves the preparation and dispensing of medicines. Although pharmacists today are rarely called on to actually prepare drug products, they are a useful source of drug information for both the clinician and the patient. *Toxicology* is that aspect of pharmacology dealing with poisons, their actions, their detection, and the treatment of conditions produced by them. The importance of toxicology to modern life is continually underscored by new discoveries of chemical hazards in the environment. As the various disciplines of science and medicine have continued to evolve, fruitful areas of inquiry have emerged from the union of fields with overlapping interest. For example, study of the interrelationships between drugs and heredity, aging, and the immune system has led to the respective development of *pharmacogenetics, geriatric pharmacology,* and *immunopharmacology.* A final subdivision of pharmacology, *pharmacognosy,* has gained new relevance. Essential at a time when most drugs were derived from plants, it literally means "drug recognition" and deals with the characteristics of plants and how to identify those with pharmacologic activity.

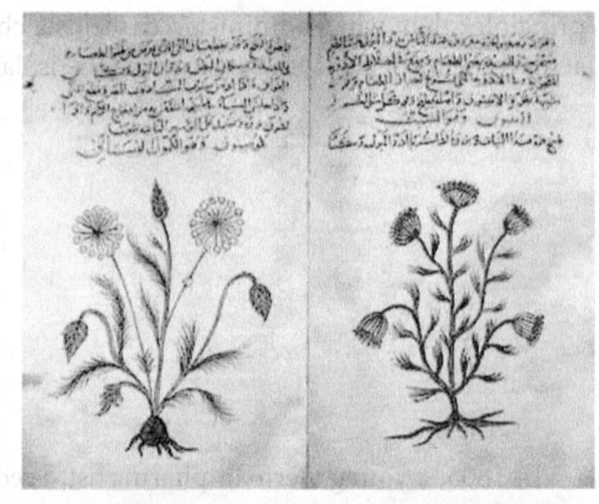

Although most drugs today are synthesized chemically, phytochemistry, especially the synthesis of complex chemical structures by plants, remains of interest. Furthermore, herbal medicine as a discipline of pharmacognosy has gained significant importance since 1994. The use of products in this area has spurred interest in the active components of herbal medicines, their clinical efficacy, and their potential liabilities.

After a description of how the study of drugs is classified, it is appropriate to discuss what is meant by the word *drug.* To the pharmacologist, a drug is any chemical agent that has an effect on the processes associated with life. This definition is obviously broad and ill-suited for many parties who define the term more restrictively to better serve their particular needs. The therapist, for example, considers drugs as those chemicals that are effective in treating disease states. To the lay public, drugs generally connote those substances that cause mental and psychological alterations. Finally, governmental agencies are concerned with the revenue derived from the taxes levied against the sale of certain substances or with public health problems associated with their use. Some of these agents, such as tobacco and alcohol, are legally sequestered—that is, by law they are considered "nondrugs."

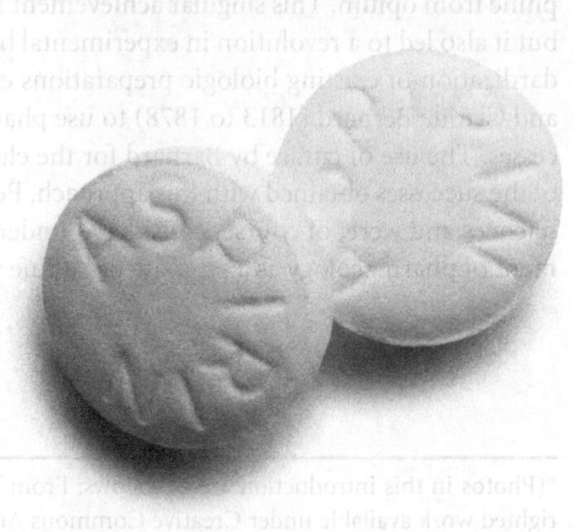

Although pharmacologists have long recognized these agents as potent drugs, they are exempted from the usual governmental restraints and are not subject to normal scrutiny by the U.S. Food and Drug Administration. There are other substances that have gained such special status not by historical accident, as did some of those previously mentioned, but by considerations of public health. Examples of these include chlorine and fluoride added to community water supplies and iodides mixed with table salt. Lawsuits over the question of whether these public measures constitute an illegal form of "mass medication" have been resolved by the courts, at least in part through the categorization of these chemicals as legal nondrugs when they are used in a specific manner for the public good.

Drugs discussed in this book almost exclusively include only those substances with a known therapeutic application. Even so, the potential number of agents for consideration is large: several thousand drugs marketed in a multiplicity of dosage forms and, in some instances, in a bewildering variety of combinations. To limit confusion, emphasis is placed on single, prototypical agents that represent their respective drug classes. By this approach, an understanding of the properties of related agents can be more readily achieved; at the same time, differences that may exist between them can be highlighted. Finally, it is important to recognize that there are certain generalizations that apply to all drugs. These principles of drug action are the subject of the first four chapters in this book. A mastery of the concepts presented in these chapters is necessary for a thorough understanding of pharmacology, for the rational use of therapeutic agents, and for the objective evaluation of new drugs.

NEW TO THE 7TH EDITION

The 7th Edition of *Pharmacology and Therapeutics for Dentistry* is substantially different from previous editions. Some of the chapters from the previous edition (e.g., those not directly related to, or only narrowly focused upon, dental practice) have been removed. Furthermore, the chapters in this edition have focused on content that is pertinent to the dental student. This has resulted in a reduction in chapter and book length. Appendices have been expanded to provide additional reference information. Other changes to the 7th Edition include the following:

(1) updated pharmacologic information
(2) revised and expanded illustrations
(3) dentally related case studies and subsequent discussions
(4) outlines at the beginning of each chapter
(5) bolded words and phrases in the text to focus the reader on key concepts and drugs
(6) color use for the first time

It is our hope that this concise, contemporary, and authoritative edition of *Pharmacology and Therapeutics for Dentistry* will be a great benefit to the pharmacology student and faculty member.

CONTENTS

PART I

Principles of Pharmacology

1

Pharmacodynamics: Mechanisms of Drug Action*

Frank J. Dowd and Peter W. Abel

KEY INFORMATION

- Most drugs bind to, and act through, receptors.
- The vast majority of drug receptors are proteins.
- Five different families of receptors are presented.
- Binding of a drug to a receptor is selective, and the affinity of the binding is measured by its K_d.
- The effect of the drug after binding to a receptor is called signal transduction. This occurs through a number of steps.
- Drug agonists at a given receptor can be distinguished based upon affinity of binding, potency (EC_{50}), and intrinsic activity (maximal effect, also called ceiling effect or E_{max}).
- Partial agonists have lower E_{max} values than full agonists.
- Antagonists are drugs that bind to receptors and block the effects of agonists.
- Antagonists whose blockade of the receptors can be overcome by adding higher concentrations of an agonist are called competitive antagonists.
- Conversely, receptor blockade by a noncompetitive antagonist is not surmountable by adding higher concentrations of the agonist.
- Tolerance to a drug (reduced response to a drug despite continued treatment) can occur by a number of mechanisms, which include desensitization and downregulation of the receptors.
- Receptors are not static structures and can cycle through more than one configuration.

CASE STUDY

Joe B, your dental patient, takes medication for chronic asthma. He has been given a drug preparation which includes salmeterol, a bronchodilator, and the adrenal corticosteroid fluticasone. His physician has indicated to Joe that he may need a rescue inhaler at times, but the rescue inhaler should not be used unless necessary to reverse an acute asthma attack. In reading about this drug combination, you see there is a "black box" warning that it may increase the risk of death from asthma. Why does it have this warning, and why was Joe warned about the frequency of use of a rescue inhaler?

DRUGS, RECEPTORS, AND SIGNAL TRANSDUCTION

Pharmacodynamics, which is the heart of pharmacology, is the study of how drugs act to achieve a response. Drugs are chemical substances that are administered to alter or modify existing physiologic or pathologic processes. In conventional doses, most therapeutic agents are generally selective in their action and influence a narrow spectrum of biologic events. How does this happen? Tissue elements to which drugs bind are called **receptors**. They have highly ordered physiologic/biochemical properties that permit only a very few particular compounds to combine with them, while prohibiting all others from doing so. Once bound, the receptor/drug complexes initiate other events to occur at the cellular level.

The existence of receptors that respond to exogenously administered drugs implies that drugs often mimic or inhibit the actions of endogenous ligands (chemicals that bind) for these receptors. These receptors existed long before drugs were developed. They originally evolved to respond to specific endogenous ligands such as hormones and neurotransmitters. Their great specificity of binding to both endogenous ligands and exogenous drugs suggests that simple molecular modifications of a drug may drastically affect the activity of the drug. This can be beneficial or detrimental to the clinical use of the drug.

Receptor Classification

For many years after their postulation more than a century ago, receptors remained an enigma to pharmacologists. Little was known about them other than the probability that they were complex macromolecules possessing a ligand-binding site to interact with specific drugs and an effector site to initiate the pharmacologic response. With the development of biochemical methods for the isolation and characterization of proteins, enzymes became available as model systems for the early study of drug–receptor interactions. Enzymes exhibit many of the properties that are ascribed to receptors. They are macromolecules having measurable biologic functions that possess specific reactive sites for selected substrates. The close association between enzymes and receptors was underscored in the early 1940s when it became apparent that some enzymes serve as drug receptors. The list of drugs that alter known enzymatic activities is extensive and includes such examples as angiotensin-converting enzyme inhibitors, anticholinesterases, protease inhibitors, reverse transcriptase inhibitors, statin cholesterol synthesis inhibitors, and various antimetabolites used in cancer chemotherapy, among others.

In addition to enzymes (including coenzymes), other receptors have been identified that are of clinical significance. The most common receptors are those located on and within the various membranes of the cell. Their study has been greatly aided in recent years by

* The authors wish to recognize Dr. John A. Yagiela for his past contributions to this chapter.

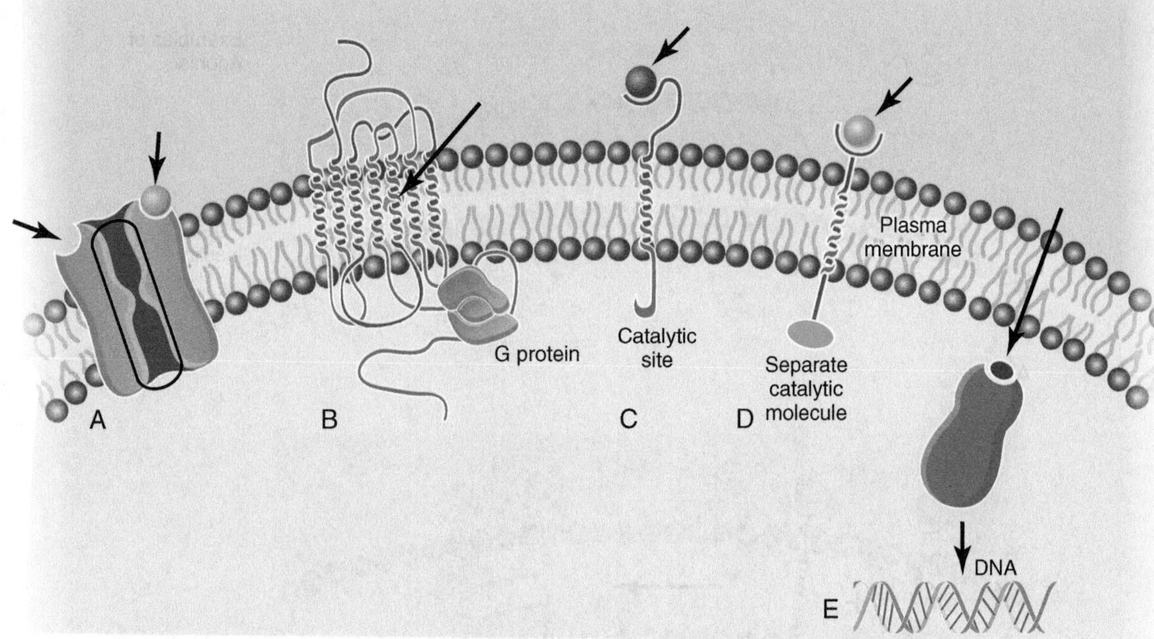

FIG 1-1 Examples of five major classes of receptors. *Arrows* denote the receptor ligand-binding sites. **A**, Ion channel–linked receptors. Drugs such as nicotine can activate ligand-gated ion channels, leading to depolarization (or hyperpolarization) of the plasma membrane. **B**, G protein–coupled receptors. Many drugs can activate G protein–linked receptors, causing release of the α and $\beta\gamma$ subunits of the G protein. **C**, Transmembrane receptors that have enzymatic cytosolic function. Agents such as insulin and epidermal growth factor activate this type of receptor. **D**, Transmembrane receptors that bind a separate cytosolic enzyme. Cytokines bind to this type of receptor. **E**, Intracellular receptors. Lipophilic substances (dark oval) such as steroids can cross the plasma membrane and activate intracellular receptors.

developments in genomics and proteomics. Many integral membrane proteins function as receptors for endogenous regulatory ligands, such as neurotransmitters, hormones, and other signaling molecules. In addition, membrane transporter proteins and metabolic enzymes, described in Chapter 2 for their influence on drug disposition, are also targets of drug action.

Nucleic acids serve as receptors for a limited number of agents. Certain antibiotics and antineoplastic compounds interfere with replication, transcription, or translation of genetic material by binding, sometimes irreversibly, to the nucleic acids involved. Other drugs, including thyroid hormones, vitamin D analogues, sex steroids, and adrenal corticosteroids, also modify transcription, but here the affected DNA becomes activated or inhibited as a consequence of drug interaction with a separate receptor protein in the cytosol or nucleus of the cell, as will be described subsequently.

Receptors involved in physiologic regulation can be grouped by molecular structure and functional characteristics into several superfamilies. Most of these receptors are membrane bound and have one or more extracellular ligand-binding domains linked by one or more lipophilic membrane-spanning segments to an effector domain often, but not always, located on the cytoplasmic side of the membrane. This arrangement is ideal for the translation of an extracellular signal into an intracellular response. Usually, the endogenous ligand "signal" (upon binding to the receptor) is hydrophilic and incapable of passive diffusion through the cell membrane. The same is true for most drugs that bind to these same receptors. For lipophilic regulatory ligands, such as thyroid hormone and various steroids, a separate superfamily of intracellular receptors exists. Commonly, when these drugs bind, they expose a DNA-binding site on the receptor protein, allowing the receptor to interact with DNA and alter transcription. These five major classes of receptors are illustrated in Figure 1-1 and described in the following text.

Ion channel–linked receptors

There are two general classes of ion channels: voltage-gated and ligand-gated (see Figure 1-1, *A*). **Voltage-gated ion channels** are activated by alterations in membrane voltage. Voltage-gated Na^+ channels open when the membrane is depolarized to a threshold potential and contribute to further membrane depolarization by allowing Na^+ influx into the cell. As described in Chapter 14, local anesthetics such as lidocaine bind to voltage-gated Na^+ channels, leading to blockade of neuronal depolarization. Specific voltage-gated ion channels also exist for several other ions, particularly K^+, Ca^{2+}, H^+, and Cl^-.

In contrast, ligand-gated ion channels (see Figure 1-1, *A*) are activated in response to the binding of specific ligands or drugs. Another name for ligand-gated ion channels is **ionotropic receptors.** (This term should not be confused with inotropic.) Many neurotransmitters, drugs, and some cytoplasmic ligands activate membrane-bound ligand-gated ion channels. These include several types of glutamate receptors, at least one 5-hydroxytryptamine (5-HT_3) receptor promoting Na^+, K^+, or Ca^{2+} movements, and certain γ-aminobutyric acid and glycine receptors promoting Cl^- influx. Depending on the ionic charge and the direction of flow, ligand-gated ion channels can either depolarize or hyperpolarize the cell membrane.

The nicotinic receptor, the first membrane-bound drug receptor to be fully characterized, is an important example of a ligand-gated ion channel (see generic example in Figure 1-1, *A*). An oligomeric structure, the polypeptide constituents of the nicotinic receptor subunits are arranged concentrically to form a channel through which small ions can traverse the plasma membrane when the receptor is activated

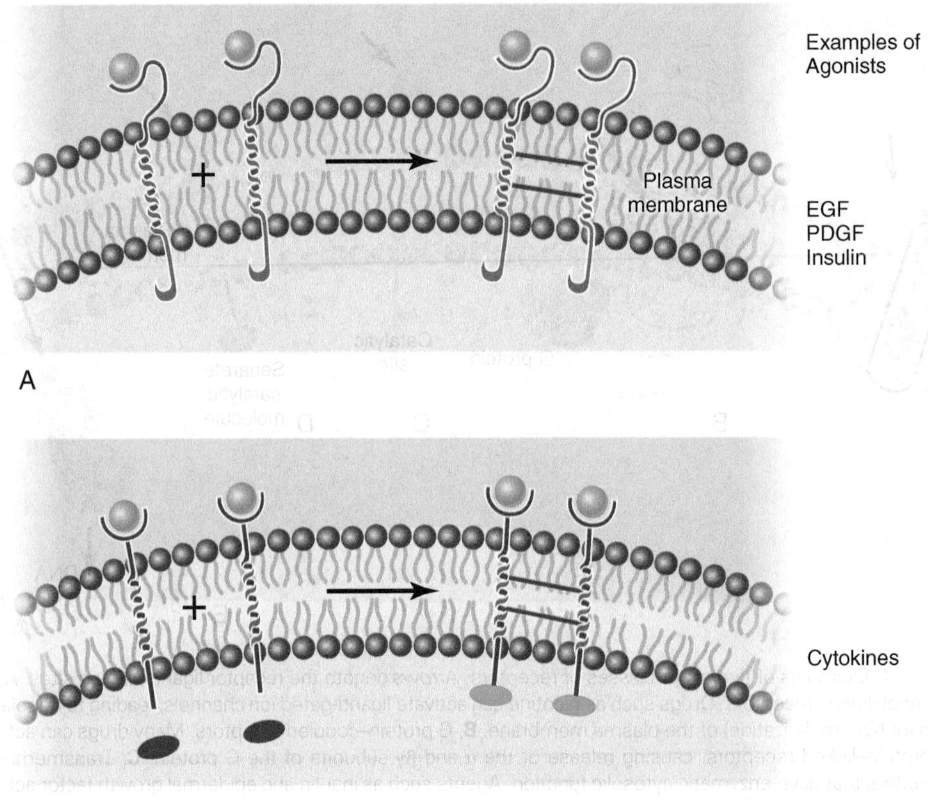

FIG 1-2 Dimerization of two membrane-bound receptor types that activate cytosolic enzymatic activity. Drugs (*blue spheres*) bind to the receptors, leading to dimerization and activation of enzymatic activity on the cytoplasmic side of the receptor (illustrated by conversion of the enzyme from *red* to *green ovals* in **B**). Examples of drugs and other ligands that work through these receptors are shown. **A**, The receptor contains enzyme activity as part of the cytoplasmic end of the receptor. *EGF*, Epidermal growth factor; *PDGF*, platelet-derived growth factor. **B**, The receptor binds and activates a separate enzyme located in the cytoplasm.

by the binding of two acetylcholine (ACh) molecules. As is the case with other ion channels, numerous subtypes of nicotinic receptors exist expressing differing affinities for specific ligands.

G protein–coupled receptors

G protein–coupled receptors, sometimes referred to as metabotropic receptors, constitute the largest superfamily of integral membrane proteins, and collectively serve as targets for approximately half of all non-antimicrobial prescription drugs (see Figure 1-1, *B*). The basic structure of these receptors includes a common seven-membered transmembrane domain. Generally, metabotropic receptors greatly amplify extracellular biologic signals because they activate G proteins, which activate ion channels or, more commonly, other enzymes (e.g., adenylyl cyclase), leading to the introduction or formation of a host of internal second messengers for each extracellular signal molecule detected.

G proteins are heterotrimers consisting of α, β, and γ subunits. After receptor activation, guanosine diphosphate (GDP, attached to the α subunit) is replaced by guanosine triphosphate (GTP), and the heterotrimer splits into the α monomer and βγ dimer. Many, but not all, of the observed cellular actions are caused by the α subunit. As an example, $G_{\alpha s}$, the specific α subunit for the G protein associated with β-adrenergic receptors, activates adenylyl cyclase, which catalyzes the synthesis of cyclic adenosine 3′,5′-monophosphate (cAMP). cAMP activates protein kinase A, which catalyzes the phosphorylation of serine and threonine residues of certain intracellular proteins, leading to a complex alteration in cellular function.

The G protein system is very complex. One receptor subtype may activate different G proteins, several receptor subtypes may activate the same G protein, and the ultimate target proteins can exist in tissue-specific isoforms with differing susceptibilities to secondary effector systems. The different G protein pathways can also interact with one another. The complexity of G protein signal transduction provides a sophisticated regulatory system by which cellular responses can vary, depending on the combination of receptors activated and the cell-specific expression of distinct regulatory and target proteins. Several specific membrane-bound G proteins are discussed beginning in Chapter 5 and continuing thereafter with regard to several clinical drugs discussed in the text.

Transmembrane receptors that have enzymatic cytosolic function

Enzyme-linked receptors have only one transmembrane domain per protein subunit, with an enzymatic catalytic site on the cytoplasmic side of the receptor (see Figure 1-1, *C*). For many of these receptors, dimerization activates the receptor to provide the conformational change required for expression of enzymatic activity. The most important cytoplasmic sites have one of the following functions: (1) tyrosine kinase activity, (2) tyrosine phosphatase activity, (3) serine or threonine kinase activity, or (4) guanylyl cyclase activity. For types 1 and 3, autophosphorylation of the receptor also occurs at tyrosine sites and at serine/threonine sites, respectively. Figure 1-2 shows how some of these receptors dimerize after a drug agonist binds.

TABLE 1-1 Receptor Types, Examples, and Approximate Time Until a Noticeable Response Occurs After Receptor Stimulation

Receptor Type	Some Receptor Examples	Time
Ion channel	Nicotinic cholinergic $GABA_A$ Glycine	Milliseconds
G protein–linked	Muscarinic cholinergic Adrenergic (α and β) Opioid Histamine	Seconds
Transmembrane with cytosolic enzyme domain	Epidermal growth factor Platelet-derived growth factor Insulin	Minutes to hours
Transmembrane that binds to a separate cytosolic enzyme	Cytokines (e.g., interleukins, interferons, tumor necrosis factors)	Minutes to hours
Intracellular (nuclear target)	Thyroid Estrogen Vitamin D	Hours to days

Many forms of cancer seem to involve mutant variants of enzyme-linked receptors in which the catalytic site or associated nonreceptor protein kinase is continuously activated. Approximately half of all oncogenes discovered to date encode for continuously activated protein kinases.

Transmembrane receptors that bind to a separate cytosolic enzyme

Another type of transmembrane receptor is one that has a noncatalytic domain that activates a separate cytosolic tyrosine kinase, called Janus kinase (JAK), that phosphorylates separate cytosolic proteins. This receptor dimerizes after binding to the kinase (see Figure 1-2) and is the type of receptor to which cytokines bind (see Figure 1-1, *D*).

Intracellular receptors

Lipophilic substances capable of crossing the plasma membrane may activate intracellular receptors (see Figure 1-1, *E*). Sex steroids, mineralocorticoids, glucocorticoids, thyroid hormones, and vitamin D derivatives all activate specific nuclear receptors that influence DNA transcription. When a drug (or hormone) binds to the receptor, it folds into the active configuration and dimerizes with a partner receptor. The conformational change results in a dramatic increase in binding to specific DNA sequences. Binding of thyroid hormone to its receptor produces more than a tenfold increase in receptor affinity for binding to DNA. DNA binding of the activated receptor often initiates transcription, leading to increased production of specific proteins. Because this type of signal transduction requires protein synthesis, drugs that activate intracellular receptors typically have a delay of several hours before the onset of their pharmacologic effect. (This is the reason glucocorticoids cannot be used as primary drugs for the management of anaphylaxis.) In some systems, the binding of the drug-receptor complex inhibits transcription. Regardless of the specific mechanism involved, however, the intensity and duration of drug effect are temporally independent of its plasma concentration.

Table 1-1 indicates the relative speed of response for the various types of receptors.

In addition to these intracellular receptors, other enzymes and proteins involved in cell function and gene expression are receiving increasing scrutiny as potential targets for drug therapy. Nitric oxide, which stimulates guanylyl cyclase directly to form cyclic guanosine 3′,5′-monophosphate (cGMP), and sildenafil, which inhibits the breakdown of cGMP by cGMP-specific phosphodiesterase-5, are two examples of currently available agents acting intracellularly on regulatory enzymes. Finally, structural proteins such as tubulin, which are assembled to form microtubules, are targets for several drugs used in the treatment of cancer, gout, and fungal infections.

Drug-Binding Forces

Implicit in the interaction of a drug with its receptor is the chemical binding of that drug to one or more specific sites on the receptor molecule. Multiple bond formation often accompanies the interaction between a drug and receptor. Four basic types of binding are pictured in Figure 1-3. Drug-binding forces vary in strength. Hydrophobic binding is often very weak, whereas covalent binding can be quite strong (e.g., the acetylation of a receptor shown in Figure 1-3).

Most drugs reversibly bind to their receptors. As described in Chapter 2, the duration of action of drugs is related to how long an effective drug concentration remains in the vicinity of the drug receptors. This time may vary from a few minutes to many days, but usually it is on the order of minutes to hours. If a drug irreversibly binds to a receptor, new receptor synthesis is usually required to reverse the effect of the drug.

Structure–Activity Relationships

Examination of structure–activity relationships (SARs) is a time-honored method of studying drug–receptor interactions. In SAR investigations, specific features of the structure of a drug molecule are identified and then altered systematically to determine their influence on pharmacologic activity. SAR studies of closely related agents (congeners) led to an understanding of the chemical prerequisites for pharmacologic activity and, on a practical level, made possible the molecular modification of drugs to provide enhanced or even novel therapeutic effects, while reducing the incidence and severity of toxic reactions. In addition, SAR studies serve to illustrate how the combined action of the various binding forces described earlier are necessary for maximal drug activity. This yields certain clues concerning the physicochemical properties of the receptor sites involved that are of value to investigators seeking to unravel the exact structure of these sites. X-ray crystallography techniques have shed light on not only the structure of receptors but the different functional conformations of the receptor and their relation to drug binding. All of the drug-binding forces shown in Figure 1-3, as well as drug size and conformation(s) (see following), are important contributors to drug structure–activity relationships.

Drug Size, Shape, and Isomerism

Most clinically useful drugs are organic compounds that have molecular weights less than 1000 and greater than 100. Exceptions include drugs such as the inorganic compound lithium carbonate and some of the newer biologic proteins, which can have molecular weights in the range of 150,000. Selectivity of a drug for a receptor is dependent on the three-dimensional structure of the drug. Thus, conversion of a *cis*- to a *trans*- conformation of a drug can have dramatic effects on affinity. Optical isomers of drugs often have very different affinities for the same receptor. Norepinephrine, for instance, is supplied in a dex trorotary (*d*) and a levorotary (*l*) form. (The two are often combined.) The *l* conformation has a tenfold higher affinity for adrenergic receptors than the *d* conformation, reflecting the importance of the three-dimensional structure as seen in mirror images.

Events Following Drug Binding: Signal Transduction

The combination of a drug with its receptor represents the first event in a series of reactions that culminate in a pharmacologic effect. An

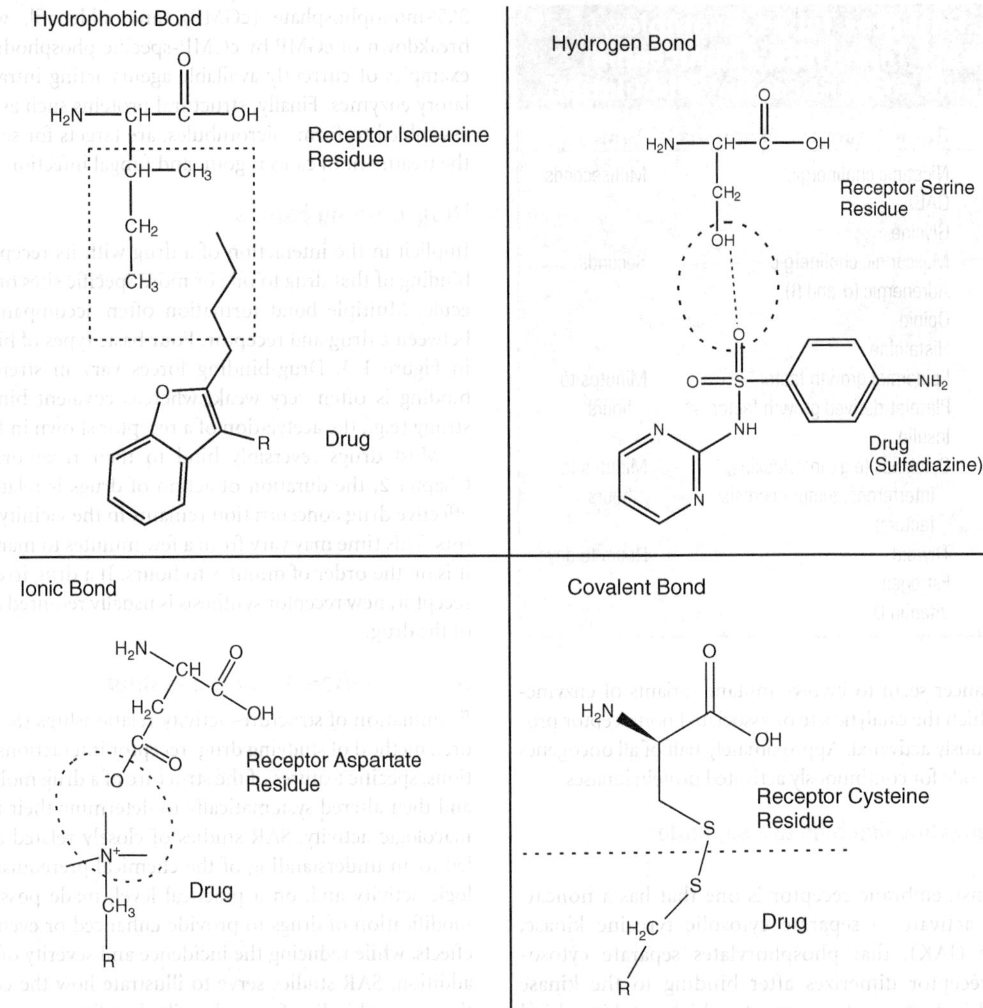

FIG 1-3 Four chemical bonds associated with drug–receptor interactions. Dotted areas indicate the region of the bonds.

important second step in this chain is the receptor response to drug binding. Drugs generally are not highly reactive compounds in the chemical sense; they exert their influences indirectly by altering, through their receptor attachment, the activity of an important regulator of a biologic process. The mechanism of action of a drug refers to this perturbation of normal function.

Activation of a receptor by a drug leads to a cascade of events that eventually results in an observable pharmacologic effect. These events constitute the **signal transduction pathway**, which is also called **stimulus–response coupling.** Individual receptor types have different signal transduction pathways (Figure 1-4).

Ion channel receptors

Ion channel receptors react to drugs by either increasing or decreasing their conductance. Channels are usually selective for a single ion. The increase or decrease in conductance of an ion leads to a cell event such as depolarization of the cell, hyperpolarization of the cell, or calcium signaling (see Figure 1-4, *A*). Nicotinic receptors and chloride channel receptors are examples of this class of receptors.

G protein–linked receptors

G protein–linked receptors encompass a variety of signaling pathways. G proteins are classified based on the nature of their α subunit. Three different types of G protein–coupled receptors are shown in Figure 1-4, *B* and *C*. The G protein complex is inactive when GDP is bound to the α subunit, which happens when the receptor is not stimulated by an agonist. Receptor stimulation leads to dissociation of GDP from the α subunit and the replacement binding of GTP (Figure 1-4, *B* and *C*). When this happens, the α subunit dissociates from the βγ subunit complex and then affects the activity of a nearby enzyme. In the case of $G\alpha_s$ the effect is to stimulate the enzyme adenylyl cyclase. Alpha subunits possess GTPase activity, which allows the G protein subunits to reassociate and return to an inactive state when the receptor is no longer stimulated. The activated function of adenylyl cyclase is to convert ATP to cyclic AMP (cAMP), which leads to activation of cAMP-dependent protein kinases (PKA) and resulting cell changes. The opposite effect, (i.e., inhibition of adenylyl cyclase) occurs when a different type of G protein–linked receptor releases α_i, bound to GTP. A third type of G protein–linked receptor involves the release of α_q. Alpha_q activates phospholipase C (PLC), which converts phosphati dylinositol-bisphosphate (PIP_2) to inositol 1,4,5-trisphosphate (IP_3) and diacylglycerol (DAG). Both are important for calcium signaling. IP_3 causes the release of calcium from intracellular stores, and DAG stimulates protein kinase C (PKC). In several cases the βγ subunit also participates in signal transduction, for instance, by affecting ion channels. Drugs that act through α_s are said to act through G_s (the G protein containing α_s) and include drugs that stimulate the β-adrenergic receptor. Likewise, drugs that act through G_i include drugs

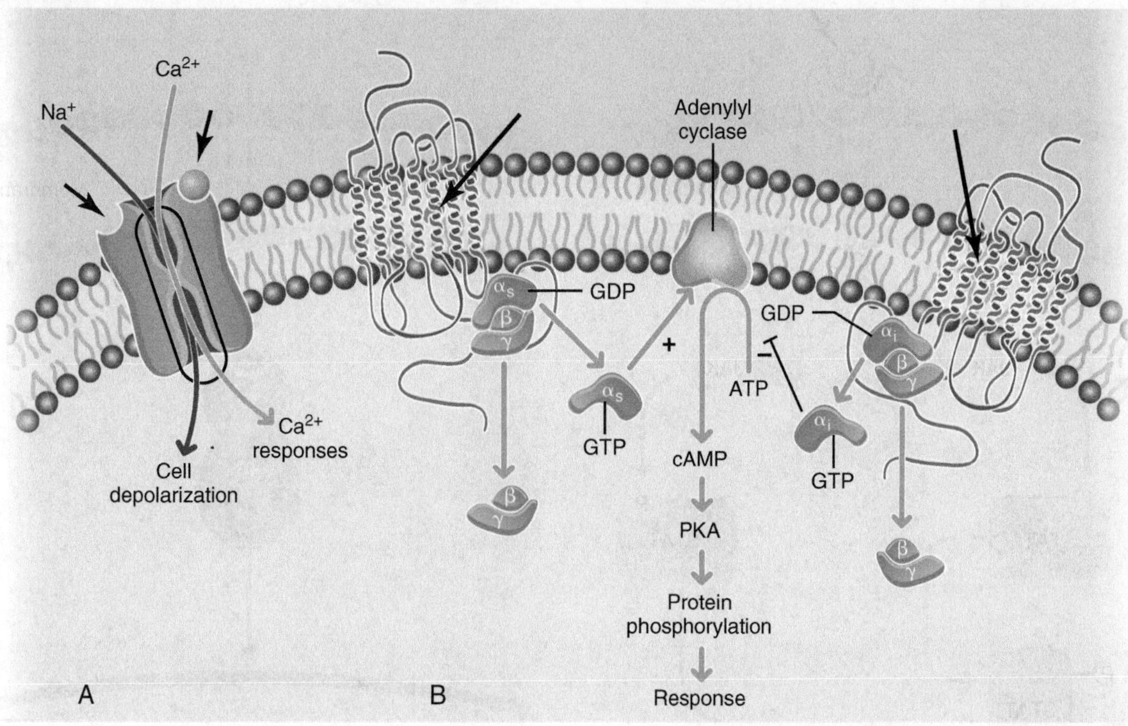

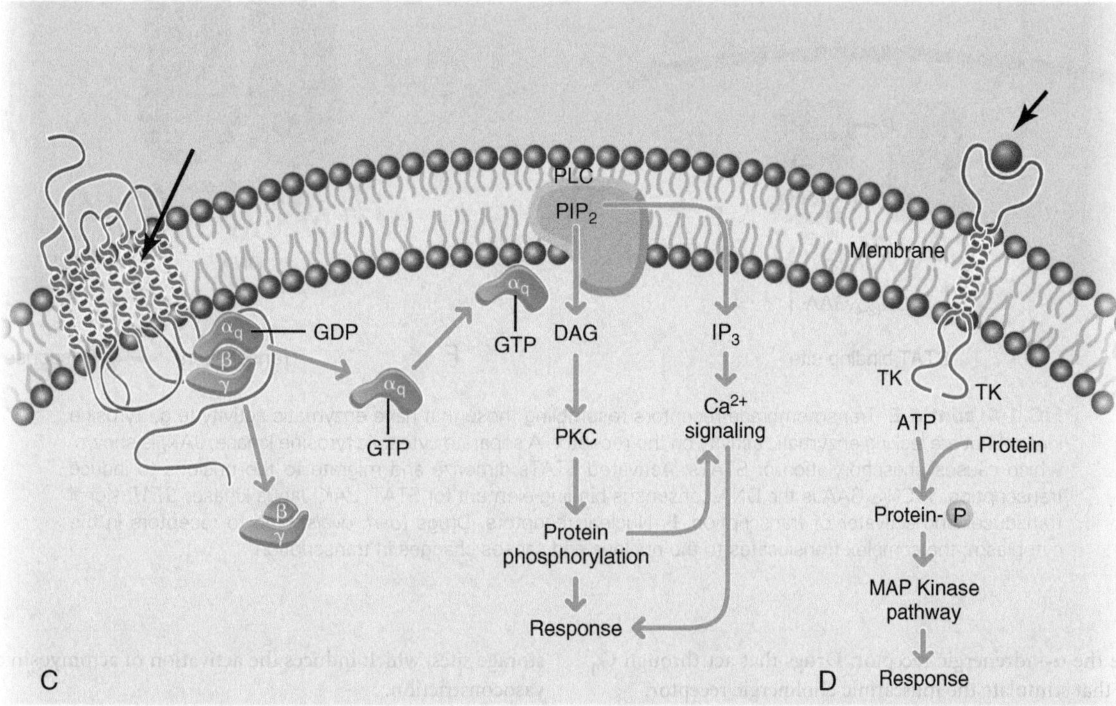

FIG 1-4 Signal transduction pathways. **A**, Ion channel receptors react to drugs by either increasing or decreasing their conductances. Although the conductances for Na^+ and Ca^{2+} are shown in the same channel, typically channels are more selective for one type of ion. Channels vary as to their selectivity for cations or anions. Drug-binding sites are indicated by *arrows* on either side of the channel. **B and C**, Three different types of G protein–coupled receptors are shown: receptors coupled to G_s, G_i, and G_q. The pathways are explained in the text. *Arrows* indicate the sites of drug binding on the receptor. *GDP*, Guanosine diphosphate; *GTP*, guanosine triphosphate; *PLC*, phospholipase C; *PIP_2*, phosphatidylinositol-bisphosphate; *IP_3*, inositol 1,4,5-trisphosphate; *DAG*, diacylglycerol; *PKA*, cyclic AMP-dependent protein kinase; *PKC*, protein kinase C. **D**, Transmembrane receptors that have enzymatic cytosolic activity. In the example given, tyrosine kinase causes the phosphorylation of a separate substrate (as well as autophosphorylation, not pictured). *TK*, Tyrosine kinase.

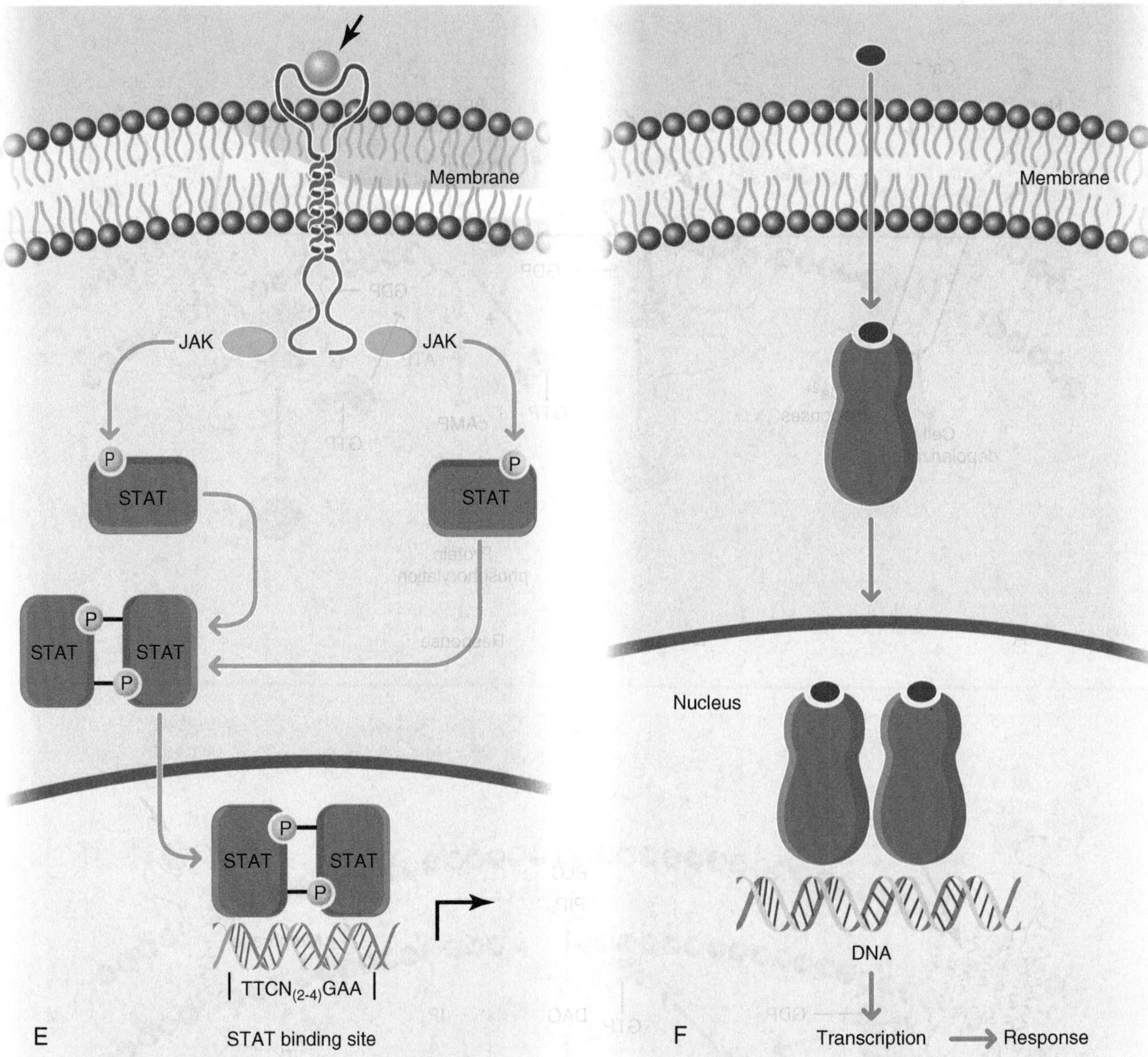

FIG 1-4, cont'd E, Transmembrane receptors resembling those that have enzymatic activity (e.g., tyrosine kinase) but are lacking enzymatic activity on the receptor. A separate cytosolic tyrosine kinase, JAK, is shown, which causes phosphorylation of STATs. Activated STATs dimerize and migrate to the nucleus to induce transcription. $TTCN_{2-4}GAA$ is the DNA consensus binding element for STAT. *JAK*, Janus kinase; *STAT*, signal transducer and activator of transcription. **F**, Nuclear receptors. Drugs (*dark ovals*) bind to receptors in the cytoplasm; the complex translocates to the nucleus and causes changes in transcription.

that stimulate the α_2-adrenergic receptor. Drugs that act through G_q include those that stimulate the muscarinic cholinergic receptor.

Epinephrine provides a useful illustration of the complex downstream consequences of drug binding. Incorporated into local anesthetic solutions to prolong the duration of pain relief, epinephrine mimics the action of the neurotransmitter norepinephrine. As a result of epinephrine attachment to α_1-adrenergic receptors on vascular smooth muscle cells, the G protein known as G_q is activated, phospholipase C_β activity is stimulated, and the membrane lipid phosphatidylinositol-4,5-bisphosphate is broken down to yield the second messengers diacylglycerol and inositol-1,4,5-trisphosphate (IP_3). Diacylglycerol initiates a cascade of metabolic events that support muscle contraction. IP_3 causes the release of Ca^{2+} from intracellular storage sites, which induces the activation of actomyosin and initiates vasoconstriction.

Transmembrane receptors that have enzymatic cytosolic activity

Insulin and several growth factors act through this type of receptor. Enzymatic activity on the cytosolic aspect of the receptor catalyzes changes that lead to the characteristic cell changes. In the example given in Figure 1-4, *D*, after insulin binds extracellularly, intracellular tyrosine kinase causes the phosphorylation of a separate substrate (as well as autophosphorylation, not pictured). Activation of several subsequent pathways such as the MAP kinase pathway follows, leading to further changes such as transcription in the nucleus.

Transmembrane receptors that bind to a separate cytosolic enzyme

Various cytokines act through these receptors. These receptors require a separate cytosolic tyrosine kinase to complete their function as receptors (see Figure 1-4, *E*). Typically, this enzyme is a JAK, which phosphorylates a group of proteins called signal transducers and activators of transcription (STATs). Activated STATs dimerize and migrate to the nucleus to induce transcription of selective genes. As can be surmised, many other steps are involved in the complex array of secondary signaling pathways.

Intracellular (nuclear) receptors

Steroid hormones, vitamin D, and thyroid hormone act through this type of pathway. Drugs that bind to these receptors diffuse into the cell and bind to intracellular receptors (see Figure 1-4, *E*). Dimerization with a co-receptor protein usually occurs after drug binding, followed by movement of the entire complex into the nucleus and induction of transcription of selective genes by binding to specific response elements (promotors/enhancers) on the DNA. Other steps are involved in the signaling pathways, and several other proteins, including co-activators and co-inhibitors, are involved in shaping the final transcription process.

CONCENTRATION–RESPONSE RELATIONSHIPS

A fundamental aspect of drug action is the relationship between the dose administered and the effect obtained. As one would expect, the magnitude of a chemical's effect on a system is positively correlated with the quantity or concentration of that chemical. For example, to increase the saltiness of a food, more salt must be added. Within certain limits, the addition of salt yields a graded and (nearly) linear response. However, with repeated additions of salt, the increase in saltiness becomes less and less until finally, further additions do not increase the sensation of greater saltiness. The dose–effect relationship of a drug is similar and is not a linear function throughout the entire dose range. Below a minimum threshold, there will be no observable effect. Above a certain ceiling, even a large dose would exert no additional effect because the maximal effect has already been reached.

Occupation Concept

Clark attempted in the 1920s to quantify drug effects through application of the law of mass action. Out of his efforts, and the contributions of others, emerged the occupation concept of drug action. The occupation concept holds that the magnitude of a pharmacologic response elicited by a drug that reversibly combines with its receptor is directly proportional to the number (or fraction) of receptors occupied by the drug. The relationship can be written as follows:

$$D + R \underset{k_2}{\overset{k_1}{\rightleftharpoons}} DR \rightarrow \text{Effect}$$

where *D* is the drug, *R* is the receptor, and k_1 and k_2 are rate constants. At equilibrium $k_2/k_1 = K_d$ (the dissociation constant). The K_d is a measure of the **affinity** of the drug for the receptor: the smaller the K_d, the greater the affinity.

After binding (DR) has occurred, an effect (*E*) follows, usually after several intervening signal transduction steps following binding, as described earlier. These intervening steps are represented by a single arrow in the preceding equation. A derivative of the Michaelis-Menton equation can be used to quantify drug effects as follows:

$$E = \frac{E_{max} \times [D]}{K_d + [D]}$$

(where E_{max} = maximal effect or ceiling effect)

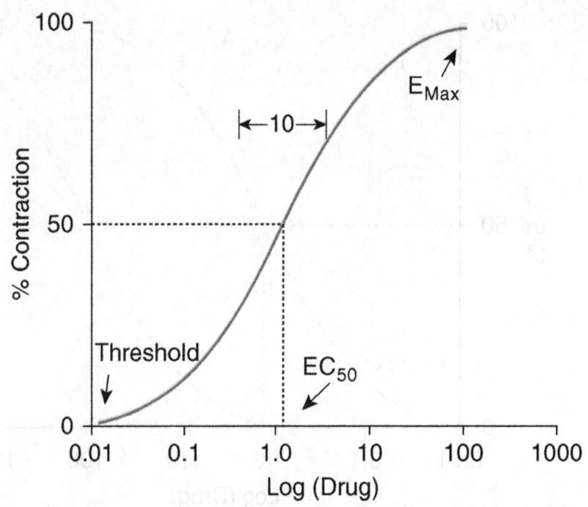

FIG 1-5 Theoretical concentration-response curve (log scale) for a smooth muscle stimulant. As shown, the linear portion of the sigmoid curve, extending from approximately 25% to 75% of the maximal effect, is encompassed by a tenfold concentration range. A range of 10,000 times is required, however, to depict the curve in its entirety (from 1% to 99% of the maximal effect). The concentration yielding 50% of the maximal response (EC_{50}) is also shown. E_{max}, ceiling effect = intrinsic activity.

Based upon this equation, the effect of the drug is predictably and quantitatively dependent on the drug concentration. Moreover, a geometric relationship (rectangular hyperbola) exists when graphing E versus [D]. The drug concentration is usually expressed in $\log_{10}$ units. This mathematic relationship between the concentration of a drug and its response may be shown visually by an experiment in which an isolated muscle is exposed to increasing concentrations of a drug while the force of contraction is measured (Figure 1-5).

When a drug is introduced into a tissue, it binds to its receptor in accordance with the K_d for that drug at that receptor. Each muscle cell may require a minimal number of receptors to be occupied before it contracts. The lowest concentration to elicit a measurable response is termed the **threshold concentration**. As higher concentrations are used, the number of receptors occupied increases, as does the intensity of response. An increase in the fraction of receptors occupied necessarily reduces the number available for subsequent binding so that at high concentrations each increment of drug produces progressively smaller additions to the magnitude of contraction. At very high concentrations, the receptor population becomes saturated, and further drug administration no longer influences contraction. A maximal muscle response for the drug, termed the **ceiling effect**, or $\boldsymbol{E_{max}}$, is achieved.

The useful concentration range for a drug falls between the threshold and the ceiling (E_{max}). By expressing data as the logarithm of the concentration versus the degree of response, this important and normally hyperbolic segment of the concentration–effect relationship becomes a sigmoid curve with the linear central portion typically extending over a tenfold concentration range. The concentration of a drug that produces a half-maximal response (**EC_{50}**) is often used to compare potencies of various drugs. The EC_{50} depends in part on the K_d, but it is not necessarily equal to the K_d. When data from several experiments are expressed on a single graph with the log concentration of the drug, this value can be accurately determined for each drug from the linear portion of the respective curve. Notice that the log concentration of the drug is plotted against a graded response in the tissue. A graded response is one in which the magnitude of the response increases incrementally as the drug concentration is increased. The curves generated are therefore called **graded log concentration**

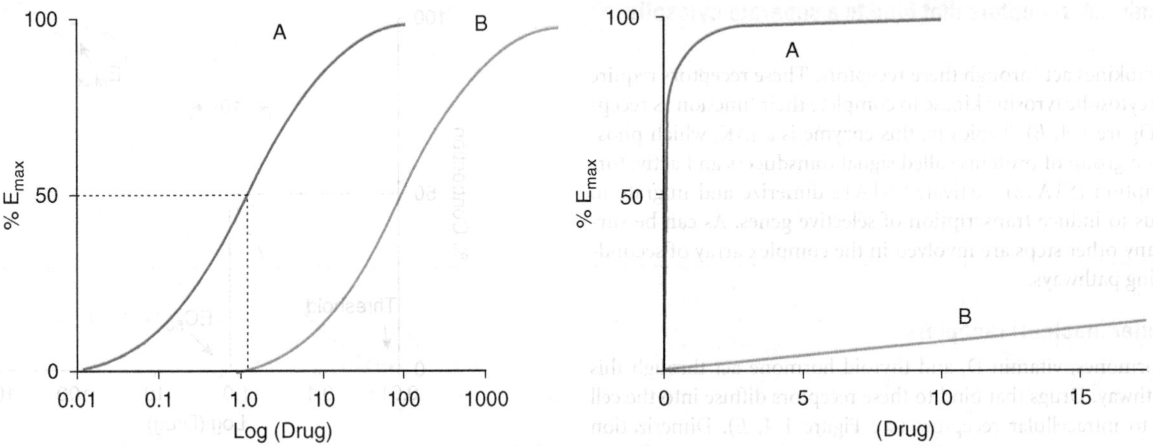

FIG 1-6 Concentration-effect curves for two drugs differing in receptor affinity by a factor of 100. *Left*, A log scale. Note the identical shapes of the two concentration–effect relationships. *Right*, An arithmetic scale. The lack of correspondence between the two curves hinders the drug comparison of the two drugs. Note that the units on the ordinate are percentages of E_{max}.

response curves. If the concentration data were not logarithmically transformed, graphical analysis would become more complex. Figure 1-6 illustrates the difficulties encountered if two drugs differing only in receptor affinity are examined on an arithmetic scale. The curve for drug A is so compressed that the concentration yielding the EC_{50} cannot be easily ascertained; for drug B, it cannot even be represented on the same page.

Agonists

Drugs, or other ligands, that bind to a receptor and elicit a response from a tissue are known as **agonists.** Agonists that produce ceiling effects—effects that are not exceeded by other drugs—are called **full agonists,** and drugs whose maximal effects are less than those of full agonists are referred to as **partial agonists.** The distinction between full and partial agonists is unrelated to differences in receptor affinity; rather, it is due to differences in their abilities to activate signal transduction changes after binding. The difference between these two classes of agonists lies in their unequal **intrinsic activities.** E_{max} is the measure of the **intrinsic activity** of a drug. Intrinsic activity is the ability of a drug to activate a receptor after the drug–receptor complex has formed. Incorporating intrinsic activity into the concentration- effect equation yields:

$$E = \text{intrinsic activity} \cdot \frac{E_{max}[D]}{K_d + [D]}$$

Thus, drugs with a low intrinsic activity are **partial agonists.** The log concentration-response curve of a partial agonist has a lower maximum and a reduced slope compared to that of a full agonist (Figure 1-7).

Two drugs (A and B) with the same intrinsic activity are shown in Figure 1-7, in which two agonists of muscle contraction are compared. The muscle was removed from the animal, placed in a bath containing an oxygenated physiologic salt solution, and attached to a strain gauge to measure contractions. In such experiments, conditions can be manipulated to ensure that each drug tested has equal access to the receptor in question. This condition greatly simplifies the interpretation of experimental results and cannot readily be duplicated in whole-animal investigations.

In addition to intrinsic activity, one other term is important in Figure 1-7: **potency.** Potency is the concentration (or dose) of the drug needed to achieve a given level or amount of response. The potency of drugs is reflected in their position on a concentration-response curve; the further to the left the drug response curve lies, the more potent the drug. The potency of a drug is usually expressed as the concentration of the drug required to achieve a half-maximal stimulation of the response (**EC_{50}**). The lower the EC_{50}, the greater the potency. In Figure 1-7, drug C has a lower intrinsic activity than either A or B; however, its potency is the same as that of drug A (because the EC_{50} values for both A and C are equal). The potency of drug C is greater than that of drug B. Because drug C has a lower intrinsic activity than either drug A or B, drug C is termed a **partial agonist.**

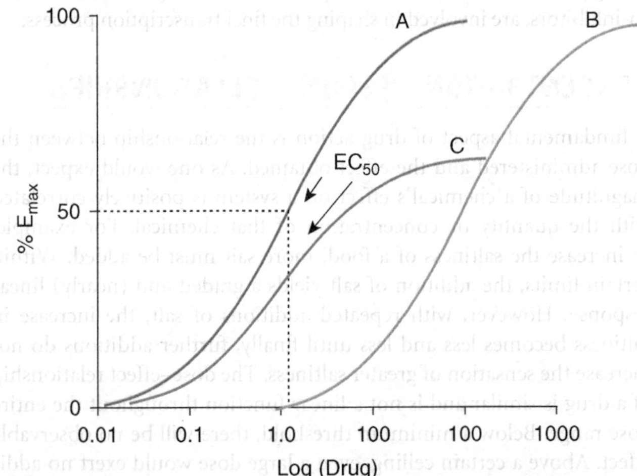

FIG 1-7 Theoretical concentration-response curves for three agonists acting at the same receptor. Drugs A and B have the same intrinsic activity (E_{max}), but B has less potency than A. Drug C has a lower intrinsic activity than either A or B, but it has the same potency as drug A (as measured by the EC_{50}.).

The terms affinity, intrinsic activity, and potency are conceptualized in Figure 1-8. This figure shows the equation linking a drug to an effect, and how affinity, intrinsic activity, and potency are related. Potency is related to affinity but is not the same as affinity. Affinity relates only to binding to a receptor; potency requires binding and achieving a response. Clinically however, the potency of a drug is also influenced by additional factors such as the drug's ability to reach the receptor (determined by the rate of absorption and the patterns of distribution and elimination). Since the concentration of a drug at the receptor is not known, clinical potencies are based on dose and are usually measured as the **ED_{50}** (effective dose to achieve 50% of the maximal response).

Notice that the term affinity relates only to the binding of the drug to its receptor, whereas intrinsic activity and potency **encompass both binding and subsequent signal transduction events leading to a response. Full agonists** are those that have an E_{max} that is the highest for any agonist at that receptor. **Partial agonists** have lower E_{max} values and therefore have lower intrinsic activity.

Figures 1-5, 1-6, and 1-7 show tissue responses to drugs and therefore are the types of graphs from which intrinsic activity and potency can be derived. On the other hand, the K_d of a drug is derived solely from binding data such as that obtained from a radioligand binding experiment, in which experiments are conducted using a radiolabeled drug in the presence of a receptor. Analysis of responses to drugs is often complicated by the fact that more than one drug molecule may bind simultaneously to a given receptor, one binding event may influence another, and the pharmacologic response may not be proportional to the number of receptors occupied by an agonist.

Indirect agonists

The discussion about agonists (full or partial) has to this point been about drugs that act directly on receptors: **direct agonists. Indirect agonists** are those that increase the level of direct agonists often by reducing the rate of metabolism of the direct agonist. A good example is the use of cholinesterase inhibitors to increase endogenous levels of acetylcholine, thereby increasing the effect of acetylcholine at its receptors.

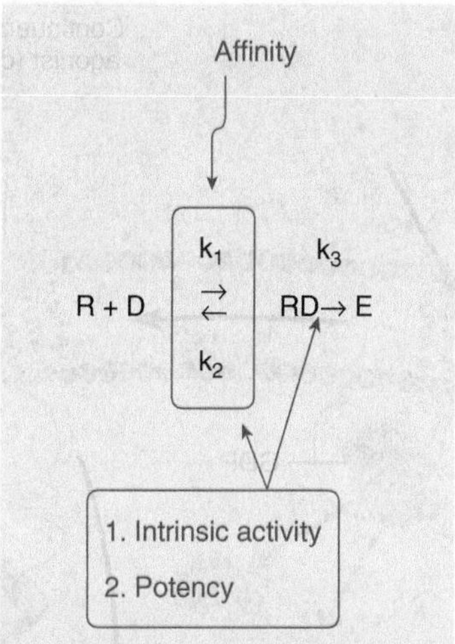

FIG 1-8 Depiction of drug characteristics. Affinity relates solely to drug binding, whereas intrinsic activity and potency encompass both binding and the events that follow leading to an effect.

Antagonists

Drugs that inhibit the effects of agonists are called **antagonists.** Pure antagonists have an intrinsic activity of zero because they bind to receptors but do not activate signal transduction pathways. Antagonists that bind reversibly to a receptor at the same site as the agonist are **competitive antagonists.** By making receptors less available for agonist binding, a competitive antagonist depresses the response to a given dose or concentration of agonist. The result is a parallel shift to the right of the agonist concentration-response curve (see Figure 1-9). An important aspect of this type of inhibition is that it is completely surmountable by a sufficiently high concentration of agonist. The presence of a competitive antagonist produces an apparent reduction in the affinity of an agonist for its receptor. The affinity of a competitive antagonist is measured as the K_i, which is equivalent to the K_d for an agonist. Competitive antagonists are common in pharmacology, and numerous examples are cited in succeeding chapters: antihistamines versus histamine, naloxone versus morphine, propranolol versus epinephrine, to name a few. By virtue of its small intrinsic activity, a partial agonist can also serve as a competitive antagonist of a full agonist. The aggregate receptor–stimulated event from the combination depends on the relative drug concentrations, receptor affinities, and intrinsic activities of the two agents.

Another type of antagonism commonly encountered is **noncompetitive.** The noncompetitive blockade is insurmountable in that the ceiling effect of an agonist can never be reattained, regardless of the concentration of the agonist that is administered. One way a noncompetitive antagonist can act is to decrease the effective number of receptors by irreversibly binding to the receptor site. The result of noncompetitive inhibition is a downward displacement of the agonist log concentration-response curve. Figure 1-9 reviews the dissimilarities between the two classic types of drug blockade. Competitive antagonists increase the EC_{50} of the agonist but do not affect the intrinsic activity of the agonist. Noncompetitive antagonists decrease the apparent intrinsic activity of the agonist with little effect on its EC_{50}.

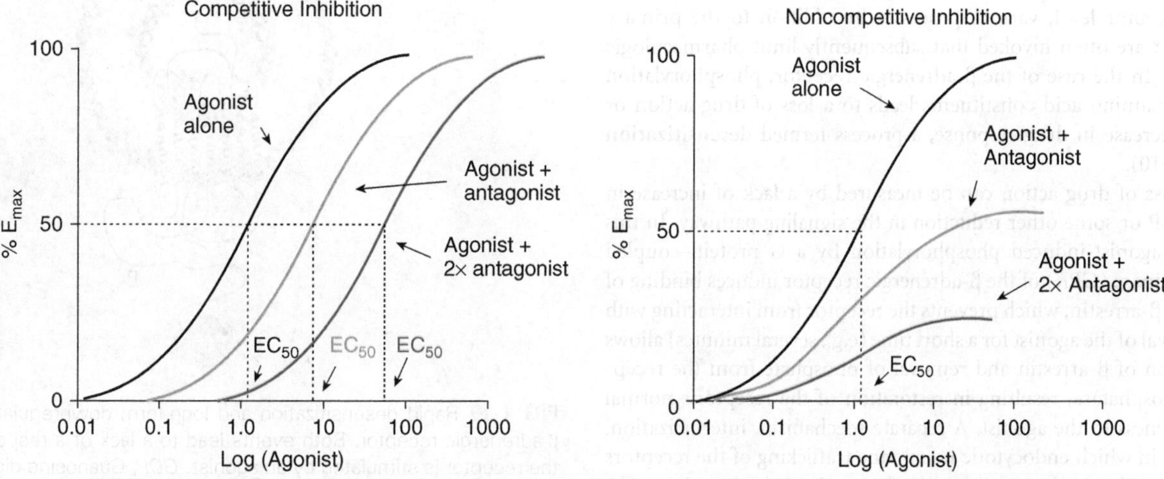

FIG 1-9 Effect of drug antagonism on a concentration response profile of an agonist. The left panel shows the effect of a competitive antagonist. Note that the EC_{50} values for the agonist increase with increasing concentrations of the antagonist. The right panel shows the effect of a noncompetitive antagonist. Note that the EC_{50} values for the agonist do not change with the antagonist.

Allosteric effects

Drugs that bind to receptors and affect the function of the receptor but do so at a site that is different from the usual ligand are said to act at an **allosteric** site. Drugs that act allosterically can either increase or decrease the receptor response. Allosteric inhibitors are another mechanism of noncompetitive inhibition.

Spare receptors

It is quite common for full agonists to achieve their maximal effect without occupying all of the relevant receptors of a cell. This is because extra receptors are present. This phenomenon is called the **spare receptor** concept or **receptor reserve.** It is demonstrated experimentally by achieving the E_{max} at a concentration of a drug that does not bind all of the receptors. It is also demonstrated by the effect of a noncompetitive antagonist. Instead of the predictable decrease in E_{max} when the noncompetitive antagonist is added, there is a shift to the right of the agonist response curve until all spare receptors have been bound by the noncompetitive antagonist. At that point, adding more antagonist generates the predictable decrease in E_{max} of the agonist.

Receptor Diversity

In addition to the fact that pharmacologic responses are often not linearly related to receptor occupancy, situations exist in which the receptors for a drug are not identical to one another. A repeating theme in the elucidation of the autonomic nervous system has been the division of receptor classes into an increasing array of types and subtypes with differing drug sensitivities. Part of the explanation for the unusual pharmacology of tamoxifen was made clear by the discovery that there were two subtypes of estrogen receptors in various tissues that responded differently to this agent. Individuals may even harbor differences in receptor structure based on single point mutations. An important example is the β_2-adrenergic receptor, for which numerous single nucleotide polymorphisms have been identified that may alter drug responsiveness in diseases such as asthma.

Pharmacodynamic Tolerance

The preceding discussion of concentration–response relationships is further complicated by the fact that the drug effect on the receptor can change with the passage of time. **Pharmacodynamic tolerance** is a general term for situations in which drug effects dissipate with time despite the continued presence of the agonist at a fixed concentration. At the receptor level, various processes in addition to the primary drug effect are often invoked that subsequently limit pharmacologic responses. In the case of the β-adrenergic receptor, phosphorylation of specific amino acid constituents leads to a loss of drug action or a large decrease in drug response, a process termed **desensitization** (Figure 1-10).

The loss of drug action can be measured by a lack of increase in cyclic AMP or some other reduction in the signaling pathway. In this example, agonist-induced phosphorylation by a G protein–coupled receptor kinase (*GRK*) of the β-adrenergic receptor induces binding of a protein, β-arrestin, which prevents the receptor from interacting with G_s. Removal of the agonist for a short time (e.g., several minutes) allows dissociation of β-arrestin and removal of phosphate from the receptor by phosphatase, resulting in restoration of the receptor's normal responsiveness to the agonist. A separate mechanism, internalization, can occur in which endocytotic membrane trafficking of the receptors takes place. This is also promoted by β-arrestin and takes place after longer exposure to an agonist. After internalization, receptors can either be shuttled back to the plasma membrane or destroyed by lysosomal enzymes. Internalization accounts for **downregulation** of the receptors.

Pharmacodynamic tolerance may also occur independently of any change in the drug receptor or stimulus–response system. As an illustration of this point, consider a drug that increases blood pressure by causing vasoconstriction in selected vascular beds. In response to the increase in blood pressure, various cardiovascular reflexes are evoked that reduce blood pressure, including activation of the parasympathetic nervous system, which causes bradycardia. The buildup of lactate and other metabolites in the affected tissues also limits vasoconstriction. Eventually, additional changes, such as decreased salt and water retention, may also reduce drug-mediated increases in blood pressure responses even further. These and other mechanisms of drug tolerance are described more fully in Chapter 3.

Multistate Model of Drug Action

Receptors may exist in more than one conformation. According to the multistate model of drug action, these forms of receptors are in equilibrium, and drugs act by altering their relative distributions. Figure 1-11 illustrates a simple two-state version in which the receptor can exist in an active or inactive conformation.

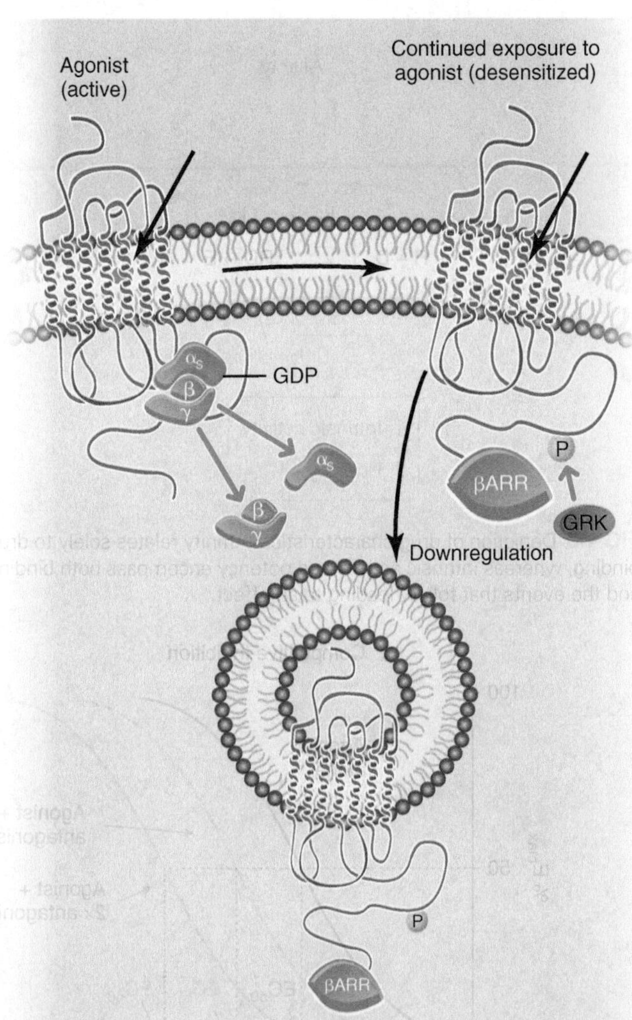

FIG 1-10 Rapid desensitization and long-term downregulation of the β-adrenergic receptor. Both events lead to a lack of a response when the receptor is stimulated by an agonist. *GDP*, Guanosine diphosphate; *GTP*, guanosine triphosphate; Ⓟ, phosphorylation on carboxyl terminal hydroxyl groups; *GRK*, G protein–coupled receptor kinase; *βARR*, β-arrestin which prevents the receptor from interacting with G_s. Refer to text above for further details.

In this model, full and partial agonists increase the proportion of receptors that exist in the active state. Receptors, in the absence of a ligand, tend to be in the inactive state. The degree to which they exist in the active state without an agonist corresponds to a level of activity which is called **constitutive activity**. Drug agonists bind to the receptor, converting the receptor to the active state. This is reflected in the difference in sizes of the reaction arrows (see Figure 1-11). Partial agonist binding produces an insufficient active form of the receptor to yield a maximal response (Figure 1-12). Competitive antagonists associate with receptors regardless of—and without influencing—their conformational state. Therefore Figure 1-12 shows no change in the active form of the receptor as a result of binding of a competitive antagonist. Noncompetitive antagonists limit the ability of agonist binding to elevate the number of receptors in the active state by reducing the total number of available receptors.

The major attractions of the multistate model are that it gives a solution for differences in the magnitude of the response between structurally related drugs, and that it affords a simple mechanism for the pharmacologic response elicited by drug binding. It also provides an explanation for drugs known as **inverse agonists**. An inverse agonist causes an effect opposite to that of the agonist, in contrast to a competitive antagonist, which simply blocks the agonist (or the inverse agonist) but has no inherent effect by itself (see Figure 1-12). In a tonically active pathway, in which the receptor has constitutive activity (without drug), a drug that preferentially binds to the inactive configuration or induces its formation would behave as an inverse agonist. In other words, inverse agonists inhibit endogenous activity of a receptor. For example, flumazenil, a competitive antagonist of the benzodiazepine receptor, reverses the effects of both agonists and inverse agonists. Additional examples of inverse agonism have been shown for various G protein–coupled receptors overexpressed in cells experimentally or after neoplastic transformation. Inhibition of constitutionally active oncogenes by inverse agonists may provide a new strategy for cancer chemotherapy.

A final advantage of the multistate model is that it can accommodate desensitization and time-dependent actions of drugs such as nicotine. Nicotine exhibits a complex pharmacologic profile. Initially, this natural alkaloid acts like an agonist: it stimulates ACh receptors at autonomic ganglia and in skeletal muscle. The stimulation is temporary, however, and in minutes the action of nicotine transforms from that of excitation to one of antagonism. This metamorphosis can be adequately explained if one assumes that a third, or "desensitized," configuration of the receptor exists to which active receptors are slowly converted and from which they even more slowly recover. Nicotine, by increasing the proportion of active receptors, causes an initial stimulation and a subsequent prolonged loss of activity as receptors are progressively trapped in the desensitized state. Ion channel desensitization is a different mechanism of desensitization from that depicted in Figure 1-10.

RECEPTOR-INDEPENDENT DRUG ACTIONS

No description of drug action would be complete without a consideration of agents that exert pharmacologic effects through receptor-independent mechanisms. Aside from the fact that these drugs act without the benefit of receptor intermediaries, there are no common traits serving to link this miscellaneous array of compounds. It has also proved impossible to derive a quantitative description of drug responses akin to that presented for receptor-based agents. The very diversity of these drugs precludes any unifying relationship between concentration and effect. Nevertheless, concentration-effect curves similar to those previously discussed are often obtained with these drugs, and general concepts such as potency and efficacy still apply. For the sake of discussion, these drugs are grouped arbitrarily into three categories: chemically reactive agents, physically active agents, and counterfeit biochemical constituents.

Chemically Reactive Agents

Chemically reactive drugs include a wide variety of compounds, some of which interact with small molecules or ions, whereas others attack proteins and other macromolecules. Gastric antacids and metallic ion chelators are two kinds of drugs that combine with inorganic substances within the body. Of particular importance to dentistry are the systemic and topical fluorides used to increase tooth resistance against dental caries. Also of interest is dimercaprol, a chelating agent capable of forming coordination complexes with mercury and other heavy metals. Drugs affecting macromolecules

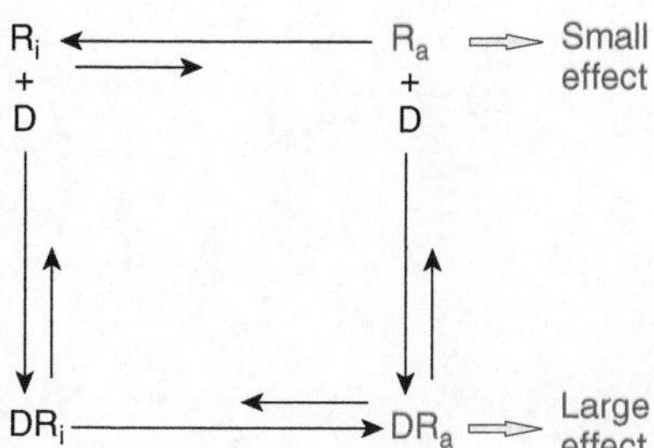

FIG 1-11 Two-state model of drug–receptor interaction. The receptor can exist in an active (R_a) or inactive (R_i) state. Unless the receptor mediates a tonically active process, without any drug, only the inactive state is present. Drugs (*D*) may bind to R_a, R_i, or both. Agonist binding favors the formation of DR_i and DR_a. The ratio of DR_a/DR_i influences the degree of response to the drug. The level of R_a corresponds to the degree of constitutive activity of the receptor.

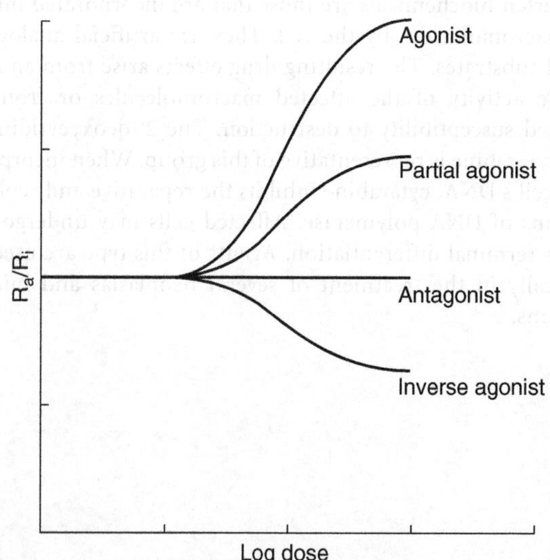

FIG 1-12 Concentration–effect relationships according to the two-state model. In this example, a tonically active process (constitutive activity) is depicted. Full agonists give the maximal ratio of active to inactive receptors (R_a/R_i). Notice that what is being plotted is the log concentration of the drug versus the ratio, R_a/R_i. Partial agonists also increase the ratio, but to a lesser degree. Antagonists bind without disturbing the existing R_a/R_i ratio, and inverse agonists exert an opposite effect by reducing the R_a/R_i ratio and inhibiting a normally partially active pathway. In this example, all the drugs are assumed to have the same receptor affinity.

include most germicides and the antineoplastic alkylating agents. Sodium hypochlorite solutions provide antisepsis and facilitate canal debridement during endodontic therapy because they release hypochlorous acid, a potent chemical disrupter of biologic matter. Generally, these compounds can be readily distinguished from drugs whose effects are receptor mediated. With the exception of certain chelating agents, they lack specificity and may individually react with various substances, organic or otherwise. Minor structural modifications also do not usually influence activity of these drugs. Finally, the reactions of these drugs rely heavily on covalent bonding or on strong ionic attachments; they do not usually depend on hydrophobic or weak electrostatic interactions.

Physically Active Agents

Physically active agents, in contrast, are often useful therapeutically because they are chemically inert and can safely be used for their colligative properties. Magnesium sulfate is an effective cathartic because it is not absorbed from the gastrointestinal tract and exerts an osmotic effect, causing retention of large amounts of water within the intestinal lumen. The colon becomes distended and is stimulated to undergo expulsive contraction. Through a similar osmotic mechanism, mannitol helps reverse cerebral edema in a patient with traumatic brain injury. A totally unrelated physical mechanism is evoked by hydrogen peroxide. Although highly reactive, hydrogen peroxide is useful in wound debridement because of its effervescent action. The release of gas bubbles promotes the physical removal of debris from injured tissues.

The physically active agents generally exhibit a surprising lack of structural specificity. For many agents, the major requirements for activity seem to be a certain pharmacologic inertness coupled with the ability to be administered in high concentrations (compared with most other drugs) without causing undue toxicity.

Counterfeit Biochemical Constituents

Counterfeit biochemicals are those that are incorporated into specific macromolecules by the cell. They are artificial analogues of natural substrates. The resulting drug effects arise from an altered biologic activity of the affected macromolecules or from their increased susceptibility to destruction. The 2′-deoxycytidine analogue cytarabine is representative of this group. When incorporated into a cell's DNA, cytarabine inhibits the reparative and replicative functions of DNA polymerase. Affected cells may undergo apoptosis or terminal differentiation. Agents of this type are used therapeutically in the treatment of several neoplasias and microbial infections.

CASE DISCUSSION

Salmeterol is an agonist at β_2-adrenergic receptors. By stimulating these receptors, it causes bronchodilation. Salmeterol is used chronically and has a long duration of action. Rescue inhalers act on the same receptors but are more effective in providing a quick and more pronounced effect than salmeterol. However, repeated administration of a rescue inhaler can cause these receptors to desensitize and downregulate, a mechanism discussed earlier. This results in a reduced ability of the drug to cause bronchodilation, which is one reason there is the warning against overuse of the rescue inhaler. The warning against overuse of salmeterol is based on a similar but less pronounced effect on the β_2-adrenergic receptors. Therefore, a glucocorticosteroid (e.g., fluticasone) is usually given with salmeterol to reduce the risk of a breakthrough asthma attack. Nonetheless, salmeterol administration needs to be given for as limited duration as possible.

GENERAL REFERENCES

1. Ariëns EJ, Simonis AM, van Rossum JM: Drug-receptor interactions: interaction of one or more drugs with one receptor system. In Ariëns EJ, editor: *Molecular pharmacology: mode of action of biologically active compounds*, New York, 1964, Academic Press.
2. Bhattacharya S, Hall SE, Li H, et al.: Ligand-stabilized conformational states of human β2 adrenergic receptor: insight into G-protein-coupled receptor activation, *Biophys J* 94:2027–2042, 2008.
3. Clark AJ: The reaction between acetyl choline and muscle cells. Part II, *J Physiol* 64:123–143, 1927.
4. Heng BC, Aubel D, Fussenegger M: G Protein-coupled receptors revisited: therapeutic applications inspired by synthetic biology, *Annu Rev Pharmacol Tox* 54:227–249, 2014.
5. IUPHAR/BPS Guide to Pharmacology (contains receptor classifications and nomenclature) (on the web) http://www.guidetopharmacology.org/ (accessed 2015).
6. Katritch V, Cherezov V, Stevens RC: Diversity and modularity of G protein-coupled receptor structures, *Trends Pharmacol Sci* 33:17–27, 2012.
7. Kenakin T: Principles: receptor theory in pharmacology, *Trends Pharmacol Sci* 25:186–192, 2004.
8. Kobilka BK: Structural insights into adrenergic receptor function and pharmacology, *Trends Pharmacol Sci* 32:213–218, 2011.
9. Rosenbaum DM, Rasmussen SG, Kobilka BK: The structure and function of G protein-coupled receptors, *Nature* 459:356–363, 2009.
10. Urban JD, Clarke WP, von Zastrow M, et al.: Functional selectivity and classical concepts of quantitative pharmacology, *J Pharmacol Exp Ther* 320:1–13, 2007.
11. Wenthur CJ, Gentry PR, Mathews TP, Lindsley CW: Drugs for allosteric sites on receptors, *Annu Rev Pharmacol Tox* 54:165–184, 2014.

2

Pharmacokinetics: The Absorption, Distribution, and Fate of Drugs*

Frank J. Dowd

KEY INFORMATION

- Drugs are able to penetrate membrane barriers by several mechanisms.
- The more lipid-soluble a drug is, the more likely it is to penetrate the lipid environment of membranes.
- Distribution of weak acids and weak bases depends on pH and the pK_a of drugs.
- Drug transporters play notable roles in the small intestine, liver, kidneys, and capillaries.
- Each route of drug administration has its own absorption characteristics.
- The blood–brain barrier is effective in keeping many drugs out of the brain.
- Drug distribution in saliva reflects plasma concentrations for several drugs.
- The liver is the most important organ for drug metabolism, employing many key enzymes, most notably the cytochrome P450 enzymes.
- Many factors, including drug inhibitors and drug inducers, can affect cytochrome P450 enzymes.
- The kidneys are the most important organs for excreting drugs.
- First-order kinetics refers to a process (e.g., elimination of a drug) in which a constant percentage of drug is eliminated per unit time.
- Zero-order kinetics refers to a process (e.g., elimination of a drug) in which a constant amount of drug is eliminated per unit time.
- Drugs differ from one another in their volumes of distribution, elimination half-times, and clearances.
- Four equations can be used to calculate drug transit in the body: volumes of distribution, half-times, clearance values, and steady-state plasma concentrations (for multiple dosing).

CASE STUDY

As a result of oral surgery that you performed on your patient, you prescribe acetaminophen plus codeine #3 (300 mg acetaminophen with 30 mg codeine), two tablets initially and one tablet every 4 hours thereafter (6 doses maximum) as needed for pain. Your patient mentions that due to gastric reflux, he also intends to begin using an over-the-counter histamine-2 blocker. He mentions that he has a bottle of Tagamet (cimetidine) with more pills in it from a previous use. Assuming the cimetidine is not out of date, would you offer any advice to your patient based on this information?

We learned in chapter one (Pharmacodynamics), that the magnitude of the effect of a drug is directly related to the concentration of the drug at the relevant receptors. When a drug is administered to a patient, however, several factors contribute to achieving the drug concentration at the receptors. Drug concentrations are rarely static; they increase and decrease as dictated by the processes of absorption, distribution, metabolism, and excretion. This chapter examines these processes (**pharmacokinetics**, Fig. 2-1) and how they influence the passage of drugs through the body.

PASSAGE OF DRUGS ACROSS MEMBRANES

For a drug to be absorbed, reach its site of action, and eventually be eliminated, it must cross one or more biologic membrane barriers. Because such barriers to drugs behave similarly, the cell membrane can serve as an example for all. The cell membrane is composed of a bimolecular sheet of lipids (primarily phospholipids and cholesterol) with proteins interspersed throughout and extending beyond the lipid phase of the membrane (Fig. 2-2). The presence of protein molecules spanning the entire thickness of the membrane provides a necessary link between the extracellular environment and the cell interior, which is consistent with the concept that drug activation of a membrane-bound receptor on the external surface of a cell can be directly translated into an intracellular response. Specific transmembrane proteins also provide important pathways for the uptake and extrusion of drugs.

Passive Diffusion

The passage of drugs across biologic membranes can involve several different mechanisms. Of these, passive diffusion is the most commonly encountered. The defining characteristic of passive diffusion is that the drug moves down its electrochemical gradient when crossing the membrane. The gut epithelial barrier is a good example of how drugs can permeate cell barriers.

Simple diffusion

One way that hydrophilic drugs may penetrate a cell barrier is by aqueous diffusion, by permeating between epithelial tight junctions or through aqueous pores. This avoids the lipid barrier of the cell membrane, but it is limited by drug size and other restrictions. More commonly, lipophilic drugs will diffuse directly through the lipid barrier of the cell membrane (**lipid diffusion**). The rate of transfer of nonelectrolytes across a membrane is directly proportional to the lipid/water partition coefficient. (The partition coefficient is a measure of the relative solubility of an agent in a fat solvent, such as olive oil or octanol, vs its

* The author wishes to recognize Dr. John A. Yagiela for his past contributions to this chapter.

solubility in water [Fig. 2-3].) A drug with a high partition coefficient (i.e., a *lipophilic* drug) readily enters the lipid phase of the membrane and passes down its concentration gradient to the aqueous phase on the other side. More molecules are then free to enter the membrane and continue the transfer process. With poorly lipid-soluble compounds, however, only a few molecules enter the membrane per unit of time, and the rate of passage is depressed.

The absence of an ionic charge is one major factor favoring lipid solubility. Conversely, drugs with an ionic charge, such as those containing a quaternary nitrogen atom, permeate membranes slowly if at all. The term **hydrophobic bonding**, introduced in Chapter 1, refers to the tendency for water-insoluble molecules to be drawn together; this behavior is responsible for the preferential tendency of lipid-soluble drugs to penetrate cell membranes by way of the lipid components. Many other therapeutic agents are weak electrolytes; depending on the pH of their aqueous environment, they can exist in ionized and neutral forms. Because charged molecules penetrate membranes with considerable difficulty, the rate of movement of these drugs is governed by the **partition coefficient** of the neutral species versus the **ionized species**. As illustrated in Figure 2-4, acidic conditions favor the transport of weak acids, and the opposite holds true for basic compounds.

The same concept of water interaction used to explain the aqueous solubility of ions also applies to many nonionic molecules. Although unsubstituted aliphatic and aromatic hydrocarbons have little or no tendency to react with water, affinity for water molecules is not restricted to structures with a formal charge. Organic residues possessing electronegative atoms such as oxygen, nitrogen, and sulfur can interact with water through the formation of hydrogen bonds to provide some degree of aqueous solubility.

Figure 2-3 shows that lipid solubility is not the only factor influencing the simple diffusion of uncharged drugs across cell membranes; molecular size is also important. Water, glycerol, and some other very small molecules permeate much more readily than would be predicted from their respective partition coefficients. Figure 2-3 also shows that some large organic molecules diffuse more slowly than expected, indicating that some degree of water solubility is necessary for the passive diffusion of drugs across membranes. No matter how lipid soluble an agent is, it will never cross a membrane if it cannot first dissolve in the extracellular fluid and be carried to the membrane structure. Benzocaine, an active local anesthetic when applied directly to nerves, is ineffective after injection because its water insolubility precludes significant diffusion away from the administration site and toward its locus of action within the neuronal membrane.

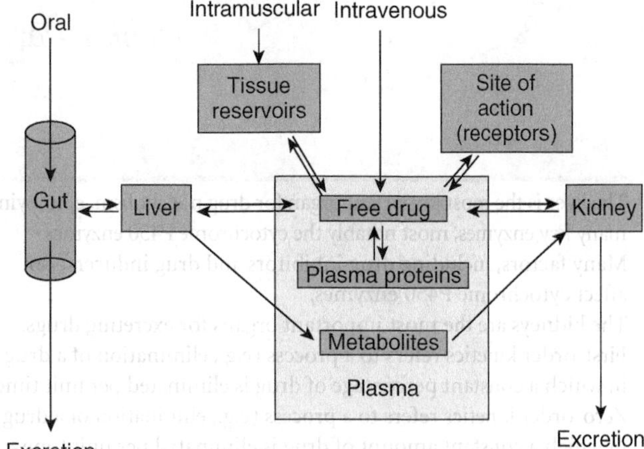

FIG 2-1 Outline of the major pathways of absorption, distribution, metabolism, and excretion of drugs. Compounds taken orally must pass through the liver before reaching the systemic circulation. When in the bloodstream, agents are distributed throughout the body and come in contact with their respective sites of action. Drugs are filtered by the kidney, only to be reabsorbed if lipid soluble. Metabolism of many drugs occurs primarily in the liver, after which the metabolites are excreted in bile or via urine. Some agents eliminated in the bile are subject to reabsorption and may participate in an enterohepatic cycle.

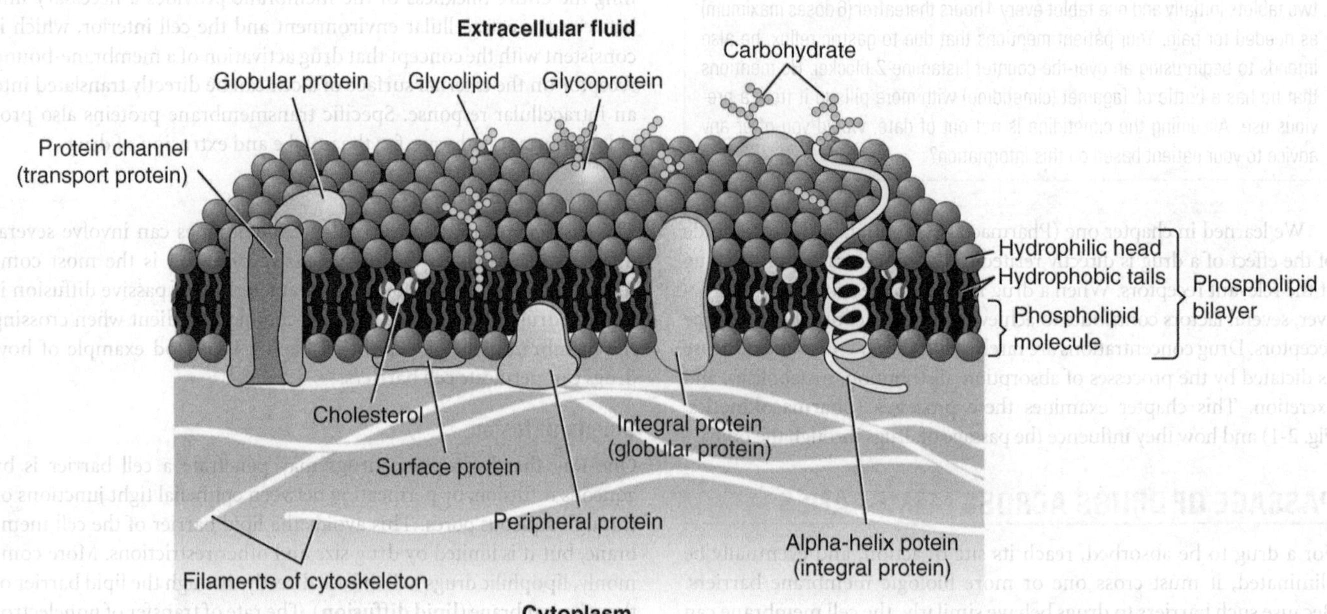

FIG 2-2 Cells are surrounded by a plasma membrane composed of a phospholipid bilayer, cholesterol, proteins, and carbohydrates. Modified from VanMeter KC, et al.: *Microbiology for the Healthcare Professional,* St Louis, ed 2, 2016, Mosby.

Similarly, when inside a membrane, a drug with an extremely high partition coefficient may be so soluble in the lipid phase that it has little tendency, despite moderate solubility in water, to diffuse out of the membrane down its concentration gradient. This is commonly called "lipid trapping."

Simple diffusion across capillary walls warrants special comment. In addition to the transcellular pathway of drug diffusion just described for lipid-soluble agents, an aqueous **paracellular pathway** formed by 10-nm to 15-nm clefts between the endothelial cells of most capillaries permits the aqueous diffusion of water-soluble drugs between the plasma and extracellular space. Hydrophilic molecules up to small proteins in size can use this route; fixed negative charges along the diffusion pathway tend to promote the movement of positively charged macromolecules while restricting movement of those with net negative charges.

Facilitated diffusion

Water, small electrolytes, and hydrophilic molecules of biologic importance generally move across plasma membranes much more readily than would be predicted by simple diffusion. In these instances,

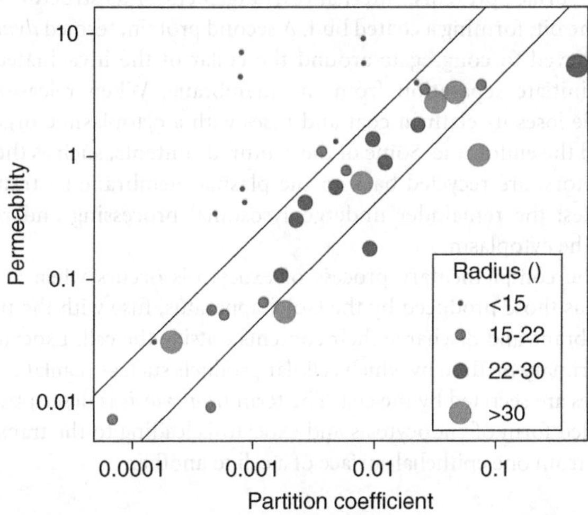

FIG 2-3 Relationship between membrane permeability and lipid (olive oil)/water partition coefficient in *Chara certatophylla*. Each *circle* represents a single nonelectrolyte with a molecular radius as indicated in the key. Small compounds permeate more readily than their partition coefficient would indicate; the reverse is true for large molecules. (Adapted from Collander R: The permeability of plant protoplasts to small molecules, *Physiol Plantarum* 2:300-311, 1949.)

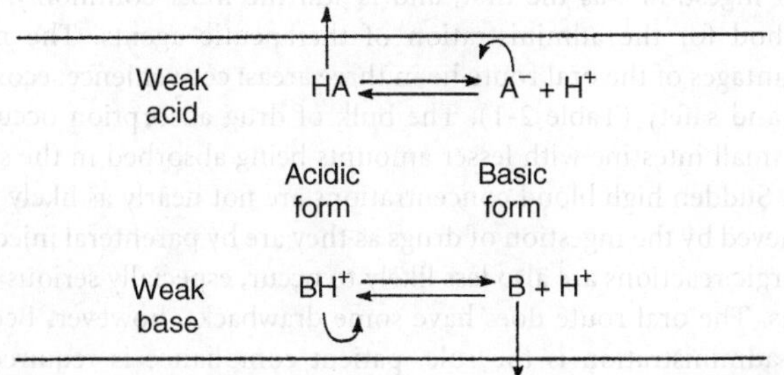

FIG 2-4 Membrane penetration by weak electrolytes. The nonionic species of drugs (*HA, B*) permeate membranes much more efficiently than do the charged forms (A^-, BH^+). Acidic conditions shift the dissociation curves to the left, favoring the diffusion of weak acids. An increase in pH favors the loss of hydrogen (H^+) and the diffusion of weak bases.

transmembrane proteins serve to circumvent the lipid bilayer and facilitate diffusion. The simplest mechanism involves a transmembrane pore (porin), such as aquaporin 1. Discovered in 1991, aquaporin 1 is a 28-kDa polypeptide that forms a 3-Å channel through which water can enter or leave cells. More than 10 variants of aquaporins have been discovered in mammalian tissues and are especially prominent in cells and organs involved with the transcellular movement of water: kidneys, capillaries, secretory glands, red blood cells, choroid plexus, brain glia, eyes, and lungs. Some aquaporins are selective for water only, increasing membrane permeability by a factor of up to 100 times; others permit the passage of glycerol and several other small molecules in addition to water.

The movement of specific ions (e.g., Na^+, K^+, and Ca^{++}) across the cell membrane is facilitated by the presence of transmembrane channels, such as the nicotinic receptor described in Figure 7-4 and the Na^+ channel illustrated in Figure 14-4. The opening of these gated channels (in contrast to porins, which are always open) is regulated by the electric potential across the membrane or by the presence of specific ligands, such as neurotransmitters. When a channel is open, passive diffusion of an ion capable of traversing it depends on the electric potential across the membrane and the chemical gradient of the ion. Boosting the electrochemical gradient by manipulating the voltage across the cell membrane is an effective method of increasing ionic flow. Even in the absence of specific ion channels, the transport of fixed ions and weak electrolytes across tissue barriers can be facilitated by the appropriate use of electric current (as in iontophoresis, discussed subsequently).

Numerous lipid-insoluble substances are shuttled across plasma membranes by forming complexes with specific membrane constituents called **carriers** or **transporters.** Carriers are similar to receptors in many ways; they are proteins, often quite selective about the agents with which they combine, and subject to competitive inhibition. Because the number of transporter molecules is finite, carrier-mediated diffusion can be saturated at high drug concentrations. The GLUT family of glucose transporters is representative of carrier proteins that facilitate the movement of hydrophilic solutes across cell membranes. The initial step in the facilitated diffusion of glucose is its binding to the exposed active site of the transporter protein. This binding sequentially causes an external barrier or gate to close and interior gate to open, after which the glucose is released into the cell. The release of glucose causes the internal gate to close and the external gate to open, re-exposing the active site and completing the cycle.

Active Transport

Active transport is the term given to the carrier-mediated transfer of a drug against its electrochemical gradient. In addition to exhibiting selectivity and saturability, active transport requires the expenditure of energy and may be blocked by inhibitors of cellular metabolism. Active transport permits the efficient absorption of substances vital for cellular function (and certain drugs that resemble them structurally) and the selective elimination of waste products and foreign chemicals, including many drugs. Approximately 2000 genes—7% of the total human genome—code for transporters and associated proteins. Two superfamilies of transporters are of special significance to pharmacokinetics: **ATP-binding cassette (ABC) transporters** and **solute carrier (SLC) transporters.**

ABC transporters hydrolyze adenosine triphosphate (ATP) to provide the energy directly needed for molecular transport and are referred to as **primary active transporters.** The most extensively researched representative is **P-glycoprotein** ("P" for altered permeability). Originally identified in 1976 for its ability to expel numerous antineoplastic drugs from mutated cells that overexpress it,

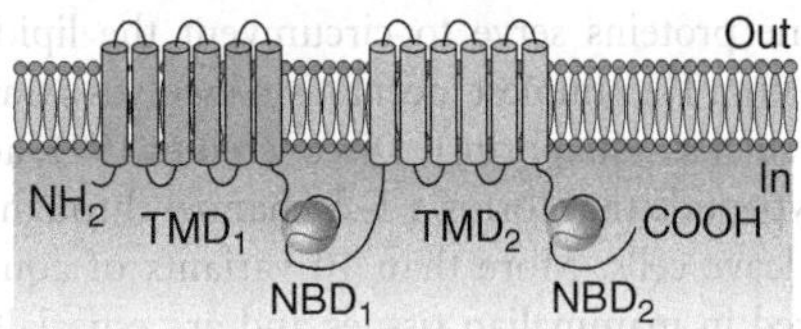

FIG 2-5 Two-dimensional topology of P-glycoprotein. Two transmembrane domains (*TMDs*) provide the transport mechanism and are powered by the nucleotide-binding domains (*NBDs*) that hydrolyze ATP. (Adapted from Sarkadi B, Homolya L, Szakács G, et al.: Human multidrug resistance ABCB and ABCG transporters: participation in a chemoimmunity defense system, *Physiol Rev* 86:1179-1236, 2006.)

P-glycoprotein is a complex 170-kDa glycoprotein with transmembrane domains that form the pump itself and a nucleotide-binding domain that hydrolyzes ATP to power the transport (Fig. 2-5). P-glycoprotein preferentially promotes the cellular extrusion of large (300 to 2000 Da) hydrophobic substances and neutral or positively charged amphiphilic molecules. Transported drugs include numerous anticancer agents (e.g., doxorubicin, vinblastine, and paclitaxel), antiviral compounds (e.g., ritonavir), Ca^{++}-channel blockers (e.g., diltiazem), digoxin, antibiotic and antifungal drugs (e.g., erythromycin and ketoconazole), hormones (e.g., testosterone), and immunosuppressants (e.g., cyclosporine).

Drug binding to active transporters occurs within the plasma membrane near the cytoplasmic surface, limiting transport to drugs with good lipid solubility or sufficient length to reach the active site. P-glycoprotein is expressed in various cells, but the highest concentrations are located in intestinal epithelial cells; renal proximal tubular cells; canalicular membranes of hepatocytes; the capillary endothelium of the brain, choroid plexus, testes, and placenta; placental trophoblasts; adrenocortical cells; and stem cells. Other ABC transporters important in pharmacokinetics include the multidrug resistance-associated protein (MRP) family. Collectively, the MRP transporters are also widespread and involved in the vectorial (one-way) movement of drugs and other xenobiotics. In contrast to P-glycoprotein, the MRP transporters pump amphipathic molecules with at least one negative charge. These substrates include bile salts, nucleotide analogues, and conjugates of glutathione, glucuronic acid, and sulfate.

In contrast, SLC transporters do not directly use ATP as an energy source for transport and are referred to as **secondary active transporters.** These transporters require an electrochemical gradient down which solutes can move. The Na^+ pump (Na^+,K^+-ATPase) a **primary active transport** process, is the main driving force for secondary active transport. By maintaining a large electrochemical gradient for Na^+ across the plasma membrane, movements of molecules that are energetically coupled to Na^+ (or another ion with a strong electrochemical potential difference across the membrane) can occur against their own concentration gradients. Secondary active transporters that move the coupled substances in the same direction as the linked ion are termed **cotransporters** or **symporters**. In contrast, **antiporters or exchangers** move the coupled substances in the opposite direction. Many SLC transporters (including the GLUT family described previously) allow the transmembrane movement of specific chemicals down their own electrochemical gradients and therefore support facilitated diffusion. In contrast to the ABC transporters, SLC transporters can facilitate bidirectional movement of substrates based on their existing concentrations across the cell membrane.

Organic anion transporters (OATs) and organic anion–transporting polypeptides (OATPs) are important subfamilies of SLC transporters involved in pharmacokinetics. As a group, they promote the cellular uptake of acidic drugs into the liver, kidney, intestine, lung, and brain, as well as their excretion via the bile and urine. An analogous family of organic cation transporters (OCTs) provides similar handling of positively charged drugs.

Endocytosis and Exocytosis

The processes of endocytosis and exocytosis are together the most complex methods of drug transfer across a biologic membrane. The term *endocytosis* refers to a series of events in which a substance is engulfed and internalized by the cell. (A similar term, *phagocytosis* or "cell eating," is a variant of endocytosis associated more with the removal of particulate matter by macrophages than with drug transport.)

Endocytosis usually begins with the binding of a compound to be absorbed, usually a macromolecule, by its receptor on the membrane surface. Several mechanisms exist. A good example is the attachment of low-density lipoprotein (LDL) to its respective receptor. With time, the bound agent–receptor complex is concentrated in an indentation of the membrane called a coated pit. *Clathrin*, a cytoplasmic protein that attaches to the internal surface of the plasma membrane, serves to capture the receptors within the pit while excluding other surface proteins. Internal rearrangement of its structure deepens the pit, forming a coated bud. A second protein, termed *dynamin*, is believed to congregate around the collar of the invaginated bud and initiate separation from the membrane. When released, the vesicle loses its clathrin coat and fuses with a cytoplasmic organelle called the endosome. Some of the captured contents, such as the LDL receptors, are recycled back to the plasma membrane by transport vesicles; the remainder undergo lysosomal processing and release into the cytoplasm.

The complementary process of exocytosis occurs when vesicles, such as those produced by the Golgi apparatus, fuse with the plasma membrane and discharge their contents outside the cell. Exocytosis is the primary method by which cellular products such as regulatory hormones are secreted by the cell. The term *transcytosis* is descriptive of a coupled form of endocytosis and exocytosis leading to the transfer of drug from one epithelial surface of a cell to another.

ABSORPTION

Absorption refers to the transfer of a drug from its site of administration into the bloodstream. The particular route of administration selected greatly influences the rate and perhaps the extent of drug absorption.

Oral Ingestion

Oral ingestion was the first, and is still the most commonly used, method for the administration of therapeutic agents. The major advantages of the oral route lie in three areas: convenience, economics, and safety (Table 2-1). The bulk of drug absorption occurs in the small intestine with lesser amounts being absorbed in the stomach. Sudden high blood concentrations are not nearly as likely to be achieved by the ingestion of drugs as they are by parenteral injection. Allergic reactions are also less likely to occur, especially serious reactions. The oral route does have some drawbacks, however. Because self-administration is the rule, patient compliance is required for optimal therapy. Drug absorption is likely to be delayed (on a clinical average of 30 to 60 minutes) and may be incomplete. Metabolic inactivation or complex formation may also occur before the drug has a chance to reach the systemic circulation. These limitations to the oral route translate into an increased variability in patient response (Table 2-1).

TABLE 2-1 Characteristics of Routes of Drug Administration

Route of Administration	Absorption Characteristics	Advantages	Disadvantages
Oral	Variable; depends on rate of gastric emptying; dosage forms affect rate	Convenient, economical, self-administration, low cost, relatively safe	Requires patient compliance; unsuitable for poorly absorbed drugs; rapid inactivation for some drugs
Sublingual, buccal	Rapid for some drugs	Avoids first-pass metabolism; predictable effect for some drugs	Drug must be kept in contact with absorption site
Intravenous	Immediate	Ideal for emergencies; rapid titration is possible; the fastest way to achieve predictable plasma drug concentrations; large volumes can be given over time	Adverse effects appear rapidly and are difficult to reverse; suspensions cannot be given; pain, vasculitis, extravasation may occur; not usually for self-administration
Intramuscular	Rapid for aqueous solutions; slow for suspensions or depot forms	More predictable response than for oral drugs; rate of absorption can be manipulated; useful for noncompliant patients	Painful; may cause muscle damage; bleeding risk with patients on anticoagulants; may interfere with some diagnostic tests that measure organ or tissue damage
Inhalation	Rapid absorption for anesthetics; some inhaled drugs (e.g., antiasthma drugs) stay in the respiration tract	Useful for bronchodilators and inhaled steroids; useful for gaseous or volatile liquid anesthetics, titration of anesthetic	Coughing; bronchodilator and steroid self-administration require patient education
Subcutaneous	Rapid for aqueous solutions; slow for suspensions or depot forms	Aqueous or depot forms can be used	Pain, tissue necrosis

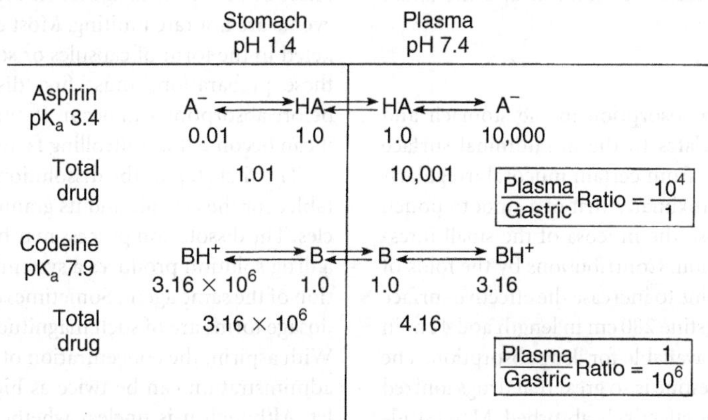

FIG 2-6 Gastric absorption of aspirin, a weak acid, and codeine, a weak base. The absorption of aspirin is promoted by ion trapping within the plasma; the low pH of stomach fluid favors gastric retention of codeine. (The actual 3.49 pK_a of aspirin is truncated to 3.4 for purposes of illustration.)

Influence of pH

Absorption is favored when the drug ingested is lipid soluble. For weak electrolytes, the pH of the surrounding medium affects the degree of ionization and drug absorption. Because the H^+ concentrations of the stomach and small intestine diverge widely, the two structures seem to be qualitatively dissimilar in their respective patterns of drug absorption. Figure 2-6 illustrates this difference and its effect on the analgesic combination of aspirin plus codeine. Aspirin is an organic acid with a pK_a (negative log of the dissociation constant) of 3.49. In gastric juice (pH 1 to 3), aspirin remains largely nonionized, and its passage across the stomach mucosa and into the bloodstream is favored. The plasma has a pH of 7.4, however, and upon entering this environment, the aspirin becomes ionized to such an extent that return of the drug to the gastrointestinal tract is prevented by the low lipid solubility of the anionic species. When equilibrium is established, the concentration of nonionized aspirin molecules on both sides of the membrane is the same, but the total amount of drug (ionized plus neutral forms) is much greater on the plasma side. The relative concentration of drug in each compartment can be calculated with the Henderson-Hasselbalch equation, as follows:

$$\text{Log}\ \frac{\text{base}\ (A^-)}{\text{acid}\ (HA)} = pH - pK_a$$

This unequal distribution of drug molecules based on the pH gradient across the gastric membrane is an example of ion trapping. The biologic process that sustains this partitioning is the energy-consuming secretion of H^+ by the gastric parietal cells. Because few organic acids have a pK_a low enough to permit significant ionization at stomach pH, almost all acidic drugs should theoretically be effectively absorbed across the gastric mucosa.

For bases such as codeine (pK_a 7.9), the opposite applies. Codeine is almost completely ionized in the acidic environment of the stomach; absorption is negligible, and virtually all the drug remains within the stomach. Only very weak bases are nonionized at gastric pH and available for absorption. In this case, the ion trapping occurs before absorption within the gastric lumen. (Interestingly, this is sometimes useful in forensic medicine. Many drugs subject to abuse are organic bases (e.g., heroin, cocaine, and amphetamine). Even when injected intravenously, they tend to accumulate in the stomach by crossing the gastric mucosa in the reverse direction. Questions of intravenous overdosage can often be answered from the analysis of stomach contents.)

When the acidic gastric fluid passes into the small intestine, it is quickly neutralized by pancreatic, biliary, and intestinal secretions. The pH of the proximal one-fourth of the intestine varies from 3 to 6, but it reaches neutrality in more distal segments. Under these more alkaline conditions, aspirin converts to the anionic form, whereas a significant fraction of the codeine molecules give up their positive charge. Although basic drugs are favored for absorption over acids in the small intestine, ion trapping is not as extensive because the pH differential across the intestinal mucosa is small. Differences in intestinal absorption based on pH are more concerned with the rate of uptake than with its extent. As one might expect, neutralization of gastric contents by the administration of antacids or ingestion of food temporarily removes the qualitative disparity in electrolyte absorption normally observed between the stomach and the small intestine.

Mucosal surface area

A second major difference between absorption in the stomach and absorption in the small intestine relates to the intraluminal surface areas involved in drug uptake. Aside from certain mucosal irregularities (rugae), the stomach lining approximates that of a smooth pouch with a thick mucus layer. In contrast, the mucosa of the small intestine is uniquely adapted for absorption. Contributions by the folds of Kerckring, villi, and microvilli combine to increase the effective surface area 600-fold. Assuming a small intestine 280 cm in length and 4 cm in diameter, approximately 200 m^2 are available for drug absorption. The surface/volume ratio in the small intestine is so great that drugs ionized even to the extent of 99% may still be effectively absorbed. Many studies have shown that acidic drugs with a pK_a greater than 3.0 and basic compounds with a pK_a less than 8.0 readily pass from the intestinal fluid into the plasma. As a result, although pH considerations favor the gastric absorption of aspirin, as much as 90% of the drug is actually absorbed from the small intestine in vivo. Experimentally, nonelectrolytes such as ethanol are also absorbed from the intestine many times faster than from the stomach.

Gastric emptying

Because almost any substance that can penetrate the gastrointestinal epithelium is best absorbed in the small intestine, the rate of gastric emptying can significantly affect drug absorption, particularly for organic bases that are not absorbed at all from the stomach. Gastric emptying is accomplished by contraction of the antrum of the stomach. A cyclical pattern of activity occurs in fasting patients where periods of quiescence (about 1 hour each) are followed by contractions that increase in intensity over a 40-minute period before terminating in a short burst of intense contractions that migrate from the stomach to the distal ileum. Ingesting a tablet or small volume of liquid may result in gastric retention of the drug for 1 hour or longer. After eating a meal, sustained antral and pyloric contractions help break up the ingested food and permit the extrusion of liquid into the duodenum while retaining particles more than 1 mm in diameter within the stomach. A mixed meal of solids and liquids usually begins to enter the duodenum in about 30 minutes and requires about 4 hours to leave the stomach completely. Conversely, a glass of water ingested on an empty stomach is moved into the small intestine in a more rapid fashion, with half of the water expelled from the stomach in 15 minutes, and essentially all of the liquid removed by 1 hour.

A major variable in delaying gastric emptying is the presence of fat. Normally, most oral medications should be taken in the absence of food but with a full glass of water. This procedure speeds drug entry into the small intestine and provides maximum access to the gastrointestinal mucosa. Occasionally, the presence of a fatty meal promotes the absorption of a drug that has a high lipid but low water solubility. The protease inhibitor saquinavir and the fat-soluble vitamins are examples of substances that are better absorbed in the presence of lipids. In these instances, the delay in gastric emptying produced by the high fat content of the chyme is compensated for by a more complete absorption. Because gastric emptying is often a limiting factor in the rate of drug absorption, many unrelated drugs exhibit latency periods (the lag phase between oral ingestion and onset of drug effect) of a similar magnitude.

Influence of dosage form

Although the times required for gastric emptying and for diffusion across the mucosal barrier undoubtedly contribute to the delayed onset of action of drugs taken orally, situations exist in which these events are not rate limiting. Most drugs intended for oral use are marketed in the form of capsules or solid tablets. In contrast to solutions, these preparations must first dissolve in the gastrointestinal fluid before absorption can occur. If dissolution is designed to be very slow, it can become the controlling factor in drug absorption.

The first step in the dissolution process is the disintegration of the tablet (or the capsule and its granules) to yield the primary drug particles. The dissolution process may be considered rate limiting whenever a drug solution produces a systemic effect faster than a solid formulation of the same agent. Sometimes discrepancies in absorption between dosage forms are of such magnitude that clinical differences are noted. With aspirin, the concentration of drug in the plasma 30 minutes after administration can be twice as high for a solution as for a solid tablet. Although it is unclear whether this difference results solely from drug dissolution or from other factors, such as the more rapid gastric emptying typical of liquids, dissolution is probably at least partially responsible.

The influence of dosage form on drug absorption is often taken advantage of by drug manufacturers. To avoid release of certain drugs within the stomach, they are often prepared in the form of enteric-coated tablets. An enteric coat consists of a film of shellac or some polymeric substitute. The covering is insoluble under acidic conditions, but it does break down to permit tablet disintegration in the more alkaline environment of the small intestine. Although these preparations are often beneficial, their usefulness nevertheless is negatively affected by an increased variability in patient response. Because drug absorption cannot begin until the tablet passes into the duodenum, the time required for gastric transit becomes an important variable. The passage of a single insoluble tablet from the stomach into the intestine is a random event that can take several minutes to more than 6 hours.

Sustained-release preparations represent another method of capitalizing on the influence of formulation on drug absorption. These products are usually designed to release a steady amount of drug within the gastrointestinal tract for 12 to 24 hours. Some preparations also provide an initial loading dose that is readily available for absorption. Sustained release may be accomplished by using a porous matrix, with the drug located in the interior spaces and on the external surface. An alternative is to make spheres of drug that dissolve at different rates because of various coatings.

The sensitivity of gastrointestinal absorption to variations in drug formulation is best exemplified by the concern over **bioavailability**. In many instances, chemically identical drugs have proved in the past to be biologically nonequivalent because of differences in formulation. In one study of tetracycline hydrochloride, nine preparations from different manufacturers were compared with an aqueous solution of the same drug. Although seven brands produced blood concentrations ranging from 70% to 100% of the reference solution, two products exhibited relative bioavailabilities of only 20% to 30%. Differences in bioavailability are more clinically important with drugs that are poorly absorbed, have low margins of safety, and are inactivated by capacity-limited processes. Since 1977, federal law has required that bioequivalence testing be performed on all new drugs, and the FDA has mandated such testing of existing products for which a problem of nonequivalence is known to exist. Bioavailability considerations related to drug selection are considered further in Chapter 42.

Active transport

Most drugs intended for oral use are absorbed by passive diffusion. Active transport systems do exist, however, for specific dietary constituents that sometimes increase the absorption of certain drugs. The absorption of levodopa and baclofen from the intestine is enhanced because they are amino acid analogues that are actively transported into intestinal cells by the large neutral amino acid transporter (an SLC transporter). Valacyclovir is, likewise, much better absorbed than is its congener acyclovir because it is a substrate for PepT-1, another SLC transporter.

Active transport mechanisms can also inhibit drug absorption. P-glycoprotein is highly expressed along the luminal surface of intestinal epithelial cells, where it exports xenobiotics that would otherwise be absorbed. This function is in concert with the "chemoimmunity defensive" role P-glycoprotein plays in protecting cells from exposure to potentially toxic compounds. Although P-glycoprotein may delay the absorption of many drugs and prevent altogether the uptake of pharmaceuticals of low absorptive potential, it is probably of minor significance regarding the extent of absorption of most drugs intended for oral use, whose concentrations in the chyme are sufficient to overwhelm the capacity of P-glycoprotein to export them. Figure 2-7 depicts the active transport of drugs into and out of intestinal cells and at other important sites.

Drug inactivation

A shortcoming of oral ingestion is the inactivation of drugs before they reach the systemic circulation. The destruction of some agents (e.g., epinephrine and insulin) is sufficiently great to preclude their administration by this route. With other drugs (e.g., penicillin G), losses may be smaller but still large enough to make oral administration inefficient. Gastric acid is one of the principal causes of drug breakdown within the gastrointestinal tract, but degradation also results from enzymatic activity. Vasopressin, insulin, calcitonin, and other polypeptides are subject to hydrolysis by pancreatic and intestinal peptidases. Intestinal cells also contain intracellular enzymes for metabolizing drugs. Of particular importance are the presence of monoamine oxidase for the inactivation of biogenic amines and the presence of CYP3A4/5 enzymes (described later) for the oxidation of numerous compounds. Enteric bacterial enzymes may also destroy certain ingested agents, such as chlorpromazine. Finally, intestinal contents can alter the effectiveness of many orally administered drugs. Binding to constituents of chyme, chelation with divalent cations, or formation of insoluble salts may decrease the amount of drug available for absorption.

A special fate exists for substances that are successfully absorbed from the gastrointestinal tract. The venous drainage of the stomach, small intestine, and colon is routed by the hepatic portal system to the liver. A **first pass** of high drug concentration through this enzyme-laden organ can significantly reduce the quantity of agent reaching the systemic circulation. For example, lidocaine is metabolized so rapidly in the liver that virtually all of an oral dose is destroyed during its first pass. Although less pronounced, disparities in opioid analgesic and antibiotic efficacies observed between the oral route and other modes of administration are of clinical importance to the practice of dentistry.

Other enteral routes

The oral and rectal mucosa are occasionally used as sites of drug absorption. Sublingual administration, in which a tablet or troche is allowed to dissolve completely in the oral cavity, takes advantage of the permeability of the oral epithelium and is the preferred route for a few potent lipophilic drugs, such as nitroglycerin and oxytocin, and even the commonly used oral sedative triazolam. One reason for selecting the sublingual route is to avoid drug destruction. Because gastric acid and intestinal and hepatic enzymes are bypassed, sublingual absorption can be more efficient overall for certain drugs than intestinal uptake. The onset of drug effect may also be quicker than with oral ingestion. In dentistry, triazolam generally reaches peak effect in 20 to 30 minutes sublingually, as compared to 30 to 45 minutes orally.

Rectal administration may be used when other enteral routes are precluded, as in an unconscious or nauseated patient. Although a significant fraction of absorbed drug enters the circulation without having to pass through the liver, uptake is often unpredictable. For many patients, aversion to rectal introduction of drugs prohibits administration by this route.

Inhalation

The alveolar membrane is an important route of entry for some drugs and many noxious substances. Although the alveolar lining is highly permeable, it is accessible only to agents that are in a gaseous state or are inhaled in sufficiently fine powders or microdroplets to reach the deepest endings of the respiratory tree. Gaseous agents include the therapeutic gases, carbon monoxide, inhalation anesthetics, and numerous volatile organic solvents. The second category of alveolar membrane penetrants is collectively known as **aerosols**. This term refers to liquid or solid particles small enough (usually ≤10 μm in diameter) to remain suspended in air for prolonged periods. Any such finely divided material, when inhaled, reaches some portion of the respiratory tree and is affected by the processes of sedimentation and inertial precipitation. Most aerosols contain a mixture of particle sizes.

Therapeutic use of aerosols is not widespread, but some emergency medications are prepared in this form. Because the onset of effect is extremely rapid after inhalation of an aerosol drug, this route can provide a means of quick self-medication for individuals in danger of acute allergic reactions to venoms or drugs. Epinephrine is one such emergency agent that is marketed as an aerosol. Many respiratory drugs are also prepared in aerosol form because they are highly effective by this route while minimizing systemic exposure. The rapidity and efficiency of alveolar membrane absorption can occasionally pose problems for therapy, however, as illustrated by the use of aerosols containing isoproterenol. Although 97% of an isoproterenol spray is swallowed under normal conditions and inactivated by various enzymes,

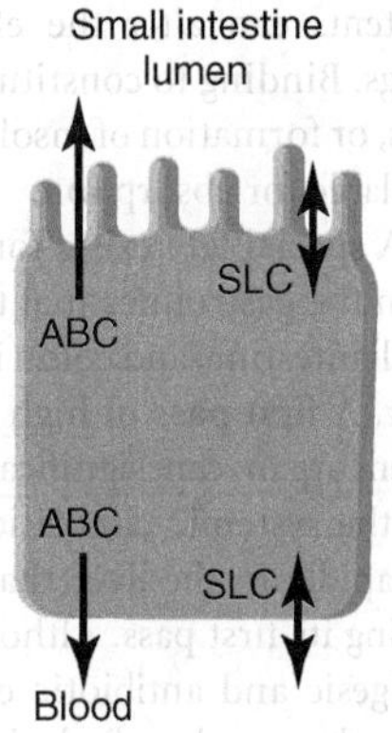

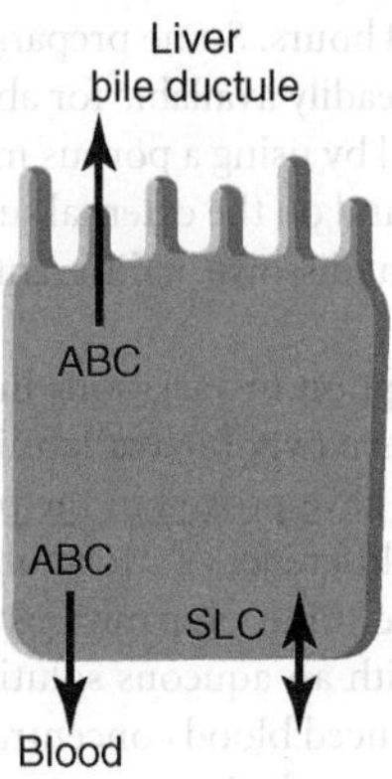

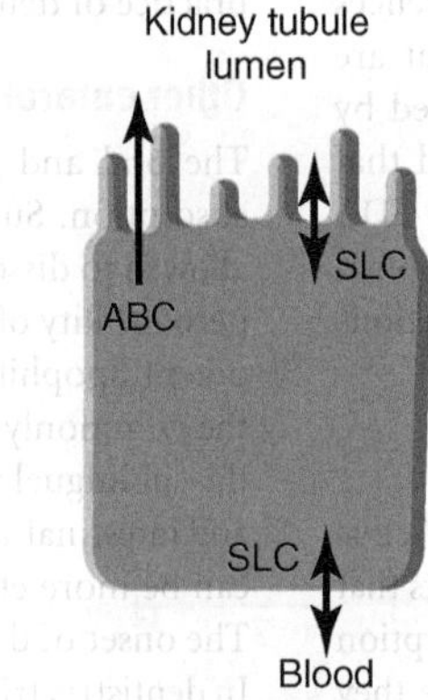

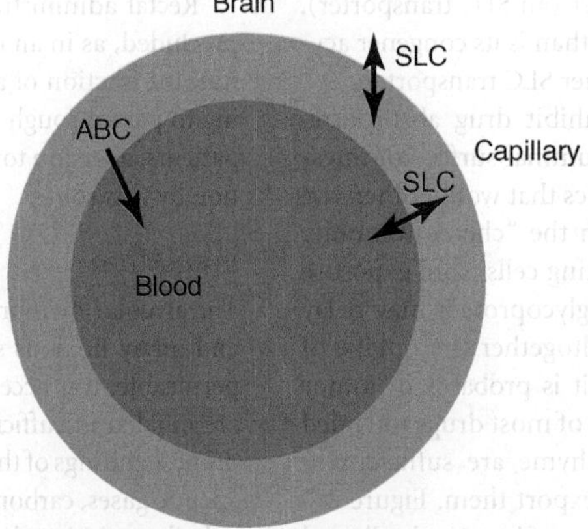

FIG 2-7 Transepithelial or transendothelial transport of drugs across the small intestine and the liver (absorption), brain capillaries (distribution), and liver and kidneys (elimination). *ABC*, ATP-binding cassette transporter; *SLC*, solute carrier transporter.

overmedication can produce toxic effects. This reflects the hazards of aerosols when abused and provides a caveat for uncontrolled self-medication with any potentially dangerous drug. Concern over aerosols is also related to questions of toxicology, such as the absorption of heavy metal dusts by industrial workers.

Parenteral Injection

Drugs are frequently given by parenteral injection when oral ingestion is precluded by the patient's condition, when a rapid onset of effect is necessary, or when blood concentrations greater than those obtainable with the enteral route are required. The method of injection selected varies with the particular drug and therapeutic need of the patient (Table 2-1).

Intravenous route

The administration of drugs by infusion or injection directly into the bloodstream is particularly useful when immediate effects or exact blood concentrations are desired. Also, through the technique of titration, the intravenous route provides an avenue for the controlled administration of drugs that have a very narrow margin of safety between therapeutic and toxic concentrations. The infusion of lidocaine to prevent ventricular arrhythmias and the incremental injection of antianxiety drugs during intravenous sedation are two examples in which titration is used to achieve a desired effect while avoiding adverse reactions. Most IV drugs should be administered over a period of 1 minute, which approximates the circulation time of blood through the body. This procedure avoids high, transient concentrations and permits discontinuance if any untoward effect is observed during the course of injection. Other characteristics of intravenous injections are given in Table 2-1.

Intramuscular route

The intramuscular route is often selected for drugs that cannot be given orally because of slow or erratic absorption, high percentage of drug inactivation, or lack of patient cooperation (Table 2-1). The rate of absorption from an intramuscular site is governed by the same factors influencing gastrointestinal uptake, such as lipid/water partition coefficient, degree of ionization, and molecular size. Many drugs are absorbed at approximately the same rate, however, regardless of these factors. Muscles with high blood flows (e.g., deltoid) provide faster absorption rates than muscles with lesser flows (e.g., gluteus maximus). Generally, 5 to 30 minutes is required for the onset of drug effect, but this latency period can be controlled to some extent. Exercise markedly speeds absorption by stimulating local circulation. Conversely, uptake may be minimized by the application of ice packs or (in an emergency) tourniquets.

Subcutaneous route

Injection of drugs into the subcutaneous connective tissue is a widely used method of administration for agents that can be given in small volumes (≤2 mL) and are not locally damaging. Subcutaneous absorption is similar to that of resting muscle, and onset times are often comparable. As with the intramuscular route, absorption can be delayed by diminishing blood flow, either through the application of pressure or by surface cooling. Pharmacologic interruption of circulation with vasoconstrictors is also a common strategy, especially in local anesthesia. Because of the ease of subcutaneous implantation, compressed pellets of drugs, sometimes mixed with insoluble matrix material, can be inserted to provide nearly constant drug release for weeks or months. Testosterone and several progestational contraceptive agents (e.g., levonorgestrel) have been successfully administered by this approach.

When subcutaneous administration is chosen for a systemic effect, the hastening of drug absorption is sometimes advantageous. Toward this end, warming the tissue promotes drug uptake by improving local circulation. Massage of the injection site, in addition to stimulating blood flow, helps spread the drug and provides an increased surface area for absorption.

Other parenteral injection routes

Intraarterial injections are occasionally performed when a localized effect on a particular organ or area of the body is desired. Injections of radiopaque dyes for diagnostic purposes and antineoplastic agents to control localized tumors are the most commonly encountered examples. Intrathecal administration is used when the direct access of drug to the central nervous system (CNS) is necessary. Indications for injection into the subarachnoid space include the production of spinal anesthesia with local anesthetics and the resolution of acute CNS infections with antibiotics. The intraperitoneal infusion of fluids is a useful substitute for hemodialysis in the treatment of drug poisoning. Although intraperitoneal injection is commonly used in animal experimentation, the risk of infection usually precludes such use in humans. Last, intraosseous (anterior tibial) injection of emergency drugs can be used when intravenous access cannot be obtained quickly.

All these specialized injection techniques are potentially dangerous to the patient. They should be performed only when expressly indicated and then only by qualified personnel.

Topical Application

Drugs are often applied to epithelial surfaces for local effects and less frequently for systemic absorption. Penetration of drugs across the epithelium is strongly influenced by the degree of keratinization.

Skin

The epidermis is a highly modified tissue that isolates the body from the external environment. The outer layer of skin (stratum corneum) is densely packed with the protein keratin. This layer is impervious to water and water-soluble drugs, and its relative thickness and paucity of lipids in contrast to other biologic membranes retard even the diffusion of even some lipophilic agents. However, certain compounds may readily penetrate the skin to cause systemic effects. These drugs include organic solvents, organophosphate- and nicotine-based insecticides, and some nerve gases. Severe poisoning has also resulted from the excessive application of sunburn creams containing local anesthetics. Even lipid-insoluble substances such as inorganic mercury can diffuse across skin if exposure is prolonged.

The benefits of improving and sufficiently controlling percutaneous absorption to make it a reliable route of drug administration have prompted several marketing strategies. A "transdermal therapeutic system" has been developed to provide continuous systemic uptake of nitroglycerin, scopolamine, fentanyl, and nicotine for prophylaxis of angina pectoris, prophylaxis of motion sickness, management of chronic pain, and assistance with smoking cessation, respectively. The system is a complex patch that consists of an outer impermeable backing, a reservoir containing the drug in a suspended form, a semipermeable membrane, and an inner adhesive seal. Another approach to improving drug penetration through the epidermis is the use of occlusive dressings. These dressings retain moisture and break down the horny layer through the process of maceration. A final technique, iontophoresis, is discussed subsequently.

Mucous membranes

The topical application of drugs to mucous membranes offers several potential advantages for local therapy as was discussed with sublingual or buccal administration. The tissues can often be visualized by the clinician, permitting accurate drug placement. The use of this route generally minimizes systemic effects while providing an optimal concentration of drug in the area being treated. In contrast to the case with skin, drugs have little trouble permeating mucous membranes to affect localized conditions. Systemic absorption of lipophilic drugs from mucous membranes readily occurs. Before this fact was widely appreciated, the topical application of tetracaine to the pharyngeal and tracheal mucosa was a leading cause of local anesthetic overdosage. In dentistry, the use of corticosteroids to ameliorate inflammatory conditions has also led to systemic responses, such as the suppression of adrenocortical function by triamcinolone. Although these effects are generally mild and transient, they can create problems for patients with hypertension, diabetes mellitus, or peptic ulcer. Local therapies can also affect systemic health by serving as antigenic stimulants and, in the case of antibiotics, by disturbing the normal microbial ecology and promoting the emergence of resistant microorganisms.

The nasal mucosa offers a suitable avenue for the uptake of certain agents. Desmopressin, used in the treatment of diabetes insipidus, and butorphanol, a potent analgesic, are examples of drugs that can be given intranasally.

Iontophoresis

Iontophoresis is the electric transport of positively or negatively charged drugs across surface tissues. The technique involves passing a direct electric current of appropriate polarity through the drug solution and patient. Permeation of mucous membranes, skin, and hard tissues is possible with this approach, yet the total dose delivered is small, and systemic toxicity is unlikely. In dental therapeutics today, iontophoretic applications of drugs are rarely used, although many of our chronic pain patients have narcotic delivery systems that use this technique of administration.

DISTRIBUTION

Distribution refers to the movement of drugs throughout the body. The rate, sequence, and extent of distribution depend on many factors: the physicochemical properties of the drug, cardiac output and regional blood flow, anatomic characteristics of membranes, transmembrane electric and pH gradients, binding to plasma proteins and tissue reservoirs, and carrier-mediated transport. For all but the very few drugs that act intravascularly, the capillary membrane constitutes the first tissue barrier to be crossed in the journey of a drug from the bloodstream to its site of action.

Capillary Penetration

After a drug gains access to the systemic circulation, it becomes diluted by the plasma volume of the entire vascular compartment. For a compound administered intravenously, this process requires only several minutes for completion; for drugs given by other routes, intravascular distribution occurs concurrently with absorption. The transfer of drugs out of the bloodstream is governed by the same factors that control its entrance. Lipophilic drugs diffuse across the capillary membrane extremely rapidly. The transfer is so expeditious that equilibrium with interstitial fluid is practically instantaneous. Under these conditions, the rate of drug uptake is determined by the blood flow through the tissue under consideration. Well-perfused organs are saturated with drug long before many other tissues have had a chance to reach even a fraction of the equilibrium concentration. Water-soluble drugs diffuse through gaps located between adjacent endothelial cells. With these agents, transcapillary movement is slower than for drugs that have high lipid/water partition coefficients and is inversely proportional to molecular weight. As molecular size increases beyond 20 to 30 kDa, aqueous paracellular diffusion ceases to be quantitatively important. Current evidence suggests that caveolae-based transcellular movement takes over as the primary transport method for large drugs. Convection may also be important in vascular beds with large gaps between endothelial cells, and it assumes special prominence when inflammatory signals cause paracellular pathways to widen.

Entry of Drugs into Cells

As previously discussed, the cell membrane acts as a semipermeable barrier, admitting some drugs into the cell, while excluding others. Nonpolar, lipid-soluble compounds distribute evenly across plasma membranes, but distribution of weak electrolytes at equilibrium is more complex. The intracellular pH is approximately 7.0, differing slightly from the 7.4 pH of extracellular fluid. Acids with a pK_a less than 8.0 tend to remain outside the cell, whereas basic drugs with a pK_a greater than 6.0 tend to accumulate within it. Because the concentration differential across the cell membrane based on a pH gradient of 0.4 can equal 2.5:1, the acid–base status of a patient can significantly affect the dose response of weak electrolytes acting intracellularly. (The influence of pH on the distribution of local anesthetics across nerve membranes is described in Chapter 14.) Ions, unless very small in size (molecular weights of ≤60 Da) or transported by membrane-bound carriers, penetrate cell membranes with difficulty, if at all. Charged drugs that do gain access to the cell by passive diffusion are distributed at equilibrium according to their electrochemical gradient across the membrane.

Restricted Distribution

In some tissues or organs, anatomic relationships and membrane transporters sequester interstitial or transcellular fluids from the general extracellular space and restrict intracellular access to drugs. The most important examples for therapeutics include the CNS and the fetal circulation.

Central nervous system

Entry of drugs into the CNS is unusually dependent on lipid solubility. Most drugs with high lipid/water partition coefficients are taken up very quickly, as exemplified by the immediate onset of general anesthesia after the intravenous injection of thiopental. The rapid distribution of lipophilic drugs into the brain and spinal cord arises from the fact that the CNS receives approximately 15% of the cardiac output yet composes only 2% of total body weight. Despite this favorable blood supply, drugs that are sparingly lipid soluble are largely excluded from the extracellular space of the brain. There are four reasons why there is an added barrier in the brain constituting the **blood–brain barrier**. These are shown in Figure 2-8. First, the capillaries of the brain do not have fenestrations and are characterized by tight junctions. Transcytosis is not characteristic of these capillaries. Second, a cellular sheath composed of processes extending from connective tissue astrocytes surrounds the capillaries. Third, P-glycoproteins actively transport drugs out of the brain. Fourth, choroid plexus cells provide an avenue to pump drugs out of the cerebrospinal fluid.

The selective distribution of compounds into the CNS has several important therapeutic ramifications. Some alkaloids intended for peripheral nervous system effects may cause central disturbances on entry into the brain. Conversion of such drugs (e.g., scopolamine) to positively charged quaternary ammonium derivatives (e.g., methscopolamine) prevents CNS influences yet allows essential peripheral nervous system activity. Conversely, drugs used for their central effects may benefit by molecular modifications that enhance their entry into the brain. Lower total doses can be given and peripheral effects minimized.

Sometimes the blood–brain barrier is a hindrance to therapy. Penicillin G, a water-soluble organic acid with a pK_a of 2.6, diffuses slowly into the CNS and is subject to active removal by the choroid plexus. For patients with bacterial encephalitis, this lack of drug penetration can complicate treatment. (Fortunately, capillary permeability in the brain often increases during meningeal inflammation.) A clever approach to circumventing the blood–brain barrier is embodied in the treatment of parkinsonism. This condition is associated with a deficiency of dopamine within selected portions of the brain. Replacement therapy with dopamine is ineffective because the drug is excluded by the blood–brain barrier. To avoid this problem, levodopa, the amino acid precursor of dopamine, is used instead. Levodopa readily enters the brain, where it is subsequently decarboxylated to the active drug.

Placental transfer

Fetal blood vessels projecting into sinuses filled with maternal blood are covered by a single syncytium of cells called **trophoblasts**. The movement of drugs across the placenta is limited by the trophoblastic membrane, which is qualitatively similar to plasma membranes elsewhere. Although trophoblasts are known to secrete amino acids and other vital nutrients actively into the fetal circulation, the entry of most drugs depends on passive diffusion across the lipid barrier. For highly lipophilic drugs such as thiopental, distribution is retarded only by the rate of maternal blood flow through the placenta and by peculiarities in the fetal circulation that limit tissue perfusion. Even so, it has been calculated that 40 minutes are required for fetal tissues to attain 90% equilibration with a constant maternal arterial concentration. Limited by a sluggish transmembrane diffusion, the transfer of water-soluble compounds is so inefficient that virtually no drug from

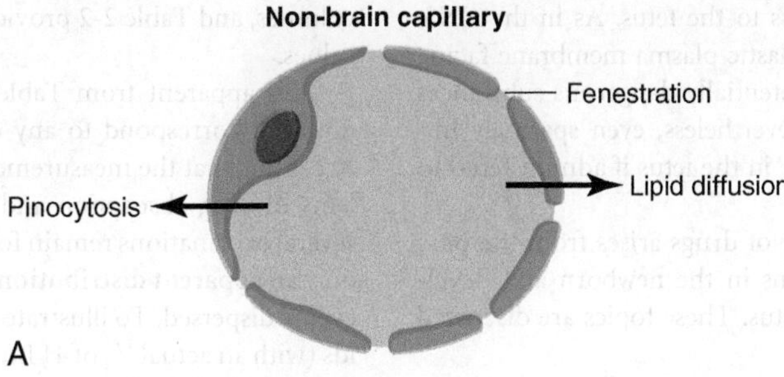

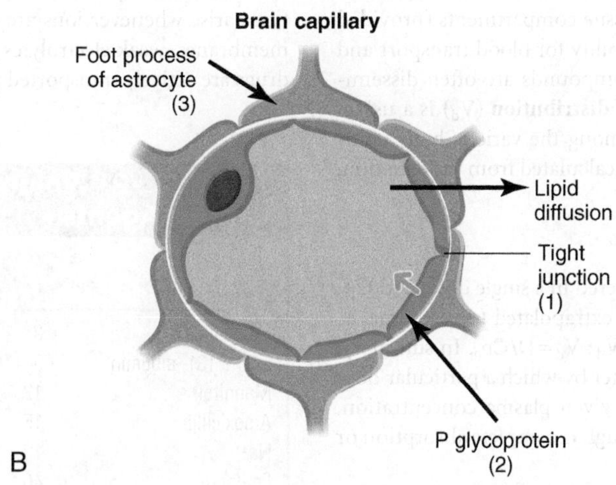

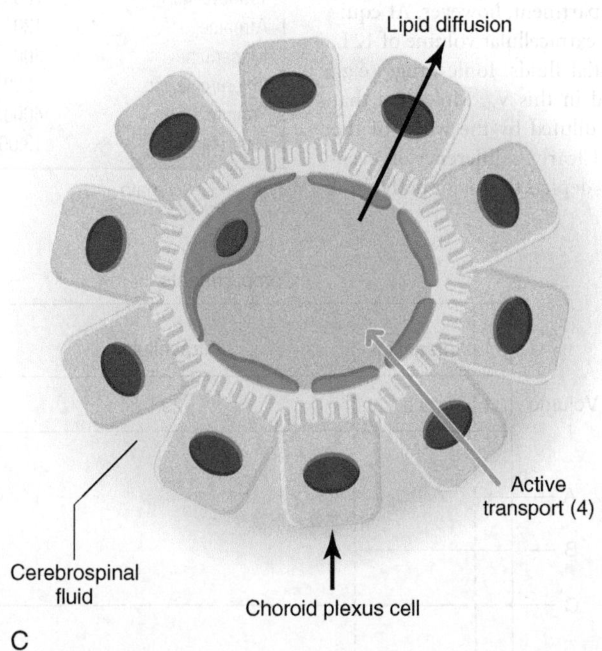

FIG 2-8 The contributors to the blood–brain barrier. The following four factors are shown. A brain capillary is compared to capillaries elsewhere in the body. (1) Tight junctions characterize the capillaries in the brain. (2) Astrocytes (glial cells) surround brain capillaries, providing an additional lipid barrier. (3) P-Glycoproteins pump drugs out of capillary cells. The third illustration shows cells of the choroid plexus surrounding a capillary. (4) These cells have SLC pumps that transport drugs from the CSF into the capillary lumen. *SLC,* Solute carrier transporters; *CSF,* cerebrospinal fluid.

a single administration may gain access to the fetus. As in the CNS, P-glycoproteins located in the trophoblastic plasma membrane facing the maternal blood tend to prevent potentially dangerous substances from entering the fetal circulation. Nevertheless, even sparingly lipid-soluble agents eventually accumulate in the fetus if administered to the mother in multiple doses.

Concern over the placental transfer of drugs arises from the possibility of inducing toxic manifestations in the newborn and developmental defects in the embryo and fetus. These topics are discussed further in Chapter 3.

Volume of Distribution

Drugs are not distributed equally throughout the body. Although lipophilic substances tend to penetrate all tissue compartments (provided that they have a modicum of water solubility for blood transport and are not actively ejected), hydrophilic compounds are often disseminated more restrictively. The **volume of distribution (V_d)** is a useful indicator of how drugs are dispersed among the various body compartments. In its simplest form, the V_d is calculated from the equation:

$$D = V_d \times Cp_0$$

where D is the quantity of drug administered in a single dose, and Cp_0 is the plasma concentration of the drug extrapolated to zero time, as shown later in Figure 2-14. Solving for V_d: $V_d = D/Cp_0$. In summary, the V_d is the **hypothetical** amount of water by which a particular dose would have to be diluted to produce a given plasma concentration, assuming that no drug has been lost through incomplete absorption or by metabolism or excretion.

As a practical matter, drugs confined within the blood have a V_d of approximately 3 L. This value represents the total plasma volume of a 70-kg man of average build. Most compounds pass readily from the vascular tree into the interstitial compartment, however. At equilibrium, these drugs are distributed in an extracellular volume of 12 L, which includes the vascular and interstitial fluids. Ionic drugs (e.g., aminoglycosides) are generally contained in this V_d. Molecules that can freely penetrate all membranes are diluted by the water of the entire body, which is approximately 41 L. Clearly, a difference of 3 versus 12 versus 41 L is significant. Figure 2-9 depicts the major body fluid volumes, and Table 2-2 provides a list of agents with representative V_d values.

It is apparent from Table 2-2 that the V_d of many compounds does not correspond to any definable anatomic fluid compartment. Accepting that the measurements were made correctly, and that problems in drug absorption and elimination were successfully avoided, several explanations remain for these results. The V_d equation provides only an **apparent distribution**, partly because it assumes that drugs are evenly dispersed. To illustrate this point, Na^+ is present in all body fluids (with an actual V_d of 41 L), but the apparent (calculated) V_d for Na^+ is only 18 L. This discrepancy arises because Na^+ is actively but incompletely extruded from intracellular water. Dissimilarities between true and calculated V_d values based on unequal compartment concentrations arise whenever ions are distributed across electrically polarized membranes, weak electrolytes are present in fluids of different pH, or drugs are actively transported into or out of a water space.

TABLE 2-2 Volumes of Distribution of Various Agents

Agent	V_d (L)*	Corresponding Fluid Compartment
Evans blue	3	Plasma water
Iodine 131–albumin	3	
Mannitol	12	Extracellular water
Amoxicillin	15	
Na^+	18	
Enalapril	40	
Urea	41	Total body water
Lidocaine	77	
Tetracycline	100	
Atropine	120	
Meperidine	300	
Chlorpromazine	1500	
Propofol	4000	
Chloroquine	13,000	

*For a 70-kg male.

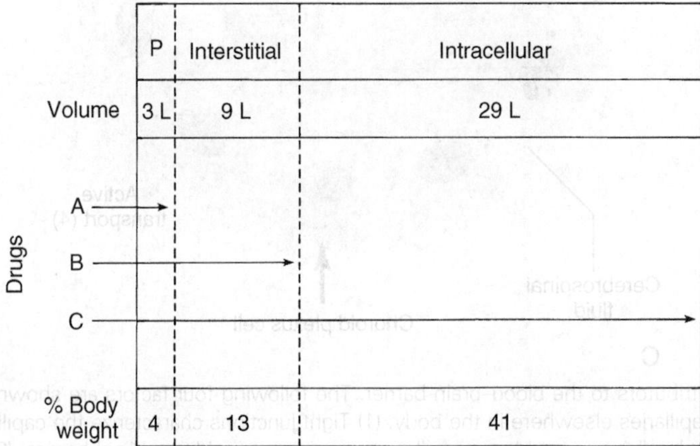

FIG 2-9 Body water compartments. The membrane barriers that separate plasma from interstitial fluid and interstitial fluid from intracellular water are indicated by *dashed lines*. The upper set of figures represents the respective volumes for a 70-kg man; the lower set are percentages of total body weight. Of the drugs shown, *A* is restricted to the plasma, *B* is distributed within the extracellular compartment (plasma + interstitial fluid), and *C* is disseminated throughout the total body water.

The enormous V_d values recorded for drugs such as propofol and chloroquine generally result from tissue binding. The sequestration of compounds within cells or certain tissues necessarily reduces the concentration of drug in the plasma, leading to an abnormally high calculation of V_d. (No drug can have a true V_d>41 L in the typical adult.) Plasma protein binding can also affect V_d determinations. Because the total drug in plasma is usually measured, binding artificially inflates the drug concentration and depresses V_d. If free drug is measured, significant binding by plasma proteins has the same effect as binding at extravascular sites. The point of the V_d is to help understand how drugs sequester and cluster in the body based on many influences.

Drug Binding and Storage

The sojourn of drugs in the body is considerably influenced by binding to proteins and other tissue components. Reducing the concentration of free solute causes a decrease in the rate of passage across membrane barriers and may alter drug distribution at equilibrium, as reflected in V_d determinations. Drug sequestration can also affect the processes of absorption, metabolism, and elimination.

Plasma protein binding

Numerous drugs become associated with plasma proteins, especially albumin. The predominant protein in plasma, albumin contains roughly 200 ionized functional groups per molecule and has the capacity to bind many different substances concurrently. A second plasma protein, α_1-acid glycoprotein (also known as orosomucoid), is a major "acceptor" of basic, or cationic, agents. Transcortin (which is specific for corticosteroids and a few other agents), other globulins, and various lipoproteins play more limited roles in drug binding.

The reversible attachment of drugs to plasma proteins is reminiscent of drug-receptor combinations in that the reaction obeys the law of mass action, as follows:

$$\text{Drug} + \text{Protein} \rightleftharpoons \text{Drug-protein complex}$$

The percentage of bound drug usually does not change over the dosage ranges used clinically, and assigning most drugs a fixed value is permissible (e.g., 99% for diazepam). Drugs differ tremendously in their affinity for plasma proteins; the percentage of binding of individual agents ranges from 0% to approaching 100%.

The binding of agents within the vascular compartment removes available free drug and therefore reduces the concentration gradient of free drug across the capillary membrane and slows egress from the plasma into the extravascular space. As free molecules leave the circulation, the bound drug begins to dissociate according to the law of mass action and becomes available for further egress.

Glomerular filtration and passive hepatic uptake involve only free drug; significant binding may depress the metabolism and excretion of drugs. When compounds are actively or otherwise rapidly taken up by organs of elimination, however, the instantaneous reversibility of binding can lead to a faster-than-normal elimination rate. Penicillin G is secreted into the urine so efficiently that blood flowing through the kidney is almost completely cleared of the antibiotic in a single pass. Because albumin binding presents the kidney with more total drug per unit time, secretion is quicker than would be the case if the drug were more evenly distributed throughout the body.

Two potential clinical concerns related to plasma protein binding involve patient variability in binding efficacy and the possibility for drug interaction. Individual differences in drug binding affect the concentration of free drug within the bloodstream and may lead to insufficient therapy in one patient and overdosage in another. The unusual susceptibility to diazepam exhibited by patients with hypoalbuminemia should be considered when the drug is used for intravenous sedation. Inasmuch as the attachment of drugs to plasma proteins is generally less selective than are drug-receptor associations, competition between drugs for binding sites is relatively common. Such interactions may reach clinical significance, however, only when the drugs are highly bound, are administered in large doses, and have a narrow margin of safety or a small V_d.

Tissue binding

As previously mentioned, drugs capable of associating with plasma proteins are also likely to bind to tissue protein constituents. Such binding does not impede the movement of drugs out of the bloodstream, but it does slow the rate of elimination. Various tissues have different affinities for drugs. By virtue of its aggregate size, muscle tissue is a significant reservoir for many drugs. Fat is also quantitatively important, especially for highly lipid-soluble compounds. Although uptake into fat is slow due to limited blood supply, adipose tissue constitutes 10% to more than 50% of total body weight, and most of an administered dose of a lipophilic drug may accumulate in fat over the course of several hours. Some tissues display unusual affinities for particular drugs; for example, the antimalarial agents chloroquine and quinacrine are heavily concentrated in the liver. Guanethidine and other quaternary ammonium compounds adhere to negatively charged residues in mucous secretions of the gastrointestinal tract.

The attachment of drugs to drug receptors warrants special comment. Important in the pharmacologic sense, the contribution of drug-receptor interactions to the total amount of binding is usually quite small. When distribution throughout the body and the various types of sequestration are considered, the percentage of drug administered that actually reaches its receptor to evoke a response is quantitatively very small.

Storage

The association between drugs and tissue elements is sometimes so stable that it is better to think of them as stored rather than transiently bound. When drugs are stored, they are not readily available for release and generally do not prolong the duration of action. Some of the most common examples of storage involve mineralized tissues and fat. Bone-seeking ions such as F^- and lead, and Ca^{++} chelators such as the tetracyclines, may be deposited with bone salts during mineralization or become associated with existing hydroxyapatite crystals. Essentially in an insoluble state, these substances are difficult or impossible to remove completely. Bone and tooth mineralization may benefit from appropriate concentrations of F^-, but most drug-induced alterations are detrimental. In the case of radioactive metals (e.g., strontium 90), storage in bone can lead to the development of leukemia, osteogenic sarcoma, and other forms of neoplasia. Zoledronic acid is exceptional in that storage in bone does lead to an extended duration of action. Given once a year for the treatment of postmenopausal osteoporosis, zoledronic acid is taken up by new bone formed during remodeling and is sequestered. Later, as osteoclasts restart bone turnover in the same area, zoledronic acid is released to inhibit further activity.

Redistribution

Strongly lipophilic drugs, especially when administered intravenously in bolus form, characteristically go through several phases of distribution: an initial transfer into vessel-rich organs (brain, heart, kidneys, liver, and lungs) followed by progressive redistribution to less highly vascularized tissues (muscle, skin, and eventually fat). When the target organ of a drug happens to have a high blood flow per unit mass, redistribution can result in the abrupt termination of drug effect. Thiopental has been extensively studied in this regard (Fig. 2-10). The onset of anesthesia with thiopental is almost instantaneous; however, consciousness is lost only temporarily, and the patient normally awakens in approximately

15 minutes. The quick onset and brief duration of thiopental reflect the rapidity by which the agent equilibrates between the blood and the CNS. Soon after a peak brain titer is reached (in 30 to 90 seconds), the concentration begins to decrease as thiopental continues to be absorbed by the relatively large mass of muscle. Consciousness returns at about the same time muscle reaches equilibrium with the blood. Thereafter, the brain and muscle concentrations parallel the plasma decay curve as the drug slowly passes into adipose tissue. With a metabolic half-time of approximately 10 hours, thiopental would be a relatively long-acting drug if not for redistribution. When repetitive injections saturate the fat reservoir, thiopental assumes the characteristics of a long-duration anesthetic.

Saliva

The transfer of drugs into saliva can be thought of as a form of redistribution because the drugs regain access to the systemic circulation after the saliva is swallowed. Although not involved in drug elimination, the entry of agents into the saliva is of pharmacologic interest in two other respects. First, drugs gaining access to the oral environment from the systemic circulation can affect microorganisms or tissue surfaces within the mouth. Although these influences are usually undesirable, a drug developed for a local effect, such as caries prevention, could conceivably be administered systemically to achieve a sustained therapeutic concentration in the saliva, while obviating the necessity of intraoral application. Drugs such as fluoride and antiplaque agents are examples of orally applied medications. Several unique factors are important in determining the clinical efficacy of medications on oral surfaces. One is substantivity of the preparation. Substantivity is the ability of a drug to remain for an extended time, due to the preparation itself or ability to form a retentive reservoir on hard or soft tissue. Salivary flow rate is important in determining the distribution of the medication. The second pharmacologic interest in saliva stems from the fact that salivary drug determinations can provide a noninvasive measure of the free plasma concentration of drugs. Because the free drug concentration in plasma is normally the primary determinant of patient response, the benefit of salivary drug quantitation to therapeutics is potentially great. Clinical studies have documented that saliva can be used to determine plasma levels of drugs, based on estimates of ratios of plasma to saliva drug concentrations. An example is shown in Table 2-3, in which the saliva concentrations reflect those of the plasma during the time period leading up to the peak concentration in the plasma. However, some drugs are not detected in saliva, even though with newer sensitive analysis methods it is possible to determine the concentration of many drugs in saliva. Moreover, the time and manner of sampling of saliva have to be controlled because salivary flows rates, which can alter drug concentrations, vary depending on several conditions. Given the fact that saliva has several advantages including its ease of collection, its noninvasive collection, and ease of storage, interest remains in using it for diagnostic purposes.

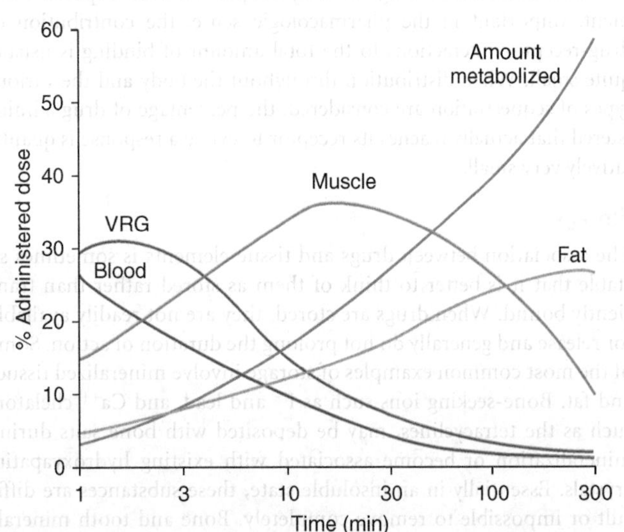

FIG 2-10 Redistribution of thiopental. *VRG,* Vessel-rich group tissues, including the brain, heart, lungs, kidneys, and liver. (Redrawn from Saidman LJ: Uptake, distribution and elimination of barbiturates. In Eger E II, editor: *Anesthetic uptake and action,* Baltimore, 1974, Williams & Wilkins.)

Drugs may enter the oral fluids from several sources: (1) passive diffusion across the alveolar and ductal cells of salivary glands, (2) active transport into saliva, (3) passive diffusion across the oral epithelium, and (4) bulk flow of fluid from the gingival crevice. Of these avenues, the first is the most important, and the fourth is the least important (except for drugs that cannot gain entry by any of the other routes). Drugs fit into different categories based on their levels in saliva. As shown in Table 2-3, the ratio of saliva/plasma concentrations varies among drugs taken from different classes. For the drugs shown in Table 2-3, there are good correlations between saliva and plasma concentration. Agents that are relatively lipid soluble (e.g., diazepam) or very small in size (e.g., ethanol) normally encounter little difficulty in equilibrating with saliva.

Active transport is a wild card with respect to predicting drug entry into saliva based on physicochemical characteristics. Digoxin is actively secreted into saliva by P-glycoprotein, effectively doubling the expected saliva/plasma ratio of 1/1 for a neutral drug with good lipid solubility. Coadministration of P-glycoprotein inhibitors significantly reduces the saliva/plasma ratio, as do polymorphisms that alter P-glycoprotein activity.

TABLE 2-3 Saliva/Plasma Values for Seven Representative Drugs

Drug	AUC (Saliva/Plasma)	C_{max} (Saliva/Plasma)	T_{max} (Saliva/Plasma)	Correlation Coefficient
Sitagliptin	0.16	0.19	4.00	0.99
Tolterodine	0.21	0.31	1.53	0.99
Hydrochlorothiazide	0.41	0.79	1.12	0.83
Metformin	0.11	0.12	2.23	0.87
Cloxacillin	1.76	2.61	1.00	0.99
Azithromycin	5.61	16.89	1.03	0.99
Rosuvastatin	0.08	0.17	1.05	0.89

The data in columns 2 to 4 are ratios (drugs present in saliva/drugs present in the plasma). *AUC,* Area under the curve (see later discussion of AUC); C_{max}, peak concentration of drug; T_{max}, time to peak concentration of drug. The correlation coefficients are the degree of linear relationship between drug concentration in saliva and drug concentration in plasma up to T_{max} for plasma.

Data taken from Idkaidek N, Arafat T: Saliva versus plasma pharmacokinetics: theory and application of a salivary excretion classification system, *Mol Pharmaceutics* 9:2358-2363, 2012.

METABOLISM

Metabolism is a major pathway for the termination of pharmacologic effects of drugs, and it is often a prerequisite for the excretion of lipid-soluble chemicals. Historically, the term **detoxification** was used in reference to drug metabolism. Typically, compounds are rendered **pharmacologically inactive** by metabolic attack; however, this is not always the case. Numerous drugs yield metabolites with full or partial activity, and some provide derivatives with novel or highly toxic drug effects. An increasing number of agents require chemical activation to be of therapeutic benefit (e.g., cyclophosphamide, mercaptopurine, methyldopa, and sulindac). The other typical effect of drug metabolism is the conversion of the parent drug to polar, relatively **lipid-insoluble compounds** that are susceptible to renal or biliary excretion or both.

Drug metabolism can be categorized according to the types of reactions involved and where they occur. Non-synthetic reactions include the various transformations of molecular structure: oxidation, reduction, and hydrolysis. These events are also called **phase I reactions** because they often represent the initial stage of biotransformation. A common outcome of phase I reactions is the addition or uncovering of one or more functional groups: —COOH, —NH_2, —O, —OH, or —SH. Synthetic, or **phase II, reactions** consist of the conjugation of drugs or their metabolites with functional groups provided by endogenous cofactors. Drugs may be metabolized by virtually any organ of the body, but quantitatively the most important enzyme systems for the biotransformation of exogenous substances are located in the liver.

Hepatic Microsomal Metabolism

Each hepatocyte contains an extensive network of **smooth endoplasmic reticulum** that catalyzes the metabolism of various endogenous chemicals (e.g., bilirubin, thyroxine, and steroids). Studies of fragmented reticular elements isolated along with other membrane structures in the form of **microsomes** have shown that numerous drugs are also chemically altered by enzymes located within this subcellular organelle. The greatest number of reactions involve oxidation; however, reduction, hydrolysis, and conjugation with glucuronic acid also occur.

Oxidation

The oxidation of drugs results in compounds that tend to be more polar, relatively more hydrophilic, and less likely to penetrate cells and bind to tissue elements. Microsomal oxidations are catalyzed by a set of mixed-function oxidases, so named because one atom of an oxygen dimer is incorporated into the drug, while the other is converted to water through the addition of two hydrogen atoms. Of particular significance to microsomal oxidation is the enzyme that actually binds the drug during metabolism: **cytochrome P450 (CYP).** This hemoprotein—actually a group of closely related isoenzymes—was designated P450 because of its absorption peak at 450 Å when combined in the reduced state with carbon monoxide. Multiple distinct CYP families have been identified in humans; the major enzymes involved in drug metabolism are shown in Figure 2-11.

In aggregate, the CYP superfamily constitutes up to 20% of the total protein content of liver microsomes. It acts as the terminal acceptor of electrons in a transport chain that also includes the reduced coenzyme nicotinamide adenine dinucleotide phosphate (NADPH) and the flavoprotein NADPH–cytochrome P450 oxidoreductase (Fig. 2-12). A unique ability of the CYP enzymes is their collective capacity to react with a diverse array of chemicals. The only identified requirement for microsomal oxidation is that the drug sufficiently penetrates the cell membranes to reach the hemoprotein. Table 2-4 lists the major CYP enzymes in humans along with some drugs that are metabolized by them and drugs that can inhibit or induce their activities.

The general pathway for oxidation of drugs by the hepatic microsomal enzyme system is depicted in Figure 2-13. The drug initially attaches to an oxidized (Fe^{+++}) CYP enzyme. This complex accepts an electron from the flavoprotein-catalyzed oxidation of NADPH. A ternary structure is produced next by the inclusion of molecular oxygen; the addition of a second electron and subsequently two protons causes the complex to break down, yielding the CYP enzyme, a water molecule, and the oxidized drug.

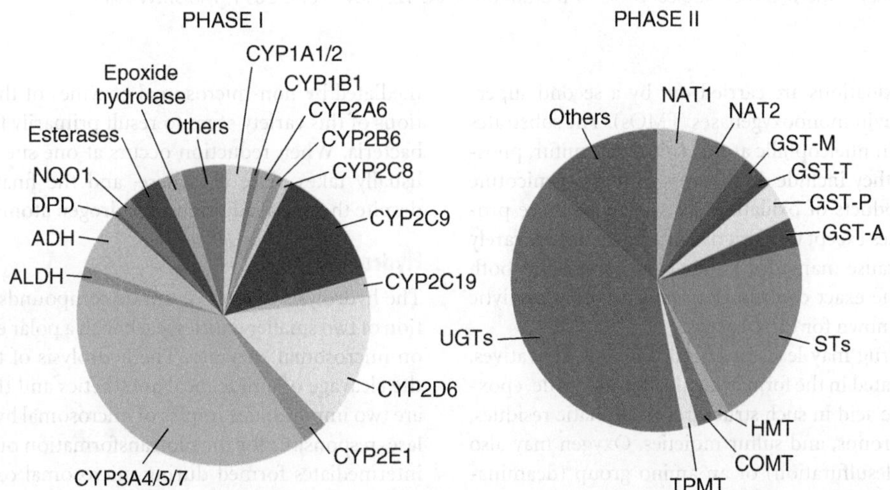

FIG 2-11 Major enzymes involved in drug metabolism. The percentage of phase I and phase II metabolism of drugs contributed by each enzyme is represented by the relative size of each section of the corresponding chart. *ADH,* Alcohol dehydrogenase; *ALDH,* aldehyde dehydrogenase; *CYP,* cytochrome P450; *DPD,* dihydropyrimidine dehydrogenase; *NQO1,* NAD(P)H:quinone oxidoreductase (or DT diaphorase); *COMT,* catechol-*O*-methyl transferase; *GST,* glutathione-*S*-transferase; *HMT,* histamine methyltransferase; *NAT,* N-acetyltransferase; *STs,* sulfotransferases; *TPMT,* thiopurine methyltransferase; *UGTs,* uridine diphosphate glucuronosyltransferases. (Adapted from Evans WE, Relling MV: Pharmacogenomics: translating functional genomics into rational therapeutics, *Science* 286:487-491, 1999.)

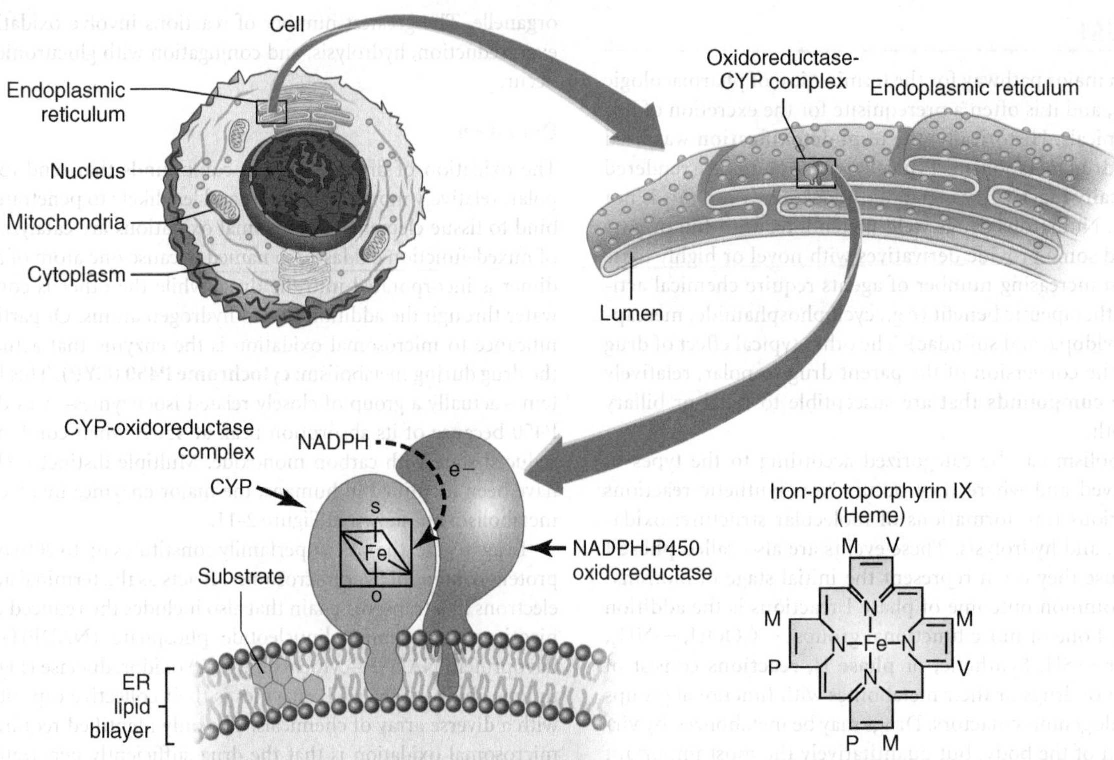

FIG 2-12 Location of cytochrome P450 (*CYP*) in the endoplasmic reticulum (*ER*). The figure shows increasingly microscopic levels of detail, sequentially expanding the areas within each black box. CYPs are mostly embedded in the cytoplasmic surface of the ER membrane. A second enzyme, NADPH–cytochrome P450 oxidoreductase, transfers electrons to CYP, where it can, in the presence of molecular oxygen, oxidize xenobiotic substrates, many of which are hydrophobic and dissolved in the ER. A single oxidoreductase species transfers electrons to all CYP isoforms in the ER. Each CYP contains an iron-protoporphyrin ring that binds and activates the oxygen. Substitutions on the ring are methyl (*M*), propionyl (*P*), and vinyl (*V*) groups. (From Gonzalez FJ, Coughtrie M, Tukey RH: Drug metabolism, In Brunton LL, Chabner B, Knollman B, editors: *Goodman & Gilman's the pharmacological basis of therapeutics*, ed 12, New York, 2011, McGraw-Hill.)

Some microsomal oxidations are carried out by a second superfamily of enzymes: the flavin monooxygenases (FMOs). The substrates for these enzymes contain nucleophilic atoms (nitrogen, sulfur, phosphorus, and selenium); they include such common drugs as nicotine and cimetidine. The products of oxidation are similar to those produced by the CYP enzymes except that reactive intermediates are rarely produced by FMOs. Because many drugs may be substrates for both enzyme superfamilies, the exact contribution made by each catalytic pathway is generally unknown for these agents.

The oxidation of a drug may lead to several different derivatives. Oxygen may be incorporated in the form of an alcohol, aldehyde, epoxide, ketone, or carboxylic acid in such structures as aliphatic residues, aromatic rings, amino groups, and sulfur moieties. Oxygen may also replace a sulfur atom (desulfuration) or an amino group (deamination), or it may not appear in the metabolite at all but become attached to a hydrocarbon unit released during the dealkylation of nitrogen, oxygen, or sulfur. The various types of microsomal oxidations are reviewed along with other phase I reactions in Table 2-5.

Reduction

The microsomal reduction of drugs is limited to molecules with nitro or carbonyl groups or azo linkages. Similar reactions may also be mediated by non-microsomal enzymes of the body, but most reductions of this variety seem to result primarily from the action of enteric bacteria. When reduction occurs at one site in a molecule, oxidation usually takes place elsewhere, and the final product is more polar despite the initial addition of hydrogen atoms.

Hydrolysis

The hydrolysis of ester or amide compounds resulting in the production of two smaller entities, each with a polar end, occasionally depends on microsomal enzymes. The hydrolysis of the ester meperidine and the cleavage of amide local anesthetics and their oxidized metabolites are two important examples of microsomal hydrolysis. Epoxide hydrolase, responsible for the biotransformation of highly reactive and toxic intermediates formed during microsomal oxidation reactions, yields inactive dihydrodiol products.

Dehalogenation

Various compounds, such as chlorophenothane and some volatile general anesthetics (e.g., halothane and sevoflurane), are dehalogenated by microsomal enzymes. The reactions are complex, may involve both oxidative and reductive steps, and may result in the formation of potentially toxic metabolites.

TABLE 2-4 Major Cytochrome P450 Enzymes and Representative Substrates, Inhibitors, and Inducers

CYP	Substrates	Inhibitors	Inducers
1A1/2	Acetaminophen, amitriptyline, caffeine, clozapine, estradiol, haloperidol, imipramine, mexiletine, naproxen, ondansetron, propranolol, ropivacaine, tamoxifen, theophylline, R-warfarin, zileuton	Amiodarone, cimetidine, ciprofloxacin, clarithromycin, erythromycin, grapefruit juice, insulin, ticlopidine	Benzo[*a*]pyrene, broccoli, char-grilled meat, modafinil, nafcillin, omeprazole, rifampin
2A6	Acetaminophen, halothane, nicotine, nitrosamines, valproic acid	Azole antifungals, pilocarpine, tranylcypromine	Barbiturates, dexamethasone, rifampin
2B6	Bupropion, cyclophosphamide, ifosfamide, methadone	Amlodipine, methimazole, thiotepa, tretinoin	Barbiturates, dihydropyridines, ifosfamide, lovastatin, rifampin
2C8/9	Amitriptyline, celecoxib, fluoxetine, fluvastatin, losartan, nonsteroidal antiinflammatory drugs, oral hypoglycemics, phenobarbital, phenytoin, sulfaphenazole, S-warfarin, tamoxifen	Amiodarone, azole antifungals, fluvastatin, lovastatin, metronidazole, paroxetine, ritonavir, sertraline, trimethoprim, zafirlukast	Barbiturates, dihydropyridines, ifosfamide, rifampin
2C18/19	Amitriptyline, citalopram, diazepam, indomethacin, naproxen, phenobarbital, phenytoin, primidone, progesterone, propranolol, proton pump inhibitors	Chloramphenicol, cimetidine, fluoxetine, fluvoxamine, ketoconazole, modafinil, omeprazole, paroxetine, ticlopidine, topiramate	Aspirin, barbiturates, carbamazepine, norethindrone, rifampin
2D6	Amphetamine, β-adrenergic blockers, chlorpheniramine, clomipramine, clozapine, codeine, dextromethorphan, flecainide, fluoxetine, haloperidol, hydrocodone, metoclopramide, mexiletine, ondansetron, oxycodone, paroxetine, propoxyphene, risperidone, selegiline, thioridazine, tramadol, tricyclic antidepressants, venlafaxine	Amiodarone, antipsychotics, celecoxib, cimetidine, cocaine, fluoxetine, methadone, metoclopramide, paroxetine, quinidine, ritonavir, sertraline, terbinafine, ticlopidine, venlafaxine	Dexamethasone, rifampin
2E1	Acetaminophen, ethanol, sildenafil, theophylline, volatile inhalation anesthetics	Disulfiram, propofol, tricyclic antidepressants	Colchicine, ethanol, isoniazid, tretinoin
3A4/5/7	Acetaminophen, alfentanil, alprazolam, amiodarone, atorvastatin, buspirone, chlorpheniramine, cocaine, cortisol, cyclosporine, dapsone, diazepam, dihydroergotamine, dihydropyridines, diltiazem, dronabinol, ethinyl estradiol, fentanyl, indinavir, lidocaine, lovastatin, macrolides, methadone, miconazole, midazolam, mifepristone, modafinil, ondansetron, paclitaxel, progesterone, quinidine, ritonavir, saquinavir, sildenafil, spironolactone, sufentanil, sulfamethoxazole, tacrolimus, tamoxifen, testosterone, trazodone, triazolam, verapamil, zaleplon, zolpidem	Amiodarone, atazanavir, chloramphenicol, cimetidine, ciprofloxacin, clarithromycin, dihydroergotamine, diltiazem, doxycycline, erythromycin, felodipine, fluoxetine, fluvoxamine, glucocorticoids, grapefruit juice, HIV antivirals, itraconazole, ketoconazole, nefazodone, sildenafil, verapamil	Barbiturates, carbamazepine, glucocorticoids, ifosfamide, modafinil, nevirapine, phenytoin, rifampin, St. John's wort, troleandomycin

HIV, Human immunodeficiency virus.

Glucuronide conjugation

The combination of compounds with glucuronic acid is the only phase II reaction catalyzed by microsomal enzymes (in this case, by a group of glucuronosyltransferases). Originally derived from glucose, glucuronic acid is transferred from its donor, uridine diphosphate, to an appropriate reactive center on the drug molecule (Table 2-6). The **glucuronide conjugate** produced is excreted, often with the help of active secretion, into the bile or urine (see Fig. 2-7). In contrast to many phase I reactions, conjugation with glucuronic acid almost invariably results in a total loss of pharmacologic activity. An important exception to this rule is morphine-6-glucuronide, which is 100 times more potent than morphine as an analgesic when injected into the CNS. Some glucuronides excreted in the bile are subject to hydrolysis by bacterial and intestinal β-glucuronidase enzymes. If it has sufficient lipid solubility, the released drug may be absorbed again. Glucuronidation is a quantitatively significant metabolic pathway for many drugs and their metabolites; for agents such as morphine, it represents the primary mode of metabolism.

Non-Microsomal Metabolism

The pattern of drug metabolism mediated by non-microsomal enzymes is considerably different from that of the microsomal system. Although important, the liver is not always predominant in non-microsomal biotransformations. The various major types of non-synthetic reactions already described take place, but their relative frequencies of occurrence are dissimilar. Generally, drugs must resemble natural substrates to be metabolized by most non-microsomal enzymes; the lack of specificity displayed in microsomal oxidation is not characteristic of non-microsomal oxidation. Although cytosolic enzymes are most commonly involved, enzymes associated with the nucleus, mitochondria, and plasma membrane also play limited roles. Plasma esterase is an important example of an extracellular enzyme involved in drug metabolism.

Oxidation

Non-microsomal enzymes are responsible for the oxidation of numerous compounds. Selected alcohols and aldehydes are oxidized by dehydrogenases present in the cytosol of the liver. Other oxidation reactions include the oxidative deamination of drugs such as tyramine and phenylephrine by mitochondrial enzymes found in the liver, kidneys, and other organs, and the hydroxylation of the purine derivatives theophylline and allopurinol by xanthine oxidase.

Reduction

Non-microsomal enzymes promote the hydrogenation of double bonds and, through a reversal of the normal dehydrogenase pathway, the removal of oxygen atoms. The reduction of chloral hydrate to

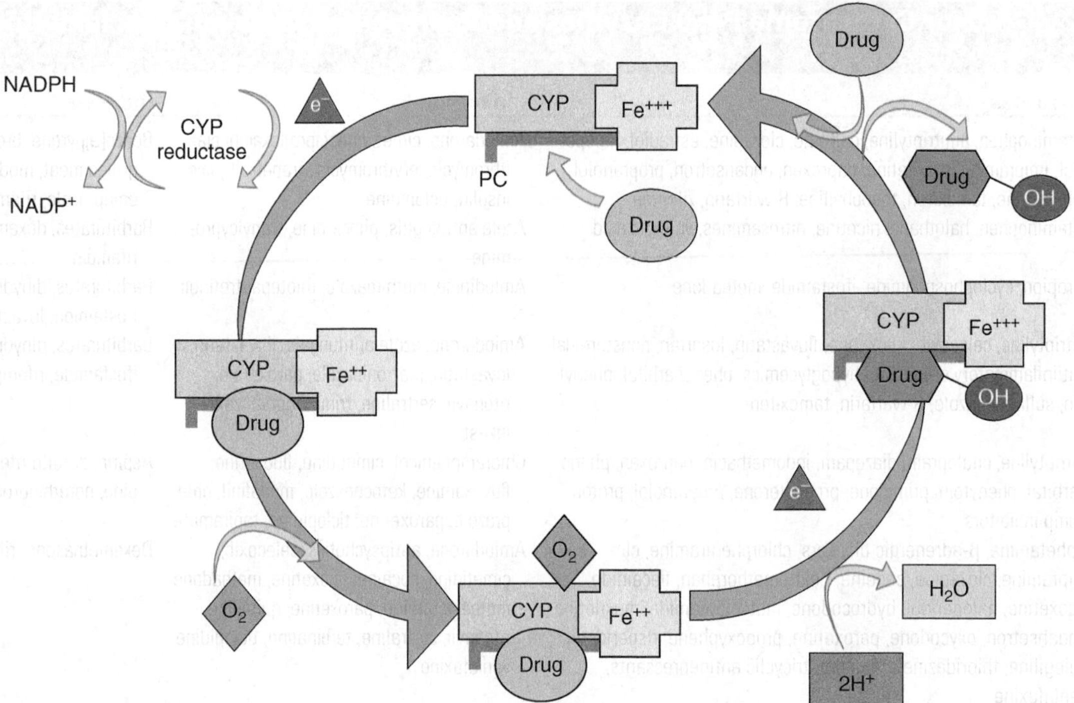

FIG 2-13 Microsomal oxidation. Free drug enters the cycle (*upper right*) and is complexed in the presence of phosphatidylcholine (*PC*) to CYP with its heme in the oxidized (*Fe+++*) state. The Fe+++ is reduced (*Fe++*) by an electron (*e−*) generated in the oxidation of NADPH to NADP+ by the enzyme NADPH–cytochrome P450 oxidoreductase (CYP reductase, *upper left*). The reduced complex absorbs molecular oxygen (*O_2, lower middle*). Addition of a second e− and two protons (*2H+, lower right*) results in the generation of one molecule of water (*H_2O*), oxidation of the drug (hydroxylation in this case), and oxidation of Fe++ to Fe+++. The cycle is complete with release of the oxidized drug. (Adapted from Markey SP: Pathways of drug metabolism, In Atkinson AJ Jr, Abernethy DR, Daniels CE, et al. editors: *Principles of clinical pharmacology*, ed 2, Amsterdam, 2007, Elsevier.)

trichloroethanol by alcohol dehydrogenase is an often-cited example of this latter type of reaction.

Hydrolysis

Most hydrolytic reactions of foreign substances depend on non-microsomal esterase and amidase enzymes. Nonspecific esterases are found throughout the body, but the two most important sites, by virtue of their hydrolytic capacity and availability to drugs, are the liver and plasma. Ester local anesthetics such as procaine and benzocaine are hydrolyzed by these enzymes. Except for blood and other tissue peptidases responsible for the breakdown of pharmacologically active polypeptides, most amidase activities reside in the liver.

Conjugation reactions

A number of synthetic reactions are catalyzed by non-microsomal transferase enzymes. As with the microsomal synthesis of glucuronides, the body usually supplies an acidic moiety (e.g., sulfate, acetate, cysteine, glycine, glutamine, or riboside phosphate) attached to a particular cofactor or carrier molecule. The quantitative contributions of the various phase II reactions are illustrated in Figure 2-11.

Conjugation with glutathione is unusual because it is directed against highly reactive metabolites, such as epoxides and quinones, and may occur with or without enzymatic support. Although a quantitatively minor pathway, glutathione conjugation is often of major importance in preventing metabolism-induced drug toxicity.

Phase II reactions can be expected whenever a drug carries one or more of the reactive centers listed in Table 2-6. Such conjugations generally result in the termination of drug effect, restriction in the apparent V_d, and acceleration of drug excretion through active secretory processes.

Non-Hepatic Metabolism

Although focusing on the liver when considering biotransformation is appropriate generally, other organs contain drug-metabolizing enzymes (including members of the CYP family) and contribute to the microsomal and non-microsomal metabolism of drugs. This ability is occasionally taken advantage of by preparing prodrugs that become metabolically activated in target tissues. The aforementioned use of levodopa to circumvent the blood–brain barrier is an example of this approach; administration of acyclovir, an antiviral prodrug that is converted to the active nucleotide form in diseased cells (see Chapter 34), is another. By virtue of location and blood supply, certain organs play special roles in drug metabolism. As previously discussed in the context of bioavailability, the intestine, working alone or in concert with the liver, can metabolize some drugs so completely that the oral route cannot be used for their administration. CYP3A4 is the principal enzyme involved in intestinal drug metabolism as well as liver metabolism. The kidney is well suited for drug metabolism because it has a well-developed microsomal enzyme system and receives a bountiful blood supply. Glucuronidation is an especially prominent activity.

In recent years, the role of the lung in drug disposition has been an active area of investigation. By means of the pulmonary circulation, virtually all the blood is exposed to lung tissue with each circulation. Studies have shown that the lung is a primary site for metabolism of endogenous blood-borne compounds such as bradykinin, angiotensin I,

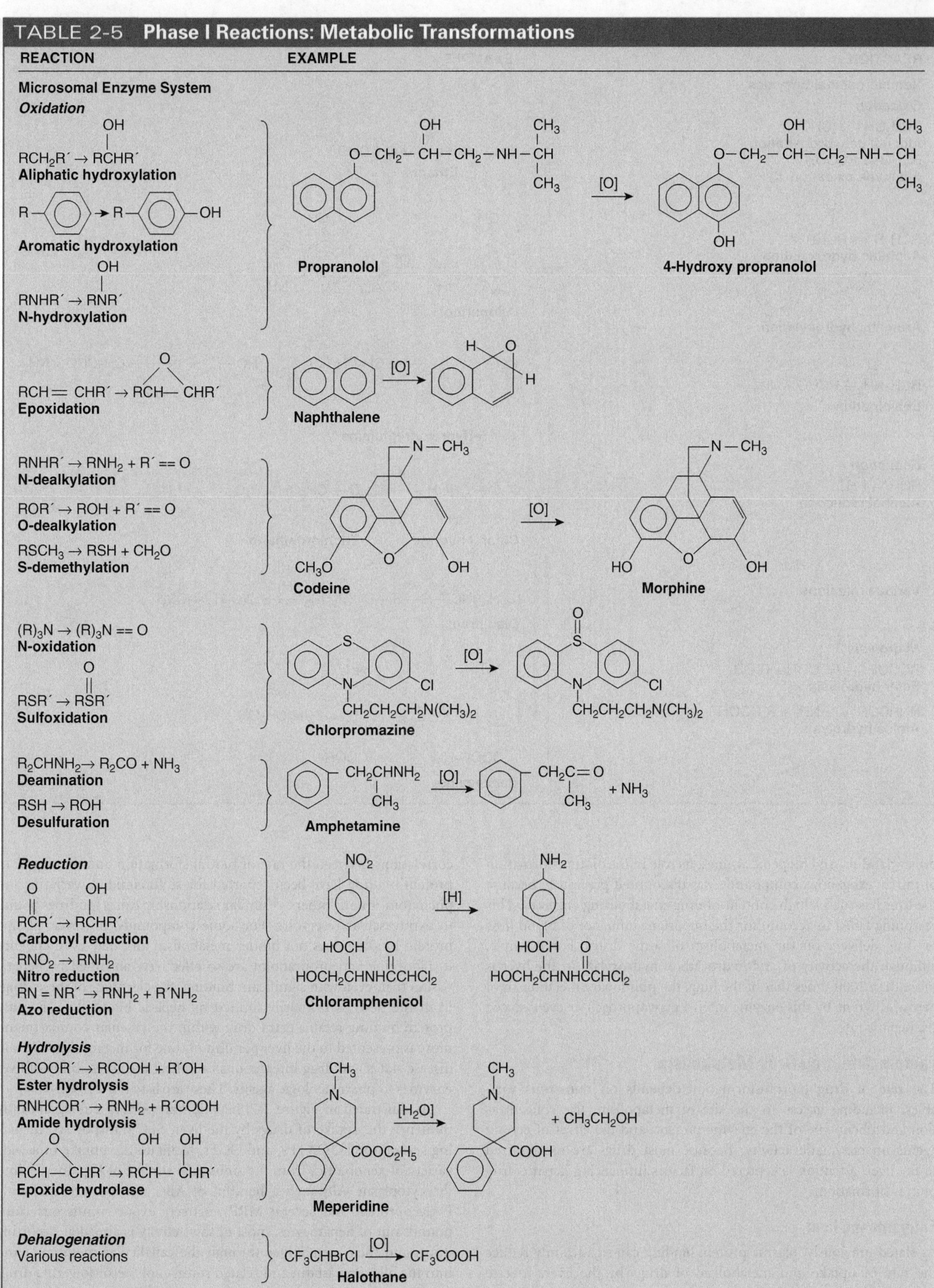

TABLE 2-5 Phase I Reactions: Metabolic Transformations

REACTION	EXAMPLE
Microsomal Enzyme System	
Oxidation	
$RCH_2R' \rightarrow RCH(OH)R'$ **Aliphatic hydroxylation** $R-C_6H_5 \rightarrow R-C_6H_4-OH$ **Aromatic hydroxylation** $RNHR' \rightarrow RN(OH)R'$ **N-hydroxylation**	**Propranolol** $\xrightarrow{[O]}$ **4-Hydroxy propranolol**
$RCH{=}CHR' \rightarrow RCH{-}CHR'$ (epoxide, bridged by O) **Epoxidation**	**Naphthalene** $\xrightarrow{[O]}$ (epoxide)
$RNHR' \rightarrow RNH_2 + R'{=}O$ **N-dealkylation** $ROR' \rightarrow ROH + R'{=}O$ **O-dealkylation** $RSCH_3 \rightarrow RSH + CH_2O$ **S-demethylation**	**Codeine** $\xrightarrow{[O]}$ **Morphine**
$(R)_3N \rightarrow (R)_3N{=}O$ **N-oxidation** $RSR' \rightarrow RS(=O)R'$ **Sulfoxidation**	**Chlorpromazine** $\xrightarrow{[O]}$ (sulfoxide)
$R_2CHNH_2 \rightarrow R_2CO + NH_3$ **Deamination** $RSH \rightarrow ROH$ **Desulfuration**	$C_6H_5CH_2CH(NH_2)CH_3 \xrightarrow{[O]} C_6H_5CH_2C(=O)CH_3 + NH_3$ **Amphetamine**
Reduction	
$RC(=O)R' \rightarrow RCH(OH)R'$ **Carbonyl reduction** $RNO_2 \rightarrow RNH_2$ **Nitro reduction** $RN{=}NR' \rightarrow RNH_2 + R'NH_2$ **Azo reduction**	**Chloramphenicol** $\xrightarrow{[H]}$ (amine)
Hydrolysis	
$RCOOR' \rightarrow RCOOH + R'OH$ **Ester hydrolysis** $RNHCOR' \rightarrow RNH_2 + R'COOH$ **Amide hydrolysis** $RCH{-}CHR'$ (epoxide) $\rightarrow RCH(OH){-}CH(OH)R'$ **Epoxide hydrolase**	**Meperidine** ($COOC_2H_5$) $\xrightarrow{[H_2O]}$ ($COOH$) $+ CH_3CH_2OH$
Dehalogenation	
Various reactions	$CF_3CHBrCl \xrightarrow{[O]} CF_3COOH$ **Halothane**

Continued

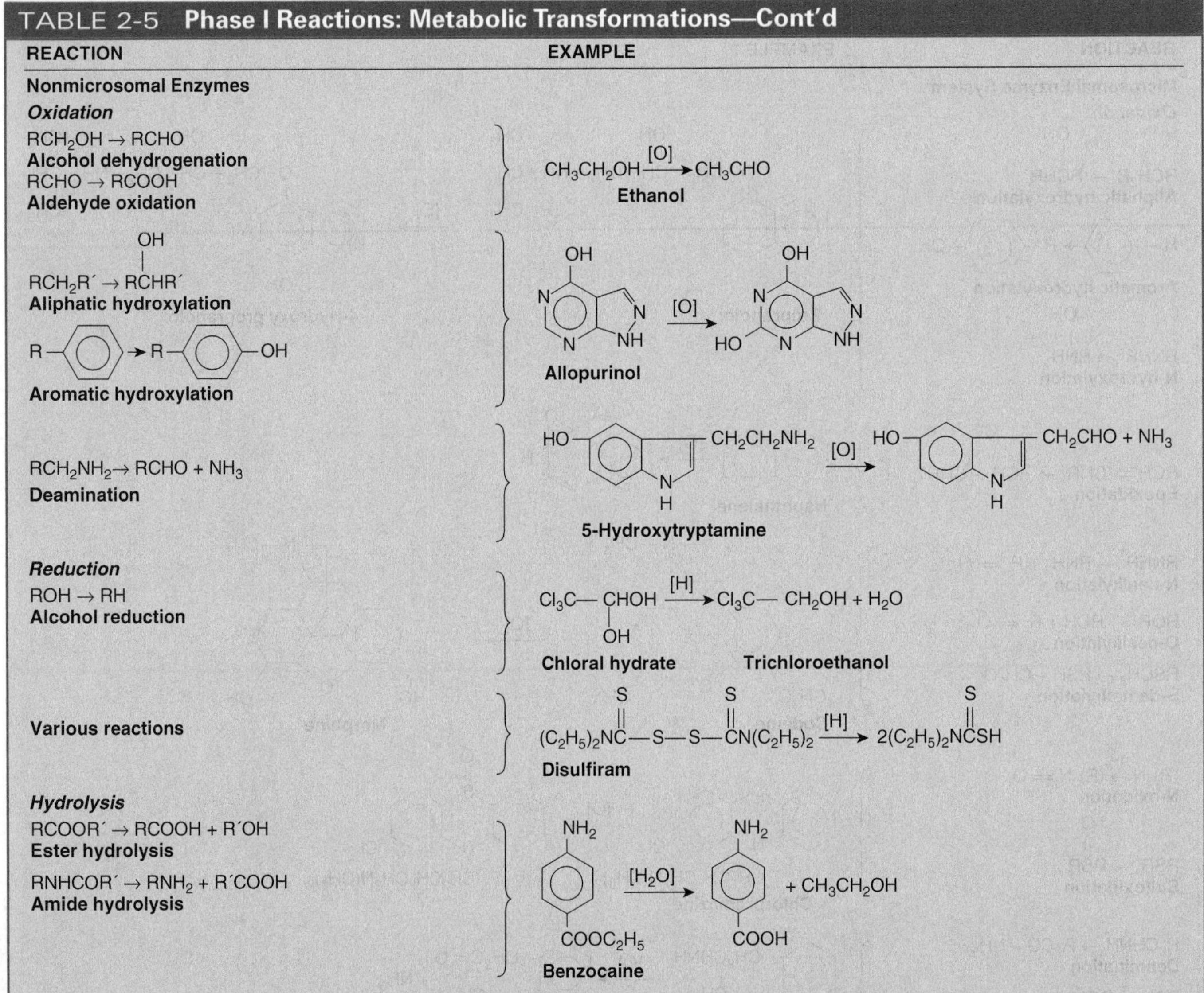

TABLE 2-5 Phase I Reactions: Metabolic Transformations—Cont'd

REACTION	EXAMPLE
Nonmicrosomal Enzymes	
Oxidation	
$RCH_2OH \rightarrow RCHO$ **Alcohol dehydrogenation** $RCHO \rightarrow RCOOH$ **Aldehyde oxidation**	$CH_3CH_2OH \xrightarrow{[O]} CH_3CHO$ **Ethanol**
$RCH_2R' \rightarrow RCH(OH)R'$ **Aliphatic hydroxylation** R–C₆H₄ → R–C₆H₄–OH **Aromatic hydroxylation**	OH, N, N, NH, N → [O] → OH, N, N, NH, HO, N **Allopurinol**
$RCH_2NH_2 \rightarrow RCHO + NH_3$ **Deamination**	HO–(indole, N–H)–$CH_2CH_2NH_2$ $\xrightarrow{[O]}$ HO–(indole, N–H)–$CH_2CHO + NH_3$ **5-Hydroxytryptamine**
Reduction	
$ROH \rightarrow RH$ **Alcohol reduction**	$Cl_3C—CH(OH)OH \xrightarrow{[H]} Cl_3C—CH_2OH + H_2O$ **Chloral hydrate** **Trichloroethanol**
Various reactions	$(C_2H_5)_2NC(=S)—S—S—C(=S)N(C_2H_5)_2 \xrightarrow{[H]} 2(C_2H_5)_2NC(=S)SH$ **Disulfiram**
Hydrolysis	
$RCOOR' \rightarrow RCOOH + R'OH$ **Ester hydrolysis** $RNHCOR' \rightarrow RNH_2 + R'COOH$ **Amide hydrolysis**	NH_2–C₆H₄–$COOC_2H_5$ $\xrightarrow{[H_2O]}$ NH_2–C₆H₄–$COOH$ + CH_3CH_2OH **Benzocaine**

prostaglandins, and biogenic amines. Its role in the biotransformation of purely exogenous compounds was discounted previously because the liver has such a high content of drug-metabolizing enzymes. This reasoning failed to account for the important influence of blood flow or drug delivery on the metabolism of some drugs. For example, although the activity of aryl hydrocarbon hydroxylase in the liver is more than 1000 times that of the lung, the pulmonary metabolism of benzo[*a*]pyrene by this enzyme in vivo may approach or even exceed the hepatic rate.

Factors Affecting Drug Metabolism

The rate of drug biotransformation depends on numerous variables, including access to the site of metabolism, the concentration and phenotype of the enzyme present, and the effect of certain agents on enzymatic activity. Because most drugs are metabolized in the liver, attention is centered on factors influencing hepatic drug biotransformation.

Entry into the liver

As stated previously, plasma protein binding can significantly reduce the rate of uptake and metabolism of drugs by the liver. Inverse correlations between the rate of biotransformation and the degree of protein binding have been reported for sulfonamides, warfarin, and phenytoin, among others. A similar relationship exists for drugs bound to extravascular reservoirs. For some compounds, however, plasma protein binding does not hinder metabolism and may even enhance it. Lidocaine and propranolol are so effectively absorbed by hepatic tissues that, even with significant binding, the clearance of these drugs from the body is primarily limited by hepatic blood flow. Because protein binding retains extra drug within the vascular compartment, more is presented to the liver per unit of time for metabolism. Certain disease states and drug interactions can affect the accessibility of liver enzymes to pharmacologic agents. These are listed in Table 2-7.

As illustrated in Figure 2-7, hepatic transporters can significantly influence the uptake of drugs by the liver. SLC transporters, including several OATs, OATPs, and OCTs, facilitate the uptake of a wide variety of xenobiotics from the sinusoidal surface of hepatocytes into the cytoplasm. Although a handful of ABC transporters, including P-glycoprotein and several MRPs, actively export numerous compounds out of hepatocytes, most of this activity is aimed at exporting drugs and their metabolites through the canalicular membrane and into the bile. Pravastatin and related statin cholesterol-lowering drugs

TABLE 2-6 Phase II Reactions: Conjugations

Conjugation Reaction (Cofactor)	Substrates	Example
Glucuronide synthesis (uridine diphosphate)	Amines Carboxylic acids Alcohols Phenols Mercaptans	Salicylic acid — UDP-glucuronide →
Acetylation (coenzyme A)	Amines Hydrazines	Sulfanilamide — Acetyl-CoA →
Glycine conjugation (coenzyme A)	Carboxylic acids	Salicylic acid — CoA + Glycine →
Methylation (S-adenosyl-methionine)	Amines Phenols Mercaptans	Norepinephrine — SAM →
Sulfate addition (3′-phosphoadenosine-5′-phosphosulfate) (PAPS)	Aromatic amines Alcohols Phenols	Acetaminophen — PAPS →
Other reactions (various)	Purines Pyrimidines Epoxides and other reactive metabolites	Naphthalene epoxide — Glutathione →

TABLE 2-7 Conditions That Can Affect Hepatic Drug Metabolism

Condition	Effect on Drug Metabolism	Mechanism
Disease		
Uremia	Increase	Reduces binding capacity of albumin; increase free drug delivery
Stress, inflammation	Decrease	Increases α_1-acid glycoprotein; reduces free drug delivery for some basic drugs
Cirrhosis	Decrease	Reduces hepatic blood flow and damage to hepatic cells
Cardiac insufficiency	Decrease	Reduces hepatic blood flow
Some infections	Decrease	Reduce hepatic blood flow
Hypothyroidism	Decrease	Reduces synthesis of metabolic enzymes
Hyperthyroidism	Increase	Increases synthesis of metabolic enzymes
Other Factors		
Reduced hepatic blood flow from drugs and other factors	Decrease	Reduces hepatic blood flow
Neonatal, elderly population	Decrease	Reduced liver enzymes in both age groups
Genetic factors	Increase or decrease	Increase or decrease in liver enzyme activity

provide excellent examples of the critical importance of active transport to hepatic uptake. Pravastatin is a hydrophilic drug that nevertheless is taken up efficiently into the liver by OATP transporters. This sequestration of pravastatin reduces the drug's systemic bioavailability to 17%, while focusing the drug's effect within the liver. This action is beneficial in two respects: (1) it augments the ability of pravastatin to depress hepatic synthesis of cholesterol; (2) it minimizes the toxic effects of pravastatin on skeletal muscle and other tissues.

Enzyme inhibition

Drug-metabolizing enzymes are subject to competitive and noncompetitive antagonism (Table 2-4). Because so many drugs are acted on by the CYP system, competitive inhibition of microsomal oxidation is easily shown in the laboratory. Drug interactions of this type are usually not clinically important. In many instances, the rate of biotransformation is limited not by the CYP electron transport chain but by the movement of drugs into the smooth endoplasmic reticulum. Some compounds exhibit saturation kinetics, however, and are restricted in metabolism by the rate of binding to specific CYP enzymes. Competition involving these agents (e.g., phenytoin and dicumarol competing for CYP2C9) is of practical significance.

Clinically useful drugs that **inhibit** the **metabolism** of numerous other agents by inactivating various CYP enzymes include the macrolide antibiotics (other than azithromycin), chloramphenicol, certain imidazole derivatives (cimetidine and the azole antifungals), and amiodarone (see Table 2-4). These drugs—or their metabolites—react covalently or otherwise strongly with specific sites on the CYP molecule. Gingko biloba and grapefruit juice are herbal and dietary constituents that powerfully inhibit certain classes of CYP enzymes.

Several drugs are used specifically as inhibitors of selected non-microsomal enzymes. When the enzyme affected happens to be responsible for the inactivation of other therapeutic agents, drug interactions are likely to develop. Examples of such enzymes are monoamine oxidase, pseudocholinesterase, and xanthine oxidase. The inhibition of aldehyde dehydrogenase by disulfiram is exceptional because that drug's primary indication is to interrupt the metabolism of another foreign compound, ethanol (see Chapter 39).

Enzyme induction

Microsomal CYP drug-metabolizing enzymes are inducible; under an appropriate chemical stimulus, catalytic activity increases. Many chemicals, including therapeutic agents and environmental toxins, are capable of stimulating their own biotransformation and the biotransformation of closely related compounds. In addition, some chemicals can augment the breakdown of a host of diverse substances. Phenobarbital illustrates this latter type of induction. On reaching the interior of the hepatocyte, phenobarbital activates a nuclear transcription factor termed the **constitutive androstane receptor**, which then migrates into the nucleus to activate genes with the appropriate response elements. Several hours thereafter, an elevation in hepatic protein synthesis becomes apparent. Reductions in the metabolic half-lives of affected drugs are paralleled by increases in microsomal weight and in the concentrations of NADPH–cytochrome P450 oxidoreductase and several CYP enzymes (most importantly, CYP2B6, CYP2C8/9, CYP2C18/19, and CYP3A4/5). The liver eventually hypertrophies, and hepatic blood flow and bile secretion are likewise enhanced. Rifampin, another broad-spectrum inducer, binds to a closely related transcription factor termed the **pregnane X receptor** to initiate a similar response.

By way of contrast, benzo[*a*]pyrene exemplifies agents with a more restrictive form of induction. Although benzo[*a*]pyrene requires new enzyme formation for its stimulation of metabolism, structural changes in the smooth endoplasmic reticulum are not prominent and may be undetectable. Enzyme induction in this case principally involves the CYP1 gene family (CYP1A1/2 and CYP1B1). The transcription factor for benzo[*a*]pyrene and many other aromatic hydrocarbons and heterocyclics is the aryl hydrocarbon receptor.

Regardless of the pattern of induction, the rate of metabolism of affected compounds may be enhanced experimentally by seven times the baseline. Stimulation is usually less pronounced clinically; nevertheless, enzyme induction has many important therapeutic ramifications. It is a major cause of drug interactions. A classic example of this form of drug interaction is the stimulation by phenobarbital of the metabolism of the anticoagulant dicumarol, which causes standard doses of the anticoagulant to be ineffective. Induction of microsomal enzymes leading to a loss of pharmacologic responsiveness is referred to as **pharmacokinetic tolerance**. Finally, enzyme induction may affect the function of endogenous chemicals metabolized microsomally. Acceleration of vitamin D oxidation to yield inactive products is the leading cause of rickets and osteomalacia in epileptic patients receiving medications such as phenytoin and phenobarbital.

It would seem an obvious outcome that enzyme induction should decrease drug toxicity in concert with any reduction in drug potency. This is not always the case, however. Of strong concern in the field of toxicology is the potential danger posed by highly reactive intermediary substances produced during microsomal oxidation of drugs such as acetaminophen, halothane, and benzo[*a*]pyrene. These substances are normally synthesized in such limited quantities that succeeding reactions, including hydrolysis and glutathione conjugation, inactivate them before cellular injury can ensue. Selective microsomal enzyme induction may sufficiently increase their synthesis that subsequent protective reactions become overwhelmed. In agreement with this thesis is a report in which cigarette smokers who exhibited high inducibility of aryl hydrocarbon hydroxylase activity, which converts benzo[*a*]pyrene and related polycyclic hydrocarbons into epoxide intermediates, were estimated to have a 36-fold increased risk of developing bronchogenic carcinoma than individuals having low inducibility.

Transporter inhibition and induction

Interactions that result in decreased or increased active transport of drugs to and from their sites of metabolism show many similarities to those described earlier for drug-metabolizing enzymes. P-glycoprotein is the most conspicuous example. Biologically, P-glycoprotein and CYP3A4 seem to act in a coordinated fashion to protect cells from toxic compounds. Both proteins share considerable overlap in substrate specificity. Most of the inhibitors for CYP3A4 listed in Table 2-4 also block P-glycoprotein transport, and drugs that activate the pregnane X receptor (e.g., rifampin) induce the formation of both proteins. Although P-glycoprotein exports drugs in the intestine back into the luminal space, it exposes the drugs to CYP3A4 metabolism during the process. In the liver, the principal action of P-glycoprotein is to convey drugs and their metabolites into the bile. This action ensures that the compounds either are excreted via the feces or are subjected again to intestinal and hepatic biotransformation.

The SLC transporters responsible for the active and facilitated uptake of drugs by the liver are subject to inhibition by various agents. With regard to the previously mentioned pravastatin, the antidiabetic drug repaglinide can completely block pravastatin uptake by OATPB1 in vitro. Potential consequences of this inhibition include loss of therapeutic effect within the liver and increased systemic toxicity elsewhere. A case report of acute myopathy in a women taking pravastatin and colchicine underscores the potential for this interaction. In contrast to P-glycoprotein, little is known about induction of SLC transporters other than complex patterns of induction and inhibition have been reported for drugs that activate transcription factors such as the pregnane X receptor.

Genetic factors

Individuals vary in their ability to metabolize drugs. Although differences can result from the environmental induction of microsomal enzymes (as seen in chemical factory workers and cigarette smokers), studies comparing identical and fraternal twins have conclusively established the preeminent influence of heredity on the rate of biotransformation (see Chapter 4). For some drugs, in nonrelated individuals, the range in metabolic half-time may exceed an order of magnitude, but usually this figure is restricted to a value of two or three. Normal individuals exhibiting the lowest microsomal metabolism rates are the most likely to undergo profound enzyme induction after phenobarbital treatment, however.

Age

Neonates, especially premature infants, often lack certain functional drug-metabolizing systems. The relative inability to conjugate bilirubin with glucuronic acid and the resultant development of hyperbilirubinemia is a commonly observed example of this deficiency in biotransformation. In contrast to newborns, children are often more adept at metabolizing drugs on a weight basis than are young adults. Thereafter, biotransformation capacity seems to diminish with age; elderly individuals may often exhibit retarded rates of drug metabolism.

EXCRETION

Foreign substances, including therapeutic medications, are prevented from building up in the body by the combined action of metabolism and excretion. Drugs and their metabolites may be eliminated by numerous routes including urine, bile, sweat, saliva, gastrointestinal secretions, pulmonary exhalation, tears, and breast milk. Quantitative considerations make the **kidney** the major organ of **drug excretion.**

Renal Excretion

Three processes—glomerular filtration, tubular reabsorption, and active transport—control the urinary elimination of drugs. Although all drugs are subject to filtration, the percentage filtered varies inversely according to the degree of plasma protein binding and to the V_d. Once filtered, agents tend to be reabsorbed in relation to their lipid/water partition coefficients. These considerations favor the renal excretion of highly polar compounds, but the exact rate of elimination also depends on whether active transport into (or, rarely, out of) the tubular fluid occurs.

Glomerular filtration

Each day, the kidneys filter approximately 180 L of plasma. Arterial blood entering Bowman's capsule is routed through a tuft of capillaries called the glomerulus. These capillaries are uniquely modified for filtration, having large numbers of pores up to 80 Å penetrating through the endothelium. Because these pores are sufficiently large to allow passage of all but the cellular elements of blood, the actual filtration barrier is provided by a thick basement membrane. Large amounts of negatively charged glycosaminoglycans help to repel albumin and other plasma proteins from entering the nephron. Approximately one-fifth of the plasma entering the glomerular apparatus is actually removed (filtered) from the blood; the remainder exits by way of efferent arterioles to supply other portions of the nephron. Generally, molecules smaller than albumin (molecular weight 69 kDa) appear in the tubular fluid. Because plasma proteins are almost completely retained within the bloodstream, bound drugs are not subject to filtration.

Tubular reabsorption

Because of the kidney's ability to concentrate tubular fluid, a chemical gradient is set up for the diffusion of drugs back into the systemic circulation. Agents with a favorable lipid/water partition coefficient readily traverse the tubular epithelium and return to the bloodstream.

For electrolytes, reabsorption from renal tubular fluid is pH dependent. Depending on the rate of H^+ secretion, the urinary pH may vary from 4.5 to 8.0. Weak acids such as aspirin are reabsorbed more effectively under acidic conditions; the reverse is true for weak bases such as amphetamine and ephedrine. Occasionally, the influence of pH on drug excretion is used to clinical advantage. A common strategy in the face of aspirin toxicity is to promote salicylate elimination through alkalization of the urine by the systemic administration of sodium bicarbonate. For the sulfonamides (also weak acids), alkalization of the urine may reduce the plasma half-time by 50% and prevent the development of crystalluria by increasing aqueous solubility. Attempts to enhance renal excretion are of little value for agents whose inactivation depends largely on biotransformation.

Active secretion

Numerous organic anions and cations are actively secreted into the urine by cells of the proximal convoluted tubule (see Fig. 2-7). The anionic transport system, responsible for the secretion of amphiphilic anions and conjugated metabolites (e.g., glucuronides, sulfates), relies primarily on two basolateral antiporters—OAT1 and OAT3—to take up anions (and some neutral and even cationic drugs) from the interstitial fluid in exchange for intracellular α-ketoglutarate. Transfer of the now intracellular organic anions into the urine principally involves the Na^+/phosphate transporter-1 (NPT-1) and two ABC transporters. Because each transport carrier is nonselective, competition of drugs for binding sites is sometimes observed.

Vectorial transport of organic cations also involves SLC transporters on the basolateral side of the tubular epithelium and a mix of transporters on the luminal side. Because of a favorable electrochemical gradient for cations, energy is not required for facilitated transport of these extracellular cations. Once inside, the compounds are pumped into the urine by one or more transporters, including P-glycoprotein, and SLC transporters.

Specific transport systems of the kidney, found principally in the distal convoluted tubule, also exist to reabsorb specific agents actively. The most important example of active reuptake of organic ions by this mechanism involves uric acid. Normally reuptake of uric acid is beneficial, but when it builds up in excess, it will crystalize and cause gout. Because the drug probenecid can compete with urate ions, it has an application in gout as a promoter of uric acid excretion.

Active secretion of substances into the urine is not adversely affected by plasma protein binding. The transporters are often so effective that drug dissociation occurs instantly, making available more drug for secretion, until all the drug has been cleared from the local blood supply. Binding to extravascular tissues does reduce the rate of renal elimination, however, regardless of the mechanisms involved.

Clearance

Clearance of drugs from the body is the sum of clearance from every organ (renal clearance + hepatic clearance + clearance from other organs). The kidney is the major organ for removing drugs from the body. The amount of drug removed per unit of time is often evaluated as a function of the plasma water "cleared" of drug, referred to as "clearance" **(CL)**. Mathematically, the volume of plasma cleared per minute (CL) can be written as follows:

$$CL = k_e \times V_d,$$

where k_e is the first-order rate constant of elimination and V_d is the apparent volume of distribution for the drug. Since first-order rate constants are given in reciprocal time (1/time) (see later), clearance for a first-order rate of elimination is given in units of volume/time. In practical terms, agents that are filtered but not reabsorbed or secreted yield a clearance of ~130 mL/min (assuming no plasma protein binding), and they serve as a measure of the glomerular filtration rate. With a V_d of 12 L, this clearance rate translates into a plasma half-time of 64 minutes. Conversely, compounds actively secreted into the urine and not reabsorbed, such as penicillin G, may approach a clearance of 650 mL/min, which is the rate of total plasma flow through the kidneys. Assuming a similar V_d of 12 L, such a drug would have a plasma half-time of approximately 13 minutes (see the later discussion on pharmacokinetic equations and calculations). By way of contrast, drugs that are highly bound and subject to passive reabsorption may exhibit clearance rates approaching 0.

Biliary Excretion

Numerous cationic, anionic, and steroid-like molecules are selectively removed from the blood for excretion into the bile and eventually the feces. Generally, these substances have molecular weights exceeding 500 Da. The transport process is an active one in which the dissolved substance is transferred from the plasma to the hepatocytes and then to the bile, as described previously for drugs that are metabolized. The bile is also a route of excretion for metabolized drugs, especially drugs that have undergone phase II reactions such as glucuronidation.

Biliary excretion is responsible for all but a small portion of the fecal elimination of drugs. The feces may also contain a variable amount of unabsorbed drug. Reabsorption of molecules excreted through the bile can occur, known as enterohepatic recycling. It can **prolong the duration** of action and may continue for an extended period of time until the system is interrupted (e.g., by metabolism, curtailment of bile flow, or ingestion of a drug chelator). Interestingly, some glucuronide conjugates secreted via bile into the gut can be metabolized by gut bacterial enzymes back to the active parent drug, which can then be reabsorbed.

Other Routes of Excretion

Pulmonary excretion is a primary route for the elimination of gases and some volatile compounds. Elimination of drugs by breast milk is important, not because of any quantitative significance, but because it represents a potential danger to the nursing infant. Drugs of particular concern include lithium, various anticancer agents, and isoniazid. The primary variable influencing the passage of drugs into milk is lipid solubility.

Other minor routes of excretion include sweat, tears, saliva, and gastric/pancreatic/intestinal secretions. In all cases, excretion is limited by the lipid/water partition coefficient. For saliva and related gastrointestinal fluids, drugs are deposited into the gastrointestinal tract after secretion and are available for reabsorption into the systemic circulation.

TIME COURSE OF DRUG ACTION

The close correspondence between the plasma concentration of an agent and its magnitude of effect has already been emphasized. Because drug administration usually encompasses the linear midrange of the log dose–response curve, the relationship between plasma titer and patient reaction is often straightforward. A temporal description of drug concentration on the basis of pharmacokinetic principles is useful in illustrating how absorption, distribution, metabolism, and excretion influence drug effects in concert and provide guidance for adjusting dosage schedules to achieve therapeutic results with a minimum of drug toxicity.

Kinetics of Absorption and Elimination

The rates of most biologic events involving the fate of drugs can be described in simple kinetic terms, that is, either zero-order or first-order kinetics. Most of the emphasis in this discussion is on rate of elimination, which is the major factor governing duration and level of drug action after the initial absorption.

Zero-order kinetics

Zero-order kinetics define processes that occur at a **constant amount per unit of time**. Mathematically, this can be written as $dC/dt = k_0$, where dC/dt is the rate of change in concentration, and k_0 is a constant in units of amount per time. A good example of zero-order absorption of drugs is the continuous intravenous infusion in which the quantity of compound entering the bloodstream each minute is held constant (e.g., 5 mg/min). An example of zero-order rate of elimination is one in which the body can only eliminate a certain amount of drug no matter what the quantity of drug is in the body. Ethyl alcohol, even in moderately intoxicating doses, is metabolized at a constant rate of approximately 6 g/hr for an adult. Only when the concentration decreases to far less than that producing any observable effect does alcohol dehydrogenation assume a first-order rate.

Another example of zero-order kinetics is the situation with toxic doses of aspirin. Aspirin is quickly deacetylated to salicylate, the anion responsible for much of the drug's pharmacologic activity. Salicylate is active and is eliminated through several metabolic pathways and by renal excretion, yielding an overall elimination half-time of approximately 3 hours at most therapeutic doses. Some of the inactivation routes are easily saturated, however, so that when an overdose is ingested, the toxicity problem is compounded by a relative loss in elimination efficiency. Elimination half-times increase continuously according to the drug concentration (Table 2-8). Salicylate has a

TABLE 2-8 Approximate Half-Time of Common Drugs

Drug	Elimination Half-time (hr)
Antibiotics	
Amoxicillin	1.7
Clindamycin	3
Erythromycin	1.5
Penicillin G	0.5
Tetracycline	10
Analgesics	
Acetaminophen	3
Aspirin (as salicylate)	3-20*
Codeine	3†
Meperidine	3
Morphine	2†
Local Anesthetics	
Articaine	0.4
Bupivacaine	2.4
Lidocaine	1.8†
Procaine	0.01
Sedative Agents	
Ethyl alcohol	1.4-20*
Diazepam	45†
Pentobarbital	30
Triazolam	3

*Capacity-limited metabolism.
†Converted to active metabolite.

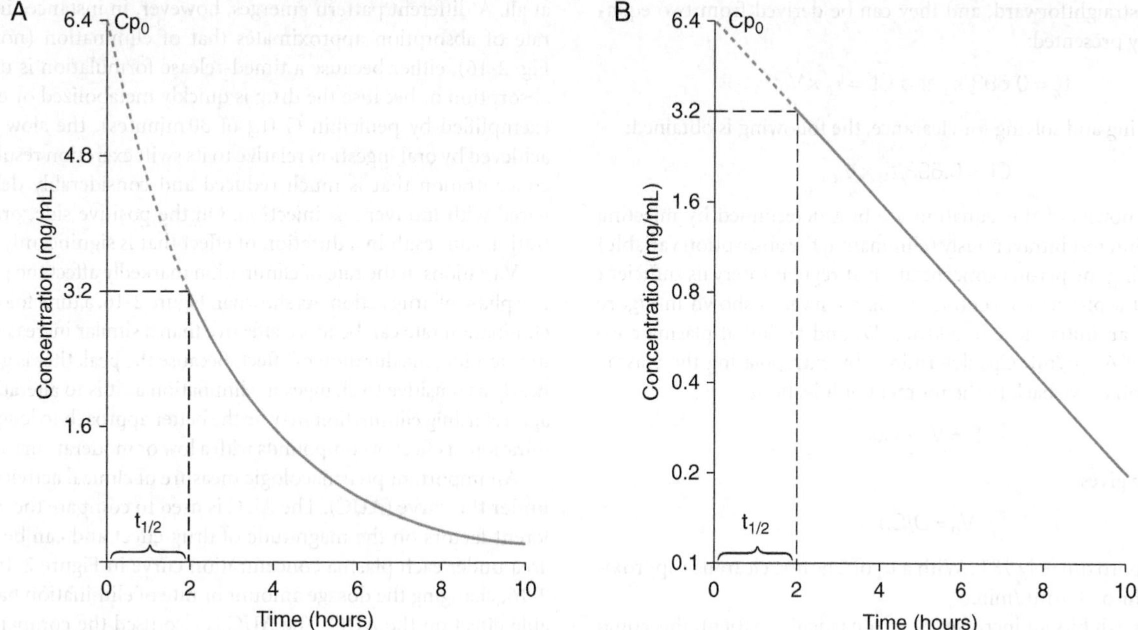

FIG 2-14 First-order elimination of a drug given as an intravenous bolus. In this example of a plasma concentration–time curve, it is assumed that the body behaves as a single compartment and that the distribution of the drug is essentially instantaneous. **A,** The plasma concentration is plotted on an arithmetic scale. **B,** A logarithmic scale is used to yield a straight line. The elimination half-time ($t_{½}$) is determined by the time interval required (2 hours in this case) for the plasma concentration to decrease by 50%. The Cp_0 indicates the interpolated concentration of drug (from line extension of drug disappearance curve in *B*) immediately after drug injection.

plasma half-time of ~20 hours when a very high concentration is present in the bloodstream. As the salicylate titer decreases into the therapeutic range, the elimination half-time decreases back to the constant of 3 hours (first-order rate of elimination).

First-order kinetics

First-order kinetics relate to events that occur at a **constant fractional rate per unit of time** (e.g., 5%/min). Here $dC/dt = k_1Cp$, where k_1 is the fractional first-order rate constant in units of time, dC/dt equals the change in drug concentration with respect to time, and Cp is the plasma drug concentration. The absorption, distribution, and elimination of compounds commonly exhibit this type of kinetics because they generally rely on processes that are first-order in character: passive diffusion, blood flow, or drug transport and metabolism operating well below saturation. Because the fraction of drug affected per unit of time is independent of concentration, as drug load increases, the amount of drug eliminated per unit time increases. Thus the **half-time ($t_{½}$) of elimination** is useful in determining the rate of drug disappearance and the concentration of drug remaining after a given period of time. Notice the relationship between the $t_{½}$ and the first-order rate constant of elimination:

$$t_{½} = 0.693/k_e$$

In first-order rate reactions, the change in drug concentration is an exponential function. Thus, after distribution has equilibrated, the disappearance curve is linear on a semi-log plot (Fig. 2-14). (The former equation contains the constant 0.693, which is the natural log of 2, since at $t_{½}$, a twofold difference in drug plasma concentration is being compared.) Also in the previous equation, it can be seen that the greater the rate constant, the shorter the $t_{½}$ and the faster the reaction. Moreover, it is easily shown that first-order processes are essentially complete (94%) after four half-times. Figure 2-14 provides an example of the first-order elimination of a drug with a $t_{½}$ of 2 hours, and Table 2-8 lists the elimination half-times of some commonly used categories of drugs in dentistry.

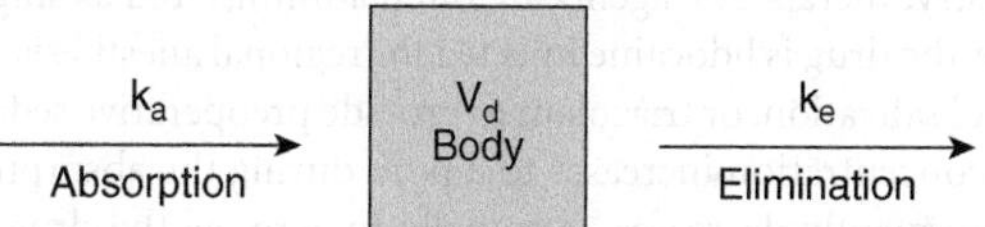

FIG 2-15 Single-compartment model of drug kinetics. Absorption into and elimination from the body are each assigned a single first-order rate constant. Distribution, assumed to be rapid compared to absorption and elimination, is not considered.

Capacity-limited reactions

Capacity-limited reactions refer to rates (in this case elimination), which display first-order kinetics at lower doses but zero order at higher doses. Higher doses thus saturate the elimination process(es). As already stated, most drug dosages used clinically are less than the doses required for saturation.

Single-Compartment Model

In its entirety, the body's disposition of an administered drug involves such a complex temporal interplay of biochemical and physiologic processes, each with its own unique set of kinetic parameters, that a full quantitative description of the time course of drug action may be impossible to achieve. For practical purposes, however, the sojourn of many agents can be described by a simple model system (Fig. 2-15) in which the body is depicted as a single compartment whose size corresponds to the V_d and whose elimination is based on first-order kinetics. In this model, which assumes rapid distribution and slower absorption/elimination, the relationships among elimination $t_{½}$, total body clearance (CL, or the volume of blood "cleared" of the drug per unit of time by the combined processes of metabolism and excretion), and V_d are straightforward, and they can be derived from two equations already presented:

$$t_{½} = 0.693/k_e \text{ and } CL = k_e \times V_d;$$

By substituting and solving for clearance, the following is obtained:

$$CL = 0.693/t_{½} \times V_d$$

The unknowns of this equation are best determined by injecting the drug of interest intravenously (eliminating the absorption variable) and measuring the plasma concentration at regular intervals sufficient to construct a plasma concentration–time curve, as shown in Figure 2-14. Given an initial dose of 500 mg (D) and an initial plasma concentration of 6.4 µg/mL Cp_0 determined by extrapolating the plasma concentration curve back to the moment of injection,

$$D = V_d \times Cp_0$$

Rearranging gives:

$$V_d = D/Cp_0$$

V_d equals approximately 78 L. With a $t_{½}$ of 2 hours, clearance approximates 27 L/hr or 450 mL/min.

If a drug exhibits an increased $t_{½}$ in a particular patient, this could mean that tissue binding of the drug is greater than normal, or it could just as easily indicate a reduction in the rate of metabolism or excretion of the agent. Similarly, a significant reduction in V_d, which occurs in some diseases, may have the curious result of reducing the $t_{½}$ of a drug even in the face of impaired clearance.

Plasma concentration: single doses

In dentistry, therapeutic agents are often administered as single doses. Whether the drug is lidocaine injected for regional anesthesia, atropine to control salivation, or triazolam to provide preoperative sedation, the plasma concentration increases to a peak during the absorptive phase and subsequently decreases, eventually to zero, as the drug is eliminated from the bloodstream. By using the single-compartment model, it is possible to construct theoretic plasma concentration curves and observe how modifications of dosage, absorption, or elimination can alter drug concentrations and, presumably, drug effects. As shown in Figure 2-16, the plasma concentration is at all times directly proportional to the dose. This relationship does not exist for agents that are capacity-limited in absorption, binding, metabolism, or excretion.

As long as absorption is several times faster than elimination, changes in the rate of drug uptake have little effect other than to alter the peak concentration. The duration of action is hardly influenced at all. A different pattern emerges, however, in instances in which the rate of absorption approximates that of elimination (not shown in Fig. 2-16), either because a timed-release formulation is used to slow absorption or because the drug is quickly metabolized or excreted. As exemplified by penicillin G ($t_{½}$ of 30 minutes), the slow absorption achieved by oral ingestion relative to its swift excretion results in a peak concentration that is much reduced and considerably delayed compared with intravenous injection. On the positive side, oral administration can result in a duration of effect that is significantly prolonged.

Variations in the rate of elimination markedly affect the post-absorptive phase of drug action. As shown in Figure 2-16, a threefold decrease in elimination rate can be more effective than a similar increase in the dose in extending the duration of effect. Because the peak titer is generally not nearly as sensitive to changes in elimination as it is to alterations in dosage, retarding elimination may be the better approach to lengthening the duration of effect of compounds with a low or moderate margin of safety.

An important pharmacologic measure of clinical activity is the **area under the curve (AUC)**. The AUC is used to compare the effect of different factors on the magnitude of drug effect and can be seen as the area under each plasma concentration curve in Figure 2-16. In Figure 2-16, changing the dosage amount or rate of elimination has a predictable effect on the AUC. The AUC is also used the compare the effectiveness of different routes of administration. For instance, the AUC for drugs that are poorly absorbed orally will be some fraction of an IV dose. The AUC can also be used to determine the extent of distribution of drugs in different body fluids, such as saliva shown in Table 2-3.

Plasma concentration: repeated doses

Whenever a drug is administered more than once per every four elimination half-times accumulation of the compound occurs within the body. Figure 2-17 shows the result of continued use of a drug given either by intravenous infusion or repeated administration. Regardless of the administration format (assuming first order of elimination), a **plateau (or steady-state) average plasma concentration** is reached in approximately **four elimination half-times**, assuming no change in the dosing rate. The periodic fluctuations obtained with intermittent administration are a function of the absorption rate and the dosage interval. These fluctuations can be minimized by increasing the frequency of administration or retarding the rate of absorption.

The average steady-state concentration relative to the peak value obtainable after an initial dose can be determined by multiplying the number of doses administered per elimination $t_{½}$ by 1.44. The steady-state concentration of a drug given once every $t_{½}$ equals 144% of the initial peak concentration. For diazepam (assuming a $t_{½}$ of 2 days)

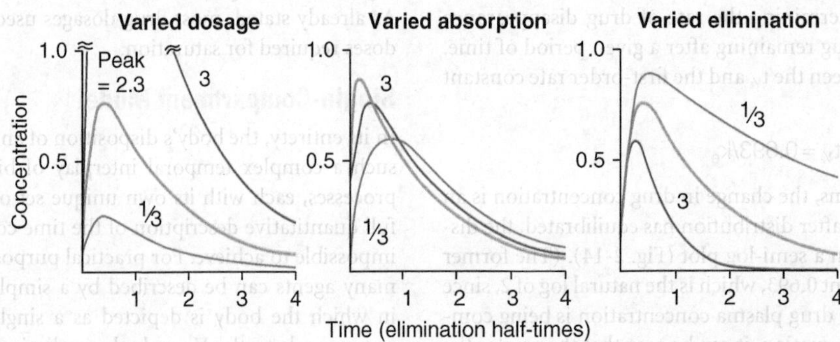

FIG 2-16 Time course of plasma concentration after single doses of drug. The various curves illustrate the influence of threefold increases (*3*) or decreases (*1/3*) of dosage, rate of absorption, and elimination on drug titers. The standard curve reproduced in all three graphs represents an agent whose first-order absorption rate is 10 times faster than elimination. A concentration of 1.0 is the value that would result if the drug were absorbed instantaneously, as with an intravenous injection.

ingested three times per day (i.e., six doses per half-time), the average plateau concentration approximates 1.44×6, or 8.6 times the peak concentration of a single dose. At least 8 days (four half-times) are required to reach this final drug plasma plateau level for diazepam.

The gradual approach to steady-state concentrations associated with slowly eliminated drugs can either benefit or hinder therapy. On the positive side, a long $t_{½}$ permits the clinician to administer the drug at convenient intervals, perhaps once a day, without having to be concerned with wide swings in plasma concentration. If patient monitoring reveals an unusual buildup of drug because of impaired metabolism or excretion or some other cause, time is available to adjust the dose before toxic effects ensue. On the debit side, the attainment of a therapeutic effect is delayed by the time required for drug accumulation to proceed. If an immediate pharmacologic effect is needed, a loading dose of the drug must be administered. A loading dose is a large, initial quantity of drug substituted for the normal amount to quickly produce a concentration approximating the steady state. For an agent given once each $t_{½}$, the loading dose is approximately twice the maintenance dose; for drugs given more frequently, the loading dose is larger. Dividing a loading dose into several smaller fractions is often wise. The sacrifice of some speed in attaining a therapeutic concentration is usually more than compensated for by the ability to evaluate patient responses during the early phase of therapy. The fact that elimination rates, which help regulate steady-state concentrations, can vary greatly among individuals should dictate caution whenever cumulative drug effects are sought.

The **maintenance dose** of a drug replaces drug loss due to elimination. The equation for the maintenance dose is similar to a previous equation:

$$MD = Cp_{ss(ave)} \times CL$$

By substituting for CL we get the equation:

$$MD = Cp_{ss(ave)} \times k_e \times V_d$$

where MD is the maintenance dose and $Cp_{ss(ave)}$ equals the average steady-state (plateau) concentration.

A Two-Compartment Model

For many drugs, the simple single-compartment model does not adequately describe the early time course of plasma concentration. Larger discrepancies are particularly likely to be observed when a relatively lipophilic drug is given intravenously, as in the use of CNS depressants for conscious sedation. In that situation, the effects of one or more additional drug reservoirs are more obvious.

The value of assuming a two-compartment model is that it takes into account the early distribution phase (α phase in Fig. 2-18) when observing drug plasma profiles. With time, a quasi–steady state is established between the central and peripheral reservoirs in which net redistribution back into the central compartment occurs as the drug is metabolized or excreted. A terminal $t_{½}$ is determined from the log-linear portion of the curve, indicating a first-order rate of elimination. The V_d is determined by extrapolating the log-linear portion of the curve (β phase in Fig. 2-18) back to the "y" axis to obtain the Cp_0 and solving for V_d. As we saw before:

$$D = V_d \times Cp_0$$

The **two-compartment model** is also useful in understanding how the duration of a drug's effect after a single injection during the α phase may be largely independent of the clearance rate or elimination $t_{½}$. In Figure 2-18, if the threshold concentration for a sedative effect of the drug was 10 µg/mL, a patient would recover from the sedation within 30 minutes, even if metabolism and excretion were completely blocked, simply by redistribution into less well-perfused tissues.

Review of Equations Used in This Chapter

The discipline of pharmacokinetics employs several equations relevant in both understanding pharmacokinetics and in performing calculations. This chapter has concentrated on a limited number of the most important equations. With the following list, it is important to see the relations between equations and how substitutions can be used to do therapeutic drug calculations based on the information provided.

1) $k_e \times t_{½} = 0.693$
2) $D = V_d \times Cp_0$ (for single drug dose)
3) $CL = k_e \times V_d$
4) $MD = Cp_{ss(ave)} \times CL$ (for maintenance dosing)

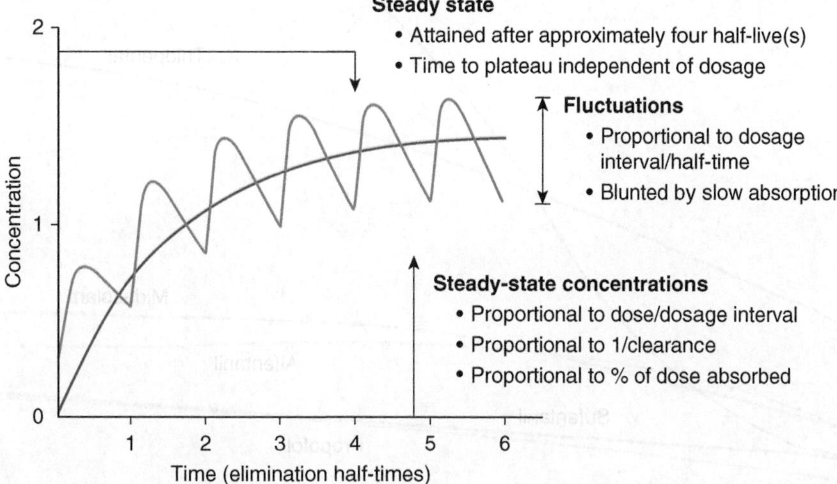

FIG 2-17 Time course of plasma concentration involving drug accumulation. The *wavy blue line* reflects the pattern of accumulation observed during the repeated administration of a drug at intervals equal to its elimination half-time when drug absorption is 10 times as rapid as elimination. The *smooth red line* depicts drug accumulation during the administration of an equivalent dosage by continuous intravenous infusion. (Adapted from Buxton ILO, Benet LZ: In Brunton LL, Chabner BA, Knollmann BC, editors: *Goodman & Gilman's the pharmacological basis of therapeutics*, ed 12, New York, 2011, McGraw-Hill.)

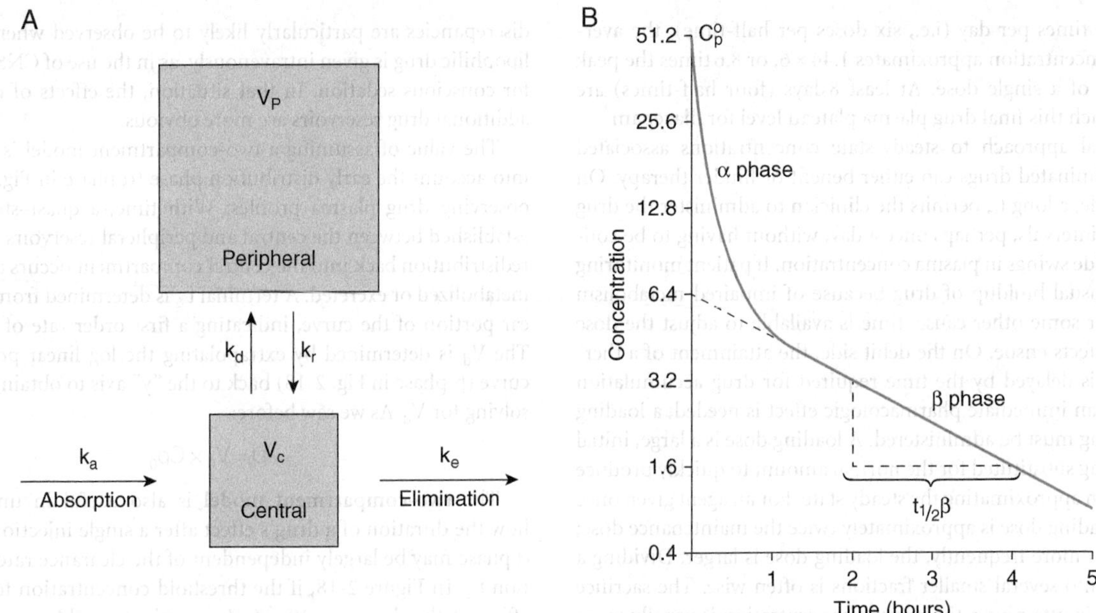

FIG 2-18 Two-compartment model of drug kinetics. **A,** In this model, drugs are absorbed into and eliminated from a central compartment that is linked by distribution processes (having rate constants of k_d and k_r) to a second, peripheral compartment. The central compartment includes the blood, from which drug determinations are taken. **B,** The plasma concentration–time curve consists of two phases: an early distribution or *α phase,* during which the concentration decreases largely as a result of distribution out of the central compartment, and a late elimination or *β phase,* during which metabolism and excretion predominate. The terminal half-time ($t_{1/2}\ \beta$) is calculated from the log-linear portion of the elimination curve. The Cp_0 is determined from the extension of the β phase line to the "y" axis. The Cp_0 is therefore an extrapolated value since a direct measurement of Cp_0 is impossible.

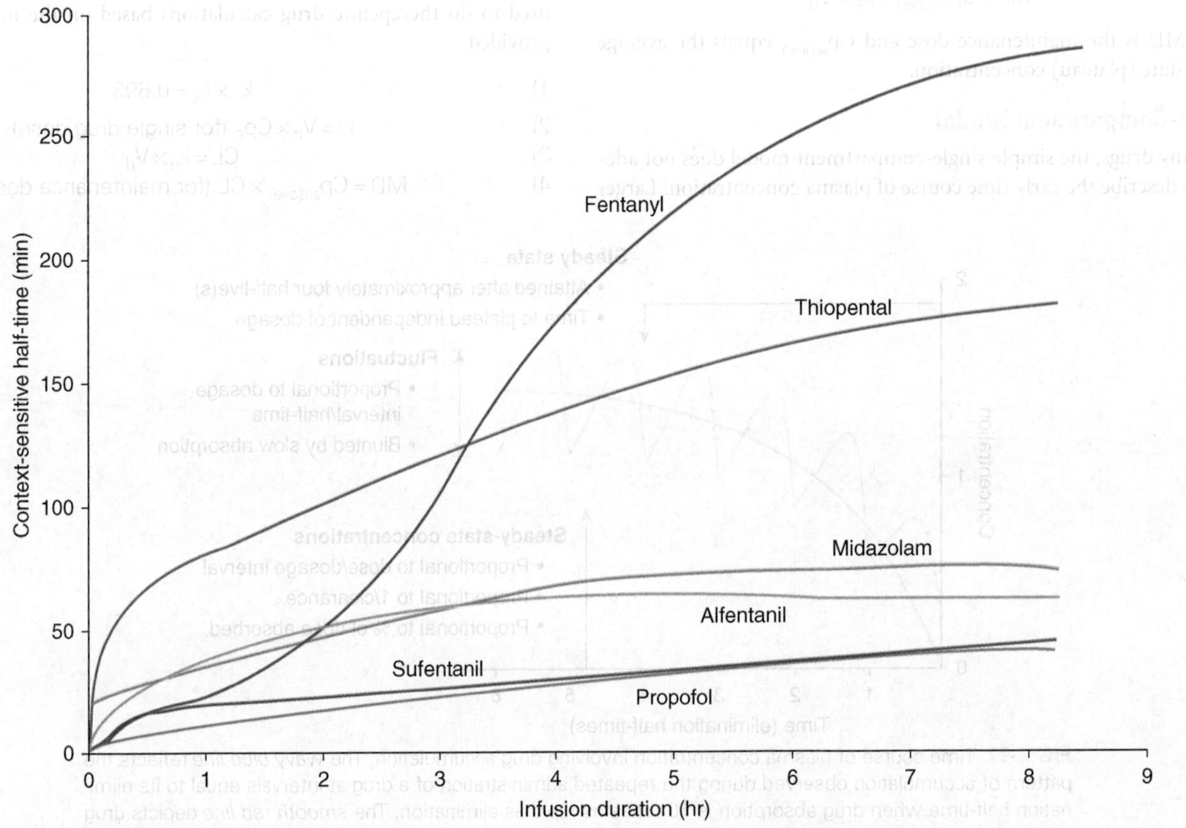

FIG 2-19 Context-sensitive half-life. (Redrawn from Hughes MA, Glass PSA, Jacobs JR: Context-sensitive half-time in multicompartment pharmacokinetic models for intravenous anesthetic drugs, *Anesthesiology* 76:334-341, 1992.)

Context-Sensitive Half-Times

The numerous variables of the multi-compartment model make it impossible to predict intuitively the influence of individual pharmacokinetic parameters such as half-times, V_d values, and clearance rates on the plasma concentration profile of a highly lipid-soluble drug given repeatedly or continuously for a period of time. This situation poses a problem when intravenous agents are administered by continuous infusion for anesthesia or sedation. A partial solution involves the use of computer modeling to estimate context-sensitive half-times. The context-sensitive $t_{½}$ is the time required for the plasma concentration of a drug to decrease by 50% when consideration is given to how long the drug has been infused. As illustrated in Figure 2-19, fentanyl shows a significant increase in this parameter as the duration of infusion exceeds 2 hours. This phenomenon is the result of saturation of redistribution sites. Conversely, propofol, with its enormous capacity for redistribution, experiences only a slow increase over time. Such information is useful clinically in selecting the appropriate agent for use and in estimating the changing duration of drug effect. Similar context-sensitive curves can be generated for recovery to different percentages (e.g., 25%) of the plasma concentration, depending on what value best predicts recovery of function. Further advances in computer modeling will undoubtedly help address other limitations of the multi-compartment model, such as the oscillations in arterial plasma concentrations that occur with bolus injection of drug and errors associated with the fact that some drugs are metabolized in more than a single compartment.

DISCREPANCIES BETWEEN PLASMA CONCENTRATIONS AND RECEPTOR ACTION

Two basic assumptions underlying pharmacokinetic studies are that the plasma concentration of a drug is predictive of the concentration around the site of drug action and the magnitude of drug effect depends on this concentration. Although these assumptions generally hold, important exceptions to them do exist. As previously stated, drugs that bind covalently to their receptors produce effects that far outlast the drugs' passage in the bloodstream. Drugs that rely on transcription and protein synthesis are delayed in effect because of the time required for these processes to occur. Additional discrepancies between plasma concentration and drug effect arise because of delays in reaching the site of action and temporal changes that occur in receptor responsiveness.

CASE DISCUSSION

It is wise to consider the possibility of a drug–drug interaction whenever two or more drugs are taken together. In this case, codeine is a drug that gets metabolized by cytochrome-P450 2D6, which converts it to morphine, a more active opioid drug. This conversion is needed to lead to the expected analgesic effect of the administered codeine. Cimetidine is an inhibitor of several cytochrome P450 enzymes, including cytochrome-P450 2D6. The combination of the two drugs would be expected to decrease the analgesic effect of codeine, because less morphine would be produced. The effect on acetaminophen by cimetidine would be expected to be less than that of codeine in part because the conjugation reactions would be less affected by cimetidine. Although the result of this interaction may be mild, the use of cimetidine is not recommended. Other histamine-2 blockers, which do not have these effects on cytochromes, are available. One recommendation would be to use an alternate histamine-2 blocker. Male patients are also at risk with cimetidine because of the antiandrogenic effect of the drug. Finally, cimetidine also poses a risk with some other opioids due to effects on cytochromes. These effects of cimetidine limit its clinical use.

GENERAL REFERENCES

1. Daneman R, Prat A: The blood–brain barrier, *Cold Spring Harb Perspect Biol* 7:1943–2064, 2015.
2. DeGorter MK, Xia CQ, Yang JJ, Kim RB: Drug transporters in drug efficacy and toxicity, *Ann Rev Pharmacol Toxicol* 52:249–273, 2012. Drug–drug interaction table: http://medicine.iupui.edu/clinpharm/ddis/clinical-table/. Accessed on January 1, 2015.
3. Duckworth RM: Pharmacokinetics in the oral cavity: fluoride and other active ingredients, *Monogr Oral Sci* 23:125–139, 2013.
4. Fan J, deLannoy IA: Pharmacokinetics, *Biochem Pharmacol* 87:93–120, 2014.
5. Gallardo E, Barroso M, Queiroz JA: Current technologies and considerations for drug bioanalysis in oral fluid, *Bioanalysis* 1:637–667, 2009.
6. Rees DC, Johnson E, Lewinson O: ABC transporters: the power to change, *Nat Rev Mol Cell Biol* 10:218–227, 2009.
7. Suetsugu S, Kurisu S, Takenawa T: Dynamic shaping of cellular membranes by phospholipids and membrane-deforming proteins, *Physiol Rev* 94:1219–1248, 2014.
8. Zakeri-Milani P, Valizadeh H: Intestinal transporters: enhanced absorption through P-glycoprotein-related drug interactions, *Expert Opin Metab Toxicol* 10:859–871, 2014.

3

Pharmacotherapeutics: The Clinical Use of Drugs*

Frank J. Dowd

KEY INFORMATION

- Quantal dose–response curves are used to measure responses to drugs in populations.
- Hyperreactive patients are those that react to lower doses of a drug than do most of the population.
- Body weight, age, gender, genetic factors, disease status, pregnancy, and lactation are important factors in a patient's response to drugs and adverse effects.
- Tolerance and rapid tolerance, tachyphylaxis, occur with certain drugs.
- The placebo effect is real, especially in treatments like pain therapy.
- Drug–drug interactions can lead to unexpected adverse effects.
- Adverse drug effects include extensions of the therapeutic effect, side effects, idiosyncratic reactions, and allergies.
- Other problematic potential effects of drugs include carcinogenesis, drug abuse, poisoning, and fetal changes including teratogenic effects.
- Drugs are derived from a number of sources including natural sources, organic synthesis, and recombinant technology.
- The safety of a drug can be estimated in several ways. One common method is to measure the therapeutic index, defined as the LD_{50}/ED_{50} from animal studies.
- Testing of new drugs begins with the preclinical phase, followed by three human clinical testing phases, and finally postmarketing surveillance.
- Among the several name designations for drugs, the nonproprietary (generic) and the proprietary are the most commonly encountered.
- Several sources of drug data are available, including books on comprehensive drug information, textbooks, and online media.

CASE STUDY

Your regular dental patient calls your office reporting that he has dental pain and swelling in the upper right side of his face. You see him on an emergency basis and diagnose a cellulitis resulting from an acute dental abscess. You prescribe amoxicillin, initial dose 2 g followed by 500 mg every 8 h. The patient gets the prescription filled at a pharmacy a short distance from your office and takes the 2 g of amoxicillin at the pharmacy. Upon leaving the pharmacy, the patient notices an urticarial rash on his arm that appears to be getting worse. He decides to return to your office. When he enters your office, he is also having some trouble breathing. You begin by administering oxygen, which appears to help the breathing. What is the likely cause of the rash and difficulty breathing? What, if anything, should be done next?

Numerous factors that complicate the attainment of therapeutic responses and the avoidance of unwanted effects should be considered when drugs are properly selected and administered. As stated in Chapter 1, drugs are often selective in the effects they produce because they activate or inhibit specific drug receptors. However, even the most selective agents generally evoke a spectrum of reactions rather than a single pharmacologic outcome. There are several reasons why this occurs. First, a drug is often used to target a given receptor in a particular organ, but these same receptors are usually located in other tissues and organs as well. Second, although a drug is selective, it often is not specific and may have effects at another receptor(s), especially at higher doses. Third, the drug may have nonselective effects, such as gastrointestinal upset. Fourth, a therapeutic dose of drug for one person may be ineffective for a second person and toxic to a third person. Therefore it becomes necessary to measure the effects of drugs in populations to determine the range of responses and to gauge their levels of safety.

MEASURING DRUG RESPONSES IN POPULATIONS; QUANTAL DOSE–RESPONSE CURVES

Figure 3-1 is a **quantal dose–response** graph illustrating the percentage of subjects responding to an agent as a logarithmic function of the dose. The graph is constructed by counting the number of animals or patients exhibiting a specified effect at various doses. With low amounts of drug, very few individuals within the population react; as the dose is increased, more are affected until a dose is reached at which the response is universal, a cumulative distribution. This is across a population average. In contrast, when looking at a frequency of response, each person will fall more on a classic bell-shaped curve. On a quantal dose–response curve, the **median effective dose** (ED_{50}) is the amount of drug required to produce a particular effect in 50% of treated individuals. Patients who are unusually sensitive to a drug are said to be **hyperreactive** or **hypersusceptible**, or perhaps **drug intolerant**. Individuals unexpectedly

*The author wishes to recognize Dr. John A. Yagiela for his past contributions to this chapter.

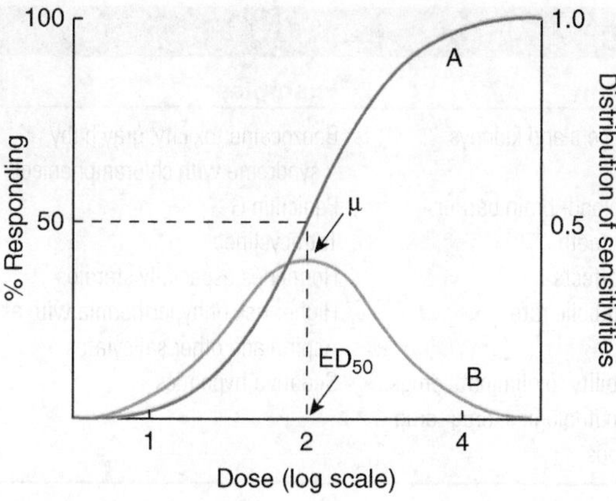

FIG 3-1 Quantal dose–response curves (dose on a log scale). Curve A represents the cumulative distribution, and curve B represents the frequency distribution of patient responses in a normal population. As shown, the mean (μ) and median (50% responding) sensitivities fall on the same dose (median effective dose, ED_{50}). (Adapted from Goldstein A, Aronow L, Kalman SM: *Principles of drug action: the basis of pharmacology*, ed 2, New York, 1974, John Wiley & Sons.)

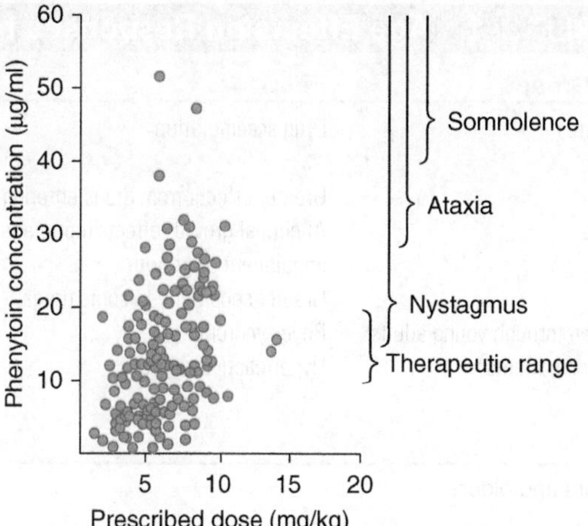

FIG 3-2 Plasma phenytoin concentration as a function of the prescribed dose. Each *circle* represents a single patient ($n = 294$). *Closed bracket* indicates the accepted therapeutic concentration range for phenytoin in plasma; *open-ended brackets* denote concentrations at which the various toxic manifestations listed may occur. (Data from Lund L: Effects of phenytoin in patients with epilepsy in relation to its concentration in plasma. In Davies DS, Prichard BNC, editors: *Biological effects of drugs in relation to their plasma concentrations*, Baltimore, 1973, University Park Press; and Kutt H, Winters W, Kokenge R, et al: Diphenylhydantoin metabolism, blood levels, and toxicity, *Arch Neurol* 11:642-648, 1964.)

resistant to conventional doses of drug are referred to as being **hyporeactive**. Many variables influence the responsiveness of individuals to drugs. Because it is impossible to predict how a given patient will respond to a particular agent, appropriate monitoring of drug effects is usually necessary to achieve optimal therapy. The use of quantal dose–response curves to estimate drug safety is discussed later in this chapter. Notice that quantal-dose response curves record the presence of the response to a dosage range of a drug, Graded dose-response curves, on the other hand as seen in Chapter 1, record the **magnitude** of the response to a range of concentrations of the drug.

FACTORS INFLUENCING DRUG EFFECTS

Differences between patients in reaction to a therapeutic agent may arise from disparities in drug concentration obtained with a standardized dose (**pharmacokinetic differences**), from variations in individual responsiveness to a given drug concentration (**pharmacodynamic differences**), or from secondary factors, such as the failure of patients to take their medication as prescribed (e.g., **noncompliance**). Figure 3-2 shows the lack of correlation that can develop clinically between the prescribed dose of a drug—in this case the anticonvulsant phenytoin—and the resultant plasma concentration and pharmacologic response. Even with the daily dose corrected for body weight, the steady-state concentration of phenytoin differed twentyfold or more. A small percentage of patients experienced nystagmus, an early indication of drug toxicity, at plasma concentrations barely sufficient to control convulsions in other patients. It is apparent that given a widely accepted therapeutic concentration range of 10 to 20 μg/mL (the plasma concentration of phenytoin supposed to provide seizure protection with minimal adverse effects), most patients in reality ended up with either an insufficient medication dose or an overdose. Although pharmacokinetic dissimilarities account for many differences in patient responsiveness, the fact that phenytoin has a **therapeutic range**, rather than a single effective concentration, indicates that there also exists some variation in pharmacodynamic sensitivity to the anticonvulsant.

Patient Factors

Many factors that can influence drug effects clinically are highly variable in individual patients. Size, age, and genetic makeup must be taken into account whenever drug therapy is planned.

Body weight and composition

Adults may differ three-fold or more in weight. Because the volume of distribution of a drug is a function of body mass, extremes in patient size may result in significant differences in plasma concentration when drugs are administered in the form of a "standard adult dose." Body composition is also an important variable. Two equally heavy patients, one obese and the other muscular, may react quite differently to certain agents. Because adipose tissue contributes very little to body water, the obese person will be more susceptible to a drug distributed essentially within one or more body fluid compartments. The same person may show unusual resistance to a highly lipophilic agent such as, diazepam, especially when it is given in repeated doses.

Age

Pediatric patients generally cannot be given adult dosages of drugs. The primary reason is their smaller body size, and various formulas have been devised to calculate pediatric fractions of the adult dose. For the following reasons, however, children must not be thought of as merely miniature adults. First, even with the size differential taken into account, neonates display an unusual hyperreactivity to drugs. Some of the reasons for this are given in Table 3-1. Immature hepatic and renal systems during the first weeks of life tend to promote drug accumulation, and the relative inefficiency of drug binding by albumin (sometimes because of competition for binding sites by bilirubin) may also lead to abnormal concentrations of drug in the vicinity of receptors. In addition, distribution of compounds into the central nervous system (CNS) may be enhanced by an incomplete maturation of the blood–brain barrier. Second, in contrast to neonates, children and infants older than 6 months often require larger milligram-per-kilogram body weight doses of drugs during therapy. This relative hyporeactivity is mostly attributable to an enhancement in the rate of elimination. Dosage adjustment on the basis of surface area rather than body weight is empirically a useful strategy in correcting for age-related differences in elimination.

There is no method of pediatric dosage calculation suitable for all drugs and therapeutic situations. In older children, adjustments based on age, weight, or (preferably) surface area may be satisfactory, but no

TABLE 3-1 Age Effects on Responses to Drugs

Age Group	Effect	Mechanism	Examples
Neonates	Drug accumulation	Immature livers and kidneys	Benzocaine toxicity, gray baby syndrome with chloramphenicol
	Greater effects from drugs entering the CNS	Immature blood–brain barrier	Penicillin G
Children	Abnormal growth effects (up to age 8 yrs)	Staining of teeth	Tetracyclines
	Impairment of growth	Hormonal effects	Hormones especially steroids
	Greater sensitivity to some drugs	Higher metabolic rate	Higher risk of hyperthermia with atropine
Children through young adults	Reye syndrome	?	Aspirin and other salicylates
Geriatric patients*	Hyperreactive to drugs	Reduced ability to eliminate drugs, existing pathologies, drug–drug interactions	Sedative-hypnotics

*65 years and older.

general guide is possible for very young children. Dosages for neonates, infants, and young children should be based on clinical trials; however, pediatric dosage schedules for older drugs are often unavailable.

Geriatric patients are frequently hyperreactive to drugs, thus careful selection of drug and dosage schedules is necessary, especially with drugs of low safety. Geriatric pharmacology is becoming increasingly important to the dentist as the general population ages.

Genetic influences

Genetic variables contribute greatly to the differences in drug responsiveness illustrated in Figure 3-1. Although the importance of heredity is underscored by the evolution of pharmacogenetics into a recognized field of study, the elucidation of multigenetic factors that lead to log-normal distributions in drug reactivity has proven difficult (see Chapter 4). Now, studies of gene expression and polymorphisms are helping to uncover an increasingly broad array of genetically determined differences in drug responsiveness (Chapter 4).

Sex, pregnancy, and lactation

The sex of a patient is sometimes important with respect to drug effects. As with children, information is lacking for many drugs because of the historic exclusion of female subjects from most drug studies. Dosage adjustments may be necessary for some drugs simply because women tend to be smaller than men and to have a higher percentage of body fat. Hepatic disposition of drugs seems not to be influenced by sex when variables such as age, size, body composition, and drug use are taken into account. Side effects such as hirsutism are less tolerable in women, and gynecomastia is more disconcerting in men.

Women seem to be more susceptible to drug-induced blood dyscrasias, and women taking systemic contraceptives may be more prone to some drug interactions. Drug-induced torsades de pointes is a potentially life-threatening arrhythmia with a significant sex bias. Women may be more likely to develop torsades because the QT interval of the electrocardiogram (see Chapter 19) is longer in women after puberty. The antiarrhythmic sotalol, one of the many drugs that can prolong the QT interval, is associated with a three times higher incidence of torsades in women. Because the preapproval clinical trials of sotalol enrolled only men, the relatively common side effect of QT prolongation was not recognized before the drug was released for general use.

Pregnancy is a major concern in pharmacotherapeutics. Alterations in liver function are common, and the hepatic toxicity of tetracycline and certain other compounds is markedly accentuated by pregnancy. The metabolism of numerous drugs is increased because of the ability of the high estrogen and progesterone concentrations to stimulate the pregnane X receptor (see Chapter 2) and cause enzyme induction. Renal excretion is likewise increased because of the elevated cardiac output and glomerular filtration. When present, pregnancy toxemia may increase drug effects by reducing the binding capacity of albumin, which is already reduced in a healthy pregnancy.

Of primary importance are the actions of drugs on the fetus. Spontaneous abortion, teratogenesis, mental retardation, drug dependence, and cancer have resulted from drug administration during pregnancy. Because few, if any, agents have been proved to be totally safe for the fetus, it is best to avoid all medications when possible. Drug administration should also be conservative in women of childbearing age because pregnancy is often undiagnosed during the first trimester, the most critical period of fetal development. Many drugs (e.g., methadone) are excreted in the milk. Because some of these agents may cause unwanted effects in the nursing infant, it is advisable to review carefully drug exposure during lactation as well. Nursing is contraindicated in women taking anticancer drugs, immunosuppressants, radioactive chemicals, ergot alkaloids, drugs of abuse, lithium salts, gold, iodine, and various antibiotics. Toxicologic concerns related to pregnancy are discussed in more detail later in this chapter.

Environmental factors

Factors such as ambient temperature, sunlight, and altitude are capable of influencing responses to certain drugs. Children given atropine on a warm day are especially susceptible to drug-induced hyperthermia, toxic skin reactions to sulfonamides increase with exposure to sunlight, and nitrous oxide loses efficacy in mountainous regions. Probably the most important environmental factor influencing drug effects is diet. The timing of meals and the types of food eaten can markedly affect drug absorption. The gastrointestinal absorption of most tetracyclines is impaired when taken with milk or other dairy products.

Numerous chemicals that are ingested, inhaled, or absorbed through the skin can influence the body's disposition of, or response to, various drugs. Patients receiving monoamine oxidase inhibitors risk severe hypertension and death if they eat foods containing tyramine (e.g., certain cheeses, beers, and wines). The therapeutic effects of levodopa in parkinsonism may be prevented by pyridoxine (vitamin B_6), present in foods and multivitamin supplements. Grapefruit juice contains substances that inhibit the CYP3A enzymes responsible for metabolizing a host of drugs (see Chapter 2). Finally, the use of insulin must be carefully matched to the patient's dietary intake to avoid complications associated with both hypoglycemia and hyperglycemia.

The indigenous microflora represents a special kind of environmental variable. Several drugs given orally are metabolized by bacterial enzymes to such an extent that absorption may be significantly impaired. The blood dose of the anticoagulant coumarin is partially governed by the amount of vitamin K produced by enteric bacteria and consumed in the diet. During antibiotic therapy, the type and number of microorganisms surviving play a large role in determining whether the patient will have significant swings in their clinical anticoagulation.

Physiologic variables

Numerous physiologic factors can modify clinical responses to drugs. Fluctuations in gastric, plasma, and urinary pH may alter the pharmacokinetics of weak electrolytes. Salt and water balance, exercise, sleep, body temperature, blood pressure, and many other factors also influence patient reactions. The effects of blocking agents are particularly sensitive to variations in physiologic or biochemical events. Isoproterenol, an adrenergic agonist, increases heart rate regardless of autonomic nervous system tone, but atropine, an acetylcholine antagonist, increases heart rate only in the face of tonic vagal activity.

Pathologic factors

Diseases may influence pharmacotherapeutics by modifying drug disposition or tissue responsiveness. Pathologic states most commonly associated with altered patient reactivity involve the organs of absorption, distribution, metabolism, and excretion. Achlorhydria, diarrhea, malabsorption syndromes, and other disturbances of the gastrointestinal tract may depress the absorption of ingested agents.

Hepatic dysfunction, whether caused by specific hepatic disease, infection, or other conditions, can markedly retard the metabolism and biliary excretion of drugs. Reduced transport capabilities can inhibit the uptake of drugs into the liver and export of metabolites from it. Reduced blood flow to the liver slows delivery of drugs to the liver, reducing the rate of metabolism (see Chapter 2).

Renal disease is a common modifier of drug effects. The plasma half-times of agents eliminated in the urine are often greatly prolonged by renal failure. Even for compounds completely inactivated in the liver, inadequate excretion of metabolites may increase the incidence of untoward reactions. A good measure of renal status is provided by the endogenous creatinine clearance. A 50% decrease in creatinine clearance should theoretically indicate a twofold increase in the elimination half-time of a drug that is removed from the blood solely by glomerular filtration. For a drug partially eliminated in the urine, the increase in plasma half-time should be correspondingly less. The customary approach to avoiding excessive drug accumulation in patients with renal disease is to lengthen the dosage interval in accordance with the degree of impaired elimination. Table 3-2 lists the approximate dosage intervals for several drugs (including some commonly used in dentistry) indicated for

TABLE 3-2 Dosage Adjustments in Renal Failure

		DOSE INTERVAL IN HOURS (AND PERCENTAGE OF NORMAL DOSE) ACCORDING TO DEGREE OF RENAL FAILURE*		
Drug	**Route of Elimination**	**Normal Function**	**Moderate Impairment**	**Severe Impairment**
Antibiotics				
Cefoxitin	Mainly renal	6	8-12	24
Erythromycin	Hepatic	6	6	12
Penicillin G	Mainly renal	4-6	4-6 (50%)	8 (33%-50%)
Tetracycline[†]	Renal/hepatic	12	12-24	Avoid use
Analgesics				
Acetaminophen[†]	Hepatic	4	6	6
Aspirin[†]	Hepatic/renal	4	4-6	Avoid use
Codeine[‡]	Mainly hepatic	4-6	4-6 (75%-100%)	4-6 (25%-50%)
Meperidine[‡]	Hepatic	3-4	3-4 (50%-100%)	Avoid use
Cardiovascular Agents				
Diltiazem	Hepatic	8	8	8
Furosemide	Renal/hepatic	12	12	12
Lisinopril	Fecal/renal	24	24 (50%-75%)	24 (25%-50%)
Propranolol	Hepatic	8	8	8 (75%-100%)
CNS Depressants				
Alprazolam	Hepatic	8	8	8
Lorazepam	Hepatic	12	12	12
Pentobarbital	Hepatic/renal	8	8	8
Phenobarbital	Hepatic/renal	8	8	8 (75%-100%)
Others				
Diphenhydramine	Hepatic	6-8	6-8	6-8
Insulin	Hepatic/renal	Variable	Variable (75%)	Variable (50%)
Prednisone	Hepatic	12	12	12
Ranitidine	Renal/hepatic	8	12	24

Data from St. Peter WL, Halstenson CE: Pharmacologic approach in patients with renal failure. In Chernow B, editor: *The pharmacologic approach to the critically ill patient,* ed 3, Baltimore, 1994, Williams & Wilkins.

*The degree of renal failure as defined by creatinine clearance: normal function to minimal impairment, >50 mL/min; moderate impairment, 10 to 50 mL/min; severe impairment, <10 mL/min.

[†]Drugs that may accentuate renal damage.

[‡]Accumulation of active metabolite limits dosing.

CNS, Central nervous system.

patients with moderate or severe renal failure. An insidious form of interaction between pathologic factors and drug effects occurs with agents potentially toxic to their primary organs of elimination. Acetaminophen accumulation permitted by liver disease may result in hepatic necrosis and further impairment of drug metabolism. A similar vicious cycle involving the kidney has been observed with various drugs.

Exaggeration of the systemic effects of epinephrine and reduction in the analgesic potency of morphine in uncontrolled hyperthyroidism are two examples of drug effects modified by disease states through non-pharmacokinetic means. Although pathologic factors may influence drug–receptor interactions directly, as in myasthenia gravis (in which receptor reactivity to acetylcholine is reduced), most alterations of patient response occur indirectly through the augmentation of overt disease or the unmasking of latent physiologic deficits. Agents that promote hyperuricemia may cause an acute exacerbation of gout, and propranolol may induce heart failure in patients with a severely compromised myocardium.

Drug Factors

In addition to individual variations in patient reactivity, certain drug factors, namely the formulation and dosage regimen of an agent and the development of tolerance, can markedly influence the success of drug therapy.

Variables in drug administration

Of all factors influencing pharmacologic responses clinically, only those involved with drug selection and administration are totally under the control of the clinician. Some of these variables—dose, drug formulation, route of administration, and drug accumulation—are discussed in detail in previous chapters. Two factors that have not yet been mentioned are the timing of administration and the duration of therapy. For example, many disturbing side effects are minimized if a sedative agent can be given shortly before sleep, including the autonomic effects of the belladonna alkaloids, the vestibular component of nausea associated with opioid analgesics, and the sedative properties of the antihistamines. Conversely, agents producing mild CNS stimulation are better tolerated in the daytime. The scheduling of doses with or between meals to limit gastrointestinal upset or to enhance absorption is discussed in Chapter 2.

The duration of therapy has several important ramifications. The duration of administration should be monitored especially carefully when drugs capable of producing physical or psychological dependence are being used or when using drugs that can have cumulative effects over time, such as chemotherapeutic agents.

Drug tolerance

In pharmacology, **tolerance** to a drug, as discussed in Chapter 1, refers to a state of decreased responsiveness that develops on repeated or continuous exposure to the agent or one of its congeners. Two major categories of tolerance are recognized: **pharmacokinetic or drug-disposition tolerance**, in which the effective concentration of the drug is diminished, and **pharmacodynamic or cellular tolerance**, in which the reaction to a given concentration of the drug is reduced. Pharmacodynamic tolerance and its mechanisms are described in Chapter 1. Other types of drug tolerance are listed in Table 3-3.

Specific mechanisms of tolerance have been established for certain drugs that evoke a rapidly developing form of tolerance termed **tachyphylaxis.** Histamine offers an example of tachyphylaxis. Because endogenous stores of histamine can be quickly depleted but take a long time to be replenished, drugs that cause histamine release (e.g., morphine and tubocurarine) can generate rapid tolerance. Tachyphylaxis is also characteristic of amphetamine use.

Factors Associated with the Therapeutic Regimen

Some factors influencing drug effects are related to the therapeutic context in which the agent is administered or prescribed. Attitudes toward the drug regimen or practitioner may determine whether an agent proves effective in a patient (or even if the drug is taken). Concurrent use of other medicines may alter drug effects directly through pharmacologic mechanisms or indirectly by promoting errors in drug administration.

Placebo effects

A placebo effect is any effect attributable to a medication or procedure that is not related to its pharmacodynamic or specific properties. The term **placebo** is derived from the Latin verb *placere*, meaning "to please." In pharmacotherapeutics, a placebo is a preparation that is pharmacologically inert (e.g., a lactose tablet).

Placebo responses to drugs arise from expectations by the patient concerning their effects and from a wish to obtain benefit or relief. Expectations develop at the conscious and subconscious levels and are influenced by many factors. The symbolic association of receiving medication in a therapeutic environment generates placebo reactions. Several important similarities and differences between placebo and specific effects of drugs must be remembered if clinicians are to avoid being deceived by the preparations they use. Therapeutic responses to placebos and to active agents may resemble each other in magnitude and duration. The pain relief and cough suppression afforded by a placebo may parallel that of codeine. Toxicities can also overlap. Pure placebos are associated with many common side effects: nausea, drowsiness, sweating, and xerostomia. However, there are many classes of drugs, such as the general anesthetics and the antibiotics, whose effects placebos cannot duplicate. Placebos are valid and often necessary inclusions in clinical trials, especially in studies such as analgesic drug trials, in which the placebo effect is well documented. However, there seems to be no justification for the therapeutic use of placebo medication in routine dental practice.

Patient noncompliance

The reasons for noncompliance are varied. They include a lack of understanding of the drug, the purpose for which it was prescribed,

TABLE 3-3 Types of Tolerances to Drugs

Type	Mechanism	Examples
Pharmacodynamic	Cell tolerance due to receptor change and/or other cell changes	Downregulation of the β-adrenergic receptor, decrease in response to mood-changing drugs
Immune	Antibodies bind to drug	Antibodies to digoxin reduce its effect
Pharmacokinetic (drug disposition)	Induction of enzymes of metabolism	Decreased half-life* of carbamazepine with continued use
Cellular distribution	Therapy results in changes in cells that make up a tissue	Anticancer drug therapy leads to cell resistance due to overexpression of P-glycoprotein
Learned tolerance	Individual uses coping skills to compensate for drug effects	Ability of alcoholics to disguise the effects of ethanol

*due to a decrease in elimination half-time

or how it is to be administered; economic factors; negative feelings toward the drug, prescriber, or medical care in general; development of adverse reactions; forgetfulness or carelessness; and perceived resolution of the problem before the drug regimen is complete or, conversely, failure to notice any therapeutic benefit. Even with serious illnesses such as essential hypertension, chronic infection, or hyperlipidemia, compliance is generally poor (approximately 50%) when the benefits of therapy are not superficially apparent. Drugs that produce unwanted side effects are especially likely to be discontinued. Deviations in self-administration tend to increase progressively with drugs that are taken long-term. Also, the more complex the therapeutic regimen in terms of doses and drugs, the higher the incidence of drug defaulting. The quality of the doctor–patient relationship is important in several respects. Patients who trust and respect their dentist or physician are more likely to take their prescribed medications. Effective communication further promotes compliance and reduces the possibility of a patient unilaterally terminating the drug if adverse effects occur. Measures that the clinician may use to enhance patient compliance are discussed in Chapter 42.

Drug interactions

The effect of a drug may be increased, decreased, or otherwise altered by the concurrent administration of another compound. Because agents routinely used in dental practice have been implicated in drug interactions, the topic is of considerable interest to the clinician and is addressed separately in Appendix 4.

ADVERSE DRUG REACTIONS

According to the Institute of Medicine, at least 1.5 million preventable adverse drug events occur annually in the United States. Up to 20% of patients hospitalized in the United States each year are admitted because of adverse reactions to drugs. Estimates of the annual cost of managing these reactions range from $3 to $7 billion.

The introduction of new, highly efficacious compounds into pharmacotherapy during the past few decades has led to a disturbing increase in the incidence of adverse reactions; drug toxicity is now considered a major cause of iatrogenic disease. Reductions in mortality rate associated with certain drugs (e.g., aspirin) show, however, that toxic responses to therapeutic agents can be minimized through concerted efforts by health professionals, the pharmaceutical industry, government, and lay public.

Classification of Adverse Drug Reactions

Drug toxicity may come in many forms: acute versus chronic, mild versus severe, predictable versus unpredictable, and local versus systemic. Therapeutic agents also differ widely in their tendency to elicit adverse reactions. Acetaminophen used to relieve headache rarely causes undesired responses, but many agents used in cancer chemotherapy invariably produce some degree of toxicity. Agents that are safe for some individuals may be life-threatening to others. Penicillin V, which normally has an exceptionally high margin of safety, can in small doses initiate fatal anaphylaxis in severely allergic patients. Adverse drug reactions can be classified according to their onset (acute, subacute, or delayed), degree (mild, moderate, or severe), or predictability (predictable and dose related; unpredictable and not necessarily dose related such as idiosyncratic and immunologic reactions). Although no classification of adverse drug reactions is universally accepted, a taxonomy based on mechanism of toxicity is the most useful in promoting the recognition, management, and prevention of untoward responses to drugs.

Extension effects

Many drugs are used clinically in dosages that provide an intensity of effect that is submaximal. The reason for this conservatism is simple: increasing drug effects beyond a certain point (**extension effects**) may be dangerous. The anticoagulant warfarin is a typical example of a drug whose therapeutic action must be held in check to avoid serious toxicity. For the treatment of peripheral vascular thrombosis, warfarin is administered in doses that sufficiently increase the prothrombin time to yield an international normalized ratio (see Chapter 26) of 2 to 3. Warfarin could be given in larger amounts to inhibit clotting further, but the risk of spontaneous bleeding would be unacceptably high. Even with conventional therapy, hemorrhage—the toxic extension of warfarin's anticoagulant effect—occurs in 2% to 4% of the patients treated. Inadvertent overmedication is one cause of warfarin toxicity; however, many additional factors influencing drug effects may also be involved, such as diet; heredity; gastrointestinal ulceration; genetic differences in drug metabolism; renal, hepatic, or cardiac insufficiency; drug interactions; and variable patient compliance. "Normal dose" has little meaning regarding warfarin because a therapeutic dose to one patient may represent an overdose to another.

Adverse responses arising from an extension of the therapeutic effect are dose related and predictable. Theoretically, they are the only toxic reactions that can be avoided without loss of therapeutic benefit by properly adjusting the dosage regimen. Table 3-4 provides additional examples of drugs that display this form of toxicity.

Side effects

Predictable, dose-dependent reactions unrelated to the goal of therapy, and often at therapeutic doses, are referred to as **side effects.** As illustrated in Table 3-5, drugs can produce a huge array of deleterious side effects. Although many such reactions are associated with only a single agent or class of drugs, others seem to be almost universal in occurrence. It is questionable, however, whether frequently noted side effects, such as nausea and drowsiness, are always drug related; similar symptoms are also commonly observed in patients after placebo administration and are reported by individuals receiving no medication whatsoever.

Side effects may be produced by the same drug–receptor interaction responsible for the therapeutic effect, differing only in the tissue or organ affected. In these instances, the categorization of

TABLE 3-4 Examples of Drug Toxicity as an Extension of the Therapeutic Effect

Drug	Medical Indication	Therapeutic Effect	Toxic Extension of Therapeutic Effect
Furosemide	Edema	Diuresis	Hypovolemia
Heparin	Thromboembolic disorders	Inhibition of coagulation	Spontaneous bleeding
Insulin	Diabetes mellitus	Reduction of blood glucose concentration	Hypoglycemia
Modafinil	Narcolepsy	Wakefulness	Insomnia
Vecuronium	Abdominal surgery	Skeletal muscle relaxation	Prolonged respiratory paralysis
Zolpidem	Insomnia	Hypnosis	Unconsciousness

TABLE 3-5 Side Effects of Drugs

Drug	Effect
Oral Cavity	
Diphenhydramine	Xerostomia
Griseofulvin	Black hairy tongue
Phenytoin	Gingival hyperplasia
Tetracycline	Pigmentation, hypoplasia of the teeth
Skin and Hair	
Amoxicillin	Dermatitis
Cyclophosphamide	Alopecia
Methandrostenolone	Acne
Minoxidil	Hypertrichosis
Bone and Joints	
Ciprofloxacin	Arthralgia
Hydralazine	Arthralgia
Phenobarbital	Osteomalacia
Prednisolone	Osteoporosis
Sensory Apparatus	
Baclofen	Blurred vision
Digoxin	Yellow vision
Gentamicin	Ototoxicity
Thioridazine	Pigmentary retinopathy
Blood	
Cytarabine	Pancytopenia
Prilocaine	Methemoglobinemia
Valproic acid	Thrombocytopenia
Zidovudine	Granulocytopenia
Metabolic Effects	
Aspirin	Metabolic acidosis
Furosemide	Hyperglycemia
Nadolol	Hypoglycemia
Rifampin	Jaundice
Neuromuscular System	
Atorvastatin	Myalgia
Chlorpromazine	Tardive dyskinesia
Dantrolene	Weakness
Lidocaine	Convulsions
Theophylline	Tremors
Central Nervous System	
Clonidine	Drowsiness and lethargy
Dexamethasone	Mental depression
Diazepam	Confusion
Levodopa	Mania
Cardiovascular System	
Bupivacaine	Bradycardia
Propofol	Hypotension
Propranolol	Cardiac failure
Respiratory System	
ACE inhibitors, e.g., lisinopril	Cough
Isoflurane	Cough
Ketamine	Laryngospasm
Meperidine	Respiratory depression
Propranolol	Bronchospasm
Gastrointestinal Tract	
Aspirin	Melena
Erythromycin	Nausea and vomiting
Lithium	Diarrhea
Morphine	Constipation
Genitourinary System	
Guanethidine	Impotence
Sulfadiazine	Crystalluria
Testosterone	Priapism

ACE, Angiotensin converting enzyme.

TABLE 3-6 Useful Side Effects of Drugs

Drug	Original Use	Subsequent Use
Amantadine	Antiviral	Parkinsonism
Amphetamine	CNS stimulant	Attention-deficit/hyperactivity disorder
Chlorothiazide	Diuretic	Antihypertensive
Diphenhydramine	Antihistaminic	Sedative
Lidocaine	Local anesthetic	Antiarrhythmic
Methadone	Analgesic	Heroin substitute
Metronidazole	Antiparasitic	Antibacterial
Phenytoin	Anticonvulsant	Antiarrhythmic
Probenecid	Inhibition of penicillin excretion	Uricosuric
Quinidine	Antimalarial	Antiarrhythmic

CNS, Central nervous system.

drug responses as toxic or therapeutic may depend on the purpose of treatment. Xerostomia induced by atropine is a side effect during the management of gastrointestinal hypermotility but is a desired effect when the drug is used to control excessive salivation. Side effects unrelated pharmacodynamically to the therapeutic action are also quite common, and they too may occasionally be useful. Table 3-6 lists some drugs whose side effects were found sufficiently noteworthy to provide new and unanticipated indications for therapeutic use.

Many side effects, particularly the more dangerous forms, develop only with drug overdose. Careful alteration of the administration regimen usually resolves these problems while maintaining effective treatment. Many other side effects occur at therapeutic or even subtherapeutic concentrations, and they cannot be avoided by dosage adjustment without loss of drug benefit. Such reactions can be tolerated, however, if they are mild, brief in duration, reversible, and compatible with therapy. Occasionally, even disturbing side effects are accepted if the need for medication is great. Drugs used in the treatment of various cancers often produce severe toxic effects that must be tolerated because no therapeutic alternative is available.

When two drugs share a common desired effect but cause different side effects, it is sometimes possible to limit toxic responses by using reduced doses of the agents in combination. Another pharmacologic approach to avoiding side effects is to add a secondary agent that is capable of blocking or otherwise compensating for the unwanted activity of the principal drug. These strategies presuppose that no additional toxicity will be generated by the combination over that produced by a single effective drug. The most fruitful pharmacologic approach to eliminating undesired side effects is through the development of more selective drugs. Studies of structure–activity relationships have proved invaluable in removing side effects unrelated to therapeutic actions and in reducing side effects that are related.

Idiosyncratic reactions

An **idiosyncratic reaction** may be defined as a genetically determined abnormal response to a drug. Often a genetic abnormality has been identified, and an enzyme change occurs (Chapter 4). Although dose dependent, such reactions are unpredictable in most instances because very few patients given an agent respond idiosyncratically and because the genetic trait responsible for an atypical reaction may be completely "silent" in the absence of drug challenge. When confronted with an unexpected response to a drug, it is a common, although erroneous, practice to describe the event as an idiosyncrasy. Most responses lying outside the normal range of drug reactivity are not truly idiosyncratic in nature but represent allergic manifestations or reflect extension or side effects in patients intolerant to the drug by virtue of factors such as age, weight, or existing disease. In dentistry, most falsely described "idiosyncratic" reactions to local anesthetics are the result of accidental intravascular injections or anxiety reactions to the process of injection.

An idiosyncratic reaction is often manifested as abnormal drug sensitivity in which the agent produces its characteristic effect at an unconventional dose. Drug effects may be unusually strong or weak in intensity or brief or prolonged in duration. In most such instances (e.g., involving succinylcholine, isoniazid, vitamin D, or phenytoin), altered drug metabolism is responsible for the abnormal responses; however, additional mechanisms have been identified, such as abnormal distribution (iron, thyroxine) and unusual receptor affinity (warfarin). In addition to perturbing characteristic drug responses, genetic singularities can produce novel drug effects that, regardless of dose, may never occur in normal individuals. One example of a novel drug effect is hemolytic anemia caused by the antimalarial drug primaquine. Red blood cells of sensitive individuals are deficient in glucose-6-phosphate dehydrogenase, an enzyme involved in the intermediary metabolism of glucose. Lacking the ability to produce normal amounts of reducing equivalents, these erythrocytes are susceptible to oxidative destruction by primaquine and several dozen other compounds. The genetic basis of primaquine hemolysis is clear: the reaction occurs almost exclusively in men of certain racial and ethnic groups (e.g., African Americans, Sardinians, Sephardic Jews, Iranians, and Filipinos).

Various idiosyncrasies are known to be associated with drugs. Some examples are listed in Table 3-7. If an adverse response is suspected to have a genetic basis, it becomes important to determine whether the patient has a personal or familial history of atypical reactivity to the drug. Because idiosyncratic reactions are quite reproducible within any individual, a single episode of serious toxicity should preclude future use of the inciting compound. Examination of the patient's family is helpful in establishing the hereditary nature of the reaction and identifying other individuals at risk. Figure 3-3 demonstrates how an enzyme deficiency in the heme synthesis pathway can lead to an attack of acute intermittent porphyria when the affected patient is challenged with a drug that stimulates an early event in that pathway.

TABLE 3-7 Some Idiosyncratic Reactions to Drugs

Genetic Abnormality	Drugs Affected	Idiosyncratic Response
NADH-methemoglobin reductase deficiency	Benzocaine, prilocaine	Methemoglobinemia
Glucose-6-phosphate dehydrogenase deficiency	Aspirin, primaquine, sulfonamides	Hemolytic anemia
Abnormal heme synthesis	Barbiturates, sulfonamides	Porphyria
Low plasma cholinesterase activity	Procaine and other ester local anesthetics, succinylcholine	Local anesthetic toxicity, extended paralysis
Altered muscle calcium homeostasis	Volatile inhalation anesthetics, succinylcholine	Malignant hyperthermia
Prolonged QT interval	Cisapride, some antipsychotics, and antiarrhythmics	Torsades de pointes

NADH, Reduced nicotinamide adenine dinucleotide.

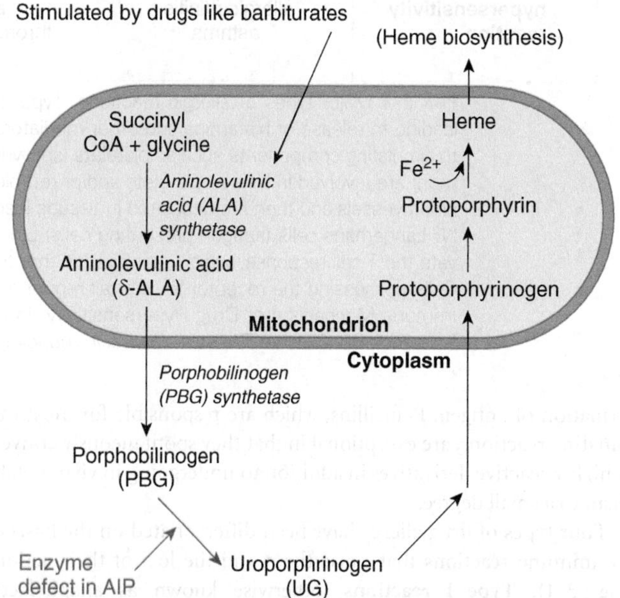

FIG 3-3 Heme synthesis and acute intermittent porphyria (AIP). The genetic basis for AIP is a deficiency in the enzyme, porphobilinogen deaminase, which catalyzes the reaction step shown in the figure. Several drugs such as barbiturates stimulate δ-aminolevulinate (ALA) synthase causing toxic levels of δALA and PBG, resulting in acute symptoms. Other porphyrins in the pathway are not pictured.

Drug allergy

Adverse responses of immunologic origin account for approximately 10% of all untoward reactions to drugs. **Allergy** can be distinguished from other forms of drug toxicity in several respects. First, prior exposure to the drug or a closely related compound is necessary to elicit the reaction. Second, the severity of response is seemingly dose independent. Third, the nature of the unfavorable effect is a function not of the offending drug but of the immune mechanism involved. Finally, the reaction is unpredictable; it usually occurs in a small portion of the population, sometimes in patients who had been previously treated with the inciting drug on numerous occasions without mishap.

Drugs differ enormously in antigenic potential. Certain compounds (e.g., caffeine and epinephrine) never cause drug allergy; others (e.g., phenyl-ethyl-hydantoin) have proved too allergenic for human use. With drugs commonly implicated clinically in allergic reactions (e.g., penicillins, sulfonamides, quinidine), the incidence of such responses is approximately 5%. Occasionally, another substance in a preparation besides the active drug (e.g., a preservative or coloring agent) causes the allergy.

Aside from agents of high molecular weight (insulin, dextran, polypeptides), drugs are usually not antigenic in the free state but must be covalently linked to endogenous carrier molecules such as albumin to generate immunologic responses. Because these therapeutic agents are often chemically inert, they generally require activation by metabolism or by sunlight (photoallergy) before serving as haptens in the

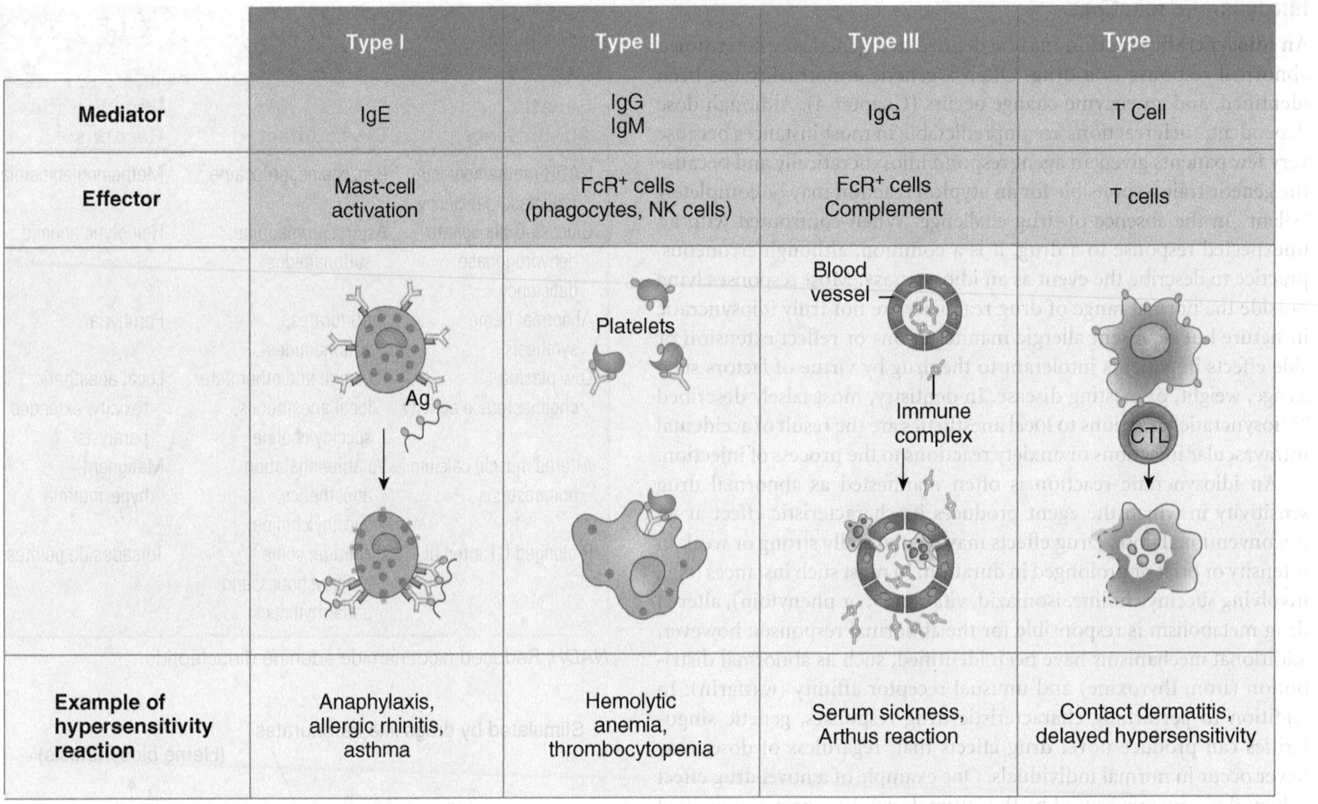

	Type I	Type II	Type III	Type
Mediator	IgE	IgG IgM	IgG	T Cell
Effector	Mast-cell activation	FcR⁺ cells (phagocytes, NK cells)	FcR⁺ cells Complement	T cells
	Ag	Platelets	Blood vessel Immune complex	CTL
Example of hypersensitivity reaction	Anaphylaxis, allergic rhinitis, asthma	Hemolytic anemia, thrombocytopenia	Serum sickness, Arthus reaction	Contact dermatitis, delayed hypersensitivity

FIG 3-4 Major types of allergic reactions. Type I: The antigen cross-links antibodies attached to mast cells leading to release of histamine and other mediators. These are immediate reactions. Type II: Antigen attaches to circulating components such as platelets (shown) or red blood cells. Cytotoxic T cells (CTL cells) and complement are involved in lysis of platelets and/or red blood cells. Type III: Antigen–antibody complexes form within blood vessels and then are deposited in tissues leading to macrophage and complement-mediated attack. Type IV: Langerhans cells (antigen presenting cells) bind the antigen, then migrate to lymph nodes. Here they activate the T cell response, which is delayed. Other types of Type IV allergic reactions are not shown. *FcR+cells,* Cells possessing the receptor for the tail region of the antibody. NK, natural killer. (Modified from Pichler WJ: Immune Mechanism of Drug Hypersensitivity, Immunol Allergy Clin North Am 24:373-397, 2004. In Modified from Rich RR, Fleisher TA, et al: *Clinical immunology: principles and practice,* ed 3, Philadelphia, 2008, Mosby.)

formation of antigen. Penicillins, which are responsible for most fulminating reactions, are exceptional in that they spontaneously convert to highly reactive derivatives in addition to undergoing in vivo metabolism to a small degree.

Four types of drug allergy have been differentiated on the basis of the immune reactions that cause them and the loci of their actions (Fig. 3-4). **Type I reactions**, otherwise known as anaphylactic responses, include the immediate forms of drug allergy, in which disturbances appear within minutes or hours of taking the drug. The underlying immune reactions are initiated by the attachment of antigen to IgE antibodies bound to the surface of mast cells and basophils. Subsequent cellular degranulation and release of histamine, leukotrienes, cytokines, and other mediators are responsible for the undesired effects. Major signs and symptoms of type I allergy involve the gastrointestinal tract (cramps and diarrhea), skin and mucous membranes (erythema, urticaria, angioneurotic edema), lungs (bronchoconstriction), and blood vessels (vasodilation, increased permeability). In its most severe form, anaphylaxis can cause death by airway obstruction or by cardiovascular collapse within a few minutes after drug exposure. Parenteral injection of the drug is more likely than oral or topical use to produce life-threatening reactions. Nevertheless, patients have died from topical application of less than 1 μg of penicillin. It is believed that patients with a history of hay fever or bronchial asthma are more prone to develop serious type I reactions. The immediate anaphylactic response is the only type of drug allergy that the dentist may be forced to treat without the benefit of medical backup. Epinephrine is the drug of choice to reverse the manifestations of a severe response; antihistamines and adrenal corticosteroids are useful as adjunctive medications (see Chapter 41).

Type II, or cytotoxic, reactions are caused by circulating antibodies (IgG and IgM). When a plasma membrane constituent serves as the hapten carrier, or when a complete antigen is adsorbed on the membrane surface, the binding of immunoglobulin is followed by complement fixation and lysis of the cell. Many forms of drug-induced hemolytic anemia, leukopenia, and thrombocytopenia are the result of this form of immunologic destruction. Type II responses are usually delayed and manifest from several hours to days after drug administration.

Type III, or immune complex, reactions occur when soluble antigen–antibody complexes form in intravascular or interstitial spaces. Eventual deposition of the complexes on the walls of small blood vessels is followed by activation of complement and migration of neutrophils into the area. These cells degranulate in attempts to remove the complexes, releasing lysosomal enzymes that cause local tissue damage and promote thrombosis of the affected vessels. Type III reactions can induce many unpleasant sequelae, some of which can be quite serious (e.g., neuropathy, glomerulonephritis, serum sickness). Reactions indistinguishable from disease states such as lupus erythematosus and erythema multiforme are also observed. Finally, soluble antigen–antibody complexes can attach to cell membranes and cause cytotoxicity indistinguishable from type II reactions.

Type IV reactions are synonymous with cell-mediated immunity. Sensitized **T lymphocytes** exposed to the drug hapten or its conjugate release lymphokines that attract additional cells (lymphocytes, macrophages cytotoxic T cells) to the antigenic site. Lysozymes and other substances (including toxic lymphokines) elaborated by the recruited cells produce local tissue necrosis. Type IV reactions are usually delayed because of the time required for effector cells to concentrate in the area involved. Historically for dentists, an important cellular immune reaction was the contact dermatitis acquired from repeated exposure of the hands to ester local anesthetics such as procaine. Before the availability of amide anesthetic drugs, allergy to procaine markedly complicated clinical practice.

Although drug allergies cannot always be prevented, their frequency of occurrence can be minimized by observing the following precautions:

1. **Take an adequate medical history**. If a patient has a presumptive history of drug allergy, it is important to discover the identity of the inciting preparation and to determine whether the reaction is consistent with an immunologic cause. Patients often complain of local anesthetic "allergy," but their complaint centers around tachycardia and anxiety. These are much more likely side effects of either the injection pain or the normal effect of the epinephrine that is usually present. They are not true antigen–antibody allergic reactions.
2. **Avoid the offending drug and likely cross-reactors**. A patient truly allergic to a drug should not receive the agent or congener again unless need for the particular medication is great. If the drug must be given, means to reverse an allergic reaction should be immediately available.
3. **Avoid inappropriate drug administration**. Do not give a drug if there is no clear indication.
4. **Promote oral use and limit topical exposure**. With the penicillins, the oral and topical routes are the least (oral) and most (topical) allergenic avenues of drug administration.
5. **Request allergy testing when appropriate**. Although such methods may be unreliable and can be dangerous, skin tests for penicillin allergy have proved predictive. Success has also been claimed regarding local anesthetics. Allergy testing may be necessary when suitable alternatives to the drug in question are unavailable.

Adherence to these recommendations will reduce the incidence of allergic reactions to drugs. The more prudent use of penicillin in recent years has undoubtedly led to a decline in the drug's mortality rate.

Pseudoallergic and secondary reactions

Pseudoallergic reactions are adverse drug responses caused by mediators of allergy that are released through antibody-independent processes. In the case of macromolecules, the alternate pathway of complement fixation may lead to various cytotoxic and immune complex reactions. Much more common are anaphylactoid reactions that mimic one or more aspects of anaphylaxis. Some opioid analgesics, neuromuscular blocking drugs, and intravenous anesthetic agents can cause independent release of histamine from mast cells. Aspirin, ibuprofen, and related inhibitors of prostaglandin synthesis can result in the overproduction of bronchospastic leukotrienes. As with true allergies, these reactions are unpredictable; however, they seem to be dose dependent, do not require prior sensitization, and may occur on initial exposure to the drug.

Secondary reactions are indirect (and often unpredictable) consequences of a drug's primary pharmacologic action. Antibiotics provide the best examples. One possible outcome of antibiotic administration is the development of superinfection, a secondary microbial disease made possible by the antibiotic-induced suppression of the normal microflora (see Chapter 33). Alternatively, the rapid lysis of susceptible bacteria may result in the Jarisch-Herxheimer phenomenon, a serum sickness–like syndrome caused by the rapid release of microbial antigens, endotoxins, or both.

Carcinogenesis

One aspect of drug toxicity that has had a strong impact on public awareness is **carcinogenesis**. Although most attention has been focused on environmental pollutants, including chemicals that pose an occupational hazard, the association of leukemia with various anticancer agents and uterine neoplasia with diethylstilbestrol underscores the tumorigenic potential of certain therapeutic drugs. The most pervasive cancer-producing substances in our society are derived from a "social" drug mixture: tobacco.

Virtually any agent capable of altering the structure of DNA is a potential carcinogen. Agents known to be carcinogenic include radioactive substances, alkylating agents, nitrosamines, and various aromatic amines and polycyclic aromatic hydrocarbons. Neoplastic transformation occurs when mutations develop in genes regulating cellular growth. Cancer is normally a multistage phenomenon involving multiple genetic mutations. Two groups of genes are implicated in chemical carcinogenesis: **oncogenes and tumor suppressor genes**. Oncogenes are derived from normal genes, or proto-oncogenes, whose function is to promote growth and development. Several mechanisms for neoplastic transformation of proto-oncogenes have been discovered, including point mutation, which would seem to be the most likely candidate for chemical carcinogenesis. Tumor suppressor genes code for proteins that normally inhibit cell growth.

Certain compounds cause tumors only after prior treatment with another agent. The first chemical seems to initiate the neoplastic transformation, and the second promotes tumor growth. Major difficulties are encountered, however, in assessing the carcinogenicity of agents intended for human use. First, the latency period between the initiation and clinical appearance of neoplasia may span years to decades. Second, although the incidence of tumor induction is dose dependent, it is not established whether a dose or duration of exposure below which tumors will not be produced can be found for any drug. Third, because an administered agent usually requires metabolism for activation, interspecies differences in biotransformation severely limit the use of animal testing in such instances. Without a foolproof method of screening drugs, continued appraisal of cancer rates regarding drug intake is a necessary, if not ideal, approach to identifying carcinogenic compounds. In view of the prolonged latency of cancer development and the flood of agents introduced into pharmacology in recent decades, it would be surprising not to witness the discovery of new carcinogens among therapeutic agents now in use.

Special Problems

Hazards of medication pertaining to abuse, poisoning, and effects on the unborn child warrant special comment because the individuals affected are generally not exposed to the agent for therapeutic purposes. In these situations, the prevention and management of adverse reactions can be complicated by matters such as the intent of the person taking the drug, an inability to identify the offending agent, and the unique susceptibility of the embryo to drug toxicity.

Drug abuse

Typified by persistent and excessive self-administration, drug abuse refers to the inappropriate and deviant use of any drug. Drug abuse presents a special problem in toxicology because of the hazards of taking pharmacologically active agents in questionable doses without proper medical supervision. This subject is discussed further in Chapter 39.

Drug poisoning

As revealed by data from the American Association of Poison Control Centers, of the more than 2400 poisoning deaths nationwide in 2013, about 30% were believed to be the result of suicide. Drug poisoning accounts for a significant percentage of reported episodes and is a major concern for health professionals and laypersons alike. Drugs most commonly implicated in fatal poisonings are analgesics, antidepressants, alcohol, CNS stimulants, and cardiovascular agents.

Children younger than 5 years of age account for most poisonings and approximately 2% of the deaths from poisoning. Aspirin, historically the leading cause of drug toxicity in small children, provides a noteworthy example of how unintentional poisoning can be controlled. Recognizing the special hazard of flavored baby aspirin, the pharmaceutical industry voluntarily limited the number of aspirin tablets per bottle to a (normally) sublethal total of 36. Safety packaging, which became mandatory after the passage of the Poison-Prevention Packaging Act of 1970, reduced the incidence of fatal ingestion further. Finally, increased public awareness concerning the danger of aspirin overdose, engendered in part by the proliferation of poison control centers throughout the United States, led to safer storage of aspirin in the home. Further decrements in the aspirin mortality rate have occurred, aided partly by the increased reliance on liquid acetaminophen and ibuprofen preparations for analgesia and antipyresis. As one might predict, however, acetaminophen and ibuprofen poisonings, previously quite rare, are now more common. The principles of toxicology and the prevention and management of drug poisoning are discussed in Chapter 40.

Drugs and pregnancy

The hazard to the unborn child of administering drugs during pregnancy has received considerable attention in the lay and professional literature. Over the years, certain compounds have been implicated in the development of congenital abnormalities. These teratogens disturb organogenesis in the developing embryo so that defects in one or more structures are produced. If the defects are incompatible with life, fetal death and either resorption or spontaneous abortion ensues; if they are less severe, the result is a malformed child.

Very little is known about the teratogenic potential of most drugs in humans, but the thalidomide disaster of 1960-1962 proved that an ordinary drug, extremely safe in adults, could induce extensive malformation prenatally. Thalidomide is a sedative-hypnotic that was released for clinical use in Europe and elsewhere in the late 1950s. The drug quickly gained wide acceptance and was commonly used by women to relieve the nausea of "morning sickness." Shortly after its introduction, an epidemic occurred of infants born with phocomelia, or "seal limb" malformation of the arms and legs. Retrospective studies determined that phocomelia was caused by thalidomide when the agent was taken 24 to 29 days after conception. Other defects were also produced by thalidomide (e.g., absence of external ears, cranial nerve dysfunction, anorectal stenosis), depending on the time of administration. Removed from the worldwide market for many years, thalidomide has made a comeback in therapy. It is currently approved for treating certain forms of leprosy; it is also used clinically to manage various sequelae of human immunodeficiency virus (HIV) infection, to treat multiple myeloma and aphthous ulcers, and as an immune modulator in disorders such as Crohn disease. Strict prescribing controls are in place to prevent its use in pregnant women.

Laboratory experiments in animals and investigations of accidental teratogenesis in humans have found that drug-induced malformation is governed by the sequential pattern of embryonic and fetal development. From fertilization to approximately 20 days, an embryo either survives or succumbs to a chemical insult. No malformations occur, however, because the cells remain undifferentiated during this period. Beginning at day 21 (when the somites appear) and continuing until the end of the first trimester (when differentiation and organogenesis are well established), teratogenic malformations are possible. The defects produced vary with the toxic action of the agent and with the time of administration. Certain malformations, such as cleft palate, may be produced by various substances; some teratogens, such as antifolate drugs, can evoke a wide spectrum of structural defects. Selective toxicity of drugs to the fetus does not end after 3 months' gestation. Although gross malformation may not occur, normal development may be retarded or otherwise affected throughout pregnancy. Immaturities in physiology and biochemistry may promote adverse reactions in the fetus at doses safe to the mother. The administration of drugs at the time of delivery is commonly associated with exaggerated effects in the neonate.

Table 3-8 lists several agents known to elicit toxic effects during pregnancy and indicates when their administration is most dangerous to the embryo or fetus. In 2015, the FDA changed from the Pregnancy Risk Categories of A, B, C, D, and X, to a new system that applies to all new drugs immediately and will apply to all drugs on the market over the next 4 years. The older classification will be abandoned in favor of a system that indicates specific types of risks and the evidence supporting the risks. One emphasis of the new system is to present more information related to risks in pregnancy and lactation. The new system is divided into a Pregnancy Subsection and a Lactation Subsection. Notable items in each are given in Table 3-9.

Despite uncertainties concerning most drugs and the unborn child, many pharmacologic agents have been used extensively by pregnant women. The major drug categories include iron supplements, analgesics, vitamins, sedative-hypnotics, diuretics, antiemetics, antimicrobials, cold remedies, hormones, "tranquilizers," bronchodilators, and appetite suppressants. Drugs vary widely in their relative risk during pregnancy. Although women and health care professionals are now more aware of the risks posed by drugs, the admonition to restrict usage of therapeutic agents, especially during the first trimester, bears reiteration. For dentistry, there are no clear data regarding the use of local anesthetics in the first trimester. In light of the possibility that local anesthetics may pose a small risk to the unborn child, prudence dictates that only urgent or emergent treatment be rendered during this critical period of fetal development. Benzodiazepine sedatives, which are known to be human teratogens, must be avoided throughout the pregnancy. Regular dental care need not be postponed, however, during the second trimester as long as reasonable attention and care are given to avoiding undue physical and emotional stress in the patient and avoiding drugs that pose a known risk to the fetus.

DEVELOPMENT OF NEW DRUGS

Advances in pharmacotherapy ultimately depend on the discovery, evaluation, and marketing of new drugs. The past several decades have witnessed an unprecedented proliferation of medicinal agents, and major revisions in how drugs intended for human use are evaluated have contributed to the manufacture of safer and more effective compounds. As a prescriber of drugs, however, the practitioner should be aware of the attendant problems and costs of developing therapeutic agents and of the unavoidable limitations in assessing drug safety before widespread use. Only with this knowledge can the clinician arrive at a balanced attitude toward new drugs and claims made for them.

TABLE 3-8 Toxic Effects of Some Drugs During Pregnancy

		MOST SUSCEPTIBLE PERIOD*			
Drug	**Toxic Effect to Fetus**	**First Trimester**	**Second Trimester**	**Third Trimester**	**Term**
ACE inhibitors	Renal toxicity		✓	✓	✓
Anticancer drugs	Cleft palate, extremity defects, severe stunting, death	✓			
Carbamazepine	Neural tube defects	✓			
Chloramphenicol	Gray syndrome, death				✓
Cortisone	Cleft palate	✓			
Coumarin anticoagulants	Hemorrhage, death				
Diazepam	Cleft palate, respiratory depression Neonatal dependency				
Local anesthetics	Bradycardia, respiratory depression				✓
Lysergic acid diethylamide	Chromosomal damage, stunted growth	✓			
Opioid analgesics	Respiratory depression, neonatal death				✓
Potassium iodide	Goiter, mental retardation				
Quinine	Deafness, thrombocytopenia			✓	✓
Sex steroids	Masculinization, vaginal carcinoma (delayed)				
Streptomycin	Eighth cranial nerve damage, micromelia, multiple skeletal abnormalities				
Tetracyclines	Inhibition of bone growth, tooth discoloration, micromelia, syndactyly				
Thalidomide	Phocomelia, multiple defects	✓			
Thiazide diuretics	Thrombocytopenia, neonatal death			✓	✓

Adapted from Underwood T, Iturrian EB, Cadwallader DE: Some aspects of chemical teratogenesis, *Am J Hosp Pharm* 27:115-122, 1970.
*Coumarins and other drugs with no indication mark are approximately evenly toxic throughout pregnancy.

TABLE 3-9 Pregnancy Risk

1. Pregnancy Exposure Registry	Contains contact information to enroll or acquire information on specific drugs.
2. Risk Summary	Statements about the drug include the likelihood of causing any of the four types of fetal developmental abnormalities: structural, fetal and infant mortality, impaired physiologic function, and alterations in growth. Specific details of the abnormality, to the extent known, are given, the nature of the evidence will be stated, and whether it comes from human or animal studies.
3. Clinical Considerations	This section covers three areas. a) Risk early in pregnancy (inadvertent exposure) b) Prescribing decisions for pregnant women: disease- associated risks, dosage adjustments during pregnancy and postpartum, fetal and maternal adverse reactions to the drug, effects of the drug during labor and delivery
4. Data	A description of the method and results of human and animal data are given. The mechanism of the adverse effect is discussed.
Lactation Risk Subsection	
1. Risk summary	Contains information on the effect of the drug on milk production, whether the drug is present in breast milk and the effect of the drug, if any, on the breast-fed child.
2. Clinical considerations	Discusses how to minimize exposure of the drug to the breast-fed child, dosing adjustments during lactation, the possible drug effects on the child, and how to monitor and respond to these effects.
3. Data	List the data supporting the risk and clinical implications

Sources of New Drugs

For several centuries, considerable effort in pharmacology was devoted to the purification of active constituents from natural plant and animal products previously used for medicinal purposes. Many new therapeutic agents are discovered by empiric screening. In screening tests, thousands of compounds from natural materials or synthetic chemistry are examined for a particular pharmacologic activity. Microplate, microarray, and other types of high-throughput technology have made screening an important method of finding new drugs capable of producing a defined drug effect. With the exception of penicillin, virtually all of the antibiotic groups have been isolated by the screening of soils and other materials for antimicrobial activity. In recent years, advances in synthetic chemistry and molecular biology have led to a proliferation of screening tests in which cells engineered to express receptors of interest and easily measured biologic responses to receptor activation are exposed to large collections of chemicals and examined for activity.

One productive technique of finding new drugs is to alter the molecular structure of an existing agent. Structure–activity relationship studies are intimately involved in this approach. When derivatives are produced, they are frequently little more than "me too" drugs: agents that, although similar in activity to the parent compound, offer no therapeutic advantage but are marketed anyway for economic reasons. That said, some drugs are developed not because their end-activity is better or different, but because they differ substantially from their predecessor in pharmacokinetic properties. Penicillin V, which is nearly identical in antimicrobial activity to its precursor, penicillin G, is preferred for oral use because its absorption is two to five times better. Pharmacokinetic differences are especially prominent among the benzodiazepine congeners, with elimination half-lives ranging from several hours to several days. The least common but usually most desirable outcome of molecular modification is the synthesis of a derivative that differs qualitatively from the parent drug in pharmacodynamic effect. Such discoveries are generally the result of attempts to enhance one aspect of an agent's spectrum of activity over all others. The observations that sulfonamides used in chemotherapy of bacterial infections could decrease blood glucose concentrations and promote urine flow under appropriate conditions eventually led to the manufacture of several new classes of drugs: carbonic anhydrase inhibitors, thiazide diuretics, and sulfonylurea hypoglycemic agents.

Increasingly, discoveries of new drugs are evolving from advances in understanding of basic physiology, biochemistry, and the human genome. These discoveries have led to the synthesis of drugs such as antimetabolites for antiviral and cancer chemotherapy and the development of drugs to modify immune reactions. **Recombinant DNA** technology, by which bacteria or even transformed mammalian cells can be altered genetically to synthesize foreign proteins, is fulfilling its promise in two ways. Recent studies have shown that stem cells can be engineered to make toxins that kill some kinds of tumor cells. Clearly, as this technology improves, it will make for great changes in cancer therapy. Recombinant technology is also used for the large-scale production of human-derived agents (e.g., interferons, insulin, calcitonin, growth hormone, hematopoietic growth factors, and monoclonal antibodies) that were previously obtainable only in small amounts. These sources of drugs will continue to grow, and it is expected that hitherto unknown agents will become available for pharmacotherapy as a result of progress in understanding the human genome.

A burgeoning source of new pharmaceutical products comes from the development of novel delivery systems for existing drugs. More complex approaches, such as various lipid formulations of drugs, may provide a safer parenteral delivery of drugs such as amphotericin B, a highly toxic antifungal agent. Conjugated monoclonal antibodies are now being used in cancer patients as vehicles for cytotoxic substances (e.g., diphtheria toxin) and radioactive isotopes. The antibody attaches to surface antigens expressed only by the tumor and delivers the active ligand so that it can provide the tumoricidal effect. Similar drug-carrying monoclonal antibodies directed against discrete cellular elements of the immune system have found use in preventing transplant rejection and in the treatment of autoimmune diseases. Attaching drugs, often covalently, to polymeric carriers is proving effective in localizing and prolonging drug effects, either because the controlled release of free drug from the immobilized matrix permits only local effects or because the drug is active in the bound state. In either case, the distribution of drug action is determined by the properties of the carrier.

Recent advances in molecular biology and other fields have led to better knowledge of individual susceptibilities to various drugs (see genomics in Chapter 4). This includes not only genomics but also other **"omics"** like proteomics (protein characterization), metabolomics (metabolism characterization), microbiomics, and others. Knowledge of the unique "omics" profile of an individual will enable the tailoring of drug selection and dose for each patient, to improve response rates and reduce adverse effects.

The last major source of new drugs is serendipity. Probably the greatest single breakthrough in pharmacotherapeutics in the twentieth century was the isolation of penicillin, made possible by the chance but astute observation of Fleming that bacteria in a culture dish were lysed by a mold contaminant of the genus *Penicillium*. Other classes of agents that originated by accident include the antiarrhythmic drugs (quinine) and the oral anticoagulants (dicumarol). Table 3-6 lists several drugs for which new therapeutic applications were fortuitously discovered after marketing.

Evaluation of New Drugs

Before a drug can be released for general use, it must pass a rigorous evaluation program established by the FDA (Figure 3-5). This program, although subject to some modification depending on the drug's intended use, invariably includes a series of animal and human investigations to ensure the product's safety and efficacy. (See Appendices 7 and 8 for reviews of drug regulations pertaining to the FDA and the development of new drugs.)

Preclinical testing

The first step in evaluating a newly discovered compound is to ascertain its pharmacologic activity in animals. Initially, laboratory animals such as rats may be given several different doses of the chemical and observed for any disturbances that may occur in physiology or behavior. If the drug is being developed for a given purpose (e.g., to reduce blood pressure), it would be tested for that particular effect as well. Agents that seem to have a useful action are enrolled in more extensive examinations. Graded dose–response curves are constructed to determine the potency and intrinsic activity of the compound (see Chapter 1). When a specific therapeutic effect is identified, quantal dose–effect relationships are drawn to estimate the compound's relative safety. As shown in Figure 3-6, quantal dose–effect curves, as described earlier in the chapter, can be prepared to compare therapeutic versus toxic responses.

When working with laboratory animals, one of the most convenient toxic effects to monitor is lethality. Death is universal, all drugs are capable of producing it, and it represents a definite end point that can be quickly and unequivocally recognized. The dose causing death in 50% of the test animals in a given period is designated as the **median lethal dose (LD_{50})**. The **ratio** of this dose to the **median effective dose** (LD_{50}/ED_{50}) defines the **therapeutic index**, a crude but useful measure of drug safety. Other things being equal, a drug with a large therapeutic index is safer than an agent with a smaller value. When many congeners are being tested concurrently, those with the most favorable therapeutic indexes are given preference in further investigations and are considered the most promising candidates for clinical application. The LD_{50}/ED_{50} ratio is not fully predictive of relative safety. Drugs produce many toxic effects besides death that can prevent their use in humans. An agent that is quite safe regarding one adverse reaction may fare poorly in regard to another type of toxicity. In that case, a **TD_{50}/ED_{50}** ratio, where TD = toxic dose, for each adverse effect should be calculated. Table 3-10 compares a group of local anesthetics in their propensity to elicit two separate toxic effects—death and local tissue irritation—as a function of the anesthetic concentration. Each test was performed in a different species: lethality in mice, irritability in rabbits, and anesthesia in guinea pigs. With procaine used as a standard, propoxycaine was 4.6 times safer regarding tissue irritation, but essentially

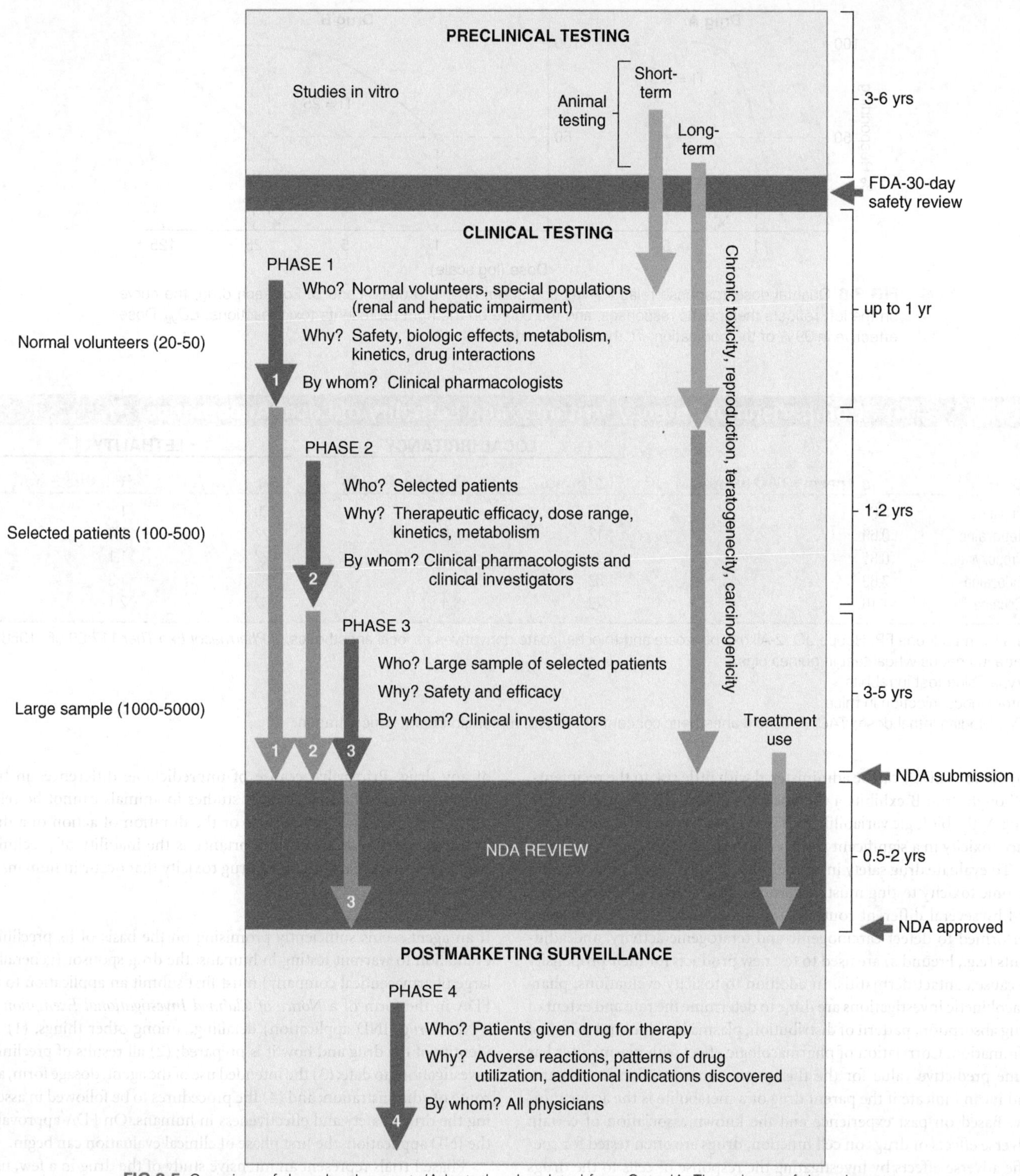

FIG 3-5 Overview of drug development. (Adapted and updated from Oats JA: The science of drug therapy. In Brunton LL, Lazo JS, Parker KL, editors: *Goodman and Gilman's the pharmacological basis of therapeutics*, ed 11, New York, 2006, McGraw-Hill.)

equivalent in relation to lethality. From these data, cocaine would seem to be the safest local anesthetic for human administration; however, cocaine has some additional liabilities—CNS stimulation and abuse potential—not shared by the other agents that severely restrict its medical usefulness. A limitation to the therapeutic index is the fact that it only compares two end points: a therapeutic response and death. It does not include nonlethal adverse effects.

A second limitation of the therapeutic index is that biologic variability is not taken into account. In Figure 3-6, drug B has a larger therapeutic index than drug A, but it is nevertheless clinically inferior. The goal of pharmacotherapy is to achieve a desired effect in virtually all patients without producing toxicity in any. Because the slopes of the quantal dose–effect curves of drug A are steep (indicating little variation in responsiveness to the drug), a dose effective in 99% of the

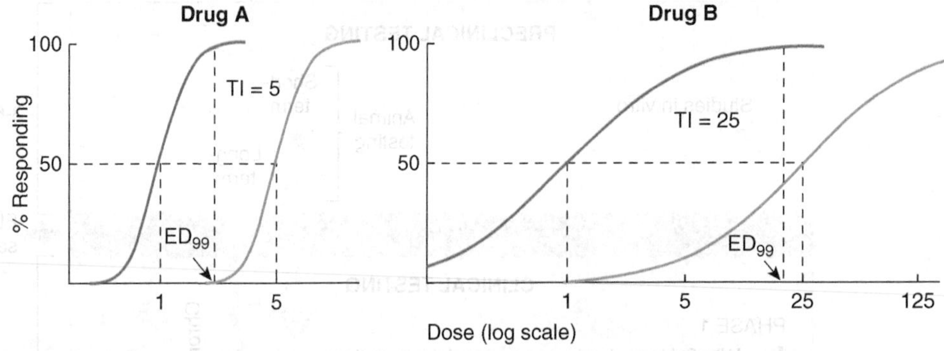

FIG 3-6 Quantal dose–response relationships (log scale) of two drugs, *A* and *B*. For each drug, the curve on the left reflects therapeutic responses, and the curve on the right represents toxic reactions. *ED_{99}*, Dose effective in 99% of the population; *TI*, therapeutic index.

TABLE 3-10 Comparison of Potency, Irritancy, and Lethality of Local Anesthetics

		LOCAL IRRITANCY†		LETHALITY‡	
Drug	**Anesthesia* TAC (mmol/L)**	**TIC (mmol/L)**	**Relative Safety**	**LD_{50} (μmol/L)**	**Relative Safety**
Procaine	8.8	176	1	220	1
Tetracaine	0.69	12	0.9	27	1.6
Propoxycaine	0.81	75	4.6	22	1.1
Lidocaine	2.69	62	1.2	85	1.3
Cocaine	1.16	79	3.4	62	2.1

Data from Luduena FP, Hoppe JO: 2-Alkoxy benzoate and thiol benzoate derivatives as local anesthetics, *J Pharmacol Exp Ther* 117:89-96, 1956.
*Intracutaneous wheal test in guinea pigs.
†Trypan blue test in rabbits.
‡Intravenous injection in mice.
LD_{50}, Median lethal dose; *TAC*, threshold anesthetic concentration; *TIC*, threshold irritant concentration.

population (ED_{99}) can be administered with little risk to the recipients. Although drug B exhibits a therapeutic index five times greater than drug A, the biologic variability to it is so great that an ED_{99} would produce toxicity in a significant fraction of the population.

To evaluate drug safety in animals thoroughly, acute, subacute, and chronic toxicity testing must be carried out in several different species and by several different routes of administration. Special studies are performed to detect carcinogenic and teratogenic activity, and adjuvants (e.g., Freund's) are used to test new products for their propensity to cause contact dermatitis. In addition to toxicity evaluations, pharmacokinetic investigations are done to determine the rate and extent of drug absorption, pattern of distribution, plasma half-life, and routes of elimination. Correlation of pharmacologic effect with plasma titer has some predictive value for the therapeutic concentration in humans, and it can indicate if the parent drug or a metabolite is the active moiety. Based on past experience and the known association of certain adverse effects of drugs on cell function, drugs are often tested for specific adverse effects by investigating the response of cells to the drugs in vitro or in whole animals. A good example is effect on the potassium channel, hERG. This channel is blocked by a number of drugs resulting in lengthening of the QT interval on the electrocardiogram, leading to **torsades de pointes** (Chapter 19). It is common practice to test the effects of experimental drugs on the hERG channel using electrophysiologic approaches and animal telemetry. Moreover, genetic polymorphisms (Chapter 4) in the hERG gene make some individuals hypersusceptible to these arrhythmias, especially with certain drugs. Such testing of drugs can give an early indication of relative drug safety.

Regardless of the number, size, or sophistication of animal tests used, studies in humans are necessary to establish the clinical worth of any drug. Primarily because of unpredictable differences in biotransformation, pharmacokinetic studies in animals cannot be relied on to determine the correct dose or the duration of action of a drug in humans. Of even greater importance is the inability of preclinical studies to detect many forms of drug toxicity that occur in humans.

Clinical trials

If an agent seems sufficiently promising on the basis of its preclinical evaluation to warrant testing in humans, the drug sponsor (generally a large pharmaceutical company) must first submit an application to the FDA in the form of a *Notice of Claimed Investigational Exemption for a New Drug* (IND application) detailing, among other things, (1) the identity of the drug and how it is prepared; (2) all results of preclinical investigations to date; (3) the intended use of the agent, dosage form, and route of administration; and (4) the procedures to be followed in assessing the drug's safety and effectiveness in humans. On FDA approval of the IND application, the first phase of clinical evaluation can begin.

Phase I trials represent an intensive study of the drug in a few, usually healthy, volunteers. The safe or tolerable human dose is arrived at by cautiously administering increasing increments of the drug to subjects until the desired response is obtained or a toxic side effect intervenes. Pharmacokinetic data from single and repeated administrations are collected to determine the bioavailability of the compound, its time course of action, and how it is eliminated from the body. Careful attention is given to any adverse effects that may occur. As with subsequent clinical studies, informed consent must be obtained from all subjects involved in phase I trials. Regulations by the FDA involving human experimentation conform to the principles incorporated in the Nuremberg Code and Declaration of Helsinki of the World Medical Association.

The second phase of clinical evaluation involves administration of the drug to a few targeted patients. The major goals of investigation are to establish efficacy and safety in patients and to arrive at the therapeutic dose. Phase II trials are the first real attempt to establish therapeutic efficacy, and many drugs are withdrawn from further investigation at this point. The exact studies made during phase II are determined in large measure by the drug. These first two phases are conducted exclusively by professionals trained and experienced in clinical pharmacology.

The decision to proceed to phase III trials commits the drug sponsor to a large-scale, controlled study of the drug. In phase III, the agent must be proved to be relatively safe and effective in a clinical setting. Proper controls (i.e., placebos when appropriate, active approved drugs when available) must be run concurrently to provide the necessary comparisons of drugs, and sufficient numbers of subjects must be used in the study to make such comparisons meaningful. The assignment of subjects to control and test categories must be unbiased. This unbiased assignment generally requires either a randomly assigned allotment of patients, in which each volunteer has an equal chance of being in any treatment group, or a crossover design, in which every subject receives each treatment in a balanced order. Bias in reporting drug effects also must be avoided; this can often be accomplished only by performing the trial under "blind" conditions. In a single-blind study, patients are not informed of which drug they receive; in a double-blind investigation, the identity of the medication is concealed from all individuals directly engaged in the study. Finally, appropriate statistical methods must be used to verify any conclusions reached about the drug.

Drug approval and continued surveillance

At the conclusion of phase III, a considerable body of information will have been gathered about the drug. These data are submitted to the FDA in the form of a *New Drug Application* (NDA). If accepted as "complete," the drug is approved for marketing as a prescription drug or as an over-the-counter item, depending on the need for professional supervision to ensure user safety. More often than not, the NDA is labeled "incomplete," however, and the sponsor is advised of additional evaluations that must be performed for it to be accepted. Even with approval of the agent, the sponsor must continue to submit reports to the FDA at regular intervals describing the quantity of drug distributed and detailing any unusual responses to the preparation, such as allergic reactions, idiosyncratic responses, or unanticipated drug interactions. This review constitutes phase IV of the clinical investigation. Continued surveillance of the drug after general release is often the only method available for identifying uncommon or delayed toxic effects.

Impact of FDA regulations on the development of new drugs

Regulations by the FDA governing the development and marketing of therapeutic agents exist largely as a result of public concern over the adverse effects of drugs. Had similar regulations been in force in Europe before 1959, the thalidomide disaster affecting approximately 10,000 children probably could have been averted. There are, however, several disadvantages to the present evaluation system used in the United States. It may take an average of 15 years for a new chemical entity (an agent unrelated to other drugs) to successfully negotiate the obstacle course of preclinical and clinical testing. The development expenses, including those associated with unfruitful compounds, may exceed $1 billion.

The delay in introducing new drugs into pharmacotherapeutics after 1962 opened up a "drug lag" between the United States and other countries. In response to this problem (and more specifically

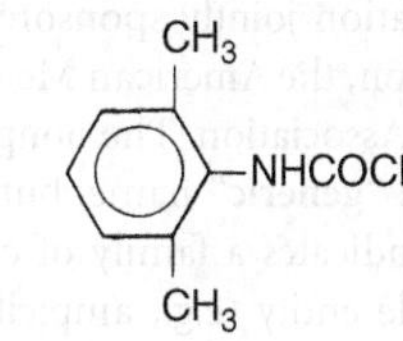

CH_3 / C_2H_5 / $-NHCOCH_2-N$ / C_2H_5 / CH_3

Chemical name (IUPAC): 2-(diethylamino) N-(2,6-dimethylphenyl acetamide)
Code name (Astra): LL 30
Nonproprietary name (USANC): Lidocaine
Official name (USP): Lidocaine
Nonproprietary name (BAN) Lignocaine
Trade names (selected): Xylocaine, Dilocaine, Lignospan, Nervocaine, Octocaine

FIG 3-7 Full nomenclature of a local anesthetic. *BAN*, British Adopted Name; *IUPAC*, International Union of Pure and Applied Chemistry; *USANC*, United States Adopted Name Council; *USP*, United States Pharmacopeia.

in response to pressure from acquired immunodeficiency syndrome advocates), the FDA established new regulations that allowed patients to receive investigational drugs targeted against serious or life-threatening disease outside clinical trials when no satisfactory alternative therapy was available. In the most extreme example, several promising drugs against HIV were made available to patients immediately after completion of phase I trials. Other strategies were instituted within the FDA to speed the review process. The FDA Modernization Act of 1997 incorporated these and other additional changes to streamline drug development.

The uncertainty and expense of bringing new drugs to market in recent years have had a striking influence on the pharmaceutical industry. Only the largest drug manufacturers have the resources to meet FDA guidelines for new drugs. Because pharmaceutical companies are profit-oriented enterprises, the enormous cost of developing a drug is incurred only if a reasonable return on the investment can be anticipated. Without some additional incentive, the development of drugs for rare diseases has been priced out of consideration. It is also to be expected that agents under patent protection will be highly priced and heavily promoted.

Two laws pertaining to drug development have been enacted in an effort to stimulate therapies for "orphan" diseases and to reduce the cost of pharmaceuticals. The **Orphan Drug Act** of 1983 provided tax incentives and other considerations to companies for the development of drugs for rare disorders (affecting <200,000 people in the United States) and for more common diseases in which there is no reasonable expectation for recovery of development costs. Future advances in genetics and genomics are likely to increase the need for orphan drugs, which are likely to be "tailor-made" to fit the genetic traits of individual patients.

Drug Nomenclature

During the course of development and marketing, a drug acquires various names or designations (Figure 3-7). The first identification of a drug is the formal chemical name. Although descriptive of the molecular structure of the compound, the chemical name is usually too unwieldy for practical purposes. A newly synthesized drug is often given a simple code name by the parent pharmaceutical firm to denote the agent during the various stages of drug evaluation. If the drug manufacturer intends to request approval by the FDA for distributing the agent, a **nonproprietary name**, or United States Adopted Name, is assigned to the drug by the United States Adopted Name

Council (USANC), an organization jointly sponsored by the United States Pharmacopeial Convention, the American Medical Association, and the American Pharmacists Association. The nonproprietary name is commonly referred to as the "**generic**" name, but by strict definition, the generic designation indicates a family of compounds (e.g., penicillins), rather than a single entity (e.g., ampicillin). If the drug is eventually admitted to the *United States Pharmacopeia (USP)*, its nonproprietary name becomes the official name. The USANC works in cooperation with the World Health Organization to standardize nonproprietary names; drugs introduced before harmonization efforts began may have different nonproprietary names.

Much confusion over drug nomenclature arises because a single drug may be marketed under many different trade names. A **trade or proprietary name** is given to a drug by the manufacturer when the agent is approved for general release. In contrast to the nonproprietary name, which is publicly owned, a trade name receives copyright protection and is the sole property of the drug company. Occasionally, a manufacturer may distribute the agent under several different trade names to promote separate uses of the drug. In addition, the manufacturer may arrange with other pharmaceutical firms to sell the drug, each using its own trade name. A profusion of trade names may develop when the drug patent expires, and all companies are permitted by law to produce the agent. Assignment of trade names to drug combination products contributes yet further to the proliferation of drug names.

Throughout this book, nonproprietary names are emphasized in discussions of the various drugs. This practice reduces confusion and equips the reader to use other sources of drug information to the best advantage. The benefits and debits of using nonproprietary designations in prescription writing are discussed in Chapter 42.

SOURCES OF DRUG INFORMATION

The continued development of new drugs and the acquisition of new information about existing agents make pharmacology a discipline requiring continual study. Various resources are available to aid the clinician in keeping abreast of advances in pharmacotherapeutics.

Official Compendia

The *USP-NF* (*United States Pharmacopeia–National Formulary*) is an official compendia of drugs in the United States. It provides an invaluable service to the practitioner by defining criteria for the manufacture of pharmaceutical preparations. It ensures that when a prescription is written for an official drug, the medication supplied to the patient meets certain standards of strength, purity, and chemical and physical properties. It is not meant to be a source of information about the clinical use of drugs.

The *American Hospital Formulary Service Drug Information* (*AFHS DI*) is a compendium recognized by the federal government for determination of medically accepted but not FDA-approved indications of drugs. Published by the American Society of Health-System Pharmacists, a nonprofit organization, the *AFHS DI* is independent of the FDA and the pharmaceutical industry. It relies upon peer review by more than 500 physicians, pharmacologists, and other health care professionals to ensure information is accurate and evidence-based. The *AFHS DI* contains information on more than 100,000 drug products and includes extensive off-label use information. Updates are available online.

Many other nations have their own official compendia. In addition, the *International Pharmacopoeia* is issued by the World Health Organization. Although not official in the sense of the *USP*, the *International Pharmacopoeia* is instrumental in promoting the standardization and unification of the various national compendia.

Unofficial Compendia

The *Physicians' Desk Reference* (*PDR*) is perhaps the most widely distributed source of prescribing information available to health professionals. The *PDR* is published annually (with interim revisions as necessary) in cooperation with more than 200 pharmaceutical manufacturing and distributing concerns. More than 2400 drugs are listed by proprietary name in an alphabetical arrangement according to drug distributor. (The cost of including a drug deters many companies from listing all their products.) Although the *PDR* is well indexed, its organization makes the comparison of similar agents difficult. The product information, which is largely derived from phase III trials and must legally conform to FDA regulations, contains concise summaries of the uses, dosage forms, and schedules, contraindications, and adverse effects of the drugs listed. Nevertheless, the lack of critical appraisals of, or relative comparisons between, the various preparations included in the *PDR* limits its use as a reliable guide for the rational selection of drugs in therapy. The *PDR* does have a useful drug identification section. The *PDR for Nonprescription Drugs, Dietary Supplements, and Herbs* and the *PDR Guide to Drug Interactions, Side Effects, and Indications* are specialized sources of information. These books are also available on compact disc (CD) format, and an electronic site called PDR.net provides World Wide Web access to these resources for health care personnel (including dentists) free of charge.

A suitable alternative to the *PDR* is *Facts and Comparisons.* Published independently of the pharmaceutical industry, *Facts and Comparisons* contains monographs in a format designed to facilitate comparisons between drugs. *Facts and Comparisons* is available in a hardcover edition, a loose-leaf version, on CD-ROM, and online. Besides information from *Facts and Comparisons*, eFacts subscriptions online also include extensive drug–drug interaction information. *A2Z Drugs* in electronic format is a quick reference guide to drugs online and for handheld devices.

Mosby's Drug Reference for Health Professions is a concise compilation of monographs for more than 850 nonproprietary drug entries (including almost 4000 proprietary name products). Because drug entries in *Mosby's Drug Reference* are not paid for by pharmaceutical companies, the book contains information specifically for health care providers and not necessarily to be in compliance with FDA-approved drug information. The book also offers a color pill atlas and online updates.

Lexi-Comp has teamed up with Wolters Kluwer to provide book, online, and mobile versions of their drug information database. Similar to *Mosby's*, it is a clinically based information system that provides "need to know" information about different drugs for the clinical practitioner. They have a version of their database that is written by, and for, dental professionals in particular.

Books on Pharmacology and Therapeutics

Textbooks of general pharmacology usually present basic principles of drug action and pharmacologic profiles of the various classes of therapeutic agents. Descriptions of relationships between pathophysiologic characteristics and drug effects contained in textbooks significantly contribute to the understanding of pharmacotherapeutics. Textbooks can provide the best overview of pharmacology and detailed coverage of key individual agents in each drug category for an organized approach for understanding drug classes. However, for clarity of presentation and because of limitations of space, detailed coverage of every available drug is not possible. However many textbooks, including this one, provide a comprehensive list of drugs in each drug class. Printed textbooks are limited in that they cannot include information on the most recent advances in pharmacotherapeutics, such as the introduction of new drugs. For this reason, most textbooks provide an online resource with updated drug information.

The *Handbook of Nonprescription Drugs*, published by the American Pharmacists Association, is one of the few sources of information concerning over-the-counter drugs. The handbook presents critical evaluations of the various preparations available to the public. Of special interest to dentists are the chapters on headache and muscle and joint pain, herbal remedies, and oral pain and discomfort.

Periodicals

Numerous journals and reviews are devoted to pharmacology and therapeutics. The *Journal of Pharmacology and Experimental Therapeutics* and *Molecular Pharmacology* offer in-depth treatment of all areas of pharmacology. These journals are primarily concerned with the experimental aspects of pharmacodynamics. *Trends in Pharmacological Sciences* is published monthly and offers in-depth articles with summary content covering all areas of pharmacology. *Clinical Pharmacology and Therapeutics* has articles dealing with drug effects in humans. Journals that review pharmacologic information of direct clinical relevance include *Drugs* and the *Annual Review of Pharmacology and Toxicology*. Although not restricted in scope to drugs, the *New England Journal of Medicine* is noteworthy for its excellent coverage of pharmacotherapeutics. Specialty journals of significance to dentistry include *Anesthesiology*, *Anesthesia and Analgesia*, and *Pain*.

The *Medical Letter on Drugs and Therapeutics* provides a unique service to practitioners in the United States. Published biweekly, the *Medical Letter* offers current, concise, and critical reviews of new drugs and pharmaceutical preparations. Expert opinion is also provided regarding the therapeutic and toxic effects of established drugs. In this respect, the periodic updates on drug interactions and on clinical selection of antimicrobial agents are especially helpful.

Dental Sources of Information

The *American Dental Association Guide to Dental Therapeutics* is published by the American Dental Association. This resource has information on drugs listed in tabular form, with more extensive coverage of drugs pertaining predominantly to dentistry. It uses the *PDR* database for much of its information. In addition, chapter authors provide specific details pertinent to clinical dental practice.

Mosby's Dental Drug Reference and *Lexi-Comp's Drug Information Handbook for Dentistry* are reference handbooks useful for the quick identification of drugs and their dental implications. Both sources are published annually; the latter is now available online and for downloading to computers and handheld electronic devices.

Although there is currently no dental periodical solely concerned with pharmacology, numerous journals feature articles dealing with drugs in dental practice. *Anesthesia Progress* is the official journal of the American Dental Society of Anesthesiology. It publishes articles on drugs useful in pain and anxiety control, and it prints abstracts from other periodicals of related articles of interest. The *Journal of the American Dental Association* is also a good source of information about dental pharmacotherapeutics. In addition to publishing original contributions and review articles, the *Journal of the American Dental Association* provides evaluations from the Council on Scientific Affairs on issues pertaining to drugs and dentistry. The *Journal of Dental Research*, which features *Critical Reviews in Oral Biology and Medicine*, occasionally publishes articles and reviews relating to drug therapy in dentistry. Specialty journals, such as the *Journal of Oral and Maxillofacial Surgery* and the *Journal of Periodontology*, also publish articles on dental pharmacotherapeutics.

Electronic Media

Most of the sources of information described previously, or the databases from which they are derived, are now available on CD, and several are available online. These formats permit the use of Boolean descriptors and hypertext links to facilitate searches within a single source or among several sources at the same time. Digital book systems, incorporating one or more sources of information in handheld devices, facilitate immediate access to drug information in all clinical settings. ePocrates Rx (www.epocrates.com) is a free resource on drugs that includes concise information ranging from pharmacodynamics to cost of drugs. It is available online and for download to Palm, Windows Mobile, iPhone, iPad, and BlackBerry devices. It is also available in a handy printed copy.

The Internet is increasingly becoming a vital source of drug information. Numerous sites on the World Wide Web provide information regarding specific issues pertaining to dental therapeutics. Some of these are free; others charge a monthly or connect fee. Many of the book titles listed previously are also available online. Some other sources are as follows. PubMed (www.ncbi.nlm.nih.gov/PubMed) is the National Library of Medicine's interface to MEDLINE and other information sources. It provides access, for a fee, to numerous scientific journals. Free access to numerous journal articles may be obtained through PubMed Central (www.pubmedcentral.gov). Uptodate.com is a medical database that keeps refereed articles on most known diseases and conditions. Heavily used in the medical community, it is considered one of the finest medical databases available. It also has information on pertinent drug therapies for the various maladies. Subscriptions, while expensive, provide excellent coverage of the most recent information on drugs and diseases. Micromedex (www.micromedex.com) is a reference that provides useful drug information for health care professionals. Lexi-Comp ONLINE (www.lexi.com) has a useful drug identification and vocal pronunciation guide for drugs and information on pharmacokinetics, adverse effects, and drug interactions. It is also available as a *Drug Information Handbook* (as mentioned earlier). eMedicine (www.emedicine.medscape.com) is an extensive online resource that presents a discussion of disorders and treatment options. RxList (www.rxlist.com) is a handy and valuable online resource concentrating on the clinical aspects of drugs.

It should be mentioned that many practitioners simply use Google (or similar) to get basic information about medications. Wikipedia is often included in the search results. While these resources are fine for extremely basic data about a drug, caution must be used at all times because these are not formally reviewed for accuracy. At no time should clinical decisions be based upon Internet data that is not from a known reliable source. Drug manufacturers' home pages will have areas where health care providers can get detailed information about their products including dosing and side effects. Medicolegally, it is always best to use a recognized information resource when making clinical care decisions for your patients.

CASE DISCUSSION

The nature of the adverse reactions, hives, and difficulty breathing suggest an allergic reaction. The time of onset after taking amoxicillin suggests a type I allergy. These are mediated by an antigen binding to IgE antibodies that are attached to mast cells and basophils. This results in the release of histamine and other inflammatory mediators. Blood pressure and heart rate monitoring must be carried out. The administration of oxygen is appropriate, but it will not block the effect of these mediators. Therefore, strategies need to be employed to block these mediators and/or their effects. At this time, the symptoms of the patient do not appear to be life-threatening; however, his condition could

Continued

CASE DISCUSSION—cont'd

worsen. Treatment depends on the type of reactions that occur, the severity of the reactions and the rapidity of the onset of symptoms. If symptoms remain mild, an antihistamine can be administered initially.

1. An H-1 blocking antihistamine such as diphenhydramine (25-50 mg IM) should be administered as soon as possible.
2. If available, an H-2 blocking antihistamine such as ranitidine (50 mg IM) should also be administered, if GI symptoms occur.
3. If bronchoconstriction is present, administer an albuterol (or similar) inhaler: one to four puffs.
4. If the blood pressure begins to fall rapidly, and the breathing is very labored, epinephrine (300 mcg SQ or IM) (0.3 ml of 1:1000) must be administered immediately. It may need to be repeated every 3 to 5 minutes. (See chapter 41).
5. Glucocorticosteroids are helpful for longer term management. If the reaction is anything but mild, consider dexamethasone (6 to 8 mg IM).
6. If the patient stabilizes (return of near-normal blood pressure and breathing), he or she may need to be continued on both oral antihistamines and oral steroids for another 2 to 3 days. However emergency help should be summoned if the reaction was initially severe.

GENERAL REFERENCES

1. Chen M, Bertino JS Jr, Berg MJ, et al.: Pharmacological differences between men and women. In Atkinson AJ Jr, Abernethy DR, Daniels CE, et al.: *Principles of clinical pharmacology*, ed 2, Amsterdam, 2007, Elsevier.
2. Cohen AF, Burggraaf J, van Gerven JMA, Moerland M, Groeneveld GJ: The use of biomarkers in human pharmacology (Phase I) studies, *Ann Rev Pharmacol Toxicol* 55:55–74, 2015.
3. Froget LM: Overview of safety pharmacology, *Curr Protoc Pharmacol* 63, 2013. Unit 10.1.
4. Ivanov M, Barragan I, Ingelman-Sundberg M: Epigenetic mechanisms of importance for drug treatment, *Trends Pharmacol Sci* 35:384–396, 2014.
5. Meissner K, Distel H, Mitzdorf U: Evidence for placebo effects on physical but not on biochemical outcome parameters: a review of clinical trials. *BMC Med* 5(3), 2007. Available at: http://www.biomedcentral.com/1741-7015/5/3. Accessed January 10, 2010.
6. Michalowicz BS, DiAngelis AJ, Novak MJ, et al.: Examining the safety of dental treatment in pregnant women, *J Am Dent Assoc* 139:685–695, 2008.
7. Mowry JB, Spyker DA, Cantilena LR, McMillan N, Ford M: 2013 Annual report of the American Association of Poison Control Centers' National Poison Data Systems (NPDS): 31st Annual Report, *Clin Toxicol* 52:1032–1283, 2014.
8. Price DD, Finniss DG, Benedetti F: A comprehensive review of the placebo effect: recent advances and current thought, *Ann Rev Psychology* 59:565–590, 2008.

Pharmacogenetics: Pharmacogenomics

David W. Hein and Denis M. Grant

KEY INFORMATION

- Pharmacogenetics/Pharmacogenomics is the investigation of variations of DNA and RNA sequence/characteristics as related to drug response and toxicity.
- All proteins are gene products and many (perhaps most) exhibit genetic polymorphism. Single-nucleotide polymorphisms (SNPs), gene deletions, and gene amplifications determine protein structure, configuration, and/or concentration.
- The consequences of genetic polymorphisms can translate into either increased or decreased clinical efficacy and into increased or decreased toxic effects.
- Personalized medicine includes rational targeting (e.g., restricting the use of trastuzumab (Herceptin)) based on disease phenotype (i.e., only in those whose tumors overexpress HER2).
- Epigenetic factors in drug responses and toxicity add additional complexity to personalized medicine.
- Drugs that produce severe adverse reactions in combination with other drugs or certain conditions (e.g., pregnancy) are used today with appropriate warnings and legal accountability to the drug prescriber. In the future, a similar accountability will be extended to the appropriate use of pharmacogenetic information.
- The U.S. Food and Drug Administration (FDA) has issued labeling regulations and posts updated pharmacogenetic information for an ever-expanding listing of drugs.
- Informed, individualized selection of drug or drug dose based on patient's genetic information will replace the paradigm of one drug and/or one dose fits all.
- Effective drugs previously discarded because of toxicity in some patients will be useful when targeted to patients with an appropriate genetic profile. This will lower the costs of drug development and should ultimately lower drug cost.
- The Clinical Pharmacogenetics Implementation Consortium (CPIC) formulates and distributes practice guidelines to enable translation of pharmacogenetic information into actionable prescribing decisions.

CASE STUDY

A 62-year-old man visiting from North Africa is scheduled for tooth extraction in your dental practice. His only medication was valproic acid (1500 mg daily), which he had been taking for several years after he had a posttraumatic generalized seizure. The tooth extraction under local anesthesia was successful and unremarkable. The patient was discharged with care instructions and a prescription for Tylenol with codeine #3 tablets (three times a day) to relieve pain.

Four days following the tooth extraction, the patient's level of consciousness rapidly deteriorated and he became unresponsive and was taken by ambulance to the local hospital. His last tablet of Tylenol with codeine #3 had been taken 12 hours earlier. Arterial blood gas measurements revealed a partial pressure of oxygen of 56 mm Hg, with a fraction of inspired oxygen of 0.5 and a partial pressure of carbon dioxide of 80 mm Hg. The patient was treated with noninvasive ventilation and was transferred to the intensive care unit. Initial neurologic examination showed a score of 6 on the Glasgow Coma Scale (no eye opening, no verbal response, and no limb withdrawal after pain stimulation). The patient's pupils were miotic, and no focal deficits were detected.

Ninety minutes after the initiation of noninvasive ventilation, repeated measurements of arterial blood gases showed that the partial pressure of oxygen was 68 mm Hg and the partial pressure of carbon dioxide was 56 mm Hg, but no neurologic improvement was observed. The serum urea nitrogen and creatinine levels were elevated, at 45.4 mg per deciliter (16.2 mmol per liter) and 2.06 mg per deciliter (182 µmol per liter), respectively; the levels were subsequently normalized with hydration. The serum level of valproic acid was 62.4 mg per liter (433 µmol per liter; normal range, 50.4 to 101 mg per liter [350 to 700 µmol per liter]) on the patient's usual dosage. The blood level of ammonia was normal.

1. How and why did this adverse event occur?
2. What should be the patient's treatment and why?

(Modified from Gasche, et al: *N Engl J Med* 351:2827-2831, 2004.)

Individual patient differences in drug responsiveness are well recognized by health care professionals. Understanding the basis for these differences is of major clinical and economic importance because of the high frequency of both therapeutic failure and adverse reactions to drugs. Patients may receive inadequate or suboptimal benefit and/or suffer adverse effects from drug treatment. In this chapter, we highlight pharmacogenetic/pharmacogenomic principles and provide illustrative examples where these principles can be applied to optimize therapeutic benefit and minimize adverse effects.

Pharmacogenetics is the branch of pharmacology that seeks to understand the genetic basis for differences in drug responsiveness among the human population. The ability to select the safest and most effective drug and dose for a patient based on the patient's pharmacogenetic profile should simplify the process of adjusting the therapeutic regimen to achieve the desired clinical response. Pharmacogenetics is defined by the U.S. FDA as the investigation of the role of variations in DNA sequence on drug response. The term **pharmacogenomics**—sometimes used interchangeably with pharmacogenetics—is defined by the FDA as the investigation of variations in DNA and RNA characteristics as related to drug response. Pharmacogenomics may also refer to the application of genomic information toward the discovery and development of drugs with new and more specific targets. The broader field of "personalized medicine" also includes more rational targeting of drugs, such as restricting the use of trastuzumab (Herceptin) to treat tumors based on the tumor phenotype (i.e., only those that overexpress HER2). MicroRNAs influence disease susceptibility and progression and therapeutic response. Single-nucleotide polymorphisms (SNPs) in the microRNA target sites can abolish existing binding sites or create illegitimate binding sites in mRNA. Genetic polymorphisms in microRNAs themselves also may have effects. The pediatric population presents a unique pharmacogenetic challenge as children have the additional complexity of ontological phenotypes that impact their drug response.

FDA labeling regulations now stipulate the following:

> ***If evidence is available to support the safety and effectiveness of the drug only in selected subgroups of the larger population with a disease, the labeling shall describe the evidence and identify specific tests needed for selection and monitoring of patients who need the drug.***

A comprehensive listing of FDA-approved drugs with pharmacogenomic information in their labeling is posted at www.fda.gov/drugs/scienceresearch/researchareas/pharmacogenetics/ucm083378.htm.

Pharmacogenetic biomarker information posted by the FDA includes germ-line or somatic gene variants, functional deficiencies, expression changes, and chromosomal abnormalities. The labeling for many of the approved drugs includes specific actions to be taken based on the pharmacogenetic biomarker information.

Both pharmacogenetics and pharmacogenomics are areas of intense interest and development within the biotechnology and pharmaceutical industries. Many pharmaceutical companies are beginning to genotype patients in premarket clinical trials to exclude individuals who are predicted to experience adverse effects or therapeutic failure. This concept is illustrated in Figure 4-1. A high-density map of the SNPs that exist throughout the human genome has been assembled to facilitate the construction of pharmacogenetic profiles that predict drug responsiveness. SNPs occur, on average, about once every 1000 bases in the three billion base human genome. A Website (www.ncbi.nlm.nih.gov/SNP) sponsored by the National Institutes of Health (NIH) National Center for Biotechnology Information maintains an updated listing of these SNPs.

This chapter presents basic principles and information resources describing pharmacogenetic differences in drug therapy and toxicity. The pharmacogenetic examples included are of historical and/or clinical interest; they are not intended to be exhaustive. Adoption of pharmacogenetic information into drug prescribing has been modest, in part due to the lack of clear, curated, and peer-reviewed pharmacogenetic guidelines for drug prescribing. A **Clinical Pharmacogenetics Implementation Consortium (CPIC)** (https://www.pharmgkb.org/page/cpic) formed in partnership with the FDA, **the Pharmacogenomics Knowledge Base (PharmGKB;** www.pharmgkb.org**)**, and the NIH Pharmacogenetics Research Network develops and posts practice guidelines to enable translation of pharmacogenetic information into actionable prescribing decisions. PharmGKB posts **very important pharmacogene (VIP)** summaries (www.pharmgkb.org/view/vips.jsp) that provide an overview of a significant gene involved in metabolism of or response to one or several drugs. Often VIPs either play a role in the metabolism of many drugs or contain variants that potentially contribute to a severe drug response. VIP summaries typically include background information on the gene including any disease associations, as well as in-depth information on the gene's pharmacogenetics. VIP genes are chosen through extensive review of a variety of sources, including the U.S. FDA biomarker list and drug labels with pharmacogenetic information, and CPIC nominations. Additionally, VIPs may be created if a gene is associated with a large number of variant

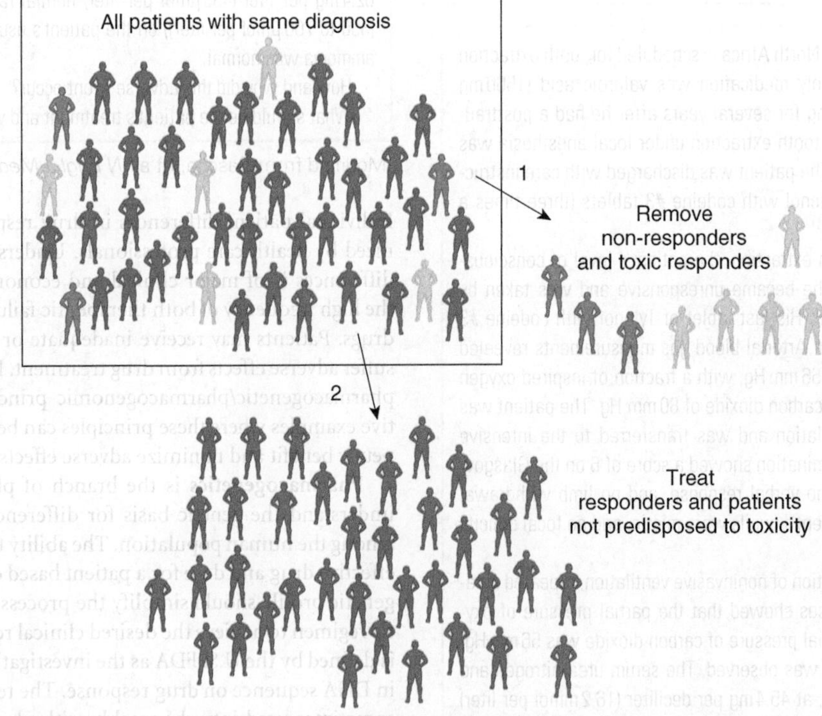

FIG 4-1 Diagram illustrating the strategy of selecting patients for drug therapy based on response to the drug. *Red figures,* Responders who lack a genetic predisposition for toxicity; *yellow figures,* inadequate responders; *green figures,* patients predisposed to toxicity because of a genetic trait.

annotations and is part of high-level clinical annotations. The CPIC publishes guidelines for gene–drug pairs that emphasize clinical relevance and applicability. Each gene–drug pair has its own page with interactive therapeutic recommendations (i.e., specific therapeutic recommendations based on pharmacogenetic information). The CPIC is also working to position the guidelines to incorporate pharmacogenetic information into drug prescribing via electronic medical records. CPIC drug prescribing guidelines are posted at www.pharmgkb.org/view/dosing-guidelines.do?source=CPIC.

The genome determines the structure, configuration, tissue distribution, subcellular compartmentalization, and concentration of endogenous proteins. In most cases, for a drug to produce a therapeutic or toxic response, it must interact with one or more proteins, which in turn are subject to genetic variation in the human population. For example, genetic differences in plasma proteins may affect the affinity and the extent of drug binding. Genetic differences in the enzymes that metabolize a drug may confer differences in the concentrations of the parent compound, its active metabolites, and toxic derivatives. Genetic differences in cell membrane proteins or drug transporter proteins may influence drug absorption, distribution, and excretion. Finally, patients may have cell surface or intracellular drug receptors mediating therapeutic or adverse effects that are genetically more or less abundant or sensitive than is the norm.

The influence of genetic differences on drug response and toxicity has been highlighted in the popular press:

> *Every year, more than 100,000 people die in the U.S. because they carry "misspelled" genes that make medications either ineffective or deadly. Now doctors can test for the genes before prescribing. . . Imagine, a lawyer asking: "Doctor, did you know this drug would kill your patient? Did you know there is a test that would have predicted that? And why did you not give your patient the test?"*
>
> ***Newsweek, February 8, 1999***

Such statements widely read by the lay public (and their lawyers) underscore the need for dental professionals to understand the role of pharmacogenetic factors in drug responsiveness. Indeed, patient malpractice claims have already alleged negligence in the use of pharmacogenetic information.

PHARMACOKINETICS/PHARMACODYNAMICS

Proteins affect both drug concentration (pharmacokinetics) and response (pharmacodynamics). Historically, genetic variation most often has been identified in pharmacokinetics, particularly in drug-metabolizing enzymes. Genetic variation in the pharmacokinetic profile often necessitates a change in the dosage regimen of a drug but not in its selection. Pharmacogenetic differences in drug target responsiveness are less well understood, but potentially they will also have a significant impact on patient outcomes in the years ahead. In these instances, certain drugs will be contraindicated for patients with particular genotypes. Just as drug prescribers are currently responsible for avoiding adverse "drug–drug" interactions as described in other chapters and in Appendix 4, they increasingly will be held accountable for avoiding "gene–drug" interactions in clinical practice. Genetic differences in both pharmacokinetics and pharmacodynamics are anticipated for many if not most drugs, yielding important consequences for drug responsiveness, especially for agents with a narrow therapeutic index. Figure 4-2 illustrates the **separate** and **combined influences of genetic polymorphisms** in pharmacokinetics and pharmacodynamics.

There are many gene–drug interactions with importance to dentistry. For example, **codeine**—one of the mostly commonly prescribed opioid analgesics for relief of pain—depends on its activation to morphine by **CYP2D6**, a drug-metabolizing enzyme that is known to exhibit a common genetic polymorphism in humans. Thus codeine is an ineffective analgesic in a significant genetic subset (up to 10%, depending on the ethnic group) of the population. As illustrated in the case presentation at the beginning of this chapter, codeine use is associated with significant toxicity in CYP2D6 ultrarapid metabolizers (UMs) and also has been reported in infants of CYP2D6 UM mothers who breastfeed. (See also Chapter 16.) Genetic polymorphisms in opioid receptors or in second messenger systems mediating opioid receptor actions have also been observed. If a patient inherits deficiencies in both CYP2D6 and the μ-opioid receptor, it is very unlikely that codeine will be of any therapeutic benefit. However, increasing the dose of codeine to compensate for the genetic deficiency in CYP2D6-mediated activation in a patient who also has the deficient μ-opioid receptor will most likely not result in analgesia but rather in an adverse reaction mediated by overstimulation of an alternative receptor that may also be responsive to codeine.

PHENOTYPE/GENOTYPE

A person's **genotype** is a genetic trait defined by the DNA sequences (i.e., alleles) inherited from the mother and the father. An individual can inherit two copies of the same allele (homozygous genotype) or a different allele from each of the parents (heterozygous genotype). The **phenotype** is a biologic or measurable expression of the genetic trait that is dependent upon the level of penetrance of the gene, the accuracy and selectivity of the method used to measure it, and the influence of environmental factors in the expression of the trait. Historically, one of the most easily measured phenotypes was plasma drug concentration, which is probably why most of the initially identified pharmacogenetic traits were pharmacokinetic phenotypes. Determination of drug concentration, however, is relatively invasive, requiring administration of a drug or surrogate chemical and collection of blood samples over time. The drug concentration also is dependent to a varying degree on patient age, general health, nutritional status, and other factors such as exposure to enzyme inducers and inhibitors. Determination of a patient's genotype is much less invasive because it does not require administration of a test drug or collection of blood samples over time. Instead, the genotype is determined from a **small sample of DNA** obtained easily from a buccal swab, hair follicle, or other ready source and is not affected by age, general health, nutritional status, or other factors. On the other hand, for these same reasons the prediction of drug response from a genetic test may not always be accurate or reproducible because of the influence of such nongenetic factors on drug response. Many methods to determine the genotype rely on DNA amplification techniques based on the polymerase chain reaction that yields millions of copies of the specific target gene. New high-throughput methods make the simultaneous determination of multiple genotypes readily available to health care professionals.

MONOGENIC VERSUS POLYGENIC PHENOTYPES

A discussion of genetic polymorphisms in enzymes and receptors would be incomplete without consideration of the differences inherent between **monogenic and polygenic phenotypes. Monogenic** phenotypes derive from genetic variations in a single gene. Thus monogenic variation often separates populations into discontinuous (bimodal or trimodal) distributions of the phenotype. Moreover, if the least commonly occurring phenotype arising from the monogenic variation has a frequency of greater than 1% in a population, it

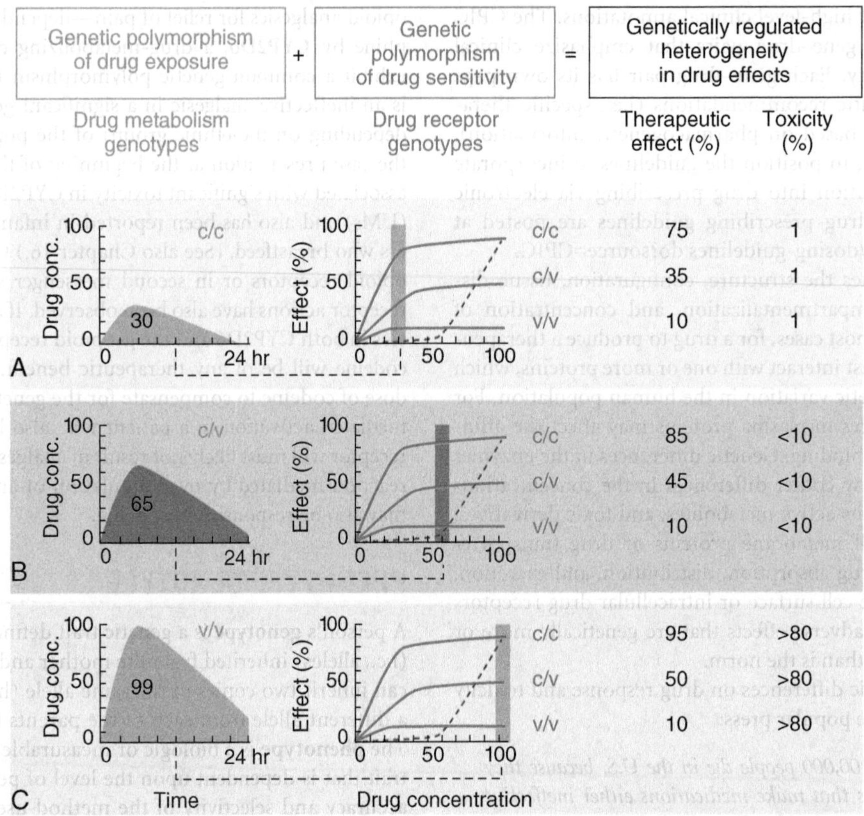

FIG 4-2 The potential consequences of administering the same dose of drug to individuals with genetic polymorphisms in both pharmacokinetics (drug-metabolizing enzymes) and pharmacodynamics (drug receptors). Active drug concentrations in the systemic circulation (columns) are determined by the individual's drug metabolism genotype, with (**A**) homozygous common (*c/c*) genotype converting 70% of a dose to the inactive metabolite, leaving 30% to exert an effect on the target receptor. **B,** For the patient with heterozygous (*c/v*) drug metabolism genotype, 35% is inactivated, whereas (**C**) the patient with homozygous variant (*v/v*) drug metabolism inactivates only 1% of the drug dose, yielding the three drug concentration time curves. The drug response is further influenced by drug receptor genotypes. Patients with a c/c receptor genotype exhibit a greater therapeutic effect (*solid lines*) at any given drug concentration in comparison to those with a c/v receptor genotype, whereas those with v/v receptor genotypes are relatively refractory to drug effects at any plasma drug concentration. The combination of genetic polymorphisms in drug metabolism and receptor yields nine different theoretical patterns of drug effect. The therapeutic ratio (efficacy versus toxicity) ranges from very favorable in a patient with c/c genotypes for drug metabolism and drug receptor to very unfavorable in the patient with v/v genotypes. (It is assumed here that the toxic dose–response curve, shown in *dotted lines,* is not influenced by these polymorphisms.) (Redrawn from Evans WE, Relling MV: Pharmacogenomics: translating functional genomics into rational therapeutics, *Science* 286:487-491, 1999.)

is termed a **polymorphism**. Different drugs or dosing regimens may be appropriate for specific phenotypes. **Polygenic** traits, in contrast, are phenotypes that derive from some combination of variations in multiple genes. In this case, clearly distinct or discontinuous phenotypes are not observed in a studied population. Instead, there is a unimodal, continuous, normal (Gaussian) distribution of the phenotype. A unimodal distribution of drug response is observed for most drugs metabolized by multiple enzymes and/or transported by multiple proteins and/or acting through multiple receptors and/or second messenger systems. This does not necessarily mean an absence of genetic variation in one or all of these proteins but rather that multiple genes contribute to the overall drug response phenotype. Since each of the genes is potentially subject to genetic variation, the utility of genetic information in predicting therapeutic and toxic responses is considerably more complicated. Until recently, polygenic phenotypes were too complex to consider in optimizing drug therapy.

ETHNIC DIFFERENCES IN PHARMACOGENETICS

The frequency of alleles, genotypes, and phenotypes for drug-metabolizing enzymes varies widely with ethnic origin. A similar variance is expected for drug receptors. Thus clinical trials are best conducted either with ethnically diverse study populations to capture differences among ethnic groups or in ethnically defined subgroups to precisely define effects in these groups. Some genotyping methods were designed originally to identify only alleles prevalent in Caucasians. However, with the documented ethnic heterogeneity within the human population, genotyping tests need to identify all relevant alleles of a particular gene regardless of ethnic frequency.

PHARMACOGENETICS OF DRUG METABOLISM

As indicated earlier, the majority of the pharmacogenetic traits identified to date occur in genes encoding drug-metabolizing enzymes.

It is anticipated that genetic polymorphisms may be identified in all drug-metabolizing enzymes. A number of these genetic polymorphisms are already known to be important in therapeutics, and selected examples of historical and clinical interest are highlighted next.

Acetylation Polymorphisms (www.pharmgkb.org/gene/PA18)

N-**acetylation** is an important **phase II conjugation reaction** for many drugs that possess an aromatic amine (e.g., procainamide, dapsone, many sulfonamides) or hydrazine (e.g., isoniazid, hydralazine) moiety. Human populations can be distinguished as **rapid and slow acetylator phenotypes** by measuring the production of *N*-acetylated metabolites after administration of drugs such as isoniazid, dapsone, or caffeine. As is the case for most drug-metabolizing enzyme polymorphisms, the frequencies of SNPs, genotypes, and acetylator phenotypes vary markedly with ethnic origin. Slow acetylator phenotypes exhibit higher plasma concentrations of parent drug and higher incidences of peripheral neuropathy from isoniazid and systemic lupus erythematosus syndrome from procainamide or hydralazine. In contrast, rapid acetylator phenotypes exhibit greater myelosuppression after treatment with amonafide.

Oxidation Polymorphisms

The cytochrome P450 (CYP) system, as described in Chapter 2, is a family of microsomal enzymes with selective but frequently overlapping substrate specificities. CYP-mediated oxidation is the predominant pathway for phase I metabolism (both activation and deactivation) and is responsible for the metabolism of a very large diversity of therapeutic drugs and environmental carcinogens. Genetic polymorphisms in many of the CYP enzymes have been identified in human populations (http://www.cypalleles.ki.se/). Variant alleles possess gene deletions, gene conversions with related pseudogenes, and/or SNPs yielding frameshift, missense, nonsense, and/or alternative splice sites. The phenotypic consequences of variant alleles and genotypes include absent, diminished, qualitatively altered, and enhanced CYP enzymatic activities. Three drug oxidation polymorphisms that have received the most clinical attention involve CYP2D6, CYP2C9, and CYP2C19. The different CYPs are products of separate genes. Thus genetic deficiency in one CYP does not imply genetic deficiencies in the others.

The oxidation polymorphism in CYP2D6 (www.pharmgkb.org/gene/PA128) was originally discovered by the toxic responses observed in some patients following administration of debrisoquine and sparteine. However, human populations with this genetic defect differ in their capacity to oxidize not only debrisoquine and sparteine but up to 25% of all currently used drugs. **Poor metabolizer (PM) CYP2D6** phenotypes result from defective splicing causing inactive enzymes, gene deletion resulting in absence of protein, and missense SNPs yielding enzymes with reduced stability or reduced substrate affinity. An **ultrarapid (UM) phenotype** resulting from **gene duplication** has also been identified. PM phenotypes experience higher concentrations of parent drug following administration and consequently suffer greater adverse effects. On the other hand, when CYP2D6 is required for prodrug activation to a more efficacious metabolite (e.g., codeine to morphine), PMs often experience therapeutic failure. The opposite effects can occur in the UM phenotype. For example, severe abdominal pain attributable to morphine has been observed in a UM patient who was treated with codeine, and as indicated in the clinical case at the beginning of this chapter, that can lead to life-threatening CNS depression.

Similarly, tamoxifen is biotransformed to the potent antiestrogen endoxifen by CYP2D6. Genetic variation and inhibitors of CYP2D6 markedly reduce endoxifen plasma concentrations in tamoxifen-treated breast cancer patients. Patients with decreased metabolism have significantly shorter time to cancer recurrence and worse relapse-free survival relative to patients with extensive metabolism. Thus the PM phenotype is an independent predictor of breast cancer outcome in postmenopausal women receiving tamoxifen for early breast cancer. Because genetically determined, impaired tamoxifen metabolism results in worse treatment outcomes, genotyping for CYP2D6 alleles can identify patients who will have little benefit from adjuvant tamoxifen therapy.

CYP2C9 (www.pharmgkb.org/gene/PA126) catalyzes the oxidation of the vitamin K antagonist warfarin, as well as other drugs including phenytoin, tolbutamide, and losartan. Over two million patients in the United States receive warfarin treatment to prevent blood clots, heart attacks, and stroke. Warfarin is a difficult drug to use because the optimal dose varies widely and depends on many factors, including genetic polymorphisms in CYP2C9 and vitamin K epoxide reductase (VKORC1 www.pharmgkb.org/gene/PA133787052, patient age, diet, and concurrent drug therapy). Allelic variants of *CYP2C9* encode enzymes with reduced or altered affinities. Individuals homozygous for certain variant *CYP2C9* alleles may exhibit up to a 90% reduction in *S*-warfarin clearance, resulting in bleeding complications during warfarin therapy. The FDA has recommended labeling changes to advise patients and health care providers regarding the effects of CYP2C9 genetic polymorphism on initial dose and response to warfarin.

CYP2C19 (www.pharmgkb.org/gene/PA124) catalyzes the oxidation of drugs including clopidogrel. Patients with poor or intermediate CYP2C19 phenotypes may experience inadequate therapeutic effects from clopidogrel therapy.

Thiopurine *S*-Methyltransferase Polymorphism (www.pharmgkb.org/gene/PA356)

Thiopurine *S*-methyltransferase (TPMT) catalyzes the **deactivating *S*-methylation** of the anticancer and antiinflammatory drugs 6-mercaptopurine, 6-thioguanine, and azathioprine. The gene encoding this enzyme exhibits genetic variation in human populations, such that the frequency of the homozygous deficient phenotype is approximately 0.3% and that of heterozygotes is about 10% in Caucasians and African Americans. Over 10 variant alleles have been identified that encode enzymes with reduced stability and/or catalytic activity. Treatment of acute lymphoblastic leukemia often requires long-term treatment with 6-mercaptopurine. Individuals with the homozygous deficient phenotype frequently develop severe hematopoietic toxicity when treated with standard doses of 6-mercaptopurine, requiring substantial reductions in dose. Individuals with heterozygous genotypes experience milder levels of toxicity. Long-term outcome studies suggest that relapse-free survival is longer in patients whose chemotherapy dosing schedules were set according to prior testing for TPMT function. 6-Mercaptopurine package inserts now provide detailed information and advice regarding pharmacogenetic *TMPT* deficiencies.

Dihydropyrimidine Dehydrogenase Polymorphism (www.pharmgkb.org/gene/PA145)

5-Fluorouracil is used extensively in the chemotherapy of solid tumors. Dihydropyrimidine dehydrogenase catalyzes the rate-limiting step in the **deactivation of 5-fluorouracil**. Patients with genetic deficiency of this enzyme have a 90% lower clearance of 5-fluorouracil and may suffer severe toxicity from even modest doses. The toxicity is dependent on the route of administration but involves rapidly dividing tissues such as bone marrow and the mucosal lining of the gastrointestinal tract. Life-threatening neurotoxicity also has been observed.

Uridine Diphosphate Glucuronosyltransferase Polymorphism (www.pharmgkb.org/gene/PA420)

Uridine diphosphate glucuronosyltransferase (UGT) catalyzes the glucuronidation of bilirubin as well as various drugs and xenobiotics. The UGT1A family of enzymes is represented in the genome by a series of four invariant exons, and the transcribed product may by spliced to any one of nine exons representing different substrate-binding domains. The family members are designated UGT1A1, 1A2, etc. UGT1A1 is the enzyme primarily responsible for bilirubin glucuronidation. UGT enzyme levels are regulated primarily through transcriptional control, and genetic variation in promoter structure influencing transcription rate. A series of thymine, adenine (TA) repeats in the proximal promoter vary in number from five to eight in populations. The lower the number of repeats, the more efficient is the transcriptional activity of the gene. The *UGT1A1*28* allele has seven TA repeats and is associated with Gilbert syndrome. The frequency of the homozygous *UGT1A1*28* genotype varies with ethnic origin but is about 10% in Caucasian and African populations and 5% in Asian populations.

Irinotecan is a topoisomerase I inhibitor that is effective against several cancers, particularly colon cancer. It is a prodrug that is converted to its active metabolite SN-38. This active metabolite is inactivated by glucuronidation catalyzed by UGT1A1. Individuals with genetic polymorphism in UGT1A1 have been shown to suffer increased toxicity (myelosuppression and diarrhea) with the use of irinotecan both alone and in combination with other anticancer drugs.

Drug Transporter Polymorphisms

A number of families of specific small-molecule transport proteins are now known to mediate the distribution of endogenous and exogenous substances across cellular membranes, thus influencing their tissue distribution and concentration. Genetic variants of many of these proteins have been identified, with consequences for drug pharmacokinetics and response. For instance, SLCO1B1 (www.pharmgkb.org/gene/PA134865839) facilitates the hepatic uptake of statins, as well as numerous endogenous compounds (e.g., bilirubin). Changes in the function of this transporter (as occur during drug–drug interactions or as a result of genetic polymorphisms in *SLCO1B1*) can markedly increase the severity of statin-related muscle damage. Simvastatin is among the most commonly used prescription medications for cholesterol reduction. A single coding single-nucleotide polymorphism in *SLCO1B1* increases systemic exposure to simvastatin and the risk of muscle toxicity.

PHARMACOGENETIC POLYMORPHISMS IN DRUG TARGETS

Since therapeutic response is often more difficult to quantify than plasma drug concentration, genetic polymorphisms in drug targets have been less extensively characterized. However, there is little doubt that genetic polymorphisms exist in most if not all proteins, including drug receptors. Several genetic polymorphisms reported in recent years are provided here as examples. It is anticipated that many more clinically relevant genetic polymorphisms in drug receptors will be discovered in the near future.

β-Adrenergic Receptor Polymorphisms

β-Adrenergic receptors mediate critical sympathetic responses in the cardiovascular, pulmonary, metabolic, and central nervous systems. β_2-Adrenergic agonists such as albuterol are potent bronchodilators widely used in the treatment of asthma. Other β-adrenergic agonists are administered to increase cardiac output in the emergency management of cardiogenic shock and decompensated congestive heart failure. Antagonists of β-adrenergic receptors are used to treat several disorders including hypertension and heart failure.

Genetic polymorphisms in both β_1 and β_2 receptors have been identified in human populations. β_2-Adrenergic receptor genotype variation has been shown to affect therapeutic response to β_2-selective agonists such as albuterol. Polymorphisms in β receptors potentially influence drug treatment of cardiovascular diseases in two ways. The primary effect is alteration of agonist or antagonist efficacy because of a variant β_1 or β_2 receptor. However, the influence on drug efficacy also may be secondary to an effect of the polymorphism on cardiovascular function. For example, a β_2-receptor variant is associated with lower systemic vascular resistance and a greater vasodilatory response. Thus individuals with this β_2-receptor variant might be more sensitive to a vasodilator (such as captopril) acting via another mechanism, secondary to the altered systemic vascular tone.

Dopamine and Other Receptor Polymorphisms

Genetic polymorphisms in **dopamine receptors** have been associated with drug abuse liability and the reinforcing effects of alcohol, cocaine, and nicotine. Genetically variant dopamine receptors are also associated with increased incidence of tardive dyskinesias following long-term treatment of schizophrenia with dopamine receptor antagonists. Schizophrenia is itself a complex set of diseases that is not adequately managed in many patients. Accordingly, both typical and atypical antipsychotic drugs have been found to be effective in some but not all patients with schizophrenia. Genetic polymorphisms in antipsychotic medication receptor targets (dopaminergic, adrenergic, serotoninergic, and/or histaminergic receptor subtypes) have been associated with different clinical responses. Combinations of drug target polymorphisms and drug metabolism variants may eventually form the basis for targeting genetic subgroups of patients with schizophrenia for effective treatment with both typical antipsychotics and newer atypical antipsychotic drugs.

IMPLICATIONS FOR DENTISTRY

The elucidation of the human genome—coupled with advancements in DNA array technology, high-throughput genotyping, and bioinformatics—will soon enable rapid elucidation of complex genetic factors necessary for better optimization of drug therapy. Pharmacogenomics will increasingly result in the development of drugs that are targeted to specific, genetically identifiable subgroups of the population. Some drugs previously abandoned for clinical use because they proved toxic in some patients may return to clinical use, but with restrictions for specific genetic subgroups. Health care providers, including dentists, will be accountable for **prescribing drugs appropriately to genetic subgroups**. For example, recent **FDA black box warnings** regarding prescribing **codeine** for tonsillectomy and/or adenoidectomy may affect prescription of codeine by dentists to alleviate tooth pain. **Automated genotyping systems** and easily accessible genetic information will provide critical information necessary for optimal drug therapy in the individual patient. Although the determination and accessibility of human pharmacogenetic information has potential ethical and legal concerns, patient-specific pharmacogenetic information is already being incorporated into patients' electronic health records. For example, St. Jude's Children's Research Hospital is preemptively determining patient genotypes for over 200 genes, and this information is released into the patient electronic health records to guide prescribing of selected drugs.

CASE DISCUSSION

1. This patient is a genetically ultrarapid-metabolizer (UM) at the CYP2D6 gene locus, possessing additional functionally expressed copies of the gene and thus elevated levels of its enzyme product. The UM phenotype occurs more frequently in individuals from North Africa. CYP2D6 is responsible for the conversion of codeine into its active analgesic metabolite morphine, and in UMs, excessive CYP2D6-mediated production of morphine leads to symptoms of morphine overdose, of which respiratory depression is the most serious.
2. Intravenous administration of naloxone (0.4 mg), repeated two times, resulted in a dramatic improvement in the patient's level of consciousness. Subsequent titration of naloxone (by continuous IV perfusion of 0.4 mg per hour for 6 hours) resulted in a normal level of consciousness and resolution of the respiratory failure. Two days after the acute event, the patient had recovered completely. Naloxone is a competitive antagonist of the μ-opioid receptor, and it is therefore able to reverse the respiratory depression produced by the agonist action of morphine at this receptor. (See Chapter 16.)

GENERAL REFERENCES

1. Eichelbaum M, Ingelman-Sundberg M, Evans WE: Pharmacogenomics and individualized drug therapy, *Annu Rev Med* 57:119–137, 2006.
2. Ma Q, Lu AY: Pharmacogenetics, pharmacogenomics, and individualized medicine, *Pharmacol Rev* 63(2):437–459, 2011.
3. McDonagh EM, Boukouvala S, Aklillu E, Hein DW, Altman RB, Klein TE: PharmGKB summary: very important pharmacogene information for N-acetyltransferase 2, *Pharmacogenet Genomics* 24(8):409–425, 2014.
4. Nebert DW, Zhang G, Vesell ES: From human genetics and genomics to pharmacogenetics and pharmacogenomics: past lessons, future directions, *Drug Metab Rev* 40(2):187–224, 2008.
5. Roden DM, Altman RB, Benowitz NL, Flockhart DA, Giacomini KM, Johnson JA, Krauss RM, McLeod HL, Ratain MJ, Relling MV, Ring HZ, Shuldiner AR, Weinshilboum RM, Weiss ST: Pharmacogenomics: challenges and opportunities, *Ann Intern Med* 145(10):749–757, 2006.
6. Rollason V, Samer C, Piguet V, Dayer P, Desmeules J: Pharmacogenetics of analgesics: toward the individualization of prescription, *Pharmacogenomics* 9(7):905–933, 2008.
7. Roses AD: Pharmacogenetics in drug discovery and development: a translational perspective, *Nat Rev Drug Discov* 7(10):807–817, 2008.
8. Sillon G, Joly Y, Feldman S, Avard D: An ethical and legal overview of pharmacogenomics: perspectives and issues, *Med Law* 27(4):843–857, 2008.
9. Weaver JM: New FDA black box warning for codeine: how will this affect dentists? *Anesth Prog* 60(2):35–36, 2013.
10. Weinshilboum RM, Wang L: Pharmacogenetics and pharmacogenomics: development, science, and translation, *Annu Rev Genomics Hum Genet* 7:223–245, 2006.
11. Zhou SF, Di YM, Chan E, Du YM, Chow VD, Xue CC, Lai X, Wang JC, Li CG, Tian M, Duan W: Clinical pharmacogenetics and potential application in personalized medicine, *Curr Drug Metab* 9(8):738–784, 2008.

PART II

Pharmacology of Specific Drug Groups

5

Introduction to Autonomic Nervous System Drugs

Peter W. Abel and Michael T. Piascik

KEY INFORMATION

- The autonomic nervous system regulates the function of smooth muscles, the heart, and certain secretory glands.
- Sympathetic division nerve pathways originate in thoracic and lumbar regions of the spinal cord.
- Parasympathetic division nerve pathways originate in cranial and sacral regions of the spinal cord.
- Norepinephrine is the neurotransmitter released from most postganglionic sympathetic nerves; whereas both norepinephrine and epinephrine are released from the adrenal medulla.
- Acetylcholine is the neurotransmitter released from all nerves in the parasympathetic nervous system.
- Norepinephrine and epinephrine produce their effects by activating α- and/or β-adrenergic receptors on organs and tissues.
- Acetylcholine produces its effects by activating nicotinic or muscarinic receptors on nerves, organs, or tissues.
- Although the autonomic nervous system can function autonomously, the central nervous system can contribute a significant regulatory effect to autonomic function.

CASE

Your patient, Mr. K, arrives early for his appointment at noon for removal of impacted third molars. He seems impatient because he cannot be seen immediately for his procedure. You notice that he is sweating and seems anxious about his visit. When preparing him for his procedure, you notice his face becomes flushed; he reports he can feel his heart beating in this chest. What is a likely cause of the signs and symptoms shown by Mr. K? What factors could contribute to this reaction? What drugs or other treatments would be helpful to reduce or prevent this reaction?

AUTONOMIC NERVOUS SYSTEM

The autonomic nervous system (ANS) and the endocrine system are the major regulatory systems for controlling homeostatic functions. These two systems collectively regulate and coordinate the cardiovascular, respiratory, gastrointestinal, renal, reproductive, metabolic, and immunologic systems. This chapter introduces the pharmacology of the ANS. An understanding of the pharmacology of agents affecting the ANS rests on two basic foundations: a knowledge of the structural and functional organization of the ANS and an understanding of where certain neurotransmitters are located and how these neurotransmitters affect cellular function.

The ANS, also referred to as the visceral, vegetative, or involuntary nervous system, regulates the function of smooth muscle, the heart, and certain secretory glands. These structures function in the absence of neuronal input, but the ANS contributes a regulatory and coordinating function. Most of our knowledge of the ANS is restricted to efferent functions; much less is known about the afferent limb. Sensory afferent fibers carry impulses that are received and organized centrally, often at an unconscious level. A person is unaware of impulses generated at the baroreceptors, although these impulses may trigger a generalized body response, such as a reflex decrease in blood pressure, which the person may sense. It has been estimated that approximately 80% of the vagus nerve consists of primary afferent fibers; nevertheless, most currently available ANS drugs influence efferent activity.

Anatomy

In contrast to the somatic nervous system, the ANS consists of a two-neuron system in which preganglionic nerves emanate from cell bodies in the cerebrospinal axis synapse with postganglionic nerves originating in autonomic ganglia outside the CNS (Figure 5-1). The ANS is divided into two parts on the basis of the anatomic characteristics of each division. The sympathetic division includes nerve pathways that originate in the thoracolumbar regions of the spinal cord, whereas the parasympathetic division includes nerve pathways from the craniosacral regions of the cerebrospinal axis.

Sympathetic nervous system

The organizational anatomy of the two divisions of the ANS is shown in greater detail in Figure 5-2. The sympathetic division originates from neurons with cell bodies located in the **intermediolateral columns of the spinal cord**, extending from the first thoracic to the third lumbar segments. The myelinated preganglionic fibers emerge with the ventral roots of the spinal nerves and synapse with second neurons in one of three possible types of ganglia: paravertebral, prevertebral, or terminal. The paravertebral ganglia are composed of 22 pairs of ganglia lying on either side of the spinal cord. The superior cervical ganglia (the topmost pair) innervate structures in the head and neck, including the submandibular glands; whereas the superior, middle, and inferior cervical ganglia all innervate the heart. The prevertebral ganglia are located in the abdomen and pelvis and include the celiac, superior mesenteric, and inferior mesenteric, which innervate the stomach, the small intestine, and the colon. The few terminal ganglia lie near the organs they innervate, principally the urinary bladder and rectum.

A striking anatomic aspect of the sympathetic nervous system, and one that has great functional significance, is that a single preganglionic

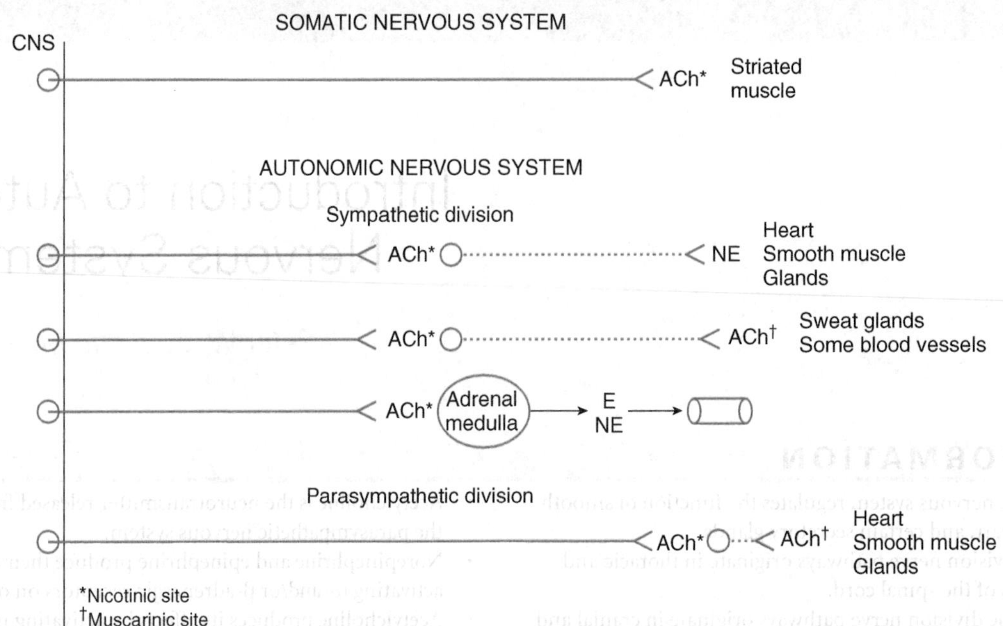

FIG 5-1 Functional organization of the somatic nervous system and the autonomic nervous system, with the structures innervated by the different nerves and the chemical mediators responsible for transmission at the various sites. *Solid lines* indicate somatic motor or preganglionic autonomic nerves; *dashed lines* indicate postganglionic autonomic nerves. *ACh,* Acetylcholine; *E,* epinephrine; *NE,* norepinephrine.

nerve may contact 20 or more postganglionic nerves. Impulses arising in one preganglionic neuron of the sympathetic nervous system may ultimately affect many postganglionic neurons, which explains the diffuse and widespread character of sympathetic nervous system responses. Stimulation of the sympathetic nervous system also activates nerves that innervate the adrenal medulla and cause it to release a mixture of the catecholamines epinephrine and norepinephrine. This release provides an additional basis for the widespread effects of the sympathetic nervous system.

Parasympathetic nervous system

The parasympathetic nervous system, or **craniosacral division,** has its origin in neurons with cell bodies located in the brainstem nuclei of four cranial nerves—the oculomotor (cranial nerve III), the facial (cranial nerve VII), the glossopharyngeal (cranial nerve IX), and the vagus (cranial nerve X)—and in the second, third, and fourth segments of the sacral spinal cord. The preganglionic nerves arising from the brainstem form part of the cranial nerves and travel with them to synapse with postganglionic neurons located in ganglia near or actually within the structures innervated. The midbrain outflow from the nucleus of the oculomotor nerve synapses in the ciliary ganglion located in the orbit. The ganglion gives rise to nerves that supply the ciliary muscle and the sphincter muscle of the eye. Neurons of the facial nerve that synapse in the sublingual and submandibular ganglia form the chorda tympani and provide innervation to the sublingual and submandibular glands. Other neurons of the facial nerve synapse in the sphenopalatine ganglion; postganglionic nerves terminate in the lacrimal gland and in mucus-secreting glands of the nose, palate, and pharynx. Nerves originating in the glossopharyngeal nuclei synapse in the otic ganglion; its postganglionic neurons innervate the parotid gland. A major component of the cranial outflow is the vagus nerve, which originates from vagal nuclei in the medulla oblongata. Preganglionic nerves pass to ganglia located within the heart and the viscera of the thorax and abdomen. Postganglionic nerves, very short in length, arise from these ganglia to terminate in the aforementioned structures. Neurons originating from sacral segments form the pelvic nerves, which synapse in terminal ganglia lying near or within the uterus, bladder, rectum, and sex organs.

In contrast to the arrangement in the sympathetic nervous system, there is little divergence in the parasympathetic nervous system. Responses are more focused. The parasympathetic nervous system is characterized by long preganglionic and very short postganglionic nerves and, with only a few exceptions, an absence of well-defined, anatomically distinct ganglia.

Functional Characteristics

Most organs are dually innervated by the sympathetic and parasympathetic nervous systems, such as most salivary glands, the heart, and abdominal and pelvic viscera, whereas other organs receive innervation from only one division. The **sweat glands, adrenal medulla, piloerector muscles**, and most **blood vessels** receive innervation from only the **sympathetic nervous system.** The parenchyma of the parotid, lacrimal, and nasopharyngeal glands are supplied only with parasympathetic nerves. Table 5-1 lists the organs to which nerve fibers of the parasympathetic and sympathetic nervous systems are distributed, the effects of stimulation of these nerves, and the autonomic receptors that are activated by neurotransmitters released from autonomic nerves.

To understand or predict the effects of autonomic drugs on a specific organ, it is necessary to know how each division of the ANS affects that organ, whether the organ is singly or dually innervated, and, if dually, which of the two systems is dominant in the organ. In most circumstances, one or the other of the two divisions of the ANS will provide the dominant influence, but often neither division is totally dominant in many of the dually innervated organs. The fact that both divisions of the ANS modulate the intrinsic activity of the various tissues cannot be overemphasized.

The anatomic and functional characteristics of the two divisions of the ANS show that there are striking differences between the

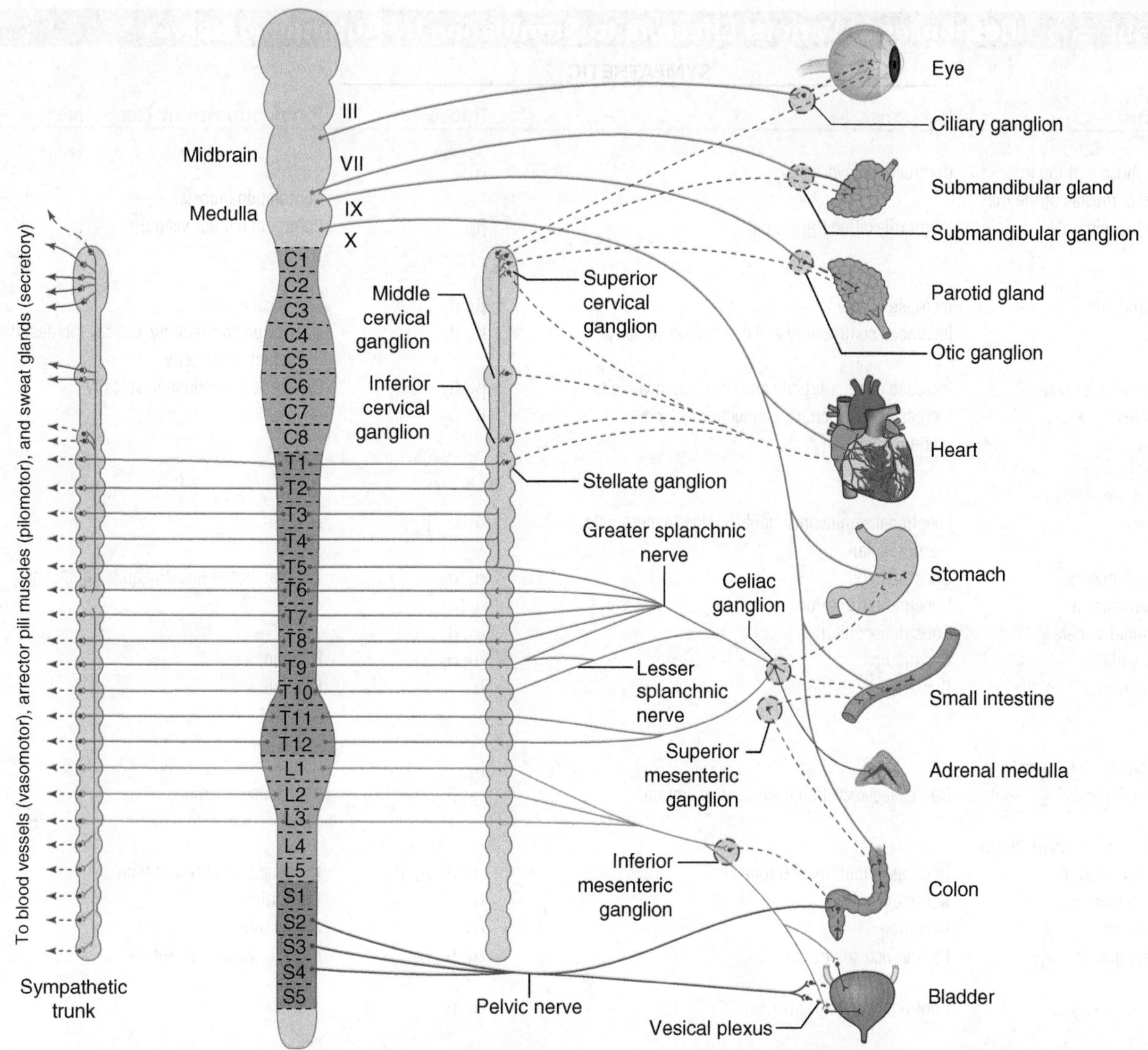

FIG 5-2 General arrangement of the autonomic nervous system showing one side of the bilateral outflow. On either side of the spinal cord (*C1* to *S5*) are pictured the two chains of the paravertebral sympathetic ganglia. Preganglionic nerves of the sympathetic nervous system are indicated by *light solid lines;* postganglionic nerves of the sympathetic nervous system are indicated by *light dashed lines.* Preganglionic nerves of the parasympathetic nervous system, originating from the brain and sacral spinal cord, are shown by *bold solid lines;* postganglionic nerves of the parasympathetic nervous system are shown by *bold dashed lines.* (Adapted from Kelly DE, Wood RL, Enders AC: *Bailey's textbook of histology,* ed 18, Baltimore, 1984, Williams & Wilkins.)

sympathetic and parasympathetic nervous systems. The sympathetic nervous system can produce a widespread and massive response that would enable an organism confronted with a stressor (e.g., pain, asphyxia, or strong emotions) to mount an appropriate response (**"fright, fight, or flight"**). In dental patients, oral surgical procedures constitute physiologically significant stressors that can stimulate the sympathetic nervous system. The parasympathetic division is primarily concerned with the conservation and restoration of bodily resources. These differences in function are subserved by some of the anatomic characteristics that have already been mentioned, including the involvement of the adrenal medulla and the high ratio of postganglionic to preganglionic nerves in the sympathetic, but not the parasympathetic, nervous system.

NEUROTRANSMITTERS

The concept of chemical mediators of neurotransmission of information emerged at the end of the nineteenth century. **Acetylcholine** was identified as the primary neurotransmitter released from **preganglionic nerves** and from **postganglionic nerves** in the **parasympathetic nervous system.** Norepinephrine was found to be the neurotransmitter released from most postganglionic sympathetic nerves, whereas norepinephrine and epinephrine are released after sympathetic stimulation of the adrenal medulla. Although acetylcholine, norepinephrine, and epinephrine have come to be recognized as the principal mediators of ANS activity, evidence exists that other molecules, including dopamine, adenosine triphosphate (ATP), neuropeptide Y, and calcitonin

TABLE 5-1 Responses of Various Effectors to Stimulation by Autonomic Nerves

	SYMPATHETIC		
Effector	**Response**	**Receptor**	**Parasympathetic Response***
Eye			
Radial muscle of the iris	Contraction (mydriasis)	α_1	—
Sphincter muscle of the iris	—		Contraction (miosis)
Ciliary muscle	Slight relaxation (far vision)	β_2	Contraction (near vision)
Heart†			
Sinoatrial node	Increase in rate	β_1, β_2	Decrease in rate
Atria	Increased contractility and conduction velocity	β_1, β_2	Decreased contractility, usually increased conduction velocity
Atrioventricular node	Increase in automaticity and conduction velocity	β_1, β_2	Decrease in conduction velocity
Ventricles	Increased contractility, conduction velocity, and automaticity	β_1, β_2	—
Blood Vessels‡			
Coronary	Functional significance doubtful due to metabolic autoregulation	$\alpha_1, \alpha_2, \beta_2$	—
Skin and mucosa	Constriction	α_1, α_2	Dilation, but of questionable significance
Skeletal muscle	Constriction; dilation	α, β_2§	—
Abdominal viscera	Constriction; dilation	α_1, β_2	—
Salivary glands	Constriction	α_1, α_2	Dilation
Erectile tissue	Constriction	α	Dilation
Lungs			
Bronchial smooth muscle	Relaxation	β_2	Contraction
Bronchial glands	Decreased secretion; increased secretion	α_1, β_2	Increased secretion
Gastrointestinal Tract			
Smooth muscle	Decreased motility and tone	$\alpha_1, \alpha_2, \beta_1, \beta_2$	Increased motility and tone
Sphincters	Contraction	α_1	Relaxation
Secretion	Inhibition	α_2	Stimulation
Salivary glands	Protein-rich secretion‖	$\alpha_1, \beta_1, \beta_2$	Profuse, watery secretion
Spleen capsule	Contraction; mild relaxation	α_1, β_2	—
Urinary Bladder			
Detrusor	Relaxation	β_2, β_3	Contraction
Trigone and sphincter	Contraction	α_1	Relaxation
Ureter			
Motility and tone	Increased	α_1	Increased (?)
Uterus	Variable, depending on species, endocrine status	α_1, β_2	Variable
Miscellaneous			
Pilomotor muscles	Contraction	α_1	—
Sweat glands	Secretion¶		—
Liver	Glycogenolysis, gluconeogenesis	α_1, β_2	Glycogen synthesis
Adipose tissue	Lipolysis	$\alpha_1, \beta_1, \beta_3$	—

*All parasympathetic responses are mediated by activation of muscarinic receptors. Most responses are mediated by predominantly M_3-muscarinic receptors, except in the heart where M_2-muscarinic receptors dominate.

†Norepinephrine released from sympathetic nerves activates primarily β_1 receptors; epinephrine released from the adrenal medulla stimulates β_1 and β_2 receptors. The predominant adrenergic receptor in the heart is β_1.

‡In most smooth muscles, including blood vessels, α_1 receptors contract (constrict), whereas β_2 receptors relax (dilate). Prejunctional α_2 receptors on sympathetic nerve terminals inhibit norepinephrine release, which relaxes blood vessels and causes vasodilation; postjunctional α_2 receptors cause vasoconstriction.

§Blood vessels in skeletal muscle are innervated by some sympathetic nerves that release acetylcholine, which acts on muscarinic receptors to cause vasodilation. However, their functional significance is doubtful.

‖The human parotid glands do not receive sympathetic innervation.

¶The sweat glands receive sympathetic innervation, but with few exceptions (e.g., the sweat glands of the palms of the hands, which are activated by α_1 receptor stimulation), the transmitter is acetylcholine, and the receptors activated are muscarinic.

gene–related peptide, may also serve as chemical transmitters for specific neuronal circuits.

Location of Adrenergic and Cholinergic Junctions

Figure 5-1 showed the sites at which the neurotransmitters acetylcholine and norepinephrine and the hormone epinephrine act as chemical mediators. With the exception of effectors (smooth muscle, the heart, and secretory glands) that are innervated by postganglionic sympathetic nerves where the neurotransmitter is norepinephrine, all other sites are innervated by cholinergic nerves, including the ganglia of the ANS, the adrenal medulla, a few effectors of the sympathetic nervous system, and all the effectors of the parasympathetic nervous system. At cholinergic junctions, cholinergic nerves release acetylcholine, which acts on cholinergic receptors to produce an effect. Cholinergic receptors are composed of two structurally unrelated types, called muscarinic and nicotinic, which are located at specific sites in the ANS. Muscarinic receptors are located on effectors innervated by cholinergic nerves; this includes effectors at postganglionic parasympathetic junctions and a few postganglionic sympathetic junctions (**most sweat glands** and some blood vessels). Nicotinic receptors are found at different anatomic sites, including postganglionic nerve cell bodies at all autonomic ganglia, the adrenal medulla, and skeletal muscle in the somatic nervous system. There are also different types of structurally related **adrenergic receptors** (α_1, α_2, β_1, β_2, β_3) that are found at postganglionic sympathetic junctions where norepinephrine is released from postganglionic sympathetic nerves. These adrenergic receptors do not have a precise anatomic distribution, however; some effector organs have only a single adrenergic receptor, whereas other organs have two or more adrenergic receptor types. Research has revealed the existence of additional subtypes of these adrenergic and cholinergic receptors, however; there are few clinically used drugs that selectively interact with these receptor subtypes.

ADRENERGIC NEUROTRANSMISSION

Catecholamine Synthesis

The catecholamines norepinephrine and epinephrine are the primary neurotransmitters and hormones released after stimulation of the sympathetic nervous system. The synthesis and storage of the catecholamines can be modified by a number of clinically useful drugs. The synthetic process, shown in Figure 5-3, involves numerous enzymes that are synthesized in the nerve cell body and carried by axoplasmic transport to the nerve endings. The enzyme **tyrosine hydroxylase**, which catalyzes the conversion of tyrosine to dihydroxyphenylalanine, is the rate-limiting enzyme in this process; any drug that inhibits the function of tyrosine hydroxylase reduces the rate at which norepinephrine is produced in the nerve terminal. The concentration of norepinephrine in the cytoplasm is one of the factors that regulates its own formation, principally by feedback inhibition on tyrosine hydroxylase activity. The enzyme **phenylethanolamine N-methyltransferase**, which catalyzes the conversion of norepinephrine to epinephrine, occurs almost exclusively in the chromaffin cells of the adrenal medulla and is missing in peripheral nerve terminals. Norepinephrine is the final product in most adrenergic nerves, whereas mainly epinephrine (80%), with some norepinephrine (20%), is produced in adrenal chromaffin cells in humans.

Catecholamine Release

Evidence suggests that 95% of intracellular norepinephrine is stored in vesicles, where it is protected from intracellular enzymatic destruction until it is released by depolarization; the other 5% is found in the cytoplasm. Most norepinephrine is stored in vesicles complexed with the protein chromogranin, the enzyme dopamine β-hydroxylase, and ATP. There are two different norepinephrine pools inside the neuron: a mobile pool and a reserve pool. Membrane depolarization causes release of transmitter from the mobile pool. A diagrammatic representation of the adrenergic nerve terminal is shown in Figure 5-4.

Autonomic neuroeffector junctions are less structurally organized than the neuromuscular junction. The autonomic axon resembles a string of beads as it passes among smooth muscle fibers in blood vessels and other sites (see Figure 5-4). The beaded varicosities release neurotransmitter near directly innervated effector cells. As the nerve impulse passes down the axon, and depolarization successively involves each varicosity, extracellular Ca^{2+} enters into the nerve terminals, and norepinephrine is released into the junctional cleft by the process of exocytosis. After crossing the junctional cleft by passive diffusion, the

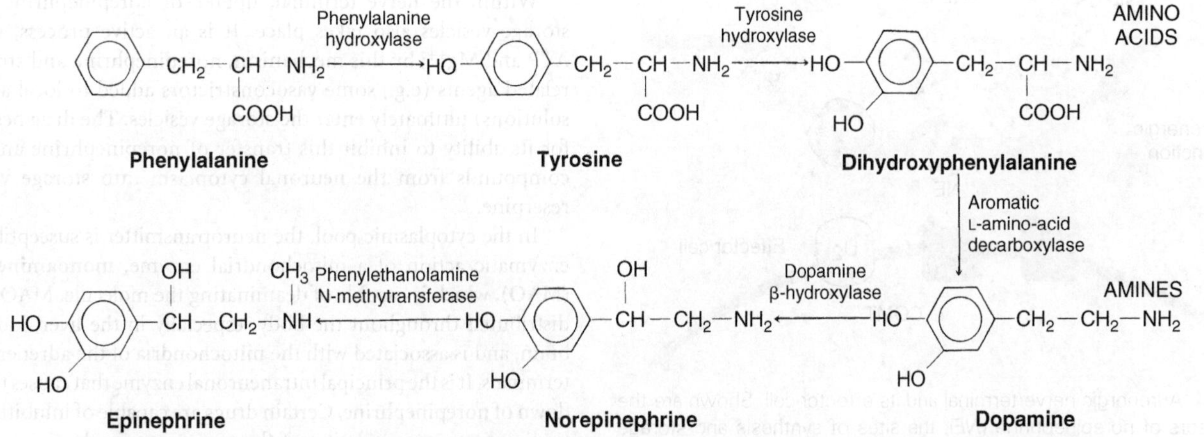

FIG 5-3 Biosynthesis of adrenergic transmitters. The amino acids in the top row can penetrate the blood–brain barrier, whereas the amines in the bottom row cannot. Conversion of dopamine into norepinephrine occurs in the storage vesicles of adrenergic nerves and the adrenal medulla, whereas conversion of norepinephrine to epinephrine occurs only in storage vesicles in the adrenal medulla and in some neurons of the central nervous system. The enzyme tyrosine hydroxylase is the rate-limiting regulatory enzyme in the synthesis of catecholamines and is a target for the enzyme inhibitor metyrosine.

transmitter binds to receptor sites on the effector organ and elicits an appropriate response.

Adrenergic Receptors

In 1948, Ahlquist first proposed the existence of two kinds of adrenergic receptors. He called these alpha (**α**) and beta (**β**). Two types of the β-adrenergic receptors, called $\boldsymbol{\beta_1}$ and $\boldsymbol{\beta_2}$, were next identified, followed by two different α-adrenergic receptors: α_1, the predominant postjunctional receptor, and α_2, located prejunctionally and postjunctionally. The presence or absence of these different adrenergic receptors, identified in part by experiments using synthetic drugs (agonists and antagonists) highly selective for individual adrenergic receptor types, provides an explanation for the seemingly contradictory (or opposing) actions of the adrenergic transmitters (e.g., vasodilation in some vascular beds and vasoconstriction in others; see Table 5-1).

More recent molecular cloning and pharmacologic studies have shown the existence of multiple subtypes of adrenergic receptors. The α_1-adrenergic receptor family consists of three subtypes, classified as $\boldsymbol{\alpha_{1A}}$, $\boldsymbol{\alpha_{1B}}$, **and** $\boldsymbol{\alpha_{1D}}$. Similar studies have shown the existence of multiple subtypes of the α_2 receptors ($\boldsymbol{\alpha_{2A}}$, $\boldsymbol{\alpha_{2B}}$, $\boldsymbol{\alpha_{2C}}$) and the β-adrenergic receptors ($\boldsymbol{\beta_1}$, $\boldsymbol{\beta_2}$, $\boldsymbol{\beta_3}$). The human β_2 receptor is a protein of 413 amino acids, with seven transmembrane-spanning domains (see Chapter 1). This heptahelical structure is a general characteristic of many cell surface neurotransmitter receptors. Because many of these receptors seem to have substantial differences in tissue distribution and function, considerable research is being directed toward the development of drugs with selectivity at individual receptor subtypes. These drugs may possess greater specificity of action compared with currently used adrenergic agonists or antagonists.

As can be seen in Table 5-1, some organs express only one type of adrenergic receptor, whereas others have several types. α_1-Adrenergic receptors mediate smooth muscle contraction and stimulate metabolic functions such as, glycogenolysis and lipolysis. The function of α_2 receptors at postjunctional sites includes vascular smooth muscle contraction. Norepinephrine acts on prejunctional α_2 receptors to inhibit neurotransmitter release. Centrally, α_2 receptors are known to be involved in the regulation of blood pressure. Although several important exceptions exist, β_1 receptors are often associated with excitatory cellular responses, and β_2 receptors are associated with relaxation. β_3 Receptors stimulate lipolysis in fat cells and relax the detrusor muscle in the bladder.

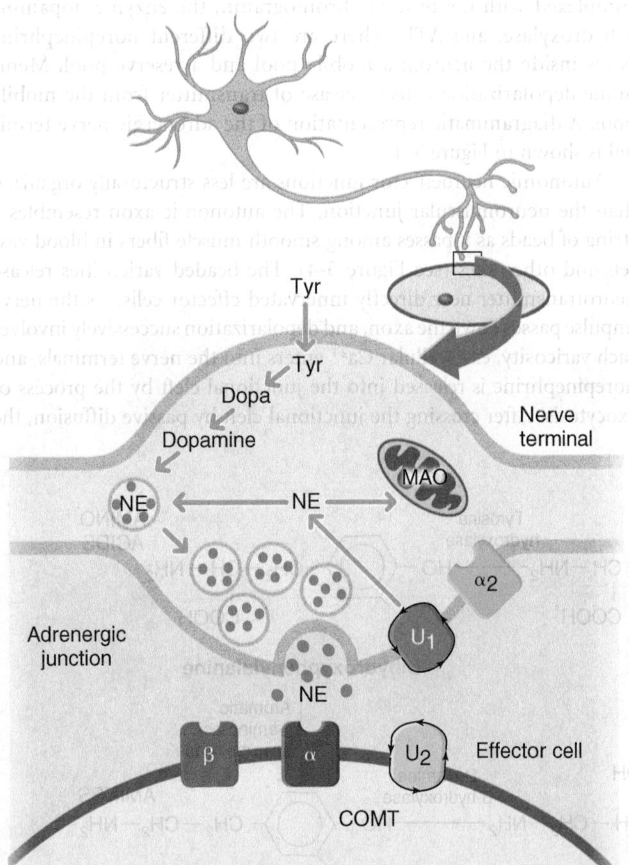

FIG 5-4 Adrenergic nerve terminal and its effector cell. Shown are the precursors of norepinephrine (*NE*), the sites of synthesis and storage of dopamine and NE, and the location of prejunctional and postjunctional adrenergic receptors (α_2, α, β). It also shows the enzymatic (catechol-O-methyltransferase [*COMT*], monoamine oxidase [*MAO*]) and neuronal (uptake-1, U_1) and extraneuronal (uptake-2, U_2) mechanisms by which the action of NE is terminated. *Dopa,* Dihydroxyphenylalanine; *Tyr,* tyrosine.

Catecholamine Fate

The fate of the released catecholamines and systems responsible for termination of their action are quite different from mechanisms of neurotransmitter termination at cholinergic junctions. At adrenergic junctions, uptake of the transmitter accounts for the greatest proportion of transmitter loss, with enzymatic breakdown and diffusion away from the junction responsible for only a small percentage of the total. As depicted in Figure 5-4, uptake can be neuronal (**uptake-1,** U_1) or extraneuronal (**uptake-2,** U_2). Neuronal uptake by the **norepinephrine transporter** requires energy and extracellular Na^+ and exhibits stereospecificity. Amphetamines, tyramine, and levonordefrin (α-methylnorepinephrine) are examples of drugs that are taken up by this transporter system. Inhibitors of neuronal uptake include cocaine and imipramine. Extraneuronal uptake by the *extraneuronal transporter*, also called *organic cation transporter 3,* has a greater capacity but lower affinity than neuronal uptake. At high concentrations of norepinephrine, extraneuronal uptake results in the rapid removal of the transmitter. Extraneuronal uptake is insensitive to neuronal uptake inhibitors such as cocaine.

Within the nerve terminal, uptake of norepinephrine into the storage vesicles also takes place. It is an active process, requiring ATP and Mg^{++}; by this mechanism, norepinephrine and structurally related agents (e.g., some vasoconstrictors added to local anesthetic solutions) ultimately enter the storage vesicles. The drug best known for its ability to inhibit this transfer of norepinephrine and related compounds from the neuronal cytoplasm into storage vesicles is reserpine.

In the cytoplasmic pool, the neurotransmitter is susceptible to the enzymatic action of a mitochondrial enzyme, **monoamine oxidase (MAO)**, which is capable of deaminating the molecule. MAO is widely distributed throughout the body, especially in the liver, kidney, and brain, and is associated with the mitochondria of the adrenergic nerve terminals. It is the principal intraneuronal enzyme that causes the breakdown of norepinephrine. Certain drugs are capable of inhibiting MAO, leading to an accumulation of the transmitter in the nerve terminal, an effect that has physiologic and therapeutic implications. A second enzyme that causes the breakdown of norepinephrine is **catechol-O-methyltransferase (COMT)**. It is widely distributed in many tissues and is the principal extraneuronal enzyme involved with the metabolic inactivation of norepinephrine.

CHOLINERGIC TRANSMISSION

Synthesis, Release, and Fate of Acetylcholine

The general concept of transmitter synthesis, storage, and removal also applies to acetylcholine at cholinergic junctions of the ANS. As shown in Figure 5-5, the synthesis of acetylcholine begins with the conversion of choline to acetylcholine in the nerve terminal. This is accomplished by the enzyme **choline acetyltransferase**, which uses the mitochondrial cofactor acetyl coenzyme A as the acetyl group donor for the reaction. The newly synthesized acetylcholine is then transported into and stored in vesicles. Like the adrenergic neurotransmitter release process described earlier, depolarization of the nerve terminal triggers a Ca^{2+}-dependent vesicular transported to the prejunctional membrane to make contact with specialized docking proteins and releases the contents of the vesicles by exocytosis. Acetylcholine crosses the junctional cleft and attaches reversibly to the postjunctional receptors, which exist in close proximity to a highly specific enzyme, **acetylcholinesterase (AChE)**. Acetylcholine becomes bound to the enzyme at two primary sites (see Chapter 6) and is hydrolyzed to choline and acetate at such a rapid rate that the nerve can respond to another stimulus milliseconds later. The choline produced by the action of AChE is returned to the nerve terminal by a carrier membrane transport mechanism and is used again in the synthesis of acetylcholine.

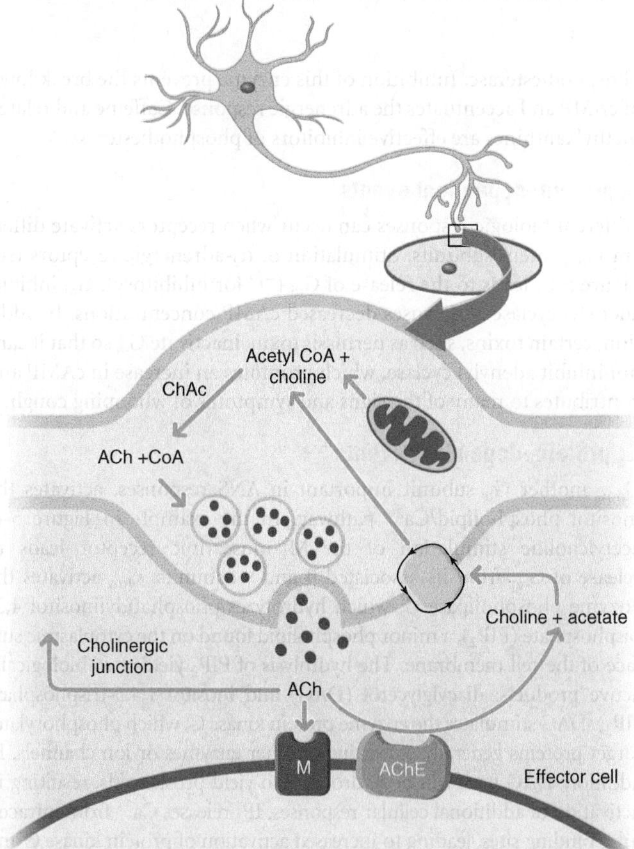

FIG 5-5 Cholinergic nerve terminal and its effector, in which are shown the intraneuronal synthesis of acetylcholine (*ACh*), the vesicles containing ACh, the release of ACh into the junctional cleft, its removal by the action of acetylcholinesterase (*AChE*) and diffusion, and the subsequent reuptake of choline back into the nerve terminal. *CoA,* Coenzyme A; *ChAc,* choline acetyltransferase; *M,* muscarinic receptor. (Adapted from Hubbard JI: Mechanism of transmitter release from nerve terminals, *Ann N Y Acad Sci* 183:131-146, 1971.)

Even in the total absence of AChE activity, the action of acetylcholine can also be terminated quickly by pseudocholinesterase, a nonspecific plasma enzyme also known as butyrocholinesterase, which is found in many tissues, including blood. Clinically, a subpopulation of patients lacks plasma pseudocholinesterase activity and can have prolonged paralysis with muscle-relaxing agents such as succinylcholine, which is metabolized primarily by this enzyme (see Chapter 7). Acetylcholine is also removed from the junctional cleft by the process of diffusion.

Cholinergic Receptors

As with the adrenergic receptors, receptors for acetylcholine can be separated into two major categories: nicotinic and muscarinic. The anatomic distribution and functional significance of these receptors have been described (see Table 5-1 and Figures 5-1 and 5-2). Nicotinic receptors outside the CNS are located on postganglionic nerves in autonomic ganglia, on chromaffin cells in the adrenal medulla, and on skeletal muscle in neuromuscular junctions. Nicotinic receptors on postganglionic neurons and in the adrenal medulla are classified as **N_N (nerve) receptors; N_M (muscle) receptors** are found on skeletal muscle in neuromuscular junctions. In contrast to adrenergic receptors and muscarinic receptors, nicotinic receptors are ion channel receptors composed of an allosteric protein containing four different subunit types—α, β, δ, and γ—gathered together in a transmembrane pentamer. Each of the subunits has an intracellular and extracellular exposure, and together they surround a central channel. Recognition sites for acetylcholine and other agonists, cholinergic antagonists, and certain bacterial toxins are located primarily on the α subunits.

Muscarinic receptors of the ANS are located primarily on effector cells—smooth muscle, the heart, and secretory glands—that are innervated by postganglionic parasympathetic nerves. Molecular cloning studies have deduced the amino acid sequence of **five subtypes of muscarinic receptors** classified as M_1 to M_5. As with adrenergic receptors, muscarinic receptors all have seven transmembrane-spanning domains and display the same general structure as the adrenergic receptors.

SIGNAL TRANSDUCTION AND SECOND MESSENGERS

The binding of an autonomic neurotransmitter to its receptor on the plasma membrane surface of a target cell initiates a signaling cascade that alters the physiologic activity of the cell. The exact response elicited depends not on the neurotransmitter per se, but on the type of receptor activated. There are two general classes of membrane-bound receptors that interact with autonomic drugs: ion channel–linked and G protein–linked receptors.

Ion Channel–Linked Receptors

Ion channel–linked receptors, otherwise known as ionotropic receptors, are ligand-gated ion channels that undergo binding-dependent conformational changes leading to an opening of the ion channel (see Chapter 7). The nicotinic receptor is a ligand-gated ion channel that, when activated, leads to rapid membrane depolarization as a result of the net inward passage of positively charged ions through the channel. The nicotinic receptor increases the permeability of the cell membrane to Na^+, producing an excitatory postsynaptic potential that activates neurons.

G protein–linked receptors

Adrenergic and muscarinic receptors belong to a large family of receptors characterized by their functional dependence on **G proteins**

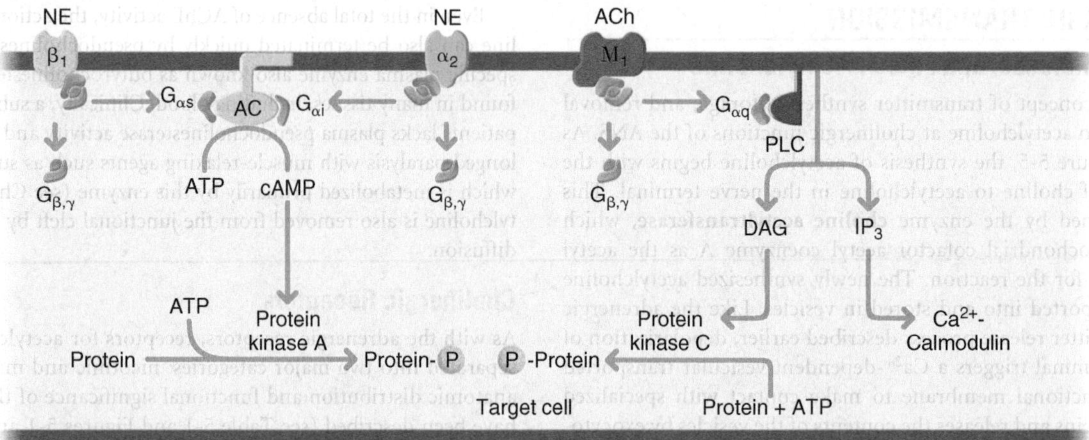

FIG 5-6 Sites of action of primary messengers, such as norepinephrine (*NE*) and acetylcholine (*ACh*), and their role in regulating the formation of second messengers in target cells. The binding of the agonist to its receptor (in this example, β_1-adrenergic or α_2-adrenergic, or M_1-muscarinic) leads to release of the α subunit of the associated G protein ($G_{\alpha s}$, $G_{\alpha i}$, or $G_{\alpha q}$). $G_{\alpha s}$ activates adenylyl cyclase (*AC*), leading to the production of cAMP. Elevated cAMP activates protein kinase A, which catalyzes the phosphorylation of numerous target proteins. $G_{\alpha i}$ inhibits AC, leading to a reduction in cAMP. Receptor activation of $G_{\alpha q}$ leads to stimulation of the enzyme phospholipase C (*PLC*). PLC catalyzes the hydrolysis of phosphatidylinositol 4,5-bisphosphate in the cell membrane, yielding diacylglycerol (*DAG*) and inositol 1,4,5-trisphosphate (*IP_3*). DAG activates protein kinase C, which catalyzes the phosphorylation of numerous target proteins. IP_3 increases intracellular Ca^{2+} release from intracellular storage sites, resulting in activation of calmodulin and other Ca^{2+}-dependent events.

(shorthand for guanine nucleotide-binding proteins) to initiate cellular signaling. G proteins are heterotrimers, so named because they consist of three different proteins: the α subunit, which activates target proteins (enzymes, ion channels) and hydrolyzes guanosine triphosphate (GTP) to guanosine diphosphate (GDP), and the β and γ subunits, which attach the G protein to the cell membrane and have signaling properties distinctly different from the α subunit. G proteins are signal transducers in that they convert the external signal of neurotransmitter binding into an alteration of cellular function. Molecular cloning studies suggest that there are many different types of G protein heterotrimers consisting of different varieties of α, β, and γ subunits.

As an immediate result of G protein actions, intracellular signaling molecules are generated that serve as "**second messengers**" for the neurotransmitters, which are the primary messengers. Figure 5-6 depicts two major second messenger pathways: the cyclic 3′,5′-adenosine monophosphate (**cAMP**) and the **Ca^{2+}/inositol phospholipid pathway.** These two pathways mediate many of the actions of the G protein–coupled adrenergic and muscarinic receptors.

G_s protein–dependent events

In the example illustrated in Figure 5-6, activation of the β_1-adrenergic receptor by norepinephrine leads to the receptor's association with a membrane-bound G protein heterotrimer called G_s ("s" implies a stimulatory effect). This binding activates G_s, causing free $G_{\alpha s}$ complexed with GTP to bind to and activate effector enzymes such as adenylyl cyclase, leading to the production of cAMP. cAMP then activates protein kinase A, which phosphorylates numerous target proteins. This phosphorylation step alters the ongoing activity of the cell because many of these target proteins are either enzymes or ion channels. Protein kinase A can activate the enzyme glycogen phosphorylase, leading to increased glycogen breakdown and release of glucose. Some other responses linked to increased cAMP synthesis include relaxation of vascular smooth muscle, increased contractile force of the myocardium, and secretion of amylase and other proteins by salivary glands. cAMP is subject to breakdown by a second enzyme, cAMP phosphodiesterase. Inhibition of this enzyme prevents the breakdown of cAMP and accentuates the adrenergic response. Caffeine and related methylxanthines are effective inhibitors of phosphodiesterase.

G_i protein–dependent events

Different biologic responses can occur when receptors activate different G_α protein subunits. Stimulation of α_2-adrenergic receptors (see Figure 5-6) leads to the release of $G_{\alpha i}$ ("i" for inhibitory). $G_{\alpha i}$ inhibits adenylyl cyclase and causes decreased cAMP concentrations. In addition, certain toxins, such as pertussis toxin, inactivate $G_{\alpha i}$ so that it cannot inhibit adenylyl cyclase, which promotes an increase in cAMP and contributes to many of the signs and symptoms of whooping cough.

G_q protein–dependent events

$G_{\alpha q}$, another G_α subunit important in ANS responses, activates the inositol phospholipid/Ca^{2+} pathway. In the example in Figure 5-6, acetylcholine stimulation of the M_1-muscarinic receptor leads to release of $G_{\alpha q}$ from its associated β and γ subunits. $G_{\alpha q}$ activates the enzyme phospholipase C, which hydrolyzes phosphatidylinositol 4,5-bisphosphate (PIP_2), a minor phospholipid found on the cytoplasmic surface of the cell membrane. The hydrolysis of PIP_2 yields two biologically active products: diacylglycerol (DAG) and inositol 1,4,5-trisphosphate (IP_3). DAG stimulates the enzyme protein kinase C, which phosphorylates target proteins generally consisting of other enzymes or ion channels. In addition, DAG itself can be hydrolyzed to yield prostanoids, resulting in activation of additional cellular responses. IP_3 releases Ca^{2+} from intracellular binding sites, leading to increased activation of protein kinase C and to other biologic responses, including activation of calmodulin-mediated events. M_1-muscarinic, M_3-muscarinic, and α_1-adrenergic receptors all activate the inositol phospholipid/Ca^{2+} pathway.

Additional second messenger systems

Other second messenger systems exist besides those mentioned earlier, and the roles of cyclic 3′,5′-guanosine monophosphate, Ca^{2+}, calmodulin, nitric oxide, prostanoids, peptides, and other mediators of cellular function are currently under extensive investigation.

OTHER AUTONOMIC NEUROTRANSMITTERS AND CO-TRANSMITTERS

Dopaminergic Transmission

Dopamine receptors exist outside the CNS, in the kidney (where their activation leads to vasodilation), the mesenteric vascular bed, and other sites. The discovery of dopamine receptors in the periphery has led to the use of dopamine to treat cardiogenic shock and renal failure, where it has the capacity to increase cardiac contractility (by stimulating β_1-adrenergic receptors) and renal blood flow. There are five subtypes of dopamine receptors (D_1 to D_5), all of which resemble adrenergic receptors in overall structure and use G protein–mediated second messenger systems.

Purinergic Transmission

Evidence has accumulated that there are noncholinergic, nonadrenergic nerves, designated as purinergic, that are found in the gastrointestinal tract, vasculature, lungs, bladder, and CNS. ATP is stored in vesicles in purinergic nerve endings and, when released, directly activates purinergic receptors of the P2 type, or it is broken down to adenosine, which activates P1 receptors, also called adenosine receptors. There are four types of adenosine receptors and two major groups of P2 receptors: P2X and P2Y receptors. Aden osine and other nucleotides can inhibit norepinephrine release from adrenergic nerves indicating that they can act as neuromodulators, regulating the release of norepinephrine through a feedback mechanism. ATP can also act as a co-transmitter with norepinephrine and acetylcholine (Fig. 5-7).

Co-release of Neurotransmitters

Certain neurons release more than one neurotransmitter, such as norepinephrine with ATP. In recent years, it has become increasingly clear that various peptide co-transmitters are released with classic ANS transmitters. When co-transmitter release occurs, it is thought that the two substances may have slightly different functions, with one substance functioning as a neurotransmitter and the other functioning as a neuromodulator, or that they act cooperatively as transmitters to elicit some physiologic response. Cholinergic neurons in the cat submandibular gland contain and release vasoactive intestinal peptide, a co-transmitter that potentiates the salivary secretion induced by acetylcholine. Similarly, neuropeptide Y enhances vasoconstriction by a direct action on the vasculature and by potentiating the effects of norepinephrine (see Fig. 5-7). The recognition of the existence of multiple co-transmitters affecting the ANS offers additional new targets for drug development.

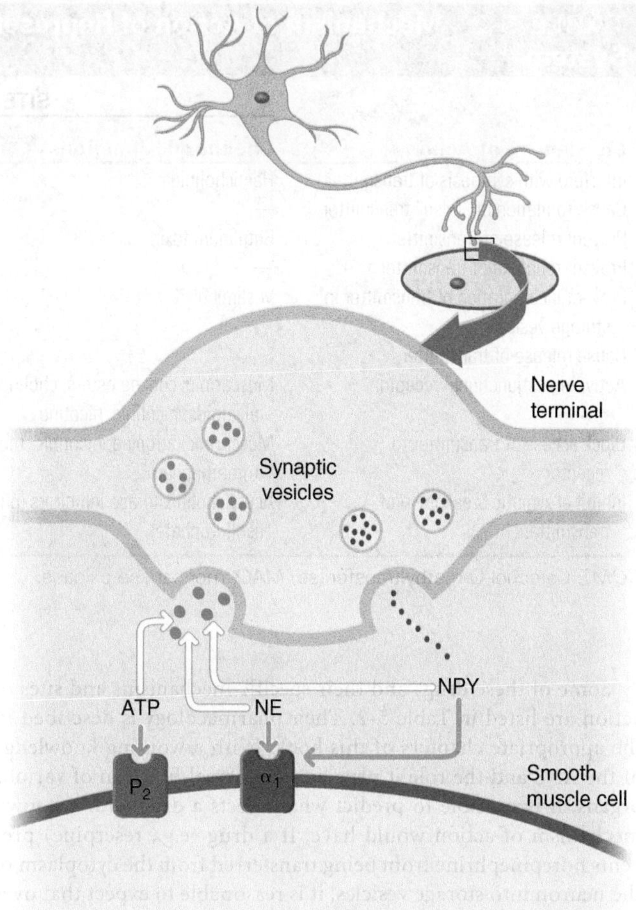

FIG 5-7 Co-release of neurotransmitters and neuromodulators. Norepinephrine (*NE*) and ATP, stored in the same storage vesicles, are released together from the sympathetic nerve varicosity to stimulate (*solid arrows*) their respective α_1 and P_2 receptors on smooth muscle. Neuropeptide Y (*NPY*), stored in separate vesicles, is also released during sympathetic nerve stimulation. Here, NPY serves as a neuromodulator (*dashed arrows*), increasing the activity of NE. All three agents inhibit further release (*open arrowheads*) through effects on prejunctional receptors (not shown).

CENTRAL CONTROL OF AUTONOMIC FUNCTION

Virtually all levels of the CNS contribute significantly to the regulation of the ANS; this includes the spinal cord and brainstem, where reflexes regulating blood pressure are integrated, and the higher centers in the hypothalamus, limbic system, and cerebral cortex, which integrate highly complex autonomic responses involved in behavior, reproduction, and emotional states. The locations of centers in the CNS that directly regulate autonomic functions such as blood pressure, respiration, micturition, and sweating are known. The ANS modulates the activity of these centers through the hypothalamus, which plays a crucial role in the integration of responses to changes in temperature, emotional states, and patterns of sexual and reproductive activity, all of which involve integration of the endocrine, autonomic, and other systems. The limbic system has been shown through stimulation experiments to cause changes in blood pressure, sexual activity, rage-like responses, and a host of other reactions characteristic of ANS stimulation. Thus the limbic system plays an important role in patterns of sexual activity and states of rage and fear, and its effects may be superimposed on the effects exerted by the hypothalamus. The cerebellum and the cerebral cortex also make contributions to patterns of autonomic activity, but their importance is less than that of the hypothalamus.

SPECIFIC SITES AND MECHANISMS OF ACTION OF AUTONOMIC DRUGS

The foregoing discussion in this chapter has shown that neurotransmission in the ANS—and normal function of the two divisions of the ANS—depends on many integrated steps, including synthesis of transmitter, release of transmitter, combination of the transmitter with the receptor, and destruction by highly specific enzymes or reuptake and reuse of the transmitter in the nerve terminal. The explosion of knowledge about the function of the ANS at the neuronal and molecular levels has been accompanied by the discovery and development of drugs that interfere with one or several steps in the complex processes described in the earlier sections on cholinergic and adrenergic transmission.

TABLE 5-2 **Mechanism of Action of Representative Drugs Affecting the Autonomic Nervous System**

	SITE OF ACTION	
Mechanism of Action	**Cholinergic Junctions**	**Adrenergic Junctions**
Interfere with synthesis of transmitter	Hemicholinium	Metyrosine
Cause formation of "false" transmitter	—	Methyldopa
Prevent release of transmitter	Botulinum toxin	Guanethidine
Prevent reuptake of transmitter	—	Imipramine, cocaine
Prevent incorporation of transmitter in storage vesicles	Vesamicol	Reserpine
Cause release of transmitter		Tyramine, amphetamine
Activate postjunctional receptor	Muscarinic: choline esters, cholinomimetic alkaloids; nicotinic: nicotine	α_1 Receptor: phenylephrine; α_2 receptor: clonidine; β_1 and β_2 receptors: isoproterenol; β_2 receptor: albuterol
Block access of transmitter to receptor	Muscarinic: atropine; nicotinic: tubocurarine, trimethaphan	α_1 and α_2 Receptors: phentolamine; α_1 receptor: prazosin; α_2 receptor: yohimbine; β_1 and β_2 receptors: propranolol; β_1 receptor: metoprolol
Inhibit enzymatic breakdown of transmitter	Acetylcholinesterase inhibitors (physostigmine, isoflurophate)	MAO inhibitors (selegiline); COMT inhibitors (entacapone, tolcapone)

COMT, Catechol-O-methyltransferase; *MAO*, monoamine oxidase.

Some of these drugs and their specific mechanisms and sites of action are listed in Table 5-2. Their pharmacology is described in the appropriate chapters of this book. With a working knowledge of the ANS and the role it plays in the normal function of various organs, it is possible to predict what effects a drug with a known mechanism of action would have. If a drug (e.g., reserpine) prevents norepinephrine from being transferred from the cytoplasm of the neuron into storage vesicles, it is reasonable to expect that over time (a relatively short time) the stores of norepinephrine will be reduced, leaving adrenergic nerve terminals throughout the body depleted of norepinephrine. It is now possible to predict that the depletion of norepinephrine throughout the sympathetic nervous system will place the organism under the unopposed control of the parasympathetic nervous system. The pupils are constricted, postural hypotension occurs, and gastrointestinal motility and secretion are increased. Thus knowledge of autonomic drug mechanism of action is important to understand the actions of and therapeutic uses of the various types of autonomic drugs.

CASE DISCUSSION

In dental patients, oral surgery constitutes physiologically significant stressors that can stimulate the sympathetic nervous system. Activation of the sympathetic nervous system increases sympathetic nerve activity with noticeable increases in circulating catecholamine concentrations observed in patients during oral surgery and with the development of postsurgical pain. This is shown in Figure 5-8.

In addition to prescribing a sedative like a benzodiazepine to be taken before stressful procedures, the dentist should encourage patients to share their concerns about dental visits and tell the dentist if they feel nervous or anxious about dental care. Affected patients should be treated during times of the day when they are less pressured or rushed. In addition, patients may find using headphones for listening to their favorite music or other distractions can reduce stress.

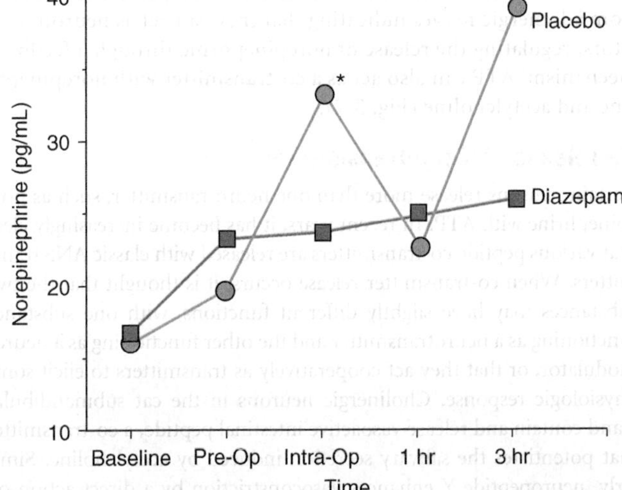

FIG 5-8 This figure shows the response of the sympathetic nervous system to the stress of oral surgery, as indicated by the circulating concentration of norepinephrine. Plasma norepinephrine was measured 1 week before surgery (baseline) and on the day of surgery at the indicated time points. Patients were randomly injected intravenously with either placebo or diazepam (0.3 mg/kg), followed by intraoral injections of 2% lidocaine with 1:100,000 epinephrine before surgical removal of impacted third molars. Placebo-treated patients showed significant increases (asterisks) in norepinephrine at the intraoperative and 3-hr postoperative periods, whereas diazepam-treated patients did not. The stress of oral surgery is mediated by the CNS because drugs that reduce anxiety (e.g., diazepam) reduce the sympathetic response to surgical stress and postoperative pain. This finding emphasizes the role of the CNS in initiating and coordinating sympathetic responses to stress. (Adapted from Hargreaves KM, Dionne RA, Mueller GP, et al: Naloxone, fentanyl, and diazepam modify plasma β-endorphin levels during surgery, *Clin Pharmacol Ther* 40:165-171, 1986.)

GENERAL REFERENCES

1. Burnstock G, Ralevic V: Purinergic signaling and blood vessels in health and disease, *Pharmacol Rev* 66:102–192, 2013.
2. Biasi MD: Nicotinic mechanisms in the autonomic control of organ systems, *J Neurobiology* 53:568–579, 2002.
3. Birdsall JM, Caulfield MP: International union of pharmacology. XVII. Classification of muscarinic acetylcholine receptors, *Pharmacol Rev* 50:279–290, 1998.
4. Eglen RM: Muscarinic receptor subtypes in neuronal and non-neuronal cholinergic function, *Auto Autocoid Pharmacol* 26:219–233, 2006.
5. Goldstein DS: Adrenaline and Noradrenaline, *Encyclopedia of Life Sciences*, John Wiley & Sons, 2010.
6. Dionne RA, Hargreaves KM, Mueller GP, et al.: Naloxone, fentanyl, and diazepam modify plasma β-endorphin levels during surgery, *Clin Pharmacol Ther* 40:165–171, 1986.
7. Avramopoulou V, Kalamida D, Poulas K: Muscle and neuronal nicotinic acetylcholine receptors. Structure, function and pathogenicity, *FEBS Journal* 274:3799–3845, 2007.
8. Changeux J-P, Lukas R, le Novère N, et al.: International Union of Pharmacology. XX. Current status of the nomenclature for nicotinic acetylcholine receptors and their subunits, *Pharmacol Rev* 51:379–401, 1999.
9. Perez DM, Piascik MT: α1-Adrenergic receptors: new insights and directions, *J Pharmacol Exp Ther* 298:403–410, 2001.
10. Westfall DP, Westfall TC: Neurotransmission: the autonomic and somatic motor nervous systems. In Brunton LL, Chabner B, Knollman B, editors: *Goodman and Gilman's the Pharmacological Basis of Therapeutics*, ed 12, McGraw-Hill, 2011.

6

Cholinergic Agonists and Muscarinic Receptor Antagonists

Frank J. Dowd

KEY INFORMATION

Cholinergic Agonists

- Acetylcholine stimulates both muscarinic and nicotinic receptors.
- Agonists at cholinergic receptors are either directly acting or indirectly acting.
- Muscarine, pilocarpine, and cevimeline are directly acting at muscarinic agonists.
- Carbachol is directly acting and nonselective but used for its muscarinic effects.
- A number of tissues respond to muscarinic receptor agonists.
- Indirectly acting cholinergic agonists are drugs that inhibit acetylcholinesterase.
- Neostigmine and physostigmine are reversible inhibitors of acetylcholinesterase.
- Organophosphates are irreversible inhibitors of acetylcholinesterase.
- Drugs that inhibit acetylcholinesterase increase acetylcholine at both muscarinic and nicotinic sites.

Antagonists at Muscarinic Receptors

- Atropine and atropine-like drugs (antimuscarinic drugs) (e.g., benztropine, ipratropium, solifenacin) block muscarinic receptors.
- The therapeutic and adverse effects of antimuscarinic drugs are the result of inhibition of the effect of acetylcholine, or other agents that stimulate muscarinic receptors, in various tissues and organs.
- Common effects of antimuscarinic drugs include (roughly in order of occurrence or magnitude and depending on route of administration) the following: xerostomia, dry eyes, lack of sweating, urinary retention, reduced overall GI activity, antiparkinsonian effects in CNS, mydriasis, cycloplegia, bronchodilation, and cardiac effects including tachycardia. (These effects are opposite of those from muscarinic receptor agonists.)
- Atropine-like drugs are used for their effects on the respiratory system, GI tract, genitourinary tract, central nervous system, and to block excessive stimulation of muscarinic receptors.
- The indications for atropine-like drugs are the following: to produce mydriasis, overactive bladder, chronic obstructive pulmonary disease, to reduce salivary secretion, sinus node tachycardia, as a preanesthetic medication, to reduce parkinsonian tremors, to reduce bowel activity, to prevent motion sickness, and to reduce the effects of substances that stimulate muscarinic receptors, namely: cholinesterase inhibitors, drugs that directly stimulate muscarinic receptors, and poisoning from certain types of mushrooms.
- Contraindications for the use of antimuscarinic drugs include prostate hypertrophy and atony of either the urinary bladder or GI tract.

CASE

Mrs. C is your 65-year-old dental patient. It has been one year since her last dental appointment. Nine months ago, her physician prescribed solifenacin (VESIcare) for her overactive bladder. After starting at a dose of 5 mg/day, the dose was increased to 10 mg/day, and the medication has been effective in reducing her urinary urgency. She reports that she can tolerate solifenacin reasonably well; however, she occasionally has dry eyes and especially notices xerostomia that is most evident at night. She sometimes has to keep a glass of water on her nightstand at night to relieve the dry mouth. Mrs. C has had good oral health in the past and has not had active caries in the last several years. At this appointment, her oral soft tissue looks dry but, otherwise, normal. Incipient root surface carious lesions are observed on the facial surfaces of tooth numbers 4, 5, and 11. You deduce that the xerostomia may be contributing to the increase in caries. Would you include a drug sialogogue in managing Mrs. C's oral condition?

CHOLINERGIC AGONISTS

Cholinergic drugs (also called **cholinomimetic drugs**) are agents that mimic the actions of the endogenous neurotransmitter **acetylcholine (ACh)**. They are **directly acting cholinergic** drugs because they bind to and stimulate cholinergic receptors. As described in Chapter 5, ACh is the primary neurotransmitter released from the nerve terminals of (1) the preganglionic fibers of the parasympathetic and sympathetic nervous systems, (2) the postganglionic fibers of the parasympathetic nervous system (which include most of the postganglionic cholinergic neurons), and (3) some postganglionic fibers of the sympathetic nervous system (mostly fibers to the sweat glands). ACh is also the primary neurotransmitter released at somatic efferent nerves innervating skeletal muscle. The major cholinergic receptors for acetylcholine at these sites are **nicotinic receptors**. Therefore, Figure 6-1 shows that peripheral cholinergic nerves may be linked to either muscarinic or nicotinic receptors. **Review Figures 5-1 and 5-2 for important information on the anatomy and physiology of the autonomic nervous system and somatic nerves to skeletal muscles.**

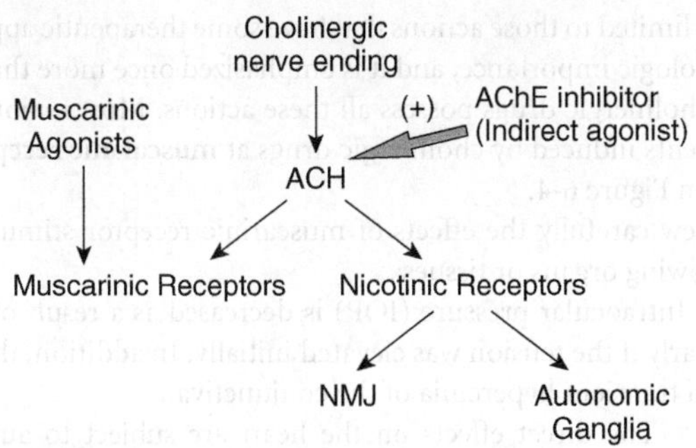

FIG 6-1 Effects of cholinergic nerve endings and muscarinic receptor agonists. *NMJ*, Skeletal neuromuscular junction.

$$(CH_3)_3\overset{+}{N}-CH_2-CH_2-O-\overset{O}{\overset{\|}{C}}-CH_3$$

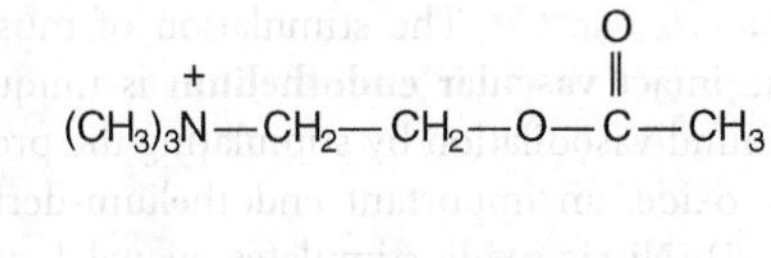

Acetylcholine

FIG 6-2 Structural formula of ACh.

Muscarine **Pilocarpine**

FIG 6-3 Structural formulas of muscarine and pilocarpine.

Most cholinergic drugs produce parasympathetic responses by stimulating muscarinic receptors located on tissues innervated by the postganglionic fibers of the parasympathetic nervous system. These drugs are often referred to as muscarinic or **parasympathomimetic** agonists. A few cholinergic agonists produce a nonselective stimulation of the parasympathetic and sympathetic branches of the autonomic nervous system by activating ganglionic nicotinic receptors located on the cell bodies of postganglionic fibers. In addition, some cholinergic agonists excite skeletal muscle by activating a separate group of nicotinic receptors located on the motor endplate of the neuromuscular junction. Finally, those synapses in the CNS that contain nicotinic and muscarinic receptors can be stimulated by cholinomimetic agonists capable of penetrating the blood–brain barrier.

Drugs that inhibit the hydrolysis of ACh (Figure 6-2), by the enzyme **acetylcholinesterase** (**AChE**) produce their cholinomimetic effects indirectly. They are therefore called **indirectly acting cholinergic** drugs. These anticholinesterases prolong the effective life of ACh released from cholinergic nerves. As a group, the anticholinesterases are less selective in effect than many directly acting cholinomimetics, and they are largely without activity in denervated tissues. Nevertheless, their dependence on ACh release confers the potential advantage of retaining neural control over their effects (Figure 6-1).

CHOLINOMIMETIC AGONISTS (DIRECTLY ACTING)

The cholinomimetic agonists directly stimulate cholinergic receptors, muscarinic or nicotinic or both, to cause a pharmacologic response in an effector. These cholinergic drugs are classified into three groups on the basis of their origin and chemical composition: choline esters, which include ACh and its synthetic congeners, the naturally occurring alkaloids, including **muscarine, pilocarpine, and nicotine,** and synthetic drugs, **cevimeline** being the major example. With few exceptions (e.g., nicotine), all these agents exert prominent muscarinic effects. The structures of muscarine and pilocarpine are shown in Figure 6-3.

Chemistry and Classification

Choline esters

The history of the discovery of ACh and its (Figure 6-2), identification are covered in Chapter 5. In 1909, Hunt synthesized the acetyl ester of choline, and earlier Hunt and Taveau reported on the pharmacology of a number of synthetic congeners of ACh. Interest in the choline esters arose, in part, out of the hope that some of these compounds would have a longer duration of action than ACh and, at the same time, a greater degree of selectivity. These characteristics were attained in some cases; however, ACh and related drugs are therapeutically or diagnostically used only in selected instances.

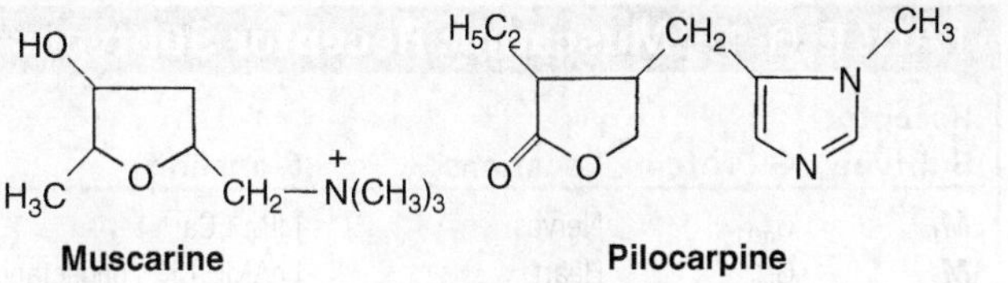

Natural alkaloids and congeners

Several alkaloids obtained from various plants possess direct cholinomimetic activity. Muscarine, the prototype muscarinic agonist, is present during certain times of the year in the mushroom *Amanita muscaria* and is especially prominent in several *Inocybe* and *Clitocybe* species. Although a quaternary ammonium compound (Figure 6-3), muscarine has a rapid onset of action after oral ingestion and produces physiologic responses characteristic of profound parasympathetic nervous system stimulation. In severe poisoning, cardiovascular collapse may occur. Pilocarpine is found in the leaves of the South American shrub *Pilocarpus jaborandi.* It is also a selective muscarinic receptor agonist. Pilocarpine remains in the armamentarium for a few specific uses and has a specific dental indication. Cevimeline, a synthetic agent, is similar in pharmacology to pilocarpine. Nicotine, an alkaloid found in tobacco leaves (*Nicotiana tabacum*), is important historically as the prototype nicotinic receptor agonist. In the form of cigarettes, nicotine is the most commonly used cholinergic agonist, and it is responsible for the physical dependence associated with smoking. This drug, as well as other drugs selective for nicotinic receptors, are discussed in Chapter 7.

Mechanism of Action

ACh is capable of stimulating both muscarinic and nicotinic receptors when administered systemically; however, although muscarinic responses are produced by low doses of ACh, effects on ganglionic and somatomotor transmission require increasingly higher doses. The choline ester bethanechol and the plant alkaloid muscarine both produce a relatively **selective activation of muscarinic receptors** located on autonomic effector tissues (especially in smooth muscle and glandular tissues) and on the cell bodies of unique populations of CNS neurons. Although these muscarinic agonists produce qualitatively similar responses in different organ systems, they vary in their relative potencies in evoking these reactions.

Parasympathomimetic responses to cholinergic drugs are mediated by the stimulation of several populations of muscarinic receptors. Muscarinic receptors belong to a large family of plasma membrane receptors whose basic structure is a peptide that consists of seven helical segments spanning the plasma membrane. (See Chapter 1.) A total of five muscarinic receptor protein subtypes (m_1 through m_5, corresponding to the pharmacologically identified receptors M_1 through M_5) have been produced from cloned muscarinic receptor genes, and it has been established that multiple receptor subtypes can coexist in the same organ or tissue. Table 6-1 describes some of the characteristics of the muscarinic receptors subtypes. **It is important to remember, however, that agonists selective for a given subtype are not used clinically, and only a few selective muscarinic receptor antagonists,**

TABLE 6-1 Muscarinic Receptor Subtypes

Receptor Subtype	G Protein	Locations	Signaling
M_1	$G_{q/11}$	Nerves	↑ IP_3, ↑ Ca^{2+}
M_2	$G_{i/o}$	Heart	↓ cAMP, ↑ K^+ conductance
M_3	$G_{q/11}$	Glands*, smooth muscle, endothelial cells	↑ IP_3, ↑ Ca^{2+}
M_4	$G_{i/o}$	CNS	↓ cAMP, ↑ K^+ conductance
M_5	$G_{q/11}$	CNS	↑ IP_3, ↑ Ca^{2+}

*Including salivary glands.
IP_3, Inositol 1,4,5-trisphosphate; *cAMP*, cyclic AMP.

with selectivity for an individual muscarinic receptor subtype, are used clinically at present.

The systemic administration of high doses of ACh also activates nicotinic receptors located on the cell bodies of postganglionic nerve fibers of the autonomic nervous system (N_N receptors) and nicotinic receptors located in the neuromuscular junction (N_M receptors). As described in Chapter 5, nicotinic receptors are composed of five glycoprotein subunits forming a rosette around a central channel spanning the plasma membrane. The α subunits contain the ACh-binding sites. When stimulated by ACh, nicotine, or another nicotinic receptor agonist, a conformational change in the protein occurs, allowing Na^+ and, to a lesser extent, Ca^{2+} ions to move down their respective concentration gradients. The net ionic movement depolarizes the postganglionic cell body or muscle endplate. Prolonged stimulation of nicotinic receptors with ACh or nicotine results in a phenomenon referred to as "depolarization blockade," in which responses to further stimulation are attenuated and then lost (see Chapter 7).

Pharmacologic Effects of ACh and Other Muscarinic Receptor Agonists

The pharmacologic effects produced by directly acting cholinergic drugs vary according to the receptors they stimulate, their distribution throughout the body, and their mode of inactivation. The duration of action of ACh and its congeners is determined by their susceptibility to hydrolysis by AChE and **pseudocholinesterase**. Methacholine, with some susceptibility only to AChE, has a longer duration of action than ACh. Bethanechol, carbachol, cevimeline, and the natural alkaloids are not affected by the cholinesterases at all and therefore also have longer durations of action than ACh.

Currently available agents exhibit significantly different affinities for muscarinic and nicotinic sites, so that carbachol has more pronounced nicotinic effects than does ACh, and bethanechol, muscarine, pilocarpine, and cevimeline have very few nicotinic properties. Differences in effect are also noted regarding various target tissues. Thus bethanechol and carbachol are very effective stimulants of the gastrointestinal and urinary tracts, whereas ACh and methacholine exert more prominent cardiovascular effects. Some of the limitations of injected ACh arise because the drug is so quickly metabolized that it gains little access to tissues that are not well perfused.

Peripheral muscarinic effects

Cholinergic agonists that stimulate muscarinic receptors produce end-organ responses that mimic parasympathetic nervous system stimulation. Table 5-1 outlines several of the physiologic responses produced by direct electrical stimulation of parasympathetic nerves. The following listing of the specific muscarinic effects of the cholinergic drugs is limited to those actions that have some therapeutic application or toxicologic importance, and it is emphasized once more that not all of the cholinergic drugs possess all these actions. Most major cholinergic events induced by cholinergic drugs at **muscarinic receptors** are shown in Figure 6-4.

Review carefully the effects of muscarinic receptor stimulation at the following organs or tissues:

Eye. Intraocular pressure (IOP) is decreased as a result of miosis, particularly if the tension was elevated initially. In addition, there may also be a transient hyperemia of the conjunctiva.

Heart. The direct effects on the heart are subject to autonomic modification. For example, a baroreceptor-mediated increase in sympathetic nervous system activity may occur if the muscarinic drug produces a significant fall in blood pressure.

Vascular smooth muscle. The stimulation of muscarinic (M_2) receptors on the intact **vascular endothelium** is unique because it produces a profound vasodilation by stimulating the production and release of nitric oxide, an important endothelium-derived relaxing factor (Figure 6-5). **Nitric oxide** stimulates guanylyl cyclase located in vascular smooth muscle, which in turn catalyzes the formation of cyclic guanosine 3′,5′-monophosphate. This cyclic nucleotide reduces intracellular Ca^{2+} concentrations, leading to vascular smooth muscle relaxation and vasodilation. The effect of agonists on the muscarinic receptors of endothelial cells accounts for the vasodilation when these drugs are administered systemically, especially intravenously. This occurs despite the lack of nerve innervation to these receptors on endothelial cells.

Bronchial smooth muscle. The smooth muscle of the bronchioles is constricted by muscarinic receptor agonists.

Gastrointestinal smooth muscle. Motility, peristaltic contractions, amplitude of contraction, and tone are all increased by muscarinic receptor agonists. Conversely, sphincter muscles are relaxed.

Secretory glands. All glands that are innervated by cholinergic fibers are potentially stimulated by cholinergic drugs. These include the salivary, lacrimal, bronchial, sweat, gastric, intestinal, and pancreatic glands. It should be noted again that the secretion by sweat glands is controlled by sympathetic nerves, which in this case have cholinergic postganglionic fibers.

Urinary tract. Muscarinic receptor agonists stimulate contraction of the detrusor muscle, which results in decreased bladder capacity and opening of the urethral orifice in the fundus of the bladder. The sphincter and trigone muscles are relaxed with muscarinic receptor stimulation.

Peripheral nicotinic effects

Several cholinomimetic drugs can stimulate nicotinic receptors. Stimulation of autonomic ganglia leads to a mixture of parasympathetic and sympathetic effects. Because these effects often oppose each other, the resultant outcome is often difficult to predict. In the case of ACh and carbachol, which also exert prominent muscarinic activity, parasympathetic effects predominate. This is likely due to the fact that these drugs have a more difficult time gaining access to nicotinic receptors. The pharmacology of nicotine, which is devoid of direct muscarinic properties, is reviewed in Chapter 7. None of these agents produces clinically useful skeletal muscle stimulation.

Central nervous system effects

As previously mentioned, there are both muscarinic and nicotinic receptors in the CNS. ACh, the choline esters, and the cholinomimetic alkaloids are all known to evoke CNS actions when applied directly to brain tissue. Central cholinergic systems have been implicated in central regulation of most physiologic systems (i.e., cardiovascular,

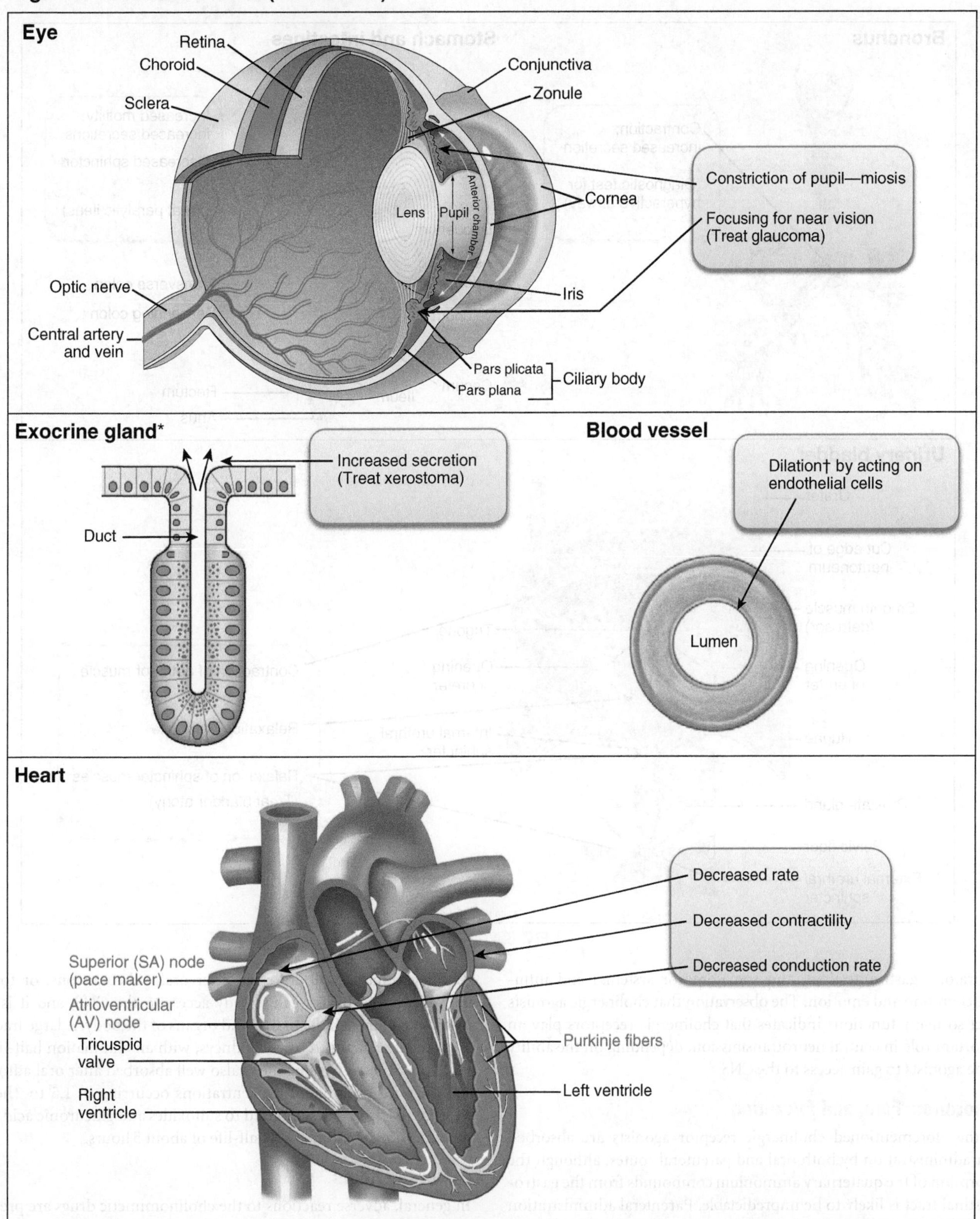

FIG 6-4 Effects of muscarinic receptor agonists. (Adverse effects are largely due to over-extension of the effects shown.) *Includes salivary, lacrimal, and sweat glands as well as several glands in the respiratory and GI tracts. †Directly acting muscarinic agonists dilate blood vessels. Blood vessels are not appreciably dilated by indirectly-acting cholinergic agonists (ACHE inhibitors) or by parasympathetic stimulation. (*Eye,* Modified from Kumar V, Abbas AK, et al.: Robbins and Cotran: Pathologic Basis of Disease, ed 9, Philadelphia, 2015, Saunders; *Exocrine glands,* Modified from Waugh A, Grant A: *Ross and Wilson Anatomy and Physiology in Health and Illness, ed 11,* Edinburgh, 2010, Churchill Livingstone; *Blood vessel,* Modified from Mahan LK, et al.: *Krauses's Food and The Nutrition Care Process,* ed 13, St Louis, 2011, Saunders; *Heart,* Modified from Patton KT, Thibodeau GA: *The Human Body in Health and Disease,* ed 6, St Louis, 2014, Mosby; *Bronchus,* Modified from Standring S: *Gray's Anatomy: The Anatomical Basis of Clinical Practice,* ed 41, Edinburgh, 2016, Churchill Livingstone; *Stomach and Intestines,* Modified from Bontrager KL, Lampignano JP: *Textbook of Radiographic Positioning and Related Anatomy,* ed 8, St Louis, 2014, Mosby; *Urinary bladder,* Modified from Patton KT, Thibodeau GA: *Anatomy and Physiology,* ed 9, St Louis, 2016, Mosby.)

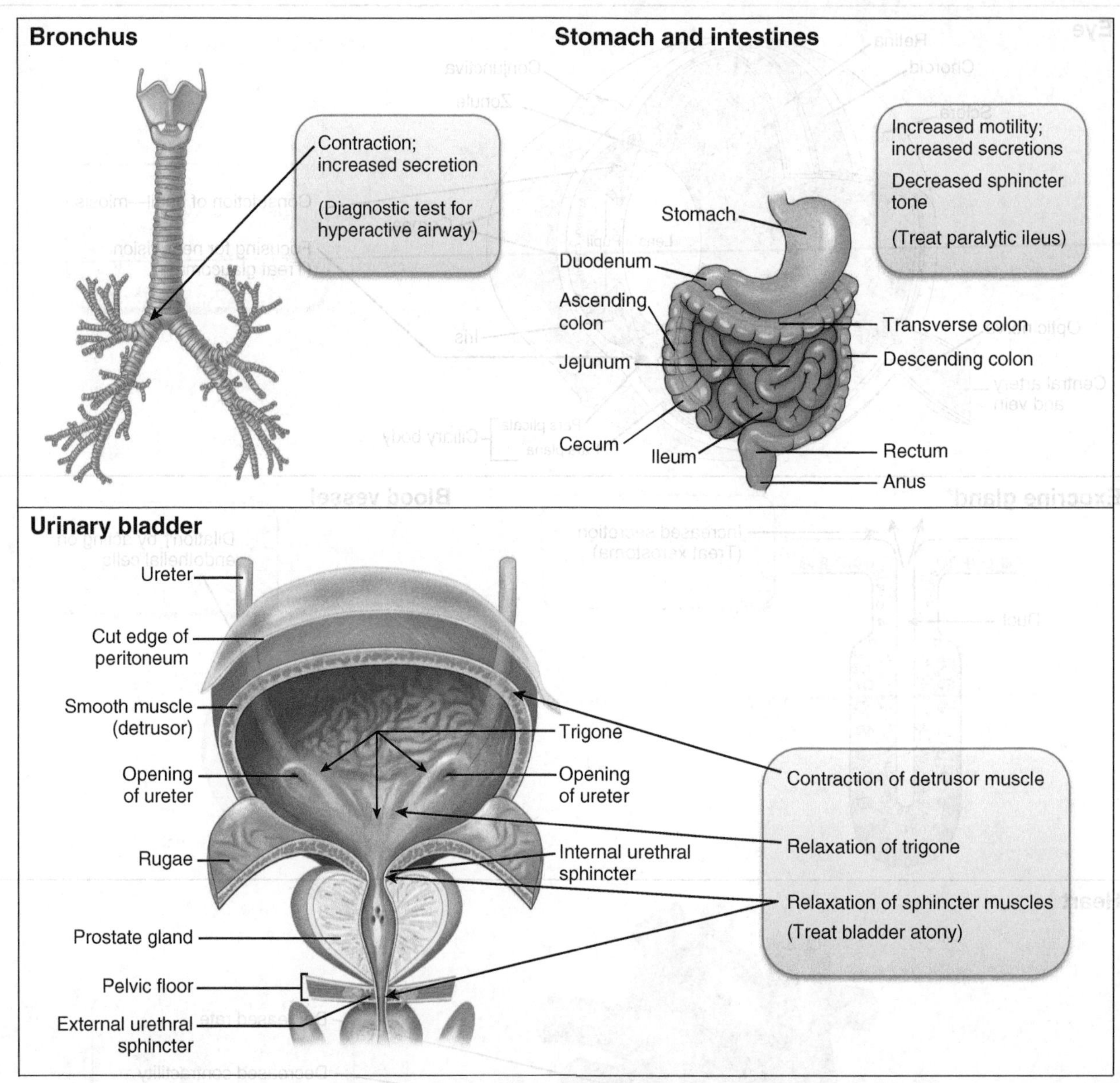

FIG 6-4, cont'd

respiratory, gastrointestinal, and somatomotor systems) and influence cognition and emotion. The observation that cholinergic agonists affect so many functions indicates that cholinergic receptors play an important role in central neurotransmission, depending on the ability of the agonists to gain access to the CNS.

Absorption, Fate, and Excretion

All the aforementioned cholinergic receptor agonists are absorbed after administration by both oral and parenteral routes, although the absorption of the quaternary ammonium compounds from the gastrointestinal tract is likely to be unpredictable. Parenteral administration of the choline esters must be carried out with extreme caution because of the profound effects they may have on cholinergic effectors. ACh is rapidly destroyed by AChE and pseudocholinesterase and exerts an effect measured in seconds if given by bolus intravenous injection. Methacholine, more slowly metabolized than ACh by AChE and immune to pseudocholinesterase, is therefore longer in duration of action. Carbachol and bethanechol are, for all practical purposes, not affected by the cholinesterases, so they have a much longer duration of action and the potential for producing widespread and prolonged cholinergic effects.

Pilocarpine is well absorbed after oral, subcutaneous, or topical administration. It also gains ready access to the CNS, and it is well distributed through the tissues and organs of the body. A large fraction is excreted unchanged by the kidneys, with an elimination half-life of 0.75 to 1.5 hours. Cevimeline is also well absorbed after oral administration, with peak blood concentrations occurring in 1.5 to 2 hours. Most of the drug is metabolized to sulfoxides and glucuronic acid conjugates, with an elimination half-life of about 5 hours.

Adverse Effects

In general, adverse reactions to the cholinomimetic drugs are predictable consequences of the stimulation of cholinergic receptors, as listed in Box 6-1.

ANTICHOLINESTERASES

Summary and Historical Development

Anticholinesterases are drugs that stimulate cholinergic transmission indirectly by inhibiting the enzyme AChE, which hydrolyzes and inactivates ACh in the synaptic clefts of the autonomic nervous system, the CNS, and the neuromuscular junction of the somatic nervous system.

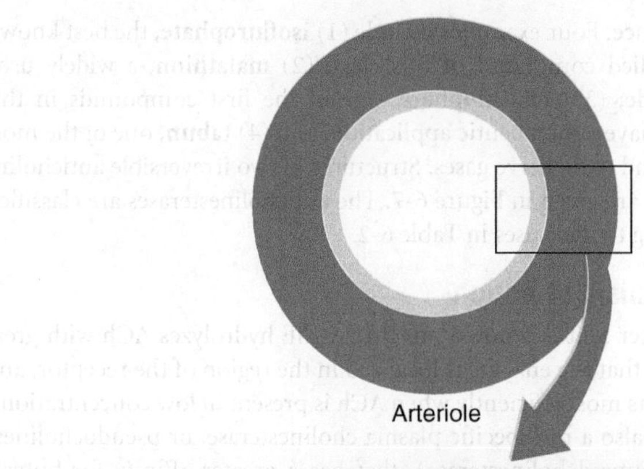

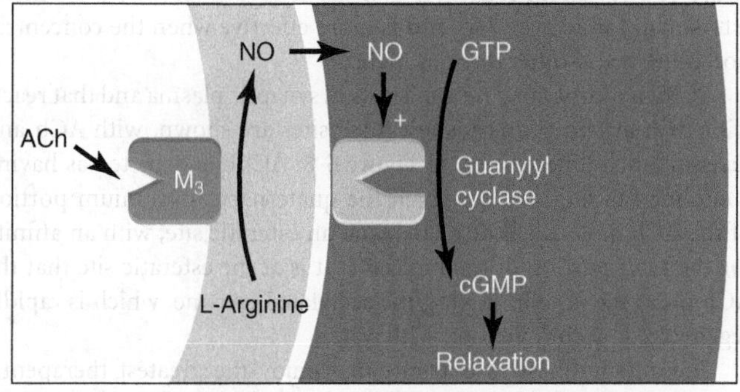

FIG 6-5 Mechanism of vascular relaxation by muscarinic receptor agonists. The muscarinic agent *ACh* binds to its receptor (*M_3*) on the intact vascular endothelium. Newly synthesized nitric oxide (*NO*) diffuses into the vascular smooth muscle, where it stimulates the formation of cyclic guanosine 3′,5′monophosphate (*cGMP*) from guanosine triphosphate (*GTP*).

BOX 6-1 Adverse Effects of Muscarinic Receptor Stimulation*

- Salivation
- Sweating
- Lacrimation
- Urination
- Defecation
- Bronchospasms
- Hypotension
- Increases gastric secretion and motility

*Patients with increased risk of adverse responses include those with asthma, cardiovascular disease, and peptic ulcer.

Agents in this class derive their pharmacologic effects from their ability to prolong the life of ACh at receptor sites. These cholinesterase inhibitors are sometimes referred to as **indirectly acting** cholinergic drugs.

Anticholinesterases can be subclassified as either **reversible** or **irreversible** cholinesterase inhibitors. Reversible inhibitors (e.g., **neostigmine** and **physostigmine**) temporarily inactivate the enzyme by forming noncovalent associations with the enzyme or covalent bonds that are readily hydrolyzed. Irreversible cholinesterase inhibitors (**organophosphates**) inactivate the enzyme by forming a permanent covalent bond with the enzyme.

Physostigmine, or eserine, the earliest known anticholinesterase, has a colorful history. An alkaloid, it is derived from a bean, or nut, known as the Calabar, ordeal, or Esére bean, and it was used in witchcraft trials by certain native tribes in West Africa. The bean was brought to England by a British medical officer stationed in Calabar in the mid-1800s, and its pharmacologic properties were investigated in a number of laboratories, including those of Fraser, who studied its toxicity in the 1860s and noted that its actions were antagonized by atropine. As early as 1877, physostigmine was used for the treatment of glaucoma, which remains one of its principal uses today. In 1914, noting the extreme brevity of the action of ACh, Dale suggested that an enzyme capable of destroying ACh must exist in the body, and in 1930, it was found that physostigmine could prevent the rapid destruction of ACh.

By the 1930s, the chemical structure of physostigmine had been elucidated, a series of synthetic analogues had been synthesized, and several researchers had reported independently that the derivative neostigmine was effective in the treatment of myasthenia gravis (MG). Until the basic mechanism of neurohumoral transmission was elucidated, however, it was not understood that these drugs acted therapeutically as anticholinesterases.

Chemistry and Classification

Reversible anticholinesterases include the truly reversible nonester quaternary ammonium compounds and the esters of carbamic acid, which react covalently with the enzyme surface. The carbamoylated enzyme is regenerated by hydrolysis in about 30 minutes; the continued presence of the anticholinesterase yields a duration of action of several hours. The reversible anticholinesterases may be classified as simple quaternary ammonium compounds (edrophonium) or carbamate ester derivatives, including tertiary amines (physostigmine), and quaternary amines (neostigmine and ambenonium). Three representative reversible anticholinesterases are shown in Figure 6-6.

Irreversible anticholinesterases are organophosphates that result in a phosphorylated enzyme not significantly regenerated by hydrolysis. They have limited therapeutic value but are of great toxicologic

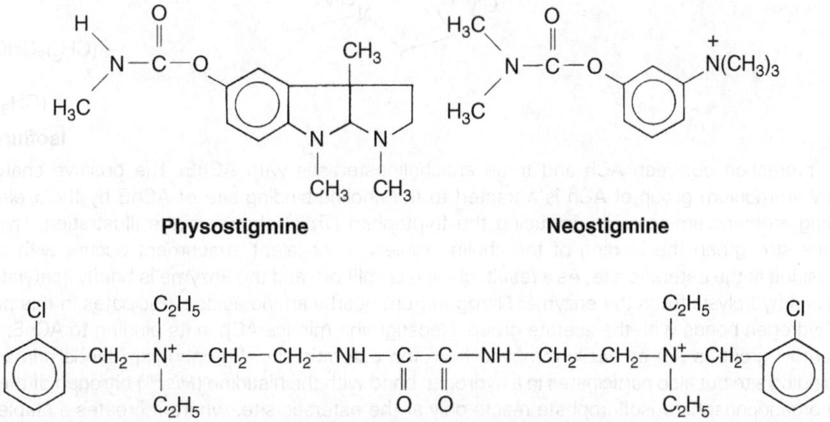

Physostigmine

Neostigmine

Ambenonium

FIG 6-6 Representative reversible anticholinesterases.

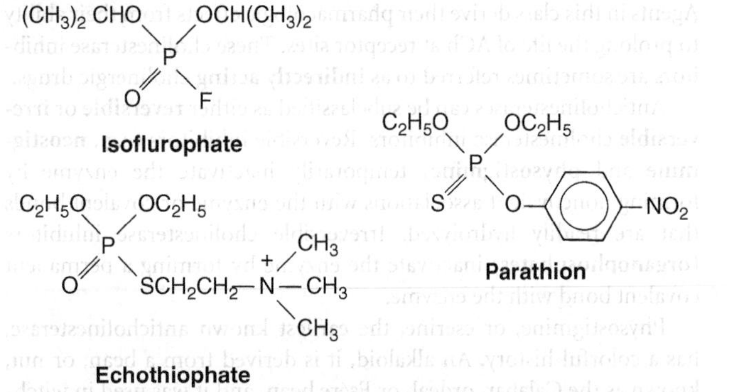

Isoflurophate

Parathion

Echothiophate

FIG 6-7 Representative irreversible anticholinesterases.

TABLE 6-2 Some Anticholinesterases and Their Uses

Use	Drugs
Treatment of glaucoma	Demercarium, echothiophate, physostigmine
Treatment of myasthenia gravis	Ambenonium, edrophonium*, neostigmine, pyridostigmine
Treatment of Alzheimer disease	Donepezil, galantamine, rivastigmine, tacrine
Reversal of nondepolarizing muscle relaxants	Edrophonium, neostigmine, pyridostigmine
Insecticides (organophosphates)	Malathion, paraoxon, parathion
Insecticides (carbamates)	Aldicarb, carbaryl, propoxur
Nerve gas	Sarin, soman, tabun

*Short acting, for diagnosis only.

significance. Four examples include (1) **isoflurophate**, the best known and studied compound of this class; (2) **malathion**, a widely used insecticide; (3) **echothiophate**, one of the first compounds in this class to have a therapeutic application; and (4) **tabun**, one of the most potent and toxic nerve gases. Structures of two irreversible anticholinesterases are given in Figure 6-7. The anticholinesterases are classified according to their uses in Table 6-2.

Mechanism of Action

In Chapter 5, it is pointed out that AChE hydrolyzes ACh with great rapidity, that the enzyme is localized in the region of the receptor, and that it acts most efficiently when ACh is present in low concentrations. There is also a nonspecific plasma cholinesterase, or pseudocholinesterase (butyrylcholinesterase), that has a greater affinity for butyric esters than for acetyl esters and is more effective when the concentration of ACh and other esters is high.

AChE is a large enzyme that exists in synaptic plasma and that reacts with ACh at two primary sites; these sites are shown, with ACh and several anticholinesterases, in Figure 6-8. AChE is depicted as having a choline-binding site, to which the quaternary ammonium portion of the ACh molecule is attracted, and an esteratic site, with an affinity for the ester portion of the molecule. It is at the esteratic site that the ACh molecule is split, leaving the acetylated enzyme, which is rapidly regenerated by combination with water.

The anticholinesterase agents that enjoy the greatest therapeutic use are those drugs, like **neostigmine** and **physostigmine**, that interact strongly with both binding sites of the AChE. As with the organophosphates, attachment of such drugs to the serine residue at the esteratic site is achieved by a covalent linkage. This bond is subject to hydrolysis, however, and these drugs are categorized as **reversible** cholinesterase inhibitors.

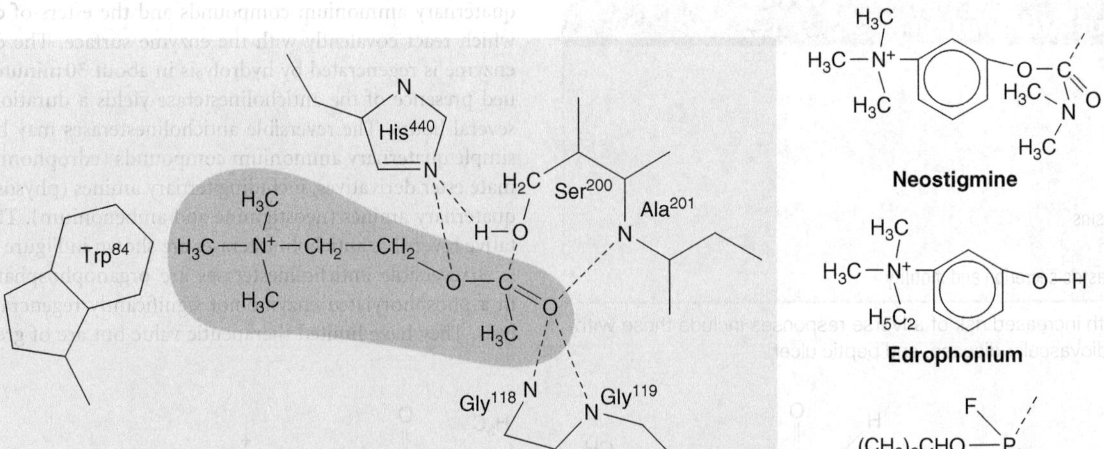

Neostigmine

Edrophonium

Isoflurophate

FIG 6-8 Interaction between ACh and three anticholinesterases with AChE. The positive charge of the quaternary ammonium group of ACh is attracted to the choline-binding site of AChE by the π electrons of surrounding aromatic amino acids, including the tryptophan (*Trp*[84]) shown in the illustration. Hydrophobic interactions strengthen the binding of the choline moiety. A covalent attachment occurs with the serine (*Ser*[200]) residue at the esteratic site. As a result, choline is split off, and the enzyme is briefly acetylated before spontaneous hydrolysis frees the enzyme. Nitrogen from nearby amino acids participates in this process by forming hydrogen bonds with the acetate group. Neostigmine mimics ACh in its binding to AChE; however, the carbamoyl group is not as easily removed from the esteratic site. Edrophonium binds primarily to the choline-binding site but also participates in a hydrogen bond with the histidine (*His*[440]) nitrogen of the esteratic site. The organophosphate isoflurophate reacts only at the esteratic site, where it creates a stable covalent bond. (Adapted from Sussman JL, Harel M, Frolow F, et al: Atomic structure of acetylcholinesterase from *Torpedo californica*: a prototypic acetylcholine-binding protein, *Science* 253:872-879, 1991.)

The **organophosphate** anticholinesterases have an affinity chiefly for the esteratic site of the AChE molecule. They produce a very stable covalent attachment; indeed, there is virtually no hydrolysis with many of these compounds, and cholinesterase activity remains depressed until new enzyme is synthesized. Because enzyme turnover may take several weeks, the organophosphates are referred to as **irreversible** in action. The terms reversible and irreversible connote differences in duration of effect, not necessarily in site of attachment.

The anticholinesterases, whether reversible or irreversible, owe their pharmacologic effects chiefly to the fact that they prolong the life of ACh at sites where it is a mediator. Thus their actions are often identical with those of ACh, although much more prolonged and, in most cases, completely dependent on the presence of endogenous ACh in the area of the effector. For this reason, most of the anticholinesterases are ineffective in denervated organs. **Exceptions** to this generalization are the quaternary ammonium compounds such as **neostigmine** and **pyridostigmine** and the bisquaternary amine **ambenonium** that also **stimulate nicotinic (N_M) receptors directly**. Neostigmine, for example, is capable of direct stimulation of the neuromuscular junction and is effective on denervated skeletal muscle. Its pharmacology is therefore the result of a combination of anticholinesterase and cholinomimetic properties.

Pharmacologic Effects

The cholinesterase inhibitors produce muscarinic effects similar to those elicited by the directly acting cholinergic agonists (described earlier and outlined in Chapter 5). These effects are mediated by increasing the concentration of ACh at the autonomic neuroeffector junctions. Nicotinic effects result from increasing ACh at skeletal muscle neuromuscular junctions and at ganglia. The activity of the anticholinesterases is greatest for those organs that receive more or less continuous cholinergic nerve stimulation. As a result, their effects are seen first in the smooth muscles of various ocular structures, the gastrointestinal tract, and the urinary bladder.

An important disparity in action between **anticholinesterases** and direct-acting muscarinic drugs is that the former **do not cause significant muscarinic receptor–mediated vasodilation** because many blood vessels receive no parasympathetic innervation, and thus no ACh is available to be protected against hydrolysis. Instead, vascular effects of high doses of anticholinesterases are largely mediated through their effects on autonomic ganglia and on medullary vasomotor centers. (The latter case occurs primarily with physostigmine, which is not permanently charged and can penetrate the blood–brain barrier.) Quaternary cholinesterase inhibitors such as neostigmine are also able to **directly** stimulate N_M receptors and, to a lesser extent, N_N receptors.

As is the case with cholinomimetic alkaloids, the anticholinesterases are also known to evoke CNS actions. The central nervous system (CNS) effects that are seen in anticholinesterase poisoning—confusion, ataxia, respiratory abnormalities, convulsions, coma, and death from respiratory paralysis—provide powerful evidence that cholinergic receptors play an important role in central neurotransmission. There are both muscarinic and nicotinic receptors in the CNS. Anticholinesterases that contain a quaternary ammonium group (such as neostigmine) are poorly absorbed after oral administration and do not readily pass through the blood–brain barrier. Predictably, they are quite effective at skeletal neuromuscular junctions but have little or no CNS effects.

Absorption, Fate, and Excretion

Physostigmine is readily absorbed after oral, subcutaneous, and topical administration, and it is destroyed principally through hydrolysis at the ester linkage by plasma esterases, including pseudocholinesterase. The other reversible cholinesterases listed in this chapter, such as neostigmine and pyridostigmine, are quaternary ammonium compounds, which means that they pass through biologic membranes with difficulty. Some of these compounds are broken down by esterases or hepatic microsomal enzymes. Both they and their metabolites appear in the urine.

The organophosphate anticholinesterases, with the exception of echothiophate, are highly lipid soluble, and they are rapidly absorbed from the gastrointestinal tract, the skin and mucous membranes, and the lungs. These characteristics explain their potential toxicity when used as aerosols, dusts, vapors, or liquids. Most of the organophosphates are metabolized by A-esterases (paraoxonases) in the plasma and liver and by microsomal oxidation; for a few drugs, enzymatic transformation results in a more toxic product than the original compound.

Adverse Effects

In humans, intoxication from anticholinesterases has resulted from overdosage with drugs used in the treatment of MG, from exposure to toxic amounts of carbamate insecticides or organophosphate in insecticides or chemical warfare agents. Organophosphate insecticides have gained wide spread use in many countries, and thousands of cases of poisoning are attributable to these compounds, especially parathion. Most of the organophosphates are volatile liquids at ordinary temperatures and are highly lipid soluble. They are readily absorbed through the skin, the respiratory tract, the gastrointestinal tract, and the eyes. The symptomatology of anticholinesterase poisoning reflects the role of ACh as a neuromediator at muscarinic and nicotinic receptors located both peripherally and in the CNS. In high doses, the reversible anticholinesterases can produce the same symptoms as the irreversible anticholinesterases; the chief difference between these two groups lies in the ready access to the circulation and the longer duration of action of the irreversible anticholinesterases. Table 6-3 summarizes the signs of poisoning with the anticholinesterases according to muscarinic, nicotinic, and CNS effects.

TABLE 6-3 Some Manifestations of Overdosage with Anticholinesterases

Muscarinic Effects (PERIPHERAL)	Nicotinic Effects*	CNS Effects
Miosis, frontal headache (brow ache), conjunctival hyperemia, blurred vision	Muscular weakness, twitching, fasciculations	Restlessness, giddiness, tension, anxiety, nausea
Rhinorrhea, nasal hyperemia	Tachycardia	Tremors, electroencephalographic changes
Lacrimation, salivation, sweating	Elevation or depression of blood pressure	Confusion, ataxia, convulsions
Increased bronchial secretions, tightness of chest, bronchoconstriction, wheezing	Death from respiratory failure	Depression of respiratory and circulatory centers, cyanosis, coma, respiratory and circulatory collapse
Anorexia, nausea, vomiting, cramps, diarrhea, involuntary defecation		Death from respiratory failure
Urinary urgency, involuntary micturition		
Bradycardia, hypotension		

*Nicotinic effects include both stimulation and inhibition of synaptic and junctional transmission.

The treatment of acute intoxication from an *organophosphate* should include the following actions:

1. Remove the victim from the source of contamination, or remove the organophosphate-containing contaminant.
2. Administer atropine. Atropine does not relieve the neuromuscular blockade produced by these agents, but it does alleviate the effects of excessive muscarinic receptor stimulation, including many of the CNS manifestations of poisoning. Repeated, often very large doses, may be required.
3. Maintain the airway and administer artificial respiration.
4. Inject a benzodiazepine such as diazepam if atropine fails to relieve the convulsions.
5. **If and only if the poisoning is from an organophosphate,** then administer **pralidoxime.** This drug is one of several oximes that were synthesized in the 1950s as cholinesterase reactivators after organophosphate poisoning. Figure 6-9 shows the structure of pralidoxime and its selective effect on regeneration of AChE after organophosphate bonding.

In some instances of organophosphate poisoning, the acute cholinergic phase may be followed by delayed peripheral neuropathy. Two types have been described. One appears 2 to 5 weeks after exposure to the organophosphate and involves phosphorylation and inhibition of an enzyme called **neurotoxic esterase.** The second neuropathy, called an *intermediate syndrome,* has been reported in approximately 10% of patients recently treated for organophosphate poisoning and appears 24 to 96 hours after exposure. This condition, which is unresponsive to atropine and pralidoxime, involves the proximal limb muscles, neck flexors, certain cranial nerves, and the muscles of respiration. These patients require respiratory support, and several have died of respiratory failure. It is theorized that the intermediate syndrome may be caused by contamination of the organophosphate or an interaction of the organophosphate with some other pesticides.

GENERAL THERAPEUTIC USES FOR DIRECTLY AND INDIRECTLY ACTING CHOLINERGIC AGONISTS

ACh itself has had very little therapeutic application because of the extreme brevity of its action. The synthesis of congeners has solved the duration problem and in addition resulted in drugs with more selective actions. Although these compounds have limited use in contemporary therapeutics, the choline esters and the alkaloid pilocarpine are still used for some important purposes, as are the reversible anticholinesterases. The irreversible anticholinesterases are principally used as laboratory tools, as insecticides, and occasionally therapeutically for ophthalmologic purposes.

Glaucoma

Glaucoma is the name given to a group of diseases characterized by an elevation of IOP, a progressive atrophy of the optic disk, and a gradual loss in the field of vision. The aqueous humor is produced in the ciliary epithelium, passes into the posterior chamber, and then through the pupil into the anterior chamber. It leaves the eye by two pathways in the anterior chamber angle. In the first, the aqueous humor passes through the trabecular meshwork across the inner wall of the Schlemm canal and then into the venous circulation. In the second route, called the *uveoscleral pathway,* aqueous humor flows across the iris and anterior face of the ciliary muscle and ultimately exits through the sclera. Most forms of glaucoma result from an interference with the drainage from the trabecular meshwork or from closure of the angle by the iris.

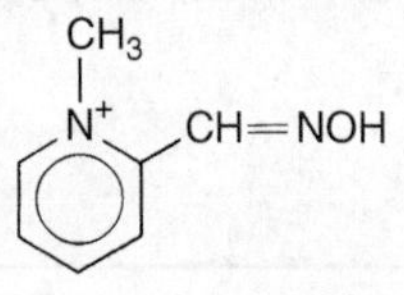

CH_3 — N^+ — CH=NOH

FIG 6-9 Structural formula of pralidoxime.

Therapy in glaucoma is directed at stimulating the musculature of the iris and ciliary body, increasing the facility of outflow of aqueous humor, reducing its formation, or extracting liquid from the eye. Although historically the cholinergic agents (in this application called *miotics*) have been the initial and principal drugs used in the treatment of chronic open-angle glaucoma, a number of other drugs are currently used, either alone or in conjunction with the cholinergic miotics (see appendix 5). In fact, β-adrenergic receptor blockers and prostaglandin preparations are now more commonly used for first-line therapy.

Pilocarpine and other drugs that stimulate muscarinic receptors lower IOP by decreasing resistance to aqueous humor outflow. Pilocarpine is available for topical administration in various solutions and in a long-acting gel formulation. Carbachol, a slightly longer-acting drug, is now only occasionally used.

The long-acting miotics—the anticholinesterases demecarium and echothiophate—are used for patients with chronic open-angle glaucoma who are refractory to the short-acting miotics and the other conventionally used drugs. These agents are quite potent and are administered in the lowest possible concentrations. Long-term administration (6 months or more) of echothiophate has been associated with the development of cataracts. Adverse effects clearly limit their usefulness in the long-term therapy of glaucoma. Refer to Appendix 5 for a list of drugs used to treat glaucoma.

Xerostomia

Xerostomia can occur at any age, but it is most often seen in the elderly population. However, xerostomia is not inevitable with aging. In fact, age-related decreases in salivary gland production are not the reason many older people have dry mouth. Dry mouth may result from several causes, including radiation to the salivary glands, therapy with antineoplastic agents, disease (e.g., Sjögren syndrome), and treatment with a variety of drugs more common in the older population. Saliva serves several functions in protecting the oral cavity. Adequate saliva volume is required for cleaning the teeth and cleansing the oral cavity. Buffers in saliva reduce the effect of acids. Proteins, including mucins, aid in mineralization of dental enamel; reduce wear on the teeth by providing lubrication; have antibacterial, antiviral, and antifungal properties; and provide growth factors for tissue repair. It is clear that reduced salivary flow rate, which is a major (but not the only) cause of the perception of dry mouth, is a risk factor for oral disease. Xerostomia can be very uncomfortable and is known to be associated with increased caries; oral pain; increased oral infection; and difficulty speaking, chewing, and swallowing. Both **pilocarpine** and **cevimeline** have been approved for the treatment of xerostomia in subjects with functional salivary gland tissue.

A 5- to 10-mg dose of pilocarpine elicits significant increases in parotid, submandibular, and sublingual secretion, with maximal flow rates being achieved in 30 minutes and a return to basal rates in approximately 3 hours. The drug is usually given three times daily. The saliva-stimulating effect depends on residual salivary gland function. Generally, at these doses, there is no significant effect on blood pressure, heart rate, or cardiac function. Sweating is a common side effect; chills, nausea, and dizziness have also been reported. Cevimeline is a selective M_1 and M_3 muscarinic receptor agonist also used for the treatment of xerostomia. Because of its receptor preference, this drug is reported to have fewer adverse effects than pilocarpine; however, clinical studies have not been carried out to confirm this claim. It is administered at a dose of 30 mg three times daily. The dentist must carefully determine whether muscarinic receptor agonists should be used to treat dry mouth.

Therapy for xerostomia must not compromise other therapy the patient may be receiving. Moreover, risk factors for muscarinic receptor agonists need to be considered.

Oral fluids, including saliva substitutes, may be added for the relief of dry mouth and should be substituted for pilocarpine and cevimeline if the drugs are not well tolerated, in patients at risk such as those with uncontrolled asthma, in patients for whom pilocarpine or cevimeline would compromise existing therapy, or where there is a complete loss of salivary function. For other contraindications, refer to the section on therapeutic uses in dentistry.

Reversal of Neuromuscular Block

The use of reversible anticholinesterases to terminate the neuromuscular block of curare-like drugs in general anesthesia is covered in Chapter 7.

Myasthenia Gravis

MG is a disease characterized by weakness and easy fatigability of the skeletal muscles, particularly ocular and oropharyngeal muscles, and by marked variations in severity of symptoms even in the course of a single day. The prevalence of the disease is about 14 to 15 per 100,000 population. Approximately 10% of patients die from the disease.

The typical patient with MG initially has ocular complaints—double vision and/or ptosis—and difficulty in chewing and swallowing. Later, dyspnea and other respiratory problems may arise. Approximately 10% of myasthenic patients have a tumor of the thymus, and approximately 75% have hyperplasia of lymphoid tissue of the thymus. MG is an autoimmune disorder in which there is continuous production of antibody to the **acetylcholine receptor (AChR)** at the neuromuscular junction. The primary defect in MG is loss of AChR through accelerated destruction of receptors and without a concomitant increase in rate of synthesis, and by complement-mediated focal lysis of the postsynaptic membrane. Other forms of MG may involve other proteins at the neuromuscular junction.

Treatment for MG is now fairly standardized. After a positive diagnosis, six methods of treatment are available. In the first, a reversible anticholinesterase (such as **neostigmine**) is used to enhance neuromuscular transmission. Also employed sometimes are the following: thymectomy, adrenal corticosteroid therapy, immunosuppressant drugs, plasmapheresis, to remove offending antibodies, and high-dose intravenous immunoglobulins.

Therapy with an anticholinesterase is likely to be complicated by side effects resulting from the accumulation of ACh at cholinergic receptor sites. Some of these effects are characteristically muscarinic—abdominal cramps, diarrhea, sweating, salivation, lacrimation—and can be well controlled by the **administration of atropine** and related drugs. Other side effects, such as muscle fasciculations and CNS symptoms, are not controllable by the muscarinic blocking drugs and may be warning signs of an impending cholinergic crisis, which results from overdosage with the anticholinesterases. Cholinergic crisis is characterized by muscle weakness, particularly of the respiratory muscles, resulting from persistent depolarization of the neuromuscular junction. **Cholinergic crisis** closely resembles **myasthenic crisis**, the latter of which may come about because of inadequate medication, and it is urgently necessary in such patients to determine quickly which of the two conditions exists. This can be done by giving, with great caution and with resuscitation equipment immediately available, a very low dose of edrophonium. If the symptoms are relieved, the problem is myasthenic weakness; if muscle strength decreases, cholinergic crisis is established.

Antidote for Atropine Poisoning

All the cholinergic drugs with muscarinic properties should theoretically be useful in antagonizing the effects of atropine, but the most effective drugs for this purpose are the anticholinesterases, and the drug of choice is physostigmine. When the diagnosis of atropine poisoning is confirmed, physostigmine is administered intravenously, and it rapidly relieves the delirium and coma. Neostigmine and other quaternary ammonium compounds are of limited use because they are incapable of counteracting the CNS effects of atropine.

A number of psychotropic agents (e.g., tricyclic antidepressants, phenothiazines, and antihistamines) share to varying degrees the antimuscarinic effects of atropine. Particularly when used in combination (for intravenous sedation or for other reasons), these agents may induce a central anticholinergic syndrome consisting of confusion, delirium, hallucination, and psychotic behavior. Intravenous physostigmine in doses of 0.5 to 2 mg is effective in reversing this syndrome. Inasmuch as the duration of action of parenteral physostigmine is 1 to 2 hours, repeated administrations may be necessary to avoid recurrence of the syndrome.

Paralytic Ileus and Bladder Atony

After abdominal and pelvic surgery, there is often a failure of normal peristalsis that leads to postoperative abdominal distention and discomfort. Neostigmine has been used to advantage in the treatment of this condition, as has bethanechol, which is preferred to other choline esters because of its reduced cardiac effect.

Bladder atony also follows surgery and sometimes parturition. It leads to urinary retention and can be treated with bethanechol or neostigmine.

Senile Dementias of the Alzheimer Type

Alzheimer disease and related senile dementias are progressive and debilitating neuropsychiatric diseases. Alzheimer disease is manifested by memory loss, language deficits, and other symptoms, and it usually terminates in death from some debilitating condition in approximately a decade. Although the cause of Alzheimer disease remains an active area of investigation, the dementia appears to be a form of amyloid encephalopathy resulting from the deposition of the protein β-amyloid in selective regions of the CNS. The deposition of this protein causes the formation of neurofibrillary tangles, oxidation, inflammation, neuronal cell death due to multiple factors, and loss of several different neurotransmitters important in cognition and memory. One central neurochemical affected by Alzheimer disease, especially early in the course of the illness, is ACh.

Deficits in ACh and in choline acetyltransferase, the enzyme responsible for the formation of ACh from choline and acetyl coenzyme A, have been identified in the brains of Alzheimer patients. The identification of these deficiencies suggested a treatment strategy for Alzheimer disease analogous to that used in the pharmacologic therapy of Parkinson disease, namely, replacement of the missing (in this case cholinergic) agonist. In fact, early experiments with physostigmine showed some transient, if variable, improvement. The AChE inhibitors that are used to treat Alzheimer disease easily penetrate the blood–brain barrier. **Donepezil** and **rivastigmine** are two examples of AChE inhibitors used to treat Alzheimer disease. The AChE inhibitors have shown modest but significant improvement in Alzheimer patients. Their benefit seems to be in temporarily slowing memory loss and loss of function. Memantine, an *N*-methyl D-aspartate receptor antagonist, and vitamin E, an antioxidant, are also sometimes used.

ANTIMUSCARINIC DRUGS

Various drugs can interfere with the transmission of nerve impulses at cholinergic junctions. As shown in Table 5-2, some drugs prevent the

TABLE 6-4 Chemical Structures of Two Antimuscarinic Drugs

Type of Compound	Example	Chemical Structure
Naturally occurring alkaloid	Atropine	H_2C—CH—CH_2; N–CH_3; CH—O—CO—CH(CH_2OH)—C_6H_5; H_2C—CH—CH_2
Synthetic but not quaternary ammonium compound	Benztropine	H_2C—CH—CH_2; N–CH_3; CH—O—CH(C_6H_5)$_2$; H_2C—CH—CH_2

uptake of choline by the nerve terminal or the release of acetylcholine (ACh) from the terminal; other drugs block at ganglia or, by a competitive or depolarizing form of blockade, at neuromuscular junctions. The drugs in this chapter block responses in muscarinic receptors and are essentially without effect, except at inordinately high doses, at nicotinic receptors. Hence, these drugs are known as **antimuscarinic** or **muscarinic receptor–blocking drugs**; the term **anticholinergic**, although often used for this class of drugs, is somewhat inaccurate because these drugs, for the most part, are selective for muscarinic receptors, not nicotinic receptors. They are also termed **atropine-like** because of their derivation from, or relation to, the oldest and best known member of the group. Because peripheral muscarinic receptors are the primary targets of ACh released by postganglionic cholinergic neurons, the effects achieved by the antimuscarinic drugs are chiefly on the smooth muscle, cardiac muscle, and glands that are innervated by these neurons.

The antimuscarinic drugs have a colorful, even sinister, history. The natural alkaloids are derived from a number of plants, including *Atropa belladonna* (deadly nightshade), *Datura stramonium*, also known as jimsonweed or Jamestown weed, *Hyoscyamus niger* (henbane), and Mandragora, among others. The Swedish botanist Linné named the shrub *Atropa belladonna* after Atropos, one of the three Fates, who cuts the thread of life. The term *belladonna* comes from the Italian "beautiful woman" and is so named because instillation of one of these drugs into the eyes was said to make women more attractive. Atropine, scopolamine, and related natural chemicals are therefore also referred to as **belladonna alkaloids**.

Chemistry and Classification

Antimuscarinic drugs fall into four categories:

1. Naturally occurring belladonna alkaloids—atropine and scopolamine—which are organic esters. **Atropine** and **scopolamine** are composed of an aromatic acid (tropic acid) and a complex organic base (tropine or scopine, respectively). Atropine is a racemic mixture of *d*- and *L*-hyoscyamine; the *L* isomer is the active form and is often used separately.
2. Semisynthetic derivatives, such as homatropine, which is produced by combining tropine with mandelic acid, and the quaternary ammonium derivatives of atropine, scopolamine, and homatropine (atropine methylnitrate, methscopolamine bromide, and homatropine methylbromide, respectively).
3. Synthetic quaternary ammonium compounds, such as, **glycopyrrolate, propantheline, ipratropium,** and methantheline.
4. Synthetic antimuscarinic drugs that are not quaternary ammonium compounds, such as **benztropine, trihexyphenidyl,** and cyclopentolate.

Structures of two (atropine and benztropine) shown in Table 6-4.

Mechanism of Action

The antimuscarinic drugs, whether the naturally occurring alkaloids or the semisynthetic or synthetic derivatives, are **competitive antagonists of ACh at muscarinic receptors.** (Review Figures 6-1 and 6-4 for location of muscarinic receptors.) They have an affinity for muscarinic receptor sites but lack intrinsic activity. Thus they occupy the receptor sites and prevent access of ACh, creating a blockade that is reversible. Reversible blockade means that the blockade by antimuscarinic drugs can be reversed by increasing the amount of ACh in the area of the receptor, as would occur after the administration of an anticholinesterase drug. Because atropine can antagonize the muscarinic effects of the anticholinesterases and vice versa, each drug can be used as an antidote for the other in case of poisoning. In effect, the antimuscarinic drugs are capable of blocking responses to parasympathetic nerve stimulation, to sympathetic nerve stimulation of thermoregulatory sweat glands, to ACh protected from hydrolysis by anticholinesterases, and to direct-acting muscarinic agents, although their capability for inhibiting the latter two is greater than for the first two.

Although atropine is a highly effective antagonist at all muscarinic receptors, five muscarinic subtypes, M_1 to M_5, have been described, each with different affinities for certain muscarinic agonists and antagonists, different anatomic distributions, and different second messenger signaling mechanisms (see Table 6-1). The relatively selective affinity of the tricyclic benzodiazepine pirenzepine for M_1 versus M_2 and M_3 receptors gives it stronger antimuscarinic properties in certain sites (e.g., corpus striatum, cerebral cortex, and enterochromaffin cells) over others (e.g., heart and ileum). Pirenzepine was the first clinically useful selective muscarinic receptor antagonist. Darifenacin is a selective antagonist at the M_3 receptor and is available for treatment of overactive bladder. The characterization of different muscarinic receptor subtypes continues to provide an impetus for development of selective antagonists.

Pharmacologic Effects

Therapeutic doses of the antimuscarinic drugs produce effects attributable to the blockade of peripheral muscarinic receptors and similar receptors in the CNS located within the medulla and higher cerebral

TABLE 6-5 The Relative Effects of Atropine and Scopolamine on Various Effectors

	Iris	Ciliary Body	Secretion: Saliva, Sweat, Bronchial	Bronchial Muscle	GI Muscle	Heart	CNS
Atropine	+	+	+	++	++	++	+
Scopolamine	++	++	++	+	+	+	++

centers. In the discussion that follows, the principal review is of atropine and scopolamine, which have always been considered the prototypes for this class of drugs, but it must be emphasized that (1) atropine and scopolamine differ in the relative intensity of their antimuscarinic effects on specific organs (Table 6-5); (2) there is a difference in the susceptibility of various effectors to antimuscarinic agents in general (Table 6-6); (3) because of differences in chemical structure, some antimuscarinic drugs pass readily into the CNS, whereas others do not; (4) there are some major differences among antimuscarinic drugs in the onset and duration of their actions (Table 6-7); and (5) muscarinic receptor subtypes have differing affinities for specific antimuscarinic drugs.

TABLE 6-6 Order of Susceptibility of Effectors to Increasing Doses of Antimuscarinic Agents

Response	Dose
Secretion (saliva, sweat, bronchial)	Low
Mydriasis, cycloplegia, tachycardia	↓
Loss of parasympathetic control of urinary bladder and gastrointestinal smooth muscle	↓
Inhibition of gastric secretion	High

TABLE 6-7 Onset and Duration of Cycloplegia Induced by Two Topical Antimuscarinic Drugs

Drug	Onset (Minutes)	Duration
Atropine	30 to 40	6 days or longer
Tropicamide	20 to 35	2 to 6 hours

Peripheral Nervous System Actions

The antimuscarinic drugs possess both peripheral and CNS actions, but the nature and intensity of these vary with the individual drug and the dose administered. Most peripheral effects are caused by an interruption of parasympathetic impulses to a given effector. This results in control of the tissue or organ by the sympathetic nervous system, which often exerts effects opposite to those of the parasympathetic nervous system. An important exception is where the sympathetic effect acts through muscarinic receptors, most notably in the sweat glands. Thus the **sympathetic effect of sweating is inhibited by antimuscarinic drugs**. The pharmacologic effects observed depend in large part on the existing activity of postganglionic cholinergic neurons. Thus inhibition of sweating and hyperthermia are likely to be observed on a hot day, but no effect on thermoregulation is apparent in a cold environment. In general, atropine-like drugs block the salivation, lacrimation, urination, and defecation response to cholinergic drugs previously described and the hypotensive and bradycardic effects of muscarinic receptor stimulation. The effects of antimuscarinic agents on specific tissues are described next (see Figure 6-4).

Eye

Atropine-like drugs block muscarinic receptors in the sphincter of the iris and in the ciliary muscle, leading, respectively, to dilation of the pupil (mydriasis) and paralysis of accommodation (cycloplegia). Photophobia and fixation of the lens occur for far vision, and thus vision for near objects is blurred. IOP is not significantly affected except in the case of narrow-angle (or angle-closure) glaucoma, for which administration of these drugs may cause a dangerous rise in IOP. The onset and duration of the mydriatic and cycloplegic effects differ, as shown for cycloplegia in Table 6-7, and the choice of an agent for an ophthalmologic procedure will be influenced by these differences.

Respiratory tract

After administration of antimuscarinic drugs, the bronchial smooth muscle is left under the sole control of the sympathetic nervous system and is therefore relaxed. This relaxation of the smooth muscle decreases airway resistance. Sometimes there is an increase in respiratory minute volume resulting from an increase in the physiologic dead space and medullary stimulation. The bronchoconstriction caused by muscarinic agonists, sulfur dioxide, and certain other bronchial spasmogens is easily reversed by atropine, but that caused by histamine, 5-hydroxytryptamine, and the leukotrienes is resistant. Secretion of all glands in the nose, mouth, pharynx, and respiratory tree is inhibited. This suppression of secretory activity in the respiratory tract is the underlying reason for the effectiveness of antimuscarinic drugs in preventing laryngospasm during general anesthesia; these agents are not capable of directly blocking contraction of the laryngeal muscle.

Salivary glands

Parasympathetically mediated salivary secretion is abolished in a dose-dependent manner, whereas salivary gland vasodilation is much less affected. The mouth and throat become unpleasantly dry, to the point that speech and swallowing may become difficult. Dry mouth or xerostomia can lead to any one of a number of adverse effects on the oral cavity.

Gastrointestinal tract

Although the antimuscarinic drugs are quite effective in preventing the expected motor and secretory responses of the gastrointestinal tract to administered cholinergic drugs, their effects on vagal stimulation are more ambiguous. Antimuscarinic drugs have a marked inhibitory effect on motility throughout the gastrointestinal tract. Thus, interference with the normal parasympathetic impulses to the gastrointestinal tract, as would occur with the antimuscarinic drugs and the ganglionic blocking agents, will cause a profound decrease in the tone of gastrointestinal smooth muscle as well as in the frequency and amplitude of peristaltic contractions. Regarding secretion, gastric secretory activity in human beings is inhibited only at very high doses of the belladonna alkaloids, when essentially all other parasympathetic function has been blocked, and the patient has an extremely dry mouth, blurred vision, an increased heart rate, and marked inhibition of gastrointestinal motility.

Cardiovascular system

The effects of antimuscarinic drugs differ according to the dose administered and whether the subject is in the erect or recumbent position. With oral doses used to limit salivation (e.g., 0.4 to 0.6 mg of atropine in adults), mild bradycardia often results. At these low doses, a selective blockade of prejunctional muscarinic receptors augments ACh release from postganglionic parasympathetic fibers innervating the heart. In most cases, however, the heart rate increases significantly in human beings given more than 0.4 mg intravenously or 1 mg orally. In the standing or upright patient, there is little or no change in cardiac output. As implied in Table 6-5, doses of scopolamine that cause mydriasis cause less tachycardia, whereas atropine administered systemically in doses sufficient to have ocular effects will inevitably accelerate the heart.

Genitourinary tract

The ureters and the urinary bladder (detrusor muscle) are relaxed by atropine. The sphincter and trigone muscles are contracted by atropine. These effects are due to muscarinic receptor blockade. Together, these changes in the bladder cause urinary retention in humans. This retention is particularly likely in the presence of prostatic hypertrophy.

Body temperature

The belladonna alkaloids suppress sweating because the sweat glands (other than the apocrine sweat glands as found on the palms of the hand) are innervated by cholinergic fibers of the sympathetic nervous system. The receptors at the neuroeffector sites in the sweat glands are therefore muscarinic. The rise in body temperature that can follow the administration of large doses of atropine or scopolamine may have a CNS component, but the primary cause is the peripheral inhibition of sweating. It is also the most serious and life-threatening result of an overdose of one of these drugs.

Central Nervous System Effects

CNS effects are produced only by those antimuscarinic drugs that can penetrate the blood–brain barrier. The quaternary amines, such as methscopolamine and propantheline, therefore have little or no effect on the CNS.

Medulla and higher cerebral centers

Both scopolamine and atropine produce complex effects on the CNS. With conventional therapeutic doses of atropine, there is stimulation of the CNS, which is generally manifested only as a mild stimulation of respiratory centers located in the vagal nuclei of the medulla. At therapeutic doses, scopolamine usually produces effects ranging from decreased psychological efficiency to drowsiness, sedation, euphoria, and amnesia, but it can also cause excitement, restlessness, hallucinations, and delirium. Atropine is much less active in this respect than scopolamine.

Antitremor activity

The belladonna alkaloids were first used in the treatment of Parkinson disease in the mid-1800s, long before their mechanism of action was understood and before the biochemical nature of the defect of parkinsonism had been elucidated. Their effectiveness in suppressing tremor was later suggested to result from a "central atropine-ACh antagonism," and more recently it has become apparent that the striatum is the site of cholinergic systems that in parkinsonism are released from an inhibitory balance mediated by dopamine (see Chapter 13).

Vestibular function

The belladonna alkaloids have since ancient times been the basis of various remedies to treat motion sickness. Scopolamine is more effective than atropine. It acts on several areas of the brain including the vestibular apparatus and the cortex.

Absorption, Fate, and Excretion

The belladonna alkaloids and their tertiary derivatives and analogues are readily absorbed from all parts of the gastrointestinal tract except the stomach, as would be expected with alkaloids that form acid salts. Absorption is more rapid from subcutaneous tissue or muscle than it is from the gastrointestinal tract. The drugs are distributed throughout the body, including the CNS. The fate of most of these drugs in human beings is not well studied, but the kidneys provide the main route for excretion of atropine or its metabolites. Within 24 hours, 27% to 94% of a dose of labeled atropine is excreted, and very little is excreted after 24 hours. A third of the atropine appears as unchanged atropine and the remainder as a metabolite of uncertain identity. Rabbits possess a genetically determined enzyme, atropinesterase, that explains their singular ability to tolerate large doses of atropine. Various idiosyncratic responses or variations in sensitivity to one or another of the actions of these drugs are not uncommon. Young people show a high incidence of idiosyncratic responses; persons with Down syndrome are more sensitive to the mydriatic effects, whereas African Americans develop more exaggerated tachycardia.

Antimuscarinics with a quaternary ammonium structure are incompletely absorbed after oral ingestion and are often given by nonenteral routes. These drugs are largely excluded from the CNS.

General Therapeutic Uses

The therapeutic uses of the antimuscarinic drugs are all based on the pharmacologic effects, both peripheral and central (Table 6-8). However, as should be clear, it is difficult to obtain a high degree of selectivity in the organ or organs to be affected because the antimuscarinic drugs tend to affect many muscarinic sites. Certain drugs, however, are more effective and therefore potentially more useful in a particular therapeutic role than others. It should also be noted that the quaternary ammonium compounds differ from atropine and scopolamine in a number of important respects. Two important differences are (1) the quaternary ammonium compounds do not readily pass the blood–brain barrier because they are ionized, and thus they have little or no effect on the CNS, and (2) they have greater ganglionic blocking properties than do the nonquaternary compounds. This latter point may explain why orthostatic hypotension and impotence are sometimes encountered in patients being treated with the quaternary ammonium compounds.

Other Uses

Antidote to anticholinesterases

Toxicity from anticholinesterases may result from their use in the treatment of MG (particularly in the early phase of therapy when the patient is not as tolerant to the muscarinic effects of these drugs) or from exposure to one of the organophosphate insecticides or anticholinesterase nerve gases. These anticholinesterases typically produce a spectrum of peripheral muscarinic and nicotinic effects as well as CNS effects. Atropine is effective in antagonizing the effects at muscarinic sites and thus will relieve the hypersecretion of salivary, lacrimal, and respiratory glands; bronchoconstriction; gastrointestinal symptoms; sweating; various other manifestations of muscarinic stimulation; and some CNS actions. Atropine does not interfere with the desired effects of anticholinesterases at **neuromuscular junctions** when these drugs are being used for MG or to reverse neuromuscular blockade induced by curare-like agents (see Chapter 7); it also does not prevent the neuromuscular stimulation, followed by respiratory failure, characteristic of excessive nicotinic stimulation. For the treatment of acute toxicity

TABLE 6-8 **Effects and Indications of Antimuscarinic Drugs**

Tissue	Effect	Indication(s)	Common Drugs Used
Eye			
Sphincter of iris	Mydriasis	To dilate pupils[a]	Tropicamide[b]
Ciliary muscle	Cycloplegia		Cyclopentolate[b]
			Homatropine
Bronchii			
Smooth muscle	Relaxation	Asthma (certain forms)	Ipratropium[c]
Secretory cells	Reduced secretion	Bronchitis	Tiotropium[c]
Salivary glands	Reduced secretion	To reduce saliva	Atropine[d]
			Glycopyrrolate
GI tract			
Smooth muscle	Reduced peristalsis	Rarely, ulcers[e]	Glycopyrrolate
Glands	Reduced secretions		Pirenzepine[g]
Heart	Tachycardia	Bradycardia[f]	Atropine
	Increased AV nodal conduction	Heart block	
Genitourinary tract			
Bladder detrusor	Relaxation	Urinary incontinence	Oxybutynin
			Flavoxate
Bladder sphincter and trigone	Constriction	Overactive bladder	Darifenacin
			Solifenacin
CNS			
Medulla and higher centers	Sedation, euphoria, amnesia[h]	Rarely, preanesthetic medication	Scopolamine
Corpus striatum	Reduced tremor	Parkinsonian tremor	Benztropine, trihexyphenidyl
Vestibular apparatus	Reduced activity	Motion sickness	Scopolamine

[a]The topical use of these drugs is strongly contraindicated in patients with a predisposition to narrow-angle glaucoma. See Appendix 5.
[b]Shorter duration of action.
[c]Quaternary compounds used by inhalation.
[d]A typical adult dose of atropine is 0.5 mg orally.
[e]Other drugs, such as proton pump inhibitors are more commonly used.
[f]Also can prevent vagal reflexes in surgery.
[g]Muscarinic M_1 receptor selective.
[h]Especially scopolamine.

with anticholinesterases, very large doses of atropine are used; for the treatment of milder symptoms of muscarinic stimulation, as in the treatment of MG, much lower doses suffice.

Antidote to poisoning by mushrooms containing muscarine

As stated previously, the mushroom *Inocybe lateraria* is poisonous because of its high content of the alkaloid muscarine. Atropine is a specific antagonist of antimuscarinic chemicals found in this and other plant sources.

Adverse Effects

Atropine and related drugs, despite wide availability and defined toxicity, have produced relatively few fatal cases of poisoning in adults. Children are more sensitive to atropine and most of the reported fatalities have involved children who accidentally ingested medicines that had antimuscarinic action. Children are more susceptible to hyperthermia and other toxic effects of atropine; dosages therefore need to be carefully controlled. The colloquialism "hot as a hare, red as a beet, dry as a bone, blind as a bat, and mad as a hatter" vividly conveys the symptoms of atropine intoxication, which are predictable extensions of the pharmacologic effects of this group of drugs. Present are dryness of the mouth, extreme thirst, a burning sensation in the throat, and difficulty in swallowing; dilation of the pupils and cycloplegia with severe impairment of vision and photophobia; flushing of the skin, vasodilation of skin vessels, absence of sweating, and a rise in body temperature in warm environments to 105 °F or more; urinary retention; and derangements of CNS activity. Mild toxic reactions may subside in a few hours; most patients require a day or more for complete recovery. Therapy for atropine poisoning involves physostigmine, which is useful in raising the amount of ACh in the vicinity of the receptors and acts rapidly to terminate the atropine blockade. The antianxiety drugs such as diazepam may be used to control CNS excitation. Therapy also includes supportive care.

A practice of drug abuse in young adults in certain locales of the United States is the chewing of seeds from the moonflower plant (*Datura inoxia*). Patients present with typical signs of antimuscarinic drug poisoning due to the high level of scopolamine in the plant. These signs include hallucinations, dry, hot and flushed skin, dry mouth, and tachycardia.

Topical use of antimuscarinic drugs in the eye is absolutely contraindicated in cases of suspected or diagnosed narrow-angle glaucoma. Systemic doses of anticholinergic drugs can be used in patients with open-angle glaucoma but not in patients with narrow-angle glaucoma. As previously mentioned, use of these drugs may precipitate the first attack of acute intraocular hypertension. In prostatic hypertrophy, anticholinergic drugs may cause urinary retention.

Drug Interactions

The anticholinergic effect of the atropine-like drugs is potentiated by antihistamines (which particularly accentuate the xerostomia), the tuberculostatic drug, isoniazid, tricyclic antidepressants and several other drugs. The phenothiazines tend to potentiate the CNS effects of the antimuscarinic drugs. When atropine is given in the presence of propranolol, or another β-adrenergic receptor–blocking drug, it is likely to antagonize the slowing of the heart and the increased duration of the atrioventricular nodal refractory period for which propranolol may have been prescribed to achieve. Atropine will also block the vagal actions of drugs such as the digitalis glycosides.

Botulinum Toxin

Botulinum toxin prevents the release of ACh from nerve endings by interrupting the action of proteins involved in fusion of ACh-containing vesicles and the plasma membrane. It is sometimes used to treat localized muscle dystonias and cerebral palsy. It is also used to reduce wrinkles, to treat migraine, and to treat overactive bladder.

THERAPEUTIC USES IN DENTISTRY

Cholinergic Agonists

All the cholinomimetic drugs that have an affinity for muscarinic sites are capable of stimulating salivation. **Xerostomia** is a common problem encountered by dentists in patients with Sjögren syndrome, those who have had head and neck radiation, and those undergoing treatment involving drugs that produce dry mouth. Muscarinic receptor agonists may be useful in stimulating salivary flow when there is functional salivary gland tissue present and when there is no contraindication for their use. Muscarinic receptor agonists should not be administered if they will compromise other therapy that the patient is undergoing. For instance, antimuscarinic therapy for overactive bladder would tend to be compromised by the administration of a muscarinic receptor agonist. (Antimuscarinic drug therapy would also reduce the clinical efficacy of pilocarpine or cevimeline.) Muscarinic receptor agonists are contraindicated in urinary tract obstruction, hyperactive airway disease, chronic obstructive pulmonary disease, acute heart failure, gastrointestinal spasms, hyperthyroidism, and acute iritis. Pilocarpine is usually taken at doses of 5 or 10 mg three times a day, 30 minutes before each meal. Cevimeline is given at doses of 30 mg three times daily.

Physostigmine may be of value in treating certain adverse reactions to antimuscarinic drugs used for intravenous sedation.

Antimuscarinic Drugs

The principal use of the **anticholinergic drugs** in dentistry is to **decrease the flow of saliva** during dental procedures. Small doses given orally approximately 30 minutes to 2 hours before the procedure are effective, but the drugs may also produce side effects that may be objectionable to some patients. The same dose may also be used to diminish salivary flow in heavy metal poisoning. Table 6-9 lists two preparations and oral dosages used in dentistry. Atropine is often selected because it is well absorbed from the GI tract. However, because it is a quaternary amine, glycopyrrolate has fewer CNS effects than the belladonna alkaloids. Compared with atropine, it is a more selective antisialagogue and less likely to promote tachycardia in conventional doses. During general anesthesia, the anticholinergics also diminish secretions in the respiratory tract, thus lessening the likelihood of laryngospasm, and they help prevent reflex vagal slowing of the heart.

Not only do dentists occasionally have reason to use antimuscarinic drugs, but dentists often encounter patients who are taking them for any one of the reasons enumerated. Moreover, drugs of several different pharmacologic classes have substantial antimuscarinic effects. The most characteristic effects of these drugs that concern dentists are xerostomia and the discomfort that this brings to the patient as well as the deterioration in oral health. In those cases in which using a muscarinic receptor agonists may antagonize therapy involving an antimuscarinic drug, patients can be advised to drink water, suck on noncariogenic lemon drops, and irrigate the mouth with saliva substitutes to alleviate xerostomia. If saliva flow is reduced, patients need to pay scrupulous attention to oral hygiene, and caries control needs to be more aggressive. If there is progressive deterioration in oral health, consultation with the patient's physician may be helpful in identifying suitable therapeutic alternatives without as much xerostomia. The use of antimuscarinic drugs should be avoided in patients with prostate hypertrophy and those with atony in the urinary or gastrointestinal tract.

TABLE 6-9 Antimuscarinic Preparations and Oral Adult Dosages Used in Dentistry

Drug	Dose	Time of Administration*
Atropine sulfate	0.4 to 0.6 mg	1 to 2 hours
Glycopyrrolate	1 to 2 mg	30 to 45 minutes

*Time before the procedure when the drug is administered.

CHOLINERGIC DRUGS (DRUGS THAT ARE SELECTIVE FOR NICOTINIC RECEPTORS ARE DISCUSSED IN CHAPTER 7.)

Nonproprietary (Generic) Name	Proprietary (Trade) Name
Cholinomimetics	
Acetylcholine	Miochol-E
Bethanechol	Urecholine
Carbachol	Miostat, Isopto Carbachol
Cevimeline	Evoxac
Methacholine	Provocholine
Pilocarpine hydrochloride	Pilocar, Pilocel, Salagen
Pilocarpine nitrate*	P.V. Carpine Liquifilm
Pilocarpine ocular therapeutic system	Ocusert Pilo-20, Ocusert Pilo-40
Pilocarpine and epinephrine	E-Pilo-1, P_2E_1
Pilocarpine and physostigmine	Isopto P-ES
Anticholinesterases	
Ambenonium	Mytelase
Demecarium	Humorsol
Donepezil	Aricept
Echothiophate	Phospholine
Edrophonium	Tensilon, Reversol
Galantamine	Reminyl, Razadyne
Isoflurophate*	Floropryl
Neostigmine	Prostigmin, Bloxiverz
Physostigmine	Eserine Sulfate, Isopto Eserine
Physostigmine salicylate	Antilirium
Pyridostigmine	Mestinon
Rivastigmine	Exelon
Tacrine	Cognex
Cholinesterase Reactivator	
Pralidoxime	Protopam

*Not currently available in the United States.

ANTIMUSCARINIC DRUGS

Nonproprietary (Generic) Name	Proprietary (Trade) Name
Naturally Occurring Alkaloids	
Atropine	Atropisol, Atropen
Belladonna (tincture and extract)	—
L-Hyoscyamine	Levsin, Levbid
Scopolamine	Isopto Hyoscine
Scopolamine (transdermal therapeutic system)	Transderm Scop
Semisynthetic Derivatives	
Atropine ophthalmic	—
Homatropine	Isopto Homatropine
Methscopolamine	Pamine
Synthetic Quaternary Ammonium Compounds	
Aclidinium	Tudorza Pressair
Clidinium	Quarzan
Glycopyrrolate	Robinul, Cuvposa
Hexocyclium*	Tral Filmtabs
Ipratropium	Atrovent
Mepenzolate	Cantil
Methantheline*	Banthine
Propantheline	Pro-Banthine
Tiotropium	Spiriva
Tridihexethyl	Pathilon
Trospium	Sanctura
Umeclidinium	Incruse Ellipta
Synthetic Nonquaternary Ammonium Compounds	
Benztropine	Cogentin
Biperiden	Akineton
Cyclopentolate	Cyclogyl
Darifenacin	Enablex
Dicyclomine	Bentyl, Byclomine
Flavoxate	Urispas
Oxybutynin	Ditropan
Solifenacin	VESIcare
Tolterodine	Detrol
Trihexyphenidyl	Artane
Tropicamide	Mydriacyl, Tropicacyl
Tricyclic Benzodiazepine	
Pirenzepine*	Gastrozepine

*Not currently available in the United States.

CASE DISCUSSION

The patient will need assistance to reduce the risk of caries due to dry mouth. Several options are available. Strategies that can be used are the following: better patient hydration, saliva substitutes, sucking on noncariogenic fruit drops to stimulate flow, fluoride therapy, and drug therapy to stimulate salivary flow. A sialogogue, pilocarpine or cevimeline, can be used in certain circumstances. The question is: is this indicated here? Muscarinic receptor stimulation by either one of these drugs would likely be effective if the patient was not on the interacting medication, solifenacin. Solifenacin blocks the very receptors targeted by either pilocarpine or cevimeline. This is because the drug does not distinguish between the muscarinic receptors in the urinary bladder and the muscarinic receptors in the salivary glands. Moreover, attempting to stimulate muscarinic receptors with either sialogogue would tend to compromise the effect of the solifenacin used to reduce urinary urgency. A knowledge of the receptor pharmacology of these drugs dictates avoiding the use of a muscarinic receptor agonist to stimulate salivary flow in this case.

GENERAL REFERENCES

1. Dale HH: The action of certain esters and ethers of choline, and their relation to muscarine, *J Pharmacol Exp Ther* 6:147–190, 1914.
2. Furchgott RF: Endothelium-derived relaxing factor: early studies, and identification as nitric oxide, *Biosci Rep* 19:235–251, 1999.
3. Ghezzi L, Scarpini E, Galimberti D: Disease-modifying drugs in Alzheimer's disease, *Drug Des Devel Ther* 7:1471–1478, 2013.
4. Guyer AC, Long AA: Long-acting anticholinergics in the treatment of asthma, *Curr Opin Allergy Clin Immunol* 13:1473–6322, 2013.
5. Jayarajan J, Radomski SB: Pharmacotherapy of overactive bladder in adults: a review of efficacy, tolerability, and quality of life, *Res Rep Urol* 6:1–16, 2013.
6. Silman I: *Cholinergic mechanisms: function and dysfunction*, New York, 2004, Taylor and Francis.
7. Silvestri NJ, Wolfe GI: Myasthenia gravis, *Semin Neurol* 32:215–226, 2012.
8. Wolff A, Fox PC, Porter S, Konttinen YT: Established and novel approaches for the management of hyposalivation and xerostomia, *Curr Pharm Des* 18:5515–5521, 2012.

7

Drugs Affecting Nicotinic Receptors*

Xi-Qin Ding

KEY INFORMATION

- Acetylcholine (ACh) is the major neurotransmitter at the peripheral nicotinic receptor sites:
  - autonomic ganglia
  - skeletal neuromuscular junctions
- Nicotine initially stimulates then inhibits nicotinic receptors.
- The only therapeutic use for nicotine is in treating smoking cessation.
- The clinically useful drugs acting at the skeletal neuromuscular junction are neuromuscular junction blockers.
- Skeletal neuromuscular junction blockers (peripherally acting) are:
  - depolarizing (succinylcholine)
  - nondepolarizing (drugs similar to tubocurarine)
- Other drugs that relax skeletal muscle do so by acting on the central nervous system (CNS) (e.g., diazepam, cyclobenzaprine) or the somatic nerve (botulinum toxin).
- Dantrolene relaxes skeletal muscle by blocking release of calcium from the sarcoplasmic reticulum in the muscle cell.
- The clinical uses of skeletal neuromuscular blockers include endotracheal intubation, surgery, tetanus, and electroconvulsive therapy.
- The main adverse effects of skeletal neuromuscular blockers are respiratory failure for all drugs, with varying risks of the following depending on the drug: hypotension, arrhythmogenic effects, muscle spasm, and malignant hyperthermia.
- The main drug interactions of neuromuscular blockers involve anticholinesterases, general anesthetics, sympathomimetics, and some antibiotics.

CASE STUDY

Ms. Miller is your 35-year-old dental patient. At her last visit, she complained of pain in her jaw and ear area. The physical exam and CT scan results suggested that the pain might be caused by temporomandibular joint (TMJ) disorders. You asked her to take some over-the-counter pain medication (ibuprofen). Today, three weeks after her last visit, she visited your clinic again, and complained that the pain was not relieved by ibuprofen, the aching facial pain was getting worse, and sometimes it was difficult to open her mouth. You decide to continue medication treatment for her condition. What drug would you choose to alleviate her TMJ pain? What precautions would you take with your choice of medication?

Early in the sixteenth century, Spanish explorers of the New World encountered a plant extract used by South American natives to poison the tips of their hunting arrows. This extract, known as *curare*, was brought back to Europe, and its lethal action was quickly found to depend on muscular paralysis. Further understanding of the actions of curare did not occur for many years.

In 1856, the French physiologist Claude Bernard reported that the site of action of curare was the junction between nerve and muscle. He found that although curare blocked neuromuscular transmission, it did not impede conduction of impulses along the motor nerve or contraction of a directly stimulated muscle. The active substance used by Bernard in his studies, *d*-tubocurarine, was subsequently purified, and in 1942 it was administered for the first time to a patient undergoing surgery for appendicitis to relax the abdominal musculature. Drugs that block neuromuscular transmission have since found widespread acceptance for their ability to produce muscular flaccidity and are frequently administered as adjuncts to general anesthesia during surgery.

In 1889, the Cambridge physiologist John Newport Langley showed that nicotine could "paralyze" transmission at autonomic ganglia, and, in 1905, he showed that nicotine could stimulate muscle when applied to the motor endplate and that curare could block this effect. These findings led to the adoption of the term *nicotinic* to refer to the receptors present at autonomic ganglia and the neuromuscular junction.

The discovery of curare led to developments in two different directions: to drugs that affect transmission at nicotinic cholinergic receptors and to drugs that interfere with the mechanisms of skeletal muscle contraction. These two topics are the subjects of this chapter.

DRUGS AFFECTING GANGLIONIC TRANSMISSION

Ganglionic Transmission

Nicotinic receptors (see Chapters 1 and 5) play a crucial role in the transmission of autonomic impulses across the ganglionic synapse. As described in Chapter 5, acetylcholine (ACh) is the primary

*The author wishes to recognize Dr. Joel D. Schiff for his past contributions to this chapter.

neurotransmitter at sympathetic and parasympathetic ganglia, where it is released by preganglionic neurons and stimulates postganglionic neurons by activating the ganglion-type nicotinic receptor (N_N). Although it is sometimes convenient to think of autonomic ganglia as simple relay stations between the CNS and effector tissues, the existence of other receptors and neurotransmitters within the ganglia indicates that some modulation of the primary nervous inputs may occur.

Various pharmacologic and electrophysiologic studies show that at least four classes of receptors are involved in autonomic ganglia: cholinergic nicotinic, cholinergic muscarinic, α-adrenergic, and peptidergic. Muscarinic and peptidergic receptors mediate slow and late slow excitatory postsynaptic potentials, which seem to facilitate the transmission of high-frequency impulses through the primary nicotinic receptor pathway. Catecholamine-containing (dopamine or norepinephrine) interneurons have been proposed for sympathetic ganglia but are not found in parasympathetic ganglia. As shown in Figure 7-1, these interneurons may be stimulated by preganglionic muscarinic activity to release catecholamines that hyperpolarize the postganglionic neuron, producing an inhibitory postsynaptic potential. These secondary events of ganglionic transmission only modulate the primary depolarization, by making it more or less likely to occur. There are two important facts in ganglionic transmission. First, the autonomic ganglia contain neuronal components that are not protected by a structure analogous to the blood–brain barrier, which means that they are affected by many drugs and chemicals that never gain access to central synapses. Second, ACh is the primary transmitter of the ganglionic synapse, and any drug that interferes with the synthesis, release, or inactivation of ACh or with its interaction with the N_N receptor has the capacity to interfere with ganglionic transmission.

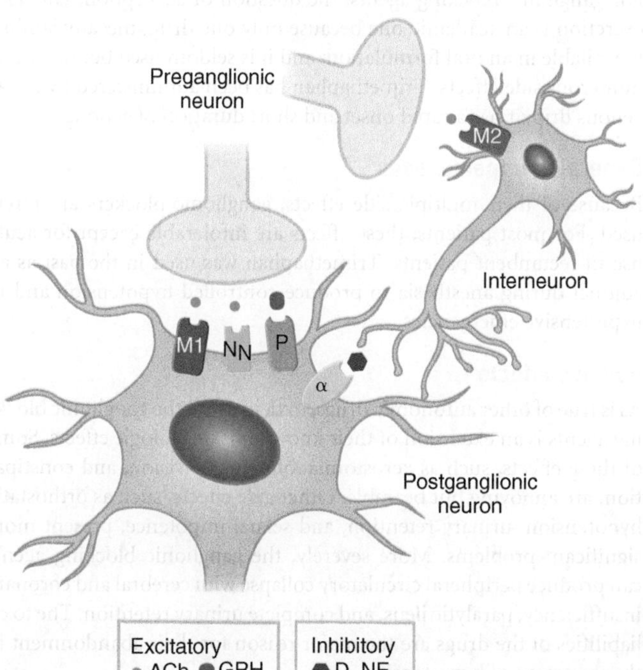

FIG 7-1 Ganglionic transmission. The principal pathway involves ganglion-type nicotinic receptor (*N_N*) transmission sensitive to conventional ganglionic blocking drugs. Muscarinic receptors (*M_1* and *M_2*), sensitive to atropine blockade, support and inhibit depolarization of the postganglionic neuron, respectively. As shown, a catecholamine-containing interneuron participates in causing inhibition. Co-release of peptides such as gonadotropin-releasing hormone (*GRH*) produces long-lasting facilitation of transmission. *α*, α-Adrenergic receptor; *ACh*, acetylcholine; *D*, dopamine; *NE*, norepinephrine; *P*, peptidergic receptor.

Nicotinic Receptor Stimulating Drugs

Nicotine

Nicotine, as indicated in Chapter 6, is the principal psychoactive ingredient in tobacco products. As a selective depolarizing drug at nicotinic receptors, this alkaloid stimulates transmission at autonomic ganglia and at nicotinic synapses in the CNS. It also activates various sensory fibers equipped with nicotinic receptors, including mechanoreceptors in the lung, skin, mesentery, and tongue; nociceptive nerve endings; and chemoreceptors in the carotid body and aortic arch. Stimulation of nicotinic receptors in skeletal muscle is easily shown in the laboratory, but it is not evident normally in humans because initial stimulation is soon followed by inhibition at these nicotinic sites. Nicotine has a dual effect on ganglionic transmission—initial stimulation and subsequent depression (see later).

An important feature of nicotinic receptors is their tendency to become **desensitized** (i.e., unresponsive) on continuous exposure to agonists or depolarizing antagonists (e.g., succinylcholine, as described later). The actions of nicotine are highly time and concentration dependent, and complex patterns of stimulation and depression are observed. The heart rate may be increased by stimulation of sympathetic ganglia and the adrenal medulla or by inhibition of vagal transmission in the heart, or both. Conversely, blockade of sympathetic transmission to the heart and stimulation of parasympathetic transmission can cause bradycardia. The heart rate may also be affected by central influences and by actions at peripheral sensory sites.

Generally, usual amounts of nicotine absorbed during cigarette smoking cause mild cardiovascular stimulation, increased gastrointestinal activity, and CNS stimulation accompanied in regular users by a feeling of well-being and decreased irritability. With long-term use, tolerance and physical dependence occur. The **addictive nature of nicotine** is thought to result from its action on the reward pathway—the circuitry in the brain that regulates feelings of pleasure and euphoria.

Acute overdose of nicotine causes nausea and vomiting, abdominal pain, dizziness and confusion, and muscular weakness. If untreated, death may ensue from cardiopulmonary collapse. Nevertheless, the primary health issues regarding nicotine stem from the chronic use of tobacco products. An increased incidence of cancer and cardiovascular and pulmonary disease has been well documented. In dentistry, tobacco use has been linked to oropharyngeal carcinoma, leukoplakia, acute and chronic periodontal disease, delayed wound healing, halitosis, and tooth staining.

The only therapeutic use of nicotine is as an adjunct in tobacco cessation programs. Nicotine is administered in multiple forms (Table 7-1) to maintain pharmacologic concentrations of the alkaloid and to prevent tobacco cessation from triggering an acute withdrawal syndrome, which includes irritability, anxiety, sleep disturbances, and cognitive impairment. The nicotine dose is reduced in a stepwise fashion over several months, during which time the patient ideally receives continued counseling and motivational assistance to remain abstinent.

Because of the deleterious effects of smoking and smokeless tobacco on health, including oral health, the dentist is encouraged to participate actively in helping patients quit tobacco use. Such participation may include, in addition to prescribing a nicotine product, procedures to promote fresh breath and tooth bleaching to remove tobacco stains from teeth, which may provide additional positive psychological feedback to encourage abstinence from tobacco use.

Varenicline

Varenicline is a partial agonist at nicotinic receptors containing $\alpha_4\beta_2$ subunits. The drug has a half-life of about 24 hours. Its receptor selectivity and long half-life provide therapeutic advantages. Headache,

TABLE 7-1 Nicotine-Containing and Varenicline Smoking Deterrents

Product	Proprietary (Trade) Name	Drug Content per Dose Form (mg)	Daily Drug Dose (mg)	Duration (wk)*
Nicotine inhalation system	Nicotrol Inhaler	4 (delivered)	≤64	≤24
Nicotine gum	Habitrol, Nicorette, Nicotrol, Thrive	2 and 4†	≤80	12
Nicotine lozenge	Commit	2 and 4†	≤80	12
Nicotine transdermal system (skin patch)‡	NicoDerm CQ	114	21	6
		76	14	2
		38	7	2
Nicotine nasal spray	Nicotrol NS	0.5§	≤40	≤14
Varenicline	Chantix	0.5 and 1	2**	12

*For the gum, lozenge, and inhalation dosage forms, the number of units used per day is gradually decreased, beginning after 6 weeks of therapy (12 weeks for the inhalation system). The transdermal system uses a sequential schedule, beginning with the strongest patch for individuals smoking more than 10 cigarettes per day (as shown). For individuals who smoke 6 to 10 cigarettes per day, the patch delivering 14 mg/day should be used for 6 weeks, followed by the 7-mg dose for 2 weeks.

†The 2-mg dose is used for individuals who smoke less than 25 cigarettes per day.

‡Patch is worn 16 to 24 hours a day.

§Dose per actuation; one to two sprays in each nostril (1-mg to 2-mg total dose) is recommended. ** A one week titration precedes this dose.

nausea and insomnia can occur. Neuropsychiatric symptoms and seizure activity have also been reported. Table7-1 provides dosage information in nicotine replacement therapy for smoking cessation.

Ganglionic Blockers

Ganglionic blocking agents can be classified on the basis of their chemical structure or mechanism of action into three groups (Fig. 7-2), as follows:

1. Depolarizing drugs, such as nicotine, which produce initial stimulation and varying degrees of subsequent block through a mechanism analogous to that of succinylcholine (see later). At higher doses, these agents can stimulate and block other cholinergic receptors, such as those at the neuromuscular junction and in the CNS.
2. Competitive drugs, such as trimethaphan and tetraethylammonium, which interfere with the binding of ACh to the nicotinic receptor.
3. Noncompetitive agents, such as hexamethonium (C6) and mecamylamine, a secondary amine. Hexamethonium interferes with ganglionic transmission by blocking ion channels that have been opened by ACh, whereas mecamylamine seems to share properties associated with both hexamethonium and the competitive blocking agents.

Pharmacologic effects

All the ganglionic blocking drugs, regardless of their structure or their mechanism of action, have the same basic pharmacology, although many of them have additional actions at sites other than ganglionic receptors. An ideal ganglionic blocking agent would be a compound that interferes only with ganglionic transmission, blocks without previous excitation, and does not influence the release of transmitter. Hexamethonium is a prototype agent that meets these criteria.

The pharmacology of the ganglionic blocking drugs is predictable because all parasympathetic and sympathetic ganglia are blocked by most of the available agents. Ganglia are not equally sensitive to the blocking drugs, however, and some effects are easier to block than others. The effects of ganglionic agents are profoundly influenced by the background tone; that is, the effect of blocking a ganglion is proportional to the rate of nerve transmission through that ganglion at any given time. If vascular tone is high, as it would be in a standing individual, the ganglionic blocking agents would produce a profound decrease in blood pressure, much greater than they would in a recumbent individual, in whom vascular tone would be lower. Finally, because these drugs block sympathetic and parasympathetic actions, the direction and magnitude of their effects are related to which autonomic division provides the dominant baseline control for a given organ. Table 7-2 summarizes the usual predominance of sympathetic or parasympathetic tone at various effector sites and the pharmacologic effects of ganglionic blockade.

Absorption, fate, and excretion

For ganglionic blocking agents, the question of absorption, fate, and excretion is an academic one because only one drug, mecamylamine, is available in an oral formulation, and it is seldom used because of its numerous side effects. Trimethaphan has been administered by intravenous drip; it has a rapid onset and short duration of action.

General therapeutic uses

Because of their multiple side effects, ganglionic blockers are rarely used. For most patients, these effects are intolerable except for acute use in recumbent patients. Trimethaphan was used in the past as an adjunct during anesthesia to produce controlled hypotension and in hypertensive emergencies.

Adverse effects

As is true of other autonomic drugs, toxicity from the ganglionic blocking agents is an extension of their known pharmacologic effects. Some of these effects, such as xerostomia, blurring of vision, and constipation, are annoying but bearable. Other side effects, such as orthostatic hypotension, urinary retention, and sexual impotence, present more significant problems. More severely, the ganglionic blocking agents can produce peripheral circulatory collapse with cerebral and coronary insufficiency, paralytic ileus, and complete urinary retention. The toxic liabilities of the drugs are the major reason for their abandonment in the treatment of hypertension.

DRUGS AFFECTING NEUROMUSCULAR TRANSMISSION

Skeletal Neuromuscular Transmission

Nervous control of skeletal muscle contraction is mediated by ACh. In response to a motor neuron action potential, ACh is released from the terminal region of the nerve fiber. The transmitter diffuses across the junctional cleft and binds to the **muscle-type nicotinic receptor** (N_M) on

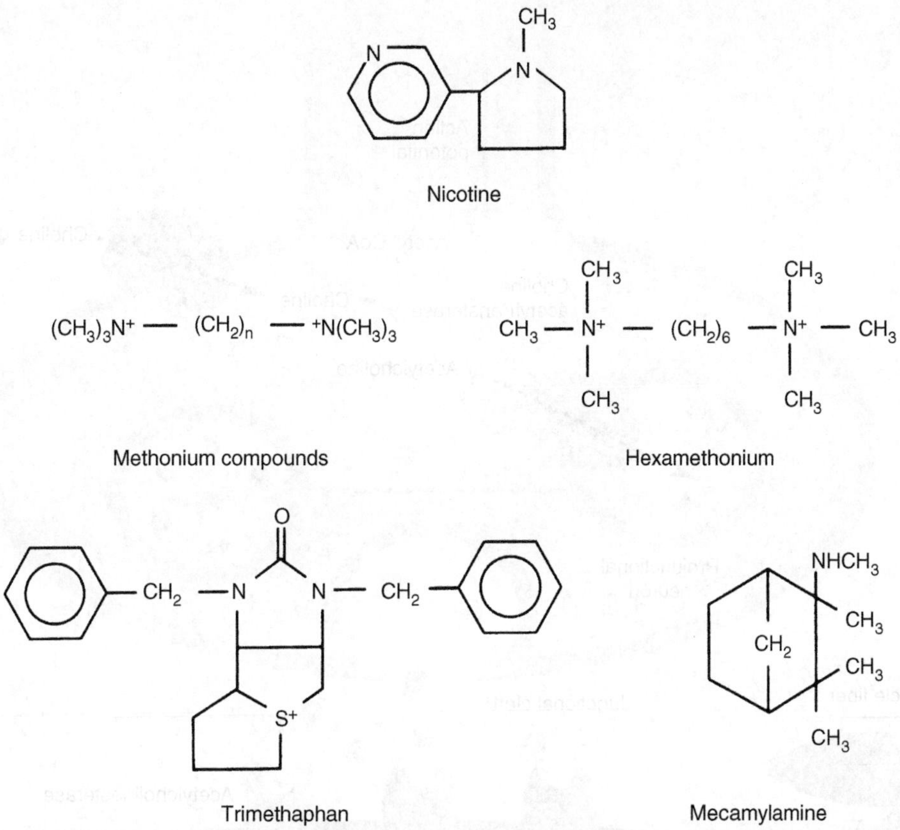

Nicotine

Methonium compounds

Hexamethonium

Trimethaphan

Mecamylamine

FIG 7-2 Structural formulas of nicotine and some nondepolarizing ganglionic blockers.

TABLE 7-2 Usual Predominance of Sympathetic or Parasympathetic Tone at Various Effector Sites and Consequences of Autonomic Ganglionic Blockade

Site	Predominant Tone	Effect of Ganglionic Blockade
Arterioles	Sympathetic (adrenergic)	Dilation; increased peripheral blood flow; hypotension
Veins	Sympathetic (adrenergic)	Dilation; peripheral pooling of blood; decreased venous return; decreased cardiac output
Heart	Parasympathetic (cholinergic)	Tachycardia
Iris	Parasympathetic (cholinergic)	Mydriasis
Ciliary muscle	Parasympathetic (cholinergic)	Cycloplegia; focus to far vision
Gastrointestinal tract	Parasympathetic (cholinergic)	Reduced tone and motility; constipation; decreased gastric and pancreatic secretions
Urinary bladder	Parasympathetic (cholinergic)	Urinary retention
Salivary glands	Parasympathetic (cholinergic)	Xerostomia
Sweat glands	Sympathetic (cholinergic)	Anhidrosis
Genital tract	Sympathetic and parasympathetic	Decreased stimulation

From Hibbs RE et al.: Agents acting at the neuromuscular junction and autonomic ganglia. In Brunton LL, Chabner BA, Knollmann BC, editors: *Goodman & Gilman's the pharmacological basis of therapeutics*, ed 12, New York, 2011, McGraw-Hill Medical.

the postjunctional membrane (endplate) of the muscle fiber (Fig. 7-3). The N_M is a pentameric complex composed of two α subunits, one β subunit, one δ subunit, and one γ subunit, and each subunit is a four-transmembrane domain peptide (Fig. 7-4). The binding of two molecules of ACh to the α subunits of the receptor causes opening of the channel and subsequent inward flow of Na^+ and a consequent depolarization of the junctional region of the muscle fiber. Under normal conditions, the depolarization is sufficient to trigger an action potential in the electrically excitable muscle fiber membrane, and muscular contraction follows.

Neuromuscular Junction Blockers

Neuromuscular blocking drugs interfere with the ability of ACh to evoke endplate depolarization at the nicotinic N_M receptor. They are generally separated into two groups according to whether the agents themselves bring about endplate depolarization in the course of their action. The depolarizing and the nondepolarizing blocking agents differ in the mechanisms through which they produce neuromuscular blockade.

Classification and mechanism of action

Nondepolarizing agents. Nondepolarizing, or competitive, neuromuscular blocking drugs include **tubocurarine** (*d*-tubocurarine) and several other benzylisoquinolines (e.g., **atracurium, cisatracurium, and mivacurium**); aminosteroids such as **pancuronium, rocuronium, and vecuronium**; and a few unrelated drugs. All contain at least one quaternary nitrogen. Often, these drugs incorporate two cationic nitrogen sites into a rigid molecular structure (Fig. 7-5).

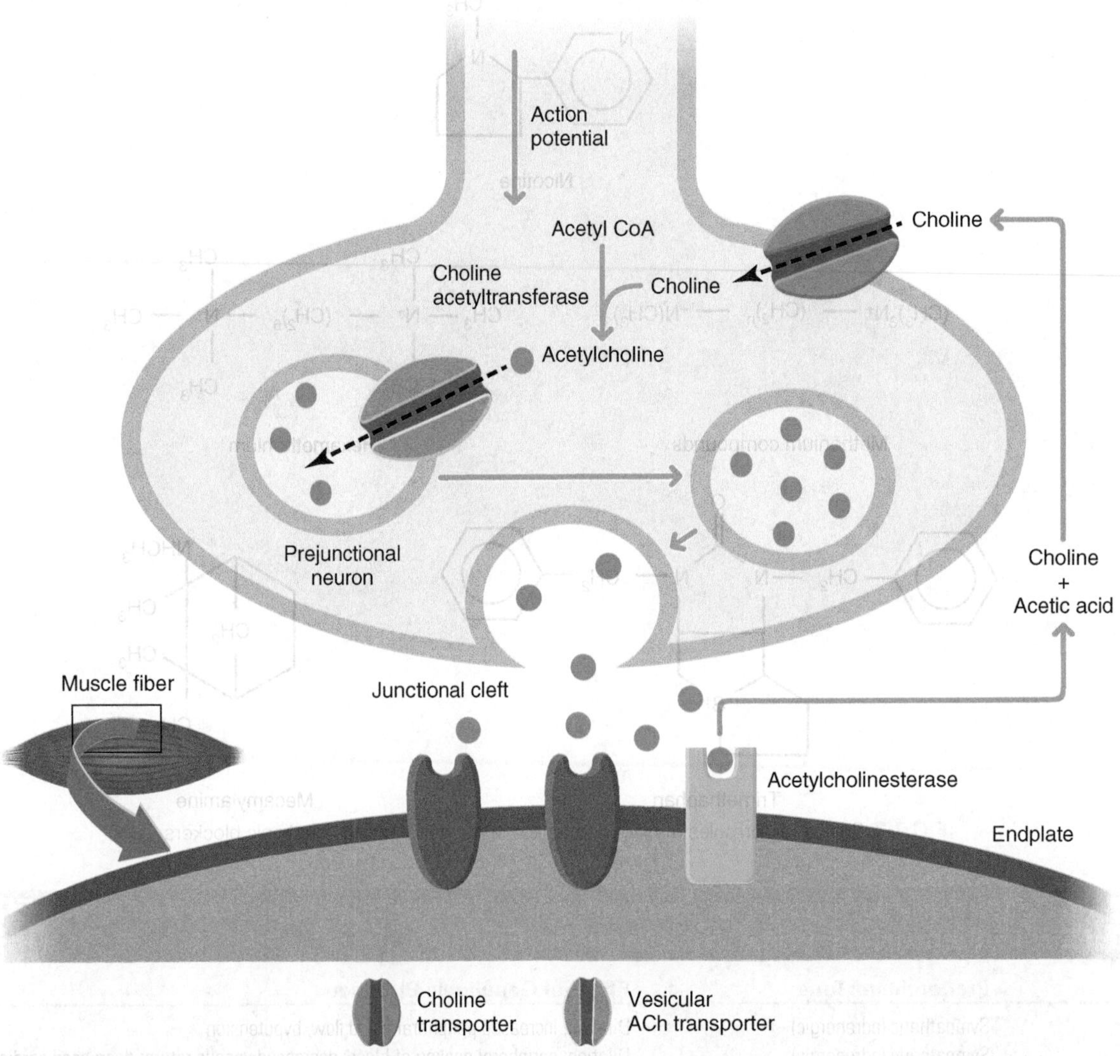

FIG 7-3 Neuromuscular transmission. ACh released from presynaptic neuron acts on muscle-type nicotinic receptor (N_M) on the motor endplate and induces depolarization of muscle fiber membranes. *ACh*, Acetylcholine.

All these drugs act by occupying the endplate N_M receptor sites of the muscle fiber, blocking access to these sites by ACh. The drugs themselves do not cause endplate depolarization. Inhibition of neuromuscular transmission is essentially competitive, with the blocking agent and ACh competing for receptor sites on the muscle fiber. By interfering with nervous excitation of muscle without themselves producing any excitation, the nondepolarizing blocking agents cause flaccid paralysis. Because of the very large safety margin in neuromuscular transmission, which results from the sixfold to tenfold excess of ACh released from the motor neuron terminal and from the large number of postjunctional receptor sites (resulting in a highly coupled stimulus-response system as described in Chapter 5), about 70% of the ACh receptors must normally be blocked to produce any clinically apparent effect on muscle function.

Tubocurarine, was first isolated as the primary active ingredient from arrow poisons used by South American Indians. It has the longest history of use and can be thought of as the prototype of this category of drugs, nevertheless, it is no longer used because of its tendency to evoke undesirable side effects. The major side effect seen with curare is hypotension. The excessive hypotension is the result of (1) blockade of autonomic ganglia and (2) release of histamine from mast cells. Histamine release may also cause bronchoconstriction in asthmatic patients.

Depolarizing agents. Similar to most nondepolarizing blockers, **succinylcholine** (also known as suxamethonium chloride), the major **depolarizing** agent, is a bisquaternary compound. In contrast to the nondepolarizing agents, succinylcholine is a much smaller molecule, composed simply of two ACh molecules attached at the acetyl ends (see Fig. 7-5). Succinylcholine has a flexible chain linkage between its cationic moieties.

Succinylcholine acts by binding to the N_M receptor. As the class name suggests, the initial effect of the binding of this agent is a depolarization of the muscle fiber. During the early phase of its action, there is a period of excitation during which the sensitivity of the muscle to ACh is increased. It is common for the drug-induced depolarization to be great enough to trigger action potentials and fasciculations (i.e., spontaneous twitching) in the muscle fibers. It is believed, however, that the fasciculations reflect activation of prejunctional N_M receptors, causing motor neuron depolarization and ACh release. Postjunctional stimulation by succinylcholine is responsible for an increased muscle tension observable with some muscles, especially the masseter. When exaggerated, masseteric tone can occasionally complicate endotracheal intubation.

The depolarization produced by the blocking agent gradually diminishes, but the endplate membrane potential does not completely return to its resting level. After the transient excitation, and during the

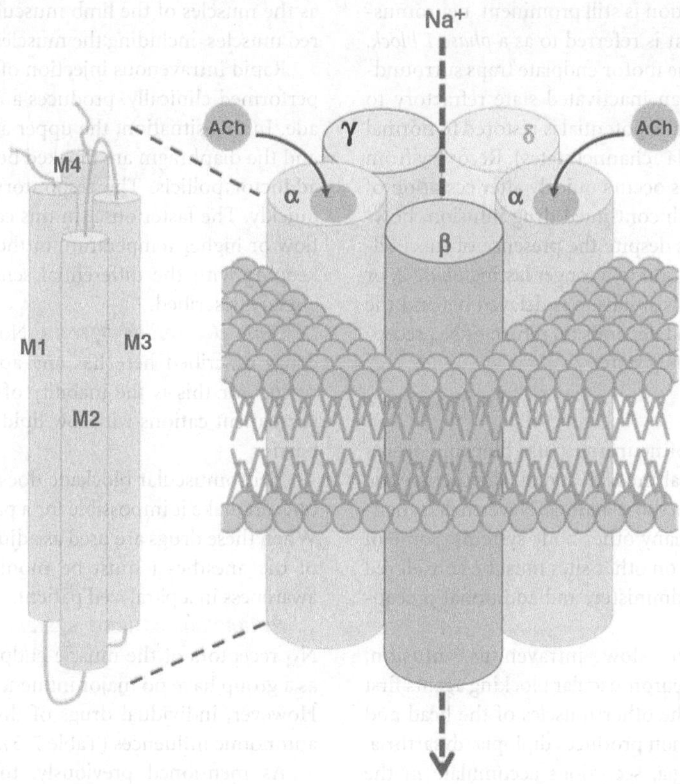

FIG 7-4 Structure of muscle-type nicotinic receptor. An α subunit is magnified to show its four membrane domains.

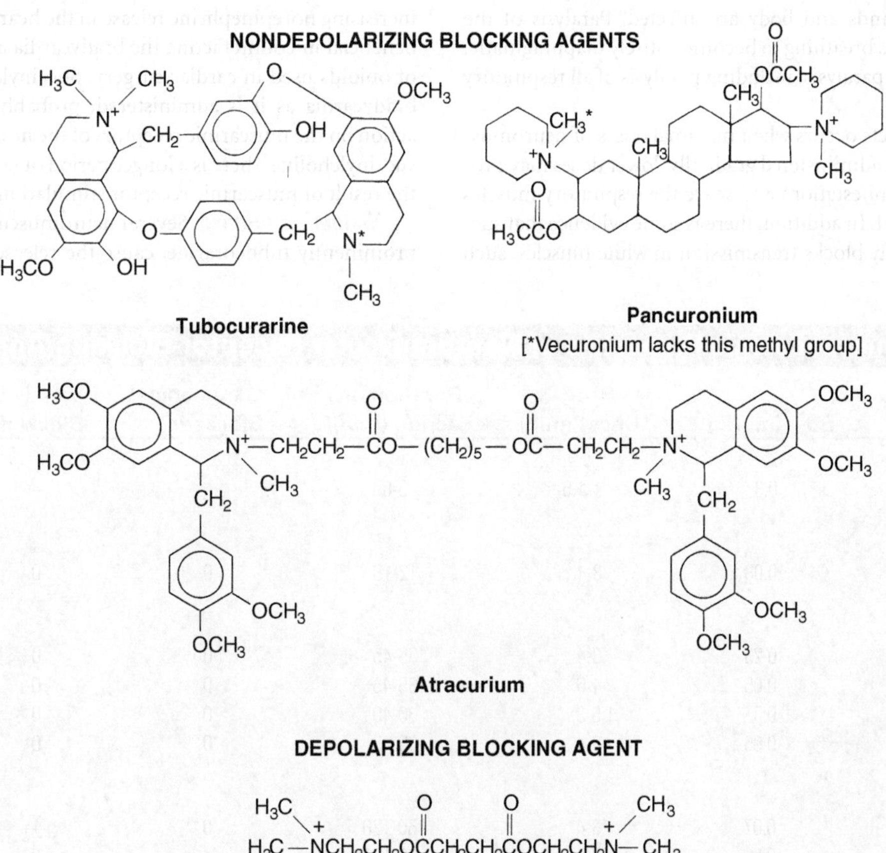

FIG 7-5 Structural formulas of some neuromuscular blockers.

period in which endplate depolarization is still prominent, neuromuscular transmission is blocked in what is referred to as a *phase 1 block.* Here, continued depolarization of the motor endplate traps surrounding voltage-gated Na^+ channels in an inactivated state refractory to further stimulation until the membrane potential is restored to normal (see Chapter 14 for a discussion of Na^+ channel states). Recovery from this form of neuromuscular paralysis occurs quickly after cessation of succinylcholine administration. With continued drug infusion, however, the endplate slowly repolarizes despite the presence of succinylcholine, and there is a gradual transition to a longer lasting *phase 2*, or *desensitization, block.* Recovery in this situation is delayed beyond the removal of the depolarizing agent and depends on return of N_M receptors from the desensitized to the resting state.

Pharmacologic effects

The major pharmacologic actions of neuromuscular blocking agents are on the motor endplate of skeletal muscle, and all the therapeutic applications of these drugs stem from those actions. Nevertheless, neuromuscular blocking agents affect many other body systems. Some of the more important of these actions on other sites must be considered when choosing blocking drugs to administer, and additional precautions in their use must be observed.

Neuromuscular junction. On slow intravenous infusion, depolarizing and nondepolarizing neuromuscular blocking agents first affect the facial muscles and then the other muscles of the head and neck. In a conscious subject, this action produces diplopia, dysarthria, and dysphagia; because of dysphagia, secretions accumulate in the throat, and breathing becomes difficult. In addition, there is an uncomfortable sensation of warmth. As the blockade progresses, the small muscles of the hands and body are affected. Paralysis of the intercostal muscles forces breathing to become entirely diaphragmatic. Finally, complete flaccid paralysis, including paralysis of all respiratory muscles, occurs.

This sequence of effects occurs when maximal doses of neuromuscular blocking agents are administered gradually; lower doses may produce only the earlier manifestations and spare the respiratory muscles from becoming paralyzed. In addition, there is some evidence that succinylcholine preferentially blocks transmission in white muscles, such as the muscles of the limb musculature, with less effect on the slower red muscles, including the muscles of respiration.

Rapid intravenous injection of full paralyzing doses, as is generally performed clinically, produces a different temporal pattern of blockade. In this situation, the upper airway muscles (larynx, tongue, jaw) and the diaphragm are blocked before peripheral muscles, such as the adductor pollicis. The respiratory muscles also recover much more quickly. The faster onset in this case may result from increased blood flow or higher temperature in these muscles; the faster recovery is in keeping with the differential sensitivity to neuromuscular blockade already described.

Central nervous system. None of the neuromuscular blocking drugs described here has any apparent influence on the CNS. The reason for this is the inability of these compounds, all of which are permanent cations with low lipid solubility, to cross the blood–brain barrier.

Neuromuscular blockade does not provide anesthesia or analgesia but can make it impossible for a patient to show outward signs of pain. When these drugs are used as adjuncts to general anesthesia, the depth of the anesthesia must be monitored closely to prevent conscious awareness in a paralyzed patient.

Autonomic nervous system. Because of their selectivity for the N_M receptors of the muscle endplate, neuromuscular blocking drugs as a group have no major influence on the autonomic nervous system. However, individual drugs of this category do exert certain specific autonomic influences (Table 7-3).

As mentioned previously, tubocurarine exerts partial blocking activity at autonomic ganglia. Pancuronium is notable for its tendency to increase the heart rate, in part by inhibiting vagal activity and by increasing norepinephrine release in the heart. This side effect has been beneficial in counteracting the bradycardia associated with high doses of opioids used in cardiac surgery. Succinylcholine causes a transient bradycardia as it is administered, probably through a vagomimetic action on the muscarinic receptors of the heart. After administration of succinylcholine, there is a longer period of tachycardia that seems to be the result of muscarinic receptor stimulation of sympathetic ganglia.

Histamine release. Several neuromuscular blocking agents, most prominently tubocurarine, cause the release of histamine from mast

TABLE 7-3 Pharmacologic Properties of Neuromuscular Receptor-Blocking Agents

Drugs	ED_{95} (mg/kg)*	Onset (min)	Duration of Action (min)†	Ganglionic Blockade	Vagal Blockade	Histamine Release
Ultrashort-Acting						
Succinylcholine	0.3	1-1.5	5-8	–	–	+
Short-Acting						
Mivacurium	0.08	3-4	12-18	0	0	+
Intermediate-Acting						
Atracurium	0.23	3-4	35-45	0	0	+
Cisatracurium	0.05	4-6	35-45	0	0	0
Rocuronium	0.3	1.5-3	30-40	0	0	0
Vecuronium	0.05	3-4	35-45	0	0	0
Long-Acting						
Pancuronium	0.07	3-4	60-120	0	++	0
Tubocurarine	0.5	2-4	60-120	++	0	++

*The ED_{95} is the dose that reduces the twitch tension in the adductor pollicis by at least 95% in 50% of individuals. Usual intubating doses are two to three times the ED_{95}.
†The duration of action is the time from onset of paralysis to return of 25% of the twitch tension in the adductor pollicis.
++, moderate effect; +, slight effect; –, opposite effect (i.e., stimulation of ganglionic and vagal transmission); 0, no effect.

cells into the circulation (see Table 7-3). These drugs are capable of producing the histamine-mediated effects of hypotension, edema, bronchospasm, and increased salivary flow. The last two actions may introduce complications during performance of controlled respiration and can be prevented by prior administration of antihistamines. Histamine-related effects can be minimized by avoiding rapid intravenous injection. Neuromuscular blocking drugs with a steroid nucleus (pancuronium, rocuronium, vecuronium) are free of this side effect; cisatracurium is the only currently available benzylisoquinoline without this clinical liability. Histamine release is generally thought to be a direct result of stimulating nicotinic receptors on the mast cell membrane.

Cardiovascular system. Although none of the neuromuscular blocking drugs has any direct effect on vascular tone, all can produce hypotension by a combination of indirect actions. The release of histamine, as described earlier, causes edema and vasodilation. The loss of skeletal muscle tone as a result of neuromuscular blockade eliminates the skeletal muscle pumping action on the veins of the extremities; there is pooling of blood in capacitance veins and a concomitant reduction in venous return to the heart. In addition to these physiologic effects on the circulation, another factor is the use of assisted or controlled ventilation during the period of muscular paralysis. The increased intrathoracic pressure produced by the respirator during its positive-pressure phase further reduces venous return to the heart. In this respect, alternating positive-pressure and negative-pressure respirators are less problematic than intermittent positive-pressure devices because of the increased venous return in the negative-pressure phase of the former. These causes of hypotension can be treated by positioning the patient with the lower extremities elevated slightly above the heart and by administering isotonic fluids intravenously, possibly in combination with sympathomimetic vasoconstrictors.

Absorption, fate, and excretion

Neuromuscular blocking agents are generally administered intravenously. Intramuscular administration of large doses is effective for most of the agents discussed and may be used in treating some pediatric patients in whom intravenous injection might present difficulties, but this route does not offer the precision of control or the rapidity of onset of action afforded by the intravenous route. The drugs discussed in this chapter are ineffective when given orally. This was known to be the case for tubocurarine by South American hunters, who readily ate prey felled by arrows laden with the drug.

All the clinically useful blocking agents show their effects within a few minutes after administration (see Table 7-3). **Succinylcholine** provides excellent **intubating** conditions (vocal cord relaxation) within 60 to 90 seconds after intravenous injection and gives its maximal effect within 2 minutes. Recovery is apparent after 5 to 10 minutes. The nondepolarizing blockers exhibit slower onsets and longer durations of action. The speed of onset for these drugs is inversely related to blocker potency, presumably because fewer drug molecules of highly potent agents are available to initiate blockade. Rocuronium, the least potent competitive blocker currently available, has been found to produce intubating conditions almost as rapidly as succinylcholine in children, and it is the best alternative to succinylcholine currently available when rapid intubation is required.

Mivacurium, a short-acting agent, has a clinical duration of action of only 15 to 20 minutes after an intubating dose. Here, the clinical duration is defined as the time from onset of muscle blockade until the point at which the twitch response of the adductor pollicis to a supramaximal electrical stimulus has returned to 25% of baseline (full recovery does not occur until much later). Comparative durations for intermediate-acting and long-acting blockers (as classified in Table 7-3) are 30 to 45 minutes and 60 to 120 minutes. With any of the drugs, blockade may be prolonged either by repeated injection or by continuous intravenous infusion.

Succinylcholine and mivacurium are hydrolyzed by plasma pseudocholinesterase, which explains their brief durations of action. Mivacurium is broken down to inactive metabolites; whereas succinylcholine is first converted to succinylmonocholine, a much weaker depolarizing blocking agent, and then to succinic acid and choline. It is possible to inhibit the plasma pseudocholinesterase with hexafluorenium, after which the action of succinylcholine is prolonged much longer.

In some individuals with atypical plasma cholinesterase, succinylcholine and mivacurium persist in the body for several hours. Some of these patients can be identified before drug administration by a cholinesterase activity assay. Purified cholinesterase has been injected intravenously before treatment to obtain a neuromuscular blockade of short duration in these patients.

Long-acting neuromuscular blockers are to a large extent excreted unchanged in the urine and bile; their actions may be greatly prolonged in patients with renal or hepatic failure, and they are largely contraindicated in such patients. Intermediate-acting neuromuscular blockers are also eliminated in the urine and bile. The primary reason for the shorter duration of action of intermediate-acting drugs compared with long-acting agents is the greater redistribution potential of the intermediate-acting drugs.

General therapeutic uses

Since the first clinical use of tubocurarine in 1942, several applications for neuromuscular blocking agents have gained wide acceptance. An ideal neuromuscular blocker would be rapid in onset, consistent in duration of action (even in patients with advanced renal or hepatic disease), and readily reversible in effect. It would be a nondepolarizing drug so that it would not cause muscle fasciculations; it would be free of autonomic and cardiovascular effects; and it would not liberate histamine from muscle or other tissues. Additionally, it would not induce tachyphylaxis, so prolonged blockade could be maintained without the need to increase the dosage over time. None of the existing neuromuscular blocking agents fulfills all these expectations; however, cisatracurium, vecuronium, and rocuronium are notable for their relative lack of effects other than neuromuscular blockade (see Table 7-3).

Endotracheal intubation. To secure a patent, protected airway, an endotracheal tube is often inserted in patients receiving general anesthesia or patients who are otherwise unconscious or in need of respiratory assistance (or both). Succinylcholine has long been the drug of choice because of its fast onset and short duration of action. It is administered intravenously to produce a depolarizing block of skeletal muscle lasting about 5 to 10 minutes (see Table 7-3). This short action is related to metabolism by plasma and liver pseudocholinesterases to succinic acid and choline. The short duration of action of this compound has made it one of the drugs of choice to relax the laryngeal muscles before intubation and as an adjuvant before electroconvulsive shock therapy. Rocuronium is the only currently available nondepolarizing blocking drug to approach the rapidity of onset of succinylcholine. This attribute is one reason why rocuronium is currently the most commonly used nondepolarizing blocking drug in clinical use. In any office where general anesthesia is used, succinylcholine should always be available to treat otherwise intractable laryngospasm.

Surgery. Neuromuscular blocking agents, especially intermediate-acting competitive blockers, are frequently used as adjuncts to general anesthesia during surgical procedures. The most common indication is to relax the abdominal wall musculature during abdominal surgery. This application is especially useful in procedures such as appendectomy, in which the underlying condition has produced reflex splinting of these muscles. During brain or cerebrovascular surgery in which the patient is sedated but conscious, neuromuscular blockade may be used to suppress cough and sneeze reflexes so that the field of operation remains immobilized.

Tetanus. In mild cases of tetanus, the patient is generally able to sustain respiration except during intermittent spasms. Here, neuromuscular blocking agents are administered to reduce the severity of these spasms. In severe cases of tetanus, in which the rigor of the patient extends to the respiratory musculature, neuromuscular blocking drugs are administered to induce flaccidity so that a mechanical respirator may be used.

Electroconvulsive therapy. In the treatment of depressive illness with electroconvulsive therapy, the therapeutic result is a consequence of the electrical stimulation of the CNS; the massive muscle spasm that accompanies such treatment is of no therapeutic benefit and has the potential for producing bodily injury. Neuromuscular blockade is induced by injection of succinylcholine before the electrical stimulation of the brain. Succinylcholine is used because of its short duration of action and lack of residual side effects.

Other uses. Succinylcholine is used to produce a short-lived muscular relaxation to permit numerous brief nonsurgical manipulations, such as bronchoscopy. In cases of laryngospasm, succinylcholine, often in subintubating doses, may be needed to relax the vocal cords and permit ventilation. Short-term infusion of cisatracurium has been shown to reduce hospital mortality in patients with acute respiratory distress syndrome.

Adverse effects

The major risk of overdosage with neuromuscular blocking agents is death from respiratory failure. When any neuromuscular blocking drug is administered, the practitioner must be prepared for the loss of respiratory function and have equipment immediately available for assisted or controlled respiration. In cases of respiratory arrest, ventilation must be maintained with external devices, generally with an endotracheal tube. Paralysis from nondepolarizing agents may be reversed to some extent through administration of an anticholinesterase (e.g., neostigmine), generally accompanied by an antimuscarinic drug (e.g., atropine) to prevent excessive muscarinic receptor-mediated sequelae to the anticholinesterase. The use of an anticholinesterase to reverse the phase 2 block of succinylcholine is also possible; however, with nondepolarizing drugs available covering a wide range of action durations, there should be no need for patient exposure to succinylcholine for a period long enough to produce a phase 2 block.

Arrhythmogenic effects of the neuromuscular blocking drugs stem from their ability to influence autonomic transmission in the ganglia and heart. Of the commonly used drugs, pancuronium is notable for its tendency to increase heart rate. Conversely, transient bradycardia is a known feature of succinylcholine, especially in small children. After a second dose of succinylcholine, bradycardia is more pronounced, and cardiac asystole has been reported. Atropine is administered before succinylcholine to ameliorate this effect. Arrhythmias have also resulted from the tendency of succinylcholine to cause hyperkalemia, especially in burn patients and patients with certain neuromuscular deficits. Sudden death may occur in children with undiagnosed muscular dystrophy. Hypotension and responses to drug-evoked histamine release have been reviewed previously.

Muscle pain is a common result of use of succinylcholine. Masseter spasm occurs in 1% of children and may complicate endotracheal intubation. In rare individuals, masseter spasm may be an early indicator of malignant hyperthermia, which is discussed in the section on dantrolene. In addition, succinylcholine tends to elevate ocular, cerebrospinal fluid, and gastrointestinal pressure and may be contraindicated in glaucoma patients, in patients suspected to have brain tumors, and in patients immediately after meals. Succinylcholine is perhaps the most likely skeletal neuromuscular junction blocking drug to cause anaphylaxis, with a reported incidence of one or two cases per 10,000 administrations.

Drug interactions

Many different classes of drugs are capable of interacting either positively or antagonistically with the neuromuscular blocking agents. The following sections describe the actions of drugs likely to be administered in conjunction with neuromuscular blockers and their effects on the activities of the blocking agents.

Anticholinesterases. Inhibitors of acetylcholinesterase, by blocking the enzymatic hydrolysis of ACh at the motor endplate, increase the amount of transmitter available at the receptor sites. These drugs antagonize the blockade produced by the nondepolarizing blocking agents, which act by competing with ACh for occupancy of receptor binding sites. Their effect when administered in conjunction with succinylcholine is more complex; after a brief period of antagonism, during which the blockade is reduced, they act to intensify the depolarizing neuromuscular blockade. Organophosphates such as echothiophate inhibit plasma cholinesterase and acetylcholinesterase. Systemic absorption of organophosphates prolongs the action of succinylcholine and mivacurium and reduces the effects of the nondepolarizing blocking agents in general. Neostigmine and pyridostigmine, but not edrophonium, also inhibit plasma cholinesterase.

Hexafluorenium, which specifically inhibits plasma pseudocholinesterase without affecting the endplate acetylcholinesterase, prolongs the presence of succinylcholine in the circulation. This action extends the duration of the neuromuscular blockade by succinylcholine, and presumably mivacurium, and decreases the dose necessary to obtain that blockade. In addition to its inhibitory effect on plasma cholinesterase, hexafluorenium is itself a weak nondepolarizing neuromuscular blocker and may slightly potentiate the blockade induced by other nondepolarizing blocking agents.

General anesthetics. Anesthetics that stabilize excitable membranes, most prominently ether and the halogenated inhalation agents, tend to interact positively with nondepolarizing blocking agents with enhanced skeletal muscle relaxation. When ether was used for general anesthesia, doses of tubocurarine had to be reduced by 50% or more. A similar reduction is necessary with isoflurane and pancuronium, but a more modest interaction occurs with sevoflurane and vecuronium.

Antibiotics. Some antibiotics, such as the aminoglycosides, reduce the amount of ACh released by the motor nerve terminal in response to an action potential and augment the muscle relaxation caused by nondepolarizing neuromuscular blocking drugs. Succinylcholine is also potentiated. Other antibiotics that may reduce dosage requirements for neuromuscular blocking agents include the tetracyclines, clindamycin, and the polymyxins.

Sympathomimetics. Catecholamines and other sympathomimetic agents may increase the amount of ACh released from the motor neuron and antagonize the blockade produced by nondepolarizing blocking agents.

Lithium. Lithium salts, used for the prophylaxis and treatment of manic-depressive illness, can slow the onset of neuromuscular blockade caused by succinylcholine but not that caused by the competitive blockers. Lithium also intensifies the blockade by pancuronium but not that by tubocurarine or succinylcholine, and it prolongs the effect of succinylcholine and pancuronium but not that of tubocurarine.

Neuromuscular blocking agents. Administration of a nondepolarizing blocking agent to a patient under the influence of the same drug or a different nondepolarizing blocking drug augments the blockade. This augmentation is usually additive; however, some combinations, such as an aminosteroid with a benzylisoquinoline, exhibit supra-additive effects. This drug interaction is used clinically; a small "priming" dose of one nondepolarizing blocker may be given to hasten the onset of the subsequent paralyzing dose of another.

Combinations of depolarizing and nondepolarizing neuromuscular blocking drugs are generally antagonistic but in a few cases have clinical value. Use has been made of this antagonism, however, in the administration of a low dose of nondepolarizing blocker before paralyzing the patient with succinylcholine. In this case, the nondepolarizing agent prevents the fasciculations normally caused by succinylcholine. It is also a frequent practice to use succinylcholine to induce a rapid blockade for tracheal intubation before the production of a long-term blockade with a nondepolarizing agent. The short lifetime of succinylcholine in the body effectively prevents any significant antagonism between the two drugs. Subsequent administration of the nondepolarizing drug generally provides evidence of enhanced neuromuscular blockade.

Other Drugs That Relax Skeletal Muscle

Many substances, synthetic and of biologic origin, have been found to act by affecting one or more of the processes involved in skeletal muscle contraction. Some of these drugs are used to treat various conditions of muscular spasms including spasms associated with stroke, multiple sclerosis, and cerebral palsy. These drugs are termed *spasmolytics*. Diazepam, methocarbamol, baclofen, tizanidine, and cyclobenzaprine are also discussed in Chapter 11.

Diazepam

Diazepam, a benzodiazepine compound, facilitates inhibition of γ-aminobutyric acid (GABA) in the CNS. It binds to the chloride channel, amplifying the effect of GABA ($GABA_A$ receptor) and acts in the spinal cord and higher centers. It is effective in treating all types of muscle spasms. The major limitation is sedation seen at muscular relaxant doses.

Baclofen

Baclofen is an orally effective agonist for the presynaptic CNS $GABA_B$ (metabotropic) receptor. When activated, the presynaptic $GABA_B$ receptor causes a decrease in release of excitatory amino acids (i.e., glutamate) and a corresponding decrease in skeletal muscle tone. Patients experience less sedation than with diazepam. This GABA analogue is used for relief of spasticity caused by multiple sclerosis, traumatic spinal cord injury, and amyotrophic lateral sclerosis.

Tizanidine

Tizanidine is a clonidine-like α_2-adrenoceptor stimulant that reduces skeletal muscle spasticity by a CNS inhibitory action, but with less hypotension than seen with clonidine. Other side effects include sedation, asthenia, and dry mouth.

Cyclobenzaprine

Cyclobenzaprine is structurally and mechanistically related to the tricyclic antidepressants. It is used for short-term (1 to 2 weeks) treatment of muscular spasms associated with musculoskeletal conditions including temporomandibular joint (TMJ) disorders. The mechanism of action of cyclobenzaprine may be to increase brainstem-mediated noradrenergic inhibition of spinal cord neurons. Side effects include atropine-like responses and effects produced by inhibition of catecholamine uptake. Cyclobenzaprine may act adversely with tramadol, antidepressants, meperidine, and MAO inhibitors. Serotonin syndrome has been reported with concurrent use of cyclobenzaprine and some of these drugs. The drug is contraindicated in patients with recent myocardial infarction, heart conduction abnormalities, heart failure, arrhythmias, and hyperthyroidism.

Other centrally acting muscle relaxants

Other drugs, such as methocarbamol and metaxalone, used to the treatment of acute muscle spasms, are discussed in Chapter 11.

Botulinum toxin

The toxin produced by *Clostridium botulinum* acts on the motor nerve terminal to prevent the release of ACh in response to the arrival of an axonal action potential (see Fig. 7-7). The toxin interferes with the influx of extracellular Ca^{2+} into the nerve terminal. Ca^{2+} influx during the action potential is necessary for ACh release. Botulinum toxin affects all peripheral cholinergic nerves.

Botulinum toxin is used in ophthalmology in the treatment of strabismus and certain ocular deviations (tropias). The toxin, applied locally, can produce long-lasting (weeks to months) paralysis of an excessively contracting extraocular muscle. The aim is that, as function gradually recovers, CNS adaptation will maintain the correction. The toxin is also used to relieve severe blepharospasm. It is injected into the orbicularis oculi, where it blocks spasmodic contractions for 3 months. Another serologically distinct form of botulinum toxin is used for certain types of skeletal muscle dystonias, such as cervical dystonias. In a cosmetic application, botulinum toxin is used to inhibit activity of certain facial muscles, such as those of the forehead, whose contractions cause skin wrinkling. Botulinum toxin is also used by intradetrusor injection to treat overactive bladder. See chapter 37 for its use in migraine.

Dantrolene

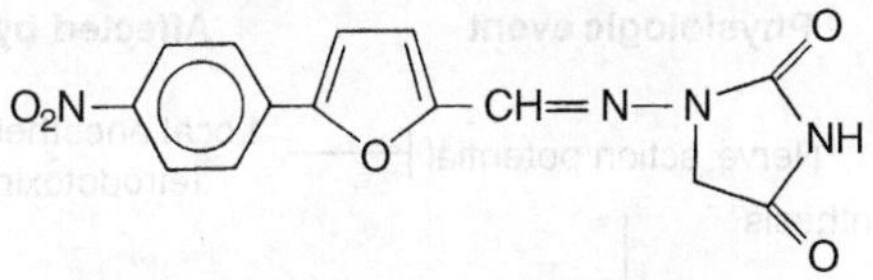

O_2N—C₆H₄—(furan)—CH=N—N(imidazolidinedione)

FIG 7-6 Structural formula of dantrolene.

Dantrolene (Fig. 7-6) is an agent that acts within the skeletal muscle fiber rather than on the neuromuscular junction. Its site of action is the sarcoplasmic reticulum ryanodine receptor Ca^{2+} channel, where it inhibits the depolarization-induced release of Ca^{2+} from the sarcoplasmic reticulum into the cytoplasm, interfering with excitation-contraction coupling. The principal therapeutic applications of dantrolene are for the relief of spasticity associated with upper motor neuron disorders and for the prophylaxis and treatment of malignant hyperthermia, a condition due to excessive release of Ca^{2+} from sarcoplasmic reticulum. Dantrolene is also used to relieve spastic movements, clonus, and rigidities that result from stroke, multiple sclerosis, or cerebral palsy.

The muscle weakness, which is simply an extension of the drug's therapeutic action, generally does not occur at dosages used for treatment of spastic movements, although doses high enough to produce

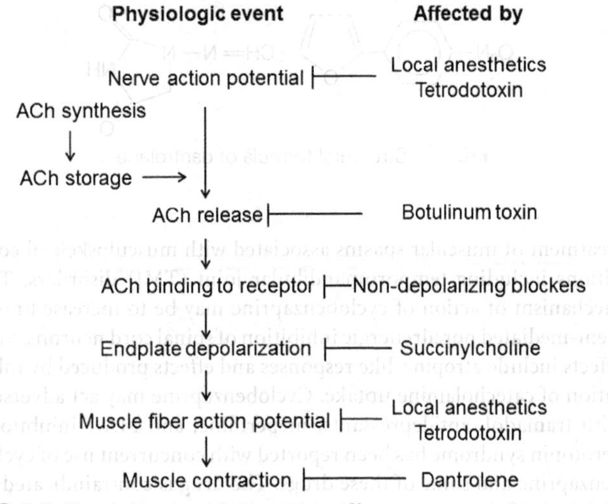

FIG 7-7 Sites of action of drugs that affect neuromuscular transmission.

this effect are sometimes needed to achieve symptom remission. Doses of dantrolene that produce muscle weakness are sometimes used in prophylaxis of malignant hyperthermia before surgery on patients with a family history of the condition. Dantrolene is strongly contraindicated in amyotrophic lateral sclerosis because the muscular weakness associated with this condition, when exacerbated by the drug, can lead to respiratory difficulty.

Adverse effects of dantrolene include muscle weakness and hepatotoxicity. Hepatotoxicity of varying degrees has been reported in approximately 1% of patients taking dantrolene for 60 days or longer. Hepatic function should be monitored during long-term therapy with dantrolene.

Dantrolene is effective when administered intravenously or orally; in the latter case, approximately 20% is absorbed, largely through the small intestine. Metabolism of dantrolene occurs in the liver, largely by 5-hydroxylation of the hydantoin moiety.

Drugs affecting nicotinic receptor transmission and other miscellaneous agents are summarized in the box shown, and sites of action of these drugs are illustrated in Figure 7-7.

APPLICATIONS IN DENTISTRY

Dental practice has few indications for the use of neuromuscular blocking agents. Among the situations in which use of these drugs might be appropriate are mandibular fractures, when muscle relaxation is needed to permit manipulation of bone fragments, and trismus, when no more conservative means exist to permit mouth opening for diagnosis and treatment. Dental anesthesiologists have a need to be well educated in the pharmacology and use of peripheral skeletal muscle relaxants.

Drugs that relax skeletal muscle by acting on the CNS are valuable in certain dental situations. These drugs can be effective in reducing contraction of skeletal muscles in TMJ disorders and the associated pain. Diazepam, and other similar drugs, may be effective in this setting. Cyclobenzaprine can also be an effective choice for the condition; however, dentists should be aware of the contraindications for its use. Muscle relaxants acting on the CNS are also sometimes prescribed to reduce patients' stress levels and to help patients stop grinding their teeth.

DRUGS AFFECTING NICOTINIC RECEPTOR TRANSMISSION AND OTHER MISCELLANEOUS AGENTS

Nonproprietary (Generic) Name	Proprietary (Trade) Name
Nicotine	See Table 7-1
Varenicline	Chantix
Ganglionic Blockers	
Hexamethonium*	–
Mecamylamine	Inversine
Trimethaphan*	Arfonad
Neuromuscular Blockers	
Nondepolarizing	
Atracurium	Tracrium
Cisatracurium	Nimbex
Mivacurium	Mivacron
Pancuronium	Pavulon
Rocuronium	Zemuron
Tubocurarine*	
Vecuronium	Norcuron
Depolarizing	
Succinylcholine	Anectine, Quelicin
Miscellaneous Agents	
Baclofen	Lioresal
Botulinum toxin type A	Botox
Botulinum toxin type B	Myobloc
Cyclobenzaprine	Amrix, Flexeril
Dantrolene	Dantrium
Diazepam	Valium
Tizanidine	Zanaflex

*Not currently available in the United States.

CASE DISCUSSION

The use of a muscle relaxant is one of the drug options to treat TMJ pain. You choose cyclobenzaprine (Flexeril). A typical dose of cyclobenzaprine is 5 mg three times per day. (A typical dose of cyclobenzaprine extended-release capsules is 15 mg once a day). The drug treatment can last for 10 days to 2 weeks. The treatment should not last longer than 2 to 3 weeks. Care must be taken to avoid excessive sedation that can occur if centrally acting muscle relaxants are given with other sedatives that the patient may be taking. These include over-the-counter first-generation antihistamines and antimuscarinic drugs. Xerostomia will likely be significant with the combination of cyclobenzaprine with one or more of these drugs. Moreover, there are contraindications that apply to cyclobenzaprine. The risk of seizures increases with the combination of cyclobenzaprine and tramadol. The effect of cyclobenzaprine is increased with drugs that inhibit cytochrome P450-1A2. Other contraindications are previously listed.

There are alternate choices for muscle relaxation, such as diazepam.

GENERAL REFERENCES

1. ADA website on nicotine replacement therapy, smoking cessation card. www.ada.org/en/~/media/ADA/Science and Research/Files/Topics_smoking_cessation_card. accessed February 2016.
2. Alhazzani W, Alshahrani M, Jaeschke R, et al.: Neuromuscular blocking agents in acute respiratory distress syndrome: a systematic review and meta-analysis of randomized controlled trials, *Crit Care* 17:R43, 2013.

3. Atherton DP, Hunter JM: Clinical pharmacokinetics of the newer neuromuscular blocking drugs, *Clin Pharmacokinet* 36:169–189, 1999.
4. Claudius C, Garvey LH, Viby-Mogensen J: The undesirable effects of neuromuscular blocking drugs, *Anaesthesia* 64(Suppl 1):10–21, 2009.
5. Crews KM, Johnson L, Nichols M: Patient management in a tobacco-cessation program in the dental practice, *Compend Contin Educ Dent* 15:1142–1155, 1994.
6. Mirzakhani H, Welch CA, Eikermann M, et al.: Neuromuscular blocking agents for electroconvulsive therapy: a systematic review, *Acta Anaesthesiol Scand* 56:3–16, 2012.
7. Moss J, Philbin DM, Rosow CE, et al.: Histamine release by neuromuscular blocking agents in man, *Klin Wochenschr* 60:891–895, 1982.
8. Oo YW, Gomez-Hurtado N, Walweel K, et al.: Essential role of calmodulin in RyR inhibition by dantrolene, *Mol Pharmacol* 88:57–63, 2015.
9. Pinder RM, Brogden RN, Speight TM, et al.: Dantrolene sodium: a review of its pharmacological properties and therapeutic efficacy in spasticity, *Drugs* 13:3–23, 1977.
10. Raghavendra T: Neuromuscular blocking drugs: discovery and development, *J R Soc Med* 95:363–367, 2002.
11. Singh YN, Marshall IG, Harvey AL: The mechanisms of the muscle paralysing actions of antibiotics, and their interaction with neuromuscular blocking agents, *Rev Drug Metab Drug Interact* 3:129–153, 1980.
12. Waud BE, Waud DR: Interaction among agents that block end-plate depolarization competitively, *Anesthesiology* 63:4–15, 1985.

8

Adrenergic Agonists

Yaping Tu, Michael T. Piascik, and Peter W. Abel

KEY INFORMATION

- Adrenergic agonists exhibit their physiologic effects through activation of adrenergic receptors.
- Agonists at adrenergic receptors are either direct-acting or indirect-acting.
- Catecholamines, norepinephrine, and epinephrine are direct-acting and nonselective adrenergic agonists.
- Indirect-acting agonists cause the release of the neurotransmitter norepinephrine from sympathetic nerve terminals.
- Adrenergic receptors are classified into three major types: α_1-, α_2-, and β-adrenergic receptors.
- Adrenergic agonists mediate functions in both the periphery and central nervous system.
- The metabolic inactivation of catecholamines largely depends on catechol-O-methyltransferase (COMT), whereas noncatecholamines are not subject to metabolism by COMT.
- A number of tissues respond to adrenergic agonists.
- Therapeutic uses of the adrenergic agonists include local vasoconstriction, vasoconstriction in the treatment of hypotension and shock, bronchodilation, relaxation of uterine smooth muscle, ophthalmic uses, relief of allergic states (including anaphylaxis), central nervous system (CNS) stimulation, and control of hypertension.
- In dental practice, epinephrine is often used in combination with local anesthetic agents to prolong the duration of anesthetic action.
- Almost all adverse effects of the adrenergic agonists on the cardiovascular system and CNS are dose dependent.

CASE STUDY

Mrs. B is an elderly patient who you have seen for routine dental care for the past 10 years. She is a friendly woman who religiously makes and keeps appointments and enjoys her visits and telling you about her grandchildren. She has Graves disease (hyperthyroidism), and over the last few years, she has developed mild hypertension. She is a fan of afternoon "talk shows" and relayed to you a story about a man who was injected with a "hypertensive drug" with his "tooth numbing medication" during a dental visit and then had a heart attack. She asks you what "hypertensive drug" is used by dentists. Because she has cardiovascular disease, she asks if you use this drug and if this could happen to her. What would you say to Mrs. B about the safe use of vasoconstrictor drugs with local anesthetics during dental procedures? What other adverse effects on the oral cavity are associated with vasoconstrictor/local anesthetic use?

HISTORY

The first recorded study of an adrenergic agent resulted in the isolation in 1887 of ephedrine from the herb *ma huang*, which had been grown and used in China for centuries. At the same time, investigators were making extracts of all the organs of the body in an attempt to discover new hormones. Studies by Oliver and Schafer in the early 1890s showed a potent vasopressor substance in extracts of the adrenal gland. The active agent, epinephrine, was soon isolated by Abel, prepared commercially, and marketed in the United States under the trade name of Adrenalin(e). In 1905, an account was published of the results of mixing procaine with epinephrine to obtain dental anesthesia. The year 1887 also witnessed the synthesis of amphetamine, which was first marketed in the 1930s and became widely abused by the mid-1950s. The addictive nature of amphetamine was soon realized and led to its designation in 1970 as a drug of high abuse potential. Concerns in more recent years regarding the potential adverse cardiovascular effects of various sympathomimetic drugs have prompted the U.S. Food and Drug Administration to increasingly regulate their use as appetite suppressants, nasal decongestants, and cold remedies. In 2004, ma huang was banned for sale as a dietary supplement.

CLASSIFICATION OF ADRENERGIC DRUGS AND RECEPTORS

One common feature of all adrenergic drugs is that their effects are mediated through activation of adrenergic receptors. **Direct-acting adrenergic agonists** bind to adrenergic receptors and activate the receptors to produce their effects. **Indirect-acting agonists** act by increasing the amount of norepinephrine available to stimulate adrenergic receptors. The most common action of indirect-acting agonists is to cause the release of the neurotransmitter norepinephrine from sympathetic nerve terminals. **Mixed-acting adrenergic agonists** have direct and indirect mechanisms of action.

Adrenergic receptors have been classified into three major types: **α_1-adrenergic, α_2-adrenergic, and β-adrenergic receptors**. In recent years, numerous receptor subtypes (**α_{1A}, α_{1B}, α_{1D}; α_{2A}, α_{2B}, α_{2C}; β_1, β_2, β_3**) have been discovered by molecular cloning and pharmacologic techniques. Several dopamine receptors have also been identified (**D_1, D_2, D_3, D_4, D_5**). These receptor subtypes are distinguished by differences in their amino acid sequences, as determined from gene-cloning experiments, and by their affinity for subtype-selective drugs. Many adrenergic agonists activate more than one of the major adrenergic receptor types. In contrast, some agonists selectively activate α receptors, others activate β receptors, and some are selective for an individual adrenergic receptor subtype (e.g., β_1 or β_2). Similarly, as discussed in Chapter 9, there are antagonists for the various adrenergic receptors, some of which are receptor type or subtype selective, and some of which are nonselective.

Although most adrenergic agonists have prominent peripheral actions that form the basis for their therapeutic applications, some of these drugs have important actions in the CNS. Adrenergic drugs such as amphetamine and ephedrine are capable of causing stimulation of adrenergic receptors in the CNS. Several drugs have been developed, including the antihypertensive agent clonidine, that have their principal action on CNS α_2 receptors, whose stimulation results in a decrease in sympathetic outflow from the brain.

CHEMISTRY AND STRUCTURE–ACTIVITY RELATIONSHIPS

The chemical structures of the three endogenous adrenergic amines are illustrated in Figure 8-1. These compounds are synthesized sequentially in adrenergic nerve terminals and adrenal chromaffin cells (see Chapter 5). These three agents, all derived from tyrosine, are also referred to as *catecholamines* because they are catechol derivatives of phenylethylamine.

Table 8-1 lists some adrenergic agonists currently in use and illustrates certain major alterations in biologic activity that occur with structural modifications. The following conclusions about the relationship between structure and activity can be drawn:

1. Direct-acting agonists generally require a hydroxyl group at positions 3 and 4 of the aromatic ring plus a hydroxyl group on the β-carbon atom of the side chain for maximal stimulation of α and β receptors.
2. Indirect-acting agonists have no β-hydroxyl group and either no or one hydroxyl group on the ring. Agents devoid of hydroxyl substitutions can penetrate the blood–brain barrier better and exert prominent CNS effects.
3. Mixed-acting agonists generally have a β-hydroxyl group and a single ring hydroxyl group.
4. Dopamine, which lacks the β-carbon hydroxyl moiety present in other endogenous catecholamines, stimulates dopamine receptors in addition to α_1 and β_1 receptors.
5. Modifications in chemical structure can confer significant differences in pharmacodynamics and/or pharmacokinetics.
6. The alkyl substitution on the nitrogen causes a shift in drug affinity toward the β_2-adrenergic receptor. The affinity of norepinephrine, with no alkyl substitution, is much greater for α-adrenergic receptors than for β_2-adrenergic receptors; the affinity of epinephrine, with a methyl group, is similar for α-adrenergic and β_2-adrenergic receptors; and the affinity of isoproterenol, with an isopropyl group, is much greater for β_2 receptors than for α receptors. All three drugs have significant β_1-adrenergic receptor effects. Changes in the position of ring hydroxyl groups lead to compounds (e.g., terbutaline and ritodrine) with selective affinity for the β_2-adrenergic receptor.

The catecholamine nucleus is extremely sensitive to oxidation. This chemical reaction results in the formation of a quinone, adrenochrome, which accounts for inactivation and color changes that may occur in solutions of catecholamines, such as in dental anesthetic cartridges. A sulfite salt (e.g., sodium metabisulfite) is incorporated in such solutions as an antioxidant to prevent catecholamine degradation.

PHARMACOLOGIC EFFECTS

The pharmacology of the adrenergic agonists is complicated by the diversity of the drugs in this group. They differ in mode of action (direct, indirect, or mixed), receptor selectivity, and relative predominance of peripheral and CNS effects. Predicting the pharmacologic activity of any adrenergic agonist is possible by knowing whether it is direct-acting or indirect-acting and what receptors it affects. The density of the receptor population in a particular organ or organ system also influences the effectiveness of adrenergic agonists. Table 8-2 summarizes the relative receptor preferences of several adrenergic drugs.

Of the many adrenergic agonists that have been isolated or synthesized and are used clinically, only a few are considered in detail here. The following discussion begins with endogenous transmitters or hormones, capable of interacting with α and β receptors, and then focuses successively on other direct-acting agonists that are more selective in receptor preference. This discussion concludes with indirect-acting and mixed-acting drugs that cause the release of norepinephrine as their primary mode of action. Where appropriate, additional drugs are mentioned in the sections on therapeutic applications and adverse effects.

Endogenous Catecholamines: Norepinephrine and Epinephrine

Vascular effects

The net effect of systemic administration of **norepinephrine or epinephrine** on the cardiovascular system depends on various factors, including the route and rate of administration, the dose given, and the presence or absence of interacting drugs. When injected locally, norepinephrine and epinephrine cause contraction of vascular smooth muscle and vasoconstriction in the surrounding tissues by stimulating α-adrenergic receptors. Systemic effects on the vasculature occurring after absorption of these catecholamines into the circulation depend on the plasma concentrations achieved and on the drugs' actions at α-adrenergic and β-adrenergic receptors. With plasma concentrations attained by an intravenous infusion of 0.2 μg/kg/min or more, the response to norepinephrine reflects stimulation of **α receptors** causing increased systolic and diastolic blood pressures. Although the same infusion of epinephrine stimulates α-adrenergic and β_2-adrenergic receptors in the vasculature, the more robust α receptor–mediated vasoconstrictor response masks the vasodilatory effect of β_2 receptor stimulation, and the net result is usually vasoconstriction, similar to that of norepinephrine. However, at low plasma concentrations, as achieved by an intravenous administration of 0.1 μg/kg/min or less, the effect of epinephrine on α-adrenergic receptors is less, allowing the **β_2 receptor vasodilator** response to become manifest. Under these conditions, mean arterial blood pressure may decrease, and the direct stimulant effect of epinephrine on the myocardium

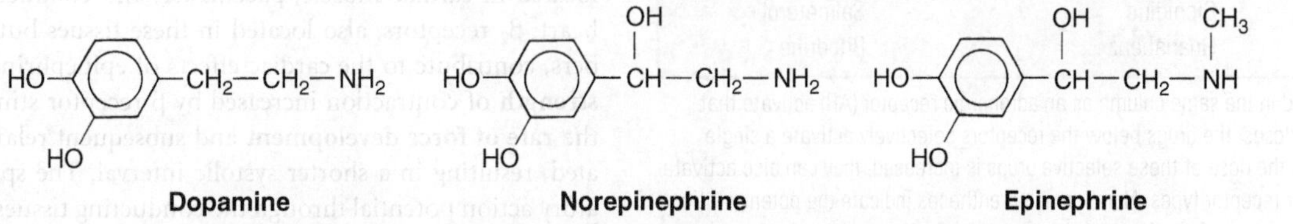

HO–C₆H₃(HO)–CH₂–CH₂–NH₂ **Dopamine**

HO–C₆H₃(HO)–CH(OH)–CH₂–NH₂ **Norepinephrine**

HO–C₆H₃(HO)–CH(OH)–CH₂–NH(CH₃) **Epinephrine**

FIG 8-1 Chemical structures of three naturally occurring adrenergic agonists.

TABLE 8-1 Structure–Activity Relationships of Selected Adrenergic Agonists

Agonist	Receptor Preference	Ring (positions 1–6)	β-Carbon	α-Carbon	Nitrogen
Structure (Phenylethylamine Nucleus)			H—Cβ—	H—Cα—	H—N—
Direct Action					
Dopamine	D*, α_1, β_1	3—OH, 4—OH	H	H	H
Dobutamine	β_1[†]	3—OH, 4—OH	H	H	CH(CH$_3$)—(CH$_2$)$_2$—C$_6$H$_4$—OH
Norepinephrine	α, β_1	3—OH, 4—OH	OH	H	H
Levonordefrin	α_2, β_1	3—OH, 4—OH	OH	CH_3	H
Epinephrine	α, β	3—OH, 4—OH	OH	H	CH_3
Isoproterenol	β	3—OH, 4—OH	OH	H	$CH(CH_3)_2$
Metaproterenol	β_2	3—OH, 5—OH	OH	H	$CH(CH_3)_2$
Terbutaline	β_2	3—OH, 5—OH	OH	H	$C(CH_3)_3$
Albuterol	β_2	3—CH_2OH, 4—OH	OH	H	$C(CH_3)_3$
Ritodrine	β_2	—4—OH	OH	CH_3	CH_2—CH_2—C$_6$H$_4$—OH
Isoetharine	β_2	3—OH, 4—OH	OH	CH_2CH_3	$CH(CH_3)_2$
Mainly Direct Action					
Methoxamine	α_1	2—OCH_3, 5—OCH_3	OH	CH_3	H
Phenylephrine	α_1	3—OH—	OH	H	CH_3
Mixed Action					
Ephedrine	α, α (CNS), β	— —	OH	CH_3	CH_3
Metaraminol	α, β	3—OH—	OH	CH_3	H
Mainly Indirect Action					
Tyramine	α, β	4—OH—	H	H	H
Hydroxyamphetamine	α, β	4—OH—	H	CH_3	H
Amphetamine	α, α (CNS), β	— —	H	CH_3	H
Methamphetamine	α, α (CNS), β	— —	H	CH_3	CH_3

CNS, Central nervous system.
*Dopaminergic.
[†]Different stereoisomers have opposing actions on β_1 receptors and β_2 receptors; thus β_1 selectivity is more apparent than real.
_ _ = no substitution on the ring

TABLE 8-2 Receptor Selectivity of Adrenergic Receptor Agonists

Epinephrine (1)	Epinephrine	Epinephrine	Epinephrine
Levonordefrin (3)	Levonordefrin	Levonordefrin	
Norepinephrine (10)	Norepinephrine	Norepinephrine	
		Isoproterenol	Isoproterenol (0.05)
α_1-AR	α_2-AR	β_1-AR	β_2-AR
Phenylephrine (20)	Oxymetazoline	Dobutamine	Albuterol
Methoxamine	Tetrahydrozoline		Terbutaline
	Brimonidine		Bitolterol
	Clonidine		Salmeterol
	Guanabenz		Ritodrine

Note: Drugs listed in the same column as an adrenergic receptor (AR) activate that receptor. At low doses, the drugs below the receptors selectively activate a single receptor type. As the dose of these selective drugs is increased, they can also activate some of the other receptor types. Numbers in parentheses indicate the potency ratio of α to β_2 receptor–mediated effects, with epinephrine having equal potency at α-adrenergic and β_2-adrenergic receptors. Potency ratios are approximate only, and they vary with the tissue and species studied.

(tachycardia) is observed. This effect is not shared by norepinephrine because it does not stimulate β_2 receptors.

Figure 8-2 shows the typical cardiovascular responses to the intravenous bolus injection of these catecholamines. The qualitatively different effects of high versus low doses of epinephrine on blood pressure and heart rate described earlier are apparent as the initially high concentration of drug declines over the course of several minutes into the low-dose range.

Cardiac effects

Norepinephrine and epinephrine stimulate β_1-adrenergic receptors located in cardiac muscle, pacemaker, and conducting tissues of the heart; β_2 receptors, also located in these tissues but in smaller numbers, contribute to the cardiac effects of epinephrine. Not only is the **strength** of contraction increased by β receptor stimulation, but also the **rate of force development** and subsequent relaxation is accentuated, resulting in a shorter systolic interval. The spread of the excitatory action potential through the conducting tissues is also increased. Pacemaker cells increase their firing rate, and automaticity is enhanced in normally quiescent muscle (latent pacemaker cells are activated).

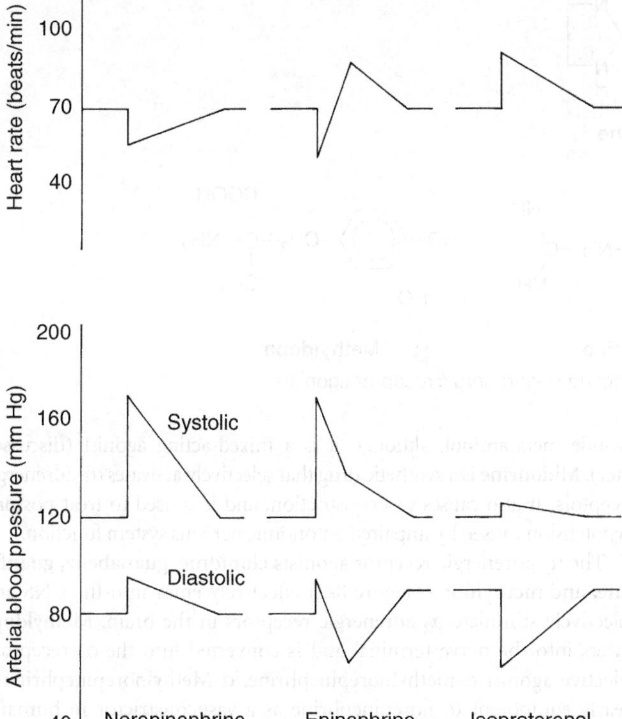

FIG 8-2 Schematic representation of the effects of three catecholamines on heart rate and arterial blood pressure in the dog. The drugs were administered intravenously by bolus injection at a dose of 1 μg/kg. Note the biphasic effect of epinephrine. Initially, the drug resembles norepinephrine by causing an increase in blood pressure and reduction in heart rate. As the concentration of epinephrine falls into the physiologic range, however, β-adrenergic receptor activation predominates. Diastolic pressure decreases, and direct cardiac effects are unmasked. The decreased heart rates seen with norepinephrine and at the beginning of the epinephrine response are produced indirectly by the baroreceptor reflex. The drug effects shown here last for approximately 5 minutes.

Stimulation of β-adrenergic receptors increases the work of the heart, which elevates cardiac oxygen consumption. Overall, cardiac efficiency (cardiac work done relative to oxygen consumption) is diminished.

Effects on nonvascular smooth muscle

The effect of adrenergic agonists on smooth muscle in the organs of the thoracic and abdominal cavities is usually relaxation. The response of the uterus varies with the species, the stage of the estrous cycle, and pregnancy. Generally, α_1-adrenergic receptor activation leads to contraction, whereas β_2 receptor activation leads to relaxation. In either case, these effects require doses of epinephrine or norepinephrine that result in significant cardiovascular stimulation and are too evanescent to be useful therapeutically.

Bronchodilation is an example of smooth muscle relaxation that is of major therapeutic importance. The **β_2-adrenergic receptors** of the bronchioles are stimulated by epinephrine. Although epinephrine is a drug of choice to counteract bronchospasm associated with hypotension, as in anaphylactic shock, β_2 receptor–selective drugs such as albuterol produce bronchodilation with less concomitant β_1 receptor stimulation of the heart and are preferred in asthmatic patients.

Effects on salivary glands

Epinephrine and norepinephrine affect secretion by salivary glands through activation of adrenergic receptors on secretory cells and by stimulation of vascular adrenergic receptors that alter blood flow to the glands. Secretory cells of the major salivary glands contain α_1-adrenergic, β_1-adrenergic, and some β_2-adrenergic receptors. The principal adrenergic receptor linked to **protein secretion is the β_1 receptor**, although α_1 receptors also play a secretory role. Salivary glands also contain myoepithelial cells, in which α_1 receptor stimulation causes contraction around secretory acinar units, contributing to secretion. Stimulation of β receptors causes a more protein-rich (eg, amylase) secretion. Overall, the predominant characteristic of epinephrine and norepinephrine stimulation of the salivary glands is a modest secretion with a high concentration of protein.

Metabolic responses

Metabolic responses to **β_2**-adrenergic and **β_1**-adrenergic receptor stimulation lead to a transitory increase in circulating blood glucose as a result of liver **glycogenolysis and increased glucagon secretion.** An **α_2** receptor–mediated **inhibition of insulin secretion** contributes to the hyperglycemia caused by epinephrine. Stimulation of α_1, β_1 and β_3 receptors is involved in the hydrolysis of triglycerides, causing an increase in triglyceride lipase activity and subsequently in the concentration of circulating free fatty acids. The specific receptors that mediate metabolic effects vary among species.

Central nervous system effects

Although the catecholamines are extensively involved in neurotransmission in the CNS, peripherally administered catecholamines gain little access to the CNS because hydroxyl groups on the aromatic ring deter passage across the blood–brain barrier. Intravenous injection of epinephrine produces a variety of apparently central effects, however, including feelings of anxiety, jitteriness, and apprehension. Most, if not all, of these effects are thought to be indirect, resulting from sensory input to the brain from the periphery.

Dopamine

Although dopamine is primarily a CNS neurotransmitter, it also has effects in the periphery, where dopamine receptors have been identified in various tissues. Molecular cloning studies have revealed at least five subtypes of the dopamine receptor (D_1 to D_5). Although the D_1 receptor subtype is thought to cause peripheral vasodilation, other dopamine receptor subtypes may also contribute to the various peripheral effects of dopamine. Peripheral dopamine-containing neurons have been found in autonomic ganglia in the form of small, intensely fluorescent cells and in kidney glomeruli. Evidence suggests that dopamine neurons help regulate sympathetic nervous system transmission, promote gastrointestinal relaxation, and cause vasodilation in some vascular beds.

Cardiovascular effects

Dopamine interacts with various receptor types to influence vascular function, and it is used therapeutically for maintaining renal function in cases of **shock** associated with compromised cardiac output. Although "low-dose" dopamine has now been used in this manner for more than 30 years, there is currently a growing body of evidence suggesting that this use for dopamine should be abandoned. Critics of low-dose dopamine have suggested that this increase in cardiac index, rather than dilation of the renal vasculature, is the primary reason for any observed increases in renal blood flow with low-dose dopamine, and that the potential for harm outweighs the benefits. With moderate doses, dopamine was thought to act at myocardial β_1-adrenergic receptors to increase contractile force. At higher doses, dopamine also stimulates α_1-adrenergic receptors, which produces vasoconstriction. As with all catecholamines, excessive doses of dopamine can cause tachycardia and generate arrhythmias. In addition to stimulating α_1 and β_1 receptors directly, dopamine in moderate to high doses causes the release of norepinephrine from sympathetic nerve terminals.

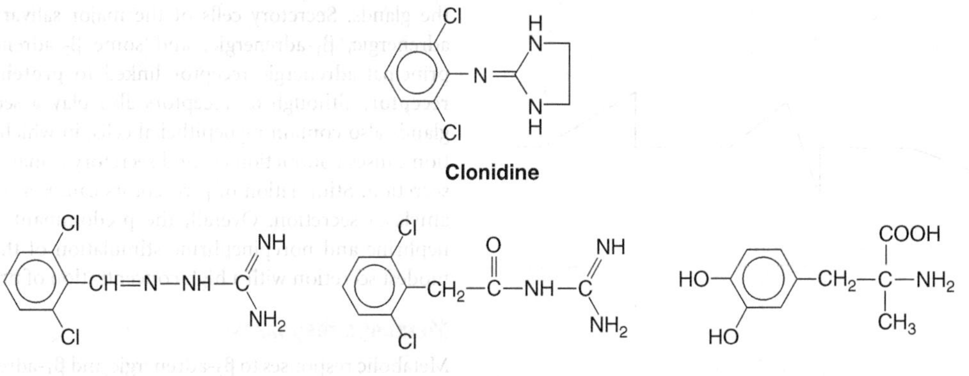

Clonidine

Guanabenz Guanfacine Methyldopa

FIG 8-3 Structural formulas of some centrally acting α_2-adrenergic receptor agonists.

Fenoldopam, a pharmacologic congener of dopamine, selectively activates D_1 receptors at therapeutic doses. It decreases mean blood pressure, increases renal blood flow, and causes diuresis and natriuresis. It is used intravenously for acute treatment of severe hypertension (see Chapter 23).

Other effects

Dopamine is involved with the sensory division of the autonomic nervous system. The high concentration of dopamine in the glomus cells of the carotid body and the effects of hypoxia on these cells suggest that dopamine is an inhibitory transmitter that modulates the frequency of discharge of the sensory fibers from that structure, which may affect cardiovascular and respiratory responses.

Dopamine itself does not penetrate the blood–brain barrier. **Levodopa**, which is converted into dopamine, does enter the CNS, however, and is used to treat Parkinson disease (see Chapter 13). Approximately 95% of an oral dose of levodopa is normally decarboxylated in the periphery to dopamine, leading to significant peripheral side effects attributable to dopamine. Dopamine can also produce nausea and vomiting as a result of excitation of the medullary chemoreceptor trigger zone, which lies outside the blood–brain barrier.

Another physiologic role for dopamine is modulation of the release of several anterior pituitary hormones. Dopamine acts as a prolactin release–inhibiting hormone by binding to D_2 receptors on the lactotrope cells of the anterior pituitary. Although dopamine itself is limited therapeutically by its inability to penetrate the blood–brain barrier, **bromocriptine** and other dopamine receptor agonists that are sufficiently lipid soluble to enter the CNS have been used successfully in the treatment of female infertility and other health problems resulting from hyperprolactinemia. Bromocriptine has also proved effective in controlling excessive secretion of growth hormone associated with pituitary adenomas. This last therapeutic application is surprising because dopamine is a stimulant of growth hormone release in the normal pituitary (see Chapter 29).

α-Adrenergic Receptor Agonists

These drugs stimulate α-adrenergic receptors, but have low affinity for β-adrenergic receptors. **Phenylephrine** and methoxamine differ from epinephrine and norepinephrine by being selective agonists at α_1-adrenergic receptors. Their primary pharmacologic effect is to cause contraction of vascular smooth muscle, resulting in an increase in systolic and diastolic blood pressures and reflex bradycardia. They are often administered either intranasally or systemically for temporary relief from nasal congestion. Because these drugs increase blood pressure, safety is always a concern. The α-adrenergic receptor agonist phenylpropanolamine was widely used in over-the-counter cold remedies until research studies showed that it increased the risk of hemorrhagic stroke in women, which led the U.S. Food and Drug Administration to mandate its removal from these medications. Other agonists with actions similar to phenylephrine and methoxamine include metaraminol, although it is a mixed-acting agonist (discussed later). **Midodrine** is a synthetic drug that selectively activates α_1-adrenergic receptors. It also causes vasoconstriction, and it is used to treat postural hypotension caused by impaired autonomic nervous system function.

The α_2-adrenergic receptor agonists **clonidine, guanabenz, guanfacine, and methyldopa** (Figure 8-3) effectively enter into the CNS and selectively stimulate α_2-adrenergic receptors in the brain. Methyldopa enters into the nerve terminal and is converted into the α_2 receptor–selective agonist α-methylnorepinephrine. α-Methylnorepinephrine is nearly equipotent to norepinephrine as a vasoconstrictor in humans. This agent has been developed as the drug levonordefrin, which is used as a vasoconstrictor in some local anesthetic solutions. An imidazoline derivative, clonidine is a selective α_2-adrenergic receptor agonist with relatively weak peripheral effects. Guanabenz and guanfacine are guanidine derivatives that, similar to clonidine, also selectively activate α_2-adrenergic receptors. These centrally acting agonists are thought to exert their antihypertensive effect by acting on α_2 receptors in the nucleus tractus solitarius of the brainstem, leading to a decrease in sympathetic outflow. Intravenous administration of these drugs may increase blood pressure acutely as a result of stimulation of peripheral vasoconstrictor α_2 receptors. This effect is not usually seen with oral administration.

Serendipity has played a role in the use of clonidine to treat the withdrawal symptoms of opioid addiction. Clonidine, when given to addicts undergoing withdrawal, blocks the nausea, vomiting, sweating, diarrhea, and other symptoms of excessive autonomic discharge (see Chapter 39). Evidence indicates that either systemic or intracerebral injection of opioids inhibits neuronal activity in the locus ceruleus of the dorsolateral pons. When the opioids are withdrawn, certain neurons are thought to be disinhibited and to release excessive norepinephrine, which gives rise to the symptoms of withdrawal. Clonidine, by stimulating presynaptic α_2 receptors on these same neurons, causes inhibition of neurotransmitter release. The current clinical practice is to follow abrupt withdrawal of the opioid with oral administration of clonidine for 2 weeks or until opioid detoxification is complete. Similarly, patients with alcohol abuse problems, certain neurologic diseases, or some forms of psychotic illness show some improvement in their condition with clonidine. Other studies have found that clonidine has analgesic and sedative effects when given alone or in combination with opioids, and clonidine has been used as an adjunct in general anesthesia and for treating some patients with chronic pain.

β-Adrenergic Receptor Agonists: Isoproterenol

Isoproterenol, a synthetic catecholamine, is a potent nonselective β-receptor agonist. It does not appreciably distinguish among the β_1, β_2, and β_3 receptor subtypes, but has very low affinity for α-adrenergic receptors, and it has no significant effect resulting from α receptor stimulation.

Cardiac and vascular effects

The actions of isoproterenol on the cardiovascular system are based solely on the stimulation of β-adrenergic receptors (see Figure 8-2). It causes a marked decrease in diastolic blood pressure from β_2 receptor–mediated vasodilation, primarily caused by relaxation of blood vessels in skeletal muscle, with some additional vasodilation in the renal and mesenteric vascular beds. There is also an increase in systolic blood pressure largely resulting from the increase in cardiac output caused by β_1 receptor stimulation of contractility. Because of the effects on systolic (slight increase) and diastolic (decrease) pressures, the mean arterial blood pressure is usually decreased. Heart rate is increased by the stimulation of β_1 receptors in pacemaker cells. The drug's ability to increase excitability and conduction velocity in the heart may induce palpitation and arrhythmias. The powerful inotropic and chronotropic actions may increase myocardial oxygen demand sufficiently to cause ischemia.

Effects on bronchial smooth muscle

As an agonist of β_2-adrenergic receptors, isoproterenol relaxes bronchial smooth muscle in the lungs to relieve or prevent bronchoconstriction. Disadvantages of the use of isoproterenol for relief of bronchospastic disorders that limit its clinical use are its nonselectivity for β-adrenergic receptor subtypes (which can result in β_1 receptor–induced tachycardia, palpitation, and arrhythmias) and the development of tolerance and refractoriness with frequent use. The introduction of selective β_2 receptor agonists has provided an important alternative class of drugs for bronchodilation. Although the β_2 receptor–selective drugs have weaker cardiac effects than isoproterenol, they still have the potential to cause cardiac acceleration and tachyarrhythmias.

Metabolic and other effects

Although the β receptor agonist activity of isoproterenol stimulates glycogenolysis and gluconeogenesis in the liver, it is not as effective as epinephrine in elevating plasma glucose. Isoproterenol stimulates the secretion of saliva that is rich in amylase and other proteins. The drug is also capable of causing CNS excitation at doses higher than are conventionally used clinically.

Dobutamine

A synthetic analogue of dopamine, **dobutamine** acts as an adrenergic receptor agonist with little or no effect on dopamine receptors. The primary action of dobutamine is to increase myocardial contractility and cardiac output without significantly increasing the heart rate. The inotropic effect results primarily from direct **β_1 receptor** stimulation in the heart, with lesser contributions from β_2 receptor activation. Peripheral vascular resistance is usually changed very little. Because blood pressure effects of this drug are a function of the combination of α_1 and β_2 receptor activation and α_1 receptor blockade, however, some patients may show a greater pressor effect; whereas others may experience a moderate reduction in ventricular filling pressure and peripheral vascular resistance. Dobutamine is used for short-term treatment of acute myocardial insufficiency resulting from congestive heart failure, myocardial infarction, or cardiac surgery.

Selective β_2-Adrenergic Receptor Agonists

Although isoproterenol and epinephrine are capable of relaxing bronchial smooth muscle, both drugs (especially isoproterenol) can also cause dangerous tachycardia and arrhythmias. These side effects limit the therapeutic use of these drugs and stimulated a search for selective agonists capable of stimulating β_2-adrenergic receptors in bronchial and uterine smooth muscle, while having less effect on the β_1 receptors of the heart. Even with the selective β_2 receptor agonists, effects on the heart are substantial, however, especially at higher doses. Metaproterenol, **terbutaline, albuterol, levalbuterol, pirbuterol,** and **salmeterol** are relatively selective β_2 receptor agonists that are effective in decreasing airway resistance without causing as much cardiac acceleration as isoproterenol. These drugs are usually inhaled; however, oral administration of metaproterenol, albuterol, and terbutaline may be useful under certain limited conditions. Systemic adverse effects are usually greater by the oral route. The use of β_2 agonists in the therapy of bronchospastic disorders is discussed in Chapter 27.

Mixed-Acting and Indirect-Acting Adrenergic Agonists

Numerous adrenergic agonist drugs produce some or all of their effects by causing the release of norepinephrine from adrenergic nerve terminals. They do so by being transported into the adrenergic nerve ending or adrenal chromaffin cells, where these drugs displace catecholamines from the vesicular storage sites into a cytoplasmic pool in the nerve endings or chromaffin cells. This cytoplasmic pool is distinct from that of the storage vesicles from which release occurs during nerve stimulation. These drugs have a pharmacologic profile similar to that of norepinephrine. In contrast to norepinephrine, these drugs are generally not subject to rapid inactivation and are usually effective by the oral route.

Ephedrine is an example of an orally active, mixed-acting drug. In addition to releasing norepinephrine, ephedrine is a direct α and β receptor agonist. It can cause bronchodilation, vasoconstriction, increased heart rate, and modest CNS stimulation. **Amphetamine**, a more lipophilic drug, is primarily an indirect-acting drug that easily enters the brain and stimulates the release of catecholamines in the CNS. Amphetamine is a potent CNS stimulant that causes numerous effects, including increased alertness, relief of fatigue, enhanced athletic performance, and euphoria. Drugs related to amphetamine include **dextroamphetamine** and **methamphetamine** that tend to have more effects on the CNS relative to the periphery. The addition of a single hydroxyl group (4-OH) to yield hydroxyamphetamine produces a drug with less CNS activity.

Acute tolerance (tachyphylaxis) is a common outcome of repeated administration of indirect-acting adrenergic drugs. Multiple doses of either mixed-acting or indirect-acting adrenergic agonists may lead to a depletion of the neurotransmitter, resulting in a reduction or loss of activity in response to nerve stimulation. These drugs are also susceptible as a class to several drug interactions. Compounds such as the tricyclic antidepressants and some adrenergic neuron-blocking drugs interfere competitively with the uptake of indirect-acting agonists into adrenergic nerve terminals and block their subsequent release of norepinephrine. The combination of a monoamine oxidase (MAO) inhibitor and an indirect-acting or mixed-acting sympathomimetic drug typically results in excessive release of catecholamines with serious consequences. Some indirect-acting compounds, such as **tyramine**, occur naturally in several foods and beverages and pose a great risk to patients taking MAO inhibitors.

ABSORPTION, FATE, AND EXCRETION

The route for administering adrenergic agonists is determined by the chemical structure. All catecholamines and certain other drugs, unless specifically modified at the α carbon of the side chain, are subject to enzymatic destruction in the gastrointestinal tract. Catecholamines are usually administered systemically by parenteral injection or intravenous infusion. Topical instillation and inhalation are the preferred routes of administration for ocular and respiratory applications, respectively.

The inactivation and metabolic disposal of catecholamines can involve many processes, as illustrated by the fate of endogenously released norepinephrine (Figure 8-4). After neuronal release, a large portion (80% in some cases) of the adrenergic neurotransmitter is returned to the nerve terminal by an active neuronal uptake process. What remains in the junctional cleft is subjected to O-methylation by **catechol-O-methyltransferase (COMT)** after uptake by postjunctional effector cells. When the transmitter is O-methylated to normetanephrine, it can no longer be transported into the adrenergic nerve terminal but is instead carried by the blood to the liver, where it is largely deaminated by hepatic **MAO**.

Of the norepinephrine that is actively transported back into the neuron, a large part is actively returned to the storage vesicles from which it can be released again on neuronal stimulation. A smaller portion is deaminated by MAO located in the outer membrane of the mitochondria to form 3,4-dihydroxyphenylglycoaldehyde. Most of the aldehyde is converted to a glycol, the remainder to an acid. Both metabolites enter the circulation and are eventually O-methylated by COMT. The major metabolic products of norepinephrine resulting from the combined action of MAO and COMT are 3-methoxy-4-hydroxymandelic acid, also referred to as vanillylmandelic acid, and 3-methoxy-4-hydroxyphenylglycol. About 90% of the total endogenous norepinephrine load excreted in the urine is in the form of vanillylmandelic acid and 3-methoxy-4-hydroxyphenylglycol. Several of these products are conjugated to the sulfate or glucuronide before being excreted by the kidney.

Exogenously administered catecholamines and endogenous dopamine and epinephrine are transported and metabolized in much the same manner as norepinephrine. Nevertheless, there are some differences. The metabolic inactivation of epinephrine and most injected catecholamines (including norepinephrine) largely depends on COMT because COMT is widely distributed throughout the body. The relative shift toward COMT for the initial enzymatic attack ensures the recovery of high concentrations of O-methylated derivatives in the urine. As with norepinephrine and epinephrine, dopamine is a substrate for MAO and COMT. The metabolite formed by the combined action of these enzymes is homovanillic acid. In contrast to the other endogenous catecholamines, dopamine, when given by intravenous infusion, is significantly potentiated by MAO inhibitors.

Noncatecholamines are not subject to metabolism by COMT and typically have durations of action significantly longer than the catecholamines. The centrally acting α_2 receptor agonists used to treat hypertension are given orally and are eliminated largely as unchanged drug (e.g., clonidine), are extensively metabolized (e.g., guanabenz), or are partly metabolized and partly excreted as the parent compound (e.g., guanfacine, methyldopa). Several of the selective β_2 receptor agonists are excreted in the urine as conjugates of sulfate or glucuronic acid.

The indirect-acting adrenergic agonists must first enter the neuron to evoke the release of the neurotransmitter norepinephrine. While in the cytoplasm, these compounds may be subjected to deamination by MAO and other enzymes. A small amount of tyramine in the neuron is oxidized at the β carbon to form octopamine. Octopamine, which has only weak adrenergic activity, can be transported into the storage vesicles, where it may act as a false transmitter. Other avenues for the metabolism of these noncatecholamines include *p*-hydroxylation, N-demethylation, deamination, conjugation in the liver and kidney, or a combination of all these. Amphetamine and ephedrine, which are resistant to the actions of MAO (also found in abundance in the gastrointestinal tract), can be administered orally.

GENERAL THERAPEUTIC USES

Clinical applications of the adrenergic agonists can be divided into eight major categories: **local vasoconstriction, vasoconstriction in the treatment of hypotension and shock, bronchodilation, relaxation of uterine smooth muscle, ophthalmic uses, relief of allergic states (including anaphylaxis), CNS stimulation, and control of hypertension**. The choice of a specific drug for each of these uses depends on the relative contribution of α-adrenergic or β-adrenergic receptors or dopamine receptors to the response in these tissues, and the drug's receptor subtype selectivity. Other factors that determine the choice of a drug include the therapeutic effect versus adverse effects profile and pharmacokinetic factors, such as the rate and routes of absorption, duration of action, and metabolic fate. Most commercially available

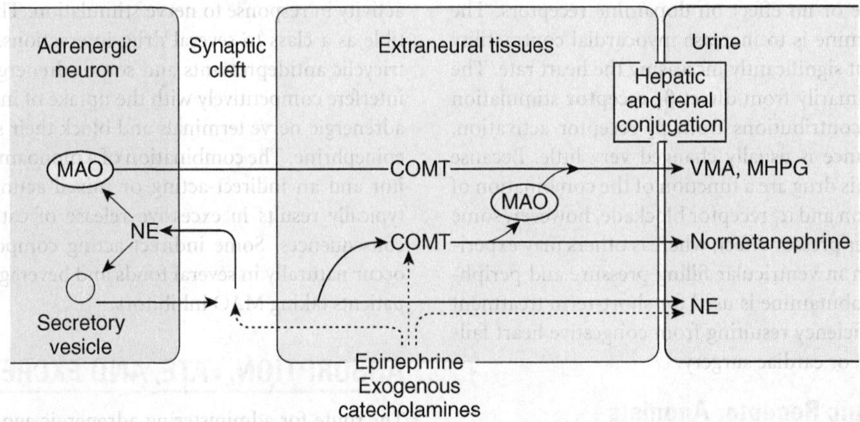

FIG 8-4 Biotransformation and excretion of catecholamines. After release, up to 80% of norepinephrine (*NE*) is taken up by a reuptake process into the nerve terminal, where most is recycled into storage vesicles, and some is metabolized by mitochondrial monoamine oxidase (*MAO*). Extraneuronal tissues metabolize endogenously released catecholamines through catechol-O-methyltransferase (*COMT*) and MAO. Excreted substances include the metabolites 3-methoxy-4-hydroxymandelic acid (*VMA*) and 3-methoxy-4-hydroxyphenylglycol (*MHPG*), and normetanephrine, small amounts of unmetabolized catecholamines, and related sulfate and glucuronide conjugates. Injected vasoconstrictors and some other adrenergic agonists are also biotransformed and excreted by some of these same pathways.

adrenergic agonists are marketed as water-soluble salts. The following section examines all of these therapeutic uses, indicating in each case one or more preferred drugs.

Local Vasoconstriction

Various drops, sprays, aerosols, and oral dosage forms of several adrenergic agonists have proved useful in providing temporary symptomatic relief of nasal congestion. These compounds are agonists at α receptors (α_1 or α_2 or both) and have minimal CNS stimulant effects. Common examples include **phenylephrine, pseudoephedrine, and oxymetazoline.**

An adverse effect associated with the local administration of nasal decongestants is rebound congestion, a chronic swelling of the nasal mucous membranes after the effect of the drugs wears off. This response is more likely with the longer acting α_2 receptor–selective nasal decongestants. Imidazoline derivatives, such as **tetrahydrozoline** and **oxymetazoline**, can paradoxically produce drowsiness, comatose sleep with hypotension, and bradycardia. These effects are thought to be caused by the entry of the drugs into the CNS, where they stimulate central α_2-adrenergic receptors. Children and infants are especially prone to these adverse effects.

Adrenergic agonists are often used to produce hemostasis for surgery and to enhance local anesthesia. Whether applied topically or administered by injection with or without a local anesthetic, adrenergic agonists can significantly improve visibility in the operative field in certain situations. Because vasoconstriction is temporary, the use of these drugs is no substitute for the adequate surgical control of bleeding. Adrenergic agonists must often be used with special caution during general anesthesia because certain inhalation anesthetics (e.g., halothane) predispose the heart to the arrhythmogenic action of the adrenergic agonists.

Treatment of Hypotension and Shock

Shock is a condition caused by inadequate tissue perfusion. It is usually associated with a decrease in arterial blood pressure and, if not treated, may quickly lead to multiorgan system failure. Adrenergic agonists may prove useful in restoring blood pressure and in correcting the distribution of blood flow, especially to the vital organs, whenever shock develops under normovolemic conditions.

α-Adrenergic receptor agonists (e.g., phenylephrine), which increase blood pressure by causing vasoconstriction, are most useful during episodes of inadequate sympathetic nervous system function that may result from spinal anesthesia or hypotensive drug overdose. Such drugs are less beneficial in other shock states associated with hypotension, however, because they may impair blood flow to the kidneys and mesenteric organs. In cardiogenic shock, which is most often caused by acute myocardial infarction, the β_1-adrenergic receptor agonists should be useful, but the improvement in tissue perfusion and coronary blood flow is often accompanied by increased myocardial oxygen demand. Dopamine has often been used for initial therapy of cardiogenic shock because it causes less generalized vasodilation than typical β receptor agonists, increases contractile force in the heart without increasing heart rate, and, through stimulation of dopamine receptors, may improve renal and mesenteric perfusion. Newer studies have cast doubt, however, on the benefits of dopamine. Dobutamine, similar to dopamine, can increase the force of myocardial contraction without producing significant changes in heart rate and is also used in patients with heart failure.

Bronchodilation

Acute and chronic obstructive pulmonary diseases are marked by increased inspiratory and expiratory resistance, and the adrenergic agonists have historically played an important role in the relief of these conditions. Currently, the adrenergic agents most useful in the treatment of bronchospastic disease are agonists with selectivity for β_2-adrenergic receptors because they produce marked bronchodilation with less effect on the heart than nonselective β receptor agonists. The selective β_2 receptor agonists used for bronchodilation include metaproterenol, terbutaline, albuterol, levalbuterol, pirbuterol, salmeterol, and formoterol. Salmeterol and formoterol have durations of action of about 24 hours. Other long-acting β_2-adrenergic receptor agonists are arformoterol, indacaterol, olodaterol, and vilanterol. These extended durations can be of significant benefit in treating patients with asthma and chronic obstructive pulmonary disease (COPD). The shorter acting drugs are used to reverse acute bronchoconstriction, whereas longer acting drugs are used prophylactically to prevent bronchoconstriction and alleviate COPD, bronchitis, and other chronic lung conditions. See Chapter 27 for a more complete discussion of the use of these agents in bronchial asthma.

Ophthalmic Uses

The two major ocular indications for adrenergic agonists are for the production of mild mydriasis and the reduction of intraocular pressure. The former is mediated by stimulation of α_1-adrenergic receptors in the radial muscle of the eye. Although muscarinic receptor antagonists such as atropine produce a much stronger pupillary dilation, adrenergic agonists are useful because they cause mydriasis without paralyzing the ciliary muscle (cycloplegia). Even greater mydriasis can be obtained if a combination of a muscarinic receptor–blocking drug and an adrenergic agonist drug is used. Phenylephrine and hydroxyamphetamine are the principal adrenergic agonists used to produce mydriasis.

The mechanisms for the reduction in intraocular pressure by adrenergic agonist drugs are not well elucidated, but several of these drugs seem to reduce the production and enhance the outflow of aqueous humor and are useful in treating wide-angle glaucoma. These drugs include the nonselective adrenergic agents epinephrine and dipivefrin (a prodrug of epinephrine), and the α_2-adrenergic receptor–selective agonists **apraclonidine** and **brimonidine.**

Treatment of Allergic States

Adrenergic agonists, especially **epinephrine**, are especially useful in reversing the effects of histamine and other mediators associated with allergic reactions. In contrast to the antihistamines, adrenergic agonists are physiologic antagonists, producing responses opposite to the acute effects produced by histamine and associated autacoids. For acute allergic reactions such as urticaria, subcutaneous injection of 0.1 to 0.5 mL of 1:1000 (i.e., 1mg/mL) epinephrine should be adequate. Fulminating disturbances such as anaphylactic shock require a faster absorption of epinephrine than provided by subcutaneous injection, especially if circulation is impaired. Intramuscular (intralingual) injection of 0.3 to 0.5 mL of 1:1000 epinephrine or, if the patient has previously been prepared for intravenous injections, slow intravenous administration of 1:10,000 epinephrine (0.1 mg in 5 minutes) is recommended. With this latter route of administration, there is a considerable risk of precipitating serious cardiac arrhythmias and ventricular fibrillation. Because of the rapid metabolism of epinephrine, reinjection at intervals of 5 to 15 minutes may be required. Subcutaneous administration generally provides the longest duration of action, and intravenous injection provides the shortest.

Central Nervous System Stimulation

For many years, selected adrenergic agonists have been used clinically because of their ability to produce stimulation of certain functions of the CNS that result in increased alertness and attention span and decreased sense of fatigue. Another potentially therapeutic effect of these agents is stimulation of the lateral hypothalamus and satiation of the food drive. The principal sympathomimetic drugs that cross the blood–brain barrier are ephedrine, amphetamines, and methylphenidate. Because of the history of abuse of amphetamine-like drugs, their procurement and use are strictly controlled by various state and federal statutes.

A major accepted use of amphetamine and related drugs is for the management of children with attention-deficit/hyperactivity disorder. The use of CNS stimulants, along with psychotherapy and family counseling, has provided remarkable relief from the restlessness, brief attention span, and impulsiveness that mark this disorder. **Methylphenidate** has been used most often for the pharmacologic treatment of attention-deficit/hyperactivity disorder. It has a relatively brief duration of action (3 to 5 hours), requiring a second dose that often must be administered by teachers or daycare providers. Alternative agents that have gained wider use in recent years include extended duration formulations of methylphenidate or the combination of amphetamine and dextroamphetamine.

Treatment of Hypertension

As mentioned earlier and discussed in Chapter 23, four centrally acting α_2-adrenergic receptor–selective agonists are used for the treatment of hypertension: clonidine, guanabenz, guanfacine, and methyldopa. They act on central α_2 receptors that are involved in the autonomic regulation of the cardiovascular system. Activation of inhibitory neurons in the brain causes peripheral vasodilation by inhibiting sympathetic outflow from the CNS and decreasing cardiac output through enhanced vagal tone and decreased sympathetic tone. Generally, these drugs do not reduce sympathetic tone as much as do peripherally acting inhibitors of the sympathetic nervous system or its receptors (see Chapter 9).

THERAPEUTIC USES IN DENTISTRY

Vasoconstrictors are widely often used in local anesthetic solutions. The vasoconstrictor most commonly used in dentistry is **epinephrine**, with **levonordefrin** (the *l* isomer of nordefrin) being used less frequently, usually with mepivacaine.

Table 8-3 lists the concentrations and amounts of adrenergic vasoconstrictors contained in commercially available dental local anesthetic cartridges. The maximum recommended strength of the vasoconstrictor is 1:100,000 epinephrine equivalency for routine nerve block anesthesia. When local tissue hemostasis is required for surgical procedures, such as periodontal surgery, the dentist may additionally choose to infiltrate the area with local anesthetic solution containing 1:50,000 epinephrine, but repeated injections of 2% lidocaine with 1:50,000 epinephrine may cause tissue necrosis and microscarring.

TABLE 8-3 Concentrations and Amounts of Adrenergic Vasoconstrictors in Dental Local Anesthetic Cartridges

Vasoconstrictor	Dilution	Amount per Dental Cartridge (μg/1.8 mL)
Epinephrine hydrochloride	1:200,000	9
Epinephrine hydrochloride	1:100,000	18
Epinephrine hydrochloride	1:50,000	36
Levonordefrin hydrochloride	1:20,000	90

Vasoconstrictors serve several useful purposes when used with local anesthetic solutions. First, they prolong the duration of local anesthesia several-fold and may improve the frequency of successful nerve block. Table 8-4 illustrates the effect of vasoconstrictors on duration of local anesthesia. Second, systemic toxicity of the local anesthetic may be minimized by reducing the peak blood concentration of the anesthetic agent. Third, when anesthetic solutions are given by infiltration, vasoconstrictors tend to reduce blood loss associated with surgical procedures (see Chapter 14).

One issue of potential toxicity is the systemic effects of vasoconstrictors after intraoral injection in patients with cardiovascular disease. Some older reports recommend that cardiac patients be given local anesthetics with vasoconstrictors if needed for adequate anesthesia because the benefits of satisfactory pain control were greater than the risks of small amounts of vasoconstrictor. The validity of this statement depends on the level of stress on the patient and the amount, rate, and manner in which the epinephrine-containing solution is injected.

It is often necessary to produce gingival retraction for operative procedures on teeth and for making impressions. Besides astringents such as zinc and aluminum salts, retraction cord impregnated with racemic (*d* and *l* isomers) epinephrine, containing as much as 1.2 mg of drug per inch of cord, is commercially available. Racemic epinephrine has approximately half the potency of *l*-epinephrine because *d*-epinephrine has approximately one-fifteenth the activity of *l*-epinephrine. Whether these large amounts of epinephrine present a hazard to a normal patient and to patients with cardiovascular disease depends on several factors. Experimental and clinical studies indicate a relatively high absorption of the vasoconstrictor if the epithelium is abraded or the vasculature is exposed, which is common in extensive restorative procedures. Systemic absorption is marked by signs of anxiety, elevated blood pressure, increased heart rate, and occasional arrhythmias. These effects can be extremely serious in a patient with cardiovascular disease or in a patient who is taking medication that reduces the uptake or otherwise enhances the activity of adrenergic agents. Because of this concern, epinephrine-impregnated retraction cord is used much less often than other types of retraction cord.

Various products are available to control capillary bleeding occurring with surgical procedures on gingival tissues. Topical epinephrine hydrochloride (1:1000) and phenylephrine (1:100) are most common. More concentrated solutions have occasionally been recommended,

TABLE 8-4 Effect of Epinephrine on the Duration of Local Anesthesia

Local Anesthetic	Vasoconstrictor	DURATION Mean (min)	DURATION Maximum (min)
Lidocaine 2%	None	44	100
Lidocaine 2%	Epinephrine 1:1,000,000	57	130
Lidocaine 2%	Epinephrine 1:750,000	67	145
Lidocaine 2%	Epinephrine 1:250,000	90	175
Lidocaine 2%	Epinephrine 1:50,000	88	210

Adapted from Keesling GG, Hinds EC: Optimal concentrations of epinephrine in lidocaine solutions, *J Am Dent Assoc* 66:337-340, 1963.

Note: Data were obtained by oral surgeons from patients undergoing exodontia. The mean and maximum duration of anesthesia was judged by luxation of the tooth and by the use of probes for soft tissue effects. All injections were inferior alveolar nerve blocks; 24 patients were included in each group.

but their use can heighten the risk of cardiovascular problems without producing any significant increased effectiveness in reducing hemorrhage.

ADVERSE EFFECTS

Almost all adverse effects of the adrenergic agonists are dose related. Toxic reactions can result from the administration of too large a dose, accidental intravascular injection, impaired uptake of the drug, a heightened sensitivity or number of adrenergic receptors, or therapeutic doses given to a patient with **preexisting cardiovascular disease.** Relatively small amounts of epinephrine can cause potentially grave effects in a highly susceptible patient. Generally, serious complications may be expected with doses of epinephrine greater than 0.5 mg, and fatalities are likely to occur with doses of 4 mg or more, although one patient is reported to have survived an injection of 30 mg. Reviews of the literature indicate that reported adverse reactions attributable to vasoconstrictors used with local anesthetics in dentistry are rare.

Most serious of the toxic effects of epinephrine are **cardiac disturbances,** with increased stimulation of the heart leading to myocardial ischemia, possibly heart attack, and arrhythmias, including ventricular fibrillation. Patients with a history of uncontrolled hyperthyroidism, hypertension, or angina pectoris are particularly susceptible. If epinephrine is administered to a patient who is taking a nonselective β-adrenergic receptor–blocking drug such as propranolol (see Chapter 9), unopposed **α-receptor** stimulation may cause **excessive vasoconstriction.** The increase in blood pressure from rapid parenteral administration can be severe enough to result in hypertensive crisis, which can cause cardiac disturbances or a cerebrovascular accident. Drugs with primarily α-adrenergic receptor stimulation can cause excessive vasoconstriction in overdose. Local tissue necrosis may result from any vasoconstrictor injected into a region where ischemia is likely, such as the digits of the hands or feet.

CNS reactions to classic sympathomimetic drugs include nervousness, excitability, insomnia, dizziness, and tremors. Long-term use of amphetamines can lead to psychotic symptoms. The most common side effects of centrally acting **α_2-agonist** antihypertensive agents are dizziness, drowsiness, and **xerostomia.** The xerostomia seems to be most severe with clonidine and guanabenz. Constipation, sexual dysfunction, CNS disturbances, bradycardia, and excessive hypotension have also been reported. A particularly troubling adverse effect of centrally acting α_2-agonists is **rebound hypertension** of serious proportions if these drugs are withdrawn abruptly.

Unique to methyldopa is the occurrence of drug-induced hepatitis, with a fever that may reach alarming levels (105 °F). Withdrawal of the drug usually allows liver function to return to normal. This reaction has been shown to be related to the transformation of methyldopa to reactive compounds that combine covalently with cellular macromolecules. Other adverse effects of methyldopa include parkinsonian signs, hyperprolactinemia, and hemolytic anemia.

ADRENERGIC AGONISTS

Nonproprietary (Generic) Name	Proprietary (Trade) Name
Ophthalmic Products	
Mydriatics	
Hydroxyamphetamine	Paredrine
Phenylephrine	Neo-Synephrine
Decongestants	
Naphazoline	Allerest, Naphcon
Oxymetazoline	Visine L.R.
Phenylephrine	Neo-Synephrine
Tetrahydrozoline	Visine
Antiglaucoma Agents (see Appendix V)	
Respiratory Tract Products	
Nasal decongestants	
Ephedrine	Pretz-D
Epinephrine	Adrenalin
Naphazoline	Privine
Oxymetazoline	Afrin, Nostrilla
Phenylephrine	Neo-Synephrine, Sudafed PE
Propylhexedrine	Benzedrex
Pseudoephedrine	Sudafed
Tetrahydrozoline	Tyzine
Xylometazoline	Otrivin
Cold remedies	
These preparations consist of antihistamines, analgesics, cough suppressants, other drugs, and one of the following adrenergic agonists:	
Phenylephrine	In Dimetapp Cold & Cough, in Dristan Multi-Symptom Nasal Decongestant
Pseudoephedrine	In Claritin-D, in Sudafed Multi-Symptom Cold & Cough
Bronchodilators	
Albuterol	Proventil, Ventolin, in Combivent
Arformoterol	Brovana
Bitolterol	Tornalate
Ephedrine	Primatene Tablets
Epinephrine	Adrenalin, Primatene Mist
Ethylnorepinephrine	Bronkephrine
Formoterol	Foradil
Indacaterol	Arcapta Neohaler
Isoetharine	Bronkosol
Isoproterenol	Isuprel, Medihaler-Iso
Levalbuterol	Xopenex
Metaproterenol	Alupent
Olodaterol	Striverdi Respimat
Pirbuterol	Maxair
Salmeterol	Serevent
Terbutaline	Brethine, Bricanyl
Vilanterol	In Anoro Ellipta
Cardiovascular System Products	
Vasoconstrictors and cardiac stimulants	
Dobutamine	Dobutrex
Dopamine	Intropin
Droxidopa	Northera
Ephedrine	–
Epinephrine	Adrenalin
Isoproterenol	Isuprel
Levonordefrin	Neo-Cobefrin

Continued

ADRENERGIC AGONISTS—cont'd

Nonproprietary (Generic) Name	Proprietary (Trade) Name	Nonproprietary (Generic) Name	Proprietary (Trade) Name
Mephentermine*	Wyamine	Dexmethylphenidate	Focalin
Metaraminol*	Aramine	Dextroamphetamine	Dexedrine, in Adderall
Methoxamine*	Vasoxyl	Diethylpropion	Tenuate
Midodrine	Orvaten, ProAmatine	Methamphetamine	Desoxyn
Norepinephrine	Levophed	Methylphenidate	Methylin, Ritalin
Phenylephrine	Neo-Synephrine	Modafinil	Provigil
Antihypertensive agents		Pemoline	Cylert
Clonidine	Catapres	Phendimetrazine	Bontril, Plegine
Fenoldopam	Corlopam	Phentermine	Adipex-P, Fastin
Guanabenz	Wytensin	Sibutramine	Meridia
Guanfacine	Tenex	**Miscellaneous Products**	
Methyldopa	Aldomet	Phenylephrine (rectal)	In Hemorid, in Preparation H
Methyldopate	—	Dexmedetomidine (α_2 agonist)	Precedex
CNS Stimulants and Anorexiants		Tizanidine (α_2 agonist)	Zanaflex
Amphetamine (+dextroamphetamine)	In Adderall	Mirabegron (β_3 agonist for overactive bladder)	Myrbetriq
Benzphetamine	Didrex		

*Not currently available in the United States.

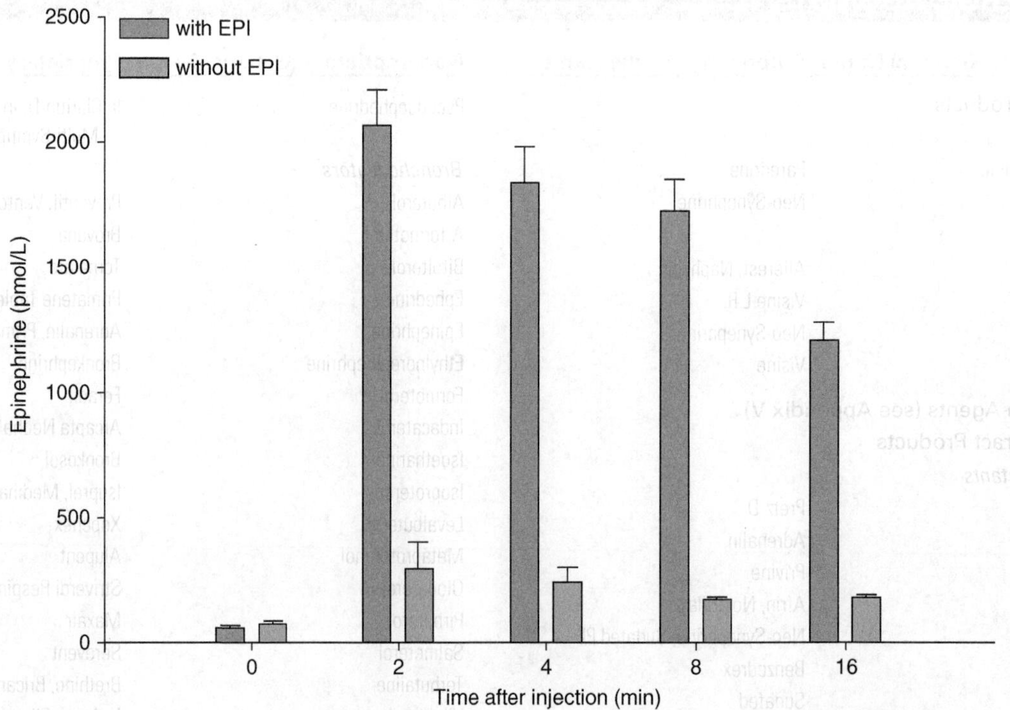

FIG 8-5 Effect of intraoral local anesthetic injections on plasma epinephrine. Unsedated oral surgery patients ($n=26$) were injected with either 14.4 mL of 2% lidocaine with 1:100,000 epinephrine (*with EPI*, 144 μg epinephrine total dose) or 3% mepivacaine without vasoconstrictor (*without EPI*) under randomized, double-blind conditions. Brackets indicate the standard error. (Adapted from Troullos ES, Hargreaves KM, Goldstein DS, et al.: Epinephrine suppresses stress-induced increases in plasma immunoreactive β-endorphin in humans, *J Clin Endocrinol Metab* 69:546-551, 1989.)

CASE DISCUSSION

Vasoconstrictors are widely used in conjunction with local anesthetic solutions in dentistry. An important issue related to potential toxicity is the systemic effects of vasoconstrictors after intraoral injection. A related question faced by the dentist is whether to administer a vasoconstrictor-containing local anesthetic solution to a patient with cardiovascular disease. Numerous well-controlled studies have shown that even the small amounts of vasoconstrictor used in dentistry significantly increase resting plasma catecholamine concentrations and affect cardiac function. As illustrated in Figure 8-5, intraoral injection of lidocaine with 1:100,000 epinephrine increased circulating epinephrine compared with injection of local anesthetic alone.

Although large therapeutic dosages were used in this study, injection of even a single cartridge of local anesthetic with 1:100,000 epinephrine can result in a temporary doubling of the plasma epinephrine concentration. With these results in mind, a joint report of the American Heart Association and American Dental Association concluded that "vasoconstrictor agents should be used in local anesthesia solutions during dental practice when it is clear that the procedure will be shortened or the analgesia rendered more profound," that "extreme care should be taken to avoid intravascular injection," and that "the minimum possible amount of vasoconstrictor should be used." Local anesthesia with vasoconstrictors has also been implicated with ischemic conditions of the pulp and alveolar bone, the latter being associated with an increased incidence of osteitis after extractions. Local tissue damage at the site of injection is related to or accentuated by the presence of vasoconstrictors.

If needed, an alternative is available; effective local anesthetic preparations without vasoconstrictor agents (e.g., 3% mepivacaine) have been shown to provide clinically effective local anesthesia, especially for nerve block procedures.

GENERAL REFERENCES

1. Bader JD, Bonito AJ, Shugars DA: *Cardiovascular effects of epinephrine in hypertensive dental patients*, Summary, Evidence Report/Technology Assessment: Number 48, AHRQ Publication No. 02-E006 Rockville, MD, 2002, Agency for Healthcare Research and Quality. Available at: http://www.ncbi.nlm.nih.gov/books/NBK11858/. Accessed February 26, 2016.
2. Bylund DB, Eikenberg DC, Hieble JP, et al.: International Union of Pharmacology nomenclature of adrenoceptors, *Pharmacol Rev* 46:121–136, 1994.
3. Cooper JR, Bloom FE, Roth RH: *The biochemical basis of neuropharmacology*, ed 8, New York, 2003, Oxford University Press.
4. Eisenhofer G, Kopin IJ, Goldstein DS: Catecholamine metabolism: a contemporary view with implications for physiology and medicine, *Pharmacol Rev* 56:331–349, 2004.
5. Gingrich JA, Caron MG: Recent advances in the molecular biology of dopamine receptors, *Annu Rev Neurosci* 16:299–321, 1993.
6. Jastak JT, Yagiela JA: Vasoconstrictors and local anesthesia: a review and rationale for use, *J Am Dent Assoc* 107:623–630, 1983.
7. Jowett NI, Cabot LB: Patients with cardiac disease: considerations for the dental practitioner, *Br Dent J* 189:297–302, 2000.
8. Kaplan EL, editor: *Cardiovascular disease in dental practice*, Dallas, 1986, American Heart Association.
9. Management of dental problems in patients with cardiovascular disease: Council on Dental Therapeutics, American Dental Association and American Heart Association joint report, *J Am Dent Assoc* 68:333–342, 1964.
10. Nelson HS: β-Adrenergic bronchodilators, *N Engl J Med* 333:499–507, 1995.
11. Nestler EJ, Hyman SE, Malenka RC: *Molecular neuropharmacology: a foundation for clinical neuroscience*, New York, 2001, McGraw-Hill.
12. Ruffolo RR Jr, Hieble JP: Alpha-adrenoceptors, *Pharmacol Ther* 61:1–64, 1994.
13. Verrill PJ: Adverse reactions to local anaesthetics and vasoconstrictor drugs, *Practitioner* 214:380–387, 1975.
14. Wong J: Adjuncts to local anesthesia: separating fact from fiction, *J Can Dent Assoc* 67:391–397, 2001.

9

Adrenergic Antagonists

Michael T. Piascik and Peter W. Abel

KEY INFORMATION

- Sympatholytics antagonize the actions of endogenously released epinephrine and norepinephrine as well as exogenously administered drugs.
- Sympatholytics can act by several mechanisms, including direct receptor antagonism, agonist action in the central nervous system, and an inhibition of the enzyme monoamine oxidase.
- Selective α_1-adrenergic receptor blockers are first-line agents in the treatment of benign prostatic hyperplasia and second-line antihypertensives.
- Common side effects of selective α_1-adrenergic receptor blockers include orthostatic hypotension and inoperable floppy iris syndrome.
- β-adrenergic receptor blockers can be classified as being nonselective, selective, and β blockers with additional properties such as the ability to generate nitric oxide, inhibit free radial formation, and inhibit hypertrophic growth.
- β-adrenergic receptor blockers have a wide versatility of cardiovascular and non-cardiovascular usage, including hypertension, ischemic heart disease, myocardial infarction, heart failure, arrhythmias, performance anxiety, open-angle glaucoma, essential tremor, and migraine headache.
- Common side effects of β blockers include bradycardia, hypotension, sedation, fatigue, and lassitude.
- Clonidine, a centrally active α_2-adrenergic receptor agonist, can be used to treat attention deficit hyperactivity disorder; alcohol, nicotine, or opiate withdrawal; neuropathic pain; or Tourette syndrome, as well as being a second-line antihypertensive.
- Common side effects of clonidine include drowsiness and xerostomia.
- Certain monoamine oxidase inhibitors can be used to treat Parkinson disease and are second-line agents in the treatment of depression.

CASE STUDY

A 54-year-old woman presents to your clinic for a routine extraction. She has a BMI of 31 and a 30-pack-year history of smoking. She also has a 15-year history of hypertension, ischemic heart disease caused by atherosclerosis, and hypercholesterolemia. She is taking hydrochlorothiazide, 12.5 mg/day, propranolol 20 mg, q.i.d., simvastatin, 20 mg/day, and nitroglycerin 0.3 mg sublingual tablets, prn. She reports she only very infrequently experiences attacks of angina pectoris. You note that her blood pressure is adequately controlled based on a reading of 120/82 mm Hg prior to beginning the extraction procedure on tooth #18 that includes treatment with two cartridges of 2% lidocaine and epinephrine 1:100,000. Fifteen minutes after injection, it is observed that her blood pressure has increased to 210/150 mm Hg. What is the most likely drug interaction to cause this elevation of blood pressure?

Our understanding of the mechanisms of transmission in the sympathetic nervous system has increased significantly. We now have a much better appreciation of the receptors utilized by the endogenous neurotransmitters and the second messenger pathways engaged by them. The consequence of this work has been the development of numerous pharmacologic agents that possess an increased degree of receptor selectivity and a high degree of therapeutic efficacy with fewer unwanted side effects. The drugs described in this chapter interfere with sympathetic nervous system transmission by diverse mechanisms of action and are collectively referred to as **adrenergic antagonists** or **sympatholytics**. Most sympatholytics are competitive antagonists of either α-adrenergic or β-adrenergic receptors. Other drugs with sympatholytic actions are agonists at central α_2-adrenergic receptors in key brain nuclei as well. Still others are inhibitors of the enzyme monoamine oxidase. The potential sites of sympatholytic drug action are presented in Figure 9-1. These drugs are used to effectively treat a variety of cardiovascular and non-cardiovascular diseases, including attention deficit hyperactivity disorder, benign prostate hypertrophy, depression, essential tremor, heart failure, hypertension, ischemic heart disease, migraine headache, myocardial infarction, open-angle glaucoma, and Parkinson disease.

HISTORY

Evidence that drugs could be used to antagonize the actions of other pharmacologic agents was obtained shortly after the isolation and synthesis of epinephrine. In 1906, Dale noticed that certain alkaloids isolated from ergot (produced by a fungus disease of rye grain) blocked the ability of epinephrine to increase systemic arterial blood pressure. Indeed, after an injection of ergot alkaloids, a hypotensive response to epinephrine was observed, and it was aptly named by Dale as the "epinephrine reversal" response. These early studies also provided the first example of selective antagonism by showing that ergot derivatives were capable of blocking some, but not all, of the actions of epinephrine.

The pioneering work of Ahlquist in delineating the **α-adrenergic and β-adrenergic receptors** provided the framework necessary to more systematically classify antagonists of sympathetic nervous system function. Nickerson and Goodman reported the development of dibenamine, an agent capable of irreversibly blocking the α-adrenergic receptor. In agreement with the work of Dale, these authors also noted that some of the responses to exogenously administered epinephrine could be antagonized by dibenamine, while others remained intact.

These classic studies established the groundwork for receptor subtypes and the idea of selective receptor agonism and antagonism, which remains a critical aspect of drug development and therapeutic use.

Phentolamine and related imidazolines were early examples of nonselective, competitive antagonists at α-adrenergic receptors. Selective antagonists of the α_1-adrenergic and α_2-adrenergic receptors have now been developed. Dichloroisoproterenol was the first β-adrenergic receptor blocker developed. The first clinically useful β blocker introduced was propranolol, which blocks β_1-adrenergic and β_2-adrenergic receptors. Selective β_1 antagonists were then discovered. We now know that there are **at least nine adrenergic receptors (α_{1A}, α_{1B}, α_{1D}, α_{2A}, α_{2B}, α_{2C}, β_1, β_2, and β_3)**. Selective antagonists against each of these receptors have been developed with the goal of obtaining drugs capable of specifically interfering with the receptor involved in a pathophysiologic condition without blockade of other receptors that could lead to unwanted side effects. These drugs are described in detail in this chapter.

In addition to sympatholytic effects due to receptor blockade, there are novel mechanisms unrelated to receptor antagonism. Direct α_2 receptor agonists produce a sympatholytic effect by activating receptors in the central nervous system (CNS). In addition, inhibition of monoamine oxidase can also produce a sympatholytic action. There are other novel sympatholytic mechanisms of action produced by a variety of drugs. However, in the 21st century, the use of these agents has been curtailed, and they have been largely relegated to historical footnotes. Brief descriptions of these drugs can be found in earlier editions of this text.

SELECTIVE α_1-ADRENENERGIC RECEPTOR ANTAGONISTS

As discussed in Chapter 5, α_1-adrenergic receptors are located predominantly on the postjunctional membranes of glands and smooth muscle. The α_1-adrenergic receptors associated with smooth muscle of arteries and veins play an important role in promoting vasoconstriction and in regulating systemic arterial blood pressure and, ultimately, blood flow. The α_1-adrenergic receptors are also important in regulating the tone of nonvascular smooth muscle, such as in the neck of the urinary bladder and capsule of the prostate. More recent evidence has suggested that the α_1-adrenergic receptor plays a role in the regulation of hypertrophic growth, the generation of reactive oxygen species, and apoptotic cell death. Antagonism of these cellular events may also be the reason that α_1-adrenergic receptor blockers are effective in the treatment of benign prostatic hyperplasia.

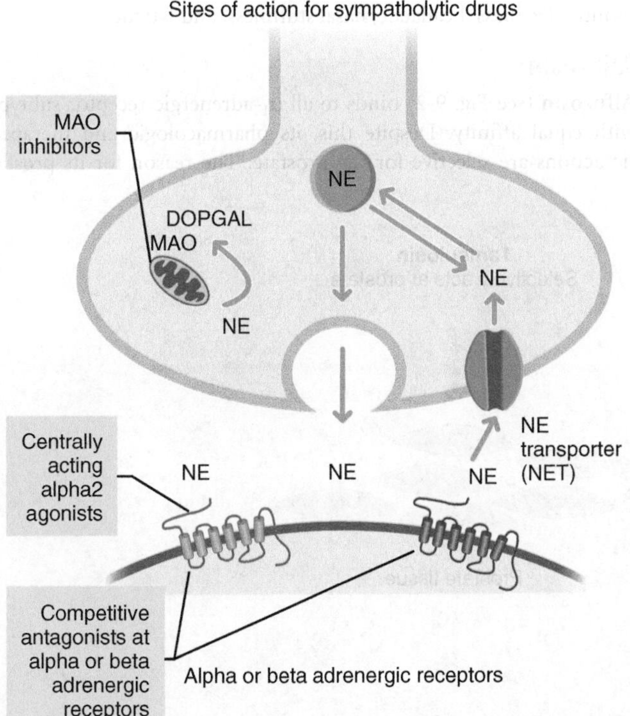

FIG 9-1 Potential sites of action for sympatholytic drugs. *MAO*, Monoamine oxidase; *DOPGAL*, 3,4 dihydroxyphenylglycolaldehyde; *NET*, norepinephrine transporter.

Prazosin and Analogues

The first antagonists that targeted the α_1-adrenergic receptor were nonselective (see later) and also blocked the α_2-adrenergic receptor. These drugs were unsuitable as antihypertensive agents, presumably because of the α_2-adrenergic receptor blockade. The disadvantages associated with the nonselective blockade of α receptors inspired a search for agents with receptor selectivity.

The first therapeutically useful α_1-adrenergic receptor antagonist developed was **prazosin** (Fig. 9-2). **Terazosin** and **doxazosin** are structural analogues that were subsequently introduced. Although these agents differ in pharmacokinetic properties, their mechanism of action is the same. The α_1-adrenergic receptor antagonists prevent the action of sympathetic neurotransmitters and exogenously administered agonists at α_1-adrenergic receptors on effector organs. Prazosin and related compounds have essentially equal affinity for all three subtypes (α_{1A}, α_{1B}, and α_{1D}) of the α_1-adrenergic receptor.

As a result of blocking smooth muscle α_1-adrenergic receptors, prazosin dilates arterioles and veins. Each of these actions contributes to the hypotension seen with this drug. Blockade of arterial smooth muscle produces hypotension by reducing peripheral resistance. The venodilation resulting from blocked venous α_1-adrenergic receptors decreases cardiac preload. Compared with the nonselective α receptor antagonists, prazosin causes less tachycardia, a smaller increase in cardiac output, and less renin release.

Absorption, fate, and excretion

Prazosin is variably absorbed, with 40% to 70% of an oral dose becoming systemically bioavailable. A large percentage of circulating drug in the plasma is bound to α_1-acid glycoprotein. The plasma half-life is approximately 2 to 3 hours, requiring dosing two to three times per day. Most of the drug is demethylated and conjugated in the liver. Some prazosin metabolites are pharmacologically active and contribute to its therapeutic effect. Metabolites are excreted in the bile.

Terazosin is almost completely absorbed after oral administration and thus has a higher bioavailability than prazosin. It is also highly bound to plasma proteins. With a half-life of approximately 12 hours, the drug can be administered once a day. It is extensively metabolized in the liver, with both active and inactive metabolites formed. Approximately 60% of the drug is eliminated in the bile and 40% in the urine.

The systemic bioavailability of doxazosin is 60% to 70% after oral administration. Similar to the other members of this class of compounds, doxazosin circulates highly bound to plasma proteins, is extensively metabolized, and is excreted in the bile and urine. Its half-life is 10 to 20 hours, giving it an extended duration of action.

Therapeutic uses

Prazosin, terazosin, and doxazosin can be used in monotherapy for the treatment of **hypertension** (see Chapter 23). Terazosin and doxazosin, which are given once a day, may have advantages over prazosin, which requires more frequent administration. Otherwise, the clinical effects are similar. Although prazosin and analogues can alleviate the signs and symptoms of congestive heart failure (because of a reduction in preload and afterload), they have not been shown to increase survival in patients with congestive heart failure. The doxazosin arm of the ALLHAT study was terminated early because, compared to chlorthalidone, there was a 25% increase in the incidence of other cardiovascular disease and a doubling of the likelihood that patients would be hospitalized for heart failure. This finding has resulted in a significant reduction in the use of prazosin analogues in the therapy of hypertension. These drugs do not have adverse effects on lipids or cholesterol and may be particularly useful in treating patients with hyperlipidemia. Prazosin and its analogues are also effective in treating **benign prostatic hyperplasia** caused by the blocking of the α_1-adrenergic receptors associated with smooth muscle of the bladder neck and prostate. This action reduces pressure on the urethra and improves urine flow. Because of their longer plasma half-lives, terazosin and doxazosin may be preferred over prazosin for this indication. Emerging data suggest prazosin is effective for treating nightmares and improving sleep and reducing the severity of posttraumatic stress disorder. The therapeutic actions of these drugs are outlined in Figure 9-3.

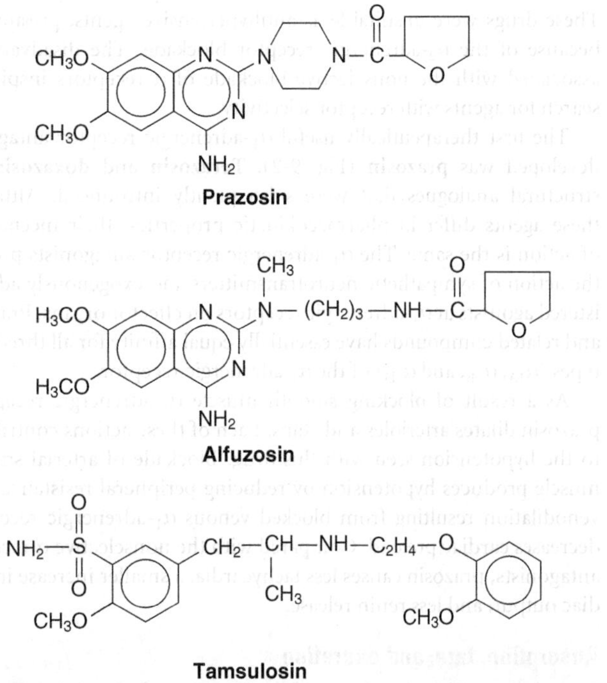

Prazosin

Alfuzosin

Tamsulosin

FIG 9-2 Structural formulas of three α_1-adrenergic receptor-blocking agents.

Adverse effects

Orthostatic or postural hypotension is a concern with prazosin analogues. The effect is most likely to occur with initial administration and is known as **"first-dose" syncope.** Hypotension ensues when the systemic arterial blood pressure decreases by more than 20 mm Hg on standing. In this situation, cerebral perfusion decreases, and an individual may become lightheaded, dizzy, or faint. In changing from the supine to the standing position, gravity tends to cause blood to pool in the lower extremities. However, several reflexes, including sympathetically mediated venoconstriction, minimize this pooling, and maintain cerebral perfusion. By blocking the α_1 receptors associated with venous smooth muscle, prazosin-like drugs inhibit the sympathetically mediated vasoconstriction associated with postural changes. This can result in **orthostatic hypotension.**

Therapy with prazosin and its analogues should be instituted initially with small doses, followed by a gradual dosage increase over time. These drugs may cause fluid retention and edema; it may be necessary to give a diuretic simultaneously. A more recently described adverse effect of the α_1 receptors blockers is **inoperable floppy iris syndrome (IFIS)** that can occur during cataract surgery. This delicate procedure requires that the pupil be dilated by administration of an α_1-adrenergic receptor agonist. This pupillary dilation is blocked in the presence of the α_1 blocker. In addition, the flaccid iris is difficult to manipulate and obstructs the surgical field. Surgery is rendered more difficult, and the risk of complications is increased. α_1-Receptor antagonists should be withheld before cataract procedures. Other adverse effects include dry mouth, dizziness, headache, nasal stuffiness, and fatigue.

Alfuzosin

Alfuzosin (see Fig. 9-2) binds to all α_1-adrenergic receptor subtypes with equal affinity. Despite this, its pharmacologic and therapeutic actions are selective for the prostate. The reason for its prostate

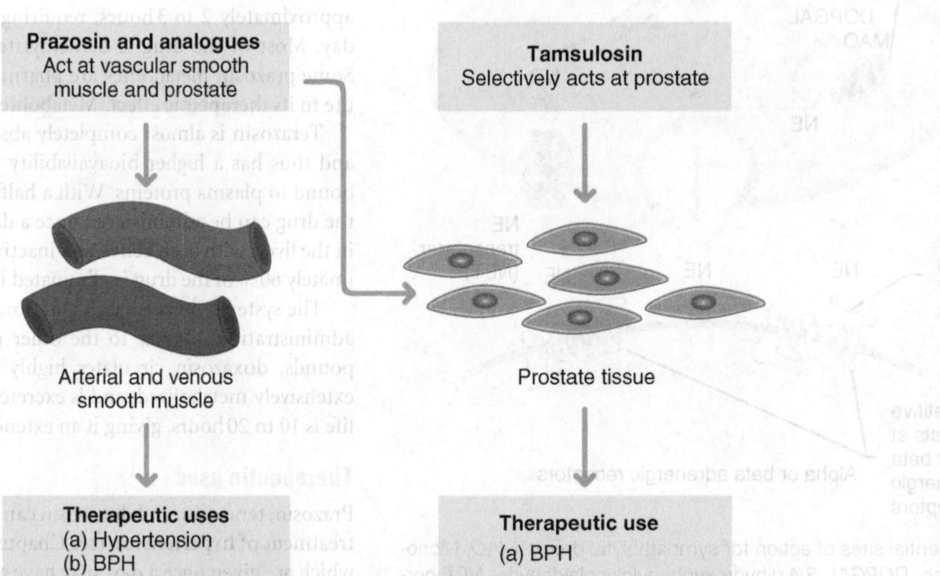

FIG 9-3 Sites of action and therapeutic uses of selective α_1-adrenergic receptor antagonists.

selectivity is not well understood. It seems to be related to the ability of alfuzosin to accumulate selectively in prostate tissue. Because of this prostate uptake, therapeutic doses of alfuzosin have little effect on systemic arterial blood pressure and are much less likely to cause syncope. IFIS remains a concern, however, with the use of alfuzosin. The drug is well absorbed and is available in a once-daily dosage form.

Tamsulosin

Tamsulosin (see Fig. 9-2) is the first clinically available antagonist that blocks specific subtypes of the α_1-adrenergic receptor: the α_{1A} and α_{1D} subtypes. The α_{1A}-adrenergic receptor has been shown to mediate the contraction of human prostatic smooth muscle. Because tamsulosin has a high affinity for the α_{1A}-adrenergic receptor, it is effectively used to treat benign prostatic hyperplasia. The selectivity of this compound for the prostate is reflected in the fact that there is little decrease in blood pressure after therapeutic doses of the drug. Tamsulosin is well absorbed after oral administration and circulates tightly bound to plasma proteins. It is extensively metabolized in the liver and excreted as inactive conjugation products in the urine. Tamsulosin is less likely to cause orthostatic hypotension and syncope than other α_1-selective antagonists. A review of the literature indicated that tamsulosin was more likely to cause IFIS than other α_1-adrenergic receptor antagonists.

NONSELECTIVE α-ADRENERGIC RECEPTOR ANTAGONISTS

The nonselective α-adrenergic receptor–blocking drugs prevent the action of adrenergic transmitters and sympathomimetic agonists at all α-adrenergic receptors. Although many drugs exhibit some α-blocking activity, only phentolamine and phenoxybenzamine are currently used clinically for their nonselective α-adrenoceptor antagonist action. Phentolamine is a competitive antagonist at α_1-adrenergic and α_2-adrenergic receptors, while phenoxybenzamine is an irreversible antagonist of these receptors. They are occasionally used to treat the rare epinephrine-secreting tumor of the adrenal gland, pheochromocytoma. For a more complete description of these drugs the reader is referred to earlier editions of this text.

More recently, **phentolamine mesylate** has been approved for the **reversal of soft tissue anesthesia** after administration of local anesthetics with vasoconstrictors for nonsurgical dental procedures. The drug is formulated in dental cartridges (0.4 mg/1.7-mL cartridge) and is injected in the same manner as the local anesthetic when pain relief is no longer needed. The median duration of posttreatment anesthesia in the upper and lower lips of adults and children is reduced by 85 minutes when phentolamine mesylate is injected at the end of restorative and dental hygiene procedures lasting about 45 minutes. Return of normal function (e.g., speaking, smiling, drinking) occurs in concert with return of normal sensation. It is unlikely that the phentolamine is acting by reversing the vasoconstrictor effect of injected epinephrine, which should have already disappeared from the local tissues. Instead, the phentolamine probably increases local blood flow by blocking sympathetic tone, which hastens the removal of the local anesthetic from local neurons. Doses of phentolamine used for this purpose (0.2 to 0.8 mg) (0.5 to 2.0 cartridges), are approximately 10 times less than doses injected intravenously for treatment of hypertensive emergencies, and adverse effects have been similar to those reported after sham injection.

β-ADRENERGIC RECEPTOR ANTAGONISTS

The β-adrenergic receptor antagonists, also called **β-adrenergic receptor blockers** or simply **β blockers** are an important and versatile class of drugs widely used in cardiovascular therapeutics. The β blockers are also used to treat numerous non-cardiovascular disorders. Several β blockers are among the most widely prescribed medicines in the United States. Certain β blockers have weak partial agonist properties, referred to as intrinsic sympathomimetic activity, as well have being weak local anesthetic agents. These actions do not contribute a significant degree to the overall action of the β-adrenergic receptor blockers, and the reader is referred to earlier editions of this text for a more complete discussion of these properties.

The β-adrenergic receptors are categorized into three subtypes: β_1, β_2, and β_3. Cardiovascular therapeutic efficacy is a result of β_1-receptor blockade. The β-adrenergic receptor blockers can be described in terms of their specific antagonist profile as outlined below and summarized in Table 9-1.

First-Generation β-Adrenergic Receptor Blockers, Nonselective Antagonists

These drugs are competitive antagonists with equal affinity at both the β_1-adrenergic and β_2-adrenergic receptors and as such are referred to as nonselective β blockers. Propranolol was the first β-blocking drug to be approved in the United States and is considered the prototype for this class of compounds. The beneficial effects of propranolol and other nonselective β blockers are mostly attributable to blockade of the β_1-adrenergic receptor. As discussed subsequently, blockade of the β_2-adrenergic receptor is associated with undesirable effects on the airways, vascular smooth muscle, and endocrine function.

Second-Generation β-Adrenergic Receptor Blockers, β_1-Selective Antagonists

Once it became apparent that there were subtypes of the β-adrenergic receptor, subtype selective antagonists were developed. **Metoprolol**, the first selective **β_1 receptor antagonist**, and its successors (e.g., **atenolol, acebutolol**, and **esmolol**) have attracted considerable attention because of their relative freedom from the unwanted effects of β_2-adrenergic receptor blockade. This β_1 selectivity is relative with existing agents, and these drugs lose much of their selectivity at higher doses. Presently, both nonselective and selective β blockers are used clinically.

Third-Generation β-Adrenergic Receptor Blockers, Antagonists with Additional Actions

As typified by **labetalol** and **carvedilol**, these drugs not only block the β-adrenergic receptors but have additional actions such as blockade of the α_1-adrenergic receptor, generation of nitric oxide, and decrease in reactive oxygen species, which contribute to their unique pharmacologic actions. Labetalol combines nonselective β-blocking properties with α_1-adrenergic antagonism. It is five to seven times more potent at blocking β-adrenergic receptors compared to α_1 receptors. These properties are the result of the different receptor-blocking characteristics of the four isomers that make up the drug formulation. Because of actions at β-adrenergic and α_1-adrenergic receptors, labetalol decreases peripheral resistance and blood pressure. The drug has some direct vasodilatory properties because at least one isomer is a partial agonist at β_2 receptors, and at least one isomer may exert vasodilator properties not mediated by interaction at adrenergic receptors. Because of these actions, labetalol can be used to treat hypertensive emergencies.

Carvedilol, a racemic mixture of two isomers, is the second drug to be marketed with α_1- and β-blocking activities. Carvedilol is also much more selective for β-adrenergic receptors than labetalol. Carvedilol was initially approved for use as an antihypertensive (because of its ability to block α_1 and β receptors), but more recent clinical studies have shown that it is particularly useful in decreasing morbidity and mortality associated with heart failure. The pharmacologic actions that

TABLE 9-1 Comparison of β-Adrenergic Receptor–Blocking Drugs

Drugs	Potency of Blockade (Propranolol = 1)	Oral Bioavailability	Half-Life (hr)	Route of Elimination	Lipophilicity	Dosing Frequency (times/day)	Therapeutic Indications
Nonselective ($\beta_1 + \beta_2$), First Generation							
Nadolol	1.0	30	10-24	Renal	Low	1	Angina pectoris; hypertension
Pindolol	6.0	80	3-4	Hepatic/renal	Moderate	1-2	Hypertension
Propranolol	1.0	30	3-5	Hepatic	High	2-3	Angina pectoris; arrhythmias; essential tremor, hypertension; hypertrophic subaortic stenosis; migraine prophylaxis; myocardial infarction; pheochromocytoma
Timolol	6.0	50	3-5	Hepatic/renal	Moderate	1-2	Hypertension; migraine prophylaxis; myocardial infarction; glaucoma
Selective (β_1), Second Generation							
Acebutolol	0.3	40	3-4	Hepatic/renal/ nonrenal	Moderate	2-3	Hypertension; ventricular arrhythmias
Atenolol	1.0	50	6-9	Renal	Low	1-1	Angina pectoris; hypertension; myocardial infarction
Esmolol*	0.02	—	0.15	Red blood cell esterase	—	—	Supraventricular tachycardias; noncompensatory tachycardias
Metoprolol	1.0	40	3-7	Hepatic/renal	Moderate	2-3	Angina pectoris; hypertension; myocardial infarction, heart failure
Third Generation, with Additional Actions							
Carvedilol	10	90	7-10	Hepatic	Moderate	2	Myocardial infarction, hypertension, heart failure
Labetalol	0.3	90	3-4	Hepatic	Low	2	Hypertension, hypertensive crisis

*Has a very brief duration of action and is given intravenously only.

make carvedilol useful in treating heart failure are probably the result of blockade of both α_1-adrenergic and β-adrenergic receptors. The vasodilatory actions of carvedilol that occur as a result of α_1 receptor blockade decrease peripheral resistance and, as a result, the workload of the heart. There is also evidence that carvedilol exerts antioxidant activity and acts as a free radical scavenger, which could provide benefit in patients with heart failure.

The pharmacodynamic and pharmacokinetic properties of propranolol and other selected β blockers are summarized in Table 9-1.

Chemistry

As exemplified by the first β blocker, dichloroisoproterenol, halogen substitution of the catechol hydroxyl groups of the β agonist, isoproterenol, results in a partial agonistic activity at the β receptor. As illustrated in Figure 9-4, the currently available β-blocking drugs all possess an ethylamino moiety similar to that seen in β-adrenergic receptor agonists attached through a methoxy linkage to a variant ring structure. β_1 Selectivity is conferred by a benzene ring with a large substitution in the *para* position.

Pharmacologic Effects

The pharmacologic effects of the β blockers occur as a result of preventing binding and subsequent receptor activation by epinephrine, norepinephrine, and exogenously administered adrenergic agonists in tissues regulated by β-adrenergic receptors.

Effects on the cardiovascular system

The β blockers **decrease the rate and force of myocardial contraction.** The major sites of action for the negative chronotropic effects are the β_1-adrenergic receptors associated with the sinoatrial (SA) node, the atrioventricular (AV) node, and the His-Purkinje system. There is a decrease in firing rate, slowed conduction, and reduced automaticity. These actions contribute to the antiarrhythmic efficacy of the β blockers. The decrease in contractile force occurs largely as a result of β_1-adrenergic receptor blockade associated with ventricular (the major site of action) and atrial muscle. Collectively, these changes result in a decrease in cardiac output. The negative inotropic and chronotropic actions lessen the oxygen consumption of the heart and contribute to the usefulness of the β blockers in treating ischemic heart disease. The effects of the β blockers are most pronounced under conditions of heightened sympathetic activity, when there are significant amounts of circulating and neuronally released catecholamines.

In normotensive patients, β blockers do not normally reduce blood pressure; however, they are highly effective in reducing blood pressure in hypertensive patients. These agents reduce blood pressure equally in the supine and standing positions, with little or no orthostatic hypotension.

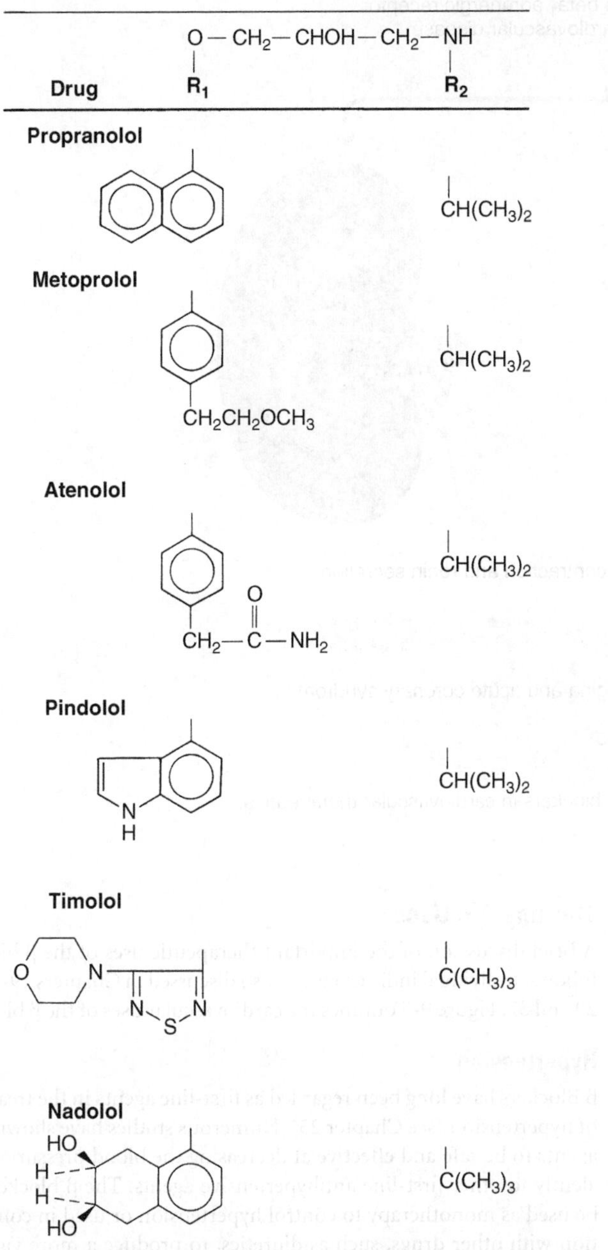

$O-CH_2-CHOH-CH_2-NH$

Drug	R_1	R_2
Propranolol		$CH(CH_3)_2$
Metoprolol	$CH_2CH_2OCH_3$	$CH(CH_3)_2$
Atenolol	$CH_2-C(=O)-NH_2$	$CH(CH_3)_2$
Pindolol	N H	$CH(CH_3)_2$
Timolol	O N N S N	$C(CH_3)_3$
Nadolol	HO H H HO	$C(CH_3)_3$

FIG 9-4 Structural formulas of some β-adrenergic receptor antagonists. All the drugs share a similar side chain, differing only in the terminal hydrocarbon group (R_2). Considerable variation exists in the ring structures (R_1).

This attribute was discovered serendipitously while β blockers were being used to treat angina pectoris. Since that time, propranolol and other β blockers, alone or in combination with other drugs, have long been among the drugs of first choice in the treatment of hypertension. However, as discussed later, this usage in hypertension is being reevaluated. Although the mechanisms by which the β blockers reduce blood pressure are not completely understood, certain facts are known. When propranolol is first administered to a patient, cardiac output decreases, and peripheral resistance increases. The latter effect may result from β_2 receptor blockade in the vasculature or from a baroreceptor-mediated increase in sympathetic tone. With continued therapy, peripheral resistance also decreases. By **blocking renal β_1-adrenergic receptors** involved in renin secretion, β blockers cause a reduction of plasma renin concentrations. The reduction in plasma renin activity eventually leads to a reduction in angiotensin II concentrations and aldosterone secretion. A decrease in heart rate and cardiac output are major contributors to a reduction in blood pressure. Other mechanisms that seem to contribute to the reduction in blood pressure include inhibition of CNS sympathetic outflow and an alteration in baroreceptor responsiveness.

Effects on smooth muscle

Pulmonary smooth muscle. By blocking the β_2-adrenergic receptors associated with airway smooth muscle, propranolol and other nonselective β blockers prevent sympathetic stimulation of bronchiolar smooth muscle, while leaving parasympathetic activity and other bronchoconstrictive influences unchecked. This imbalance can lead to a marked **increase in airway resistance** in patients with bronchospastic disorders such as asthma, chronic bronchitis, and emphysema. Propranolol and other nonselective β blockers are contraindicated in patients with bronchospastic disease. This limitation was a major impetus for development of selective β_1 receptor–blocking drugs.

Vascular smooth muscle. β_2-Adrenergic receptors are also expressed on vascular smooth muscle and account for additional unwanted side effects of nonselective β blockers. For example, these agents can exacerbate peripheral vascular disease by **blocking the vasodilatory effects** of the β_2-adrenergic receptor. In addition, they can potentiate the vasoconstrictor actions of neurotransmitters or drugs that activate the α_1-adrenergic receptor. This includes epinephrine given with local anesthetic agents.

Gastrointestinal tract effects

Similar to other adrenergic antagonists, propranolol tends to produce a relative preponderance of parasympathetic activity in the gastrointestinal tract. The net effect is related to the amount of sympathetic activity that is blocked, but it is usually of little importance.

Metabolic effects

Propranolol and other nonselective β blockers antagonize the β_2-adrenergic receptors responsible for initiating glycogenolysis in the liver and in skeletal muscle. **Hypoglycemia** may result from this action, but it is rare in the nondiabetic individual. The release of fatty acids from adipocytes by epinephrine is mediated by β_1-adrenergic or β_3-adrenergic receptors. All clinically useful β-adrenergic antagonists blunt this release. While these drugs also increase triglyceride concentrations and decrease blood concentrations of high-density lipoproteins, this does not preclude the use of β blockers in patients with elevated serum lipids, including cholesterol.

Ocular effects

While the antihypertensive effects of the β blockers were being studied, investigators noticed a **decrease in intraocular pressure** in patients with open-angle glaucoma. The production of aqueous humor is decreased by β blockers. Several β receptor blockers are commonly used topically (eye drops) in treating open-angle glaucoma (Appendix 5).

Central nervous system effects

The versatility of the β blockers is reflected in the fact that they can be used to treat a variety of disorders that have CNS involvement, including migraine headache, performance anxiety (stage fright), and benign essential tremor.

As described subsequently, the β-blocking drugs can cause various side effects related to their CNS activity. Theoretically, the most hydrophilic β blockers (e.g., nadolol and atenolol) should have the least access to the CNS and be associated with the lowest occurrence of such effects. There is evidence that more hydrophobic β blockers are more likely to produce a greater degree of sedation.

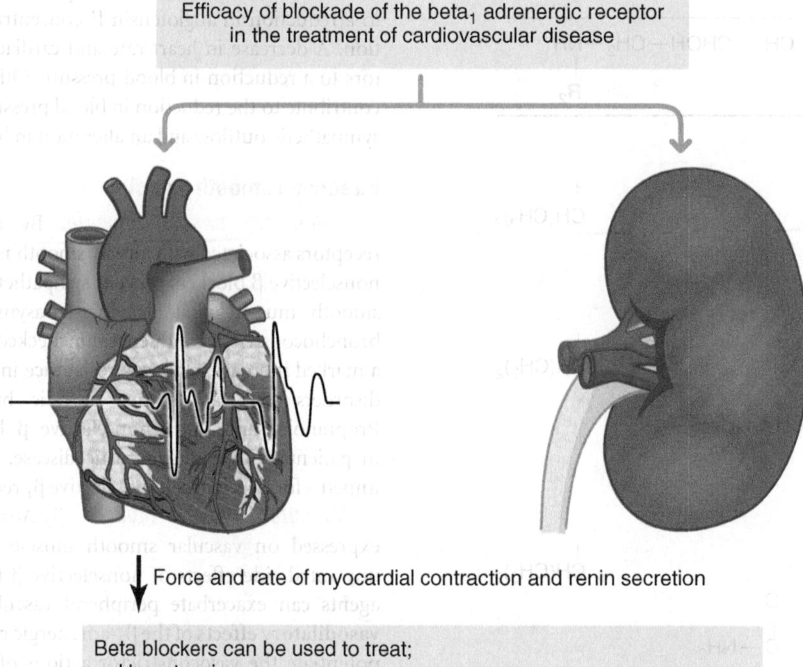
Efficacy of blockade of the beta$_1$ adrenergic receptor in the treatment of cardiovascular disease
Force and rate of myocardial contraction and renin secretion
Beta blockers can be used to treat;
• Hypertension
• Ischemic heart disease-stable angina and acute coronary syndromes
• Post MI
• Supraventricular tachyarrhythmias
• Heart failure

FIG 9-5 The uses of β-adrenergic receptor blockers in cardiovascular therapeutics.

Absorption, Fate, and Excretion

Most clinically approved β blockers are available in oral dosage forms. Esmolol, a selective β_1 receptor antagonist with a very brief duration of action, is limited to intravenous use for the treatment of acute hypertension and to control ventricular rate in patients with supraventricular tachyarrhythmias. Levobunolol and metipranolol are available only in solutions suitable for ophthalmic use. Key features of the metabolism and pharmacokinetic properties of selected β blockers are summarized in Table 9-1.

In its first pass through the liver, approximately 50% of propranolol is metabolized. The first-pass extraction can vary widely among patients, necessitating individualized dosing regimens. Peak plasma concentrations of propranolol occur approximately 90 minutes after oral administration, with 90% of the drug bound to plasma proteins. The half-life after oral administration is 3 to 5 hours; intravenous administration results in a half-life of 1.5 to 2 hours. Nadolol is unique among currently available drugs because it has an elimination half-life of up to 24 hours. The bioavailability of propranolol and metoprolol may be significantly improved if the drugs are taken after a high-protein meal, presumably because the protein reduces first-pass metabolism of the drugs. To minimize variation in drug effects, the dosing schedule should be consistent regarding meals.

Metabolism of propranolol occurs almost exclusively in the liver, with oxidative reactions involving the benzene ring and the side chain. One metabolite, 4-hydroxypropranolol, is as active as the parent compound. Less than 5% of the administered drug is excreted intact in the urine. As noted in Table 9-1, most of the other β-blocking drugs are excreted more extensively by the kidney than is propranolol.

Therapeutic Uses

A brief discussion of the important therapeutic uses of the β blockers follows. Individual indications are also discussed in Chapters 19-21, 23, 29 and 37. Figure 9-5 outlines the cardiovascular uses of the β blockers.

Hypertension

β Blockers have long been regarded as first-line agents in the treatment of hypertension (see Chapter 23). Numerous studies have shown these agents to be safe and effective at decreasing the blood pressure equivalently to other first-line antihypertensive agents. The β blockers can be used as monotherapy to control hypertension or used in combination with other drugs, such as diuretics, to produce a more vigorous antihypertensive response. Many of the side effects associated with the use of other antihypertensives, such as Na^+ and water retention or the development of tolerance, do not occur with β blockers. The effects of β blockers on blood triglycerides and glucose metabolism described previously do not preclude their use in patients with hyperlipidemia or diabetes. The only systemic β blockers not approved for use in hypertension are esmolol and sotalol. However, the first-line status of the β blockers has been questioned by several recent meta-analyses. These analyses show that there is an increased risk of stroke in patients, especially the elderly taking β blockers. Indeed, the most recent recommendations on the treatment of hypertension, JNC8, have removed β blockers from the list of the drugs of choice to treat hypertension.

Ischemic heart disease

The β blockers are first-line agents in the treatment of angina pectoris associated with atherosclerotic coronary artery disease. The overall therapeutic approach to this disease is described in Chapter 21. In this condition, there is an imbalance between the oxygen demand of the myocardium and the ability of the partially occluded coronary arteries to deliver oxygen-rich blood to the myocardial muscle. This imbalance leads to cardiac ischemia and development of the characteristic chest pain of angina pectoris. Two of the major determinants of myocardial work and oxygen consumption—the force and rate of contraction—are decreased by β blockade. Both selective and nonselective β blockers can be used effectively for this indication. Although β blocker–mediated reductions in oxygen consumption are efficacious in reducing the incidence and severity of anginal attacks, they are not helpful in managing variant angina. β blockers can be used effectively in combination with other anti-ischemics for anginal prophylaxis including nitrates, dihydropyridine calcium channel blockers, as well as ranolazine. Due to the combined negative inotropic and chronotropic actions, β blockers should not be used with the nondihydropyridines verapamil and diltiazem.

Myocardial infarction

In addition to stable angina pectoris the β blockers are also drugs of choice in treatment of acute coronary syndromes to prevent myocardial infarction and the prophylaxis of reinfarction. The favorable action for this indication is related to the decrease in cardiac work and on myocardial oxygen consumption produced by the β blockers. These drugs can limit the likelihood and reduce the severity of reinfarction. The antiarrhythmic activity of the β blockers may also contribute to reducing mortality rates after myocardial infarction.

Heart failure

As our knowledge base increases, there has been a dramatic shift in the therapeutic approaches to the treatment of heart failure. Prior to 1990 the emphasis was on positive inotropic agents, vasodilators, and diuretics, and β-adrenergic receptor blockers were not even considered as therapeutic options. However, several clinical trials demonstrated that β-adrenergic receptor blockers improve left ventricular function and the symptoms of heart failure as well as decrease the progression of the disease and, most importantly, increase patient survival. The therapeutic approaches to heart failure are discussed in Chapter 20.

The β-adrenergic receptor is rapidly engaged and disengaged by adjustments to sympathetic tone as metabolic demands change. However, in the setting of heart failure the receptor is continuously activated leading to pathophysiologic changes that ultimately contribute to the signs and symptoms of failure. For example, the increase in circulating catecholamines ultimately results in the desensitization and downregulation of the myocardial β-adrenergic receptor population, the main receptor utilized by the sympathetic nervous system to increase cardiac output. The β_1-adrenergic receptor is also a potent stimulus for the generation of reactive oxygen derivatives, hypertrophic growth, and cardiac remodeling. In addition, the β_1-adrenergic receptor regulates renin secretion. Therefore, the elevated sympathetic nervous system activity increases circulation of angiotensin II. Angiotensin II not only has the ability to increase peripheral vascular resistance and promote Na^+ retention, but it is also a positive signal for the generation of reactive oxygen species and hypertrophic growth responses. Angiotensin II also stimulates the adrenal release of aldosterone, which is a positive signal for hypertrophic growth responses. These activities impair cardiac performance further, which sets in motion a vicious cycle of increasingly compromised ventricular performance (see Chapter 20). Antagonism of this constellation of effects makes the β blockers effective in patients with heart failure.

These aforementioned results are not indicative of a class effect. Trials with several other β blockers failed to show any beneficial effect. The only β_1 blockers shown to be effective in heart failure are bisoprolol, carvedilol, and metoprolol succinate (in extended release preparations). This is in contrast to metoprolol tartrate, which has not been shown to be effective.

Treatment of arrhythmias

The β blockers can be used to treat various supraventricular tachyarrhythmias, including atrial flutter and atrial fibrillation. The sympathetic nervous system richly innervates the SA and AV nodes, and the β_1-adrenergic receptor is the major regulatory receptor at these sites. A complete discussion of antiarrhythmic drug therapy is provided in Chapter 19. In the setting of sinus tachycardia, blockade of the SA nodal β_1-adrenergic receptors results in a slowing of heart rate. In atrial fibrillation and flutter, blockade of the β_1-adrenergic receptors in the AV node slows conduction and increases the nodal refractory period. This slows AV nodal conduction time, thus protecting the ventricle from the excessive stimulation caused by the abnormal atrial depolarizations. While a member of the β blocker family, sotalol has the added action of being a K+ channel blocker (see Chapter 19) and can be used to treat atrial fibrillation and ventricular tachycardia. Esmolol has a short plasma half-life and is used intravenously for rapid action in the acute management of supraventricular tachyarrhythmias. Propranolol and acebutolol are other members of this class widely used for their antiarrhythmic action.

Non-cardiovascular uses

In addition to wide versatility in cardiovascular therapeutics, the β blockers can be used to treat a wide variety of non-cardiovascular disorders including:

- pheochromocytoma (administered with an α-adrenergic receptor–blocking drug)
- thyrotoxicosis
- migraine headache prophylaxis
- open-angle glaucoma
- performance anxiety (stage fright)
- essential tremors
- variceal bleeding prophylaxis

Adverse Effects

Many of the adverse effects of the β blockers (Table 7-2) are logical extensions of their pharmacologic actions. These effects are most prominently seen on the heart, smooth muscle, brain, and organs that mediate metabolic responses.

Effects on the heart

As an extension of their actions on SA and AV nodal function, β blockers can induce bradycardia and partial to complete AV conduction block. The abrupt withdrawal of propranolol has been linked to attacks of angina pectoris, myocardial infarction, and sudden death, especially in patients with angina. The chronic blockade of the β-adrenergic receptor may induce β receptor supersensitivity, which contributes to a rebound exacerbation of these clinical problems. Withdrawal from β-blocking drugs should be done slowly, over 1 to 2 weeks. In addition to the effects on conduction, β blockers can decrease myocardial contractility. The negative inotropic and chronotropic effects can contribute to the fatigue that is associated with the use of these drugs. As a result of the combined decease in contractility and conduction, β blockers should not be used with nondihydropyridine Ca^{2+} channel blockers such as verapamil or diltiazem.

Effects on smooth muscle

Because of the blockade of β_2 receptors in blood vessels, nonselective β blockers tend to reduce adrenergic vasodilator responses of the vasculature to epinephrine. This effect is of little consequence in most patients, even though cold hands and feet may result. In patients with peripheral vascular disease, such as Raynaud disease, worsening of the condition is likely, and β blockers, especially nonselective ones, should be used cautiously in such patients.

Bronchospasm resulting from blockade of β_2 receptors is apt to occur in patients with asthma and chronic obstructive airway diseases such as chronic bronchitis and emphysema. This is more problematic for nonselective β blockers. Selective β_1 blockers are less likely to affect bronchial smooth muscle and produce decreases in airways resistance. Nevertheless, the risk of bronchoconstriction with these drugs is still present because there is a limit to the selectivity for the β_1 receptor.

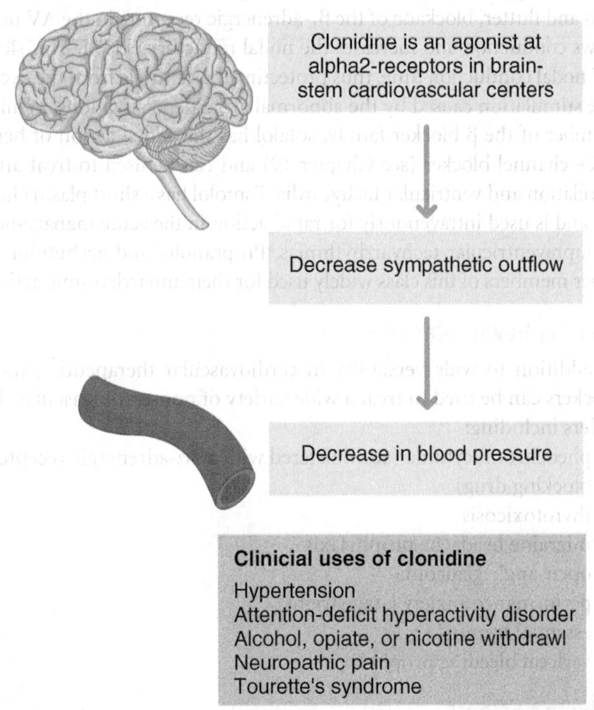

FIG 9-6 The mechanism of action and therapeutic uses of clonidine.

Metabolic effects

A common warning sign of hypoglycemia to a diabetic patient is an increase in heart rate. Because this action is largely mediated by the β_1-adrenergic receptor, this early sign of hypoglycemia is blunted by all clinically used β blockers. In addition, the effects of compensatory sympathetic stimulation and epinephrine release resulting from reduced blood glucose concentrations may be blocked in patients receiving β blockers.

Central nervous system effects

Patients receiving β blockers may experience CNS depression, weakness, fatigue, sleep disturbances including insomnia and nightmares, hallucinations, dizziness, and depression. As noted earlier, a component of the fatigue symptomatology could be due to the decrease in myocardial contraction.

DRUGS THAT REDUCE SYMPATHETIC OUTFLOW

Centrally Acting Adrenergic Agonists

Several drugs, including methyldopa, clonidine, guanabenz, and guanfacine, produce a sympatholytic action by a unique mechanism. These drugs are α_2-adrenergic receptor agonists (see Chapter 8). They interfere with sympathetic nervous system activity by stimulating brainstem regulatory α_2-receptors in the nucleus tractus solitarius, resulting in an inhibition of sympathetic outflow to cardiovascular effectors. This results in a decrease in systemic arterial blood pressure. These drugs have largely been supplanted as antihypertensives by safer, more effective therapeutic entities. Special note should be made of methyldopa which is used to treat hypertension in pregnancy. Of this class of agents, clonidine has shown the most versatility. It can be used outside the domain of cardiovascular drug therapy. The clinical uses of clonidine are summarized in Figure 9-6. Some of the major adverse effects of these drugs are summarized in Table 9-2. Of special note are the drowsiness and xerostomia produced by clonidine.

TABLE 9-2 Major Adverse Effects of Drugs That Suppress the Activity of the Sympathetic System by Actions at Adrenergic Receptors

	RECEPTOR-BLOCKING DRUGS			
Adverse Effects	**Nonselective α Receptor–Blocking Drugs**	**Selective α_1 Receptor–Blocking Drugs**	**β Receptor–Blocking Drugs**	**Selective α_2-Adrenergic Receptor Agonist Acting on the CNS (Clonidine)**
CNS Effects				
Depression		+	+	+
Drowsiness			++	+++
Dreams/insomnia			++	
Cardiovascular Effects				
Orthostatic hypotension	+++	++ (first dose)		+
Heart rate	↑	↑*	↓	↓
General Autonomic Effects				
Diarrhea	++	+		Constipation
Nasal stuffiness	++	+		
Xerostomia		+		+++
Asthma			++	
Fluid retention				++
Special reactions			Heart failure, angina withdrawal reaction	Withdrawal reaction

+, Rare; ++, occasional; +++, common; ↑, increase; ↓, decrease; *CNS*, central nervous system.
*Heart rate increase is less with selective α_1 receptor–blocking drugs compared to the nonselective α receptor–blocking drugs.

Monoamine Oxidase Inhibitors

Monoamine oxidase (MAO) inhibitors are another example of drugs that have sympatholytic actions by a unique, non-receptor action. The actions of this enzyme have been discussed in Chapter 5. MAO is the intracellular enzyme responsible for inactivation of norepinephrine by converting it to 3,4-dihydroxyphenylglycolaldehyde (DOPGAL, See Fig. 9-1). MAO is expressed in two isoforms, MAO-A and MAO-B, both in the periphery and CNS. By poorly understood mechanisms, MAO inhibitors reduce systemic arterial blood pressure and once were developed with the idea of treating hypertension. Because of the potentially serious side effects, these drugs are no longer used for this indication (see below). Phenelzine is an irreversible inhibitor of MAO-A and MAO-B and is a second-line agent for the treatment of depression. Selegiline is a selective, irreversible inhibitor of MAO-B. This enzyme is expressed in high levels in the dopamine rich regions of the brain that have been associated with the pathophysiology of Parkinson disease. Because of this expression, selegiline is used in the treatment of this disease.

MAO inhibitors are associated with a wide constellation of side effects, including orthostatic hypotension, dizziness, weakness, xerostomia, and syncope. Tremors and hallucinations have also been reported. Most serious is the hypertensive crisis that can occur after eating or drinking food stuffs containing substantial amounts of tyramine. Aged cheese, liver, beer, and wines are among the most common of these tyramine-containing foods. Hypertension is the result of three factors: (1) the metabolism of tyramine by MAO that would normally occur in the gastrointestinal tract is blocked by the MAO inhibitors; (2) tyramine is an indirect-acting amine and causes release of neurotransmitter from the cytoplasmic pool of adrenergic nerve endings; and (3) large amounts of the transmitter accumulate in the cytoplasmic pool of adrenergic nerve endings as a result of the inhibition of MAO. In addition to the typical symptoms of acute hypertension (throbbing headache, flushing, and hyperpyrexia), cerebrovascular accidents and occasionally deaths have occurred.

IMPLICATIONS FOR DENTISTRY

Considering the wide range of therapeutic indications for the drugs discussed in this chapter, dental practitioners are quite likely to encounter patients taking one or more of these drugs in their practices. Dentists must pay heed to the potential risks associated with these pathologic conditions and the therapeutic agents used to manage them.

Physical Implications

A consideration for patients being treated with certain sympatholytics is the patient's position during and after dental procedures. Suddenly standing upright after being in a supine position in the dental chair is apt to cause syncope. This problem is particularly likely for the drugs more prone to cause orthostatic hypotension (e.g., α_1-adrenergic receptor–blocking drugs and drugs with combined α-blocking and β receptor–blocking activity, MAO inhibitors). Accidents ranging from chipped teeth and restorations to fractured mandibles and worse have resulted from falls.

Drug Interactions

Because nonselective β blockers inhibit β_2-adrenergic receptor–mediated vasodilation, there is a risk of a hypertensive episode after administration of local anesthetic agents that contain vasoconstrictors. In this situation, the vasoconstrictor actions of epinephrine at α-adrenergic receptors are not opposed by the vasodilator actions of β_2-adrenergic receptors, resulting in an exaggerated increase in blood pressure that could be deleterious in patients with hypertension or ischemic heart disease. In a recent summary of case reports, patients receiving propranolol for either migraine or hypertension had a significant increase in blood pressure following the administration of local anesthetic containing epinephrine. In this report the authors concluded that certain patients could be hypersensitive to this interaction. As an example, one patient's blood pressure rose from 120/80 to 210/110 mm Hg after administration of an epinephrine containing local anesthetic (See Hersh and Giannakopoulos ref).

Clonidine is well known to cause xerostomia. The use of clonidine-like drugs may result in clinical symptoms related to dry mouth, such as difficulty in swallowing and speech. Long-term use of xerostomia-causing drugs is associated with a higher incidence of oral candidiasis and dental caries. The use of β-adrenergic receptor blockers is likely to alter the composition of salivary proteins. The effects of these changes have not been fully explored; however, there is a concern that they could adversely influence oral health. The effect of drugs that alter the function of adrenergic nerve endings on salivary proteins is also not well explored.

The use of drugs that release catecholamines should be scrupulously avoided with MAO inhibitors. Amphetamines and drugs with mixed sympathomimetic actions are absolutely contraindicated. The use of the analgesic meperidine is contraindicated in patients taking MAO inhibitors because a syndrome of CNS excitation, hyperthermia, and convulsions may commonly result. Opioid analgesics unrelated to meperidine (e.g., morphine) should be used cautiously because MAO inhibitors tend to increase the CNS depression from many opioid analgesics and sedatives.

ADRENERGIC ANTAGONISTS

Nonproprietary (Generic) Name	Proprietary (Trade) Name
α-Adrenergic Receptor Blockers (Selectivity)	
Alfuzosin (α_1)	Uroxatral
Doxazosin (α_1)	Cardura
Phenoxybenzamine (α_1, α_2)	Dibenzyline
Phentolamine (α_1, α_2)	Regitine, OraVerse
Prazosin (α_1)	Minipress
Tamsulosin (α_{1A})	Flomax
Terazosin (α_1)	Hytrin
β-Adrenergic Receptor Blockers (Selectivity)	
Acebutolol (β_1)	Sectral
Atenolol (β_1)	Tenormin
Betaxolol (β_1)	Betoptic, Kerlone
Bisoprolol (β_1)	Zebeta
Carteolol (β_1, β_2)	Cartrol
Esmolol (β_1)	Brevibloc
Levobunolol (β_1, β_2)	AKBeta, Betagan
Metipranolol (β_1, β_2)	OptiPranolol
Metoprolol (β_1)	Lopressor, Toprol XL
Nadolol (β_1, β_2)	Corgard
Nebivolol (β_1)	Bystolic
Penbutolol (β_1, β_2)	Levatol
Pindolol (β_1, β_2)	Visken
Propranolol (β_1, β_2)	Inderal
Sotalol (β_1, β_2)	Betapace
Timolol (β_1, β_2)	Blocadren
Combined α- and β-Adrenergic Receptor Blockers	
Carvedilol (β_1, β_2, α_1)	Coreg
Labetalol (β_1, β_2, α_1)	Trandate, Normodyne

CASE DISCUSSION

This patient has a history of hypertension and ischemic heart disease. Both conditions are adequately controlled by appropriate medical therapy. However, shortly after receiving an epinephrine containing local anesthetic, she experiences a significant increase in blood pressure to levels that are potentially dangerous. The fact that this patient has hypertension does not preclude the use of vasoconstrictors, as the combination of epinephrine and local anesthetics are usually well tolerated in hypertensive patients. What makes this case different is the fact that this patient was also taking propranolol, a nonselective β blocker. Blockade of the β_2-adrenergic receptor associated with the vasculature removes the vasodilatory effects of this receptor which would tend to counterbalance the vasoconstrictor activity of the α_1-adrenergic receptor. Therefore, any systemically absorbed epinephrine would induce an unopposed pressor action at the α_1-adrenergic receptor. Some patients are more susceptible to this pressor action, and this is perhaps a reason for the significant hypertensive response. Moreover, this adverse reaction is more likely to occur if the anesthetic with epinephrine is inadvertently injected intravenously. This is a definite possibility with this procedure, given the fact that a mandibular block was most likely given to achieve anesthesia. If possible, avoidance of the use of epinephrine should be the goal in this patient, but if epinephrine is needed, 0.036 mg (2 cartridges of 1:100,000) should be the maximum dose.* Each injection should be given slowly and only after aspiration. Monitoring of blood pressure is important so as to halt injection if an adverse response occurs.

*See Hersh and Giannakopoulos reference.

GENERAL REFERENCES

1. Ahlquist RP: A study of adrenotropic receptors, *Am J Physiol* 153:586–600, 1948.
2. Becker DE: Adverse drug interactions in dental practice, *Anesth Prog* 61:26–34, 2014.
3. Brodde OE, Bruck H, Leineweber K: Cardiac adrenoceptors: physiological and pathophysiological relevance, *J Pharmacol Sci* 100(5):323–337, 2006.
4. Clifford GM, Farmer RD: Medical therapy for benign prostatic hyperplasia: a review of the literature, *Eur Urol* 38:2–19, 2000.
5. Cotecchia S: The α_1-adrenergic receptors: diversity of signaling networks and regulation, *J Recept Signal Transduct Res* 30(6):410–419, 2010.
6. Cutfield NI, Tong DC: Common medications among dental outpatients: considerations in general dental practice, *NZ Dent J* 108:140–147, 2012.
7. Dale HH: On some physiological actions of ergot, *J Physiol (London)* 34:163–206, 1906.
8. Herman WW, Ferguson HW: Dental care for patients with heart failure: an update, *J A Dent Assoc* 141:845–853, 2010.
9. Hersh EV, Giannakopoulos H: Beta-adrenergic blocking agents and dental vasoconstrictors, *Dent Clin N Am* 54:687–696, 2010.
10. Hersh EV, Moore PA, Papas AS, et al.: Reversal of soft-tissue local anesthesia with phentolamine mesylate in adolescents and adults, *J Am Dent Assoc* 139:1080–1093, 2008.
11. Jang Y, Kim E: Cardiovascular effect of epinephrine in endodontic microsurgery: a review, *Restor Dent Endod* 38(4):187–193, 2013.
12. Lechat P: Clinical pharmacology of beta-blockers in cardiology: trial results and applications, *Hot Topics in Cardiol* 16:7–14, 2008.
13. Little JW, Falace DA, Miller CS, et al.: *Dental management of the medically compromised patient*, ed 8, St. Louis, 2013, Mosby/Elsevier.
14. Poirier L, Tobe SW: Contemporary use of β-blockers: clinical relevance of subclassification, *Canadian J Cardio* 30(suppl):S9–S15, 2014.
15. Popescue SM, Scrieciu M, Mercut V, et al.: Hypertensive patients and the management in dentistry, *ISRN Hypertension* 108:2014, 2013.
16. Schwinn DA, Price RR: Molecular pharmacology of human α_1-adrenergic receptors: unique features of the α_{1A}-subtype, *Eur Urol* 36(suppl 1):7–10, 1999.
17. Silvestre FJ, Miralles JL, Gascon R: Dental management of the patient with ischemic heart disease: an update, *Med Oral* 7(3):222–230, 2002.
18. Tavares M, Goodson JM, Studen-Pavlovich D, et al.: Reversal of soft-tissue local anesthesia with phentolamine mesylate in pediatric patients, *J Am Dent Assoc* 139:1095–1104, 2008.
19. Yagiela JA: Adverse drug interactions in dental practice: interactions associated with vasoconstrictors. Part V of a series, *J Am Dent Assoc* 130:701–709, 1999.

10

Psychopharmacology: Antipsychotic and Antidepressant Drugs*

Vahn A. Lewis

KEY INFORMATION

- Mental disorders and treatment of mental disorders are common in medicine.
- Treatments for mental disorders are palliative, and patient responses are variable, so use of combination therapy is common.
- Treatments for mental disorders have complex pharmacology, often acting at many receptors simultaneously.
- Antipsychotic drugs typically inhibit dopamine D_2 receptors and include phenothiazines (e.g., thioridazine), the butyrophenones (haloperidol), and newer drugs (e.g., olanzapine, quetiapine, and aripiprazole).
- Antidepressants drugs often inhibit the uptake of serotonin (5-hydroxytrypamine) (5-HT) or norepinephrine or both and include the following: the tricyclic antidepressants (e.g., amitriptyline), second-generation drugs (e.g., amoxapine, maprotiline, and bupropion), selective serotonin reuptake inhibitors (e.g., fluoxetine and paroxetine), serotonin-norepinephrine reuptate inhibitors (SNRIs) (e.g., venlafaxine, duloxetine), monoamine oxidase inhibitors (e.g., tranylcypromine), and St. John's wort.
- Drugs for manic-depressive illness include lithium, carbamazepine, and sodium valproate.
- Side effects associated with psychoactive drugs are generally complex and include actions on the brain, heart, muscle, gastrointestinal tract, the blood and immune system, and the autonomic nervous system, and they include actions on the salivary glands that may predispose patients to dental disease.
- Drug interactions with drugs commonly used in dentistry are common and may arise with local anesthetics, vasoconstrictors, antibiotics, analgesics, and anxiolytics.

CASE STUDY

Ms. B is a 42-year-old dental patient. It has been a few years since her last dental appointment, and she has numerous caries. Her medical history includes symptoms of schizophrenia but also depression, which began when she was about 24 years old. She was placed on haloperidol 5 mg three times a day and benztropine 2 mg three times a day (added to reduce extrapyramidal symptoms), and later imipramine was added to relieve a persistent depression. Last year, she was hospitalized to update her medical treatment to new therapy. She is now taking quetiapine (Seroquel) 300 mg/day, duloxetine (Cymbalta) 30 mg/day, and lorazepam (Ativan) 2 mg three times a day if needed for nervousness or panic attacks. She typically smokes about two packs of cigarettes per day and has for the last 20 years. Could Mrs. B's caries be related to her psychotropic therapy? What other medical issues might accompany the use of psychotropics, and how might you manage the dental consequences of them?

INTRODUCTION

According to the National Institutes of Mental Health, 20% of the population has a diagnosable mental disorder in their lifetime. The *Diagnostic and Statistical Manual of Mental Disorders* (DSM-V) classifies many types of mental disorders. Figure 10-1 summarizes a selection of topics discussed in the DSM-V, but a new feature of this edition is the increased recognition that psychiatric disorders show comorbidity with each other.

The DSM-V reflects greater recognition that symptoms do not fit neatly into diagnostic groups and may overlap. A gender difference, in incidence, is well known for depression but also seen in other major mental disorders. Another realization is that each of the major mental disorders has an increased incidence of suicide. These are episodic and progressive disorders, and although appropriate treatment tends to improve the course of a disorder, it rarely produces a cure.

Schizophrenia, which affects 1% of the population, is the most severe of the psychiatric disorders, and disturbances of mood (affective disorders) are the most common. Psychotic states such as schizophrenia or schizophreniform disorders are treated with **antipsychotic drugs**, sometimes also referred to as ***neuroleptics.***

Twenty percent of women and 10% of men have at least one **major depressive** episode during their lifetimes. These are treated with **antidepressant** drugs. The incidence of **bipolar disorder (manic-depressive illness)** is about 5% of the population, and it is treated with lithium salts and some anticonvulsant drugs. In daily practice, the dentist can expect to treat patients taking psychotherapeutic agents for various mental disorders.

MAJOR PSYCHIATRIC DISORDERS

Schizophrenia

Dopamine hypothesis

The classic "**dopamine hypothesis**" for schizophrenia suggests that schizophrenia is related to hyperactivity of central dopamine (DA) pathways. DA innervation is extensive and contributes to the activity

*The author wishes to recognize Dr. Leslie Felpel for his past contributions to this chapter.

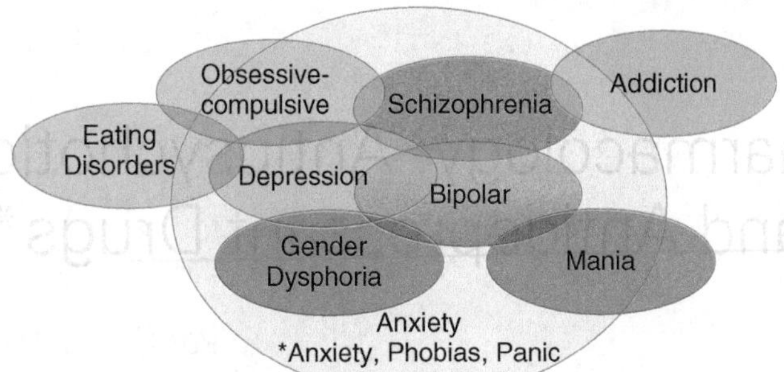

FIG 10-1 Overlap in the treatment of mental illness. Current thinking suggests that psychiatric classifications may be comorbid with each other, implying that treatments need to be customized and involve multiple drugs.

TABLE 10-1 Dopaminergic Cell Groups and Their Relationship to Actions and Side Effects of Antipsychotic Drugs

Cell Group	Relationship/Action
Mesolimbic and mesocortical	Considered the major therapeutic targets for antipsychotics, reward processing, appetite regulation
Nigrostriatal	Essential for motor function, related to the motor side effects of antipsychotics
Tuberoinfundibular	Regulation of hormones, especially inhibition of prolactin secretion; thought to mediate side effects such as amenorrhea, dysmenorrhea, gynecomastia, galactorrhea, and infertility
Chemoreceptor trigger zone	Receptors thought to mediate the antiemetic actions of antidopaminergic drugs
Medullary-periventricular	May mediate the actions of antidopaminergic drugs on appetite

in numerous brain areas (Table 10-1). Most antipsychotics are DA antagonists in various experimental conditions, and agents that release DA (e.g., amphetamine) can induce an acute psychotic state similar to schizophrenia. These findings do not explain the delay in antipsychotic effect of therapeutic agents or why some patients do not respond.

The role of DA in schizophrenia has been complicated by the identification and cloning of several DA receptor subtypes and the discovery that other neurochemicals, either independently or by regulating DA, may be involved in the disease process. Hyperactive dopaminergic neural pathways offer a simple and attractive mechanism to explain schizophrenia, but this is an incomplete explanation for the disease. It is justified to assume, however, that the Parkinson-like motor disturbances, which are common side effects of the antipsychotics, result from blockade of DA transmission in the basal ganglia. Five dopaminergic cell groups are considered important either for the therapeutic actions of antipsychotic drugs or for side effects of the antipsychotic agents. Table 10-1 summarizes these.

Other neurotransmitters

Other neurotransmitters have been implicated in psychotic behavior and are of interest regarding the cause of psychotic symptoms. **Phencyclidine**-induced psychosis is proposed to be an even better model for schizophrenia than the dopamine hypothesis. The predominant action of phencyclidine is to block of *N*-methyl-D-aspartate (NMDA)–type glutamate (glutamatergic) receptors. NMDA receptors are polyagonist receptors, involving simultaneous action of **glutamate**, **glycine**, and **polyamine** neurotransmitters. There is some interest in glycine uptake transporter blockade as a possible indirect alternative to the use of glutamate receptor agonists for therapy for schizophrenia. GABA deficiency may also play a role. Iomazenil, a benzodiazepine inverse agonist used in brain scanning, can increase the likelihood of amphetamine-induced positive schizophrenia signs, suggesting that reduced gabaminergic tone may also play a role.

Affective Disorders

The affective illnesses are expressed as dysregulations of mood. There are many types of affective disorders categorized in DSM-V, but for purposes of this discussion, it is sufficient to consider only depression and mania. Most individuals have had reactive, or secondary, depression with feelings of sadness or grief associated with a personal loss. In normal circumstances, such reactions are related to specific causes, are not incapacitating, and are generally short lived (1 to 2 weeks) (e.g., early onset postpartum depression). In contrast, for a mentally ill patient, depression is a severe, disabling disorder characterized by reclusiveness and nonverbalization that may last for extended periods (2 to 5 weeks minimum to years). The patient is sad most of the day; gains little pleasure from activities; and may have other signs, such as weight loss, irritability, insomnia, feelings of guilt, agitation, or difficulty in concentrating. This kind of depression is called primary, endogenous, unipolar, or **major depressive disorder** (MDD). A serious consequence of this disorder is an increased risk of committing suicide.

Depression is also a risk factor or is comorbid with other diseases, such as sleep disorders, weight changes, sexual disorder, pain disorders, anxiety disorders (and panic attacks), drug abuse, psychoses, myocardial infarction, and coronary artery disease.

Depression

Antidepressants are primarily indicated for the treatment of depression. Physicians are confronted with many treatments but little evidence of superiority of one treatment over another. Psychotherapy can be provided as initial therapy and is frequently beneficial; however, it usually takes longer than drug treatment to be effective. A combination of drugs and psychotherapy may be more effective than either treatment alone, but the effects are not usually dramatic. Drug selection is based on therapeutic effect, side effects, and cost.

Antidepressants may be used to treat chronic neuropathic pain. In general, agents with stronger norepinephrine reuptake blocking ability are superior in this application; some uses include diabetic neuropathy, neuralgias, and postherpetic neuralgia. Other uses for antidepressants include adjunct treatment in alcoholism and attention deficit hyperactivity disorder (ADHD).

The reduced side effects of selective serotonin reuptake inhibitors (SSRIs) has led to their employment for many new indications: obsessive-compulsive disorder, social phobia, posttraumatic stress disorder (PTSD), panic disorder, social phobia, bulimia nervosa, borderline personality disorder, autism, neurogenic orthostatic hypotension, premature ejaculation, premenstrual disorder, and others. In general, these do not represent cures but symptom management.

Mania and bipolar disorders

Patients with mania exhibit a distinct period of abnormally elevated, expansive, or irritable mood, sometimes requiring hospitalization. Three or more of the following symptoms also suggest a manic episode:

TABLE 10-2 Therapeutic and Adverse Effects Associated with Some Receptors Bound by Common Antipsychotic and Antidepressant Drugs

Receptor or Process Blocked	Therapeutic Effect of Block*	Adverse Effects Resulting from Blockade of Receptor or Protein
Histamine (H_1)	Sedation, anxiolysis, anti-allergy effect	CNS depression, hypotension, dry mouth, weight gain
Muscarinic	Reduction of extrapyramidal side effects	Xerostomia, blurred vision, hypohidrosis, sinus tachycardia, constipation, urinary retention, memory dysfunction (amnesia), hallucinations
α_1-Adrenergic		Memory dysfunction, postural (orthostatic) hypotension, reflex tachycardia, epinephrine reversal, dizziness, dry mouth, weight gain, priapism
α_2-Adrenergic	Blockade of presynaptic autoregulation, increasing CNS 5-HT, NE, and DA	Priapism, hypersalivation, hypoglycemia
Dopamine (D_2)	Amelioration of the positive signs and symptoms of psychosis	Extrapyramidal symptoms (EPS), sexual dysfunction, hyperprolactinemia, dry mouth, weight gain
Serotonin	5-HT_1-agonists reduce EPS, improve cognition, reduce negative symptoms 5-HT_1 antagonists reduce anxiety 5-HT_2 antagonists reduce EPS 5-HT_3 antagonists reduce emesis 5-$HT_{6,7}$ improve cognition	One or more receptors linked to: irritability, depression, insomnia, flu-like symptoms, nausea, weight gain, heart valve damage, and altered bone mass regulation
5-HT reuptake	Slow reversal of depression, anxiety disorders, eating disorders, PTSD, etc.	Gastrointestinal disturbance, sexual dysfunction, dry mouth, exacerbate Parkinson symptoms, bleeding
NE reuptake	Reversal of depression, reduced neuropathic pain, fibromyalgia, ADHD etc.	Dry mouth, urinary retention, erectile dysfunction, CNS stimulation, tremor, pro-convulsant, cardiovascular
Dopamine reuptake	Antimelancholy effect, hedonic, reduce sexual dysfunction	Psychomotor activation, psychosis, pro-convulsant action, dependence

5-HT, 5-Hydroxytryptamine; *CNS*, central nervous system; *NE*, norepinephrine.
*Recent work has shown that a number of agents are inverse agonists rather than classic antagonists. This may have some therapeutic consequences.

(1) inflated self-esteem, (2) decreased need for sleep, (3) talkativeness, (4) flight of ideas, (5) distractibility, (6) increased goal-directed activity, and (7) excessive interest in pleasure. There are several types of bipolar disorders; the typical type is called bipolar I disorder.

Most bipolar I patients also have alternating periods of severe depression, hence the name, manic-depressive illness. The first episode of psychopathology is often depression, sleep disorders, or anxiety, but psychopathology later progresses to include manic episodes. The incidence of bipolar disorder may be 2% to 5% of the population and 45% of community mental health patients.

Paradoxically, gene survey results suggest that bipolar disorder is more similar to schizophrenia as both are viewed as degenerative disorders. **Treatment focuses on controlling the manic symptoms first.**

Monoamine Hypothesis

As in the case of schizophrenia, various theories have been offered to explain the cause of affective disorders, with attention focusing on putative neurotransmitters. The classic monoamine hypothesis of affective disorders proposes that depression results from a deficiency of **norepinephrine (NE), serotonin (5-HT)**, or both at central synaptic sites. This hypothesis is indirectly supported by the fact that most antidepressant drugs increase synaptic concentrations of one or more monoamines, either by blocking the reuptake of monoamines into the presynaptic nerve terminal or by preventing its catabolism by the enzyme monoamine oxidase (MAO) in the nerve terminal after reuptake.

Attention is focusing on presynaptic or postsynaptic intracellular metabolism cascades. Numerous changes in secondary metabolism have been identified, but most studies have focused on other agents such as lithium. Antidepressants likely produce increases in downstream neurotrophic factors, for example, **brain-derived neurotrophic factor (BDNF)** and vascular endothelial growth factor. However, antidepressants are not the only causes of such changes, and they are seen in some common physiology such as menstruation. Changes in biochemistry of many monoamines, hormones (corticosteroids, thyroid), substance P, and omega-3 fatty acids have been shown. Depression may involve a variety of neural degenerative components.

Development of Antipsychotic and Antidepressant Drugs

The development of current psychotropic medications has involved numerous developments. The psychotherapeutic properties of early psychoactive drugs were discovered by accident. In 1950, while attempting to develop **antihistaminic** agents, the Rhône-Pauline Laboratories in France synthesized the phenothiazine **chlorpromazine**. The unusual neuroleptic property of **chlorpromazine** was noted, and the drug was used to treat schizophrenic patients in 1952. The discovery of **chlorpromazine** and other phenothiazines made possible the outpatient treatment of psychotic disorders. Antipsychotic efficacy correlated with blocking the **dopamine-2** (D_2) type receptor.

A characteristic of early antipsychotic drugs is interference with multiple neurotransmitter systems. In addition to blocking dopaminergic receptors, many block **adrenergic, muscarinic, serotonergic, histaminergic, hERG potassium channels**, and/or additional receptors or channels. These drugs have many side effects that can be related to these multiple receptor actions (Table 10-2). Blocking of cholinergic or serotonergic receptors reduced dose-limiting **extrapyramidal side effects** (EPS).

The next phase of development focused on drugs with selective DA antagonists such as **haloperidol**, but serious EPS could be treatment limiting.

Clozapine was developed in Europe in the early 1970s. **Clozapine** is remarkable because it has an "atypical" spectrum of actions: low in EPS and effective in treating both positive and negative type psychotic symptoms.

The **tricyclic antidepressants (TCAs)** were synthesized in an attempt to produce more specific antipsychotic agents (note in Figs. 10-2 and 10-7 the chemical similarity of TCAs and phenothiazines). It was soon recognized, however, that **imipramine**, a prototypic TCA, was more beneficial in treating depression than in treating schizophrenia. In some psychotic patients, the new agents triggered manic-like episodes.

Pursuing numerous leads for better antidepressants led to several novel agents termed **second-generation** or heterocyclic antidepressants. These agents vary widely in structure and actions. Today, they are employed as adjunct agents or replacements to circumvent problems with other agents.

Efforts to develop more selective agents were rewarded with newer classes of drugs: **SSRIs** (e.g., **fluoxetine**) with many fewer adverse effects than TCAs and fewer drug and food interactions than MAO inhibitors. These drugs have revolutionized the use of antidepressant medication due to their improved tolerability. This has also greatly increased the indications for the use of antidepressant medication.

Vortioxetine and **Vilazodone** block serotonin transporter (SERT) but also several 5-HT receptor types, combining certain actions found in some second-generation agents with those in the SSRIs.

The success of SSRIs led to the development of other selective agents: selective **serotonin-noradrenalin reuptake inhibitors (SNRIs**, e.g., **duloxetine**). They are more effective in some patients.

St. John's wort is a botanical remedy with a long history of use for mild to moderate depression. It is now thought that the active principle is the compound **hyperforin.**

The antidepressant properties of **monoamine oxidase inhibitors (MAOIs)** were discovered when it was observed that isoniazid, an antituberculosis drug, produced a euphoric state in patients and was found to be an MAOI.

Treatment for **bipolar disorder** was improved with the promotion of **lithium** therapy, in particular through the work of John Cade, to treat the manic component. More recently, anticonvulsant agents (in this use, referred to as "mood stabilizers") and atypical **antipsychotic drugs** are also employed. Lithium carbonate is being used in combination with or replaced by these newer therapies.

Because of new insights into the treatment of mental illness, the increased use of combinations of drugs is likely. This may improve therapy but may also lead to more side effects and drug interactions.

ANTIPSYCHOTIC DRUGS

In schizophrenia, the patient's ability to function is markedly impaired because of disturbances in thought processes. These disturbances increase the likelihood of adverse social outcomes, such as unemployment, poverty, social isolation, and suicide.

Schizophrenic patients may have positive symptoms, negative symptoms, and cognitive symptoms disorders. **Positive symptoms** include hallucinations (false perceptions), delusions (false beliefs), and agitation. **Negative symptoms** include interpersonal withdrawal, loss of drive, and flattened affect (restricted range of emotions). **Cognitive symptoms** include attention deficit and memory problems.

Positive symptoms respond to the antipsychotic drugs that were developed first (**typical** or "classic" antipsychotics), whereas negative symptoms tend to be more responsive to newer "**atypical**" antipsychotic drugs.

The principal drugs effective in the treatment of schizophrenia are dopaminergic receptor antagonists. Five dopamine receptors (D_1 through D_5) have been cloned. The possibility that each of these receptors may subserve a different physiologic function illustrates the complexity of the dopaminergic system. D_1 and D_5 have similar actions and are linked to an increase in cyclic 3′,5′-adenosine monophosphate synthesis, whereas D_2, D_3, and D_4 decrease cyclic 3′,5′-adenosine monophosphate synthesis. Interest has now focused on the relative specificity and affinity of the antipsychotic agents for each of the DA receptors. Clinical potency of typical antipsychotic drug relates most closely to **blocking D_2 receptors** (Table 10-3). In postmortem brain samples from schizophrenic patients, there is an increase in the number of D_2 receptors but not D_1 receptors.

Newer antipsychotic drugs affect other receptors as well as or in preference to the D_2 receptor.

Other receptor actions in antipsychotic drugs

Although there is little doubt that DA is involved in schizophrenia, other neurotransmitter systems may also play a role in treatment of the disease. In addition to DA, neurotransmitters such as 5-HT (serotonin), glutamate, NE, glycine, and GABA have been implicated in schizophrenia.

Psychotropic medications may interact with receptors in a number of ways. Many of these agents block other receptors. However, newer research suggests that some cases are **inverse agonists** and actually reduce constitutive activity. However, studies have not been done for all older drugs to differentiate between these possibilities, so in this chapter, antagonism might result from either of these mechanisms. Other agents are **partial agonists**, which produce a submaximal stimulation of the receptor (which can reduce the risk of motor side effects) but simultaneously limit endogenous transmitter from "overactivating" the receptors.

Antipsychotics that have anticholinergic or block **5-HT$_{2A}$** receptors produce fewer EPS. Older antipsychotics may be anticholinergic, while newer agents tend to block serotonin receptors. Action at some 5-HT receptors may reduce the negative symptoms of schizophrenia, Drugs that are partial agonists at the **5-HT$_{1A}$**, antagonists at 5-HT$_{6,7}$, or even inverse agonists can exhibit "atypical" properties in being more effective in reducing negative symptoms and cognitive symptoms.

Cholinergic, cannabinoid, and sigma receptor agonists are other drugs that can induce psychosis-like reactions. These receptors might be future therapeutic targets.

Chemistry and Structure–Activity Relationships

Of the several classes of antipsychotics, some are closely related structurally, others share a stereochemical resemblance, and still others seem to be chemically unrelated.

Phenothiazines and thioxanthenes

The basic ring structure of the phenothiazines is illustrated in Figure 10-2. Substitutions at R_1 divide the phenothiazine antipsychotics into three major groups. One group, represented by **chlorpromazine,** has an aliphatic chain at C_1. Compounds such as chlorpromazine with three carbons in the chain linked to an amine ($-CH_2-CH_2-CH_2-N(CH_3)_2$) have antipsychotic properties, whereas compounds with only two carbons, such as **promethazine,** are usually more antihistaminic or anticholinergic in nature and possess fewer antipsychotic effects. A second group, represented by **thioridazine,** has a piperidine ring at R_1 attached to the carbon chain. These phenothiazines are usually less sedating than the aliphatic agents but more sedating than the next group. A third group, represented by **prochlorperazine** and **perphenazine,** contains a piperazine ring on the carbon chain at R_1. Drugs in this group are the most potent of the three as antipsychotic agents but are also the most likely to produce motor side effects. Minor changes in the

TABLE 10-3 Comparison of Relative Receptor Antagonist Affinities of Some Typical and Atypical Antipsychotic Drugs

Drug	Affinity Order						
Chlorpromazine	$\alpha_1 \geq$	$5\text{-}HT_2$>	**D_2>**	D_1>	M>	α_2	
Haloperidol	sigma = **D_2>**	$D_1 = D_4$	α_1>	$5\text{-}HT_2$			
Olanzapine	$5\text{-}HT_2$>	M_1>	α_1=	**D_2=**	H_1>	D_1	
Risperidone	$5\text{-}HT_{2A}$>	**D_2=**	α_1=	α_2>>	M		
Quetiapine	α_1=	H_1=	**D_2=**	$5\text{-}HT_2$>	D_1		
Ziprasidone	$5\text{-}HT_{2A}$=	$5\text{-}HT_{1A}$ pag>	**D_2>**	α_1>	H_1		
Iloperidone	α_1>	**$5\text{-}HT_{2A}$=D_2=D_3**	D_4>	$5\text{-}HT_{6,7}$			
Lurasidone	**$5\text{-}HT_7$>**	α_{2A}>	**D_2=**	$5\text{-}HT_{2A}$>	$5\text{-}HT_{1A}$ pag>	α_{2C}>	α_1
Aripiprazole	**D_2 pag>**	$5\text{-}HT_{1A}$ pag>	$5\text{-}HT_{2A}$>	$5\text{-}HT_{2C}$>	D_4>	α_1>	H_1

The relative affinity for D_2 receptors is shown. Binding to other receptors has also been reported for some of the other drugs. D_2 receptors are bold for emphasis.

5-HT, 5-Hydroxytryptamine; *α*, α-adrenergic; *D*, dopaminergic; *M*, muscarinic; *H*, histaminergic; *pag*, partial agonist; =, equal to the following receptor type; ≥, greater than or equal to the following receptor type; >, greater than the following receptor type; >>, much greater than the following receptor type.

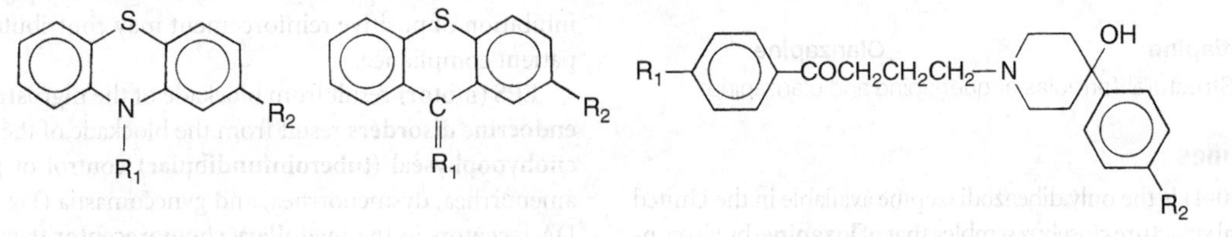

Phenothiazine nucleus **Thioxanthene nucleus** **Butyrophenone nucleus**

FIG 10-2 Structural formulas of representative antipsychotic drugs.

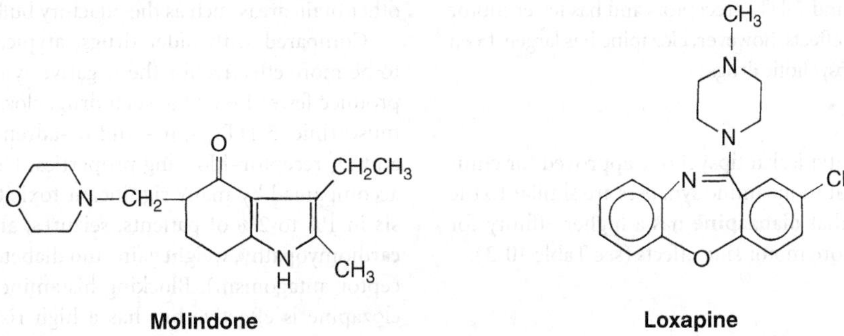

Molindone **Loxapine**

FIG 10-3 Structural formulas of molindone and loxapine.

structure of these molecules can increase or abolish antipsychotic activity. The thioxanthene antipsychotics, represented by **thiothixene**, are closely related to the phenothiazines and are formed when the nitrogen of the central ring is replaced by a carbon atom.

Butyrophenones

The butyrophenone antipsychotics are not chemically related to the phenothiazines, but they contain a stereochemically related nucleus (see Fig. 10-2). The only butyrophenone antipsychotic available in the United States is **haloperidol. Droperidol**, another butyrophenone, is marketed as an antipsychotic in some countries, but it is occasionally used in the United States primarily to reduce nausea and vomiting associated with anesthesia and surgery. Combined with the opiate fentanyl, it is also used to achieve deep sedation by **neuroleptanalgesia.**

Dihydroindolones

The structure of **molindone** is shown in Figure 10-3. This compound is not structurally related to the phenothiazines, thioxanthenes, or butyrophenones. The pharmacologic and clinical profile of molindone resembles that of the piperazine group of phenothiazines very closely.

Dibenzoxazepines

Loxapine (see Fig. 10-3) is the only dibenzoxazepine available in the United States. The structure of this compound contains seven members in its central ring. Similar to molindone, this drug has a clinical and pharmacologic profile similar to that of piperazine phenothiazines.

Diphenylbutylpiperidines

Pimozide, a diphenylbutylpiperidine derivative, is a modified butyrophenone in which the keto group has been replaced with a 4-fluorophenyl moiety. Pimozide is a selective D_2 antagonist that has antipsychotic properties and typical Parkinson-like side effects. The U.S. Food and Drug Administration approved pimozide for the treatment of Tourette syndrome, a condition characterized by phonic and motor tics, but it has been used in Europe to treat schizophrenia.

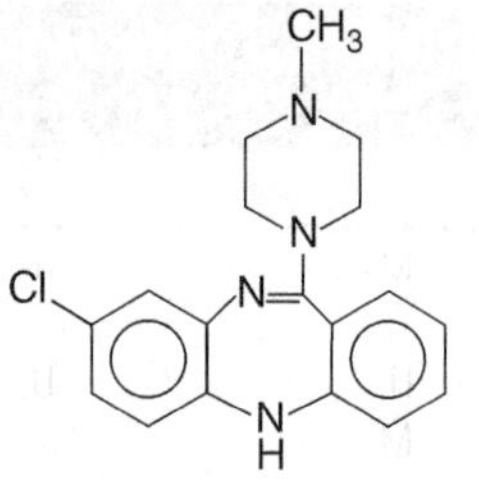

FIG 10-4 Structural formula of clozapine.

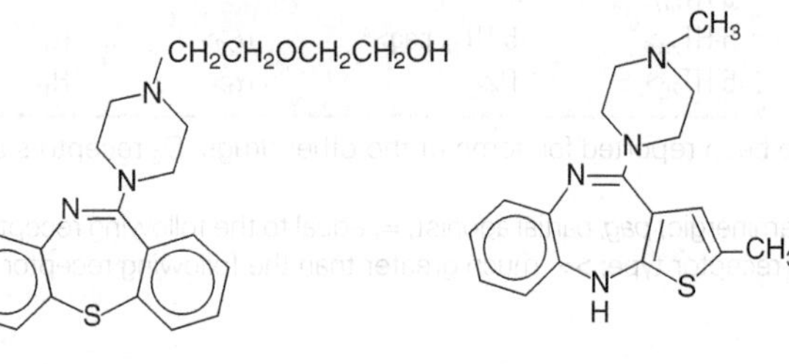

Quetiapine Olanzapine

FIG 10-5 Structural formulas of quetiapine and olanzapine.

Dibenzodiazepines

Clozapine (Fig. 10-4) is the only dibenzodiazepine available in the United States. Its chemical structure closely resembles that of **loxapine**, but in contrast to loxapine, it is a prototype for the **atypical antipsychotic drug class** in light of its low risk for producing EPS and other therapeutic advantages. Clozapine has greater affinity for the D_4 rather than for D_2 receptors. In addition, it blocks muscarinic and 5-HT_{2A} receptors and has fewer motor side effects. Because of adverse effects, however, clozapine has largely been replaced by other atypical antipsychotic drugs.

Thienobenzodiazepines

Olanzapine (Fig. 10-5) is an atypical antipsychotic approved for clinical use. Its inhibitory actions at monoamine synapses are similar to the actions of **clozapine** except that **olanzapine** has a higher affinity for D_2 receptors and produces more motor side effects (see Table 10-3).

Benzisoxazoles

Risperidone is a neuroleptic agent that combines antagonist action at D_2 and 5-HT_{2A} receptors. Risperidone has effects similar to haloperidol, but in low doses, it is considered to be an atypical antipsychotic drug with fewer motor side effects than haloperidol. **Paliperidone** is an active metabolite of risperidone with a pharmacologic profile similar to risperidone. **Iloperidone** also belongs in this group.

Other drugs expressing atypical antipsychotic activity

Other atypical antipsychotic drugs such as **quetiapine** (a dibenzothiazepine) (see Fig. 10-5) are effective for positive and negative symptoms. **Ziprasidone** (a dihydroindolone) has actions similar to risperidone. **Aripiprazole** is a dihydrocarbostyril derivative that has been found to act as a partial agonist at D_2, D_3, and 5-HT_{1A} receptors and to act as an antagonist at 5-HT_{2A} receptors. It is reported to produce minimal side effects commonly associated with antipsychotic drugs. Several others are listed next and in Table 10-4.

Benzodiazepines

The benzodiazepines are primarily used as antianxiety and hypnotic drugs, but more recently the clinical indications for this drug group have been expanded to include some psychotic disorders. **Diazepam, chlordiazepoxide, alprazolam, clonazepam, and lorazepam** all have found clinical usefulness in the treatment of some symptoms of schizophrenia, schizoaffective disorders, combativeness, agitation, and delirium. The benzodiazepines seem to have marginal antipsychotic properties when used alone but may be most useful as adjuncts to standard antipsychotic agents.

Dopaminergic Pathways as a Basis for the Effects of Antipsychotic Drugs

Although the precise mechanism of action of antipsychotic drugs is unknown, they all share the ability to block DA receptors in the brain. The **mesolimbic/mesocortical tracts** play key roles in their **antipsychotic action** (Fig. 10-6). For typical antipsychotic agents, the dose required to alleviate positive symptoms of psychosis is most closely related to affinity for blocking the D_2 receptor in the mesolimbic/mesocortical pathway(s).

The mesolimbic/mesocortical tract plays an important role in behavior, arousal, positive reinforcement, cognitive function, communication, and psychological responses. Although blocking mesolimbic/mesocortical DA is thought to be central to antipsychotic efficacy, the inhibition of positive reinforcement may contribute to the low rate of patient compliance.

EPS (motor) result from blockade of the **nigrostriatal pathway**, and **endocrine disorders** result from the blockade of the **hypothalamic-adenohypophyseal (tuberoinfundibular)** control of **prolactin** inducing amenorrhea, dysmenorrhea, and gynecomastia (Fig. 10-6). Blockade of DA receptors in the **medullary chemoreceptor trigger zone** is thought to contribute to the **antiemetic actions** of antipsychotic drugs, and blockade of DA receptors in the medulla or brainstem may play a role in appetite dysregulation (see Fig. 10-6). There are also DA interneurons in other brain areas such as the olfactory bulb and retina.

Compared with older drugs, atypical antipsychotic agents seem to be more effective for the negative symptoms of schizophrenia and produce fewer EPS. One such drug, clozapine, also has histaminergic, muscarinic, 5-$HT_{2,6,7}$, α_1- and α_2-adrenergic, and dopamine D_1, D_2, and D_4 receptor–blocking properties. However, clozapine use can be accompanied by many significant toxicities, including **agranulocytosis** in 1% to 2% of patients, seizures, and hypotension, myocarditis, cardiomyopathy, weight gain, and diabetes (possibly due to α_2 adrenoceptor antagonism). Blocking histamine H_1 improves sleep. Because clozapine is effective but has a high risk of **agranulocytosis**, newer agents have been developed that have therapeutic effects similar to clozapine but with fewer adverse effects.

The use of clozapine is restricted and is available only through the Clozaril (clozapine) National Registry. A Risk Evaluation and Mitigation Strategy program has been mandated for clozapine. This program requires special certification of prescriber and pharmacist for the use of the drug. Certification requires enrolling and assessment of both prescriber and pharmacist as well as patient enrollment to ensure proper use of clozapine, including regular blood tests to detect changes in neutrophil count and other granulocytes.

Atypical antipsychotics **olanzapine, risperidone**, and **paliperidone** have lower D_2 receptor binding and higher 5-HT_2 receptor binding and are relatively free of EPS. **Quetiapine** has a therapeutic effect and a side-effect profile similar to olanzapine. Moreover, partial DA agonists reduce EPS because they produce some dopaminergic agonist tone in the basal ganglia to avoid EPS effects.

A consequence of the improved side-effect profile for atypical antipsychotic drugs is the expansion of indications for their use. In addition to schizophrenia, some are used to treat mania associated with bipolar disorder. Risperidone has been approved for aspects of autism, irritability, aggression toward others, deliberate self-injury, temper tantrums, and labile mood. It has been approved for treatment of schizophrenia

TABLE 10-4 **Principal Side Effects of Antipsychotic Drugs**

Antipsychotic Agent	Approximate Equivalent Dose (mg)	Sedation	Extrapyramidal Symptoms	Anticholinergic Effects	Orthostatic Hypotension	Prolonged QT Interval/TdP	Weight Gain
Conventional (Typical) Agents							
Phenothiazines (Aliphatic)							
Chlorpromazine	100	+++	++	++	+++	++	+++
(Piperazines)							
Fluphenazine	2	+	+++	+	+	++	++
Perphenazine	10	++	++	+	+	+	ND
Prochlorperazine	15	++	+++	+	+	+	ND
Trifluoperazine	5	+	+++	+	+	+	ND
(Piperidines)							
Mesoridazine	50	+++	+	+++	++	+++	+
Thioridazine	100	+++	+	+++	+++	+++,TdP	+++
Thioxanthene							
Thiothixene	4	+	+++	+	++	ND	ND
Butyrophenones							
Haloperidol	2	+	+++	+	+	++,TdP	+
Droperidol*	2.5	++	ND	ND	++	+,TdP	++
Diphenylbutylpiperidine							
Pimozide	1	++	+++	++	+	++,TdP	+
Dihydroindolones							
Molindone	10	++	++	+	+	0	ND
Ziprasidone	20	+	+	+	+	++,TdP	+
Dibenzoxazepine							
Loxapine	15	+	++	+	+	ND	ND
Novel (Atypical) Agents							
Dibenzodiazepine							
Clozapine	50	+++	+	+++	++	+	++++
Thienobenzodiazepine							
Olanzapine	5	+++	+	+++	++	+,TdP	++++
Dibenzothiazepine							
Quetiapine	50	++	+	0	++	++,TdP	++
Benzisoxazole							
Risperidone	2	+	+ to ++	0	+	++,TdP	++
Paliperidone	6		+	ND	+	+	++
Iloperidone	24	+	+	0	+++	++	++++
Dihydrocarbostyril							
Aripiprazole	15	0/+	0/+	0	0/+	−/+	0
Brexpiprazole	2	+/−	0/+	+/−	0/+	0	+/−
Other							
Asenapine	5	+	+	0/+	0,+	+	++
Lurasidone	40	+	+ to ++	0/+	0,+	+	+

*Not used to treat psychosis in the United States.
Level of risk for each adverse effect is indicated by the number of + signs.
ND, No data; *TdP*, torsades de pointes.

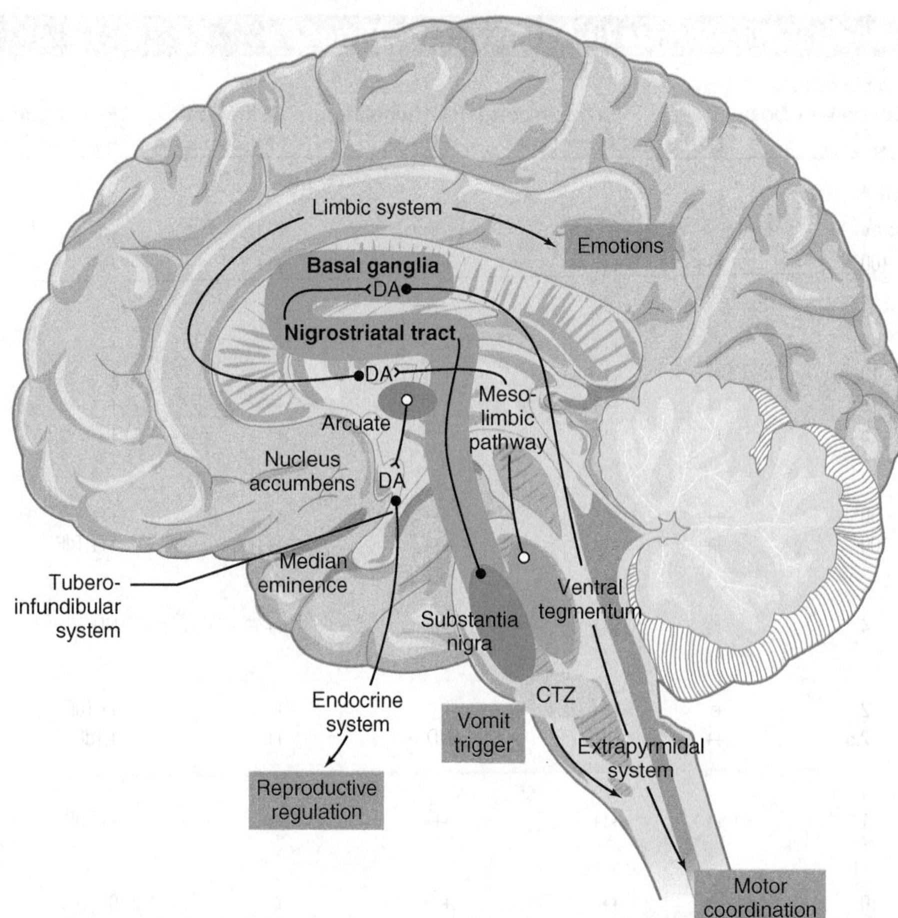

FIG 10-6 Dopaminergic pathways and sites in the brain. The role of each pathway in the action of antipsychotic drugs is shown. Tuberoinfundibular pathway is also known as hypothalamic-adenohypophyseal pathway. *CTZ,* Chemoreceptor trigger zone; *DA,* dopamine. (Modified from Kester, M. et al., *Elsevier's integrated pharmacology,* Philadelphia, Mosby, ed. 2, 2012.)

and bipolar I in children. Another trend is the use of partial DA partial agonists (aripiprazole) as an adjunct in the treatment of depression.

Extrapyramidal effects

The motor side effects, EPS, are the most difficult side effects for most patients. EPS are reminiscent of Parkinson disease with slow motor function, tremors, dystonias, akathisia, dyskinesias, and rigidity. EPS become prominent when more than 80% of the D_2 receptors in the basal ganglia are blocked or lost. EPS may develop during treatment, and tardive dyskinesia can occur when an agent is stopped. Typical antipsychotics produce EPS; in descending order of most to least potent are the butyrophenones and piperazines, aliphatics, and piperidines. For instance, fluphenazine and haloperidol have more EPS (see Table 10-4). Many newer antipsychotic drugs that have atypical properties and block 5-HT_{2A} receptors are associated with fewer EPS. Haloperidol may have some unique effects on motor function. It is metabolized to a potentially neurotoxic metabolite, which may adversely affect the dopaminergic cells in the substantia nigra, inducing Parkinson disease. Haloperidol also potently blocks sigma receptors. Sigma receptors in the red nucleus have been shown to participate in the generation of dystonias (oculogyric crisis and torticollis) associated with neuroleptic use. This observation may be particularly important for facial dystonias because sigma receptors are also expressed in cranial nerve nuclei. While tertiary amine anticholinergic anti-Parkinson agents help reduced EPS from antipsychotic drugs, DA replacement drugs like levodopa are not useful as they may exacerbate psychosis.

Tardive dyskinesia is an EPS that manifests after termination of long-term antipsychotic therapy. This condition is thought to reflect the development of supersensitive DA receptors in the basal ganglia. Tardive dyskinesia has been estimated to occur in 15% to 20% of patients receiving long-term typical antipsychotics characterized by abnormal, rapid, and alternating movements of the face and tongue and sometimes movements in the extremities and torso. Tardive dyskinesia does not regress on reduction of the dose or withdrawal of the drug. The only consistently effective treatment for tardive dyskinesia has been increasing the dose of the antipsychotic that caused it in the first place. Atypical antipsychotics, on the other hand, cause fewer EPS. Using lower doses of antipsychotics and slower dosage adjustments help reduce the likelihood of EPS. Clonazepam may be helpful in mild cases, and botulinum toxin may allow control of overactive muscle groups.

Sedative actions

Phenothiazines and related antipsychotics produce sedation on initial administration, but tolerance develops in 1 to 4 weeks. Sedation varies between drug groups. Blocking histamine, dopamine, 5-HT, or NE may contribute to sleepiness. In contrast to antianxiety agents or barbiturates, chlorpromazine does not produce a similar risk for abuse or respiratory depression. Nevertheless, when used in combination with other sedatives, these adverse effects can be potentiated.

Seizure threshold

The antipsychotics, including atypical ones, may reduce the seizure threshold. The convulsion is usually of the generalized tonic-clonic type. The incidence of antipsychotic-induced seizures is approximately 1%, but nearly 7% in epileptic patients who receive antipsychotics. Chlorpromazine is more likely to cause this effect than fluphenazine, thiothixene, or molindone.

Antiemetic action

Chlorpromazine is an effective antiemetic and previously was commonly used for this purpose. (The neuroleptics that are still used to treat nausea include prochlorperazine and droperidol.) The antiemetic action is exerted on the chemoreceptor trigger zone rather than on the vomiting center (see Fig. 10-6). Motion sickness is more responsive to anticholinergics and antihistamines.

Endocrine system

Endocrine system alterations result partly from actions on the hypothalamus (see Fig. 10-6). Most of the endocrine effects of antipsychotics are related to disturbances in the secretion of pituitary hormones. Particularly prominent is the release of prolactin (**hyperprolactinemia**) elicited by blockade of DA receptors. DA in the adenohypophysis normally inhibits prolactin release. While any antipsychotic can increase prolactin, it is most prominent with risperidone and its metabolite paliperidone. Prolactin can cause lactation and amenorrhea or delayed ovulation and menstruation in women or gynecomastia, decreased libido, and impotence in men. This can be particularly disturbing when these agents are used in children.

Weight gain and **diabetogenic** effects have been observed for several atypical antipsychotic agents. Weight control is complex and includes both hypothalamic and peripheral mechanisms. Inhibition of histamine, dopamine, serotonin, or other neurotransmitters may play a role in the weight gain effects. Clozapine and olanzapine are the most likely and molindone and ziprasidone are the least likely to cause this effect. Although this weight gain is rarely a severe side effect, it frequently leads to noncompliance.

Diuretic and antidiuretic effects have been shown in animals and humans, although a weak diuresis seems to be the predominant effect in humans.

Other central nervous system actions

Although medullary respiratory centers can be depressed by chlorpromazine, therapeutically active doses normally elicit little or no effect. If a sedative-hypnotic, antianxiety, or opioid drug is given to a patient receiving antipsychotic medication, however, summation of the depressant effects may result in clinically evident respiratory depression.

All antipsychotic drugs have a **black box warning** regarding their use in dementia. There are several areas of concern: increased death due to cardiovascular complications, increased diabetic symptoms, and increased infections. Antipsychotics may disrupt thermoregulation by an action on the hypothalamus and produce poikilothermia (either hypothermia or hyperthermia may occur) depending on the ambient temperature.

Patients taking antipsychotic medications may complain of akathisia, a restless feeling that motivates the patient to constantly move or pace. This is also seen with numerous other drugs and can be a symptom of Parkinson disease or Alzheimer dementia.

Peripheral Actions of Antipsychotics

Autonomic nervous system

The following side effects of the antipsychotics may result from their antimuscarinic properties and antiadrenergic properties (see Table 10-2). Dry mouth, associated with a series of neuroleptics, is related to their blocking potency at α_1-adrenergic, H_1-histaminergic, and D_1-dopaminergic receptors. Clozapine and olanzapine are reported to cause hypersalivation, which is most prominent at night, possibly due to altered α_2 adrenoreceptors. Although the autonomic effects of antipsychotics can be annoying, tolerance usually develops to these reactions.

Cardiovascular system

The use of antipsychotic medication is associated with a statistical doubling of the sudden cardiac death rate.

A number of drugs, including the antipsychotic and antidepressant drugs, are associated with prolongation of the QT interval, which may also lead to the development of an often fatal torsades de pointes arrhythmia. This effect has been attributed to inhibition of the hERG delayed rectifier potassium channel in the heart (see Chapter 19). hERG function can be altered by genetic as well as drug actions. Many antipsychotics are implicated to varying degrees (see Table 10-4).

Orthostatic hypotension is a result of α-adrenergic receptor–blocking actions of antipsychotics (see Table 10-2), whereas tachycardia and increased coronary blood flow derive from central compensatory cardiovascular reflexes. The aliphatic and piperidine phenothiazines and clozapine are the most likely, and the piperazines the least likely, to cause orthostatic hypotension (see Table 10-4). In the emergency treatment of phenothiazine-induced vasomotor collapse, epinephrine is contraindicated because the α-adrenergic receptor–blocking action of the phenothiazines may cause "**epinephrine reversal**" and an even greater reduction in blood pressure.

Respiratory effects

About 20% of elderly patients placed on antipsychotic medications develop respiratory tract infections. There has been little research to determine which factors are particularly important in this. There is evidence that respiratory infections can alter the clearance of some antipsychotic drugs.

Absorption, Fate, and Excretion

Numerous dosage forms are used for antipsychotic medications. Traditional tablets are common, but in addition, rapid-dissolving tablets and long-acting antipsychotic injection forms are also available. With rapidly dissolving oral tablets, some of the drug may be absorbed before encountering first-pass metabolism.

Long-acting injectable agents also reduce first-pass metabolism and may be used in patients who forget or do not consistently take their medication. **Fluphenazine enanthate, fluphenazine decanoate, haloperidol decanoate, and aripiprazole lauroxil** are long-acting forms. These injectable forms are effective for several weeks after an injection once therapeutic blood concentrations are stabilized. Generally, injection forms are safe for younger patients in good physical condition. A disadvantage to this mode of administration is that the drug cannot be withdrawn if side effects occur, and therapeutic levels are sometimes difficult to stabilize.

Most of these agents are lipid soluble and are highly tissue and plasma bound, leading to long half-lives. For example, aripiprazole has a volume of distribution of 5 L/kg and a half-life of ~75 hours.

Metabolism of antipsychotic drugs is complex. Most agents are metabolized by the P450 isoforms **CYP2D6 or CYP3A4.** Other isoforms may also participate (1A2, 2B6, 2C9), and **MAO** contributes in the liver and in the brain. The P450 isoforms CYP2D6 and CYP1A2 are known to have genetic polymorphisms, and preliminary investigations suggest that patients who are poor metabolizers may have more antipsychotic toxicity than normal metabolizers. Although metabolites for many antipsychotic drugs are active, their antipsychotic effects are usually not as potent as the effects of the parent compounds. The plasma half-lives of the antipsychotic drugs are not true indicators of their long durations of action. Half-lives for the phenothiazines range from 20 to 40 hours, yet the lipid solubility of the drugs and their metabolites allow them to remain in tissues for prolonged periods.

TABLE 10-5 Metabolism of Selected Antipsychotic Drugs

	1A2	2C9	2C19	2D6	3A4	P-gly
Chlorpromazine	S,D			S,H	S,D	
Haloperidol	S	S	S	S,H,D	S,H	
Thioridazine	S,H	H	S	S,H		
Pimozide	S		H	H	S,H	
Clozapine	S,D*	H	S,H	S	S,D	S
Risperidone			S	S,H	S,H	S,H
Olanzapine†	S	H	H	S,H	H	S
Quetiapine			S	S,H	S	—
Ziprasidone	S			H	S	H
Aripiprazole				S,H,D	S	S,H
Brexpiprazole				S	S	

S, Substrate; *H*, inhibitor; *D*, inducer.
Column headings refer to specific isozymes involved in drug metabolism.
*Clozapine-70% CYP1A2 elimination.
†Olanzapine primarily eliminated by glucuronidation.
(Data from Flockhart, D.A., Cytochrome P450 drug interaction table, Indiana University. Available at http://medicine.iupui.edu/clinpharm/DDIs/. Accessed June 3, 2016; Supercyp http://bioinformatics.charite.de/supercyp/.) Note the relative importance of CYP 2D6, 3A4 and 1A2 in metabolism of these drugs.

P-glycoproteins may also contribute to the removal of antipsychotics and antidepressant drugs. Several antipsychotic drugs are either substrates or inhibitors of the *p*-glycoprotein transporter (part of the ABC ATP transporter family) (Chapter 2 and Table 10-5). Genetic variations in either the CYP enzymes or the ABC transporters may alter the efficacy of antipsychotics or antidepressants in individual patients.

Dosing requirements of antipsychotic drugs for most patients usually fall within a general range, but dosage may vary considerably. Some of the variability has been related to genetic difference in patients. Adjustments in dose are frequently made depending on the patient's clinical response and side effects. Generally, treatment with antipsychotic agents is uninterrupted and indefinite in duration.

Adverse effects

The most troublesome side effects of the antipsychotic agents, particularly the benzothiazines and butyrophenones, are the **extrapyramidal disorders.** Therapy may have to be terminated in patients exhibiting pronounced and intractable motor disturbances. Use of atypical agents may help reduce this problem. The use of anticholinergic drugs, antihistamines, or amantadine can reduce Parkinson-like symptoms and the motor restlessness of akathisia without compromising antipsychotic therapy. Acute dystonic reactions (e.g., torticollis, facial grimacing, oculogyric crisis) are also treated with centrally acting antihistamines and antimuscarinic drugs such as diphenhydramine or benztropine or switching to a better tolerated atypical antipsychotic.

Tardive dyskinesia is a problematic neurologic disorder because of its disabling effect and resistance to pharmacologic management. The adverse effect is irreversible or only slowly reversible. The low incidence of extrapyramidal effects with clozapine and some atypical agents has given new hope that these disturbing side effects of the antipsychotics can be reduced.

Other adverse effects may also be serious enough to necessitate adjustment of the dosage or withdrawal of the medication. These reactions may be manifested as cholestatic jaundice, blood dyscrasias, or dermatologic responses. The latter may take the form of contact dermatitis, urticaria, or photosensitivity or hypersensitivity like Stevens-Johnson syndrome.

TABLE 10-6 Interactions of Antipsychotic Drugs* with Other Drugs

Dental Drug or Over-the-Counter Drug	Possible Response When Combined with Antipsychotic
Promethazine	CNS depression, extrapyramidal symptoms
Barbiturates	CNS depression, reduced efficacy of antipsychotic drug
Benzodiazepines	CNS depression
General anesthetics (inhalation and intravenous)	CNS depression (especially respiratory depression)
Ethanol	CNS depression
Opioid analgesics	CNS depression, respiratory depression, miosis
Antihistamines	CNS depression, anticholinergic effect
Epinephrine	Epinephrine reversal, orthostatic hypotension
Anticholinergics	Anticholinergic toxicity: arrhythmias, hallucinations, gastrointestinal inhibition
Drug metabolism inhibitors (amiodarone, erythromycin, clarithromycin, itraconazole) (linezolid)	Elevation of antipsychotic blood concentrations, extrapyramidal symptoms; linezolid can elevate clozapine blood levels
Protein-bound drugs	Displacement of clozapine might result in adverse reactions

*Primarily the phenothiazines, thioxanthenes, butyrophenones, molindone, and loxapine.
CNS, Central nervous system.

Clozapine can produce serious adverse reactions. It was initially withdrawn from the market because it was discovered to cause agranulocytosis in approximately 1% to 2% of the patient population. The drug was reintroduced with the provision that all patients receiving it be continually monitored. (See earlier in chapter.)

Although antipsychotic agents have been implicated with increasing seizures (but usually in epileptic patients), evidence suggests that there may be an increased propensity for seizures in mental disorders, and when studied, antipsychotics may reduce seizure frequency somewhat. Orthostatic hypotension and cardiovascular and respiratory collapse have also been documented. Some predisposing factors have been proposed. Excessive sedation and respiratory collapse may be associated with concomitant use of depressant agents, including benzodiazepines. Epinephrine reversal (caused by α-adrenergic receptor antagonism by antipsychotic drugs) can contribute to declines in blood pressure.

Normally, less severe side effects of antipsychotics include **orthostatic hypotension** and syncope, xerostomia, nasal stuffiness, urinary retention, constipation, and alterations in body temperature (usually poikilothermia). In prolonged, high-dose therapy with phenothiazines, a blue-gray pigmentation may occasionally occur in skin exposed to direct sunlight. Antipsychotic-associated dysphagia is a common cause of morbidity and mortality in elderly patients.

A rare but sometimes fatal idiosyncratic effect, usually associated with potent antipsychotics such as haloperidol and fluphenazine, is **neuroleptic malignant syndrome.** It is characterized by sustained and widespread muscular contractions, fluctuating levels of consciousness, autonomic abnormalities, and fever. Treatment for neuroleptic malignant syndrome includes immediate withdrawal of the drug and supportive measures. Some benefit may be gained from the skeletal muscle relaxant dantrolene. Bromocriptine, a dopaminergic agonist, may also be helpful. Physical cooling to reduce fever may be necessary. The risk of developing neuroleptic malignant syndrome is lower with the newer atypical drugs, but some cases have been reported. Drug interactions for antipsychotic drugs are summarized in Table 10-6.

The partial agonist antipsychotic **aripiprazole** is an example of a drug with a very good side-effect profile even among atypical drugs. It is associated with fewer extrapyramidal effects, reduced release of prolactin, minimal weight gain, and little effect on the QT interval and others (see Table 10-4).

General Therapeutic Uses

Currently, antipsychotic drugs are primarily used for the treatment of psychotic states. The wide variety of pharmacologic effects of the phenothiazines has led, however, to their use as **antiemetics** as preoperative medications to relax and calm the patient. Antipsychotics may be used to control the manic phase of bipolar disorder. Other applications of the phenothiazines include the control of hallucinations associated with acute alcohol withdrawal and the treatment of intractable hiccough. Haloperidol, pimozide, and aripiprazole are used in the treatment of **Tourette syndrome.**

Because of the perceived reduced side effects and improved efficacy of the atypical antipsychotic drugs, an expansion of indications has resulted. Indications for these drugs have increased in children, including autism and disruptive disorder, juvenile treatment-resistant schizophrenia, and have been proposed for pervasive developmental disorder of childhood. Additional indications in adult patients include borderline personality disorder, delusional disorder, first-episode schizophrenia, mood disorders with psychotic features (aripiprazole), obsessive-compulsive disorder, schizoaffective disorders, and personality problems. There is a black box warning against the use of antipsychotic agents in dementia-related psychosis in elderly due to increased risk of death.

Currently, atypical antipsychotics tend to be preferred clinically. This is due to better clinical efficacy in patients displaying negative symptoms and better side-effect profiles.

Implications for Dentistry

Many patients being treated for mental illness report poor oral health, but it is not all due to their treatments; poor oral health is also correlated to their mental disorder, older age, unemployment or financial strain, and smoking behavior. The dentist inevitably encounters these patients in practice. Because of the perceived stigma associated with psychiatric illness, the psychiatric disorder, or the effects of the psychotropic drugs, patients may forget or be reluctant to discuss their disorder with dentists or to provide complete information regarding their treatment. Many patients are receiving more than one drug for their condition, and they may be using various other drugs (e.g., alcohol, tobacco, cough remedies, aspirin, dietary supplements) that may not be revealed in a medical history questionnaire. Antipsychotics can add to the central nervous system (CNS) depressant effects of sedative-hypnotics, antianxiety agents, anesthetics, or opioid analgesics used in the course of dental treatment. Antipsychotics may potentiate the effects of general anesthetics and the respiratory depressant response to opioids (see Table 10-6). Some antipsychotic and several antihistaminic drugs have substantial antimuscarinic activity. Some antipsychotic drugs may also contribute to the long QT syndrome.

Dyskinesias and **tardive dyskinesia** have important implications in dentistry because the facial musculature is prominently involved in the disorder. The abnormal movements of tardive dyskinesia often start in the orofacial musculature, particularly the tongue, which alternately protrudes, retracts, and undergoes a rolling movement. Bruxism may also occur. Because the orofacial muscles are affected in the early development of tardive dyskinesia, the patient may believe that the dentist can correct the problem.

Dysphagia, difficulty in swallowing, is a concern, especially for elderly patients taking antipsychotic medications. Antagonism of cholinergic or dopaminergic receptors can interfere with autonomic control of the esophagus and swallowing, and it can contribute to xerostomia. These patients may also have trouble with eating, resulting in associated weight loss.

Dental issues for patients with dysphagia include difficulty with tooth brushing, swallowing, drooling, choking, aspiration, coughing, and increased respiratory pathology. Positioning the patient in a more upright position and efforts to prevent aspiration may be necessary. Because of difficulty in swallowing, the patient may not want to take medications via the oral route.

Individuals who require treatment with antipsychotic drugs usually take these drugs for an extended period or for life. Prolonged phenothiazine use can sometimes cause a reduction in leukocyte count, which rarely predisposes the patient to infection and infrequently oral candidiasis. The tendency of clozapine to cause agranulocytosis is a factor that can lead to serious susceptibility to infection.

Certain antipsychotics can lessen the vasoconstrictor action of α_1 adrenergic receptor agonists, amplify the sedation of antihistamines and other CNS depressants, pose a risk with other drugs for cardiac arrhythmias because of mutual effects on hERG channels, and worsen dry mouth when administered with antisialagogue agents.

TABLE 10-7 Some Mechanisms of Antidepressant Drugs

Mechanism	Drug Examples
Block 5-HT reuptake (SERT)	TCAs, most second-generation drugs, SSRIs, dual action drugs, SNRIs
Block NE reuptake (NET)	TCAs, some second-generation and SNRIs
Inhibit MAO	MAO inhibitors, St. John's wort*
Blocks presynaptic autoreceptors (e.g., α_2)	Mirtazapine
Blocks dopamine reuptake (DAT)	Bupropion
Partial dopamine agonist	Aripiprazole
Block serotonin receptors and SERT	Dual action drugs
Blocks reuptake of many amine neurotransmitters	St. John's wort
Neuroprotective actions	SSRIs, anticonvulsants, Li^+
Facilitate GABA	Alprazolam

*Only at high doses.
DAT, dopamine transporter; *NET*, norepinephrine transporter; *SERT*, serotonin transporter.

ANTIDEPRESSANTS

Mechanisms of Antidepressant Agents

Numerous mechanisms are responsible for the actions of the known antidepressant drugs (Table 10-7). Most clinically used antidepressants increase the synaptic concentrations of serotonin (5-HT) or NE or both by blocking the reuptake transporters, the serotonin transporter (SERT), or the norepinephrine transporter (NET) in the brain, and this relationship has given support to the monoamine hypothesis of affective disorders.

The increase in neurotransmitters, as a result of blocking their reuptake, can be measured in a few hours from the time that the antidepressants are administered. A challenge to the monoamine hypothesis is the time required for full antidepressant activity, which may take from 2 to 8 weeks in clinical practice.

Part of this delay may also be related to the pharmacokinetics of the antidepressants, which have half-lives averaging 24 hours. To reach plasma equilibrium, the drugs need, on average, to be taken for at least 4 to 5 days; however, this does not explain the entire delay.

TABLE 10-8 Key Serotonergic Pathways in the Action of Selective Serotonin Reuptake Inhibitors (SSRIs)

Midbrain (Raphe) Projection to	Possible SSRI Effect	Signs of Dysregulation
Prefrontal cortex	Relief of depression	Depression
Hippocampus, limbic cortex	Alleviation of panic disorder	Anhedonia, anxiety, panic, sexual dysfunction
Basal ganglia	Alleviation of obsessive-compulsive disorder	Agitation; extrapyramidal side effects, including akathisia, Parkinson-like tremor, and rigidity
Hypothalamus	Alleviation of eating disorder	Bulimia and binge-eating disorders
Spinal cord (pontine-medullary cell bodies)	Sexual dysfunction	Inhibited ejaculation and orgasm

A **current hypothesis** to explain the therapeutic effect of antidepressants and the time delay is as follows. Antidepressant drugs produce an increased serotonergic tone in the raphe nuclei due to blocking reuptake. Because of abundant presynaptic autoregulatory receptors (autoreceptors), however, the release of 5-HT is acutely "turned off" in the raphe nuclei. With continued exposure to the antidepressant drugs, the autoreceptors desensitize or downregulate, allowing increased 5-HT release at the synaptic terminals ("turned on"). This increased release may lead to a downregulation of some postsynaptic 5-HT receptors. Changes in postsynaptic receptor profiles appear to be a basis for the therapeutic effects of antidepressant drugs. Antidepressants and electroconvulsive therapy lead to similar changes.

An analogous course of events is thought to occur with NE. The NET is inhibited, resulting in reduced presynaptic α_2 adrenergic receptors and further release of NE. Long-term antidepressant use reduces postsynaptic β adrenergic receptors in the brain without significantly affecting postsynaptic α_1. Much of the NE in the brain is found in the locus coeruleus (LC), whose neurons project as far as the forebrain. The LC neurons not only respond to various phasic external stimuli and stress-related stimuli ("fight or flight") but also participate in tonic brain states, including the sleep–wake cycle and arousal. The LC may be involved in mediating anxiety, depression, panic attacks, and PTSD. The raphe nuclei contain the bulk of the 5-HT–synthesizing neurons in the brain, and these project to wide areas of the brain (Table 10-8).

All known antidepressant drugs also increase brain-derived neurotrophic factor (BDNF). However, two recent studies have found the relationship between plasma BDNF and depression to be less than reported earlier and that changes in BDNF have been measured in numerous non-depressive brain illnesses and other conditions. Mutant forms of BDNF may account for some of the differences in the findings.

The antidepressant drugs can be classified into the following categories: TCAs, tetracyclic and other second-generation drugs, SSRIs, SNRIs, MAO inhibitors, and the nutraceutical, St. John's wort. Refer to Box 10-1 to see actions of antidepressant drugs.

Tricyclic Antidepressants (TCAs)

TCA chemistry and structure–activity relationships

A small modification of the phenothiazine ring structure resulted in an entirely new group of drugs, the TCAs. The name of these compounds is derived from the triple-ring structure consisting of two benzene moieties connected through a seven-membered ring (Fig. 10-7).

The prototype for TCAs is **imipramine**, a dibenzazepine derivative. Structural analogues of imipramine include the dibenzocycloheptadienes, in which a carbon atom is substituted for the nitrogen of the central ring, and the dibenzoxepines, in which an oxygen atom replaces one of the methylene groups of the center ring of the dibenzocycloheptadiene molecule. A prototype drug for the dibenzocycloheptadienes is **amitriptyline**, and for the dibenzoxepines, it is **doxepin**.

BOX 10-1 Actions of Antidepressant Drugs

Drugs That Inhibit Reuptake of NE and 5-HT with Similar Potencies (Twentyfold Difference or Less)

Amitriptyline
Amoxapine*
Clomipramine
Doxepin
Duloxetine
Imipramine
Nefazodone
Nortriptyline
Protriptyline
Milnacipran

Drugs That Inhibit 5-HT Reuptake with Greater Potency (Fiftyfold More Than NE Reuptake)

Citalopram
Fluoxetine
Fluvoxamine
Paroxetine
Sertraline
Trazodone†
Venlafaxine†

Drugs That Block 5-HT Uptake and Are Agonists, Partial Agonists, or Antagonists or Inverse Agonists at Serotonin Receptors

Vortioxetine
Vilazodone

Drugs That Inhibit NE Reuptake with Greater Potency (Approximately Fiftyfold More than 5-HT Reuptake)

Maprotiline
Reboxetine
Desipramine

Drugs That Have Little Direct Effect on Either 5-HT or NE Uptake

Bupropion
Mirtazapine

*Also blocks D_2 receptors.
†Not classified as a selective serotonin reuptake inhibitor.
5-HT, 5-Hydroxytryptamine; *NE*, norepinephrine.

Substitutions at R (see Fig. 10-7) usually consist of aminopropyl groups that may be either dimethyl or monomethyl amino derivatives. Compounds such as imipramine, amitriptyline, and doxepin have two methyl moieties on the nitrogen atom of the side chain and are tertiary amines. **Desipramine, nortriptyline**, and **protriptyline** have one methyl group and are secondary amines.

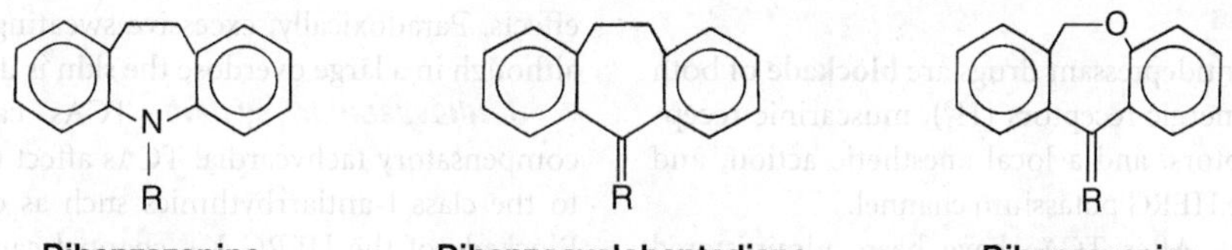

Dibenzazepine Dibenzocycloheptadiene Dibenzoxepine

FIG 10-7 Structural formulas of the tricyclic rings of the dibenzazepine, dibenzocycloheptadiene, and dibenzoxepine antidepressants.

TABLE 10-9 Elimination of Antidepressants

Drug	1A2	2B6	2C9	2C19	2D6	3A4	P-gly
Tricyclics Tertiary Amines							
Amitriptyline	S,H	S	S	S	S,H	S	S,H
Clomipramine	S,H			S	S,H	S	S,H
Doxepin	S		S	S	S,H		S,H
Imipramine	S			S	S,H	S	S,H
Trimipramine					S,H	S	S,H
Tricyclics Secondary Amines							
Desipramine	H				S,H		S,H
Nortriptyline	S,H			S	S,H	S	S,H
Protriptyline					S,H	S,H	S,H
Second-Generation Antidepressants							
Amoxapine	H				S,H	S	S,H
Maprotiline					S,H	S,H	S,H
Mirtazapine	S,H				S	S,H	S,H
Trazodone					S	S	S,H
Nefazodone				H		S	S,H
Bupropion		S			H		
Selective Serotonin Reuptake Inhibitors (SSRIs)							
Fluoxetine	H		S	H	S,H	Nor-fluoxetine* H	S,H
Paroxetine	H		H		S,H	H	S,H
Sertraline	H		H	H	S,H	S	S,H
Fluvoxamine	S,H		H	H		H	S,H
Citalopram			H	S,H	S,H	S	S,H
SNRIs							
Venlafaxine			S	S	S,H	S	S,H
Duloxetine	S,H				S,H	S,H	S,H
Dual Action Antidepressants							
Vilazodone			H	S,H	S	S	S,H
Vortioxetine			H		S		
Monoamine Oxidase (MAO) Inhibitors							
Tranylcypromine	H			H			
Phenelzine	H	H	H	H	H		

Cytochrome isozymes and *P*-glycoprotein are listed.
*The product of this enzymatic step.

TCA absorption, fate, and excretion

TCAs are readily absorbed from the gastrointestinal tract. The drugs are distributed throughout the body and are tightly bound to plasma and tissue proteins. Many pharmacologically active metabolites are formed in the liver by microsomal oxidation reactions. TCAs are metabolized by several isoforms of P450, with particular involvement of CYP1A2, CYP2C19, CYP2D6, and CYP3A4 (Table 10-9). Subsequent glucuronidation inactivates the agents and promotes their excretion. Many TCAs are substrates or inhibitors of *p*-glycoprotein transporters. Approximately two-thirds of a single dose is eliminated in the urine and one-third in the feces over several days, mostly as metabolites.

TCA pharmacologic effects

Common properties of the antidepressant drugs are **blockade** of both the **SERT** and **NET**, histaminergic receptors (H_1), muscarinic receptors, and α-adrenergic receptors, and a local anesthetic action, and many are known to block the HERG potassium channel.

Central nervous system. After TCAs have been administered for approximately 2 to 3 weeks to depressed patients, they become less confused and have an elevation of mood. Untoward CNS effects include dizziness, lightheadedness, and delirium and hallucinations. Antidepressant therapy is associated with an increase in suicide ideation, especially in those under 25 years of age.

Autonomic nervous system. TCAs are more potent **anticholinergics** than their phenothiazine analogues, especially with the tertiary amines (See Table 10-2). Amitriptyline, one of the most potent anticholinergic TCAs, is about one-eighth as potent as atropine. Anticholinergic action is usually considered in the context of an adverse quality, but this action may speed up the onset of antidepressant effects. Paradoxically, excessive sweating is also sometimes reported, although in a large overdose the skin is dry.

Cardiovascular system. TCAs can cause **hypotension** and compensatory tachycardia. TCAs affect the heart in a manner similar to the class I antiarrhythmics such as quinidine and procainamide. Blockade of the HERG K+ channel can induce prolongation of the QT interval and flattening of the T wave, and various arrhythmias have been reported (e.g., torsades de pointes). Postural hypotension, particularly in elderly patients, is common, probably because of α_1-adrenergic receptor blockade. Because TCAs block the reuptake of catecholamines and block muscarinic receptors, they can increase heart rate and blood pressure; however, chronic use tends to decrease blood pressure.

Adverse effects of TCAs

A comparison of the adverse effects of antidepressants is shown in Table 10-10. TCAs may initially cause anxiety or feelings of fatigue and

TABLE 10-10 Major Adverse Effects of Antidepressant Drugs

Drug	Anti-ACh	Sedation	Orthostatic Hypotension	Prolonged QT Interval	Sexual Dysfunction	Weight Gain or Loss
Tricyclic Tertiary Amines						
Amitriptyline	++++	++++	+++	+++,TdP	+	++
Clomipramine	+++	++	++	++		+
Doxepin	++	+++	+++	+++,TdP	+	++
Imipramine	++	++	+++	+++	+	++
Tricyclics Secondary Amines						
Desipramine	+	+	+	+++,TdP	+	+
Nortriptyline	++	++	+	+++	+	+
Protriptyline	+++	+	+	+		+
Tetracyclic and Other Second-Generation Agents						
Amoxapine	+++	++	+	+		+
Maprotiline	++	++	+	+,TdP		+
Mirtazapine	++	+++	++	+/–,TdP	+	++
Trazodone	+	++++	++	+,TdP	+	+,–
Nefazodone	0/+	++	+	++	+	0,+
Bupropion	++	0/+		—	+	+,–
Selective Serotonin Reuptake Inhibitors (SSRIs)						
Fluoxetine	0/+	0/+	0/+	++,TdP	++	0/+
Paroxetine	0	0/+	0	0/+	++	++
Sertraline	0	0/+	0	0/+,TdP	++	++
Fluvoxamine	0/+	0/+	0	0	++	+,–
Citalopram	0/+	0/+	0/+	+,TdP	+++	+
Dual Action Drugs						
Vilazodone	0/+	0	0	0	+	+/–
Vortioxetine	0/+	0	0		+	+
Serotonin-Norepinephrine Reuptake Inhibitors (SNRI)						
Venlafaxine*	0	0	0	+,TdP	++	0/–
Duloxetine	0	0	0	0	+	+
Milnacipran	0	0	0	0/+	0	0
Monoamine Oxidase (MAO) Inhibitors						
Tranylcypromine	+	+	0	+/0		+
Phenelzine	+	+	+	+/0		+

Severity of adverse effects is indicated by the number of + signs.
ND, No data; *TdP*, torsades de pointes resulting from prolonged QT interval.
*May induce hypertension.

weakness but tolerance develops to these effects. Although these agents do not elicit the EPS of the antipsychotic agents, mild tremor may sometimes occur. In some individuals, tics, ataxia, and incoordination have been reported.

In addition to their antimuscarinic effect, **alpha 1 adrenergic blockade** can contribute to **dry mouth** and orthostatic hypotension. Memory deficits may also occur. Sexual dysfunction (including loss of libido, impaired erection and ejaculation, and anorgasmy) is an additional side effect that may lead to patient noncompliance.

Acute overdosage, sometimes self-inflicted by suicidal patients, is a potentially life-threatening situation and is characterized by CNS excitation or depression and anticholinergic effects, and cardiovascular complications like **arrhythmias** are a potential consequence of acute overdose. Even in conventional doses, the incidence of sudden death from myocardial infarction or ventricular arrhythmias is increased in patients with cardiac disease. Fatalities have also occurred in children with no apparent preexisting cardiac defect. Blood dyscrasias, skin rashes, photosensitization, and cholestatic jaundice, many of which are manifestations of allergic reactions, have been reported but are less frequent than with the phenothiazines. TCAs cause a dose-related increase the risk for seizures, with clomipramine among the most likely to produce this effect.

Acute withdrawal from TCAs is characterized as a cholinergic crisis, flu-like symptoms (GI distress), vivid dreaming, and may include triggering of manic reactions.

TCA drug interactions

Adverse drug interactions are another potential problem for patients treated with antidepressants. Coadministration of TCAs with MAO inhibitors may cause anxiety, vomiting, tremor, convulsions, coma, and even death. TCAs may also obtund the antihypertensive action of guanethidine and the sympathomimetic action of amphetamine and tyramine by preventing their uptake into nerve terminals. The effects of clonidine (an α_2-adrenergic receptor agonist) are also inhibited. Other drug interactions that the dentist must consider are discussed next and are similar to interactions listed in Table 10-6 for the antipsychotic drugs.

Dental consequences of TCAs

TCAs have important dental implications. Reduced salivary flow increases the risk of dental caries, oral candidiasis, and oral functional abnormalities. Three-quarters of patients taking imipramine may report **dry mouth**. Anticholinergic agents (e.g., atropine) should not be administered with TCAs because additive effects can result not only in xerostomia but also in other toxic reactions (e.g., **confusion, agitation, hyperthermia, hallucinations, tachycardia, urinary retention**). The use of antianxiety agents, barbiturates, and other sedatives should be carefully controlled in patients receiving TCAs because of additive depressant effects on the CNS. The duration of action of barbiturates may be prolonged by TCAs, but the long-term use of hepatic metabolism inducers can reduce half-lives of TCAs by microsomal enzyme induction. Certain inhibitors of cytochrome P-450 2D6 and other cytochromes (e.g., amiodarone, erythromycin, clarithromycin, and itraconazole) can increase the likelihood of toxicity from the TCAs.

The risk of **long QT** syndrome and torsades de pointes is increased by many antidepressants, so adding other agents that increase this risk should be avoided. These include macrolide antibiotics (erythromycin, clarithromycin) and fluoroquinolone antibiotics (moxifloxacin, levofloxacin), imidazole antifungal agents (e.g., itraconazole), antihistamines, and cholinergic agonists.

Because of the cardiotoxic effects of TCAs and their potentiation of adrenergic drugs, high doses or accidental intravascular injection of local anesthetic solutions may precipitate arrhythmias and hypertension. The use of TCAs is not a contraindication, however, for the use of epinephrine with local anesthetics as long as care is taken not to inject the vasoconstrictor intravenously or in large doses. The use of the TCAs for treating depression has declined since the advent of newer drugs. They are usually reserved for depressed patients who are unresponsive to newer drugs. However, TCAs are useful in certain types of neuropathic pain and some other chronic pain syndromes.

Tetracyclic Antidepressants and Other Second-Generation Drugs

This is a heterogeneous group of antidepressants developed after the development of TCAs. **Amoxapine** (Fig. 10-8), a tetracyclic dibenzoxazepine resembling TCAs in chemical structure, is the N-demethylated metabolite of the antipsychotic loxapine. **Maprotiline** is related to the TCAs, but it contains a tetracyclic ring structure (see Fig. 10-8). **Mirtazapine** (Fig. 10-9) is also a tetracyclic compound. **Trazodone** and **nefazodone** (see Fig. 10-8) are triazole derivatives. **Bupropion** (Fig. 10-10), an aminoketone, is structurally dissimilar to all other antidepressants but similar to cathinones, found in Khat and more recently in "bath salts."

Pharmacology of second-generation drugs

These compounds differ significantly in their selectivity of action on monoamine uptake and neurotransmitter receptors. Their current use is primarily as adjuncts when SSRIs or SNRIs (see later in text) are not effective. Table 10-11 shows a comparison of receptor and transporter binding affinities. Amoxapine blocks dopamine (D_2) receptors and has **antipsychotic** properties as well as **antidepressant** effects, making it useful for patients with psychotic and mood disturbances. Maprotiline pharmacology is considered to be similar to TCAs, although its receptor binding is somewhat unique. Mirtazapine blocks histamine receptors that may increase drowsiness. Its therapeutic action on α_2 receptors may induce downregulation of SERT and NET. It produces a quicker relief of depression than most antidepressants, giving it an advantage over some other drugs. **Trazadone and nefazodone block 5-HT$_2$** receptors more strongly than SERT. Blockade of 5-HT$_{2A}$ receptors appears to be their major action as antidepressants. **Bupropion** is an unusual antidepressant. It causes the **release of NE and DA** as well as being a weak inhibitor of SERT and NET. Used as an adjunct antidepressant, it does not produce sexual side effects. Bupropion is approved for **treating tobacco dependence** and may be prescribed by dentists for this purpose.

Absorption, fate, and excretion

All second-generation agents are well absorbed from the oral route. Peak concentrations of the drugs are reached in approximately 1 to 3 hours. These drugs are metabolized with elimination half-lives ranging from 2 to 4 hours for nefazodone to up to 40 hours for maprotiline and mirtazapine.

Bupropion yields two active metabolites (including hydroxybupropion) that may accumulate and contribute to antidepressant activity by blocking NET. Peak action is seen in 3 hours, with a half-life of approximately 20 hours. Bupropion is metabolized by CYP2B6, which may cause the drug to have an important drug interaction profile. Smoking does not alter its kinetics. Nearly 80% of an orally administered dose is excreted as inactive metabolites in the urine.

Adverse effects of second-generation drugs

Amoxapine, maprotiline, mirtazapine, trazodone, and nefazodone share common side effects, including **sedation**, cardiovascular effects,

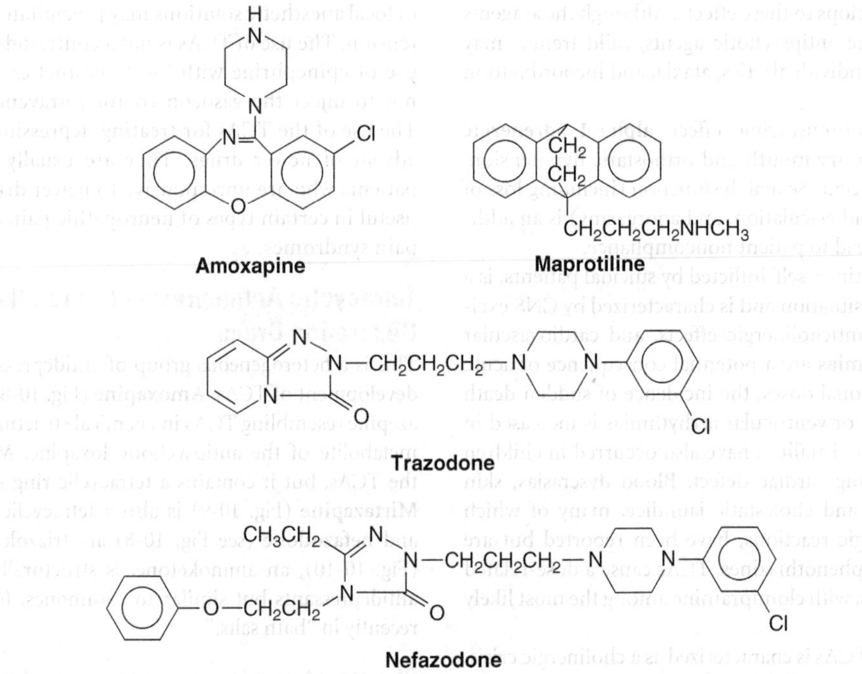

Amoxapine

Maprotiline

Trazodone

Nefazodone

FIG 10-8 Structural formulas of amoxapine, maprotiline, trazodone, and nefazodone.

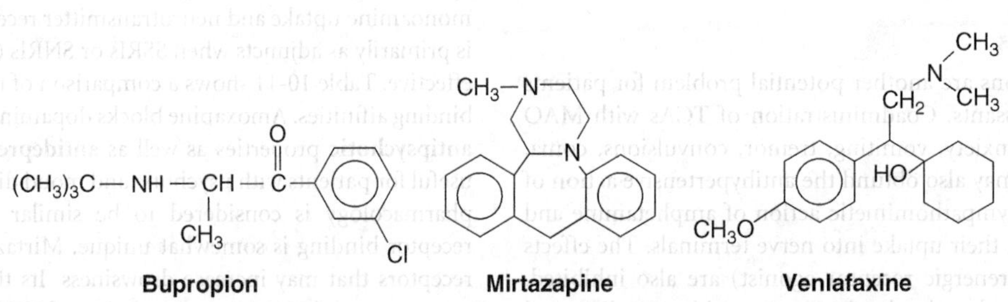

Bupropion

Mirtazapine

Venlafaxine

FIG 10-9 Structural formulas of bupropion, mirtazapine, and venlafaxine.

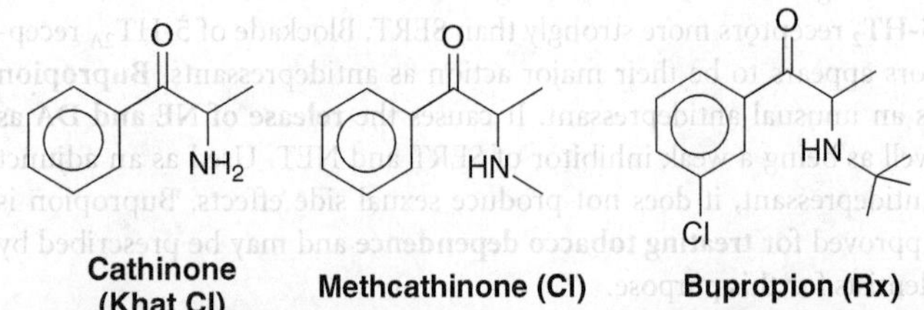

FIG 10-10 Structural formulas of cathinones compared to bupropion. *CI*, Class 1 controlled substance

TABLE 10-11 Selected Second-Generation (SG) Receptor or Transporter Binding Comparison

SG Drug	Drug Receptor Binding Hierarchy
Amoxapine	$5\text{-HT}_2 > \text{NET} = \text{D}_2 > \text{H}_1 > \alpha_1 = 5\text{-HT}_{6,7} = \text{SERT}$
Maprotiline	$\text{H}_1 > \text{NET} > 5\text{-HT}_2 >> \text{D}$
Mirtazapine	$\text{H1} > \alpha_2 = 5\text{-HT}_2 = \text{D}_4 >> \text{NET}$
Trazadone	$5\text{-HT}_2 > \alpha_1 > 5\text{-HT}_1 > \text{H}_1 > \text{SERT}$
Nafazodone	$5\text{-HT}_{2a} > \alpha_1 > 5\text{-HT}_{1A} >> \text{SERT} > \text{NET} = \text{DAT}$
Bupropion	$\text{H}_1 > \text{DAT}$ (indirect) ($> \text{NET}$ metabolite) (indirect) $>$Nicotinic $\alpha_2\beta_2$

DAT, Dopamine transporter; *NET*, Norepinephrine transporter; *SERT*, serotonin transporter.

and skin rashes. The incidence and severity of these reactions vary considerably, however, among the drugs. The second-generation antidepressants produce fewer sexual dysfunctional side effects compared with TCAs or SSRIs. **Weight gain** is an effect that may lead to noncompliance (see Table 10-10). None of these agents should be combined with MAO inhibitors.

Each of the second-generation agents has some unique side effects that can limit clinical usefulness. Because of its antidopaminergic activity, amoxapine produces EPS and can increase prolactin secretion and cause amenorrhea, gynecomastia, and galactorrhea. Amoxapine is approximately equal to TCAs in cardiotoxicity, whereas maprotiline has less effect on the heart. Maprotiline and bupropion may trigger seizure activity. Drugs that block the reuptake of catecholamines seem to have a higher incidence of seizures.

Trazodone sometimes produces persistent priapism requiring surgical detumescence, which can result in permanent impotence. Nefazodone and some of its metabolites are potent inhibitors of CYP3A4, and nefazodone is capable of blocking the metabolism of numerous drugs. **Nefazodone** has been associated with serious **hepatotoxicity** and has an associated black box warning.

Bupropion is especially likely to cause **convulsions** (black box warning). Bupropion was withdrawn from the market after its initial introduction because of seizures; it was reintroduced at lower recommended doses. Bupropion is contraindicated in patients with epilepsy and in patients who have had bulimia or anorexia nervosa because of an increased risk of seizures in these patients. Other side effects of bupropion include headache and dry mouth, tremor, **insomnia**, and the possible induction of psychosis. Bupropion is a dopamine transporter (DAT) inhibitor, but it is thought to have a low abuse potential. However, abuse of bupropion is on the rise; some are crushing tablets and snorting the drug. Bupropion has minimal cardiovascular effects and only infrequently produces orthostatic hypotension. Less commonly, bupropion generates rashes or erythema multiforme (Stevens-Johnson syndrome).

Dental consequences of second-generation drugs

Although tetracyclic and other second-generation antidepressants may have fewer side effects than TCAs, their amine blocking and sedative properties should be kept in mind. Bupropion is exceptional in that central stimulation is more likely than sedation; it is contraindicated with a patient history of seizures, anorexia nervosa, and bulimia. It may aggravate the condition of an already nervous patient. The drug is reported to produce dry mouth in approximately 25% of patients who use it, including patients in smoking cessation programs. The dentist should recognize that bupropion, although generally safe, occasionally can produce severe reactions such as seizures or Stevens-Johnson syndrome. Long-term success rates in smoking cessation programs, even with pharmacotherapy, are low. Levodopa increases bupropion toxicity. Ritonavir, an antiviral agent metabolized by CYP2B6, increases bupropion actions. Carbamazepine reduces bupropion blood concentrations. Structurally, bupropion is *m*-chloro-methcathinone, and it shares some properties with other **cathinones** such as Khat, methcathinone, and drugs found in "bath salts" (e.g., methylenedioxypyrovalerone), possibly exacerbating any stimulant actions of bupropion such as seizures (Fig. 10-10).

Selective Serotonin Reuptake Inhibitors (SNRIs)

Figure 10-11 shows five SSRIs currently approved for use in the United States: **fluoxetine, fluvoxamine, sertraline, paroxetine, citalopram.** Escitalopram, the S enantiomer of citalopram, is also approved.

Pharmacologic effects of SSRIs

The selectivity of SSRIs for **SERT** provides a theoretic basis for greater selectivity in various depressive states with fewer side effects, and the SSRIs are the drugs most commonly used for MDD. These drugs cause downregulation of presynaptic inhibitory $5\text{-HT}_{1B/D}$ autoreceptors, which facilitate 5-HT transmission; this leads to postsynaptic changes analogous to those seen with TCAs. Several serotonergic pathways account for various effects of SSRIs (see Table 10-8). SSRIs have been found to be useful for other disorders in which 5-HT is thought to play a role, such as obsessive-compulsive disorders, panic disorders, bulimia, social phobia, PTSD, generalized anxiety disorder, social anxiety disorder, premenstrual distress disorder, and some aspects of schizophrenia. In general, SSRIs are effective in about 50% of patients, and some patients need other medications or adjunct agents added.

Absorption, fate, and excretion of SSRIs

The major difference among SSRIs is their pharmacokinetic profile. The elimination half-life of fluoxetine is long, approximately 45 hours compared with 26 hours for sertraline, 21 hours for paroxetine, and 14 hours for fluvoxamine. Generally, these drugs are metabolized by CYP2D6 and CYP3A4 isozymes. Fluoxetine is metabolized to norfluoxetine, an active metabolite with an extended half-life (~200 hours) that is also an inhibitor of CYP2D6 and CYP3A4. Paroxetine has active metabolites that contribute to its pharmacologic effect, whereas the metabolites of sertraline and fluvoxamine are inactive. The long half-life of fluoxetine

Fluoxetine

Fluvoxamine

Paroxetine

Sertraline

Citalopram

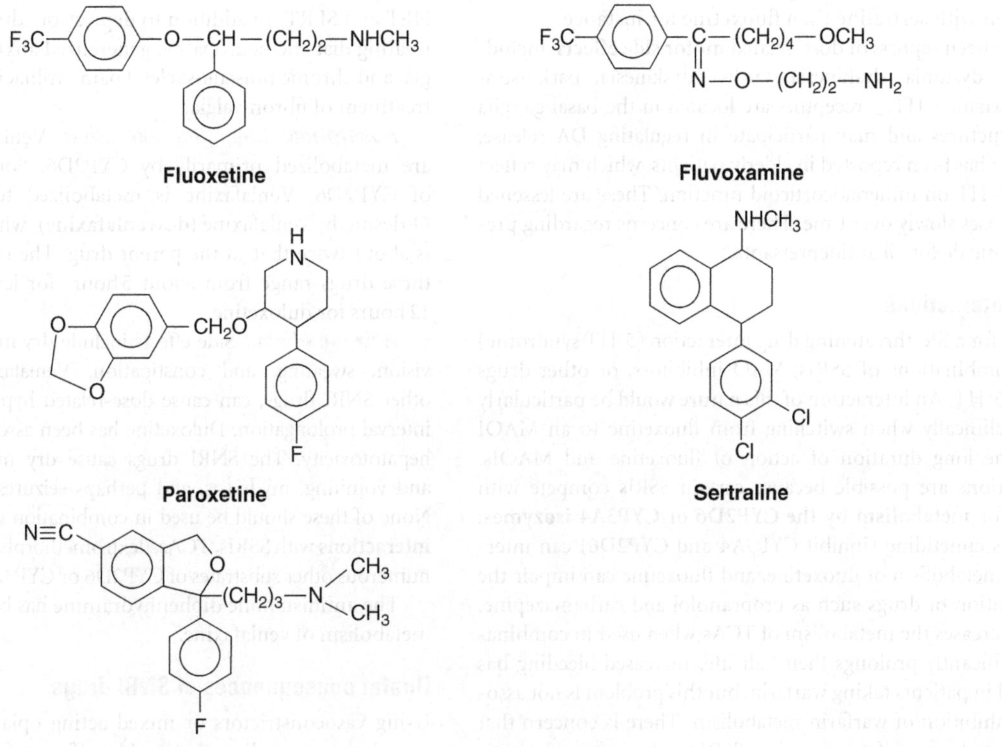

FIG 10-11 Structural formulas of the selective serotonin reuptake inhibitors fluoxetine, fluvoxamine, paroxetine, sertraline, and citalopram.

BOX 10-2 Side Effects of Selective Serotonin Reuptake Inhibitors

Early Onset, Transient
Nausea
Anxiety
Agitation
Sleep disturbance/insomnia

Late Onset
Weight gain
Asthenia
Sexual dysfunction
Withdrawal syndrome

is clinically relevant when considering drug interactions. SSRIs are substrates for *p*-glycoprotein efflux transporters (Table 10-9).

Adverse effects of SSRIs

Compared with TCAs, SSRIs have minimal anticholinergic effects and produce less sedation and less lethality in overdose, and they may be more useful in elderly patients.

Side effects have been categorized as early onset or late onset (Box 10-2). The most prominent early side effect of SSRIs is **gastrointestinal upset** (diarrhea, nausea, vomiting) reflecting the stimulatory nature of 5-HT in the enteric nervous system. Tolerance to this effect develops over 4 to 6 weeks. Patients may also have anxiety, agitation, and **insomnia**. Tolerance to sleep disturbances may not occur. Late-onset side effects include weight gain, sexual dysfunction (e.g., anorgasmy and decreased libido), asthenia (weakness), and drug withdrawal symptoms. The intensity of the long-term side effects varies among the SSRIs. Sexual dysfunction is more common with sertraline than fluoxetine for instance.

There have been reports of dose-related **motor side effects**, including akathisia, dystonia, dyskinesia, tardive dyskinesia, parkinsonism, and **bruxism**. 5-HT_{1-4} receptors are located in the basal ganglia or related structures and may participate in regulating DA release. Hyponatremia has been reported in elderly patients, which may reflect the effect of 5-HT on mineralocorticoid function. These are lessened by reducing doses slowly over time. There are concerns regarding precipitation of suicide for all antidepressants.

SSRI–drug interactions

The potential for a life-threatening drug interaction (5-HT syndrome) exists with combinations of SSRIs, MAO inhibitors, or other drugs that increase 5-HT. An interaction of this nature would be particularly problematic clinically when switching from fluoxetine to an MAOI because of the long duration of action of fluoxetine and MAOIs. Drug interactions are possible because certain SSRIs compete with other drugs for **metabolism by the CYP2D6 or CYP3A4 isozymes.** Drugs such as cimetidine (inhibit CYP3A4 and CYP2D6) can interfere with the metabolism of fluoxetine, and fluoxetine can impair the biotransformation of drugs such as propranolol and carbamazepine. Fluoxetine decreases the metabolism of TCAs when used in combination and significantly prolongs their half-life. Increased bleeding has been reported in patients taking warfarin, but this problem is not associated with inhibition of warfarin metabolism. There is concern that GI bleeding may be more frequent when SSRIs and nonsteroidal anti-inflammatory analgesics are used together. The high incidence of gastrointestinal disturbances, particularly nausea and vomiting, during initial treatment with SSRIs can pose clinical problems. Fluoxetine (or its metabolite norfluoxetine, which inhibits CYP3A4) can prolong sedation from some benzodiazepines (e.g., alprazolam, midazolam, and triazolam).

Dental consequences of SSRIs

The high incidence of gastrointestinal disturbances, particularly nausea and vomiting, during initial treatment with SSRIs can pose clinical problems. Postponement of clinical procedures to a later date may be advisable because tolerance develops to these side effects. Fluoxetine (or its metabolite norfluoxetine) prolongs the duration of action of certain benzodiazepines, probably by decreasing their metabolism. This inhibition may lead to protracted sedation, especially in light of the long half-lives of fluoxetine and its active metabolite. The interaction is most pronounced with benzodiazepines (alprazolam, midazolam, and triazolam) that are metabolized by CYP3A4-catalyzed α hydroxylation on the triazolo ring of these drugs.

Newer SERT inhibitors with dual action (dual action drugs)

Vortioxetine and Vilazodone are like SSRIs with the additional actions on 5-HT receptors. Vilazodone antagonizes SERT but is also a partial agonist at 5-HT_{1A}. Vortioxetine antagonizes SERT and 5-HT_{3A}, is a partial antagonist of 5-HT_{1A}, and has actions at other 5-HT receptors.

Serotonin-norepinephrine reuptake inhibitors (SNRIs)

The drugs in this group are venlafaxine, duloxetine, desvenlafaxine, milnacipran, and levomilnacipran. What distinguishes this group from the others is that the SNRIs have little effect on receptors and inhibit SERT and NET selectively. All are approved for MDD. Venlafaxine (see Fig. 10-9) and duloxetine inhibit SERT more than NET, whereas milnacipran and its levo enantiomer have close to equal affinity for NET and SERT. In addition to depression, duloxetine is approved for treating diabetic neuropathy, generalized anxiety disorder, fibromyalgia, and chronic musculoskeletal pain. Milnacipran is approved for the treatment of fibromyalgia.

Absorption, fate, and excretion. Venlafaxine and duloxetine are metabolized primarily by CYP2D6. Some are mild inhibitors of CYP2D6. Venlafaxine is metabolized to an active metabolite *O*-desmethylvenlafaxine (**desvenlafaxine**), whose half-life (~10 hours) is about twice that of the parent drug. The elimination half-lives for these drugs range from about 5 hours for levomilnacipran to about 12 hours for duloxetine.

Adverse effects. Side effects include **dry mouth, insomnia**, blurred vision, sweating, and constipation. Venlafaxine, more likely than other SNRI drugs, can cause dose-related hypertensive effects and QT interval prolongation. Duloxetine has been associated with **seizures** and hepatotoxicity. The SNRI drugs cause dry mouth, insomnia, nausea and vomiting, mydriasis, and perhaps seizures and sexual side effects. None of these should be used in combination with MAOIs. Other **drug interactions** with SSRIs, TCAs, dextromethorphan, pentazocine, and with numerous other substrates of CYP2D6 or CYP3A4 have been reported.

The antihistamine diphenhydramine has been found to inhibit the metabolism of venlafaxine.

Dental consequences of SNRI drugs

Using vasoconstrictors or mixed-acting opiate agents like **tramadol** may increase cardiovascular side effects of drugs like venlafaxine. Further risk may come from agents that interfere with the normal metabolic clearance of many antidepressants, especially **agents blocking**

CYP2D6 or 3A4. COMT inhibitors, such as entacapone used in the treatment of Parkinson disease, can increase the toxicity of vasoconstrictor agents and agents such as the SNRIs.

Monoamine Oxidase Inhibitors

MAOIs inhibit the metabolic degradation of the naturally occurring monoamines: epinephrine, NE, DA, and 5-HT. At least two forms of MAO (MAO-A and MAO-B) are in the brain. Selective inhibitors of MAO-A reduce the metabolism of NE and 5-HT, while MAO-B is more involved with metabolism of DA and tryptophan. Currently, three nonselective MAOI antidepressants are available: **phenelzine, isocarboxazid**, and **tranylcypromine. Selegiline** is an MAO-B inhibitor used in the treatment of Parkinson disease. **Linezolid** is a more recently developed antibiotic that also is a nonselective inhibitor of MAO.

MAOI pharmacologic effects

Similar to TCAs, **MAOIs** increase the concentration of NE and 5-HT in the CNS. By preventing the catabolic action of MAO, MAOIs allow the buildup of monoamines in the presynaptic nerve terminals (see Chapters 5 and 9). This effect apparently leads to **adaptive changes in receptors** similar to the changes seen with TCAs. Although these effects are compatible with the monoamine hypothesis of depression, MAOIs affect other enzymes and have nonenzymatic actions as well.

MAOIs are considered to be less effective than TCAs and to have serious side effects and drug and food interactions. MAOIs are seldom used and are reserved for treatment of those unresponsive to other drugs. Numerous precautions need to be taken, particularly regarding drug interactions and dietary restrictions.

MAOI adverse effects

Most of the original MAOIs have been withdrawn from the market because of their serious side effects. The important adverse reactions to the remaining MAOIs as for the original drugs are excessive **cardiovascular** stimulation with certain foods and other drugs as well as **hepatotoxicity**. MAOIs may also cause orthostatic hypotension and, in overdosage, central excitatory manifestations of insomnia, agitation, hyperreflexia, and convulsions.

MAOI drug interactions

Drug interactions are of particular concern with MAOIs because they are likely to be serious and potentially fatal. Among the drugs with which MAOIs interact are all classes of **antidepressants**, meperidine, alcohol, and other CNS depressants, indirectly acting or mixed-acting sympathomimetics such as amphetamine or ephedrine, phenylephrine (commonly used in over-the-counter preparations as a nasal decongestant), and monoamine precursors such as levodopa.

In addition to drug interactions, acute hypertensive crises have been precipitated by the ingestion of foods containing naturally occurring pressor amines, such as tyramine, which release NE from nerve endings. Patients treated with MAOIs have elevated cytoplasmic stores of NE that can be released by agents such as tyramine. In addition, ingested tyramine, which is normally metabolized by enteric and hepatic MAO, reaches the systemic circulation in increased amounts (see Chapter 9). Foods containing tyramine must be avoided. Hypertensive crises precipitated by such foods are characterized by severe headaches, often localized in the occipital region, with fever.

MAOIs are contraindicated with SERT inhibitors for an additional reason. This combination may precipitate the "serotonin syndrome," which consists of hyperthermia, facial flushing, dizziness, confusion, headache, sweating, fever, rigidity, myoclonus or tremor, respiratory disturbances, gastrointestinal upset, and mental status changes ranging from delirium to coma. This drug interaction may occur several weeks after termination of fluoxetine (a SERT inhibitor) because of its slow elimination from the body (half-life of approximately 200 hours for active metabolites). MAOIs may increase the cardiovascular effects of anti-Parkinson drugs: COMT inhibitors, MAO-B inhibitors, or direct dopaminergic agonists.

Dental consequences of MAOI

MAOIs can cause serious drug and food interactions. Interactions most relevant for the practicing dentist include the prolongation and enhancement of the CNS effects of the **opioid analgesics, barbiturates, and other CNS depressants.** MAOIs given in conjunction with **meperidine** cause potentially fatal reactions, including hyperthermia, excitement, and seizures, in addition to reactions that resemble an opioid overdose. Meperidine should not be used concurrently or for several weeks after therapy with MAOIs. Other opioids, which are not similar chemically to meperidine, may be used with caution.

Hypotension can develop with the concomitant use of general anesthetics and MAOIs. It is prudent to discontinue the use of MAOIs for 2 weeks before surgery. Neither epinephrine nor levonordefrin is potentiated by inhibition of MAO activity.

St. John's Wort

St. John's wort, a traditional herbal remedy, is helpful for treating depression. In ancient Greece and Rome, St. John's wort (*Hypericum perforatum*) was placed above icons for its mystical powers (*hyper* means "above;" *eikon* means "icon"). The drug is available as a herbal preparation from health food stores and pharmacies in the United States and outsells fluoxetine in Germany.

St. John's wort has many biologically active components, including hypericin, hyperforin, and some flavonoids. Commercially available capsules contain approximately 3% to 5% hyperforin and 0.3% hypericin. It has only more recently been understood that **hyperforin** may be the most active constituent, so labeling may still refer to hypericin as the active agent. Using products with USP certification can help assure the presence of active drug.

St. John's wort blocks the reuptake of 5-HT, NE, DA, GABA, and glycine with approximately equal potency, a unique therapeutic property. **Several mechanisms** have been proposed for hyperforin. Recent focus has been on the TRPC6 ion channel that regulates Na^+ and Ca^{2+} entry into cells. Hyperforin activates this channel. Hyperforin may reduce the Na^+ gradient on which the neurotransmitter symporters depend, decreasing neurotransmitter uptake.

St. John's wort reaches peak plasma concentrations in approximately 4 hours and has a half-life of approximately 9 hours. There is disagreement as to the relative clinical effectiveness of St. John's wort despite evidence of an antidepressant action in mild to moderate depression. In some studies it rivals fluoxetine. Some of this variation may result from poor quality herbals or outright frauds sold as St. John's wort. Commonly noted side effects include gastrointestinal upset, fatigue, dizziness, dry mouth (but less than with other antidepressants), and restlessness. The drug seems to be relatively free of the typical autonomic side effects associated with TCAs. Rare, but possibly dose-related, toxicities are phototoxicity and cataract formation.

Drug interactions are a concern with St. John's wort and can result from multiple mechanisms. **Hyperforin induces P450 isozymes** (e.g., CYP3A4), synthetic enzymes (e.g. uridine 5′-diphosphoglucuronosyl transferase), and multidrug-resistant protein (e.g., *p*-glycoproteins). At higher than therapeutic doses, St. John's wort may block MAO-A and MAO-B. Chronic use causes many drug interactions that are clinically significant, including many frequently used medical and dental drugs (e.g., reducing the effect of midazolam, erythromycin, and lidocaine). St. John's wort has been shown to reduce the effect of oral contraceptives.

Dental Implications for Depressed Patients

Untreated depression has been correlated with numerous **intraoral changes** that may predispose depressed patients to dental or oral disease. Known factors include reduced salivary flow, preference for carbohydrates (possibly because of decreased brain 5-HT), and decreased motivation and interest in oral health maintenance. Depressed patients may be more likely to have periodontitis. Chronic facial pain, burning sensations in the mouth, and temporomandibular joint disorders may be associated with depression.

All drugs used to treat depression have been reported to produce varying degrees of **xerostomia** and may increase the likelihood for dental caries and other oral health problems. Estimates of degree of dry mouth vary widely in the literature for the same drug possibly due to differences in dosage, duration of therapy, and underlying physical status among patients. Although antimuscarinic action has been a principal explanation for dry mouth, other drug actions may also contribute. Changes in salivary function can reflect actions of drugs on the salivary glands, the cardiovascular system, immune function, or the CNS centers controlling these functions. The relative likelihood of xerostomia is much greater with TCAs than with other antidepressants. Other common oral side effects of antidepressants include altered taste sensation, stomatitis, and glossitis.

Amitriptyline and certain other antidepressants are among the more commonly **used drugs for chronic facial neuralgias**, including atypical facial pain and facial arthromyalgia (Costen syndrome and temporomandibular joint dysfunction syndrome). Drug responses vary from patient to patient. Although effective doses are lower than the doses required for the treatment of depression, the same delayed onset to effect (several weeks) has been reported. The selective NE reuptake blockers such as duloxetine may also be useful in the treatment of chronic pain. Because these agents block the reuptake of NE, concurrent use of **vasoconstrictors** in dental cartridges could produce exaggerated cardiovascular responses.

Dentists have been encouraged to assist with **tobacco cessation. Bupropion** is one agent recommended for this indication. This drug is marketed (for different purposes) under two trade names, **Wellbutrin and Zyban**, so patients should not accidentally be given both because of dose-related increased risk for seizures. Some patients are abusing bupropion. Dentists should monitor the rate of prescribing this medication and consider if it is being used in excess. If so, it could lead to seizures or drug dependence issues.

Drugs for Bipolar Disorder

Manic disorder or bipolar disorder is a unique diagnostic condition. A genetic component is suspected. Bipolar disorder is characterized by mood swings with alternating cycles of depression and mania. Abnormalities on several chromosomes have been demonstrated and there is an increased rate of maternal transmission rate with several of these.

Lithium salts are important for treating mania, but Li^+ alone may be inadequate treatment for 50% of patients exhibiting bipolar disorder. In addition to the antimanic effects of Li^+, evidence suggests Li^+ may also exert neuroprotective actions that may be prophylactic in unipolar and bipolar disorders and possibly in neural degenerative disorders such as Alzheimer disease. Other agents can be used to control manic patients temporarily while Li^+ therapy is being instituted and to treat individuals for whom Li^+ alone proves ineffective. Typical and atypical antipsychotic drugs are used in most patients during initiation of therapy. More recently, valproate and carbamazepine have been used in the treatment of bipolar disorder.

Lithium Salts

Li^+ was observed to be effective for mania by Cade in 1949, but it was not generally embraced until the late 1960s. **Lithium carbonate** was chosen as the best tolerated salt.

Pharmacologic effects

The mechanism of action of Li^+ is not established. Many changes resulting from Li^+ administration have been documented, including effects on plasma membrane cation channels, plasma membrane ion pumps, and exchange systems, and positive and negative effects on neuronal release of various neurotransmitters.

Although the mechanism of action of Li^+ remains unresolved, two effects of Li^+ offer likely explanations for the therapeutic and possibly adverse effects (Fig. 10-12). The first is the inhibitory effect of the ion on phosphomonoesterases involved in inositol signaling pathways. Li^+ inhibits phosphoinositide metabolism by **inhibiting inositol monophosphatase**, the enzyme responsible for converting inositol monophosphate to inositol. Li^+ also inhibits inositol polyphosphate-1-phosphatase, which catalyzes the 1-dephosphorylation of certain inositol bisphosphates and polyphosphates. Li^+ inhibits the effect of neurotransmitters that use signaling pathways involving inositol trisphosphate.

A second effect that may play an important role in the action of Li^+ is **inhibition of glycogen synthase kinase-3β (GSK-3β)**. This inhibition can influence at least two intracellular signaling cascades: activation of β-catenin and increased glycogen synthesis. By inhibiting GSK-3β, Li^+ acts like the endogenous inhibitor of GSK-3β, which stimulates cell receptors linked to GSK-3β (see Fig. 10-12). This stimulation results in changes in cell–cell interaction, axonal remodeling, and signaling in neurons. By inhibiting GSK-3β, Li^+ also acts like insulin, which stimulates glycogen synthesis (GSK-3β inhibits glycogen synthase).

Clinically, Li^+ alleviates the manifestations of mania over 1 to 2 weeks. Sleep and appetite disturbances abate, and mood swings are prevented. Li^+ has little effect on mood in patients who do not have mania and provides a prophylactic action against future manic attacks. Patients who stop taking Li^+ may not respond as well to subsequent Li^+ treatment trials, possibly because of progression of the neurodegenerative process. Li^+ does not have anticonvulsant actions.

Absorption, fate, and excretion

Li^+ is readily absorbed from the gastrointestinal tract. The cation eventually equilibrates throughout the total body water; no particular affinity for the brain or a specific organ has been detected. Excretion of Li^+ is primarily through the kidney, and reduced kidney function is associated with greater Li^+ toxicity if blood concentrations are not carefully monitored.

Adverse effects

Some of the most common side effects of Li^+ (e.g., gastrointestinal irritation, **fine hand tremor**, muscular weakness, **polyuria**, thirst, sleepiness, a sluggish feeling) are often associated with initial therapy and usually fade within 1 to 2 weeks. Thirst, polyuria, and hand tremor occasionally may continue for several months or years. Severe intoxication results in vomiting, diarrhea, unconsciousness, and convulsions. Most adverse effects of Li^+ have been found to correlate very closely with serum Li^+ concentrations. The **therapeutic index for Li^+ is low**, and plasma titers of Li^+ must be monitored. **Li^+ inhibits** the renal response to **antidiuretic hormone** (ADH) and may cause nephrogenic diabetes insipidus. The effect on ADH is the basis for the thirst, xerostomia, and polyuria associated with the drug. Na^+ depletion leads to reduced excretion of Li^+, so dosages of Li^+ may need to be reduced during concurrent therapy with a diuretic.

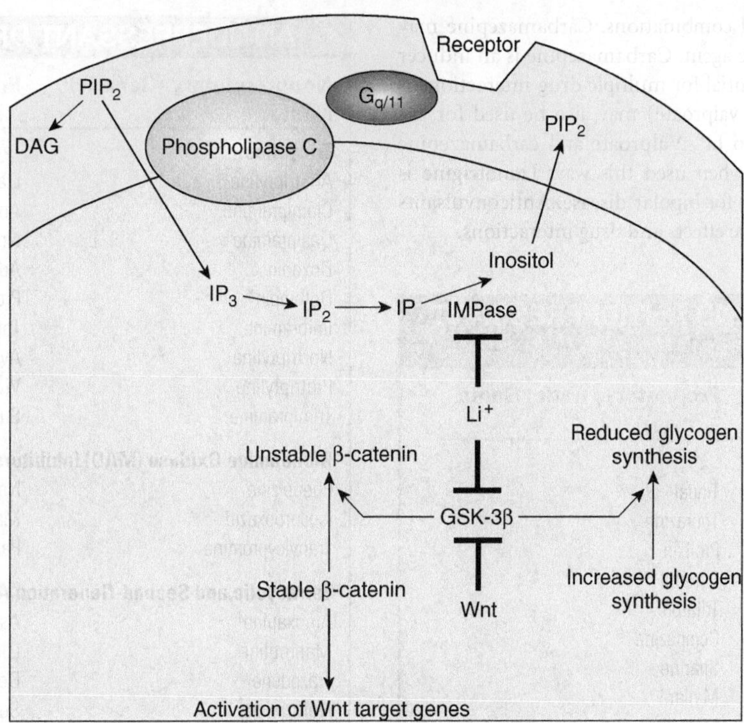

FIG 10-12 Two mechanisms by which Li^+ may mediate its pharmacologic effects. Li^+ inhibits inositol monophosphatase (*IMPase*) and glycogen synthase kinase-3β (*GSK-3β*). By the first mechanism, Li^+ inhibits signaling through the inositol pathway by depleting phosphatidylinositol bisphosphate (*PIP_2*). The result of this depletion is the inability to produce sufficient inositol-1,4,5 trisphosphate (*IP_3*). By the second mechanism, Li^+ stabilizes β-catenin, leading to changes in neuronal function, such as receptor signaling and remodeling. In addition, glycogen synthesis is promoted by Li^+. *DAG*, Diacylglycerol; *IP*, inositol monophosphate; *IP_2*, inositol bisphosphate; *Wnt*, glycoprotein that inhibits GSK-3β.

Any situation, such as a **sodium-restricted diet** or sweating, that tends to reduce the Na^+ load may increase **Li^+ toxicity.** Cardiovascular disease, renal disease, or severe dehydration can also increase the risk of toxicity from Li^+.

Li^+ may cause hypotension and cardiac arrhythmias, but changes are not usually significant if concentrations remain in the therapeutic range. Li^+ can also induce hypothyroidism in about 30% of patients. **Hypothyroidism** can be managed with thyroid replacement therapy. With continued Li^+ therapy, approximately 4% of patients develop diffuse, nontoxic **goiters.** Teratogenic effects, such as cleft palate, deformities of the ear and eye, and cardiac defects are associated with Li^+ administration during the first trimester of pregnancy.

Simple and convenient methods for measuring Li^+ have been sought that do not involve taking blood samples. One such method has been the use of salivary measurements. Although the saliva/plasma Li^+ ratio varies considerably from patient to patient, within a single patient, its variability is low. There is some promise that saliva sampling may be beneficial in **Li^+ monitoring.**

General therapeutic uses

Li^+ is used for the treatment of mania and as long-term treatment of manic-depressive illness. Initial high (therapeutic) doses are often adjusted downward to maintenance levels, which may partially explain the initial feelings of tiredness. Frequent measurements of Li^+ are required to maintain proper plasma concentrations.

Implications for dentistry

Patients with bipolar disease may have substantial dental pathology. Lithium may induce nephrogenic diabetes insipidus producing **hyposalivation** in about 70% of patients. These patients have a greater risk for poor oral hygiene, accumulations of supragingival and subgingival calculus, extensive dental caries, and numerous missing teeth. Patients taking Li^+ frequently have a metallic taste that can alter the palatability of food. Polydipsia can also contribute to caries if the patient drinks sugary or acidic beverages to relieve the sensation of dry mouth.

Chronic lithium treatment may **prolong the actions of local anesthetics.** Examples have been reported, and anesthesia may persist for up to 18 hours in some cases after typical nerve blocks.

Nonsteroidal antiinflammatory drugs may **decrease the renal excretion of Li^+** and lead to toxic plasma concentrations after several days of combined therapy. Metronidazole, angiotensin-converting enzyme inhibitors, and angiotensin II receptor blockers can increase the levels of lithium. In early phases of Li^+ therapy, **facial spasm** and transient facial paralysis, especially of the lower jaw, have occurred. Paradoxically, facial pains associated with cluster headaches may respond to treatment with Li^+.

Hyperparathyroidism, as a result of lithium therapy, may shift the balance of mandibular bone from cortical bone to more trabecular bone and increased tori.

Other Antimanic Drugs

Approximately 50% of patients who have mania do not respond to Li^+. Characteristics common to many Li^+-refractory patients include severe mania mixed with either psychotic episodes or anxiety and a history of rapid cycling. Antipsychotic agents are frequently used to help control the florid excitation and delusions early in treatment, and some atypical antipsychotics have been approved for this use.

Carbamazepine, an anticonvulsant discussed in Chapter 12, may be effective in some refractory cases. Carbamazepine has been reserved for patients who do not respond to conventional therapy and may be used in Li^+/carbamazepine fixed combinations. Carbamazepine may also be effective as a prophylactic agent. Carbamazepine is an inducer of drug metabolism, so the potential for multiple drug interactions is present. **Valproic acid** (sodium valproate) may also be used for the treatment of mania refractory to Li^+. Valproate and carbamazepine are termed "mood stabilizers" when used this way. Lamotrigine is approved as a maintenance drug for bipolar disease. Anticonvulsants can contribute a variety of adverse effects and drug interactions.

ANTIPSYCHOTIC AND ANTIDEPRESSANT DRUGS

Nonproprietary (Generic) Name	Proprietary (Trade) Name
Phenothiazines	
Acetophenazine*	Tindal
Chlorpromazine	Thorazine
Fluphenazine	Prolixin
Mesoridazine	Serentil
Perphenazine	Trilafon
Prochlorperazine	Compazine
Promazine*	Sparine
Thioridazine	Mellaril
Trifluoperazine	Stelazine
Triflupromazine*	Vesprin
Thioxanthenes	
Chlorprothixene*	Taractan
Thiothixene	Navane
Butyrophenone	
Haloperidol	Haldol
Dibenzoxazepine	
Loxapine	Loxitane
Diphenylbutylpiperidine	
Pimozide	Orap
Dibenzodiazepine	
Clozapine	Clozaril
Benzisoxazole	
Risperidone	Risperdal
Paliperidone	Invega
Iloperidone	Fanapt
Thienobenzodiazepine	
Olanzapine	Zyprexa
Dihydroindolone	
Ziprasidone	Zeldox, Geodon
Molindone	Moban
Lurasidone	Latuda
Dibenzothiazepine	
Quetiapine	Seroquel
Dihydrocarbostyril	
Aripiprazole†	Abilify
Brexpiprazole	Rexulti
Tetracyclic-dibenzo cyclohepta pyrrole	
Asenapine	Saphris

†Also used in conjunction with antidepressants.
*Not currently available in the US.

ANTIDEPRESSANT DRUGS

Nonproprietary (Generic) Name	Proprietary (Trade) Name
Tricyclics	
Amitriptyline	Elavil, Endep
Clomipramine	Anafranil
Desipramine	Norpramin
Doxepin	Adapin, Sinequan
Dothiepin*	Prothiaden
Imipramine	Tofranil
Nortriptyline	Aventyl, Pamelor
Protriptyline	Vivactil
Trimipramine	Surmontil
Monoamine Oxidase (MAO) Inhibitors	
Phenelzine	Nardil
Isocarboxazid	Marplan
Tranylcypromine	Parnate
Tetracyclic and Second-Generation Agents	
Amoxapine†	Asendin
Maprotiline	Ludiomil
Trazodone	Desyrel
Nefazodone	Serzone
Bupropion	Wellbutrin, Zyban
Mirtazapine	Remeron
Selective Serotonin Reuptake Inhibitors (SSRIs)	
Fluoxetine	Prozac
Fluvoxamine	Luvox
Paroxetine	Paxil
Sertraline	Zoloft
Citalopram	Celexa
Escitalopram	Lexapro
Serotonin-Norepinephrine Reuptake Inhibitors (SNRIs)	
Venlafaxine	Effexor
Desvenlafaxine	Prestiq
Milnacipran	Savella
Levomilnacipran	Fetzima
Duloxetine	Cymbalta
Dual Action Drugs	
Vortioxetine	Brintellix
Vilazodone	Viibryd
Bipolar	
Aripiprazole	Abilify
Carbamazepine	Tegretol
Lamotrigine	Lamictal
Lithium carbonate	Eskalith, Lithobid
Lithium citrate	Cibalith-S
Valproic acid (and derivatives)	Depakene, Depakote

*Not currently available in the United States.
†Amoxapine is listed separately from the other tricyclics because it is a second-generation or atypical antidepressant.

CASE DISCUSSION

Ms. B's diagnosed mental disorders and their treatments may increase the likelihood of dental disease. Her medical history of schizoaffective disease may be treated with one or more agents that have variable efficacy and the potential for distressing side effects, drug interactions, and orofacial and dental disorders. Although early studies of the combination of antipsychotic drugs and antidepressants led to some manic episodes, newer agents are used to treat this disorder more successfully. Her earlier medications were replaced with newer drugs to produce fewer side effects. However, for her condition, the new medications continue to have the potential for extrapyramidal symptoms but more often different side effects, such as weight gain and sexual dysfunction. Xerostomia is still a risk, and this could contribute to caries in the future. Instruct the patient on good oral hygiene, a good diet, and regular dental check-ups with possible fluoride treatment. Her medical therapy may also contribute to drug interactions with vasoconstrictors, sedative drugs, and drugs metabolized by cytochrome P450. Dental drug doses should be limited to reduce interactions. Like many psychiatric patients, she struggles with cigarette abuse and its harmful effects. You may elect to treat these patients with smoking cessation agents like nicotine replacement products, bupropion, or varenicline. Placebo-controlled trials suggest that such treatments can help and do not interfere with antipsychotic treatment; however, individual case reports note that varenicline may exacerbate schizophrenic or bipolar symptoms. In any case the patient should be urged to take steps to stop smoking. This patient needs dental therapy and can be treated, but with knowledge of the agents used. Dry mouth, caries, bruxism, oral dyskinesias, periodontal disease, and possible changes in bone formation may need treatment.

GENERAL REFERENCES

1. Dale E, Bang-Andersen B, Sánchez C: Emerging mechanisms and treatments for depression beyond SSRIs and SNRIs, *Biochem Pharmacol.* 95(2):81–97, May 15, 2015.
2. Drug Bank http://www.drugbank.ca/w/databases (an extensive database for drugs and their actions, accessed November 13, 2015).
3. Drugs for psychiatric disorders, *The Medical Letter* 130:53–64, June 11, 2013.
4. Dwoskin LP, Rauhut AS, King-Pospisil KA, et al.: Review of the pharmacology and clinical profile of bupropion, an antidepressant and tobacco use cessation agent, *CNS Drug Reviews* 10(3–4):178–207, 2006.
5. Finnerup NB, Attal N, Haroutounian S, et al.: Pharmacotherapy for neuropathic pain in adults: a systematic review and meta-analysis, *The Lancet Neurology* 14(2):162–173, February 2015.
6. George M, Amrutheshwar R, Rajkumar RP, et al.: Newer antipsychotics and upcoming molecules for schizophrenia, *Eur J Clin Pharmacol* 69(8):1497–1509, August 2013, http://dx.doi.org/10.1007/s00228-013-1498-4. Epub April 2, 2013.
7. Leucht S, Cipriani A, Spineli L, et al.: Comparative efficacy and tolerability of 15 antipsychotic drugs in schizophrenia: a multiple-treatments meta-analysis, *Lancet* 382:951–962, 2013.
8. Network and Pathway Analysis Subgroup of Psychiatric Genomics Consortium: Psychiatric genome-wide association study analyses implicate neuronal, immune and histone pathways, *Nat Neurosci.* 18(2):199–209, February 2015.
9. O'Leary OF, Dinan TG, Cryan JF: Faster, better, stronger: towards new antidepressant therapeutic strategies, *Eur J Pharmacol* 753:32–50, April 15, 2015.
10. Solismaa A, Kampman O, Seppälä N, et al.: Polymorphism in alpha 2A adrenergic receptor gene is associated with sialorrhea in schizophrenia patients on clozapine treatment, *Hum Psychopharmacol* 29(4):336–341, 2014.
11. Supercyp http://bioinformatics.charite.de/supercyp/ (Information on drugs and their cytochrome metabolism accessed November 13, 2015).
12. Warren KR, Postolache TT, Groer ME, et al.: Role of chronic stress and depression in periodontal diseases, *Periodontol 2000* 64(1):107–138, February 2014.

11

Sedative-Hypnotics, Antianxiety Drugs, and Centrally Acting Muscle Relaxants*

Joseph A. Giovannitti Jr. and Matthew R. Cooke

KEY INFORMATION

- Central nervous system (CNS) depressants relieve anxiety, produce sedation, and induce sleep, unconsciousness, and muscle relaxation.
- Benzodiazepines and benzodiazepine-like drugs are the most commonly prescribed sleep aids.
- Benzodiazepines have a wide margin of safety except when combined with other CNS depressants, such as alcohol.
- Benzodiazepines and barbiturates act at the GABA receptor complex to increase Cl^- influx with resultant membrane hyperpolarization and decreased neuronal activity.
- Benzodiazepines interact at a specific subunit of the $GABA_A$ receptor and are reversed by flumazenil.
- Benzodiazepines are subject to drug interactions involving the CYP 3A4 isoenzymes.
- Zolpidem, zaleplon, and eszopiclone are less prone to drug interactions involving CYP 3A4 isoenzymes and are reversed by flumazenil.
- Barbiturates produce dose-dependent depression of the CNS, cardiovascular, and respiratory systems and have limited use in dentistry.
- The α_2-receptor agonists clonidine and dexmedetomidine produce sedation and modulate the adrenergic stress response without loss of consciousness. Tizanidine has central muscle relaxant properties in patients with spastic disorders such as cerebral palsy.

CASE STUDY

Ms. G is a 60-year-old patient with moderate dental anxiety who presents in your office for multiple dental extractions. Her medical history is significant for hypertension, for which she takes verapamil 40 mg three times a day. Her BMI is 21.6, and her history is otherwise noncontributory. You administer an oral dose of triazolam 0.25 mg while she sits in the waiting room. After she is feeling less anxious, you accompany her to the dental operatory and begin the procedure. After about an hour, you notice that she is no longer responsive and seems to be unconscious. Her vital signs are stable, and she is breathing normally. What are the possible causes of this unexpected reaction?

The drugs discussed in this chapter have the common pharmacologic characteristic of being CNS depressants, and they are capable of inducing various clinical responses, including relief of anxiety, sedative-hypnotic effects, and centrally acting muscle relaxation. Although all such drugs induce CNS impairment, drugs in certain categories have some degree of selectivity that determines their therapeutic indications in medical and dental practice. Pharmacokinetic differences and differences in mechanisms of action often distinguish these agents.

The drugs discussed in this chapter can be viewed as having dose-dependent, CNS-depressing effects progressing through anxiolysis, sedation, hypnosis, anesthesia, and ultimately death if the dose is sufficiently high. As anxiolytics, these drugs reduce the anxiety response; as sedatives, they produce relaxation, calmness, and decreased motor activity without loss of consciousness. As hypnotics, they induce drowsiness and a depressed state of consciousness that resembles natural sleep, with decreased motor activity and impaired sensory responsiveness. As anesthetics, these drugs cause a state of unconsciousness from which the patient cannot be aroused.

Insomnia is the salient feature of the nearly 90 different forms of sleep disorders. Epidemiologic studies report that insomnia is widespread, affecting one-third of the population. Insomnia is more prevalent among women than men and is more common in elderly individuals than in younger individuals. Benzodiazepine receptor agonists are currently the most commonly prescribed sleep aids. An advantage of benzodiazepines and related drugs is their wide margin of safety.

Anxiety is one of the most common psychiatric disorders. In the United States, approximately 8% of the population has an anxiety disorder during any given 6-month period. Although most individuals have certain periods and degrees of anxiety, pharmacotherapy is indicated only when anxiety begins to interfere with daily life. Similarly, pharmacotherapy should be considered when situational anxiety, such as might be experienced by a patient in anticipation of an operative or diagnostic procedure, is judged to be sufficient to compromise clinical care.

The *Diagnostic and Statistical Manual of Mental Disorders* (DSM-V) characterizes specific anxiety disorders. These include panic disorder with or without agoraphobia, agoraphobia without panic disorder, generalized anxiety disorder, obsessive-compulsive disorder, acute stress disorder, posttraumatic stress disorder, social phobia, specific (simple) phobia, substance-induced anxiety disorder, and anxiety resulting from a general medical condition. The major emphasis in this chapter is on drugs effective against anxiety as a symptom rather than as a specific disorder. Although antianxiety drugs have applications

*The authors wish to recognize Dr. Paul A. Moore for his past contributions to this chapter.

for treatment of anxiety disorders in general, other drugs, including tricyclic antidepressants, selective serotonin reuptake inhibitors, and monoamine oxidase inhibitors are used in the pharmacotherapy of panic disorders, phobic disorders, and obsessive-compulsive disorders. These latter agents are discussed in detail in Chapter 10.

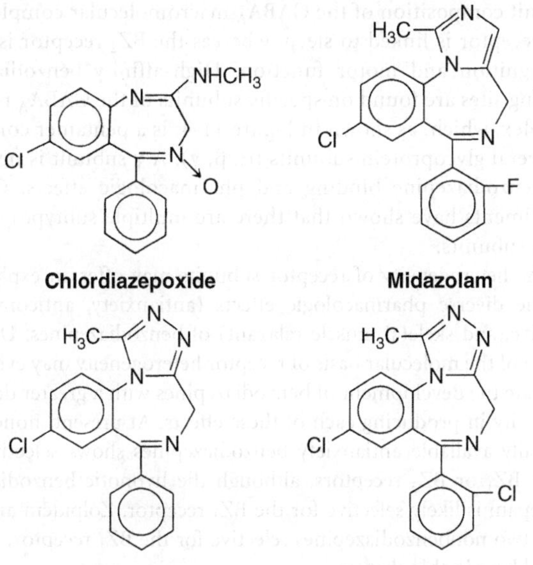

Chlordiazepoxide Midazolam

Alprazolam Triazolam

FIG 11-1 Structural formulas of chlordiazepoxide, the first benzodiazepine used clinically; midazolam, an imidazobenzodiazepine; and the triazolobenzodiazepines alprazolam and triazolam. Triazolam is derived from alprazolam by the addition of a chlorine atom on the ortho position of the phenyl group. Estazolam is formed from alprazolam by removal of the methyl group of the triazolo ring (not shown).

With their introduction in the 1960s, the benzodiazepines became extremely popular drugs because they were found to have anxiolytic selectivity and to be relatively safe even after overt overdose, unlike earlier drugs. Nonetheless, sedation is a prominent side effect of the benzodiazepines, and additive CNS depression occurs if other CNS depressants are used concurrently. The possibility that antianxiety and CNS depressant properties are pharmacologically distinguishable has been raised again with the introduction of buspirone, an azapirone derivative, which is an effective antianxiety agent with little or no sedative properties.

The usefulness and effectiveness of any given antianxiety agent varies depending on the patient, the clinical surroundings, the "chairside" manner of the dentist, the route of administration, and the properties of the chosen drug. Knowledge of the pharmacologic characteristics of the various antianxiety agents is crucial for selecting the proper drug, avoiding drug interactions, and obtaining the desired therapeutic response with minimal adverse side effects.

BENZODIAZEPINES

Benzodiazepines are among the most widely used drug classes in the history of medicine because of their selectivity and margin of safety. Currently, several dozen benzodiazepines are marketed throughout the world.

Chemistry and Structure-Activity Relationships

The structures of the pharmacologically active 1,4-benzodiazepines are shown in Figure 11-1 and Table 11-1. All benzodiazepines currently available in the United States are derived from the basic molecule shown in Table 11-1, to which are added various substituent groups. Slight modifications of the basic structure have produced

TABLE 11-1 Chemical Structures of Various Benzodiazepines

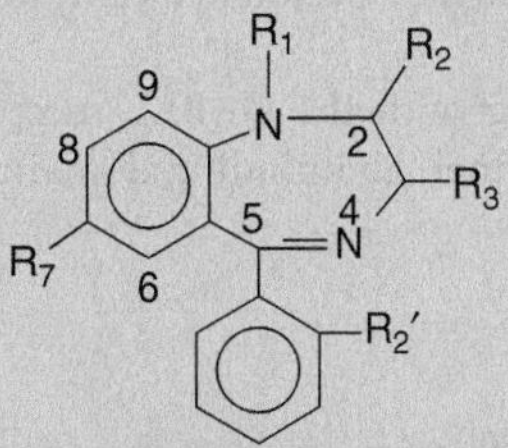

Drug	R_1	R_2	R_3	R_7	R_2'
	SUBSTITUENT GROUPS				
Alprazolam	See Fig. 11-1				
Chlordiazepoxide	See Fig. 11-1				
Clonazepam	—H	=O	—H	$—NO_2$	—Cl
Clorazepate	—H	=O	—COOH	—Cl	—H
Diazepam	$—CH_3$	=O	—H	—Cl	—H
Estazolam	See Fig. 11-1				
Flurazepam	$—CH_2CH_2N(C_2H_5)_2$	=O	—H	—Cl	—F
Halazepam	$—CH_2CF_3$	=O	—H	—Cl	—H
Lorazepam	—H	=O	—OH	—Cl	—Cl
Midazolam	See Fig. 11-1				
Oxazepam	—H	=O	—OH	—Cl	—H
Prazepam	$—CH_2—$◁	=O	—H	—Cl	—H
Quazepam	$—CH_2CF_3$	=S	—H	—Cl	—F
Temazepam	$—CH_3$	=O	—OH	—Cl	—H
Triazolam	See Fig. 11-1				

triazolobenzodiazepines (e.g., alprazolam, triazolam) and imidazobenzodiazepines (e.g., midazolam).

All benzodiazepines with psychopharmacologic activity have an electronegative group at R_7. A chlorine atom seems to confer optimal activity, whereas bromo and nitro substitutions are only weakly anxiolytic. A nitro moiety at R_7 enhances antiseizure properties, as illustrated by clonazepam, which is used as an anticonvulsant. Hydrogen or methyl groups at R_7 significantly reduce pharmacologic activity. Substitution at position 5 with any group other than a phenyl ring also reduces activity. Halogenation at R_2 increases potency; larger alkyl substitutions decrease it. Substitution on the nitrogen at R_1 with a methyl group enhances activity, as do methyl or hydrogen groups at R_3.

Mechanism of Action

Perhaps the most exciting and significant advance in the understanding of anxiety and the mechanism of action of benzodiazepines occurred with the discovery of specific benzodiazepine binding sites in the brain and the understanding that these were in some way linked to the inhibitory neurotransmitter γ-aminobutyric acid (GABA). As shown schematically in Figure 11-2, when the GABA receptor is activated, the Cl^- channel opens, allowing Cl^- influx, membrane hyperpolarization, and neuronal inhibition. Benzodiazepines, by interacting at high-affinity benzodiazepine binding sites on the GABA receptor complex, facilitate GABA action. Although the exact mechanism by which benzodiazepines accomplish this is not fully delineated, it is known that they increase the frequency at which Cl^- channels open in response to GABA.

Benzodiazepine receptors are linked to a specific GABA receptor subtype, the **$GABA_A$ receptor** (see Fig. 11-2). Figure 11-3 provides further details on binding domains associated with the $GABA_A$ receptor. Historically, GABA receptors have been classified into two subtypes: the Cl^- channel-linked $GABA_A$ receptors and the G protein-linked $GABA_B$ receptors. Benzodiazepine-sensitive $GABA_A$ receptors are activated by GABA agonists, such as muscimol (a hallucinogen), and blocked by GABA antagonists, such as picrotoxin and bicuculline (convulsants). $GABA_B$ receptors are benzodiazepine and bicuculline insensitive and are activated by baclofen, a centrally acting muscle relaxant.

The benzodiazepine receptor—along with the $GABA_A$ receptor, a barbiturate receptor, the Cl^- channel, and binding domains for other drugs—forms a single macromolecular complex. Similar to GABA receptors, benzodiazepine receptors are heterogeneous; there are at least three types: type 1 (BZ_1), type 2 (BZ_2), and the "peripheral type" benzodiazepine receptor, also known as 18K Dalton translocator protein. The function of the latter is unknown. The presence of BZ_1 and BZ_2 receptor types is determined by the subunit composition of the $GABA_A$ macromolecular complex. The BZ_1 receptor is linked to sleep, whereas the BZ_2 receptor is linked to cognition and motor function. High-affinity benzodiazepine binding sites are found on specific subunits of the $GABA_A$ receptor complex, which, as shown in Figure 11-4, is a pentamer composed of several glycoprotein subunits (α, β, γ). A γ subunit is necessary for benzodiazepine binding and pharmacologic effects. Cloning experiments have shown that there are multiple subtypes of α, β, and γ subunits.

The heterogeneity of receptor subunits may offer an explanation for the diverse pharmacologic effects (antianxiety, anticonvulsant, sedative, and skeletal muscle relaxant) of benzodiazepines. Determination of the molecular basis of receptor heterogeneity may eventually facilitate the development of benzodiazepines with a greater degree of selectivity in producing each of these effects. At present, none of the clinically available antianxiety benzodiazepines shows selectivity for either BZ_1 or BZ_2 receptors, although the hypnotic benzodiazepine quazepam is likely selective for the BZ_1 receptor. Zolpidem and zaleplon, two nonbenzodiazepines selective for the BZ_1 receptor, are discussed later in this chapter.

The benzodiazepine-insensitive $GABA_B$ receptors coupled to G proteins are associated with a decrease in Ca^{2+} conductance and an increase in K^+ conductance and could be expected to cause pharmacologic effects when stimulated or antagonized. $GABA_B$ receptors are less widely distributed than $GABA_A$ receptors but are found in high concentrations in the cerebral cortex and cerebellum. Subtypes of $GABA_B$ receptors may exist. $GABA_B$ receptors have not been studied as extensively as $GABA_A$ receptors, but they may participate in blood pressure regulation in addition to muscle activity and offer a potential site for therapeutic drug action.

The existence of subclasses of benzodiazepine receptors suggests that some agents, with specific activity for individual receptor subtypes, may be more selective than others in terms of their pharmacologic profile.

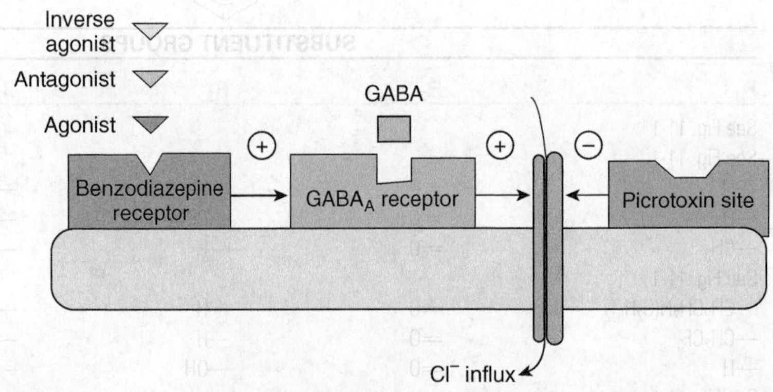

FIG 11-2 Schematic of the γ-aminobutyric acid $(GABA)_A$ receptor complex illustrating the sites of action of benzodiazepine agonists, antagonists, and GABA. The benzodiazepine receptor is coupled to the $GABA_A$ receptor so that its activation facilitates (denoted by the *plus sign*) the action of GABA on the Cl^- ionophore. Increased Cl^- influx leads to hyperpolarization (i.e., inhibition) of the neuron. Benzodiazepine antagonists inhibit the binding of benzodiazepines. Inverse agonists inhibit the constitutive activity of the benzodiazepine-$GABA_A$ receptor complex by binding to the benzodiazepine receptor. Also illustrated is the picrotoxin site, which, when acted on by picrotoxin, antagonizes (*minus sign*) the influx of Cl^- and can lead to convulsions.

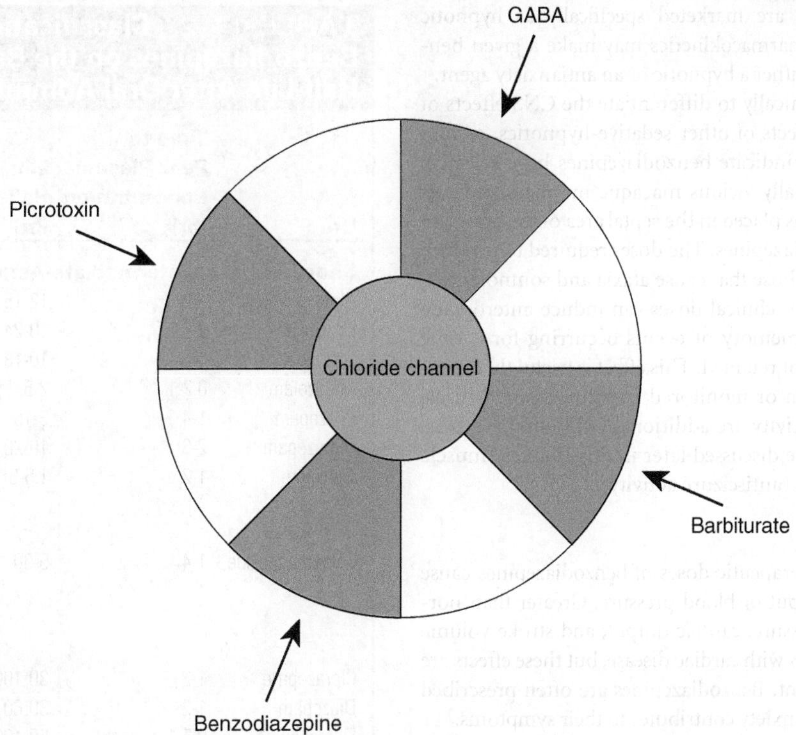

FIG 11-3 Arrangement of allosteric binding domains on the γ-aminobutyric acid *(GABA)$_A$* receptor complex. The complex is composed of five unique subunits. Multiple receptor subtypes are possible on the basis of different combinations of the subunits. Binding sites for picrotoxin (a convulsant), barbiturates, GABA, and benzodiazepines are presented for illustrative purposes. In addition, distinct binding sites for other chemical agents have been identified (shown as blank areas). The figure does not identify which receptor subunits are involved in the binding of each drug. (Adapted from Sieghart W: $GABA_A$ receptors: ligand-gated Cl^- ion channels modulated by multiple drug-binding sites. *Trends Pharmacol Sci* 13:446-450, 1992.)

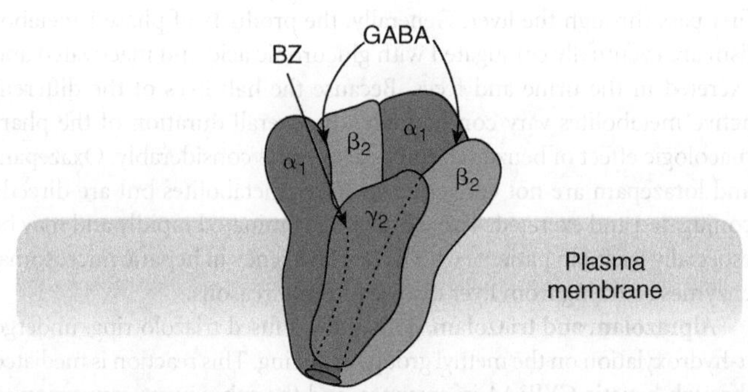

FIG 11-4 Structural model of the γ-aminobutyric acid (*GABA*)-benzodiazepine (*BZ*) receptor complex. The arrangement of the subunits (*α, β, γ*) forms the Cl^- channel. GABA binding sites are illustrated at the two analogous interfaces between the α and β subunits. The BZ binding site is associated with the interface of the α and γ subunits. (Adapted from Zorumski CF, Isenberg KE: Insights into the structure and function of GABA-benzodiazepine receptors: ion channels and psychiatry. *Am J Psychiatry* 148:162-173, 1991.)

Quazepam, a long-acting benzodiazepine hypnotic, produces sedation but seems to have little ataxic effect and may cause less tolerance than other benzodiazepines. Of all currently available benzodiazepines, only quazepam, one of its active metabolites (1-oxoquazepam), and possibly the antianxiety agent halazepam have some selectivity for the BZ_1 receptor subtype. These benzodiazepines differ chemically from other benzodiazepines by having a trifluoroethyl substituent (see Table 11-1), which may be responsible for BZ_1 selectivity. Selective activity at the BZ_1 receptor has not been associated with any special clinical benefit of quazepam, however, compared with other benzodiazepines for treating insomnia.

Although the pharmacologic actions of benzodiazepines are closely tied to GABA receptors, numerous other neurotransmitters, including glycine, norepinephrine, and 5-hydroxytryptamine (5-HT), have been suggested to play a role in their action. An interaction between GABA and 5-HT has been shown experimentally with diazepam and tryptaminergic anxiolytics. This finding is interesting in light of the mechanism of action of the nonsedating antianxiety agent buspirone (see later), a 5-HT_{1A} partial agonist.

Pharmacologic Effects

Benzodiazepines have clinically useful antianxiety, sedative-hypnotic, amnestic, anticonvulsant, and skeletal muscle relaxant properties. Benzodiazepines previously were thought to differ pharmacologically only in terms of their pharmacokinetics. However, certain benzodiazepines seem to have unique properties. Alprazolam has documented antidepressant and antipanic properties, and diazepam may be more selective as a skeletal muscle relaxant than other benzodiazepines. **Diazepam** is the only benzodiazepine approved for the treatment of skeletal muscle spasm and spasticity of CNS origin.

Central nervous system

All benzodiazepines produce a dose-dependent depression of the CNS. Drowsiness and sedation are common manifestations of this central depressant action and may be considered a side effect in some instances and therapeutically useful in others. Some benzodiazepines, such as flurazepam and temazepam, are marketed specifically as hypnotic agents. Differences in their pharmacokinetics may make a given benzodiazepine more suitable as either a hypnotic or an antianxiety agent.

Although it is difficult clinically to differentiate the CNS effects of benzodiazepines from the effects of other sedative-hypnotics, certain experimental animal models indicate benzodiazepines have selective antianxiety properties. Normally vicious macaque monkeys and rats made highly irritable by lesions placed in the septal area of the brain are tamed and calmed by benzodiazepines. The doses required to produce these effects are one tenth of those that cause ataxia and somnolence.

Certain benzodiazepines in clinical doses can induce anterograde amnesia, which means that memory of events occurring for a time after drug administration is not retained. This effect is useful therapeutically in intravenous sedation or monitored anesthesia care. Muscle relaxation and antiseizure activity are additional CNS effects of benzodiazepines. These effects are discussed later in this chapter (muscle relaxation) and in Chapter 12 (antiseizure activity).

Cardiovascular system

In a healthy adult, normal therapeutic doses of benzodiazepines cause few alterations in cardiac output or blood pressure. Greater than normal doses decrease blood pressure, cardiac output, and stroke volume in normal subjects and patients with cardiac disease, but these effects are usually not clinically significant. Benzodiazepines are often prescribed for cardiac patients in whom anxiety contributes to their symptoms.

Respiratory system

In normal doses, benzodiazepines have little effect on respiration in healthy individuals, but significant respiratory depression may occur with increasing dosages. Benzodiazepines may cause additive respiratory depressant effects with other CNS depressant drugs, especially alcohol and opioids. **Midazolam**, used primarily as an oral premedicant, and for intravenous sedation and the induction of anesthesia, can cause respiratory depression and apnea.

TABLE 11-2 Classification of Benzodiazepines on the Basis of Elimination Half-Life After Oral Administration

Drug	Time to Peak Plasma Concentration (hr)	Elimination Half-Life (hr)	Major Active Metabolites
Short-Acting to Intermediate-Acting			
Alprazolam	1-2	12-15	α-Hydroxyalprazolam
Estazolam	2	10-24	None
Lorazepam	1-6	10-18	None
Midazolam	0.2-1	2-5	α-Hydroxymidazolam
Oxazepam	1-4	5-15	None
Temazepam	2-3	10-20	None
Triazolam	1-2	1.5-5	α-Hydroxytriazolam
Long-Acting			
Chlordiazepoxide	1-4	5-30	Desmethyl-chlordiazepoxide Demoxepam Desmethyldiazepam
Clorazepate*	1-2	30-100	Desmethyldiazepam
Diazepam	1-2	30-60	Desmethyldiazepam
Flurazepam*	0.5-1	50-100	N-Desalkylflurazepam
Halazepam	1-3	14	Desmethyldiazepam
Prazepam*	2.5-6	30-100	Desmethyldiazepam
Quazepam	2	40	2-Oxo-quazepam N-Desalkylflurazepam

*Does not reach the circulation as the parent drug in clinically significant amounts. Values reflect the primary metabolite.

Absorption, Fate, and Excretion

The pharmacokinetics of individual benzodiazepines differ, and there is a wide range in speed of onset and duration of action among these compounds. Benzodiazepines frequently are classified according to their elimination half-life, as illustrated in Table 11-2; however, the elimination half-life of a given drug is only one factor affecting its clinical profile. The rates of drug absorption and tissue distribution and redistribution are often important factors in determining onset and duration of clinical effects after short-term administration. Additionally, there is a wide variation in drug half-lives among patients.

After oral administration, most benzodiazepines are rapidly absorbed and highly bound to plasma protein. **Lorazepam, oxazepam,** prazepam, and temazepam are more slowly absorbed. Peak blood concentrations are generally obtained in 1 to 3 hours. A highly lipid-soluble drug such as diazepam exerts its effect more rapidly, whereas lorazepam, which is less lipid-soluble, has a slower onset of action even after systemic absorption. Diazepam also accumulates in body fat because of its lipophilic properties, and it is slowly eliminated from these stores. This characteristic partially accounts for the prolonged half-life of diazepam, which can range from 1 to 4 days.

Many benzodiazepines are converted to pharmacologically active metabolites that have long half-lives (Fig. 11-5). Clorazepate and prazepam are nearly completely converted (in the stomach and liver) to the long-acting metabolite desmethyldiazepam (nordazepam) before they enter the systemic circulation. Desmethyldiazepam is a metabolite of many other benzodiazepines, including **chlordiazepoxide**, diazepam, and halazepam. Flurazepam is also converted to active metabolites in its first pass through the liver. Generally, the products of phase I metabolism are eventually conjugated with glucuronic acid and inactivated and excreted in the urine and feces. Because the half-lives of the different active metabolites vary considerably, the overall duration of the pharmacologic effect of benzodiazepines also varies considerably. Oxazepam and lorazepam are not converted to active metabolites but are directly conjugated and excreted. These drugs are eliminated rapidly and may be especially useful in patients who have a deficiency in hepatic microsomal enzymes resulting from liver disease or other reasons.

Alprazolam and triazolam, containing a fused triazolo ring, undergo α-hydroxylation on the methyl group of the ring. This reaction is mediated through hepatic CYP3A4 isoenzymes, and the subsequent conversion to the glucuronide occurs rapidly in the case of triazolam and accounts for the short duration of action of the drug. Midazolam, which contains a fused imidazo ring, is quickly metabolized in a similar manner. Midazolam has a rapid onset of action, a high metabolic clearance, a rapid rate of elimination, and a short duration of action. Termination of CNS activity is a result of peripheral redistribution and metabolic transformation. It is converted into several metabolites that have little pharmacologic activity; however, because of extensive first-pass metabolism, the α-hydroxy metabolite may contribute to the sedative effect when midazolam is given orally to children.

The poor oral bioavailability of triazolam, alprazolam, and midazolam of approximately 50% is believed to be due to CYP3A4 metabolism in the gut wall and hepatic first-pass metabolism. Triazolam's availability is improved when administered sublingually. Inhibition of CYP3A4 metabolism by coadministration of itraconazole, erythromycin, or grapefruit juice can significantly increase maximum blood concentrations of these short-acting benzodiazepines.

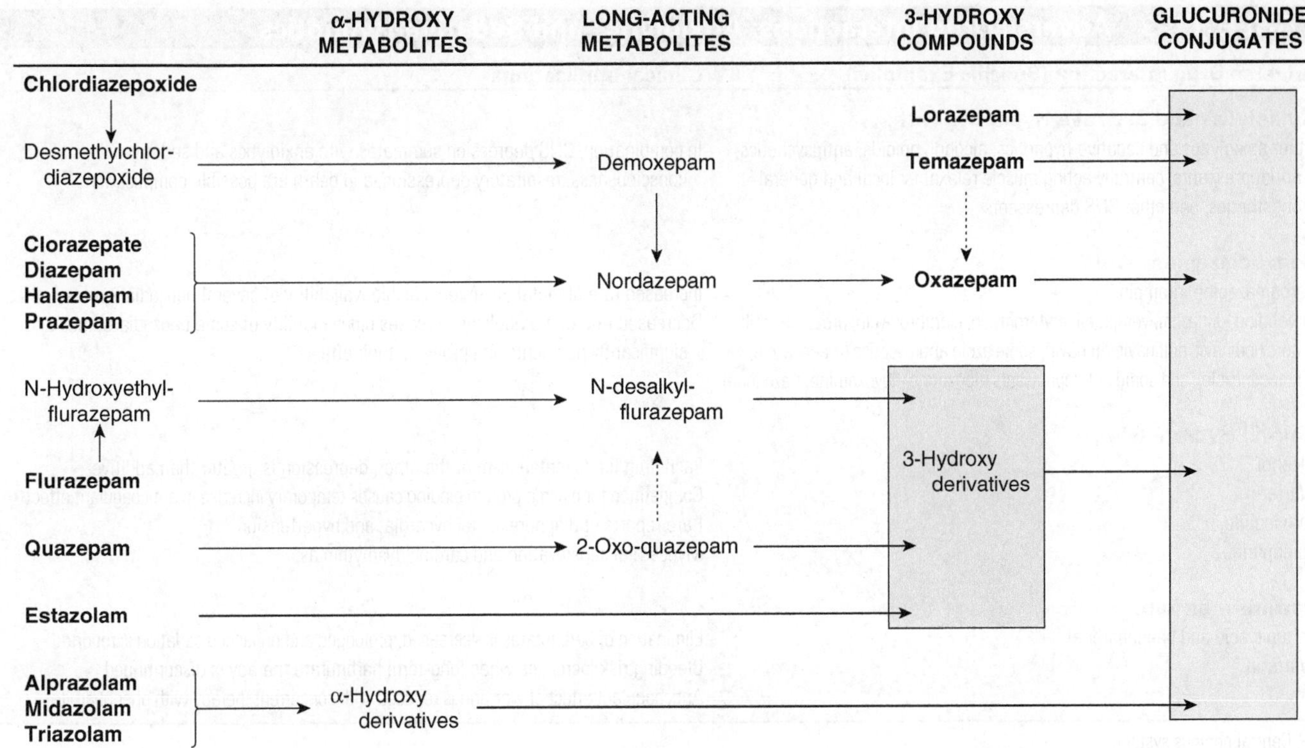

FIG 11-5 Metabolism of benzodiazepines. Drugs available for clinical use appear in **bold type**. With the exception of the prodrugs clorazepate and prazepam, only the glucuronide conjugates are inactive.

Many benzodiazepines are biotransformed to long-acting metabolites. These metabolites, which accumulate with repeated administration, are the cause of lingering residual effects. An active metabolite of flurazepam and quazepam, N-desalkylflurazepam, which accounts for some of the activity of quazepam and nearly all the activity of flurazepam, has an elimination half-life of 50 to 100 hours. In sleep laboratory studies, it has been shown that flurazepam does not reach full effectiveness until the second or third consecutive night of intake. Quazepam decreases sleep latency and facilitates sleep maintenance after a single dose.

Temazepam has a half-life of 10-20 hours, and only a very small amount of oxazepam is formed as a metabolite; estazolam has a similar half-life and forms a short-lived active metabolite. Triazolam, with a mean half-life of 2.9 hours, is converted to metabolites that, although active, are rapidly eliminated. Because of their short durations of action, temazepam and triazolam do not generally accumulate even with repeated nightly use. Triazolam is indicated for patients who have difficulty falling asleep but who stay asleep when sleep ensues.

Adverse Effects and Drug Interactions

Drowsiness is the most common side effect of benzodiazepines. This may be a therapeutic benefit in anxiety states that cause insomnia. Other signs and symptoms of dose-dependent CNS depression include ataxia, incoordination, dysarthria, confusion, apathy, muscle weakness, dizziness, and somnolence. Individuals over the age of 65 seem to be particularly susceptible, and individuals with a history of alcohol or barbiturate abuse seem to be particularly resistant to the gross CNS depressant properties of benzodiazepines.

Elderly and young patients occasionally respond to benzodiazepines with excitement rather than depression. Excitatory CNS effects may include an increased incidence of nightmares, hyperactivity, insomnia, irritability, agitation, and rage and hostility. Because these responses differ from what would be expected of a CNS depressant, they have been termed **paradoxic reactions**, similar to the disinhibition observed with alcohol.

Allergic reactions to benzodiazepines are rare and usually manifest as minor skin rashes. Because injectable formulations of diazepam contain propylene glycol and ethyl alcohol solvents, intramuscular and intravenous administration can cause local pain, phlebitis, and thrombosis. Phlebitis is more likely to occur if a vein in the hand or wrist is used and may be more common after repeated injections, especially in heavy smokers, elderly individuals, and women taking oral contraceptives. With the introduction of the water-soluble benzodiazepine midazolam, the occurrence of venous complications and pain at the injection site has diminished.

Tolerance and psychological dependence develop frequently with benzodiazepines, but true physical dependence is less common. Tolerance to the sedative-hypnotic effects of benzodiazepines is slower to develop with longer acting agents. In cases of physical dependence, the severity of withdrawal depends on the dose of the drug being used and the drug's half-life. Rapid discontinuation of benzodiazepines, especially short-acting compounds, can lead to symptoms of withdrawal. Often these symptoms are nearly identical to the symptoms for which treatment was initiated, including anxiety, irritability, insomnia, and fatigue. The symptoms become more severe with high doses and prolonged treatment. Withdrawal can be minimized by reducing the dosage very gradually (≤10% per day over 10 to 14 days) or by the use of longer acting compounds.

Mechanisms involved in the development of tolerance are unknown, but the long-term administration of benzodiazepines to animals causes downregulation of benzodiazepine receptors, which could be a contributing factor. Flumazenil, a benzodiazepine antagonist (described later), can reverse benzodiazepine overdose. Flumazenil can precipitate withdrawal in benzodiazepine-dependent patients, however.

Despite these problems, one of the major advantages of benzodiazepines compared with other sedatives is their high margin of safety. Death is

TABLE 11-3 **Adverse Drug Interactions: Anxiolytics and Sedative-Hypnotics**

Adverse Drug Interaction (Specific Examples)	Clinical Implications
Anxiolytics and Sedative-Hypnotics with:	
Other anxiolytics and sedative-hypnotics, alcohol, opioids, antipsychotics, antidepressants, centrally acting muscle relaxants, local and general anesthetics, and other CNS depressants	In combination, CNS depression summates with anxiolytics and sedatives; loss of consciousness, respiratory depression, and death are possible complications
Benzodiazepines with:	
Carbamazepine, rifampin	Increased rate of metabolism reduces bioavailability of several benzodiazepines
Cimetidine, diltiazem, verapamil, erythromycin, clarithromycin, protease inhibitors (indinavir, nelfinavir, ritonavir), some azole antimycotics (itraconazole, ketoconazole), and some antidepressants (fluoxetine, fluvoxamine, trazodone)	Decreased rate of metabolism increases bioavailability of some benzodiazepines and significantly augments and prolongs their effects
Chloral Hydrate with:	
Alcohol	Each drug limits metabolism of the other; depression is greater than additive
Warfarin	Competition for plasma protein binding causes temporary increase in anticoagulant effect
Furosemide	Rare reports of diaphoresis, tachycardia, and hypertension
Epinephrine	Myocardial sensitization and cardiac dysrhythmias
Barbiturates with:	
Valproic acid and phenobarbital	Elimination of barbiturates is decreased; prolonged and enhanced sedation is reported
Warfarin	Bleeding risk increases when long-term barbiturate therapy is discontinued Anticoagulant effect of warfarin is reduced with concurrent therapy with phenobarbital

CNS, Central nervous system.

rare in cases of overdose and is usually the result of a combination of drugs (especially alcohol) with benzodiazepines. The few deaths associated with the use of a benzodiazepine alone have primarily involved elderly patients, very young children, massive iatrogenic overdosing, or suicides.

Benzodiazepines cross the placental barrier. During the first trimester, long-term use of these drugs has been associated with increased fetal malformations, including cleft lip and cleft palate in humans. There is no clear estimate of the risk after single-dose use. All benzodiazepines are classified as pregnancy category D except triazolam, which is pregnancy category X. It is generally agreed that these drugs should be avoided during pregnancy.

Drug interactions associated with anxiolytic and sedative drugs used in dentistry are listed in Table 11-3. The **therapeutic index** for benzodiazepines is normally so **large** that wide ranges of dosing recommendations and blood concentrations do not significantly affect their safety and efficacy. Plasma concentrations after a given dose may normally vary such that a minor shift in elimination from drug interactions is unlikely to result in an overdose.

Rifampin induces metabolic enzymes in the gut and liver responsible for the metabolism of diazepam, midazolam, and triazolam. A 96% reduction in the bioavailability of midazolam has been reported. Triazolam is so rapidly and effectively metabolized in the gut that peak plasma concentrations are only 12% of normal. This **interaction between rifampin and triazolam** is one of the most pronounced alterations in drug kinetics ever reported. The almost complete loss of triazolam bioavailability and subsequent efficacy is quite significant and warrants use of an alternative anxiolytic, such as oral oxazepam, nitrous oxide inhalation, or an intravenous agent. The anticonvulsant carbamazepine can also induce hepatic enzymes for the oxidative metabolism of benzodiazepines such as alprazolam, triazolam, and midazolam. Decreased benzodiazepine plasma concentrations and greatly reduced sedative effects after oral administration of these agents may occur. This interaction may be important in medicine because of loss of seizure control. A loss of sedative efficacy in dentistry may also occur. Benzodiazepines that are metabolized solely through glucuronidation, such as oxazepam, are suitable alternative agents for sedation in these situations.

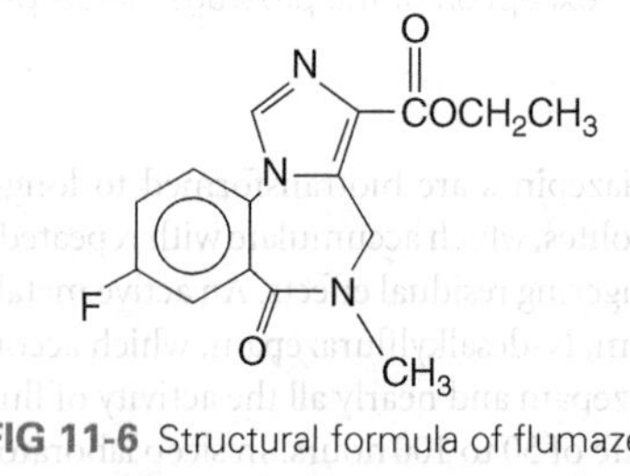

FIG 11-6 Structural formula of flumazenil.

The Ca^{2+} channel blockers verapamil and diltiazem have been shown to inhibit the CYP3A isozymes required for the metabolism of triazolam and midazolam. Peak blood concentrations of these benzodiazepines can be increased twofold to threefold and can be associated with increased sedation and performance deficits. Avoidance of this combination is recommended, particularly in elderly patients known to be sensitive to benzodiazepines.

Cimetidine and ranitidine also inhibit the oxidative metabolism of certain benzodiazepines, such as midazolam, diazepam, triazolam, and alprazolam. An increased and prolonged level of sedation after oral administration may occur because of the decreased first-pass metabolism. Benzodiazepines that are metabolized directly to the glucuronide conjugate (e.g., oxazepam) are not affected. Similarly, the antimicrobials erythromycin and clarithromycin and the azole antifungals ketoconazole and itraconazole are potential inhibitors of the hepatic isozymes required for oxidative metabolism of many benzodiazepines. By decreasing the first-pass effect and improving bioavailability, triazolam blood concentrations may increase significantly. The antiviral agents indinavir, nelfinavir, and ritonavir inhibit hepatic oxidative enzymes required for metabolism of many benzodiazepines. These significant pharmacokinetic drug interactions could potentially cause oversedation and respiratory depression.

Antagonists

The benzodiazepine antagonist **flumazenil** (Fig. 11-6) has clinical application in managing benzodiazepine overdose and in hastening

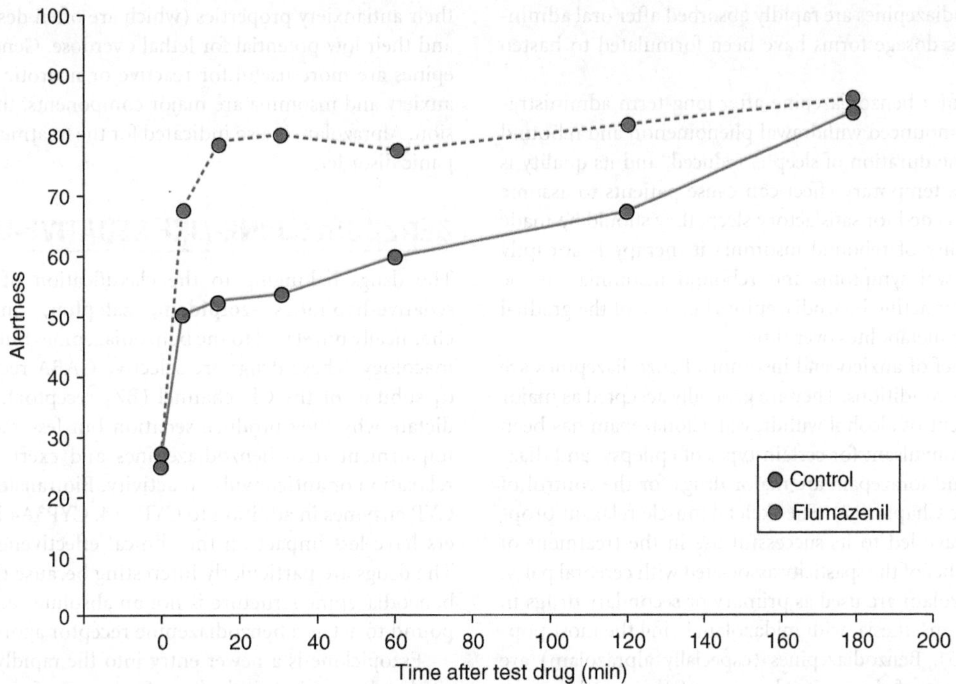

FIG 11-7 Reversal of midazolam sedation by flumazenil in patients undergoing a surgical dental extraction. Flumazenil or placebo was administered after intravenous midazolam and dental extraction. Differences between flumazenil and control groups were significant at the $P < 0.05$ level for the 5-, 15-, and 30-minute time periods. The *dashed line* represents the flumazenil group; the *solid line* represents the midazolam alone. (Adapted from Clark MS, Lindenmuth JE, Jafek BW, et al: Reversal of central benzodiazepine effects by intravenous flumazenil. *Anesth Prog* 38:12-16, 1991.)

recovery from benzodiazepine sedation or anesthesia. Flumazenil has been used successfully in reversing benzodiazepine-induced coma, but whether it should be given routinely to comatose patients when the cause of the coma is unknown is unclear. The routine use of flumazenil is not recommended in cases of mixed drug overdose, airway obstruction, or seizure disorders.

Flumazenil administered intravenously can generally reverse benzodiazepine-induced sedation in 1 to 2 minutes. In a study in which patients were sedated with midazolam before dental extraction, flumazenil significantly improved alertness compared with placebo controls (Fig. 11-7) only for the first 30 minutes after reversal. Thus, the duration of action of flumazenil (elimination half-life of 45 to 75 minutes) may likely be shorter than that of a benzodiazepine agonist, allowing for the possibility of recurrence of sedation and respiratory depression. Flumazenil is not a substitute for airway management, oxygen delivery by positive pressure when needed, and careful postoperative monitoring.

Another cautionary note is the possibility of flumazenil precipitating withdrawal in patients who are dependent on the benzodiazepines. Signs of benzodiazepine withdrawal include flushes, agitation, tremor, and seizures. In patients taking the benzodiazepine clonazepam for seizure control, flumazenil administration may initiate the onset of seizure activity.

General Therapeutic Uses

Pharmacotherapy for anxiety states is indicated only when anxiety becomes chronic or when it interferes with the individual's functioning. Benzodiazepines and other antianxiety agents are not curative; they merely treat the symptoms of anxiety. The patient then copes more effectively with the situation or responds more favorably to psychotherapy or other pharmacotherapy.

Approximately 35% of patients with a generalized anxiety disorder show marked improvement with benzodiazepines, 40% are moderately improved, and 25% remain unresponsive. These antianxiety agents are useful in the treatment of acute anxiety resulting from transient stress that is environmental, physical, or psychological in origin. For the treatment of longstanding anxiety, benzodiazepines ideally should be used only with appropriate psychotherapy. Table 11-4 lists benzodiazepines and other drugs used for the management of acute anxiety.

Although capable of selectively relieving anxiety, benzodiazepines are also capable of producing sedation and hypnosis. Some benzodiazepines—flurazepam, temazepam, triazolam, estazolam, and quazepam—are promoted specifically as hypnotics rather than as antianxiety agents. Whether a benzodiazepine is used primarily as an antianxiety agent or a hypnotic depends on a subtle interplay of the drug's pharmacodynamic properties, its pharmacokinetic characteristics, and the drug formulation.

During natural sleep, humans cycle through several stages of sleep ranging from the deepest stage, categorized as stage IV, to the most active form, known as rapid eye movement (REM) sleep. Benzodiazepines used as hypnotics increase stage II sleep at the expense of stages I, III, and IV and REM sleep. The significance of these changes is unknown, but a goal of the pharmacotherapy of insomnia is to achieve a normal sleep pattern. Sedative-hypnotic benzodiazepines may have an advantage over barbiturates with regard to REM sleep. Low doses of temazepam and flurazepam may leave REM sleep unaffected, and triazolam has such a short duration of effect that an early loss of REM cycles may be made up later in the same sleep period. Slow-wave sleep (as in stage IV) is now recognized as the most important restorative phase of sleep, and benzodiazepine suppression of slow-wave sleep may be problematic with long-term administration.

Because hypnotics are most commonly used for the treatment of patients who have difficulty falling asleep, rapid absorption is essential.

Most hypnotic benzodiazepines are rapidly absorbed after oral administration, and various dosage forms have been formulated to hasten absorption.

Discontinuation of a benzodiazepine after long-term administration can lead to a pronounced withdrawal phenomenon and rebound insomnia in which the duration of sleep is reduced, and its quality is affected. Because this temporary effect can cause patients to assume that the drug is still needed for satisfactory sleep, they should be made aware of the possibility of rebound insomnia if therapy is abruptly terminated. Withdrawal symptoms and rebound insomnia can be minimized with longer acting benzodiazepines because of the gradual decline of their active metabolites over time.

In addition to relief of anxiety and insomnia, benzodiazepines are useful for many other conditions. They are generally accepted as major drugs for the treatment of alcohol withdrawal. Clonazepam has been approved as an anticonvulsant for certain types of epilepsy, and diazepam, midazolam, and lorazepam are major drugs for the control of status epilepticus (see Chapter 12). The skeletal muscle relaxant properties of diazepam have led to its successful use in the treatment of tetanus and for the relief of the spasticity associated with cerebral palsy. Diazepam and midazolam are used as primary or secondary drugs in sedation and general anesthesia, with midazolam being the most popular (see Chapter 15). Benzodiazepines (especially alprazolam) are useful in the treatment of depression because of their rapid onset, their antianxiety properties (which are often desirable in depression), and their low potential for lethal overdose. Generally, the benzodiazepines are more useful for reactive or neurotic depression, in which anxiety and insomnia are major components, than for severe depression. Alprazolam is also indicated for the treatment of anxiety-initiated panic disorders.

TABLE 11-4 Preparations for Treatment of Anxiety

Drug	Usual Dose* (mg)	Route of Administration
Alprazolam	0.75-4.0 (adult)	Oral
	0.5-0.75 (elderly)	Oral
Clorazepate	15-60 (adult)	Oral
	7.5-15 (elderly)	Oral
Chlordiazepoxide	15-100 (adult)	Oral
	50-100 (adult)	IM, IV
	10-20 (elderly)	Oral
Diazepam	4-40 (adult)	Oral
	2-20 (adult)	IM, IV
	2-5 (elderly)	Oral
	0.3-0.6 mg/kg (children)	Oral
Lorazepam	1.5-10 (adult)	Oral
	1-2 (elderly)	Oral
	2-4 (adult)	IM, IV
Midazolam	2-10 (adult)	IM, IV
	0.25-1 mg/kg up to 20 mg (children)	Oral
Oxazepam	30-120 (adult)	Oral
	30-60 (elderly)	Oral
Triazolam	0.25-0.5 (adult)	Oral
	0.125 (elderly)	Oral
Hydroxyzine (hydrochloride and pamoate salts)†	200-600 (adult)	Oral
	25-100 (adult)	IM
	0.5-0.7 mg/kg (children)	Oral
	12.5-50 (children >6 yr)	Oral
	0.6-1.1 mg/kg (children)	IM

*Oral adult and elderly doses represent daily amounts given in divided doses (except triazolam). Parenteral, children, and triazolam doses reflect single administration.

†The pamoate salt is reported to be converted to the hydrochloride salt in the stomach, with a resultant prolonged effect, but there is no experimental evidence to support this claim.

IM, Intramuscular; *IV*, intravenous.

BENZODIAZEPINE-LIKE SEDATIVE-HYPNOTICS

The drugs belonging to the classification of benzodiazepine-like sedative-hypnotics—**zolpidem, zaleplon,** and **eszopiclone**—are chemically unrelated to the benzodiazepines but share a similar pharmacology. These drugs are selective GABA receptor agonists at the α_1 subunit of the Cl^- channel (BZ_1 receptor). This selectivity may dictate why they produce sedation but less memory and cognitive impairment than benzodiazepines and exert little skeletal muscle relaxation or anticonvulsant activity. Biotransformation is by several CYP enzymes in addition to CYP3A4. CYP3A4 inhibitors and inducers have less impact on the clinical effectiveness of this drug class. The drugs are particularly interesting because they establish that the benzodiazepine structure is not an absolute requirement for a compound to act as a benzodiazepine receptor agonist.

Eszopiclone is a newer entry into the rapidly expanding sleep-aid market. Eszopiclone is the S conformation of zopiclone. Eszopiclone is rapidly absorbed after oral administration. The drug undergoes extensive metabolism in the liver. Adverse effects of eszopiclone include altered taste and dry mouth.

Zolpidem is a novel short-acting hypnotic having an imidazopyridine structure (Fig. 11-8). Zaleplon is a pharmacologically similar drug that belongs to the pyrazolopyridine class of compounds. It has little effect on REM sleep and seems to induce a physiologic pattern of slow-wave sleep. Rebound insomnia at recommended doses, if it occurs, is mild.

Zolpidem and zaleplon have the advantage of being very rapidly absorbed after oral administration, with clinically demonstrable effects occurring in 15 to 20 minutes. Zolpidem has a half-life of approximately 2.5 hours and is metabolized in the liver to inactive metabolites. Zaleplon is similar except its half-life is about 1 hour, and zopiclone and eszopiclone have half-lives of 3.5 to 6.5 hours. Adverse effects include dizziness, drowsiness, and gastrointestinal symptoms.

Zolpidem is a sedative-hypnotic of choice for pregnant women (FDA pregnancy category B), whereas zaleplon, zopiclone, and eszopiclone are pregnancy category C. Also in contrast to benzodiazepines, zolpidem, zaleplon, and eszopiclone are not contraindicated in patients with a history of narrow-angle glaucoma. Because of their similarities with benzodiazepines, zolpidem and zaleplon show utility as enteral sedation agents for dentistry. Zaleplon has compared favorably with triazolam as a sedative during oral surgery. Flumazenil effectively reverses the CNS depression produced by the selective BZ_1 receptor agonists. These properties collectively help explain why drugs of this class are now the most commonly prescribed sedative-hypnotics in the United States.

Zolpidem

FIG 11-8 Structural formula of zolpidem.

MELATONIN RECEPTOR AGONISTS

Melatonin is naturally secreted by the pineal gland at night according to the light/dark cycle and plays a major role in the maintenance of circadian rhythms and in the regulation of the sleep/wake cycle. Activation of the MT_1 and MT_2 melatonin receptors promotes sleep, regulates reproduction and immunoresponsiveness, and inhibits aging and cancer growth. **Ramelteon** is the first melatonin receptor agonist approved by the FDA for the treatment of insomnia. It has no appreciable affinity for the GABA receptor complex, has no anterograde amnestic qualities, and cannot be reversed by flumazenil. **Tasimelteon** is also an agonist at MT_1 and MT_2 melatonin receptors. It is approved for Non-24-Hour Sleep-Wake Disorder (Non-24).

Clinical uses for ramelteon include treatment of jet lag, treatment of insomnia, treatment of sleep disturbances associated with depression, tapering of patients from hypnotics (i.e., long-term benzodiazepine use), and preoperative sedation or anxiolysis. Further comparative evaluation of ramelteon with benzodiazepines is warranted for its potential as a pretreatment anxiolytic before anesthesia or as a sole therapeutic sedative agent. Ramelteon is metabolized by various CYP enzymes and is susceptible to drug interactions involving inhibition or activation of these enzymes. Inhibitory agents such as fluvoxamine, fluconazole, and ketoconazole may increase the risk of ramelteon-related side effects. Conversely, rifampin may decrease the bioavailability of ramelteon, leading to lack of efficacy.

OREXIN RECEPTOR ANTAGONIST

Suvorexant is an orexin receptor antagonist. By blocking the effects of orexin peptides in the hypothalamus, it is able to promote sleep. It is used to treat insomnia. Dry mouth can occur as well as diarrhea and abnormal dreams.

BARBITURATES

Chemistry and Structure-Activity Relationships

The basic chemical structure of all barbiturates is barbiturate acid (Fig. 11-9). Barbituric acid, formed by the condensation of urea and malonic acid, lacks CNS depressant activity. To obtain barbiturates that have CNS depressant properties, both hydrogens at C_5 must be replaced by organic groups. Depending on the substituents added, three types of barbiturates are formed (Table 11-5). In the first group, substitutions are made only at C_5, yielding a large variety of drugs. The addition of a phenyl group at C_5 results in a drug with antiepileptic activity. If the side chain on C_5 reaches eight carbon atoms, the drug becomes more toxic and assumes convulsant properties. In the second group, when alkyl groups are substituted at N_3, the N-alkyl barbiturates are formed. The only N-alkyl barbiturates used clinically are the N-methyl derivatives (mephobarbital and methohexital).

A third group of barbiturates is formed when the oxygen at C_2 of the barbiturate nucleus is replaced with a sulfur atom. Technically, sulfur-substituted drugs are not true barbiturates because, by definition, barbiturates require oxygen at C_2. Sulfur-substituted barbiturates are commonly referred to as thiobarbiturates, whereas true barbiturates are sometimes called *oxybarbiturates*. Thiopental and thiamylal are examples of thiobarbiturates.

The clinical properties of barbiturates vary considerably depending on the lipid/aqueous partition coefficient. As lipid solubility of the barbiturate increases, hypnotic activity increases, the onset time decreases, and the duration of action decreases. With their extreme lipid solubility, thiopental and thiamylal have an extremely short duration of action and are used as intravenous anesthetics (see Chapters 15 and 38).

Mechanism of Action

The mechanism by which the barbiturates exert their CNS depressant effects bears a striking similarity to the effects of benzodiazepines. Barbiturates enhance GABA binding and **increase the duration of GABA-activated Cl^- channel** opening by acting at specific barbiturate binding sites on the $GABA_A$ receptor complex (see Fig. 11-3), leading to hyperpolarization and decreased neuronal firing. Barbiturates modulate GABA receptor function to prolong presynaptic and postsynaptic inhibition. Although benzodiazepines increase the frequency (as opposed to increasing the duration) of Cl^- channel opening, the end result (increased inhibition) is similar for the two groups of compounds. Their similar therapeutic and pharmacologic properties are not surprising. At high concentrations, barbiturates also act directly on the Cl^- channel, not requiring the presence of GABA. A third action of barbiturates is inhibition of a specific subset of glutamate receptors. These latter two actions are not shared by benzodiazepines and may help explain the **lower margin of safety** and steeper dose-response relationship for barbiturates compared with benzodiazepines.

Pharmacologic Effects

The primary pharmacologic effects of barbiturates involve the brain and spinal cord, the cardiovascular system, and the respiratory system.

Central nervous system

As with all sedative-hypnotics, barbiturates depress the CNS to varying degrees, ranging from mild sedation to respiratory arrest and death.

The behavioral effects of barbiturates indicative of general CNS depression include diminished psychological performance and responsiveness to external stimuli. Subjectively, the patient experiences

Urea Malonic acid Barbituric acid

FIG 11-9 Chemical formulation of barbituric acid.

TABLE 11-5 General Barbiturate Ring Structure with Examples of Chemical Formulas of the Three Types of Barbiturates

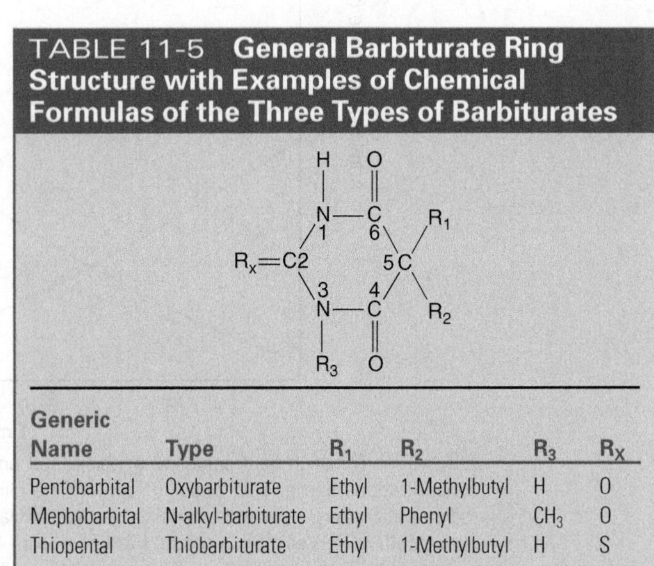

Generic Name	Type	R_1	R_2	R_3	R_X
Pentobarbital	Oxybarbiturate	Ethyl	1-Methylbutyl	H	O
Mephobarbital	N-alkyl-barbiturate	Ethyl	Phenyl	CH_3	O
Thiopental	Thiobarbiturate	Ethyl	1-Methylbutyl	H	S

relaxation, a feeling of well-being, and drowsiness. Coincident with these subjective feelings, the electroencephalogram displays an increase in fast activity (25 to 35 Hz) referred to as *barbiturate activation.*

The electroencephalogram patterns recorded after the administration of barbiturates are similar to the patterns observed during natural sleep, but there are important differences. Barbiturates decrease the time spent in REM sleep. REM sleep is the period in which vivid dreaming occurs; it is also believed to be involved in the consolidation of learning. A person deprived of REM sleep "makes up" the loss by increasing the time spent in REM sleep at a subsequent time. A typical pattern would be an increase in the frequency and duration of REM sleep subsequent to the cessation of barbiturate therapy, leading to "restless sleep." The individual may find it difficult to have a good night's sleep for several nights without readministration of a sedative-hypnotic. A vicious cycle may be started. With the exception of moderate doses of certain benzodiazepine receptor agonists, all sedative-hypnotics significantly reduce REM sleep.

Cardiovascular system

Barbiturates are cardiovascular system depressants, producing peripheral vasodilation and decreased stroke volume. At hypnotic doses, they produce mild hypotension. Due to reflexes the heart rate increases, and cardiac index is maintained or only slightly depressed. Progressive depression of the cardiovascular system develops as the dose of barbiturates is increased beyond the hypnotic range.

Respiratory system

Barbiturates are dose-dependent respiratory depressants. Medullary respiratory centers are depressed by toxic concentrations of barbiturates, and eventually even the carotid arch and aortic body receptors are depressed. Barbiturates increase respiratory reflex activity, such as cough, hiccup, sneezes, and laryngospasm, which complicates their use in anesthesia.

Absorption, Fate, and Excretion

Barbiturates are generally available as Na^+ salts, which are completely absorbed from the gastrointestinal tract and distributed to nearly all tissues of the body. Figure 11-10 is an example of the pharmacokinetic characteristics of highly lipid-soluble sedative-hypnotics like thiopental. One of the most important factors determining barbiturate distribution to the brain is lipid solubility. Thiopental, which is highly lipid-soluble, readily crosses the blood–brain barrier and, when administered intravenously, attains high concentrations in the CNS in seconds. The high blood flow to the brain also contributes significantly to the entry of drugs like thiopental (see Fig. 11-10).

Phenobarbital is metabolized by the liver, but 25% to 50% is eliminated unchanged in the urine. Most other barbiturates are transformed completely by the liver to inactive metabolites, which are excreted by the kidney. The primary mechanism by which the CNS effects of the barbiturates are terminated after a single administration is redistribution from the brain to muscle and other body tissues (see Fig. 11-10). Subsequent storage of barbiturates occurs primarily in body fat. From this depot, the drugs are slowly released, metabolized, and excreted; this slow turnover of drug accounts for the prolonged depressant effect, or hangover, after general anesthesia with thiopental and after sedation with pentobarbital or phenobarbital. On repeated administration, redistribution becomes increasingly less important, and eventually the duration of effect is determined by the elimination half-life.

Long-term use of barbiturates causes an increase in liver microsomal enzyme activity that results from increased synthesis of enzyme. Increased enzyme activity facilitates the rate of metabolism of many

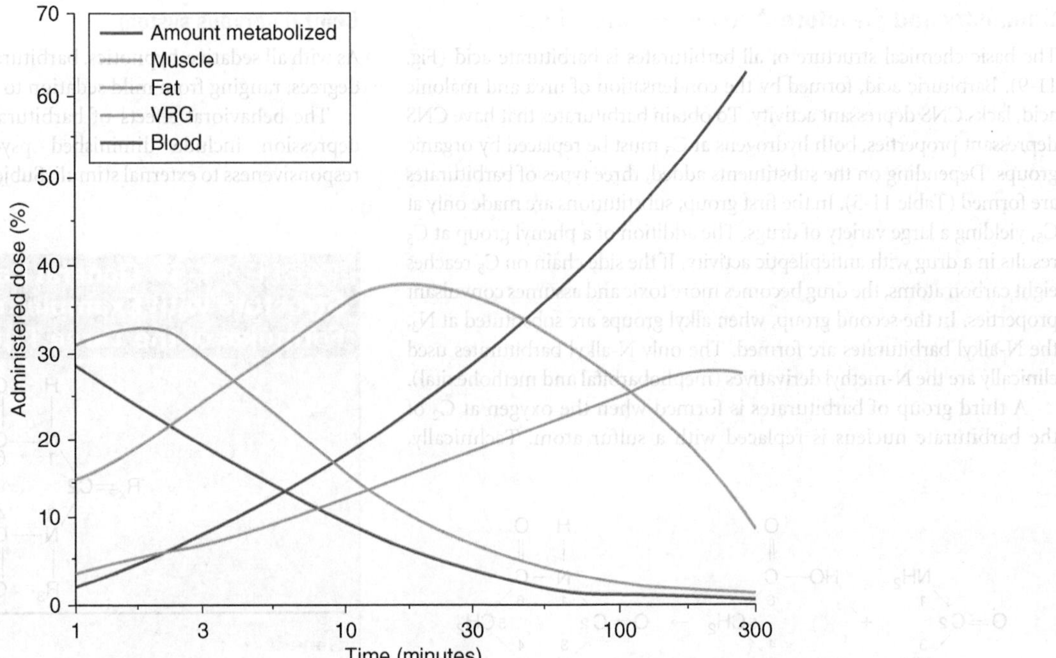

FIG 11-10 The high lipid solubility of thiopental and the high blood flow to the brain leads to high drug concentrations and a rapid onset of action. The clinical effects wane as CNS blood levels recede due to redistribution to muscle and other tissues. Accumulation in body fat creates a reservoir of drug that is slowly eliminated. *VRG,* Vessel-rich group. (Redrawn from Saidman LJ: Uptake, distribution and elimination of barbiturates. In Eger EI, editor: *Anesthetic uptake and action.* Baltimore, Williams & Wilkins, 1974. From the internet www.noranaes.org.)

drugs, including the barbiturates themselves, and it gives rise to numerous drug interactions (see Table 11-3).

The duration of action of barbiturates serves as a useful criterion for classification, as illustrated in Table 11-6.

Adverse Effects and Drug Interactions

The principal toxic reactions associated with the use of the barbiturates result from their effects on the CNS (particularly when combined with other CNS depressants), their abuse potential (see Chapter 39), and their ability to **induce hepatic microsomal enzymes**. Because barbiturates are CNS depressants, at high doses they can depress respiration and should not be administered to patients whose respiration is already compromised. Additionally, intravenously administered anesthetic barbiturates increase the incidence of respiratory complications such as laryngospasm, coughing, sneezing, and hiccup. Confusion, somnolence, and impaired psychomotor performance are other possible undesired consequences of CNS depression. As is the case with benzodiazepines, many unusual behavioral reactions have been attributed to the barbiturates. Such reactions include attitudinal depression, agitated toxic psychosis, manic behavior, increased anxiety, hostility, and rage. Careful evaluation reveals that the incidence of paradoxical responses is very small. In many cases, the response may be predictable if the patient has a history of poor impulse control or aggressive and destructive behavior.

Combining two or more CNS depressant drugs is known to produce increased levels of CNS depression. This summation reaction is the basis for some useful drug combinations in dental therapeutics, as well as for some potentially life-threatening consequences. The risk for adverse effects increases as more CNS depressants are used together. Combinations of barbiturates with opioids, benzodiazepines, antihistamines, or other CNS depressants increase the risk of oversedation, respiratory depression, and death. In like manner, alcohol consumption after general anesthesia or sedation can cause severe drowsiness and significantly impair psychomotor performance, including driving skills, and it must be restricted.

Some drugs, such as valproic acid, reduce the hepatic clearance of the barbiturates, leading to an enhanced response (see Table 11-3). Numerous drug interactions with the barbiturates arise from the ability of these agents to induce hepatic microsomal enzyme activity. Drugs used for moderate sedation may be rendered less effective and have a shorter than expected duration of action in this instance. If hepatic microsomal enzyme activity has been elevated, the effectiveness of warfarin and other drugs metabolized by this enzyme system is decreased. Many potentially dangerous drug interactions may be prevented simply by obtaining an accurate medical history, keeping a continuous record of drugs (prescribed and self-administered) taken by the patient, and consulting with the patient's physician when the patient's clinical status or drug history is uncertain.

Barbiturates augment porphyrin synthesis and are strictly contraindicated in patients with acute intermittent **porphyria**, hereditary coproporphyria, or porphyria variegata. Barbiturates increase the concentration of δ-aminolevulinic acid synthase, the initial enzyme in the synthesis of porphyrin rings found in hemoglobin and other proteins. Because these forms of porphyria are caused by defective enzymes involved in heme synthesis, blockade of the synthetic pathway downstream from δ-aminolevulinic acid causes porphyrin precursors to build up, leading to an acute exacerbation of the disease.

TABLE 11-6 Classification of Barbiturates According to Duration of Action

	Onset of Effect	Duration of Effect
Long-acting: phenobarbital	1-3 hr*	10 hr
Short-acting to intermediate-acting: pentobarbital, secobarbital	30-60 min*	3-8 hr
Ultrashort-acting: thiopental, methohexital	Immediate†	15-30 min‡

*Oral administration.
†Intravenous administration.
‡After single intravenous dose.

General Therapeutic Uses

The indications for barbiturates reflect their durations of action and selective effects of some drugs. The long-acting agent phenobarbital is used to manage tonic-clonic seizures and other types of convulsive disorders. Short-acting to intermediate-acting drugs can be prescribed for sedative-hypnotic purposes, although they are not commonly used since the advent of the benzodiazepines. In fact, the use of these barbiturates for procedural sedation has virtually disappeared. Short-acting and ultrashort-acting barbiturates are administered as intravenous sedatives and anesthetics, Their use in the United States has largely been replaced with propofol (see Chapter 15). Thiopental is not currently available, while methohexital enjoys limited use.

CHLORAL HYDRATE AND OTHER SEDATIVE-HYPNOTICS

Various drugs of diverse chemical structure, including chloral hydrate, paraldehyde, ethchlorvynol, glutethimide, and methyprylon, have sedative-hypnotic properties. Except for chloral hydrate, these agents have few if any clinical indications in dentistry.

Pharmacologic Effects

Chloral hydrate, one of the oldest nonbarbiturate sedative-hypnotics, continues to have limited dental applications. Although not approved in the United States for a specific clinical indication, it is used by several clinicians for sedation. It is supplied as a flavored syrup. Chloral hydrate is a commonly used sedative in children for technical procedures such as diagnostic imaging. Similarly, chloral hydrate has been a popular sedative-hypnotic in pediatric dentistry. Although its overall safety record is considered acceptable, the therapeutic index of the drug is actually very small.

Chloral hydrate is commonly used in combination with other drugs, such as nitrous oxide, meperidine, hydroxyzine, and promethazine. These agents are useful in augmenting the sedative effect of chloral hydrate and are valued for their antiemetic effects.

Absorption, Fate, and Excretion

Chloral hydrate is well absorbed after oral or rectal administration and is rapidly converted by the liver to trichloroethanol, which is responsible for the CNS depressant properties of the parent compound (Fig. 11-11). Plasma concentrations of chloral hydrate are nearly undetectable after administration. Trichloroethanol is conjugated with glucuronic acid and excreted in the urine. Trichloroethanol has a half-life of 4 to 12 hours. A portion of chloral hydrate and trichloroethanol is metabolized to dichloroacetic acid and trichloroacetic acid. With long-term administration, chloral hydrate can induce liver enzyme activity and compete for plasma protein binding sites, giving rise to several drug interactions.

Adverse Effects and Drug Interactions

Chloral hydrate has only minor cardiovascular effects in conventional doses. As the dose is increased beyond the therapeutic range, however, cardiovascular depression may occur. Chloral hydrate can precipitate cardiac arrhythmias in the sensitized heart and in the apparently healthy heart, and it may have been responsible for the reported death of a patient undergoing third molar extractions (see Jastak and Pallasch reference). Chloral hydrate and trichloroethanol have chemical structures (see Fig. 11-11) that resemble halothane, an anesthetic known to sensitize the myocardium to adrenergic amines. Trichloroacetic acid may also be cardiotoxic. The respiratory effects of sedative doses of chloral hydrate and the other nonbarbiturates are minimal, but become more severe as the dose is increased.

Chloral hydrate has been implicated in various drug interactions (see Table 11-3). As one might expect, chloral hydrate produces increased CNS depression when administered with other sedatives. The therapeutic advantage of this drug interaction is that it allows practitioners to decrease the dose of both CNS depressants and limit the side effects of the individual drugs. This is the rationale for a multidrug technique for pediatric sedation using chloral hydrate, meperidine, and hydroxyzine in combination. Similarly, nitrous oxide administration in conjunction with chloral hydrate deepens the level of sedation. The likelihood of oversedation and respiratory compromise increases when these drug combinations are utilized.

Chloral hydrate causes a summation of effects with other CNS depressants. However, the combination of chloral hydrate with alcohol is thought to produce a potentiation drug interaction through an alteration of alcohol metabolism. Chloral hydrate and its primary metabolite, trichloroethanol, competitively inhibit alcohol-metabolizing dehydrogenases, elevating alcohol blood concentrations (see Table 11-3). This combination, known colloquially as a "Mickey Finn" or "knock-out drops," can induce severe alcohol intoxication with stupor, coma, or death. The interaction is significant because it induces greater than additive effects and may result in a potentially life-threatening CNS depression. The dental indications for chloral hydrate are almost exclusively in pediatric sedation, and alcohol is usually not a concomitantly administered drug.

Chloral hydrate has been implicated in modifying responses to the oral anticoagulants dicumarol and warfarin. Another metabolite of chloral hydrate, trichloroacetic acid, may increase free warfarin plasma concentrations by interfering with its protein binding (normally 98% to 99%). Sedation with benzodiazepine regimens is a recommended alternative.

A potential caution concerning the widespread use of chloral hydrate in infants and children is that chloral hydrate, trichloroethanol, and trichloroacetic acid all are metabolites of trichloroethylene, an industrial solvent, environmental contaminant, and carcinogen. Chloral hydrate is also a mutagen and can cause chromosomal damage. Although no indication of human mutagenic or carcinogenic toxicity has been found with therapeutic uses of chloral hydrate, these concerns have decreased the popularity of chloral hydrate for use in pediatric dentistry.

Chloral Hydrate → Trichloroethanol

Halothane

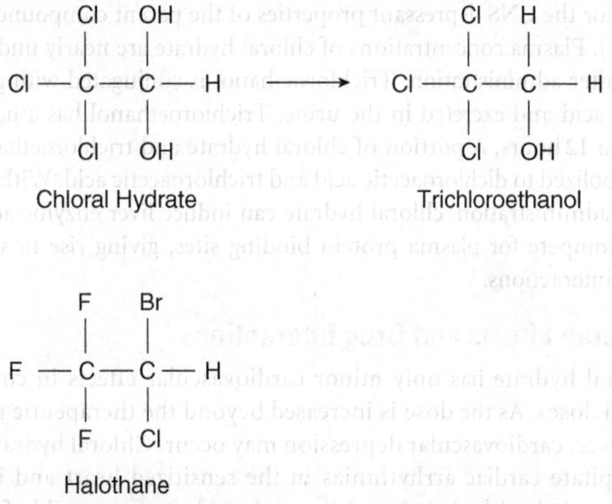

FIG 11-11 Structural formulas of chloral hydrate and its active metabolite trichloroethanol. Note the structural similarity with halothane, a known arrhythmogenic agent.

ANTIHISTAMINES

A common side effect of the first-generation H_1 antihistamines is drowsiness and sedation. This response is caused by antagonism of histamine neurotransmitter receptors within the CNS. Antihistamines such as **hydroxyzine**, a piperazine derivative, and promethazine, a phenothiazine derivative, have proved to be useful adjuncts in sedation regimens (see Chapter 38). Part of their popularity relates to their ability to augment the sedative effects of other sedative-hypnotics and to reduce the incidence of nausea and vomiting. Similarly, the ethanolamine antihistamine diphenhydramine, although used primarily for the management of allergic reactions, is also marketed as an over-the-counter agent to treat motion sickness and insomnia. Antihistamines are discussed in detail in Chapter 18.

GENERAL THERAPEUTIC USES OF SEDATIVE-HYPNOTICS

The use of barbiturate sedative-hypnotics to relieve fear and anxiety during dental procedures has been supplanted by use of benzodiazepine receptor agonists. Likewise these once popular sleep aids have virtually disappeared as newer, safer, and more effective drugs have been produced. Chloral hydrate and the antihistamine sedatives are still used in pediatric dentistry, although chloral hydrate poses more risk and its use is waning. Table 11-7 lists agents that are useful as sedative-hypnotics. The ultrashort-acting agent methohexital still has usefulness in anesthesia and intravenous sedation to deepen CNS depression for brief periods. These therapeutic indications for sedative-hypnotic agents are discussed further in Chapters 15 and 38.

AZASPIRODECANEDIONES

Buspirone (Fig. 11-12), an azapirone (short for azaspirodecanedione) derivative structurally unrelated to the benzodiazepines, represents a

TABLE 11-7 Preparations and Doses of Sedative-Hypnotics

	Route of Administration	ADULT DOSE (mg) Sedation	Hypnosis
Benzodiazepines			
Clorazepate	O	7.5-15	15-30
Diazepam*	O, IM, IV	2-10	10
Flurazepam	O	15	15-30
Lorazepam	O, IM, IV	1-3	2-4
Quazepam	O	7.5-30	7.5-30
Temazepam	O	7.5-15	15-30
Triazolam	O	0.125-0.25	0.125-0.5
Chloral Derivatives			
Chloral hydrate†	O, R		500-1000
Selective $GABA_A$ Receptor Agonists			
Zaleplon	O		5-20
Zolpidem	O		5-10
Eszopiclone	O		1-3
Melatonin Receptor Agonist			
Ramelteon	O		8

*Dose for children for preoperative sedation, 0.04-0.6 mg/kg.
†Dose for children for preoperative sedation, 50 mg/kg up to 1000 mg.
IM, Intramuscular; *IV*, intravenous; *O*, oral; *R*, rectal.

unique class of antianxiety agents. Buspirone has antianxiety effects that are therapeutically equivalent to the effects of diazepam, but it lacks the more prominent CNS depressant effects and the anticonvulsant and muscle relaxant properties of the benzodiazepines. In addition, buspirone does not augment the sedative effect of ethyl alcohol or other sedatives, and it has little effect on psychomotor or cognitive function. Physical dependence does not occur, and withdrawal does not occur at abrupt cessation. This drug has a more anxiolytic-selective profile than benzodiazepines, representing a major advance in antianxiety therapy and a useful alternative to benzodiazepines.

The antianxiety effect of buspirone is largely due to its action as a 5-HT_{1A} receptor agonist. Although buspirone does not bind to the GABA-benzodiazepine receptor complex, the benzodiazepine antagonist flumazenil can block the antianxiety effect of ipsapirone, a buspirone derivative, suggesting an interaction between benzodiazepine and tryptaminergic systems.

Peak plasma concentrations of buspirone are reached in less than 1 hour, but this may vary from patient to patient. Buspirone is extensively metabolized, with active and inactive metabolites excreted in the urine and feces. The elimination half-life is 2 to 8 hours.

Adverse effects of buspirone, such as headache, dizziness, nervousness, paresthesia, and gastrointestinal upset, are similar to the adverse effects of benzodiazepines but milder. Buspirone does not seem to produce additive sedative effects with the concomitant use of ethanol, a major advantage over benzodiazepines. Additionally, buspirone does not seem to produce significant CNS depression, which may offer a major clinical advantage for patients who cannot afford an impairment in psychomotor skills. The abrupt withdrawal of buspirone is not associated with rebound anxiety or withdrawal symptoms. There have been reports that patients taking long-term diazepam who are quickly switched to buspirone may exhibit signs of increased anxiety and withdrawal because buspirone does not suppress benzodiazepine withdrawal or show cross-tolerance with benzodiazepines. Switching a patient who is currently on long-term benzodiazepine therapy to buspirone is accomplished by initiating low doses of buspirone and gradually tapering the dosage of benzodiazepine. Another problem associated with the use of buspirone is the long delay (1 to 3 weeks) to onset of clinical effects. This limits its usefulness in clinical dentistry. The principal indication for the use of buspirone is in the management of Generalized Anxiety Disorder.

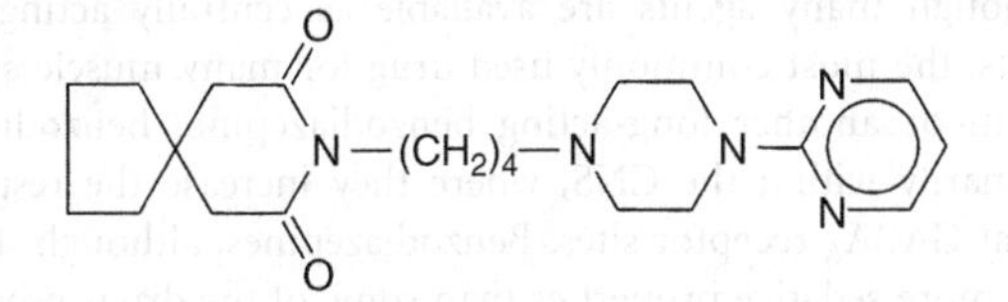

N—$(CH_2)_4$—N N N N O O

FIG 11-12 Structural formula of buspirone.

CENTRALLY ACTING MUSCLE RELAXANTS

These drugs include drugs from several different classes based on their mechanism of action or chemical group. Many have sedative effects. Diazepam, baclofen, tizanidine, and cyclobenzaprine are also discussed in Chapter 7 with respect to their use as muscle relaxers. The indications for centrally acting muscle relaxants vary depending on the drug.

Drugs Used for Treating Acute Muscle Spasms

Diazepam is a benzodiazepine used to treat acute muscle spasms. It is discussed earlier.

Cyclobenzaprine (Fig. 11-13), a structural and pharmacologic analogue of tricyclic antidepressants, is used for the short-term (2 to 3 weeks) treatment of muscle spasm associated with acute painful

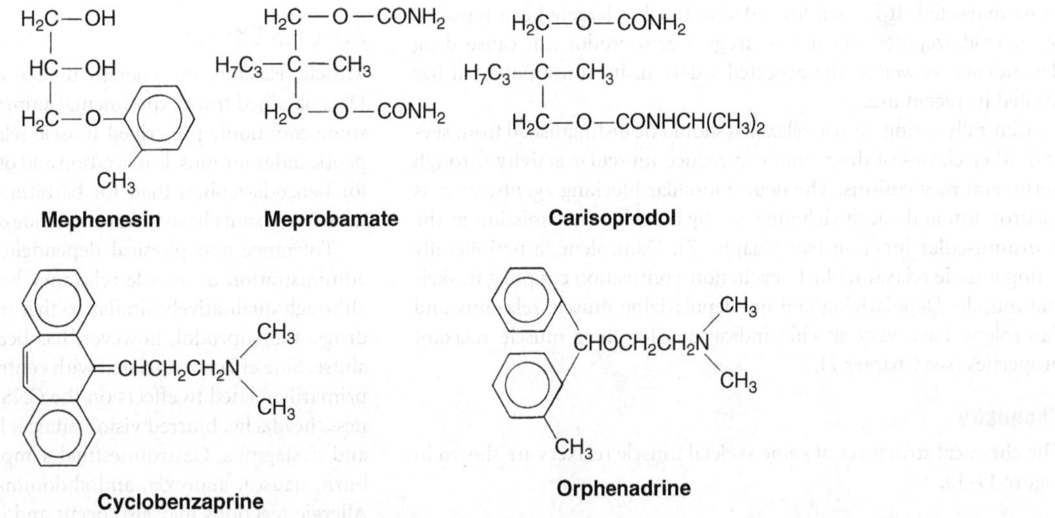

$H_2C—OH$ $HC—OH$ $H_2C—O—$ CH_3 **Mephenesin**

$H_2C—O—CONH_2$ $H_7C_3—C—CH_3$ $H_2C—O—CONH_2$ **Meprobamate**

$H_2C—O—CONH_2$ $H_7C_3—C—CH_3$ $H_2C—O—CONHCH(CH_3)_2$ **Carisoprodol**

$=CHCH_2CH_2N$ CH_3 CH_3 **Cyclobenzaprine**

$CHOCH_2CH_2N$ CH_3 CH_3 CH_3 **Orphenadrine**

O O NH Cl **Chlorzoxazone**

CH_3 N O Cl N **Diazepam**

Cl— —$CHCH_2COOH$ CH_2NH_2 **Baclofen**

FIG 11-13 Structural formulas of some centrally acting muscle relaxants.

TABLE 11-8 Pharmacologic Comparison of Centrally Acting Muscle Relaxants, Sedative-Hypnotics, Antianxiety Drugs, and Antihistamines

Pharmacologic Properties	Centrally Acting Muscle Relaxants (Propanediol Group)	Sedative-Hypnotics (Prototype Phenobarbital)	Antianxiety Drugs (Prototype Diazepam)	Antihistamines (Prototype Diphenhydramine)
Anticholinergic properties	No	No	Mild	Yes
Antihistaminic properties	No	No	No	Yes
Paradoxic low-dose excitement	Yes	Yes	Yes	No
Ataxia	Yes	Yes	Yes	No
Anesthesia	Yes	Yes	Variable	No
Arousal at high doses	Difficult	Difficult	Difficult	Easy
Lethal effect	Respiratory depression	Respiratory depression	Respiratory depression	Convulsions
Convulsant threshold	Raised	Raised	Raised	Lowered
Dependence liability	Yes, but usually mild	Yes	Yes, but usually mild	No

musculoskeletal conditions. One hypothesis for its mechanism of action is that it increases brainstem norepinephrine-mediated inhibition of ventral motor neurons of the spinal cord. Its effectiveness is similar to that of diazepam, but it produces more xerostomia, drowsiness, tachycardia, and dizziness. Many tricyclic antidepressants have significant antihistaminic effects, and the general pharmacologic properties of cyclobenzaprine are similar to those shown in Table 11-8 for the antihistamines. Cyclobenzaprine is contraindicated in those with cardiac arrhythmias or cardiac conditions such as recent myocardial infarction.

Metaxalone and **chlorzoxazone** (see Fig. 11-13) are heterocyclic carbamates that show muscle-relaxing properties. Sedation and inhibition of central polysynaptic pathways appear to contribute to muscle relaxation.

Methocarbamol and **carisoprodol** (see Fig. 11-13) are propanediol carbamates, also used primarily as centrally acting skeletal muscle relaxants. Propanediol drugs are an older type of centrally acting skeletal muscle relaxers. Meprobamate was among the first of this class to be marketed. It is used for sedation but has largely been replaced by benzodiazepines and newer drugs. Carisoprodol can cause drug dependence as well as the expected sedation. Its abuse potential has limited its recent use.

Centrally acting muscle relaxants should be distinguished from several other classes of drugs that can reduce muscular activity through peripheral mechanisms. The neuromuscular blocking agents, such as rocuronium and succinylcholine, act by blocking transmission at the neuromuscular junction (see Chapter 7). Dantrolene, a peripherally acting muscle relaxant, blocks excitation-contraction coupling in skeletal muscle. Depolarizing and nondepolarizing muscle relaxants and dantrolene have very specific indications for their muscle relaxant properties (see Chapter 7).

Chemistry

The chemical structures of some skeletal muscle relaxers are shown in Figure 11-13.

Pharmacologic effects

Table 11-8 compares pharmacologic characteristics of various classes of drugs discussed in this chapter. Qualitatively, centrally acting muscle relaxants, sedative-hypnotics, and antianxiety drugs are similar pharmacologically, whereas antihistamines produce sedation that is qualitatively different.

Centrally acting muscle relaxants cause relaxation of voluntary muscle through depression of the CNS. **Polysynaptic pathways**, which contribute to muscle activity, may be selectively inhibited. At progressively larger doses, sedation, hypnosis, unconsciousness, and even death can occur. Elevation of the convulsant threshold can be shown. The drugs are used orally.

Adequate cardiovascular performance is usually maintained at doses even higher than the doses that produce respiratory depression. The problems of shock and renal failure can complicate recovery from toxic doses of the agents, however.

Although many agents are available as centrally acting muscle relaxants, the most commonly used drug for many muscle spasms is diazepam or another long-acting benzodiazepine. Benzodiazepines act primarily within the CNS, where they increase the response to GABA at $GABA_A$ receptor sites. Benzodiazepines, although they tend to have more sedative properties than some of the drugs used almost exclusively as centrally acting muscle relaxants, have a favorable clinical profile compared with the latter agents because of their relatively strong muscle-relaxing properties and relatively low toxic and physical dependence liabilities.

Adverse Effects

Muscle relaxants are generally used at doses that cause some sedation. Data obtained from experimental animals compare the relative safety of some commonly prescribed muscle relaxants (Table 11-9). The therapeutic index for muscle relaxation and other effects is many times greater for benzodiazepines than for barbiturates. The other clinically useful muscle relaxants have therapeutic indexes between these extremes.

Tolerance and physical dependence develop with the long-term administration of muscle relaxants, but generally withdrawal is mild although qualitatively similar to that seen with other CNS depressant drugs. Carisoprodol, however, has been subject to significant recent abuse. Side effects associated with centrally acting muscle relaxants are primarily related to effects on the CNS and include drowsiness, dizziness, headache, blurred vision, ataxia, lethargy, paradoxic excitement, and nystagmus. Gastrointestinal symptoms such as vomiting, heartburn, nausea, anorexia, and abdominal distress have been reported. Allergic reactions may also occur and include skin rash, pruritus, and fever. Cyclobenzaprine has some additional side effects that stem from its actions on the autonomic nervous system. Because it has substantial anticholinergic properties, its use should be especially avoided in certain conditions (e.g., narrow-angle glaucoma, prostatic hypertrophy). Because of its effect on norepinephrine reuptake, cyclobenzaprine may also be contraindicated in patients for whom increased sympathetic activity is to be avoided (e.g., in patients with hyperthyroidism or recovering from a myocardial infarction).

Drug interactions with the centrally acting muscle relaxants are of several kinds. First, these drugs augment the depressant actions of each

TABLE 11-9 Comparison of Ataxic and Lethal Doses of Central Depressant Drugs in Mice

Agent	LD_{50} (mg/kg)	Ataxia ED_{50} (mg/kg)	Therapeutic Index
Phenobarbital	242	120	2.0
Meprobamate	800	235	3.4
Carisoprodol	980	165	5.9
Chlordiazepoxide	720	100	7.2
Diazepam	620	30	20.7

ED_{50}, Median effective dose; *LD_{50}*, median lethal dose.

other and of the opioids, other sedatives and antianxiety drugs, antihistamines, and antidepressants. Second, drug interactions can occur when these agents induce drug-metabolizing and hormone-metabolizing enzymes of the liver. Although the degree of enzyme induction varies substantially among the various sedatives, caution should be used in patients taking anticoagulants and in patients with porphyria. Third, increased skeletal muscle relaxation should be expected when centrally acting muscle relaxants are given with drugs whose primary pharmacologic activity is neuromuscular blockade (e.g., succinylcholine) or with drugs that have such an activity as a side effect (e.g., aminoglycosides or volatile general anesthetics). Fourth, cyclobenzaprine should not be given to patients taking monoamine oxidase inhibitors or guanethidine and related drugs. (Barbiturates, benzodiazepines, and other sedatives should be used with considerable caution with monoamine oxidase inhibitors.) Fifth, because the muscle relaxant actions of diazepam are partially reversed by aminophylline, patients being treated with diazepam should avoid the use of xanthine-containing foods.

General Therapeutic Uses

Centrally acting muscle relaxants are used medically as adjuncts to rest, physical therapy, and other measures for the relief of discomfort associated with acute, painful musculoskeletal conditions. They have been promoted for use in skeletal muscle spasms of local origin, multiple sclerosis, cerebral palsy, sprains, strains, fibrositis, rheumatoid spondylitis, bursitis, the urethral syndrome, and arthritis. Drugs such as salicylates and adrenocorticosteroids may be used concomitantly.

Certain conditions of skeletal muscle, such as muscle spasm or trismus, are believed to be the result of dysfunctional output patterns from the motor areas of the CNS to skeletal muscle. Drugs that could prevent or lessen these neurotropic influences on voluntary muscle would be helpful in physical medicine and dentistry. Centrally acting muscle relaxants, which overlap pharmacologically with antianxiety drugs, represent a diverse group of drugs whose pharmacologic effects include diminished output of nerve impulses to voluntary muscle. Benzodiazepines are sometimes used to alleviate abnormal muscle contractions by depressing polysynaptic CNS pathways, including polysynaptic spinal reflexes.

Centrally Acting Drugs Used for Special Cases of Skeletal Muscle Relaxation

Baclofen has been shown to stimulate $GABA_B$ receptors, which are $G_{i/o}$ protein-linked receptors and are not coupled to Cl^- channels in the nerve membrane. These $GABA_B$ receptors may inhibit motor tone, by reducing Ca^{2+} conductance and increasing K^+ conductance and by reducing the release of excitatory amino acid transmitters. Baclofen, the *p*-chlorophenyl analogue of GABA, is recommended in multiple sclerosis or traumatic spinal cord injury for the relief of spasticity. Baclofen is also used to treat trigeminal neuralgia.

Baclofen can cause drowsiness, ataxia, and confusion, which may be especially troublesome in elderly individuals. Acute toxicity may lead to respiratory depression and seizures. Sudden withdrawal from therapeutic doses is associated with a high risk of hallucinations and tachycardia. Cessation of therapy should involve tapering the doses over several days.

Antihistamine

Orphenadrine (see Fig. 11-13) is an analogue of the antihistamine diphenhydramine. The pharmacologic profile of orphenadrine, an antihistamine, differs from other skeletal muscle relaxers discussed above. Orphenadrine has been used primarily as an adjunct in the treatment of Parkinson disease. It is also indicated for acute painful skeletal muscle conditions, although it does not have a clear advantage over other drugs used for this purpose.

α_2-Adrenergic Receptor Agonist Drugs

The α_2-adrenergic receptor agonist drugs **tizanidine** and **dexmedetomidine** exert their action at central and peripheral α_2 receptors. Guanabenz, guanfacine, clonidine, which also stimulate α_2-adrenergic receptors, are discussed in Chapter 23 under antihypertensive drugs. Centrally, α_2 receptors are located in the brain (locus ceruleus) and the spinal cord. Stimulation of these receptors diminishes sympathetic outflow, which results in sedation, hypnosis, anxiolysis, analgesia, and reduced systemic blood pressure. Peripherally, α_2 receptors are located primarily at the prejunctional site of the sympathetic nerve terminal. Stimulation of these receptors impairs adrenergic transmission and results in reductions of heart rate and blood pressure.

The α_2-adrenergic receptor agonist tizanidine is a centrally acting muscle relaxant used for amyotrophic lateral sclerosis, multiple sclerosis, and spasticity arising from spinal cord injury and cerebral palsy. Tizanidine has also been used in the treatment of myofascial pain disorders of the head and neck. It appears to reduce spasticity by increasing the presynaptic, and possibly postsynaptic, inhibition in polysynaptic circuits in the spinal cord. Tizanidine has been shown to significantly reduce pain and tissue tenderness and to improve the quality of sleep in the treatment of patients with myofascial pain. In patients with infantile cerebral palsy, tizanidine was shown to significantly decrease spasticity as compared to placebo. Because of its effects at the α_2-adrenergic receptor, tizanidine may produce sedation and transient bradycardia and hypotension; however, its cardiovascular effects are usually mild.

Dexmedetomidine is a highly selective (7.3 times that of clonidine) α_2-adrenergic receptor agonist with sedative, hypnotic, and analgesic properties. It exhibits a biphasic blood pressure response in a dose-dependent fashion. Intravenous infusion of low doses results in a reduction of mean arterial pressure owing to selectivity for central and peripheral α_2 receptors. The resultant decreases in heart rate and systemic vascular resistance lead to decreases in cardiac output and systolic blood pressure. Intravenous infusion of high doses or rapid intravenous bolus administration may result in systemic hypertension because of activation of peripheral postjunctional α_2-adrenergic receptors. Dexmedetomidine has minimal, if any, effect on the respiratory system, and similar to clonidine, it significantly reduces analgesic and anesthetic requirements.

Currently, dexmedetomidine has three main clinical applications. Its primary use is as a sedative agent for critically ill patients requiring prolonged sedation and mechanical ventilatory support in a critical care setting. Dexmedetomidine possesses all of the characteristics of an ideal sedative for intensive care. It lacks respiratory depression, is analgesic and anxiolytic, has a rapid onset and is titratable, and produces sedation with hemodynamic stability. In pediatric patients, dexmedetomidine is very useful in obtunding the emergence delirium sometimes seen after general anesthesia. It produces profound calming without respiratory depression. This is a major advantage over other sedatives and opioids that have commonly been used in this situation. Finally, dexmedetomidine is used as an adjunctive sedative agent for monitored anesthesia care. It can be used with agents such as opioids, benzodiazepines, and propofol to enhance sedation and promote and maintain hemodynamic stability. Because it does not produce respiratory depression, it is very useful in patients for whom this would be a concern. Its rapid distribution half-life (6 minutes) results in fast recovery and allows for faster patient discharge.

β-Adrenergic Receptor-Blocking Drugs

The β-adrenergic receptor-blocking agent propranolol is not approved for the treatment of anxiety, but it is effective in decreasing the peripheral autonomic symptoms of anxiety (e.g., tremor, tachycardia, palpitation). Propranolol may be used for healthy patients who have disabling situational anxiety, or it may be combined with a benzodiazepine in patients who have the somatic manifestations of anxiety. Propranolol and, more recently, metoprolol have gained some popularity with performers and public speakers in preventing "stage fright." It is neither appropriate nor effective for the treatment of chronic anxiety.

Glutamate Antagonist

Riluzole is thought to act in part by blocking glutamate release and blocking the excitatory effects of this amino acid. It is approved only for the treatment of amyotrophic lateral sclerosis. Asthenia, dizziness, and nausea are among its adverse effects.

IMPLICATIONS FOR DENTISTRY

Drugs Used as Sedative-Hypnotics

Whether used by the dentist or physician, the common desired therapeutic response to these drugs is sedation or hypnosis. Additional therapeutic applications for sedative-hypnotics are discussed in detail in Chapters 12 (Anticonvulsant Drugs), 15 (General Anesthetics), and 38 (Management of Fear and Anxiety).

As a class, **benzodiazepines** are very safe and highly effective agents for producing sedation and sleep. Zolpidem and zaleplon seem to offer advantages similar to the advantages described for benzodiazepines: they are well tolerated, have a high margin of safety, and have a shallow dose-response profile. In addition, their rapid onset of action makes it possible for the patient to take the drugs immediately before bedtime.

Barbiturates are of limited usefulness in dentistry. Methohexital remains a seldom-used alternative to propofol for the induction and maintenance of deep sedation and general anesthesia. While effective and relatively inexpensive, drugs such as pentobarbital and secobarbital have been replaced by benzodiazepines and other newer drugs. Phenobarbital remains useful for the chronic control of epileptiform seizures.

The primary drugs used for their sedative-hypnotic effect in the dental setting are the benzodiazepines and the pharmacologically related benzodiazepine receptor agonists. Other less commonly used drugs are chloral hydrate, which is still used for sedation in young children, and the antihistamines, hydroxyzine, diphenhydramine, and promethazine.

The use of other sedatives is generally not warranted for dental practice because they offer no significant advantages. The clinician is best advised to recognize the names of sedative-hypnotics and to be aware of the potential for drug interactions with other CNS depressants. Preparations and doses for clinically useful sedative-hypnotics are listed in Table 11-7. These doses should be used only as guidelines because each patient has different requirements, and dosages should be individualized.

Many of the problems associated with the sedative-hypnotics, such as tolerance to sedative effects, addiction, abuse, rebound sleep disturbances, and the induction of hepatic microsomal enzyme activity, result from long-term use. Sedative-hypnotic drugs are indicated only for short-term use in dentistry; many of the usual factors limiting their use are not pertinent. This assertion is not to imply that problems do not arise with the administration of sedative-hypnotics in dental practice, but only that they are minimized. It is the clinician's responsibility to ensure that the patient is made cognizant of the danger of combining other CNS depressants, particularly alcohol, with these drugs.

Certain patients require special precautions. Elderly patients are at special risk for impaired cognitive and motor function after the administration of a sedative-hypnotic. Patients with severely impaired liver function also fall into this category. Patients with sleep apnea should be treated cautiously because any hypnotic may exacerbate this condition. The use of sedative-hypnotics is generally contraindicated in pregnant patients, especially during the first trimester. Because patients with a history of drug abuse are at a higher risk of becoming dependent on sedative-hypnotics, the minimally effective dose should be prescribed and only when absolutely necessary.

Although barbiturates produce significant depression of the CNS, to the point of unconsciousness, they are not analgesics. A patient receiving sedative doses may exhibit increased responsiveness to painful stimuli. If pain is a contributing factor to anxiety or insomnia, an analgesic is required to obtain sedation or hypnosis. Drugs that act at benzodiazepine receptors also are not analgesic drugs. Benzodiazepines do not cause hyperalgesia as can be caused by barbiturates, however.

Drugs Used to Treat Anxiety

Antianxiety agents are important in dentistry for the premedication of apprehensive adult patients, patients exhibiting mild neurosis, and uncooperative children. Antianxiety agents, particularly intravenous midazolam and diazepam, are used as adjuncts to local anesthesia. The effectiveness of intravenous diazepam in the relief of intraoperative anxiety in a patient population undergoing surgical removal of impacted third molars is illustrated in Figure 11-14. Although intravenous sedation with diazepam usually lasts approximately 45 minutes, the relief of anxiety lasts much longer. **Midazolam** and **diazepam** cause anterograde amnesia so that patients often cannot recall the procedures performed. Both drugs also depress the gag reflex and are major drugs for the treatment of seizures induced by local anesthetic overdose.

Midazolam is popular as a preoperative sedative because it is prepared in a water-soluble form and produces little irritation on injection. In contrast to diazepam, residual CNS depression and anxiety relief extending beyond the period of clinical recovery are not commonly observed when midazolam is administered as a single agent.

One of the more perplexing questions for the practicing dentist is which oral benzodiazepine to choose from the ever-expanding list. There is little doubt of the clinical effectiveness of these drugs in various dental procedures, but there are no unusual characteristics associated with any benzodiazepine that would make it clearly superior to the others. Essentially, any benzodiazepine is suitable as an antianxiety agent if the pharmacokinetics of that drug are kept in mind. The major decision to be made in the treatment of the anxious patient is which drug possesses the best pharmacokinetic profile for a given use. Although there is no simple rule of thumb, the pharmacokinetic characteristics of individual compounds to a large extent dictate the optimal dose schedule. Oxazepam and lorazepam are potentially useful drugs in patients with liver disease because they are converted to inactive glucuronides, and the conjugation reaction is often affected less by hepatic disease than other steps in drug metabolism. Although buspirone offers many advantages for the treatment of anxiety, its usefulness in dentistry is limited by its delayed onset of effect.

Because of its short half-life and rapid onset, triazolam has been recommended as a safe and effective enteral sedative. Given the large number

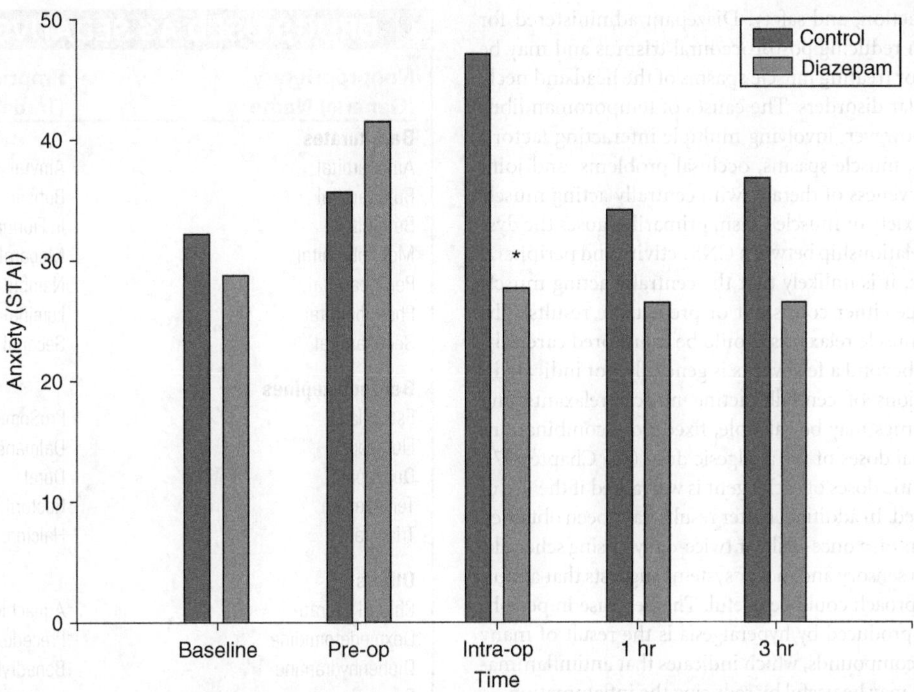

FIG 11-14 Effects of placebo and diazepam on reported anxiety with a state-trait anxiety index (*STAI*) in patients undergoing surgical removal of impacted third molars. Patients were treated with placebo solution or diazepam (0.3 mg/kg) 5 minutes before surgery. All patients also received standard local anesthesia with 2% lidocaine containing 1:100,000 epinephrine. Anxiety was assessed before ingestion and before, during, and after surgery. *Significantly different from control ($P < 0.01$). (Adapted from Hargreaves KM, Dionne RA, Mueller GP, et al: Naloxone, fentanyl, and diazepam modify plasma beta-endorphin levels during surgery. *Clin Pharmacol Ther* 40:165-171, 1986.)

of patients who avoid dental care because of fear and anxiety, dentists have found enteral triazolam to fulfill the need for a safe sedation protocol. The typical adult dose is 0.125 to 0.25 mg administered orally or sublingually 30 to 45 minutes before the dental procedures. A second dose may be needed. The maximum recommended dose of triazolam is 0.5 mg. The sublingual route for triazolam administration may be slightly more efficacious secondary to slightly higher plasma concentrations compared with the oral route. Indications and contraindications for administering oral or sublingual triazolam to anxious dental patients are discussed in Chapter 38.

The primary concern of the dentist in using an antianxiety agent should be excessive CNS depression. CNS depression may result from the antianxiety agent alone or its combination with other CNS depressants that the dentist may plan to give or that the patient may already have taken. The antianxiety agents summate with anesthetics, antipsychotics, antidepressants, opioid analgesics, and sedative-hypnotics. If CNS depressant drugs are used for deep sedation and general anesthesia in the dental clinic, suction and monitoring equipment, emergency drugs, and a means to deliver oxygen under positive pressure must be readily available. The practitioner should have appropriate advanced training in anesthesia techniques. The benzodiazepine antagonist flumazenil offers the opportunity to reverse excessive benzodiazepine-induced sedation after dental procedures, hastening postoperative patient recovery. Flumazenil is also a rapidly acting antidote for benzodiazepine intoxication. The possibility of resedation and recurrence of respiratory depression because of its short half-life has been described. The best practice in the use of benzodiazepines is to limit their administration so that an emergency antidote is never required.

The patient should be reminded that antihistamines, even the small amounts contained in over-the-counter preparations promoted as cold remedies or for insomnia, may add to the CNS depressant effect of antianxiety agents. Because of benzodiazepine-induced psychomotor impairment, the dentist should caution patients on the hazards of driving an automobile or operating potentially dangerous machinery for 24 hours after drug administration.

Chloral hydrate has been implicated in serious adverse effects when used as a sedative in dentistry. There is a risk of overdose. In addition, a prolonged recovery may occur. Chloral hydrate also increases the risk for cardiac arrhythmias. These adverse effects require special caution in its use.

Numerous factors influence the choice of an antianxiety drug. This chapter has covered some of the more important ones that the dentist should consider when making a selection. The therapeutic use of drugs for anxiety relief in dentistry is reviewed further in Chapter 38. In practice, the dentist should become familiar and comfortable with a few antianxiety drugs and select from these according to the drugs' pharmacokinetics, the particular treatment to be rendered, and the needs of the patient. The potential for the development of more specific antianxiety agents should serve as a stimulus for the practicing dentist to stay current in the field of antianxiety medication. Knowledge of the pharmacologic profile of the existing drugs may also prevent the dentist from being misled by dubious claims of specificity for newly introduced agents.

Table 11-4 lists benzodiazepine and hydroxyzine preparations and doses recommended for anxiety control. The doses indicated should be viewed only as guidelines; each patient requires individualized treatment. The minimum effective dose should be administered.

Drugs Used as Centrally Acting Muscle Relaxants

Although the indications are limited, centrally acting muscle relaxants may be valuable therapeutic agents for some dental procedures. Diazepam is generally preferred because of its good muscle-relaxing properties, prolonged action, and safety. Diazepam administered for 1 week may be useful in reducing postprocedural trismus and may be effective as an adjunct for treating muscle spasms of the head and neck, as in temporomandibular disorders. The causes of temporomandibular pain are complex, however, involving multiple interacting factors, such as patient anxiety, muscle spasms, occlusal problems, and joint dysfunction. The effectiveness of therapy with centrally acting muscle relaxants is greater if anxiety or muscle spasm primarily causes the dysfunction. Because the relationship between CNS activity and peripheral muscle tone is complex, it is unlikely that the centrally acting muscle relaxants would produce either consistent or predictable results. The use of centrally acting muscle relaxants should be monitored carefully, and long-term therapy beyond a few weeks is generally not indicated.

Although combinations of centrally acting muscle relaxants and peripherally analgesic drugs may be valuable, fixed-dose combinations often provide suboptimal doses of the analgesic drug (see Chapter 37). Prescribing full therapeutic doses of each agent is warranted if the use of a combination is indicated. In addition, better results have been obtained from longer acting agents on a once-daily or twice-daily dosing schedule. The interaction between sensory and motor systems suggests that a multiple drug treatment approach could be useful. The decrease in peripheral sensory thresholds produced by hyperalgesia is the result of many different inflammatory compounds, which indicates that antiinflammatory drugs of some kind may be useful by reducing the inflammation.

The use of analgesics to reduce peripheral and spinal (or trigeminal) hyperalgesia and centrally acting muscle relaxants to reduce brain excitation may help to reduce muscle spasm; this may explain why analgesics combined with muscle relaxants can sometimes produce a better effect than either one given alone. Centrally acting muscle relaxants generally are not the primary treatment for every type of facial pain. Trigeminal neuralgia (tic douloureux) requires specific therapies (see Chapters 12 and 37).

DRUGS USED AS ANTIANXIETY AGENTS

Nonproprietary (Generic) Name	Proprietary (Trade) Name
Benzodiazepines	
Alprazolam	Xanax
Chlordiazepoxide	Librium
Clorazepate	Tranxene
Diazepam	Valium
Lorazepam	Ativan
Midazolam	Versed
Oxazepam	Serax
Triazolam	Halcion
Azaspirodecanediones	
Buspirone	BuSpar
Propanediol Carbamates	
Meprobamate	Miltown, Equanil

DRUGS USED AS SEDATIVE-HYPNOTICS

Nonproprietary (Generic) Name	Proprietary (Trade) Name
Barbiturates	
Amobarbital	Amytal
Butabarbital	Butisol
Butalbital	In Fiorinal
Mephobarbital	Mebaral
Pentobarbital	Nembutal
Phenobarbital	Luminal
Secobarbital	Seconal
Benzodiazepines	
Estazolam	ProSom
Flurazepam	Dalmane
Quazepam	Doral
Temazepam	Restoril
Triazolam	Halcion
Others	
Chloral hydrate	Aquachloral Supprettes
Dexmedetomidine	Precedex
Diphenhydramine	Benadryl, Nytol
Eszopiclone	Lunesta
Hydroxyzine hydrochloride	Atarax, Vistaril
Promethazine	Phenergan
Ramelteon	Rozerem
Suvorexant	Belsomra
Tasimelteon	Hetlioz
Zaleplon	Sonata
Zolpidem	Ambien

DRUGS USED PRIMARILY AS CENTRALLY ACTING MUSCLE RELAXANTS

Nonproprietary (Generic) Name	Proprietary (Trade) Name
Benzodiazepines	
Diazepam	Valium
Miscellaneous	
Baclofen	Lioresal
Carisoprodol	Soma
Chlorzoxazone	Paraflex
Cyclobenzaprine	Flexeril
Metaxalone	Skelaxin
Methocarbamol	Robaxin
Orphenadrine	Norflex
Riluzole*	Rilutek
Tizanidine	Zanaflex

*For amyotrophic lateral sclerosis.

CASE DISCUSSION

Ms G has become unresponsive after taking an average (less than the maximum recommended dose) dose of triazolam. The differential diagnosis includes hyperreactivity to benzodiazepines, concomitant use of other CNS depressant drugs, and/or drug interaction. Sensitivity to the effects of benzodiazepines occurs in approximately 15% of patients and is more common among the elderly. While not considered elderly, Ms G is of an age where one would start to consider decreasing the usual dosage of a benzodiazepine. However, her pretreatment anxiety level acts as a natural antagonist to sedation, so the choice of 0.25 mg of triazolam seems appropriate. Ms G gives no history of using CNS depressants or alcohol, making drug potentiation an unlikely event. She does, however, take the calcium channel blocker verapamil for control of essential hypertension. Calcium channel blockers are known CYP3A4 inhibitors, which would make drug interaction with triazolam a real possibility. Benzodiazepines are metabolized primarily by CYP 3A4, so the concomitant use of a calcium channel blocker would result in increased bioavailability of triazolam and compound its effect. This would require a lower dose of triazolam.

GENERAL REFERENCES

1. Backman JT, Olkkola KT, Aranko K, et al.: Dose of midazolam should be reduced during diltiazem and verapamil treatments, *Br J Clin Pharmacol* 37:221–225, 1994.
2. Bowery NG: $GABA_B$ receptor pharmacology, *Annu Rev Pharmacol Toxicol* 33:109–147, 1993.
3. Clark MS, Lindenmuth JE, Jafek BW, et al.: Reversal of central benzodiazepine effects by intravenous flumazenil, *Anesth Prog* 38:12–16, 1991.
4. (DSM-V). *Diagnostic and statistical manual of mental disorders*, ed 5, Washington, DC, 2012, American Psychiatric Association.
5. Dubovsky SL: Generalized anxiety disorder: new concepts and psychopharmacologic therapies, *J Clin Psychiatry* 51(suppl):3–10, 1990.
6. Ganzberg SI, Dietrich T, Valerin M, et al.: Zaleplon (Sonata) oral sedation for outpatient third molar extraction surgery, *Anesth Prog* 52:128–131, 2005.
7. Jastak JT, Pallasch T: Death after chloral hydrate sedation: report of case, *J Am Dent Assoc* 116:345–348, 1988.
8. Krobeth PD, McAuley JW, Krobeth FJ, et al.: Triazolam pharmacokinetics after intravenous, oral and sublingual administration, *J Clin Psychopharm* 15:259–262, 1995.
9. Lopez-Rubalcava C, Saldivar A, Fernandez-Guasti A: Interaction of GABA and serotonin in the anxiolytic action of diazepam and serotonergic anxiolytics, *Pharmacol Biochem Behav* 43:433–440, 1992.
10. Malanga GA, Gwynn MW, Smith R, Miller D: Tizanidine is effective in the treatment of myofascial pain syndrome, *Pain Physician* 5:422–432, 2002.
11. Miller LG, Greenblatt DJ, Barnhill JG, et al.: Chronic benzodiazepine administration, I: tolerance is associated with benzodiazepine receptor downregulation and decreased γ-aminobutyric $acid_A$ receptor function, *J Pharmacol Exp Ther* 246:170–176, 1988.
12. Smith AJ, Simpson PB: Methodological approaches for the study of $GABA_A$ receptor pharmacology and functional responses, *Anal Bioanal Chem* 377:843–851, 2003.
13. Vasquez-Briceño A, Arellano-Saldaña ME, León-Hernández SR, Morales-Osorio MG: The usefulness of tizanidine. A one-year follow-up of the treatment of spasticity in infantile cerebral palsy, *Rev Neurol* 43:132–136, 2006.
14. Villikka K, Kivisto KT, Backman JT, et al.: Triazolam is ineffective in patients taking rifampin, *Clin Pharm Ther* 61:8–14, 1997.

12

Anticonvulsants*

Sean Flynn and M. Ali Babi

KEY INFORMATION

- The epilepsies are a group of common and complex seizure disorders.
- Seizures can be broadly classified as partial or generalized.
- Seizure can result from developmental defects, genetic mutation, or trauma generally causing an imbalance between excitatory and inhibitory drive in the brain.
- Epilepsy is most often treated with antiseizure or anticonvulsant drugs (AEDs) that act by altering ion channel conductance, GABAergic signaling, probability of synaptic vesicle release, or neuromodulation.
- First generation AEDs (phenytoin, carbamazepine, valproic acid) are still commonly used but have undesirable side effects. Newer AEDs (levetiracetam) are equally effective for some seizure types and are preferred due to more tolerable side effects.
- Alternative therapeutic strategies include surgical intervention, dietary modification, and wearable electronic stimulation devices.
- The risk of seizure-induction by dental procedures is low, but vigilance is critical.

CASE STUDY

Mrs T is a 35-year-old, right-handed woman with history of idiopathic generalized epilepsy manifesting as partial with secondarily generalized tonic-clonic seizures. Her seizures are relatively well controlled with levetiracetam (500 mg b.i.d, PO) monotherapy resulting in an occasional seizure every 4 to 6 months (latest seizure, 2 months ago). The patient has not been to see a dentist in a few years, and she is complaining of strong intermittent pain in the lower jaw. Upon examination, it is discovered that there is a clear trigger zone but no clear pathology that could account for the described pain. Acknowledging that this patient may be at a high risk for seizure due to her underlying seizure disorder and abnormal level of stress, how would you proceed to best care for this patient?

INTRODUCTION TO EPILEPSY AND SEIZURE DISORDERS

The epilepsies are a group of common and potentially devastating disorders characterized by the periodic and abnormal discharge of neurons within the brain. Approximately 65 million people worldwide (~0.5% to 1% of general population) are diagnosed with epilepsy and present clinically with more than 40 distinct forms of the disorder. Epilepsy is diagnosed if a person has experienced two or more unprovoked seizures greater than 24 hours apart. A seizure is a transient alteration in behavior resulting from the disordered, synchronous, and rhythmic firing of a population of neurons. The occurrence of a seizure during a person's lifetime may be as high as 10%; however, the occurrence of a single seizure will not result in the diagnosis of epilepsy. Many seizure disorders exist, each defined by factors including initiating event, seizure type, age of onset, and clinical manifestations. The signs and symptoms of these syndromes frequently overlap, and differential diagnosis of the form of epilepsy is sometimes difficult. Some patients prefer the term *seizure disorder*, due to the historically negative social stereotypes associated with the term *epilepsy* or *epileptic*.

Epilepsy is most often treated with antiseizure or anticonvulsant drug (AED) therapy. Treatment with monotherapy is the clinical goal; however, many patients do not achieve effective seizure control with monotherapy and require additional compounds to control seizure activity. Over 30 antiseizure drugs are approved for the treatment of seizures and act through different cellular mechanisms to restore the balance between excitatory and inhibitory drive underlying seizure generation. It is important to note that currently available antiseizure drugs do not alter the underlying pathology or alter the disease progression; as such, this approach is not curative. Antiseizure drugs are also commonly used to treat non-seizure disorders, such as chronic pain, migraine, bipolar disorder, and depression. Interestingly, but perhaps not surprisingly, these disorders also display a high level of comorbidity with epilepsy.

CLASSIFICATION OF SEIZURE TYPES

The classification proposed in 1989 by the Commission on Classification and Terminology of the International League Against Epilepsy is complex and continuously evolving due to the variable characteristics and etiologies of many epileptic syndromes. A simplified approach more suited to this discussion limits consideration to only the seizures themselves (Table 12-1). Seizures are broadly classified into two major groups: (1) **partial seizures**, which initiate as focal aberrant neuronal discharges in a single cortical site, and (2) **generalized seizures**, which initiate with abnormal neuronal activity in both cerebral hemispheres from the onset. Behavioral manifestations of both seizure types are determined based on the function of the cortical regions involved in the abnormal neuronal activity.

* The authors wish to acknowledge Dr. Vahn A. Lewis for his past contributions to this chapter.

Partial Seizures

Partial seizures can be divided into three subclassifications: (1) *simple partial*, (2) *complex partial*, and (3) *secondary generalized*. *Simple partial seizures* are characterized by seizure activity limited to specific brain regions that control muscles, somatosensation, sensory systems, higher cerebral function (psychic symptoms), or autonomic activity. Partial seizures do not impair consciousness and are often preceded by premonitory symptoms, termed *aura*. The seizure may remain localized, or it may spread to contiguous brain tissue, causing progressive symptoms as the wave of depolarization spreads along the cerebral cortex. This behavior is referred to as the Jacksonian March, after John Hughlings Jackson, who first described the phenomenon. For example, a simple partial motor seizure could begin with clonus of the face and then spread to involve the hand and arm following the organization of the motor cortex.

Complex partial seizures usually originate in the temporal or frontal lobe, but they spread to broader areas, frequently in a bilateral pattern. Consciousness is impaired; flashbacks or psychotic-like behavior may occur, and autonomic dysregulation and automatisms (involuntary, repetitive, and coordinated movements) are common.

The third type of partial seizure is a *secondary generalized seizure*. These seizures can begin as a simple and/or complex partial seizure. Following the initiation of seizure, activity spreads to the entire cortex, thalamus, and midbrain resulting in a tonic-clonic seizure. Partial seizures are often more refractory to antiseizure drugs and are often the focus of research into novel treatments.

Generalized Seizures

The most common type of generalized seizure is the **generalized tonic-clonic** (grand mal). The semiology is often described as sudden onset with loss of postural tone and tonic-clonic contractions of the arms and legs. The EEG pattern displays bilateral, synchronous high voltage polyspike activity, resulting from a bilateral generalization of seizure activity throughout the brain. Injury including head injuries, scalp lacerations, tongue biting, fracturing of teeth, and/or other bodily harms may occur due to the strong uncontrolled movements. Following a tonic-clonic seizure, patients are usually confused and lethargic, and they display headache and muscle ache. Generalize tonic-clonic seizures are responsive to pharmacotherapy.

A second common form of generalized seizure is **absence** seizure, which characteristically occurs in childhood. There are several varieties of absence seizures. The most common form (petit mal) is characterized by an abrupt but very short (5 to 10 seconds) loss of consciousness, often with minor muscular twitching (commonly restricted to the eyelids and face), and a 3-Hz spike-and-wave EEG pattern but no loss of postural control. Severe cases may involve hundreds of seizures per day. The term *absence* is appropriate because of the brief loss of consciousness and the vacant stare of the patient during a seizure. Similar to tonic-clonic seizures, absence seizures are often responsive to pharmacotherapy.

Other types of generalized seizures include (1) juvenile *myoclonic epilepsy*, characterized by sudden, brief, and violent spasms of one or more muscles or muscle groups, and (2) *atonic*, or "drop attacks," characterized by a sudden, brief loss of muscle tone. These varieties are usually associated with diffuse and severe progressive diseases of the brain and are often refractory to drug treatment.

Generalized seizures may also occur in the form of repeated or continuous seizures. When this lasts for over 5 minutes, or there is lack of return to baseline after a single epileptic seizure, this is referred to as **status epilepticus**. Tonic-clonic status epilepticus is rare but life-threatening. Status epilepticus may develop in patients with convulsive disorders, with acute disease affecting the brain (meningitis, encephalitis, toxemia of pregnancy, uremia, acute electrolyte imbalances), after abrupt withdrawal of depressant or antiseizure medication (barbiturates, benzodiazepines, opioids), or rarely after local anesthetic administration. Status epilepticus can occur in the absence of a prior history of seizures. The drugs most widely used to treat status epilepticus are intravenous benzodiazepines (lorazepam, diazepam, and midazolam), phenytoin, fosphenytoin, phenobarbital, and valproic acid. In refractory status epilepticus, the patient may have to undergo general anesthesia (e.g., midazolam, propofol, thiopental, and pentobarbital). An anesthetic dose of pentobarbital or propofol is effective and has a more rapid onset than phenobarbital. Because large doses of these drugs are usually required, there is the danger of respiratory depression and respiratory arrest, especially with barbiturates or propofol. **Status epilepticus** is best treated in a hospital setting.

TABLE 12-1 Classification of Epileptic Seizures

Classification	Clinical Aspects
I. Partial (focal, local) seizures	Involves one side of brain at onset
A. Simple partial seizures	Consciousness not impaired; specific or localized motor, sensory
B. Complex partial seizures (e.g., psychomotor, temporal lobe)	Consciousness impaired, automatisms, autonomic or psychological signs or symptoms; patients may report aura beforehand
C. Partial seizures with secondary generalization	See generalized seizures; patients may report aura beforehand
II. Generalized seizures	Involve both sides of brain at onset
A. Tonic-clonic seizures (grand mal)	Consciousness is lost; bilateral sharp tonic contraction of muscles, generalized from onset, followed by clonic contractions; patient may report aura before seizure
B. Absence seizures (e.g., petit mal)	Consciousness impaired, postural muscles not impaired, EEG spike and slow wave complexes at approximately 3 Hz
C. Myoclonic seizures	Sudden, brief contractions of individual muscles or groups producing spasms in muscles of face, trunk, and extremities
D. Clonic seizures	Repetitive clonic jerking (alternating contractions of opposing muscles)
E. Tonic seizures	Violent muscular contraction (simultaneous contraction of flexors and extensors) with limbs in strained position
F. Atonic seizures (astatic)	Sudden loss of muscle tone, consciousness sometimes lost, patients sustain fall injuries
III. Unclassified seizures	Cannot be classified because of insufficient data or atypical pattern of seizure

Adapted from Commission on Classification and Terminology of the International League against Epilepsy. *Epilepsia* 22:489-501, 1981.
EEG, Electroencephalogram.

PATHOPHYSIOLOGY

The pathophysiology of epilepsy and seizures is diverse, accounting for the many different types of seizure disorders. However, one commonality across epilepsies is a disrupted balance between excitatory (via glutamatergic signaling) and inhibitory (via GABAergic signaling) drive at the synaptic level that can result in seizure activity. Early pharmacologic studies demonstrated that $GABA_A$-receptor antagonists and glutamate-receptor (NMDA, AMPA, kainate) agonists could elicit seizure activity in normal animals. Further studies would demonstrate that interictal spikes commonly observed on EEG recordings from epilepsy patients are associated with a large depolarization and subsequent flurry of action potentials in individual neurons. The highly organized structure of cortical tissue with its laminar cell layers facilitates the flow of normal neuronal processing, while also providing a structure highly susceptible to abnormal synchronous activity that can lead to seizure generation. Under normal circumstances, excitatory synaptic activity is tightly regulated by inhibitory interneurons; however, genetic mutation, trauma, abnormal development, or a number of other insults disrupts this regulation allowing cortical networks to become hyperexcitable.

Partial epilepsies present clinically as any of the partial seizure types and account for ~60% of epilepsy patients. The etiology of partial epilepsies is broad and includes cortical lesions, tumors, developmental malformation, or acute cortical damage due to trauma or stroke. Trauma-induced epilepsy is becoming a larger issue as medical advances allow patients to survive more severe traumas that would have been fatal in previous generations. Genetics may also play a role in partial epilepsies underlying cortical malformations or tumor generation.[7] In contrast, generalized epilepsies, accounting for ~40% of patients, are usually genetic in etiology. Genetic mutations to ion channels (or channelopathies), including voltage-gated sodium channels and $GABA_A$ receptors, have been identified for many generalized epilepsies and help guide treatment strategies.

ANTISEIZURE THERAPEUTICS

Antiseizure drugs control, but do not cure, epilepsy. They may, however, play a neuroprotective role by limiting cumulative pathology that could result from uncontrolled seizure activity. The primary objective of anticonvulsant therapy is to suppress seizures while causing minimal impairment of central nervous system (CNS) function or other deleterious side effects. With the currently available anticonvulsants, seizure control can be obtained in only approximately 70% of cases, and the associated side effects, including cognitive dysfunction and hepatic failure, can be debilitating and life-threatening. Many patients with epilepsy have to take medication for life to maintain seizure control. To minimize toxicity, monotherapy is the preferred therapeutic strategy with careful monitoring of plasma drug concentrations. If seizures persist, substitution with a second drug is preferred over polytherapy. Unfortunately, for many patients, this therapeutic goal is not realized, and polytherapy or multidrug therapy is required. Antiseizure drugs work though a number of different mechanisms, and a few compounds display multiple mechanisms of action Table 12-2. Common mechanisms include:

1. alteration of conductance, through voltage and chemically gated ion channels selective for Na^+, Ca^{2+}, K^+, Cl^-, and H^+
2. enhancement of GABA signaling in the synaptic cleft
3. altered synaptic function and probability of vesicle release
4. modification of neurotransmitters with modulatory roles, including peptides and hormones

Phenobarbital, introduced in 1912, was the first synthetic organic compound used extensively to treat seizures. Subsequently, numerous anticonvulsant agents were introduced between 1938 and 1960, including the hydantoins, succinimides, and primidone. Between 1960 and 1992, several novel anticonvulsants were introduced (e.g., carbamazepine, valproic acid, clonazepam, clorazepate). With the passages of the Expedited Drug Approval Act and Prescription Drug User Fee Act in

TABLE 12-2 Mechanisms of Action and Uses for Anticonvulsant Drugs

	ION CHANNEL MODULATION					USES*			
Drug	**Na^+**	**Ca^{2+}**	**K^+**	**Increased GABA Effect**	**Decreased Excitatory Amino Acid Effect**	**Seizure Type**	**Absence**	**Other**	**Comments**
Hydantoins									
Phenytoin	X			X	X	TC, CP, SE		NP (T), rarely cardiac arrhythmias	Prompt and extended-dose forms
Fosphenytoin	X			X	X	SE			IM and IV form for injection
Iminostilbenes									
Carbamazepine	X			X		TC, CP		BI, T, other NP	
Oxcarbazepine	X					P, P-AJ			Prodrug; action similar to carbamazepine
Barbiturates									
Phenobarbital				X	X	TC, CF, SE		LA, F	
Primidone				X	X	TC, CP, focal			
Carboxylic Acid									
Valproic acid	X	TT		x (?)	x (?)	TC, SE, P	X	BI, NP, F, M, MY AD, AK	First broad-spectrum anticonvulsant
Succinimides									
Ethosuximide		TT					X		

Continued

TABLE 12-2 Mechanisms of Action and Uses for Anticonvulsant Drugs—cont'd

	ION CHANNEL MODULATION					USES*			
Drug	**Na^+**	**Ca^{2+}**	**K^+**	**Increased GABA Effect**	**Decreased Excitatory Amino Acid Effect**	**Seizure Type**	**Absence**	**Other**	**Comments**
Benzodiazepines									
Lorazepam				x	x (?)	SE		LA	
Clonazepam				x	x (?)	CP (?)	x	AK	
Clorazepate				x	x (?)	P			
Diazepam				x	x (?)	SE		LA	
Midazolam				x	x (?)	SE		F	May be effective after buccal administration but can reduce respiration rate
Carbonic Anhydrase Inhibitors									
Acetazolamide							x	CT	Rapid tolerance
Newer Agents									
Lamotrigine	x			HVA	x (?)	P-AJ, LG	x	NP, BI, AK	Restricted LG use in children <16 years old
Gabapentin		α2δ		x		P		NP (T) (PN)	May be useful for neuropathic pain
Pregabalin		α2δ		x		P		NP (D,PN), FY	
Vigabatrin				x		P-AJ, CP, LG, WS			Irreversible GABA transaminase inhibitor
Felbamate	x	HVA		x	NMDA	P-AJ, LG			Use limited by toxicity
Tiagabine				x		P-AJ			Blocks GABA reuptake
Topiramate[†]	x	HVA		x	x	P, TC		NP (M), AK	Unique monosaccharide structure
Zonisamide	x	TT		x		P-AJ			Sulfonamide-like structure, some antidepressant-like action and carbonic acid inhibition
Levetiracetam		x				P-AJ, MY, TC			SV2 protein inhibitor
Retigabine			x						

AD, Aggression in dementia; *AJ*, adjunctive use; *AK*, akinetic; *α2δ*, alpha 2 delta subunit; *BI*, bipolar disorder; *CF*, corticofocal; *CP*, complex partial psychomotor; *CT*, catamenial; *D*, diabetic neuropathy; *F*, febrile; *FY*, fibromyalgia; *HVA*, high voltage activated; *IM*, impulse disorder; *JM*, Jacksonian motor; *LA*, local anesthetic-induced seizures; *LG*, Lennox-Gastaut syndrome (children); *M*, migraine; *MY*, myoclonic; *NMDA*, *N*-methyl-D-aspartate; *NP*, neuropathic pain; *P*, partial seizures; *PN*, postherpetic neuropathy; *SE*, status epilepticus; *SV2*, synaptic vessel protein 2; *T*, trigeminal neuralgia; *TC*, tonic-clonic; *TT*, T-type; *WS*, West syndrome (children).

*Several anticonvulsants are used to treat bipolar disorder, neuralgia (and chronic pain), and impulse control disorders. They may be referred to by the term *mood stabilizers*.

[†]Derived from the sulfonamides.

1992, the approval process was facilitated, and 10 agents have since been introduced. Many of these drugs have been approved as adjunctive agents for use with earlier drugs in the treatment of "partial-onset seizures"; these indications have broadened with increased experience in their use. In some cases the newer agents are referred to as second-generation and third-generation agents, and in several cases, newer agents are related to older agents, such as phenytoin and fosphenytoin; carbamazepine and oxcarbazine; and meprobamate, felbamate, and fluorofelbamate.

Drugs are described as having characteristic spectra for treating the various forms of seizures (Fig. 12-1). Prescribing antiepileptic drugs for conditions outside their spectra may lead to problems beyond simple therapeutic failure. In particular, absence seizures can be exacerbated by many of the drugs used to treat tonic-clonic seizures (i.e., tiagabine, vigabatrin). Some children "outgrow" absence epilepsy but have a tendency to develop other forms of epilepsy in later years. The discovery of valproic acid, which displays multiple mechanisms of action, was a major breakthrough for patients in whom absence seizures convert to tonic-clonic seizures. The careful withdrawal of anticonvulsant therapy in children with a history of tonic-clonic epilepsy, but who have been seizure-free for several years, is sometimes successful. Finally, adults whose seizures were few in number before initiation of treatment and are well controlled with a single antiseizure drug may be weaned after 2 years of therapy with a reasonable expectation (~50%) of avoiding relapse.

Adverse reactions can result from the direct action of the drug or complex drug–drug interactions. Adverse reactions are diverse, and they can range from subtle cognitive dysfunction and gastrointestinal upset to more serious and life-threatening ones, such as Stevens-Johnson syndrome, toxic cardiomyopathy, and permanent blindness. Like other pharmaceutical agents, the liver is the primary site of metabolism of antiseizure drugs. Induction or inhibition of liver enzymes (cytochrome P450s, i.e., CYP34A) must be taken into consideration when prescribing medications (Box 12-1). Specific details of the effects of specific antiseizure drugs on hepatic function are discussed below.

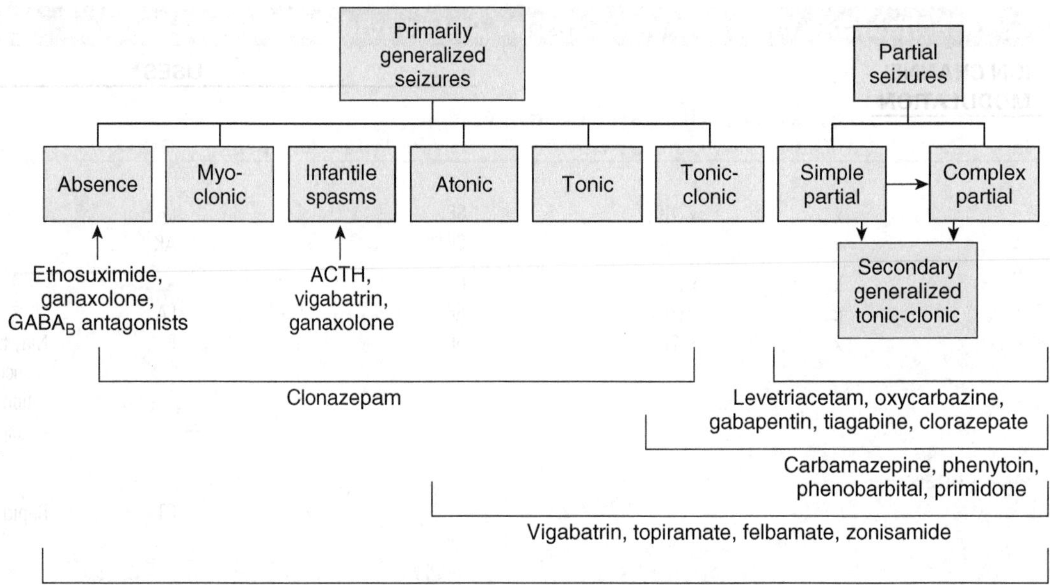

FIG 12-1 Therapeutic spectra of anticonvulsant drugs. Anticonvulsant agents need to be matched to the convulsive disorder being treated. Phenytoin, phenobarbital, carbamazepine, oxycarbazine, vigabatrin, gabapentin, and tiagabine are ineffective in, but can aggravate, absence and myoclonic seizures. Benzodiazepines and acetazolamide have broad spectra, but tolerance develops to their actions, so they cannot be used for maintenance therapy. *ACTH,* Adrenocorticotropic hormone; *$GABA_B$,* γ-aminobutyric acid type B receptor.

BOX 12-1 Adverse Effect of Antiepileptic Drugs on Liver Microsomal Enzymes

Drugs That Can Induce Liver Microsomal Enzymes

Phenobarbital
Phenytoin
Carbamazepine
Oxcarbazepine*
Lamotrigine

Drugs That Can Inhibit Liver Microsomal Enzymes

Oxcarbazepine†
Topiramate
Valproic acid
Phenytoin†

*Induces to a lesser degree than carbamazepine.
†Inhibition and induction have been reported. This is possible because different cytochrome P450 enzyme classes are involved in each effect.

CHEMISTRY AND STRUCTURE–ACTIVITY RELATIONSHIPS

Figure 12-2 shows the common structure present in all the clinically effective anticonvulsants developed before 1960. Substitution at position 1 of the ring results in the various classes of anticonvulsants indicated in Table 12-3.

A phenyl ring at R_1 or R_2, such as appears in phenytoin, is a highly desirable, although not crucial, substituent for protection against tonic-clonic epilepsy. An alkyl substituent at R_1 or R_2, such as appears in ethosuximide, is desirable (but not crucial) for control of absence seizures. A great deal of detailed structure activity information was obtained to identify opportunities for developing improved agents. More recent discoveries have included several agents with unrelated

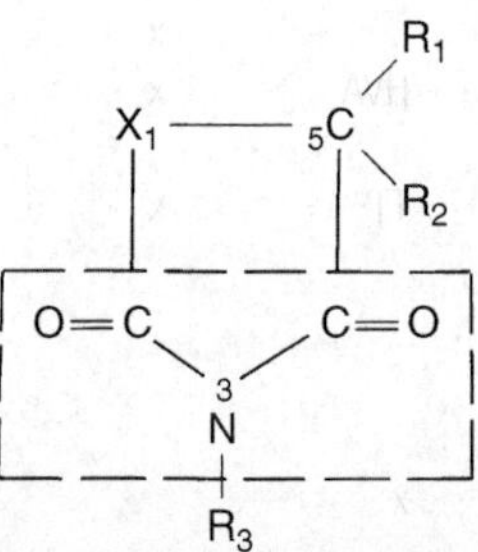

FIG 12-2 Basic ring structure common to classic anticonvulsants.

structures, however. Valproic acid is an n-dipropylacetic acid (Fig. 12-3), a simple branched-chain carboxylic acid, and carbamazepine (Fig. 12-4) is chemically related to the tricyclic antidepressants and is used in the treatment of certain affective disorders (see Chapter 10).

COMMON ANTISEIZURE DRUGS

Hydantoins: Phenytoin

Phenytoin (diphenylhydantoin) is one of the first drugs to be discovered through an organized scientific search for a therapeutically effective compound. Introduced in 1938, phenytoin was immediately recognized as a breakthrough in anticonvulsant therapy because it suppressed seizures without causing as much sedative effect as phenobarbital. Phenytoin is an effective anticonvulsant against tonic-clonic and partial seizures and an important pharmacologic tool that has increased understanding of the underlying mechanisms responsible for epileptic syndromes. Fosphenytoin (Cerebyx®, Parke-Davis) is a phosphorylated prodrug that is rapidly converted to phenytoin by endogenous phosphatase enzymes. It is water-soluble and is better tolerated by parenteral administration. The structures of phenytoin and fosphenytoin are shown in Figure 12-5.

TABLE 12-3 Classes of Anticonvulsants According to Substitution at Position X_1 of the Chemical Structure (See Fig. 12-2)

Anticonvulsant	Substitution
Barbiturates	—CO—NH—
Hydantoins	—NH—
Succinimides	—CH_2—

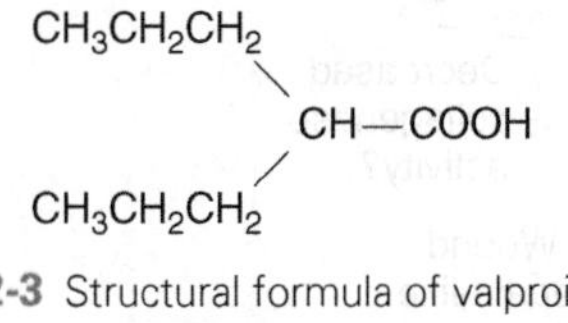

$CH_3CH_2CH_2$ \ CH—COOH / $CH_3CH_2CH_2$

FIG 12-3 Structural formula of valproic acid.

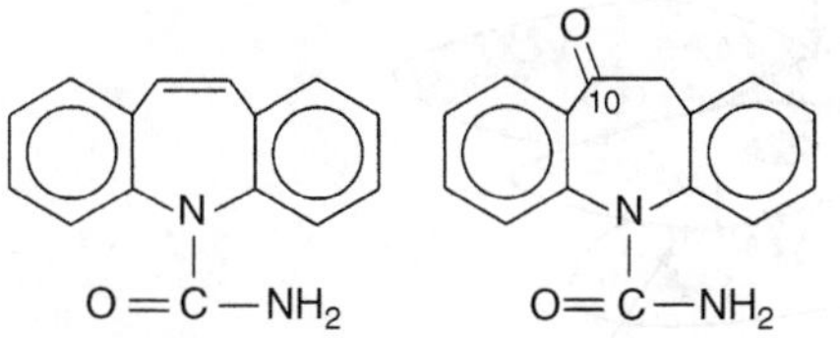

Carbamazepine Oxcarbazepine

FIG 12-4 Structural formulas of carbamazepine and oxcarbazepine.

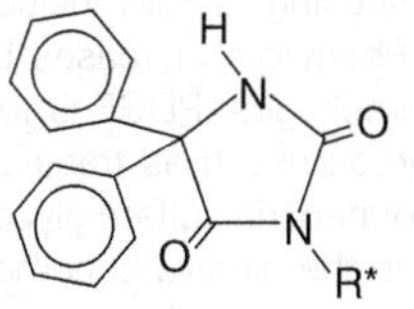

Phenytoin $R^* = H$ Fosphenytoin $R^* = \text{-}OPO_3^{--} + 2\ Na^+$

FIG 12-5 Structural formulas of phenytoin and fosphenytoin.

Mechanism of action

The major site of action of phenytoin seems to be at the Na^+ channel, and various actions have been shown at this site. Phenytoin prevents the spread of abnormal neuronal depolarization from the epileptic focus to surrounding normal neuronal populations, but spontaneous discharge at the focus is not depressed. Additionally, phenytoin suppresses the duration of neuronal afterdischarge. Phenytoin may reduce the spread of neuronal activity and afterdischarge by blocking post-tetanic potentiation, a phenomenon in which synaptic transmission is enhanced as a result of repetitive presynaptic activation (as would occur at an abnormally firing epileptic focus). The only mechanism evident at concentrations equivalent to therapeutic plasma concentrations is a reduction in sustained high-frequency neuronal firing caused by phenytoin **binding reversibly to inactivated Na^+ channels.** Phenytoin delays the neuronal recovery process whereby Na^+ channels cycle from the refractory, inactivated state to the responsive, closed configuration, which is required before an action potential can be generated again. Phenytoin binding to inactivated Na^+ channels is frequency and voltage dependent so that it becomes greater as neuronal depolarization and firing frequency increase. These properties are ideally suited for anticonvulsant activity because high-frequency neuronal discharge is characteristic of seizure disorders.

High extracellular K^+, typically found during seizures, also increases the effectiveness of phenytoin. Normal (slower) neuronal activity is unaffected by phenytoin, which may explain its minimal sedative effects. At slightly greater than therapeutic concentrations, phenytoin interferes with Ca^{2+} channel activity and the interaction of Ca^{2+} and calmodulin. These activities of phenytoin may disrupt Ca^{2+}-dependent neurotransmitter release from presynaptic nerve terminals. There are also some reports of phenytoin modulating GABA and glutamate synaptic release. Finally, phenytoin has also been found to alter the metabolism of some growth factors, which could play a role in neuroprotective actions of the drug.

Pharmacokinetics

Phenytoin is absorbed slowly from the gastrointestinal tract. The absorption rate varies with the individual, but differences in formulation of the dosage unit account for much of this fluctuation. The U.S. Food and Drug Administration (FDA) requires that phenytoin capsules be labeled as "extended" or "immediate" depending on their absorption rate. An extended-action capsule has slow absorption, with peak blood concentrations obtained in 4 to 12 hours. An immediate-action capsule has rapid absorption, with peak concentrations occurring in 1.5 to 3 hours. Because noncompliance is a major problem in anticonvulsant therapy, it is sometimes advisable to administer the total daily dose of phenytoin at one time. Once-a-day administration is inappropriate for suspensions of phenytoin (commonly used for children) because plasma concentrations may reach toxic values. Changing from one formulation or manufacturer to another has led to suboptimal plasma concentrations from differences in bioavailability.

Phenytoin given by intravenous injection can produce thrombophlebitis, arrhythmia, and hypotension. The vehicle needed to solubilize phenytoin for injection largely causes these side effects. Intramuscular injection of phenytoin may precipitate in the muscle, cause pain, and be poorly absorbed. Fosphenytoin is a water-soluble analogue that may be given intravenously or intramuscularly and is converted to phenytoin by phosphatases in the liver and red blood cells. After intramuscular administration, it produces much less pain and is absorbed rapidly.

Phenytoin is highly protein bound (90%), which may play a role in interactions with drugs that compete for plasma protein binding sites. Phenytoin is inactivated in the liver by CYP2C9/10 and to a lesser extent CYP2C19. Within the liver, phenytoin can also induce drug-metabolizing enzymes, including CYP3A4 and uridine diphosphate-glucuronosyltransferase (UGT), directly reducing the concentration of other antiseizure drugs and common medications including oral contraceptives. After conjugation with glucuronic acid, phenytoin and its metabolites are eliminated in the urine. Blood–brain barrier transporters including P-glycoprotein and multidrug resistance (MDR) proteins may facilitate phenytoin removal from the brain. Phenytoin is also secreted by the salivary glands, which may be a contributing factor in producing gingival overgrowth (hyperplasia). Peak concentrations occur at 3 to 12 hours, and the elimination half-life of phenytoin (and fosphenytoin) generally ranges from 6 to 24 hours. Near the effective dose, phenytoin often exhibits capacity-limited metabolism because the enzymes responsible for its metabolism are readily saturated. The drug's half-life can become longer, and if blood concentrations are increased beyond the saturation threshold, rapid drug accumulation may increase the likelihood of adverse reactions.

Toxicity

Ataxia, nystagmus, incoordination, and unsteadiness occur with phenytoin overdose. These sequelae may result from phenytoin-induced modulation of Purkinje cell function in the cerebellum (such changes

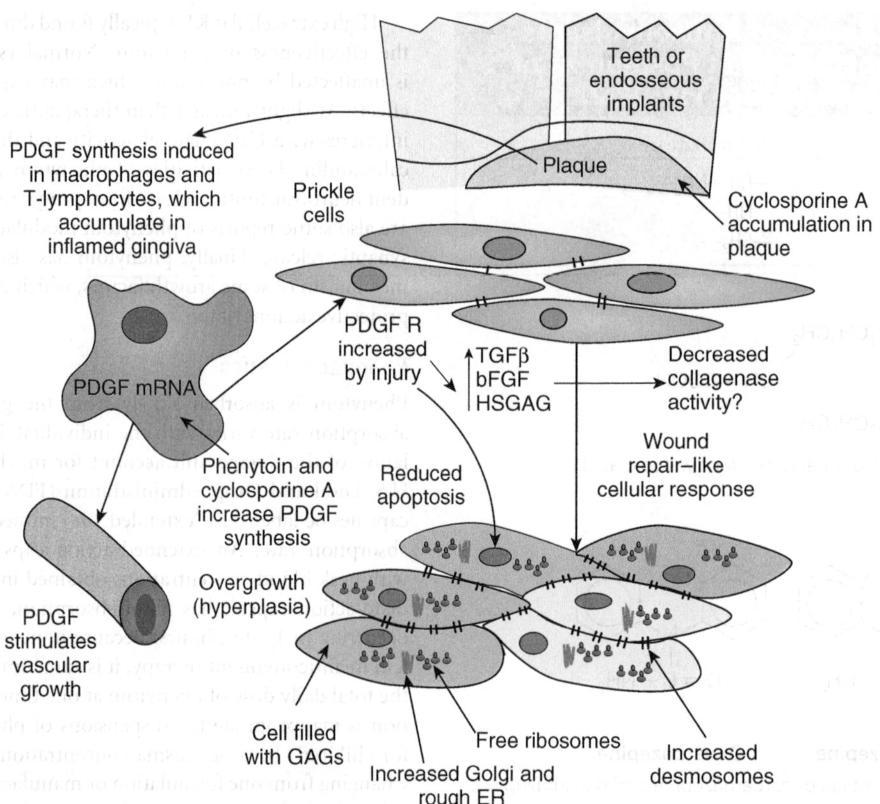

FIG 12-6 Effect of phenytoin and cyclosporine on gingival overgrowth. Predisposing factors include the presence of teeth or implants, inflammation, and overgrowth-inducing drugs. Phenytoin increases by six-fold platelet-derived growth factor (*PDGF*) mRNA in reparative/proliferative macrophages. PDGF is thought to increase angiogenesis and wound repair. Increases in fibroblastic growth factors, such as transforming growth factor-β (*TGFβ*) and basic fibroblast growth factor (*bFGF*), and production of heparin sulfate glycosaminoglycan (*HSGAG*) are induced by PDGF acting on its receptor (*R*). Prickle cells in the gingiva become filled with glycosaminoglycans (*GAGs*), rough endoplasmic reticulum (*ER*), and ribosomes, and their connective desmosomes proliferate (*bottom*).

may also be caused by repeated seizures). Drowsiness, lethargy, diplopia, confusion, and (rarely) hallucinations are other manifestations of phenytoin toxicity. Phenytoin in usual doses has little detrimental effect on the cardiovascular system; however, it can cause cardiovascular collapse, irreversible coma, and death if administered in massive intravenous doses.

Phenytoin promotes **gingival overgrowth** in approximately 10% to 30% of all patients. Gingival overgrowth is usually more severe in children, for whom its incidence may be 50%. The primary mechanism responsible for this side effect is unknown. Several factors have been proposed including inflammation, bacterial plaque, the presence of teeth or dental implants, gingival fibroblast phenotype, epithelial growth factor, collagenase activation, folic acid deficiency, Na^+/Ca^{2+} flux, and perhaps salivary delivery of phenytoin into the mouth. It has been observed more recently that phenytoin increases platelet-derived growth factor B, and its mRNA in macrophages that are thought to induce gingival fibroblast proliferation and local angiogenesis. The transforming growth factor-β pathway involving Grb1, SOS-RAS-ERK1/2, AP1, and Ca^{2+} signaling pathways has been implicated in hereditary gingival overgrowth and may play a role in drug-induced gingival overgrowth. The result is an increase in fibroblast cell growth with increased interstitial ground substance. Other drugs that induce gingival overgrowth include the immunosuppressant cyclosporine and the Ca^{2+} channel–blocking drugs. A more recent investigation has found that all of these drugs have the ability to reduce apoptosis (programmed cell death), suggesting that reduced cell loss rates could also play a role in gingival overgrowth. Figure 12-6 represents a possible model of gingival overgrowth.

Phenytoin may also cause numerous other side effects as summarized in Table 12-4. Phenytoin interferes with the metabolic activation of vitamins D and K and the absorption of Ca^{2+}. Although the resultant effect on bone metabolism is usually subclinical, overt cases of rickets and osteomalacia have been observed. Vitamin D or K supplements may prevent these conditions. Children born to mothers who have received phenytoin (often in combination with phenobarbital, carbamazepine, or valproic acid) throughout their pregnancy are at increased risk of congenital malformation. The most common anomalies are cleft lip, cleft palate, and congenital heart disease. These developmental defects, a delay in psychomotor development, prenatal and postnatal growth deficiencies, impaired intellectual performance, and genitourinary and skeletal deformations are collectively referred to as the ***fetal hydantoin syndrome.*** None of the well-studied anticonvulsants is completely devoid of teratogenic potential.

Therapeutic use

Phenytoin is one of the most widely used antiseizure agents due to its efficacy against partial and generalized tonic-clonic seizures. However, phenytoin is not effective against absence seizures. **Fosphenytoin is useful in adult patients with partial or generalized seizures that require intravenous or intramuscular administration. In addition**

TABLE 12-4 Adverse Reactions Reported for Anticonvulsant Drugs

Drug	Adverse Reactions
Phenytoin and fosphenytoin	Gingival hyperplasia, hirsutism, megaloblastic anemia, osteomalacia, sedation, ataxia, gastrointestinal disturbances, behavioral changes
Carbamazepine and oxcarbazepine	Sedation, weakness, ataxia, diplopia, gastrointestinal disturbances, skin rash, behavioral changes, aplastic anemia (rare)
Phenobarbital	Sedation, weakness, ataxia, reduced cognition, respiratory depression, blood dyscrasias, megaloblastic anemia, osteomalacia, drug dependence
Valproic acid	Sedation, weakness, ataxia, gastrointestinal disturbances, weight gain, hepatotoxicity (especially in children <2 years old), spina bifida if given during pregnancy, visual disturbances, pancreatitis, hyperammonemia
Ethosuximide	Sedation, weakness, gastrointestinal disturbances, ataxia, behavioral changes, lupus erythematosus (rare)
Diazepam	Sedation, weakness, nystagmus, ataxia, drug dependence, drug tolerance
Lorazepam	Same as diazepam
Midazolam	Same as diazepam
Chlorazepate	Same as diazepam
Clonazepam	Same as diazepam
Gabapentin	Sedation, weakness, ataxia, rash, tremor
Lamotrigine	Sedation, weakness, ataxia, diplopia, rash, headache, gastrointestinal disturbances, Stevens-Johnson syndrome (1% of children)
Topiramate	Sedation, weakness, ataxia, visual disturbances, paresthesias, kidney stones, breast pain
Tiagabine	Sedation, weakness, ataxia, gastrointestinal disturbances, tremor
Vigabatrin	Sedation, weakness, ataxia, psychotic reactions, visual disturbances, blood dyscrasias
Zonisamide	Sedation, weakness, ataxia, gastrointestinal disturbances, skin rashes, Stevens-Johnson syndrome, renal tubule acidosis, renal stones
Levetiracetam	Sedation, weakness, ataxia, exacerbation of behavioral problems, withdrawal reactions
Retigabine	Somnolence, dizziness, confusion, urinary retention, cardiac QT interval prolongation

to its use in treating epilepsy, phenytoin is useful in treating patients with **trigeminal and associated neuralgias.**

Barbiturates

Phenobarbital is one of the oldest, least expensive, and most effective anticonvulsants available. However, because of its sedative effect and the introduction of newer drugs, the use of phenobarbital for treating seizure disorders has waned in many countries. Due to its relatively low toxicity and price, it is still commonly used in developing countries and remains one of the most commonly used antiseizure drugs worldwide. Primidone, a deoxybarbiturate relative of phenobarbital, also displays antiseizure activity, but it is not often used.

Mechanism of action

The barbiturates are CNS depressants and exert a marked inhibitory effect on repetitive neuronal activity in CNS pathways. Phenobarbital enhances the binding of GABA to postsynaptic $GABA_A$ receptors and increases the time that **$GABA_A$-activated Cl^- channels** are open. At higher doses, phenobarbital may also limit sustained repetitive neuronal firing, which could facilitate its effects in treating status epilepticus. Barbiturates as a drug class can also activate Cl^- channels independently of GABA. Inhibition of the excitatory effects of glutamate (possibly kinate and α-amino-3-hydroxy-5-methyl-4-isoxazole propionate [AMPA] receptor types) may also be a major antiepileptic mechanism. Other mechanisms seem to play lesser roles. Barbiturates block the transcellular transport of Na^+ and K^+, which could explain their membrane-stabilizing properties. Similar to phenytoin, barbiturates interfere with Ca^{2+} channel function and inhibit Ca^{2+} entry into presynaptic nerve terminals.

Pharmacokinetics

Phenobarbital is completely, but slowly, absorbed from the gastrointestinal tract. About half of the drug is bound to plasma proteins. Approximately 30% of phenobarbital is excreted unchanged in the urine, and the liver inactivates the remainder, principally by CYP2C9. Phenobarbital **induces UGT enzymes CYP2C and CYP3A.** The induction of CYP3A can affect oral contraceptive concentrations. The plasma half-life of phenobarbital ranges between 50 and 140 hours. Because of its long half-life, very small fluctuations in plasma concentrations occur over a 24-hour period. Primidone is metabolized to phenobarbital, which can be detected in the plasma in approximately 24 to 48 hours. Phenylethylmalonamide, another barbiturate with anticonvulsant properties, is measurable in plasma within 1 to 2 hours after administration and has a 10- to 18-hour half-life.

Toxicity

The most common initial effect of phenobarbital and the other barbiturates is sedation; however, tolerance to this effect may develop over time. A paradoxical excitatory reaction (i.e., hyperactivity, irritability, and agitation) may also occur in children and elderly patients. Phenobarbital can cause megaloblastic anemia and osteomalacia. Phenobarbital seems to be free of teratogenic effects, but when phenobarbital is given with phenytoin (a commonly used combination), teratogenicity seems to increase.

The most common side effects of primidone are primarily a result of its CNS depressant properties. Complications include sedation, dizziness, ataxia, and nystagmus. Various blood dyscrasias and rashes similar to conditions described for phenytoin can occur.

Therapeutic use

Phenobarbital offers an appreciable spectrum of anticonvulsant activity because of its effectiveness against many generalized tonic-clonic and partial seizures. Primidone is used for generalized and partial seizures, particularly seizures refractory to other drugs. The use of primidone is limited because of its marked sedative properties immediately after administration.

Carbamazepine

Carbamazepine is an iminostilbene derivative (see Fig. 12-4) closely related chemically to the tricyclic antidepressants. It was first approved as an antiseizure agent in 1974.

Mechanism of action

Similar to phenytoin, carbamazepine reduces experimentally induced, sustained high-frequency neuronal firing at doses that produce clinically relevant plasma concentrations. This effect seems to result from carbamazepine **binding to inactivated Na$^+$ channels**, slowing neuronal recovery after activation. Carbamazepine also reduces Ca^{2+} and Na^+ flux across the neuronal membrane. The carbamazepine metabolite, 10,11-epoxycarbamazepine, also limits sustained repetitive firing in neurons and could contribute to the antiseizure properties of carbamazepine.

Pharmacokinetics

Carbamazepine is absorbed slowly following oral administration, reaching peak plasma concentrations in 4 to 8 hours. It is distributed throughout the body; highest concentrations occur in the liver, kidneys, and brain. Blood–brain barrier transporters P-glycoprotein and MDR proteins transport the drug out of the brain. Carbamazepine is metabolized by CYP3A4 and can induce CYP3A4, CYP2C9, CYP1A2, and UGT enzymes. The **induction of CYP3A4** is of particular interest as it can accelerate the metabolism of several drugs, including oral contraceptives. Carbamazepine is inactivated by further oxidation and conjugation before being excreted in the urine.

Toxicity

The most common signs and symptoms of overdose with carbamazepine are dizziness, diplopia, drowsiness, headache, ataxia, and slurred speech. Some tolerance to the neurotoxic effects is observed and effects can be minimized by initially prescribing low doses then gradually increasing dosage to reach the necessary maintenance dosage. Convulsions may be precipitated by acute intoxication with carbamazepine, and it can exacerbate absence and myoclonic seizures. Various types of involuntary motor activity in elderly patients have been reported, and hallucinations have occurred. Skin rashes have been reported. Certain Asian populations seem to have an increased risk for Stevens-Johnson syndrome. If leukopenia occurs, it is usually mild. Other hematologic reactions to carbamazepine are rare but sometimes life-threatening. Aplastic anemia is of particular concern, and agranulocytosis has also occurred.

Therapeutic use

Carbamazepine is highly effective against generalized tonic-clonic seizures and both simple and complex partial seizures. It also lacks dysmorphic side effects (e.g., gingival hypertrophy, acne, hirsutism) common to phenytoin. Similar to phenytoin, carbamazepine is indicated for the treatment of **trigeminal neuralgia**; carbamazepine has been the most commonly used drug for this disorder. Carbamazepine is also used for other neuropathic pains, such as glossopharyngeal neuralgia, postherpetic neuralgia, diabetic neuropathy, causalgia, and hemifacial spasm.

Oxcarbazepine

A keto-analogue of carbamazepine, **oxcarbazepine** (see Fig. 12-4), has a similar therapeutic profile and mechanism of action. Oxcarbazepine is a prodrug, requiring metabolic reduction to the 10-hydroxy metabolite before it becomes active. Oxcarbazepine has been approved as adjunctive or monotherapy for partial seizures in adults, monotherapy for partial seizures in children between 4 and 16 years of age, and adjunctive therapy for children 2 years old and older. It may have fewer side effects than carbamazepine and is well tolerated. Oxcarbazepine is rapidly converted to the 10-hydroxy metabolite, which exerts peak activity from 3 to 13 hours and has a 9-hour half-life. Oxcarbazepine is also a CYP3A4 inducer, but to a lesser degree than carbamazepine. Substitution of oxcarbazepine for carbamazepine will increase levels of phenytoin and valproic acid, but it will still result in decreased levels of oral contraceptives.

Valproic Acid

Valproic acid (dipropylacetic acid), approved by the FDA in 1978, is a simple branched-chain carboxylic acid with a broad-spectrum mechanism of action and antiseizure profile.

Mechanism of action

Similar to phenytoin and carbamazepine, valproic acid reduces sustained high-frequency neuronal firing at therapeutic doses by stabilizing the inactive state of **voltage-gated Na$^+$ channels**. Valproic acid is presumed to bind a different site on the Na^+ channel than phenytoin, but the final result is similar.

Experimental studies have shown that supertherapeutic doses of valproic acid increase brain GABA concentrations by interfering with enzymes involved with GABA. Valproic acid is a weak inhibitor of GABA transaminase, the first enzyme in the catabolic pathway, and a more potent inhibitor of succinic semialdehyde dehydrogenase, the next enzyme in the biosynthetic pathway. Valproic acid may also increase brain GABA by stimulating glutamic acid decarboxylase, the major synthetic enzyme for GABA. However, it has been difficult to link these activates on GABAergic neurotransmission and antiseizure effects.

The salutary effect of valproic acid on absence seizures is most likely associated with the drug's ability to inhibit Ca^{2+} influx through **T-type Ca^{2+} channels**, similar to ethosuximide. In addition to seizures, valproic acid is approved for the treatment of bipolar disorder, and its divalproex extended-release form is approved for the prevention of migraine headaches.

Pharmacokinetics

Valproic acid is completely absorbed from the gastrointestinal tract and is highly bound to plasma proteins. The absorption rate depends on the formulation (capsules, tablets, or syrup); ingestion with food may delay absorption. Divalproex sodium, a combination of valproic acid and its Na^+ salt, is supplied in capsules that are designed to be opened and sprinkled on soft food. This product is a convenient dosage form for children and elderly patients.

Valproic acid crosses membrane barriers and can be found in the fetus, milk, liver, kidney, and brain. It also accumulates in growing bone. Valproic acid is thought to enter the brain through a saturable process, and blocking MDR proteins with probenecid can increase brain concentrations. Valproic acid undergoes complex oxidation and conjugation before excretion in the urine with 10 or more metabolites. It inhibits its own metabolism and that of other drugs, such as phenobarbital. This effect can contribute to drug accumulation and drug interactions. Valproic acid inhibits the metabolism of some substrates metabolized by CYP2C9 and UGT. The half-life of valproic acid is approximately 5 to 20 hours, with peak blood concentrations at 1 to 4 hours.

Toxicity

The most common manifestations of valproic acid toxicity are appetite disturbances, indigestion, heartburn, nausea, weight change, sedation, and ataxia. The gastrointestinal reactions are usually temporary. Tremor is also a common adverse effect, especially at higher doses. Valproic acid can cause fatal hepatic dysfunction, and children are particularly susceptible. The likelihood of this apparently idiosyncratic effect decreases with age, being most common in children younger than 2 years and uncommon after age 10 years. Irreversible hepatotoxicity seems to be caused by a toxic metabolite (2-n-propyl-4-pentenoic acid). Because its production is known to be increased by enzyme-inducing antiseizure drugs, combined therapy of valproic acid and such antiseizure drugs puts the patient at increased risk of liver damage. More commonly, valproic acid may cause a reversible hepatotoxicity that is dose dependent.

Another serious toxicity associated with valproate is life-threatening pancreatitis. Pancreatitis can occur in children or adults and may follow a rapid course. This reaction may occur any time when taking the medication. Other serious side effects, such as neurologic and hematologic toxicity, are rare. High doses of valproic acid may cause platelet disorders. Valproic acid is associated with neural tube defects and its use during pregnancy results in a significantly higher risk of spina bifida. Surveys have found the teratogenic risk may be higher than that for other antiseizure drugs.

Therapeutic use

Valproic acid is a broad-spectrum antiseizure drug. It is particularly effective against absence seizures and other generalized forms of epilepsy including tonic-clonic and myoclonic seizures. Valproic acid is also used to treat partial seizures and infantile spasms. In addition to seizure disorders, valproic acid has been approved for treatment of mania in bipolar disorder and for migraine pain.

Succinimides: Ethosuximide

Ethosuximide is the major antiseizure drug in this chemical group and is used commonly to treat absence seizures in children.

Mechanism of action

The mechanism of action of ethosuximide is not firmly established; however, its administration leads to a dose-dependent inhibition of low-threshold Ca^{2+} currents carried by **T-type Ca^{2+} channels**. Low-threshold Ca^{2+} currents are an important factor in oscillatory behavior of thalamic neurons, and the thalamus is known to play an important role in generating the 3-Hz spike-and-wave rhythms that characterize absence seizures. This effect occurs at clinical concentrations and is the best explanation yet proposed for the mechanism of action of drugs effective against absence seizures.

Pharmacokinetics

Ethosuximide is absorbed from the gastrointestinal tract, metabolized in the liver by CYP3A4, and excreted as metabolites in the urine. The plasma half-life of ethosuximide is approximately 30 hours in children and 45 to 60 hours in adults. Ethosuximide passes membrane barriers rapidly and appears in cerebrospinal fluid, milk, saliva, and fetal tissues. Salivary titers accurately reflect plasma concentrations and may be useful to monitor blood levels.

Toxicity

The succinimides commonly cause gastrointestinal distress, headache, dizziness, and skin rash. Some tolerance to these effects develops over time. More serious skin reactions such as urticaria and Steves-Johnson syndrome have been reported, as well as Parkinson-like symptoms and photophobia. Blood counts are recommended at no greater than monthly intervals because potentially fatal bone marrow depression may occur. Patients with hematopoietic toxicity may exhibit fever, sore throat, and coagulopathy, as indicated by oral and cutaneous petechiae. Ethosuximide is less teratogenic than valproate, and of the two, it is preferred for pregnant women or women of childbearing age.

Therapeutic use

Ethosuximide prevents absence seizures in approximately 50% of patients and reduces their frequency in another 40% to 45%. As a result, it is often the initial pharmacologic treatment used for absence seizures. However, it is not effective against tonic-clinic seizures.

DRUGS AFFECTING γ-AMINOBUTYRIC ACID TRANSMISSION

GABAergic mechanisms seem to contribute to seizure susceptibility in numerous animal models of epilepsy. Impaired GABAergic function can be shown in rats, mice, gerbils, and baboons genetically prone to epilepsy. Although faulty GABAergic mechanisms have not been convincingly shown in humans, cerebrospinal fluid concentrations of GABA are reduced in epileptic patients, and surgically removed epileptic brain tissue exhibits decreased GABAergic activity. Drugs that are antagonists at $GABA_A$ receptors (bicuculline, picrotoxin) are potent convulsants, whereas drugs that facilitate GABAergic mechanisms (benzodiazepines) act as anticonvulsants.

Similar to other neurotransmitter pathways, the $GABA_A$ receptor system has multiple sites that may lend themselves to pharmacologic control (Fig. 12-7). Presynaptically, neurotransmitter synthesis, storage, and release mechanisms may be targeted. Additionally, GABA reuptake transporters, autoreceptors, and catabolic enzymes are found presynaptically. Some GABAergic neurons contain cotransmitters, such as enkephalin or substance P. Postsynaptically, multiple forms of $GABA_A$ receptors (ligand-gated ion channels) are found. The ligand-gated ion channel can be composed of various component isoforms. In the human, six α (1-6), three β (1-3), three γ (1-3), and individual δ, ε, π, and θ subunit isoforms have been identified. Each ion channel is a mixture of five of these subunits creating a pentamer, with the predominant isoform being two α's, two β's, and one γ subunit ($2\alpha_1$, $2\beta_2$, γ_2). Three ρ subunits have also been identified, but they do not normally interact with other subunit isoforms. Some changes in ion channel subunit composition have been seen in epileptic brain (See Chapter 11).

Benzodiazepines

Most benzodiazepines have anticonvulsant properties, but this class of drugs is used primarily as sedative or antianxiety drugs. The pharmacologic profiles of the benzodiazepines and the mechanisms by which they facilitate GABAergic transmission are discussed in detail in Chapter 11. For the treatment of epilepsy, **diazepam, clonazepam, clorazepate, midazolam, and lorazepam** are the principal benzodiazepines used.

Mechanism of action

The main antiseizure activity of the benzodiazepines results from their enhancement of GABA-mediated systems, acting as positive allosteric modulators. Specific subunit configurations of $GABA_A$ receptors allow for the presence of a selective benzodiazepine-binding site. When bound, benzodiazepines at nonsedating doses increase the frequency of **$GABA_A$ receptor activation and associated Cl^- channel** opening. At higher does, similar to those given acutely to treat status epilepticus, benzodiazepines can reduce sustained high-frequency firing in neurons, potentially due to activity at voltage-gated sodium channels.

Pharmacokinetics

The absorption, fate, and excretion of benzodiazepines are discussed in detail in Chapter 11. There are no differences in these properties when these drugs are used as anticonvulsants compared with when they are used as antianxiety agents. Both clorazepate and diazepam produce the major metabolite N-desmethyl-diazepam, which also displays anticonvulsant properties acting as a partial agonist at the $GABA_A$ receptor.

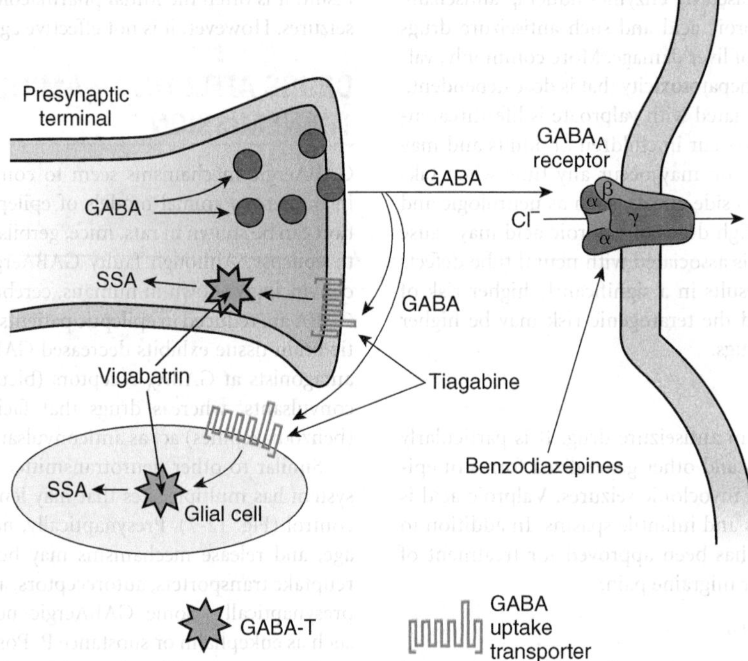

FIG 12-7 Proposed sites of actions for drugs acting at the γ-aminobutyric acid (*GABA*) synapse. GABA inhibits the postsynaptic neuron by acting on a receptor (*GABA$_A$*) on the Cl^- channel. Benzodiazepines act to facilitate the action of GABA postsynaptically by interacting with a separate site on the Cl^- channel. The action of GABA can be terminated by reuptake or catabolism. GABA is taken back into the presynaptic nerve terminals and glial cells by a Na^+-driven symporter protein. Tiagabine blocks this GABA transporter. GABA α-oxoglutarate transaminase (*GABA-T*) terminates the action of GABA by converting it to succinic semialdehyde (*SSA*). Vigabatrin inhibits GABA-T.

Toxicity

The predictable adverse effects of drowsiness, dizziness, ataxia, nystagmus, dysarthria, and hypotonia occur with all benzodiazepines. Respiratory depression can be an issue when intravenous agents are used. Serious side effects are very rare. The administration of clonazepam occasionally precipitates a different variety of seizure from the one being treated. The teratogenic potential of the benzodiazepines is discussed in Chapter 11. There is little evidence that clonazepam is teratogenic, but it is recommended that use of the compound during pregnancy be limited to cases in which the clinical situation warrants the risk.

Therapeutic use

Although the benzodiazepines are useful adjuncts to the conventional anticonvulsants for seizure prophylaxis, patients seem to develop tolerance to their antiseizure effect quickly. The benzodiazepines may have greatest clinical usefulness in short-term therapy, such as when antiseizure medication is being changed or for emergency treatment.

Midazolam, clonazepam, and lorazepam have higher affinities for the benzodiazepine receptor and may be more effective antiseizure drugs. The actions of lorazepam can be slow to develop but are longer lasting than diazepam. Intravenous midazolam has also been found to be effective in the treatment of status epilepticus and local anesthetic excitotoxicity. Buccal midazolam is also effective and can be administered more quickly and conveniently than rectal diazepam emulsion, and its actions are seen more quickly. Clonazepam is generally effective for absence seizures and childhood myoclonic epilepsy and is sometimes effective for complex partial seizures and reflex epilepsies (photosensitive epilepsy). Clorazepate is indicated as adjunctive therapy in the management of partial seizures.

Vigabatrin

Mechanism of action

Vigabatrin (Fig. 12-8) is an irreversible inhibitor of the major degradation enzyme for GABA, GABA transaminase, effectively increasing the concentrations of GABA in the brain. Its effects related to epilepsy are thought to result from an increase in GABA-mediated inhibitory activity.

Pharmacokinetics

Vigabatrin is rapidly absorbed through oral administration, reaching peak blood concentrations in 0.75 to 2 hours. It does not bind appreciably to plasma proteins. Vigabatrin has no active metabolites and is excreted by the kidneys. Its plasma half-life is 4 to 7 hours, but irreversible inhibition of GABA transaminase lasts for several days after the drug is cleared, prolonging the antiseizure effect.

Toxicity

Adverse effects of vigabatrin include sedation, fatigue, weight gain, amnesia, and visual field defects. The effects on the visual field result from irreversible atrophy of the retinal nerve. The defects may be more common in men and seem to be related to the total drug exposure. Although uncommon, psychosis may occur and is seen most often in adult patients.

Therapeutic use

Vigabatrin is considered an adjunctive therapy for drug–refractory complex partial seizures in adults. In addition, vigabatrin is approved to treat children ages 1 month to 2 years for infantile spasms, a particularly difficult to treat pediatric disease.

Tiagabine

Tiagabine (see Fig. 12-8), approved in 1996 as an adjunct for refractory complex epilepsy, is a nipecotic acid derivative that inhibits GABA uptake.

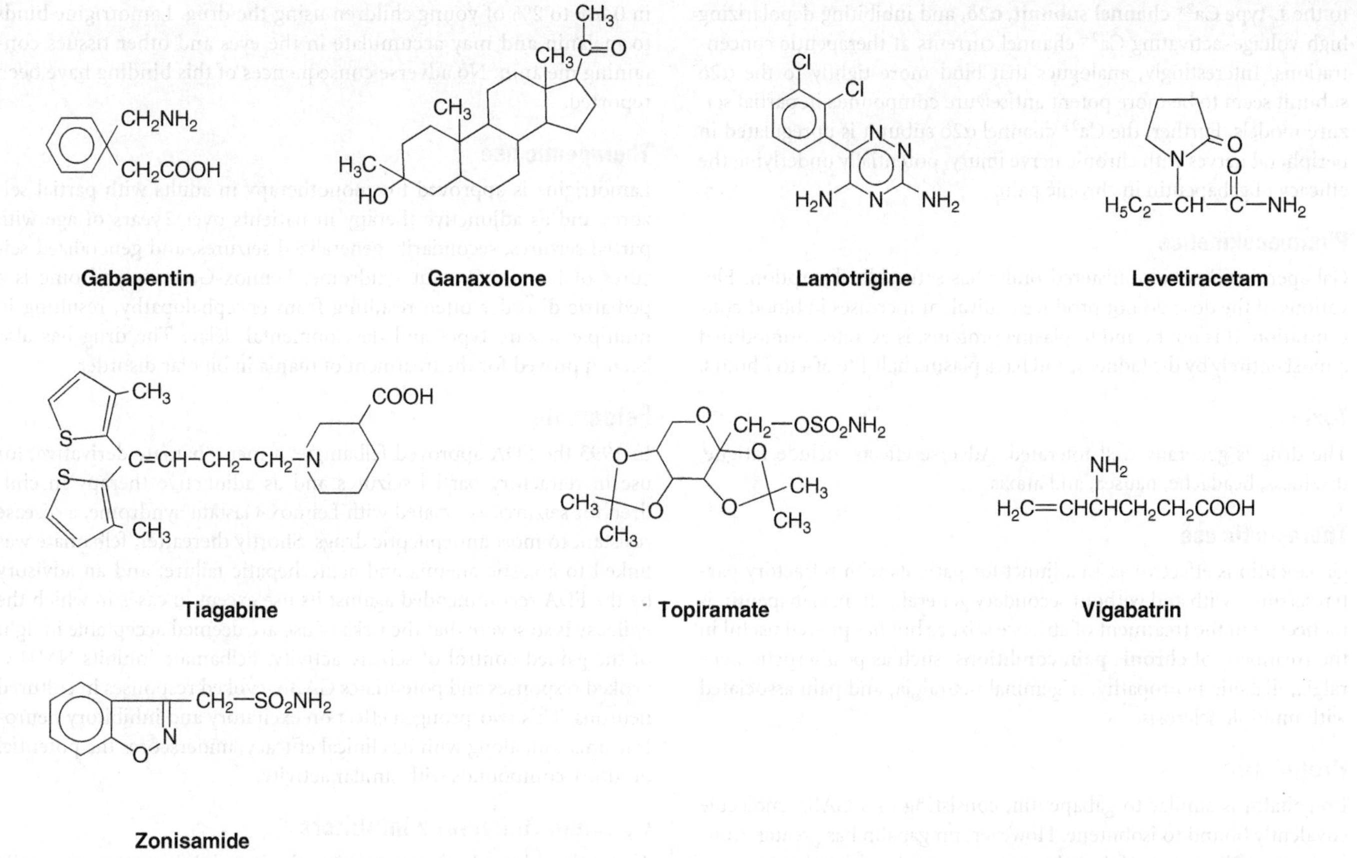

Gabapentin Ganaxolone Lamotrigine Levetiracetam

Tiagabine Topiramate Vigabatrin

Zonisamide

FIG 12-8 Structural formulas of newer antiepileptic drugs.

Mechanism of action

Tiagabine inhibits the GABA transporter, **GAT-1**, thereby increasing the concentration of GABA in the synaptic cleft and prolonging the duration of inhibitory synaptic currents.

Pharmacokinetics

Tiagabine is readily absorbed through oral administration, with a peak blood concentration reached in 45 minutes. This drug is metabolized in the liver by CYP3A4 and possibly CYP1A2, 2C19, and 2D6 to inactive 5-oxo metabolites and is also glucuronidated. Tiagabine has a half-life of 7 to 9 hours, which is shortened to 2-3 hours when administered with enzyme-inducing drugs like phenobarbital, phenytoin, and carbamazepine.

Toxicity

Principal side effects include dizziness, fatigue, sleepiness, nausea, tremor, and difficulty concentrating. Due to its increase in GABAergic neurotransmission, tiagabine can exacerbate spike-and-wave EEG discharges and is contraindicated in patients with generalized absence epilepsy. Tiagabine has also been associated with occurrence of seizure in patients without epilepsy and off-label use is discouraged.

Therapeutic use

Tiagabine is approved for adjunctive therapy in patients, 12 years or older, with refractory partial seizures with or without secondary generalization.

Neurosteroids

In addition to its receptor for benzodiazepines, the $GABA_A$ receptor complex has a separate binding site for steroid molecules. Steroid hormones generally are thought to act through steroid nuclear binding proteins that modify DNA translation in the cell nucleus. Some steroids, such as allopregnanolone, also act on these cell surface receptors to facilitate the action of GABA on the $GABA_A$ receptor.

Infantile spasm with a "chaotic" EEG is a serious epileptic condition of early life that is refractory to most anticonvulsants and has a poor prognosis. Historically, it has been effectively treated with adrenocorticotropic hormone. More recent studies have shown that vigabatrin and the neurosteroid ganaxolone are also effective for this condition. Ganaxolone (see Fig. 12-8) is a pregnenolone derivative without progestational hormonal activity. It exerts anticonvulsant activity against complex partial seizures, has an antiseizure spectrum that suggests usefulness in absence seizures, and displays antiseizure activity in an animal model of catamenial epilepsy. It is thought to act on selective $GABA_A$ component isoforms as a positive allosteric modulator. Other, newer anticonvulsant drugs that are being evaluated for treatment of infantile spasms include topiramate, lamotrigine, and zonisamide.

MISCELLANEOUS ANTICONVULSANTS

Gabapentin

Gabapentin (see Fig. 12-8) is a GABA analogue specifically designed to cross the blood–brain barrier. It consists of a GABA molecule covalently bound to a lipophilic cyclohexane ring.

Mechanism of action

Despite its design and intended effect, gabapentin does not interact with GABA receptors, GABA uptake, or metabolism. It may influence synthesis or release of GABA, and it increases GABA concentrations in certain regions of the brain. A major action of gabapentin is its binding to the **L-type Ca^{2+} channel subunit, α2δ**, and inhibiting depolarizing high voltage–activating Ca^{2+} channel currents at therapeutic concentrations. Interestingly, analogues that bind more tightly to the α2δ subunit seem to be more potent antiseizure compounds in partial seizure models. Further, the Ca^{2+} channel α2δ subunit is upregulated in peripheral nerves with chronic nerve injury, potentially underlying the efficacy of gabapentin in chronic pain.

Pharmacokinetics

Gabapentin when administered orally has saturable absorption. Elevations of the dose do not produce equivalent increases in blood concentration. It is not bound to plasma proteins, is excreted unmodified almost entirely by the kidneys, and has a plasma half-life of 4 to 7 hours.

Toxicity

The drug is generally well tolerated. Adverse effects include fatigue, dizziness, headache, nausea, and ataxia.

Therapeutic use

Gabapentin is effective as an adjunct for patients with refractory partial seizures, with and without secondary generalization. Gabapentin is ineffective in the treatment of absence seizure but has proved useful in the treatment of **chronic pain conditions**, such as postherpetic neuralgia, diabetic neuropathy, trigeminal neuralgia, and pain associated with multiple sclerosis.

Pregabalin

Pregabalin is similar to gabapentin, consisting of a GABA molecule covalently bound to isobutene. However, pregabalin has greater affinity for the α2δ subunit of the calcium ion channel and may have greater efficacy for treating neuropathic pain where these subunits are upregulated. Similar to gabapentin, pregabalin is effective as an adjunct for patients with refractory partial seizures, with and without secondary generalization. It has also been approved for the treatment of postherpetic **pain**, diabetic neuropathy, adjunctive treatment of partial-onset seizures, and **fibromyalgia**. It has been studied as a treatment of oral surgery pain and was found to produce some pain relief. It has also been studied as a treatment for general anxiety disorder.

Lamotrigine

Lamotrigine (see Fig. 12-8) is a phenyltriazine derivative originally designed as an antifolate.

Mechanism of action

Lamotrigine **inhibits Na^+ influx** in rapidly firing neurons by delaying the recovery of Na^+ channels from the inactivated state. The drug has also been shown to inhibit synaptic release of glutamate from rat cortical brain slices.

Pharmacokinetics

The drug is used orally and is well absorbed from the gastrointestinal tract. The plasma half-life is approximately 24 hours, but induction of liver microsomal enzymes by other antiseizure drugs including phenobarbital, phenytoin, and carbamazepine may decrease the half-life to approximately 12 hours. Conversely, valproic acid may increase the half-life of lamotrigine up to 60 hours by inhibiting its metabolism. In patients receiving valproic acid, addition of lamotrigine reduces valproate concentration by ~25%.

Toxicity

Lamotrigine usually has mild side effects, including ataxia, dizziness, diplopia, and rash. Stevens-Johnson syndrome has been reported in 0.8% to 2% of young children using the drug. Lamotrigine binds to melanin and may accumulate in the eyes and other tissues containing melanin. No adverse consequences of this binding have been reported.

Therapeutic use

Lamotrigine is approved for monotherapy in adults with partial seizures and as adjunctive therapy in patients over 2 years of age with partial seizures, secondarily generalized seizures, and generalized seizures of Lennox-Gastaut syndrome. Lennox-Gastaut syndrome is a pediatric disorder often resulting from encephalopathy, resulting in multiple seizure types and developmental delay. The drug has also been approved for the treatment of mania in bipolar disorder.

Felbamate

In 1993 the FDA approved felbamate, a meprobamate derivative, for use in refractory partial seizures and as adjunctive therapy in children for seizures associated with Lennox-Gastaut syndrome, a disease resistant to most antiepileptic drugs. Shortly thereafter, felbamate was linked to aplastic anemia and acute hepatic failure, and an advisory by the FDA recommended against its use except in cases in which the epilepsy is so severe that the risks of use are deemed acceptable in light of the gained control of seizure activity. Felbamate inhibits NMDA-evoked responses and potentiates GABA-evoked responses in cultured neurons. This two-pronged effect on excitatory and inhibitory neurotransmission, along with its clinical efficacy, underscores the potential of future compounds with similar activity.

Carbonic Anhydrase Inhibitors

Acetazolamide and other carbonic anhydrase inhibitors are primarily effective against absence seizures but are also useful for the control of seizures that recur at a specific time of the menstrual cycle (catamenial epilepsy). Clinical usefulness is limited due to rapid development of tolerance, so carbonic anhydrase inhibitors are primarily used as adjunctive agents.

Topiramate

Topiramate is a sulfamate-substituted monosaccharide (see Fig. 12-8).

Mechanism of action

Topiramate has a broad spectrum of antiseizure actions, including frequency-dependent blockade of voltage-gated Na^+ channels, activation of a hyperpolarizing K^+ current, benzodiazepine-like potentiation of postsynaptic $GABA_A$ receptors, inhibition of the AMPA/kainate subtype(s) of glutamate receptors, and weak inhibition of carbonic anhydrase enzyme.

Pharmacokinetics

Absorption after oral ingestion is rapid, with little (10% to 20%) binding to plasma proteins, reaching peak plasma concentration within 2 hours. A mean half-life of approximately 20 hours permits twice-daily dosing. Topiramate is not extensively metabolized and is primarily (~70%) excreted in urine unchanged. The remainder is metabolized by hydroxylation, hydrolysis, and glucuronidation with no metabolite accounting for more than 5% of the total administered dose. It may specifically inhibit CYP2C19, which can affect coadministered drugs including oral contraceptives.

Toxicity

Topiramate is reported to be more effective than several newer anticonvulsants; however, it also produces more side effects; this may reflect the dosages used to evaluate the drug rather than minimally effective doses. CNS depression is the most common side effect. Topiramate can also compromise short-term memory function.

Therapeutic use

Topiramate is a broad-spectrum anticonvulsant currently approved for partial-onset seizures, monotherapy of tonic-clonic seizures, treatment of Lennox-Gastaut syndrome, and prophylaxis of migraine headaches.

Zonisamide

Zonisamide was developed in Japan and is now available in the United States. Zonisamide is structurally related to the sulfonamides (see Fig. 12-8).

Mechanism of action

The primary antiseizure mechanisms of action for zonisamide include inhibition of T-type Ca^{2+} channels and inhibition of sustained repetitive neuronal firing by prolonging the inactivated state of the voltage-gated Na^+ channel.

Pharmacokinetics

Zonisamide is almost completely absorbed after oral administration, binding extensively to erythrocytes; peak plasma concentrations are observed at 4 to 6 hours. Approximately 85% of zonisamide is excreted in urine primarily as unchanged drug or a glucuronide metabolite. Zonisamide is primarily metabolized by CYP3A4, and it does not induce its own metabolism. However, blood concentrations may be reduced if CYP34A inducers (phenobarbital, phenytoin, and carbamazepine) are used concurrently.

Toxicity

Overall, zonisamide is well tolerated. However, it can produce numerous allergic reactions in patients who are sensitive to sulfonamides. These reactions include skin rashes, including Stevens-Johnson syndrome, epidermal necrolysis, aplastic anemia, and agranulocytosis. The incidence of these events is very low. Other unusual side effects include a propensity to produce renal metabolic acidification and kidney stones and, rarely, dehydration and hyperthermia, particularly in children during hot weather. Zonisamide is a pregnancy category C drug and had displayed teratogenicity in preclinical trials; thus zonisamide should be avoided during pregnancy if possible.

Therapeutic use

Double-blinded, placebo-controlled studies demonstrated that adjunctive zonisamide treatment with other drugs was superior to placebo in patients with refractory partial seizures. Zonisamide is currently FDA approved as an adjunctive therapy for partial seizures in adults.

Levetiracetam

Levetiracetam is a pyrrolidine derivative, the racemically pure S-enantiomer of alpha-ethyl-2-oxo-1-pyrrolidineacetamide (see Fig. 12-8).

Mechanism of action

The specific mechanism of action related to the antiseizure activity of levetiracetam remains unclear. However, there is a strong correlation between antiseizure activity and binding with the synaptic **vesicle glycoprotein (SV2A)**, a protein suggested to be involved in vesicle fusion, as well as inhibition of presynaptic calcium channels. It has been proposed that these pharmacologic actions could limit vesicle fusion effectively reducing synaptic activity.

Pharmacokinetics

Levetiracetam is rapidly and almost completely absorbed (1 hour to peak concentration) after oral administration, and it is less than 10% bound to plasma proteins. Steady state is reached in 2 days with twice-daily dosing. Levetiracetam is not extensively metabolized in humans. The major metabolic pathway is hydrolysis of the acetamide group and is not dependent on liver cytochrome P450 enzymes. Levetiracetam does not induce cytochrome P450 or glucuronidation enzymes and displays no known deleterious drug–drug interactions. The half-life is approximately 7 hours in healthy adults but 2.5 hours longer in elderly patients. It is eliminated by renal excretion with 66% eliminated as unchanged drug.

Toxicity

Levetiracetam is generally well tolerated. Typical side effects included somnolence and fatigue, coordination difficulties, and risk of suicidal thoughts. Most of the side effects were reported in the first month of therapy. Levetiracetam is currently a pregnancy category C drug.

Therapeutic use

Levetiracetam is FDA approved for adjunctive therapy for myoclonic seizures, juvenile myoclonic epilepsy, partial-onset, and primary generalized tonic-clinic seizures in adults and children as young as 4 years old. Insufficient evidence is currently available for approval of levetiracetam as monotherapy for partial or generalized epilepsy. If patients are taken off levetiracetam due to good seizure control, withdrawal should be gradual to avoid deleterious reactions.

Retigabine

Retigabine was one of the mostly widely studied drugs in the preclinical setting, before its FDA approval in 2011.

Mechanism of action

Retigabine has a novel mechanism of action for an antiseizure drug, acting as positive allosteric modulator of the **neuronal potassium channels KNCQ (Kv2 to 5)**. Under normal physiologic conditions, KNCQ channels help establish the neuronal resting membrane potential, by providing a continual hyperpolarizing influence. Retigabine increases the number of KNCQ channels open at rest, effectively limiting the overall excitability of neurons and facilitating their recovery from membrane depolarization. This activity significantly limits neuronal action potential burst firing, decreasing the probability of initiation and propagation of seizure activity.

Pharmacokinetics

Retigabine is rapidly absorbed after oral administration, reaching peak plasma concentration between 0.5 and 2 hours. It is approximately 80% bound to plasma proteins. Retigabine is extensively metabolized in humans primarily by glucuronidation carried out by UGT enzymes and acetylation. It does not induce any cytochrome P450 enzymes. The half-life is between 7 and 11 hours in healthy adults. The major route of elimination (85%) is through renal excretion with approximately 36% eliminated as unchanged parent drug.

Toxicity

Typical side effects are dose related and include somnolence, dizziness and vertigo, confusion and hallucinations, and slurred speech. Urinary retention was observed in approximately 2% of patients during clinical trials, and urologic symptoms should be closely monitored. A cardiac QT-prolonging effect was observed in healthy volunteers, and patients with known cardiac dysfunction should be closely monitored. Similar to other antiseizure drugs, there is an increased risk of suicidal behavior and withdrawal seizure if retigabine treatment is rapidly discontinued.

Therapeutic use

Retigabine is FDA approved for adjunctive therapy for partial-onset seizures in patients aged 18 years or older.

Perampanel

Perampanel is a drug approved for treating partial-onset seizures. It is a noncompetitive inhibitor of the AMPA receptor, a glutamate excitatory receptor. Serious psychiatric adverse effects have been reported, as well as dizziness and other CNS adverse effects.

NONPHARMACOLOGIC TREATMENTS

Surgical treatment of seizure disorders is possible when the seizure focus is well localized and presents in noncritical brain regions. Removal of damaged and dysfunctional brain tissue can produce good clinical outcomes in some patients. However, patients are often maintained on antiseizure drugs postsurgery to ensure seizure control. Surgical resections are performed with growing success due to improved diagnostic imaging techniques, such as 2-[^{18}F]fluoro-2-deoxy-D-glucose and [^{11}C]-flumazenil coupled with EEG allowing for better localization of seizure foci and smaller resected areas.

Implantable devices offer an additional nonpharmacologic approach to the treatment of epilepsy. Vagal nerve stimulators have been approved as adjunctive therapy for patients with partial epilepsy aged 12 and older and patients who are not helped enough by current antiseizure medications. Studies have also suggested vagal nerve stimulators may help patients with generalized seizure and children with Lennox-Gastaut syndrome. Vagal stimulation has obvious implications regarding cholinergic drugs. Responsive neurostimulation was approved in 2013 for adjunctive treatment of adults with refractory partial-onset seizure with one or two identified epileptic foci. During surgical implantation of the RNS system, electrical leads are placed in the seizure foci allowing for recording and stimulation of a specific brain region. When specific patterns of activity are detected, stimulation is delivered and hypersynchronous neuronal activity is disrupted, limiting seizure generation and spread. Deep brain stimulation has also been explored for the treatment of partial-onset seizures in patients with refractory epilepsy and has been approved in Canada, Australia, and the Europe an Union. DBS for the treatment of epilepsy focuses on regulation of the anterior nucleus of the thalamus, which is thought to regulate brain regions commonly implicated in the initiation of partial-onset seizures.

A final nonpharmacologic approach for the treatment of childhood epilepsy is dietary modification. The ketogenic diet is high in fats and low in carbohydrates and proteins. These diets must be carefully controlled but have been found effective in some patients who do not respond well to medication. This dietary regimen forces the body to use fat for its primary source of energy, resulting in an increased concentration of ketones. The increased production of ketones is thought to improve seizure control, but it remains unclear exactly how this dietary therapy works.

GENERAL ANTISEIZURE THERAPEUTIC USE

The goal of anticonvulsant therapy is to obtain complete control of epileptic seizures with the fewest drugs and at the least toxic and lowest possible dose. Approximately 70% to 80% of all patients can be seizure-free if drug plasma concentrations are properly monitored and the appropriate dose adjustments are made. Initial anticonvulsant therapy sometimes necessitates frequent alterations in dose and a trial-and-error approach until the seizures become well controlled with a specific anticonvulsant. Even after seizures are initially controlled, the continued administration of anticonvulsant drugs may lead to the development of tolerance. The addition of other anticonvulsants necessitates dosage adjustments. Anticonvulsant therapy is not static, routine, nor completely predictable but rather subject to a variety of ever-changing factors.

Febrile seizures, induced by high fevers, are the most frequent seizures in children. Propensity for these seizures may have a genetic basis, be related to particular diseases (influenza), or be caused by immaturity of CNS excitation control. Children with febrile seizures rarely develop other seizure disorders or continue to have seizures. Short-term treatment with diazepam, phenobarbital, or intranasal midazolam has been used. In some patients in whom febrile seizures are recurrent, prophylactic phenobarbital or diazepam may be prescribed to prevent seizures in future fevers. Rarely, patients may need longer term continuous phenobarbital or valproic acid treatment.

Although anticonvulsant medications have substantial toxic potential, uncontrolled seizures also carry important risks. Repeated seizures can result in loss of memory and mental function. For several of the newer anticonvulsants that facilitate GABA or inhibit excitatory amino acid function, there is the potential for additional drug-induced compromise of memory function.

Anticonvulsants can be valuable in treating patients with various chronic pain problems. Neuropathic pain results from abnormalities in nerve fiber conduction, such as neuralgia, causalgia, and phantom pain. Beneficial actions of anticonvulsants may be related to blockade of Na^+ and Ca^{2+} channels, activation of GABAergic transmission, and inhibition of NMDA and other glutamate receptors. Agents that have proved effective in these conditions include carbamazepine, phenytoin, sodium valproate, gabapentin, and clonazepam.

Traditional anticonvulsants (carbamazepine and valproic acid) and "mood stabilizers" (a synonym used in psychiatry for some newer anticonvulsants) are sometimes valuable adjuncts in treating the manic phase of bipolar disorder. Other anticonvulsant drugs may also be useful. In one study, adjunctive gabapentin was no more effective than placebo.

IMPLICATIONS FOR DENTISTRY

Dentists should expect to be confronted at some time by a seizing patient in the dental office. It is extremely helpful if an emergency plan has been previously developed and practiced before having to deal with convulsions clinically. One of the best ways to manage seizures is to prevent them. Appointments should be planned for times when a patient with a seizure disorder has high blood concentrations of anticonvulsant medication. The dentist should verify that the patient has taken his or her medications before the appointment. Careful attention to local anesthetic doses and avoiding accidental intravascular injections by practicing aspiration before administration are important. If the patient's seizure is of the reflexive type, avoiding the triggering stimuli is important. The dentist should ask the patient before treatment if he or she is aware of any triggering stimuli. Finally, attention to the patient's fear and apprehension can limit the risk of inciting an attack.

Some patients sense the onset of seizure activity in the form of auras. If a patient reports an aura, the dentist should prepare for a seizure by removing all instruments from the patient's mouth and pulling back trays or other objects from which the patient might sustain injury. The patient should be placed in the supine position. If no seizure occurs, the patient can determine when to proceed. If the patient does have a seizure, the dentist must protect the patient from injury and falls. No attempt should be made to open the patient's mouth during a tonic-clonic seizure because this can induce additional injuries. Seizures generally end in 2 to 5 minutes, after which the patient is disoriented or falls asleep for 30 or more minutes. If the patient is snoring or seems to have an obstructed airway, the head, neck, and jaw should be positioned to ensure a clear airway.

Fortunately, many local and general anesthetics have anticonvulsant properties by themselves. Should a seizure occur during anesthesia, emergency medical services should be called if multiple independent seizures occur, a single prolonged seizure occurs, or if respiration is compromised. Patients may need supportive care after a seizure, which would include treatment of any wounds that may have occurred and dealing with incontinence.

In most cases, seizures are brief and self-limiting. Occasionally, pharmacotherapy may be required. Part of the dentist's emergency plan should include a properly stocked emergency cart and staff trained in the use of the medications. Ideally, emergency administration of antiseizure medications would be delivered intravenously; however, this is not always possible in the dental office. Newer products have improved this situation. A rectal gel dosage form of diazepam (Diastat) is available that can produce anticonvulsant blood concentrations in approximately 15 minutes. This product has been formulated for use by laypeople for the emergency treatment of seizures at home and simplifies emergency treatment if an intravenous line is unavailable. The disadvantage of this approach is that many individuals are uncomfortable with the route of administration. Midazolam has been tried and found effective in the treatment of status seizures and can be administered intravenously, intramuscularly, intranasally, or intrabuccally offering an alternative emergency treatment strategy. Seizure control is almost immediate with intravenous administration. The buccal route would be natural in the dental office.

Because midazolam has a relatively short duration of action, the use of a longer acting agent, such as lorazepam, phenytoin, or phenobarbital, may be needed in the hospital to provide prolonged seizure control. Fosphenytoin may have some advantages over traditional agents, although its action is delayed. Fosphenytoin at 15 to 20 mg/kg phenytoin equivalents is tolerated better and can be effective 10 to 60 minutes after intravenous administration, which should be given no faster than 100 to 150 mg phenytoin equivalents per minute. Intramuscular administration of fosphenytoin can be done but it is not recommended for aborting seizure activity.

Common or significant adverse effects that are pertinent for the everyday practice of dentistry should be noted. The fact that some anticonvulsants alter mineral metabolism should be considered when confronted with anomalies in tooth development or advanced bone loss. Several anticonvulsants can produce teratogenic effects. The defects produced can involve the facial and oral structures. Practitioners should be alert for new drug-related adverse effects and report them to the FDA Medwatch program.

Several side effects specific to individual anticonvulsant agents are clinically relevant to dentistry. Phenytoin-induced gingival overgrowth is a well-known example. Overgrowth most commonly occurs in the anterior mandibular region, especially in the case of "mouth breathers," and develops to the greatest extent in the interdental papillae between the incisors. Edentulous areas of the alveolar mucosa do not undergo hypertrophy or do so to a lesser extent than other areas. Phenytoin-induced overgrowth may totally or partially obscure the crowns of teeth, which hampers mastication and oral hygiene, is aesthetically unpleasant, and necessitates periodic resection. Because of the angiogenesis induced, the gingival tissue is quite vascular; surgery by cautery or laser is often preferred. The rate of development of gingival overgrowth can be diminished by proper oral hygiene.

Many antiseizure drugs induce hepatic microsomal enzyme activity, which can reduce the blood concentration of other drugs metabolized by the same enzyme system. Of relevance to dentistry is the effect of enzyme induction on antibiotics (e.g., tetracycline) and other agents (midazolam, triazolam) used in clinical practice. Drugs that inhibit CYP3A4 (e.g., erythromycin) can lead to unexpected elevations of antiseizure drugs and potential toxicity. The microsomal enzyme-inducing antiseizure drugs can reduce the effectiveness of oral contraceptives. Valproic acid can inhibit CYP3A4 drug metabolism. It can also inhibit platelet aggregation, so increased monitoring of patient use of aspirin or nonsteroidal antiinflammatory drugs may be warranted.

Some short-term effects directly involve the mouth. Carbamazepine-induced taste disorders have been reported, but these apparently subside with time. Xerostomia has also been reported. Primidone is known to cause the unusual side effect of localized gingival pain. This response has led patients and dentists to assume erroneously that the pain is of pathologic rather than pharmacologic origin. Clonazepam has been reported to produce hypersalivation in some patients. A complete medical history is essential for proper dental treatment.

It is often recommended that a patient with epilepsy be treated cautiously to reduce emotional upset and to help prevent the precipitation of a seizure. Except when seizures are not well controlled, individuals with epilepsy need not be handled differently from other patients. Because of the lingering stigma associated with epilepsy, these patients may be reluctant to reveal their disease. A seizure disorder may be ascertained only by a clinician who is alert to subtle clues offered by antiseizure drug-induced side effects and by careful questioning of the patient.

Antiseizure drugs may be used in the treatment of chronic orofacial pain problems, such as trigeminal neuralgia or burning mouth syndrome. Carbamazepine has been the first-choice drug for the treatment of trigeminal neuralgia. Some patients also respond to other antiseizure drugs. Burning mouth syndrome is currently a treatment challenge and may involve pathologic and psychological components. Current treatments include clonazepam, capsaicin, and antidepressant therapy.

Finally, saliva offers a readily available and potentially useful tool for monitoring concentrations of several antiseizure drugs. Saliva/plasma correlations have been described for carbamazepine, phenobarbital, phenytoin, and ethosuximide. Stability of the samples for some drugs is high and allows the samples to be mailed to a laboratory for analysis, potentially making drug monitoring faster and less expensive.

ANTICONVULSANTS

Nonproprietary (Generic) Name	Proprietary (Trade) Name
Hydantoins	
Fosphenytoin	Cerebyx
Mephenytoin*	Mesantoin
Phenytoin	Dilantin
Barbiturates	
Mephobarbital	Mebaral
Phenobarbital	Luminal
Primidone†	Mysoline
Succinimides	
Ethosuximide	Zarontin
Oxazolidinediones	
Paramethadione*	Paradione
Trimethadione	Tridione

Continued

ANTICONVULSANTS—cont'd

Nonproprietary (Generic) Name	Proprietary (Trade) Name
Benzodiazepines	
Clobazam	Frisium
Clonazepam	Klonopin
Clorazepate	Tranxene, Gen-Xene
Diazepam	Valium, Diastat
Midazolam	Versed
Nitrazepam*	Mogadon
Lorazepam	Ativan
Others	
Acetazolamide	Diamox, Duramed
Carbamazepine	Tegretol
Felbamate‡	Felbatol
Gabapentin	Neurontin
Pregabalin	Lyrica
Lamotrigine	Lamictal
Levetiracetam	Keppra
Oxcarbazepine	Trileptal
Eslicarbazepine	Aptiom
Retigabine	Potiga
Rufinamide	Banzel
Tiagabine	Gabitril
Topiramate	Topamax
Valproic acid	Depakene, Depakote§
Vigabatrin	Sabril
Zonisamide	Zonegran
Perampanel	Fycompa

*Not currently available in the United States.
†Not a true barbiturate.
‡Restricted use.
§Divalproex, a stable compound of valproic acid, and sodium valproate.

CASE DISCUSSION

The observation that the patient's pain has a clear trigger zone but no clear pathology suggests that there may be an underlying neurologic problem. The patient will need to be referred to a neurologist for further evaluation. Upon further neurologic exam, it was demonstrated that the patient was experiencing trigeminal neuralgia and was started on gabapentin. Normally, carbamazepine would be the first choice for treatment of trigeminal neuralgia. However, given that the patient is of childbearing age and might be taking an oral contraceptive, carbamazepine should be avoided due to induction on liver enzymes affecting other drug metabolism. If gabapentin proves to be ineffective at controlling the pain, lamotrigine is another safe alternative to carbamazepine. When the patient does return for a routine appointment, ensure that you and the patient are prepared for the possibility of a seizure. Ask the patient to schedule her appointment at a time when antiseizure medications will be at a stable blood level. Develop a plan of action should the patient have a seizure or enter status epilepticus. In the event of seizure, remove all sharp objects and protect the patient's head and neck. Do not put anything in the patient's mouth, and wait for the seizure to self-terminate. If seizure persists, emergency services should be called, and buccal midazolam or rectal diazepam should be administered to terminate seizure activity. Although it is important to be prepared for the worst scenario, preventive measures including ensuring patients are taking medication properly and creating a minimal stress environment are critical to ensuring patients with seizure disorders have a safe dental experience.

GENERAL REFERENCES

1. Berg AT, Scheffer IE: New concepts in classification of the epilepsies: entering the 21st century, *Epilepsia* 52:1058–1062, 2011.
2. Brookes-Kayal AR, Bath KG, Berg AT, et al.: Issues related to symptomatic and disease-modifying treatments affecting cognitive and neuropsychiatric comorbidities of epilepsy, *Epilepsia* 54:44–60, 2013.
3. Cherubini E, Conti F: Generating diversity at GABAergic synapses, *Trends Neurosci* 24:155–162, 2001.
4. Hocker S, Wijdicks EF, Rabinstein AA: Refractory status epilepticus: new insights in presentation, treatment, and outcome, *Neurol Res* 35:163–168, 2013.
5. IOM (Institute of Medicine): *Epilepsy across the spectrum: promoting health and understanding*, 1st ed., Washington, DC, 2012, The National Academies Press.
6. Mavrogiannis M, Ellis JS, Thomason JM, et al.: The management of drug-induced gingival overgrowth, *J Clin Periodontol* 33:434–439, 2006.
7. Noebels J: Pathway-driven discovery of epilepsy genes, *Nat Neurosci* 18:344–350, 2015.
8. Schousboe A, Madsen KK, Barker-Haliski ML, et al.: The GABA synapse as a target for antiepileptic drugs: a historical overview focused on GABA transporters, *Neurochem Res* 39:1980–1987, 2014.
9. Simonato M, Brooks-Kayal AR, Engel J, et al.: The challenge and promise of anti-epileptic therapy development in animal models, *Lancet Neurol* 13:949–960, 2014.
10. Stephen LJ, Brodie MJ: Antiepileptic drug monotherapy versus polytherapy: pursuing seizure freedom and tolerability in adults, *Curr Opin Neurol* 25:164–172, 2012.

Antiparkinson Drugs*

James T. Boyd, Clayton English, and Karen M. Lounsbury

KEY INFORMATION

- Parkinson disease (PD) is a common neurodegenerative movement disorder.
- Cardinal features of PD include resting tremor, rigidity, bradykinesia, and postural instability.
- Loss of dopamine producing neurons underpin the movement impairment of PD.
- Nonmotor symptoms are common in PD, such as cognitive impairment, autonomic dysfunction (e.g., orthostatic hypotension), sleep disorders, and psychiatric manifestations (depression, anxiety, and psychosis).
- Pharmacologic therapies are based on the replacement of deficient dopamine signaling.
- Treatments reduce symptoms of PD, but do not reverse the progression of disease.
- Levodopa is a precursor drug that enhances brain levels of dopamine.
- Common side effects of levodopa include nausea, vomiting, and orthostatic hypotension.
- Carbidopa is administered concomitantly with levodopa, and it inhibits peripheral metabolism of levodopa into dopamine to reduce side effects.
- Selective type-B monoamine oxidase inhibitors (selegiline and rasagiline) delay degradation of dopamine, used as monotherapy or as adjunctive therapy with levodopa.
- Catechol-O-methyltransferase inhibitors (entacapone and tolcapone) reduce peripheral metabolism and increased brain delivery of levodopa, resulting in prolonged levodopa responses.
- Dopamine agonists (e.g., pramipexole and ropinirole) directly bind D_2 and D_3 receptors and are considered alternatives or adjuncts to levodopa.
- Medical refractory PD motor symptoms can be treated surgically with deep brain stimulation.

CASE STUDY

Mr. WP is your 70-year-old dental patient with Parkinson disease (PD). He has a 10-year history of PD, and, in recent years, he has been experiencing motor fluctuations with predictable episodes of medication wearing off and a return of stiffness and tremor. When medications are effective for his PD symptoms, he nevertheless experiences generalized involuntary twisting movements known as dyskinesias, including the head and neck. Despite being diligent about his dental care, xerostomia associated with PD and its treatments have resulted in recurrent dental caries. He will be returning in the near future for management of two recently identified new dental caries. How will you approach the peri-procedural management of PD medications to minimize jaw hypomobility and rigidity or involuntary movements during his procedure?

Parkinson disease (PD), first clearly described in 1817 by James Parkinson, is a chronic, progressive, degenerative disease of the central nervous system (CNS) and affects approximately 1% of the population older than 50 years. PD has an insidious onset, beginning with mild signs such as slight unilateral hand clumsiness, mild tremor, and subtle changes in speech and facial expression. The essential signs of clinical parkinsonism are **resting tremor, rigidity, bradykinesia, and postural instability**. Patients with PD are said to have a **"masklike" facial appearance** due to reduced spontaneous blinking and expression. Many patients exhibit a complex tremor of the hands that is reminiscent of the way pharmacists once made "pills," called a pill-rolling tremor. Progressive reduction in size, speed, and fluidity of movement along with increasing muscular rigidity result in gradually increasing loss of independence. The combination of increased muscle tone and tremor in the resting limb produces rhythmic resistance, classically described as cogwheel rigidity. Poor coordination of respiration and speaking, along with reduced control of the larynx produces monotone and low-volume speech.

Prodromal "nonmotor" symptoms can commonly be present well before the development of the cardinal motor features. These prodromal symptoms include reduced olfaction, constipation, urinary frequency and urgency, and rapid eye movement (REM) behavioral sleep disorder (enactment of dreams due to loss of typical paralysis during REM sleep). Autonomic nervous system dysfunction (e.g., orthostatic hypotension) is common, though it generally occurs later in the disease course. The patient may have various ill-defined sensory symptoms consisting of numbness, tingling, abnormal temperature sensation, and visual disturbances. Higher rates of anxiety disorders are reported in PD patients (e.g., panic disorder, generalized anxiety, and social phobia), and the anxiety issues may precede the motor symptoms. Pain in PD has been reported in up to 20% of patients, often related to dyskinesias or increased muscle tone, but they may also represent diseased central sensorimotor interactions. Sleep disturbances, including restless leg syndrome, daytime sleepiness, insomnia, and REM behavioral disorder have been identified. Drooling commonly occurs due to reduced frequency and impaired efficiency of swallowing, rather than excessive salivation. Swallowing impairment (dysphagia) is common, and it may be severe in advanced disease leading to a high risk of aspiration and pneumonia.

*The authors wish to recognize Dr. Vahn A. Lewis for his past contributions to this chapter.

Although Parkinson indicated that the senses and intellect were "uninjured" in parkinsonism, the disease is associated with mild cognitive impairment in up to 25% of cases. In addition, the incidence of dementia in those with over 20 years of disease duration is 83%. Depression (~40%) and anxiety (~30%) can be present throughout the course of PD, even before motor symptoms develop. Although the psychological and social implications of the disease contribute, deficiencies in norepinephrine and serotonin neurotransmitters likely underpin the high prevalence. Psychosis increases in prevalence with advancing disease, resulting from both escalating dopaminergic medication needs and accumulating pathology in cortical regions. Visual illusions and hallucinations are most common, though delusions and other psychotic presentations do occur. The mean age of PD onset is 60 years with escalating prevalence with advancing age. Progression of PD occurs at widely variable rates, reaching advanced motor stages as early as 10 years or as protracted as over 25 years. Growing evidence supports a complex interaction of genetic susceptibility and environmental exposures that may contribute to the development of PD. Secondary parkinsonism may result from a variety of etiologies such as vascular (multi-infarct state, hypoxia), infectious (e.g., encephalitis, toxoplasmosis), toxicity (carbon monoxide), metabolic (hepatic failure), and drug-induced and traumatic brain injury. All of these conditions are irreversible, with the exception of drug-induced parkinsonism induced by dopamine receptor antagonists (e.g., antipsychotics and antiemetics).

Atypical degenerative parkinsonian disorders (previously called Parkinson's plus disorders) are a group of maladies that have similar symptoms to PD, but they are distinguished clinically by prominent co-morbidities including cognitive impairment, autonomic dysfunction, and imbalance and falls. These disorders include multiple system atrophy, progressive supranuclear palsy, corticobasal degeneration, and Lewy body dementia. Compared with PD, prognosis is poor, with a rapid course of deterioration and absent or limited dopaminergic therapy responses.

NEUROBIOLOGY AND PATHOPHYSIOLOGY

Although the actual cause of PD remains undetermined, advances have been made in understanding of the neuropathology of parkinsonism, the central control of movement, and the role of neurotransmitters in motor control and extrapyramidal function. The classic motor signs of PD occur when there is a 60% to 80% loss of dopamine neurons in the basal ganglia. The brains of patients with idiopathic PD and some other neurologic disorders contain inclusion bodies called Lewy bodies. These inclusion bodies contain alpha-synuclein, ubiquitin, and in some leucine-rich repeat kinase 2 (LRRK2). Alpha-synuclein is localized in synapses and nuclei (sy + nuclei + n) and is thought to play a role in protein trafficking to the plasma and mitochondrial membranes, and possibly regulation of neurotransmitter reuptake transporters. Dysfunction in the regulation of synuclein by ubiquitin-mediated proteasomal degradation has also been linked to the development of Lewy bodies. Excess formation of alpha-synuclein results in synucleinopathy. **Lewy bodies** decrease neuron survival of the affected cells, which may trigger increased microglial-mediated inflammation and cell destructive activity.

By studying the pattern of alpha-synuclein inclusions, it has been observed that the common sporadic form of PD begins in the olfactory tract, dorsal motor nucleus of the vagus nerve, and lower brainstem before motor symptoms appear. The most sensitive neurons apparently are small neurons with long axons, typical of catecholamine and other autonomic neurons. Prodromal autonomic and olfactory symptoms coincide with the development and spread of alpha-synuclein accumulations. As the disorder progresses, the lesions ascend to involve brainstem, thalamus, basal ganglia, limbic, and finally cortical structures. When sufficient damage to dopamine cells occurs, clinical motor signs become evident. The overt symptoms generally progress over 10 to 20 years and may terminate in severe invalidism. Life expectancy is reduced because of the complications associated with long-term invalidism (infection, trauma due to falls, and immobility).

Hereditary PDs are familial disorders that are usually seen in patients younger than 50 years old and are associated with changes in alpha-synuclein, the ubiquitin-proteasome pathway, or mitochondrial function (Table 13-1). Autosomal dominant loci tend to induce the disease; whereas, recessive factors often contribute to expression but may not act alone. Patterns of inheritance deemed "family clustering" are seen with mutations that confer increased risk but with variable expression and age of onset, with additional presumed contributions of posttranslational genetic or environmental factors. The most common example of this clustering is the LRRK2 mutation. Mutations that affect the function of dopamine neurons can cause Parkinson's symptoms directly; whereas in other cases, accumulation of Lewy bodies leads to subsequent damage of the dopamine cells.

Environmentally induced parkinsonism is a result of a toxic agent from the environment or brain trauma that damages the basal ganglia. A dramatic upsurge of interest in environmental factors as a cause for PD occurred when several young drug abusers developed severe parkinsonian symptoms after self-administering a drug that they thought was a heroin analogue. The compound, 1-methyl-4-phenyl-1,2,3,6-tetrahydropyridine (MPTP), was a by-product of a faulty synthesis of the opiate analgesic alphaprodine. Later work established that the chemical causing the toxicity was actually 1-methyl-4-phenylpyridinium (MPP+), a metabolite of MPTP. MPP+ toxicity stems from its transportation into cells by catecholamine reuptake transporters and subsequent interference with mitochondrial energy production. Acute MPP+ selectively destroys dopamine neurons in the substantia nigra, and this replicates the motor features of PD, although not the synucleinopathy.

Environmental agents may contribute to the development of PD, and various pyridines which exhibit neuronal toxicity are present in the environment in pesticides (e.g., rotenone and paraquat) and herbicides. In contrast, some environmental exposures have been identified

TABLE 13-1 Inheritance of Parkinson Disease

Gene/Protein	Inheritance	Clinical Phenotype	Pathology
SNCA/alpha-synuclein	AD	EO-LO fast progression	Alpha-synuclein accumulation, synaptic function
PARK2/Parkin	AR	EO slow progression	Ubiquitin-E3-ligase, synucleinopathy
PARK7/DJ-1	AR	EO slow progression	Oxidative stress
PINK1	AR	EO slow progression	Oxidative stress, synucleinopathy
LRRK2	AD	LO classical	Tauopathy
VPS35	AD	LO classical	Iron transport
ATP13A2	AR	JO atypical	Lysosome dysfunction, iron accumulation
FBX07	AR	JO atypical	Oxidative stress
PLA2G6	AR	JO atypical	Lipid metabolism
DNAJC6	AR	JO atypical	Vesicle transport

Data from Verstraeten, Theuns, and Broeckhoven: Progress in unraveling the genetic etiology of Parkinson disease in a genomic era. *Trends Genet* 31:140-149, 2015.

AD, Autosomal dominant; *AR*, autosomal recessive; *JO*, juvenile onset; *EO*, early onset; *LO*, late onset.

to reduce the likelihood of developing PD, including caffeine consumption and cigarette smoking.

Changes in Brain Function in Parkinson Disease

A model of basal ganglia function is shown in Figure 13-1. Motor activity in the cerebral cortex is stimulated by thalamocortical input and modulated by many factors, including sensory feedback, memory readout, and emotional response. The basal ganglia modulates the thalamocortical processing through a γ-aminobutyric acid (GABA)–mediated inhibitory input derived from the substantia nigra pars reticulata and globus pallidus interna, nuclei whose functions seem to be similar and for this discussion are referred to as the basal ganglia/thalamic inhibitor. The output of the basal ganglia/thalamic inhibitor is influenced by both direct and indirect pathways within the basal ganglia. The direct pathway generally inhibits the basal ganglia/thalamic inhibitor and disinhibits the thalamic drive and increases motor activity. The indirect pathway, involving excitatory input from the subthalamic nucleus, inhibits movement by facilitating basal ganglia/thalamic inhibitor outflow.

Dopamine from the substantia nigra pars compacta (SNpc) innervates the **direct and indirect pathways in the striatum**. In the direct pathway, it acts on D_1 receptors, which increase GABA inhibition of the basal ganglia/thalamic inhibitor. In the indirect pathway, dopamine acts on D_2 receptors, which inhibit GABA outflow to the indirect pathway. In the case of PD, a loss of dopamine neurons from the SNpc leads to dysregulation of

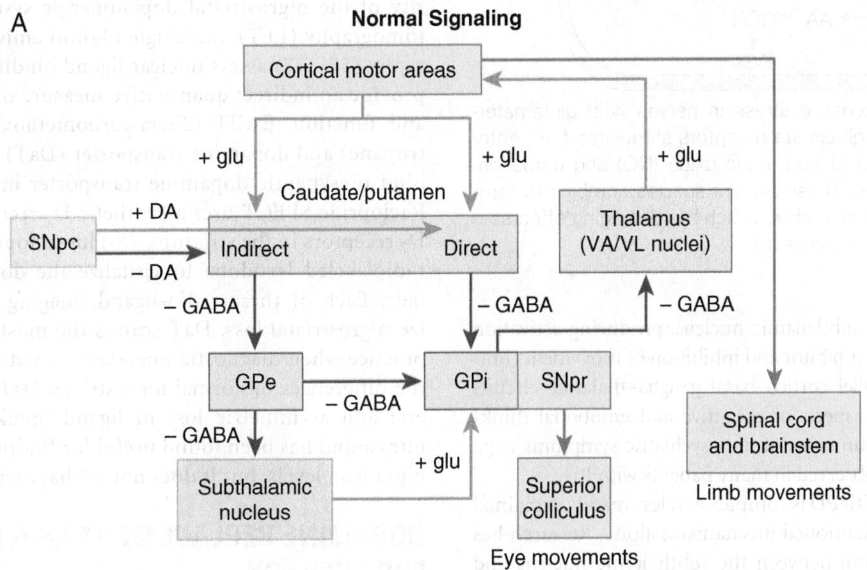

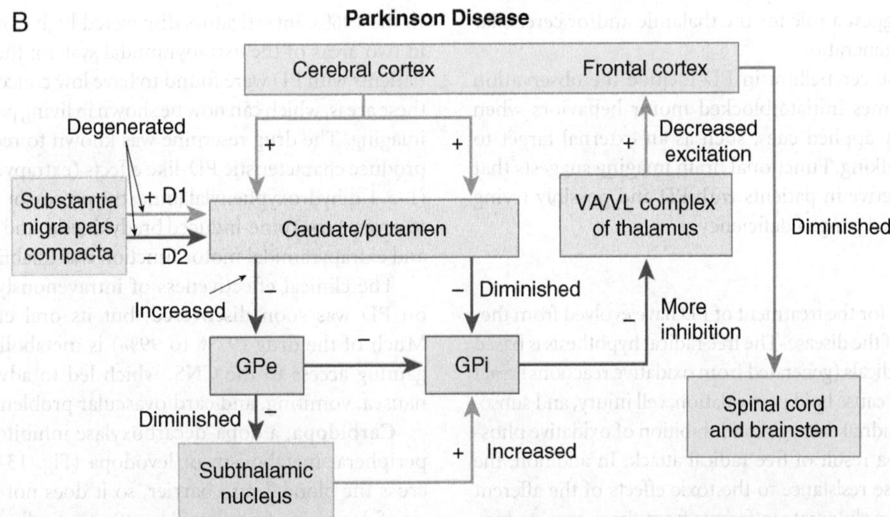

FIG 13-1 Movement controlled by the cortex under the influence of the thalamus and basal ganglia. The ventral anterior (*VA*) and ventral lateral (*VL*) nuclei of the thalamus relay excitatory input to the motor cortex. Glutamatergic (*glu*) cortical fibers project to the striatum, activating GABAergic neurons. The GABAergic output from the basal ganglia is funneled through the substantia nigra pars reticulata (*SNpr*) and globus pallidus interna (*GPi*), which exerts an inhibitory action on the thalamus. By the direct pathway, cortical input inhibits the SNpr and GPi and disinhibits the thalamus output. The indirect pathway, involving the globus pallidus externus (*GPe*) and the subthalamic nucleus, is complex but generally leads to an increase in inhibitory output from the SNpr and GPi. Excitatory D_1 dopamine receptors are believed to modulate the output of the direct pathway; whereas inhibitory D_2 receptors modulate the output of the indirect pathway. Dopamine neuron cell bodies are located in the substantia nigra pars compacta (*SNpc*). Acetylcholine (*ACh*) is found in large interneurons within the striatum and opposes the effects of dopamine. *DA*, Dopamine; *GABA*, Y-aminobutyric acid. (+) And (–) refer to stimulatory and inhibitory pathways, respectively.

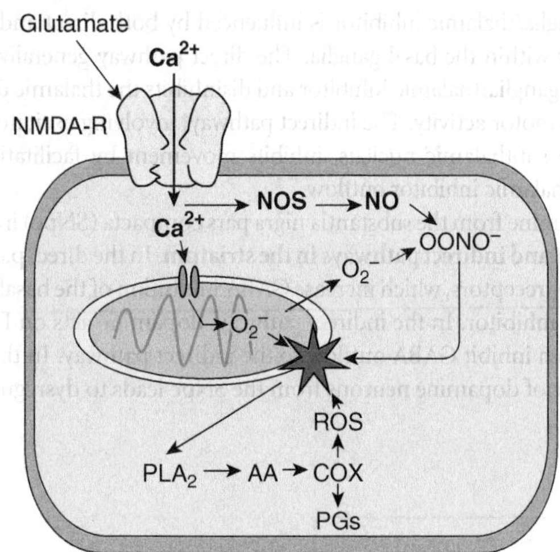

FIG 13-2 Ca^{2+}-mediated oxidative stress in nerves with glutamatergic receptors. Activation of glutamate receptors stimulates Ca^{2+} entry which stimulates production of both nitric oxide (NO) and mitochondrial reactive oxygen species. These oxidant species combine to form the highly reactive peroxynitrite radical, which has damaging effects on mitochondria and can result in cell death.

the indirect pathway by the subthalamic nucleus, producing activation of the basal ganglia/thalamic inhibitor and inhibition of movement (bradykinesia or akinesia). Parallel cortico–basal ganglia–thalamic circuits are proposed that subserve aspects of executive and emotional thinking, which may in part explain some of the psychiatric symptoms (e.g., depression, hallucinations) observed in many patients with PD.

The tremor associated with PD is complex and less readily explained by alterations in the aforementioned mechanisms alone. Research has suggested that the interaction between the subthalamic nucleus and the external segment of the globus pallidus may be one source of tremor. Other studies suggest a role for the thalamic and/or cerebellar dysregulation in tremor generation.

Hints for a role of the cerebellum in PD include the observation that patients can sometimes initiate blocked motor behaviors when presented with externally applied cues, such as an external target to guide a foot to initiate walking. Functional brain imaging suggests that the cerebellum is hyperactive in patients with PD and possibly trying to compensate for the basal ganglia deficiency.

Neuroprotection

Neuroprotective strategies for the treatment of PD have evolved from theories regarding the cause of the disease. The free radical hypothesis is based on the concept that free radicals (generated from oxidative reactions) react with membrane lipids and cause lipid peroxidation, cell injury, and subsequent cell death. Mitochondrial damage and inhibition of oxidative phosphorylation also occur as a result of free radical attack. In addition, the damaged neurons may lose resistance to the toxic effects of the afferent excitatory neurotransmitter glutamate (afferents from the cortex, pedunculopontine nucleus, and subthalamic nucleus), whose toxicity is mediated by excessive calcium flux and nitric oxide synthesis (Fig. 13-2). In the most severe case, these reactions can lead to apoptosis and cell death.

The brain is usually protected from damage caused by free radicals because it contains protective substances (e.g., glutathione, ascorbic acid, melatonin, vitamin E) and enzymes (e.g., glutathione peroxidase, superoxide dismutase) that prevent free radical buildup. The SNpc of patients with PD has reduced concentrations of glutathione and glutathione peroxidase. This decrease occurs early in the disorder and can by itself decrease mitochondrial complex 1 function.

Multiple attempts to capitalize on these potential contributing mechanisms have failed to yield a modifying effect in PD progression. These have included free radical scavenger drugs such as vitamin E, monoamine oxidase inhibitors such as selegiline and rasagiline, mitochondrial enhancers/bioenergetics such as creatine and co-enzyme Q10, and antiapoptotic agents such as pioglitazone.

Diagnostic Imaging in Parkinson Disease

Standard cerebral imaging techniques of computed tomography and magnetic resonance imaging are insensitive to any structural change in early PD, and they are only performed to identify potential alternative secondary causes of parkinsonism. Multiple tomographic imaging techniques can quantify functional changes in the integrity of the nigrostriatal dopaminergic system. Positron emission tomography (PET) and single photon emission computed tomography (SPECT) assess nuclear ligand binding within the brain and provide an indirect quantitative measure of dopaminergic cell loss and function. β-CIT (2beta-carbomethoxy-3beta-(4-iodophenyl) tropane) and dopamine transporter (DaT) (^{123}I-ioflupane) SPECT bind presynaptic dopamine transporter in the nigral projections. Raclopride SPECT uses a synthetic D_2 receptor agonist that binds D_2 receptors in the striatum. 18-Fluorodopa (FDOPA) PET utilizes radiolabeled levodopa to visualize the dopaminergic end terminals. Each of these radio-ligand imaging techniques can visualize nigrostriatal loss. DaT scan is the most widely used in clinical practice when diagnostic uncertainty exists. Figure 13-3 illustrates the differences in normal nigrostriatal DaT imaging and the bilateral and asymmetric loss of ligand uptake in PD. Transcranial ultrasound has been found useful for finding changes in substantia nigra iron levels, but it does not yet have widespread use.

DOPAMINE REPLACEMENT AS A BASIS FOR THERAPY

In the 1960s, investigators discovered high concentrations of dopamine in two areas of the extrapyramidal system: the striatum and the SNpc. Patients with PD were found to have low concentrations of dopamine in these areas, which can now be shown in living patients using tomographic imaging. The drug reserpine was known to reduce catecholamines and produce characteristic PD-like effects (extrapyramidal signs). **Levodopa** (L-3,4-dihydroxyphenylalanine, the precursor of dopamine) was shown to reverse reserpine-induced bradykinesia, and a link between dopamine and extrapyramidal motor function was established.

The clinical effectiveness of intravenously administered levodopa on PD was soon discovered, but its oral effectiveness was limited. Much of the drug (97% to 99%) is metabolized to dopamine before gaining access to the CNS, which led to adverse side effects such as nausea, vomiting, and cardiovascular problems.

Carbidopa, a dopa-decarboxylase inhibitor, prevents much of the peripheral metabolism of levodopa (Fig. 13-4). Carbidopa does not cross the blood–brain barrier, so it does not inhibit the CNS synthesis of dopamine from levodopa. Systemically administered levodopa is transported into the brain through the blood–brain barrier by a saturable amino acid transporter. Combining levodopa with carbidopa permits the use of lower doses of levodopa with greater effectiveness in parkinsonism compared with levodopa alone. It has been found that catechol-O-methyltransferase (COMT) may become upregulated in patients taking carbidopa. This discovery prompted the development of COMT inhibitors to inhibit further the peripheral metabolism of levodopa. Another enzyme important in catecholamine metabolism is MAO. MAO-B inhibitors may also help reduce the amount of levodopa required to reduce PD motor symptoms.

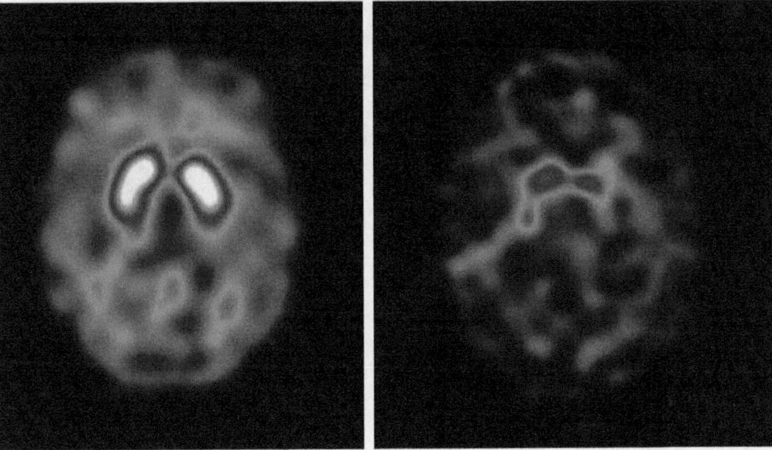

FIG 13-3 Functional imaging allows for indirect quantification of nigrostriatal dopamine neurons. In dopamine transporter SPECT imaging (also called a DaT scan), ^{123}I-ioflupane binds the presynaptic dopamine transporter in the nigral end terminals in the caudate and putamen. Normal uptake (left) produces a large comma shaped area of ligand binding. PD (right) results in an asymmetric, smaller, and circular limited binding field due to nigral cell loss.

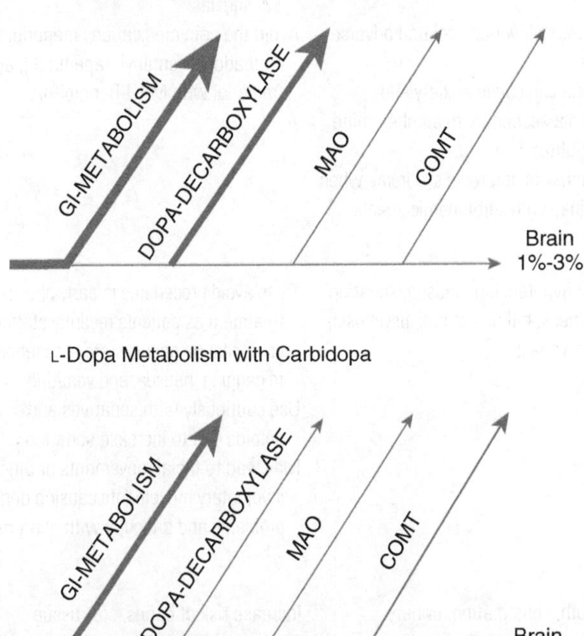

FIG 13-4 Levodopa (L-dopa) metabolism alone and with a dopa-decarboxylase inhibitor. L-Dopa can be eliminated by several mechanisms before it reaches the brain. Substantial elimination occurs in the gastrointestinal (*GI*) tract and peripheral tissues. Carbidopa reduces L-dopa metabolism outside the brain. A higher percentage (10% vs 1% to 3%) of the dose of L-dopa gets to the brain when administered with carbidopa. To reduce metabolism of dopamine further, catechol-O-methyltransferase (*COMT*) inhibitors may be added; these drugs also reduce 3-O-methyldopa competition for levodopa transport into the brain. *MAO*, Monoamine oxidase.

Dopamine is a neurotransmitter in numerous areas of the brain, and the side effects of its supplementation can be understood in the context of its actions. Dopamine can act to amplify the effects of stimulation and can modulate functions of numerous cortical and subcortical structures. Dopamine in the basal ganglia is crucial for regulating motor tone, and its loss is associated with muscle stiffness. Dopamine modulates learning and memory. The mesolimbic dopamine and basal ganglia seem to be associated with drive, salience, fear, and reward. Drugs that increase the actions of dopamine can cause dependence.

Dopamine also has multiple effects outside the basal ganglia. Dopamine inhibits the release of prolactin by an action on the hypothalamus. Dopamine modulates appetite, and it is associated with the chemoreceptor trigger zone where it produces an emetic action. Dopamine neurons are also found in the eye and olfactory tracts. Dopamine has a vasodilatory action in the kidney and is also a precursor for the neurotransmitter norepinephrine which affects blood pressure and cardiovascular function. There are five dopamine receptor subtypes ($D_{1\text{-}5}$), and nonselective stimulation of dopamine receptors through dopamine replacement (levodopa) provides antiparkinson effectiveness. However, the therapeutic effectiveness of agents with selective agonist action on the D_2 receptors provides clear evidence that reestablishing D_2 receptor signaling is key to the therapeutic actions of dopamine in PD.

DRUG THERAPY FOR PARKINSON DISEASE

Table 13-2 presents an overview of the drugs used in the treatment of PD. Dopamine replacement with levodopa is the principal treatment. Patients do not always respond uniformly to levodopa, however, and adjunct agents can be beneficial. The therapeutic effectiveness of PD medications is described based on their estimated equivalency to gold standard of levodopa, as shown in Table 13-3. In advanced disease, disabling dopaminergic nonresponsive motor features emerge, such as gait freezing and postural instability. Additional nonmotor features such as dementia, hypersomnolence, fatigue, and apathy can predominate with limited therapeutic opportunity for improvement.

Levodopa

Levodopa (Fig. 13-5) is a neutral amino acid formed from L-tyrosine, and it is a precursor of the endogenous catecholamines, including dopamine and norepinephrine. The major metabolic fate of levodopa is decarboxylation to dopamine by aromatic L-amino acid decarboxylase, commonly referred to as dopa decarboxylase (DDC). Catechol-O-methyltransferase (COMT) is an enzyme that can methylate levodopa and reduce its transport into the brain. COMT inhibitors have been developed to reduce this problem (Fig. 13-6).

TABLE 13-2 **Overview of Medications Used in the Treatment of Parkinson Disease**

Medications	Mechanism of Action	Adverse Effects	Implications for Dentists
Levodopa	Transported across blood–brain barrier and converted into dopamine in the basal ganglia	Nausea, vomiting, involuntary movements, and postural hypotension	May need to schedule treatment within 60-90 min after receiving dose to decrease movements during examination Facial movements from levodopa may lead to dental problems and difficulty with dentures. May cause taste alterations
Carbidopa (with levodopa)	Inhibits dopa-decarboxylase in peripheral circulation Allows higher concentrations of levodopa to reach the CNS and decreases peripheral adverse effects	Few adverse effects, may increase risk of involuntary movements when combined with levodopa	See levodopa
Tolcapone, entacapone	Spare levodopa from peripheral metabolism and from competition for brain amino acid transporters through inhibition of COMT, prolongs action of levodopa	Increases levodopa adverse effects Tolcapone has been associated with hepatotoxicity	Can increase risk of tachycardia, hypertension, and arrhythmias when combined with epinephrine and other vasoconstrictors. Ampicillin and erythromycin can reduce elimination of entacapone and increase risk of dyskinesias
Selegiline (also called deprenyl) and rasagiline	Block MAO-B irreversibly; increasing dopamine in presynaptic stores May reduce synthesis of reactive metabolites and slow progression of disease	Can increase levodopa-related adverse effects Selegiline can cause anxiety and insomnia secondary to amphetamine metabolites Increase risk of serotonin syndrome when combined with serotonergic agents	Avoid the pain medications meperidine, methadone, fentanyl, tapentadol, and tramadol with MAO-B inhibitors
Dopamine Receptor Agonists			
Bromocriptine, apomorphine, pramipexole (D_2, D_3), ropinirole (D_2, D_3), rotigotine (D_1, D_2, D_3)	Act directly on dopaminergic receptors to reduce symptoms of parkinsonism	Postural hypotension, nausea, sedation, sleepiness, hallucinations, psychosis, impulsiveness	Try to avoid procedures in early phases of treatment as patients recently started on dopamine agonists are susceptible to gagging, nausea, and vomiting Use cautiously with sedatives and opioids due to increase sedation May lead to facial movements or other involuntary movements causing dental problems and difficulty with dentures
Anticholinergics (Antimuscarinic)			
Trihexyphenidyl, benztropine, biperiden, diphenhydramine, orphenadrine	Balance CNS dopamine/acetylcholine ratios through inhibition of muscarinic receptors in the basal ganglia Primarily reduces tremor and rigidity	Dry mouth, constipation, urinary retention, triggering of acute-angle glaucoma, mydriasis, impaired memory, and hallucinations	Increase risk of caries, soft tissue disease, difficulties swallowing and speaking, due to dry mouth
Other			
Amantadine	Increases release of dopamine; blocks dopamine reuptake and NMDA receptors	Nausea, vomiting, dysarthria, dizziness, hallucinations, psychosis, livedo reticularis, and sleep disturbances	May worsen adverse effects and dental problems of other Parkinson disease treatments including levodopa, dopamine agonists, and anticholinergics

CNS, Central nervous system; *COMT*, catechol-O-methyltransferase; *MAO-B*, monoamine oxidase B; *NMDA*, *N*-methyl-D-aspartate.

Pharmacologic effects

The CNS and peripheral nervous system actions of levodopa are indirect and result from its conversion to dopamine. In practice, levodopa is always given with a DDC inhibitor to increase the percentage of levodopa delivered to the CNS and to reduce peripheral adverse effects of dopamine.

Central nervous system. Because PD is characterized by a dopamine deficiency, the intuitive therapeutic strategy would be to restore dopamine concentrations toward normal. Dopamine does not cross the blood–brain barrier and is thus ineffective when administered systemically. The immediate amino acid precursor of dopamine, levodopa, is readily transported into the brain and is decarboxylated to

TABLE 13-3 Selected Antiparkinson Drugs and Their Approximate Clinical Effectiveness Expressed in Levodopa Equivalent Dose

Drug Class	Drug	Total L-Dopa Equivalent Dose mg/100 mg L-Dopa
L-dopa	L-dopa	100
	Controlled-release L-dopa	133
	Duopa/Duodopa	90
COMT inhibitors	Entacapone	LD × 0.33
	Tolcapone	LD × 0.5
Dopamine agonist	Pramipexole	1
	Ropinirole	5
	Rotigotine	3.3
	Apomorphine (subcutaneous)	
MAO-B inhibitor	Selegiline 10 mg (oral)	10
	Selegiline 1.25 mg (sublingual)	1.25
	Rasagiline	1
Other	Amantadine	100

Adapted from Tomlinson CL, Stowe R, Patel S, Rick C, Gray R, Clarke CE: Systematic review of levodopa dose equivalency reporting in Parkinson's disease. *Mov Disord* 25:2649-2653, 2010.
LD, L-DOPA.

dopamine in nigrostriatal neurons. The newly synthesized dopamine is sequestered in vesicles in the neuron terminals in the striatum, where it is available for release. Despite this seemingly physiologic approach, levodopa provides a robust symptomatic relief without complete resolution of motor abnormalities.

A beneficial response to levodopa is obtained in most patients. The cardinal features of bradykinesia, rigidity, and tremor are often readily attenuated early in the disease course and allow maintenance of independence and ability to perform activities of daily living for many years. Patients receiving long-term levodopa therapy commonly experience **motor fluctuations**, a decrease in the length of time that a given dose of levodopa exerts its therapeutic effect. The relative medication states are referred to as **on and off**, respectively representing periods when levodopa is effectively controlling symptoms and when rigidity and bradykinesia are disabling. New formulations of levodopa have been developed to improve the stability and consistency of enteric delivery. Oral delayed-release carbidopa/levodopa capsules (Rytary) provide slower absorption and improved maintenance of serum levels, resulting in a more sustained clinical benefit. Carbidopa/levodopa enteral gel suspension (Duopa/Duodopa) is delivered directly to the duodenum/jejunum via an implanted intestinal tube and external delivery pump, providing a steady basal delivery throughout the day and rapidly administered rescue to stabilize clinical response and reduce motor fluctuations.

An additional complication of long-term levodopa therapy is the development of choreoathetosis (jerky, twisting, and writhing movements) caused by the treatment, commonly referred to as **levodopa-induced dyskinesias**. Dyskinesias often correlate with the maximum plasma concentration of levodopa (peak-dose dyskinesia).

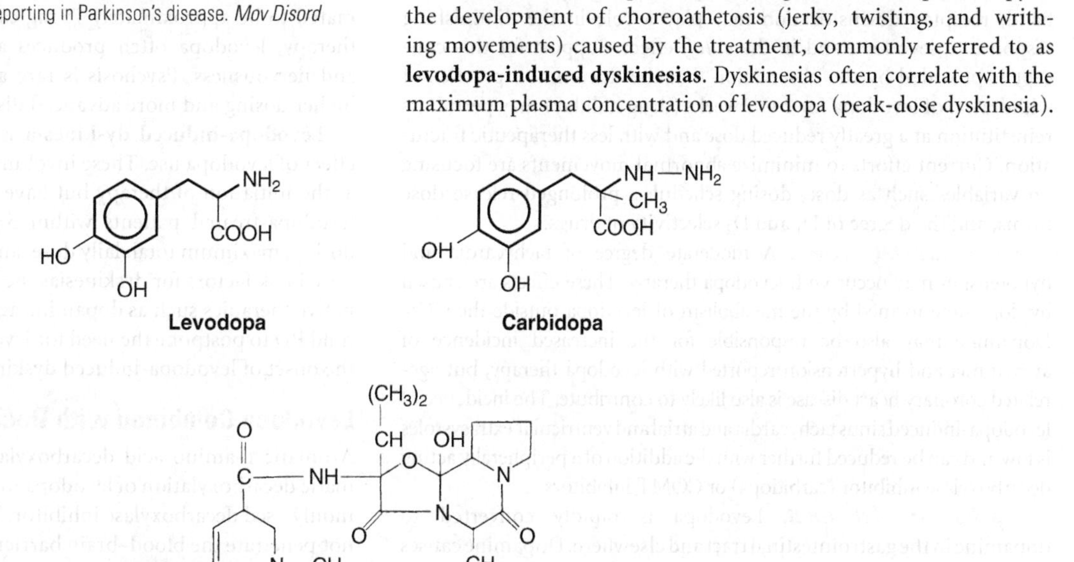

FIG 13-5 Structural formulas of drugs used in the treatment of Parkinson disease. The dopamine backbone contained within three structures is emphasized.

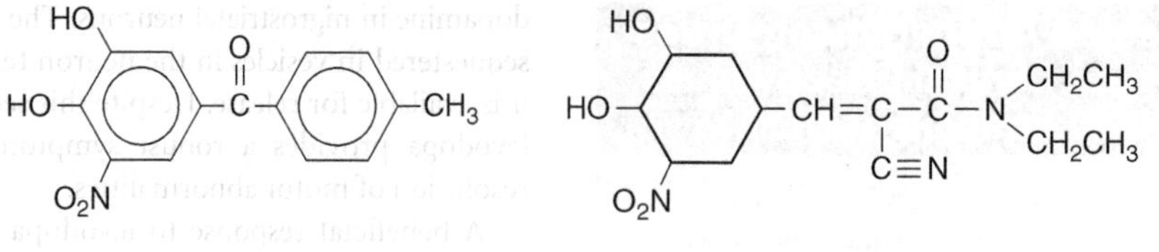

Tolcapone

Entacapone

FIG 13-6 Structural formulas of the nitrocatechol catechol-O-methyltransferase (*COMT*) inhibitors tolcapone and entacapone.

Chorea (unpredictable brief flitting movements) and athetosis (writhing serpentine-like movements) represent the most common types of hyperkinesias associated with dopaminergic therapy. Dystonia is another hyperkinetic movement, identified by the co-contraction of opposing muscles that results in sustained, abnormal, and often painful postures. Dystonia generally occurs in a low or *off* medication state, and more rarely as a form of *on* state dyskinesia.

Levodopa-induced dyskinesias are a common problem, though the mechanisms responsible are poorly understood and various factors may be involved in their generation. Loss of dopaminergic input (denervation) to the striatum produces some increased sensitivity of postsynaptic dopamine receptors (denervation supersensitivity) to dopamine. D_1 receptors and stimulated adenylyl cyclase activity are increased by denervation and by long-term levodopa. On the other hand, receptor desensitization may play a role in the diminishing response to levodopa and in the *on/off* effect. Support for this concept is provided by the observation that the uncommon practice of withdrawal of levodopa for 2 to 3 weeks (drug holiday) may permit its reinstitution at a greatly reduced dose and with less therapeutic fluctuation. Current efforts to minimize abnormal movements are focusing on variables such as dose, dosing schedules, prolonged-release dose forms, and the degree of D_1 and D_2 selectivity of drugs.

Cardiovascular system. A moderate degree of tachycardia and hypotension may occur with levodopa therapy. These effects are caused by dopamine formed by the metabolism of levodopa outside the CNS. Dopamine may also be responsible for the increased incidence of arrhythmia and hypertension reported with levodopa therapy, but age-related coronary heart disease is also likely to contribute. The incidence of levodopa-induced sinus tachycardia and atrial and ventricular extrasystoles is low and can be reduced further with the addition of a peripherally acting decarboxylase inhibitor (carbidopa) or COMT inhibitors.

Gastrointestinal tract. Levodopa is rapidly converted to dopamine in the gastrointestinal tract and elsewhere. Dopamine causes significant nausea, which can be reduced by the co-administration of peripheral decarboxylase inhibitors.

Absorption, fate, and excretion

Levodopa is absorbed from the gastrointestinal tract, but when administered alone, approximately 95% of the drug is converted to dopamine in the small intestine and liver. Individuals with reduced gastric acidity may have reduced absorption. Only 1% of orally administered levodopa reaches the brain. When the drug is combined with a peripherally acting decarboxylase inhibitor, the dose of levodopa can be reduced by 80% (see Decarboxylase Inhibitors). The enzymes MAO and COMT found in the nervous system and various tissues metabolize dopamine and levodopa, respectively, and inactive metabolites are excreted in the urine. Agents that block these enzymes are available to augment levodopa delivery to the CNS and improve the effectiveness of available dopamine. A diminished response to levodopa may occur when it is taken with a meal high in protein, perhaps related to competition for saturable amino acid carrier transport systems in the CNS. Protein-restricted diets can provide improved consistency of dose responses. Delayed gastric emptying and alterations in intestinal motility can produce variability in dose responses.

Adverse effects

Initially, many patients treated with levodopa experience **nausea, vomiting,** and **orthostatic hypotension.** Tolerance develops to these side effects, reducing the need for therapeutic intervention. These symptoms are greatly reduced if a decarboxylase inhibitor is given concurrently. During early titration, inadequate peripheral aromatic L-amino acid decarboxylase inhibition may result from the standardized ratio of decarboxylase (carbidopa or benaseride) to levodopa. Further dose escalation can paradoxically improve peripheral side effects due to necessary threshold inhibition of decarboxylase (estimated to be approximately 75 mg carbidopa total daily). On initial therapy, levodopa often produces anxiety, insomnia, nightmares, and nervousness. Psychosis is rare at initiation and increases with higher dosing and more advanced disease.

Levodopa-induced dyskinesia is the most challenging adverse effect of levodopa use. These involuntary movements are not evident at the initiation of therapy but have been reported in up to 50% of levodopa-treated patients within 5 years of treatment. Infrequent dosing, maximum total daily dose, and duration of exposure are proposed risk factors for dyskinesias. Because of these risk factors, alternative therapies such as dopamine agonists are usually considered in mild PD to postpone the need for levodopa, thus potentially delaying the onset of levodopa-induced dyskinesias.

Levodopa Combined with Decarboxylase Inhibitors

Aromatic L-amino acid decarboxylase is responsible for the enzymatic decarboxylation of levodopa to dopamine. Carbidopa is a commonly used decarboxylase inhibitor. The decarboxylase inhibitors do not penetrate the blood–brain barrier and inhibit only the peripheral conversion of levodopa to dopamine, including the conversion that occurs in the intestinal lumen. Carbidopa allows an 80% decrease in the dosage of levodopa necessary to control parkinsonian symptoms (see Fig. 13-4). Carbidopa is relatively nontoxic but is inactive as an antiparkinson drug in the absence of levodopa.

The levodopa-carbidopa combination is not recommended in pregnancy or in patients younger than 18 years. Carbidopa is available as a single agent or formulated with levodopa in a fixed ratio of 10 mg/100 mg, 25 mg/100 mg, and 25 mg/250 mg (carbidopa/levodopa) and controlled-release preparations with fixed ratios of 25 mg/100 mg and 50 mg/200 mg (carbidopa/levodopa). Packaged alone (but used in combination with levodopa), carbidopa is useful for patients who require greater amounts of the drug than provided in the standard ratios.

Catechol-O-Methyltransferase Inhibitors

Peripheral metabolism of levodopa decreases its distribution into the CNS. The addition of carbidopa eliminates peripheral metabolism of levodopa via L-aromatic amino acid decarboxylase, which constitutes the majority of levodopa metabolism in the periphery. Levodopa can be metabolized by COMT into 3-O-methyldopa, further decreasing available levodopa for the CNS. Tolcapone and entacapone are two reversible inhibitors of COMT that allow more levodopa to reach the CNS and extend the effect of levodopa in patients who have wearing off effects of levodopa on average by an hour per day.

Both therapies are given concurrently with levodopa, and each drug has minimal efficacy when given as a monotherapy. Additionally, each treatment can potentiate the adverse effects of levodopa, and both therapies are additionally associated with levodopa-independent gastrointestinal adverse effects (e.g., nausea, diarrhea).

Tolcapone inhibits both central and peripheral COMT and is dosed up to three times a day concurrently with levodopa. Due to rare but severe hepatotoxicity, tolcapone is reserved for patients who have failed to respond to other treatments. Liver function tests must be monitored every two weeks for the first year and then monthly afterward for patients receiving tolcapone. **Entacapone** is a COMT inhibitor with only peripheral activity. It has a shorter half-life relative to tolcapone and must be administered with each dose of levodopa/carbidopa up to a max of 1600 mg/day. Entacapone is not associated with hepatotoxicity; however, it can cause an orange discoloration of the urine and GI side effects (nausea, vomiting, and diarrhea). Entacapone is available in combination products with levodopa/carbidopa.

Drug interactions of concern with COMT inhibitors include the catecholamines (e.g., epinephrine), drugs that interfere with biliary excretion (including ampicillin and erythromycin), norepinephrine reuptake inhibition (e.g., tricyclic antidepressants, atomoxetine), and nonselective MAO inhibitors.

Monoamine Oxidase Type-B Inhibitors

Selegiline and **rasagiline** are "selective" irreversible inhibitors of MAO-B, the major MAO enzyme in the striatum responsible for dopamine metabolism. Because MAO-A is not inhibited, peripheral catecholamine metabolism is less affected. The rationale for using a selective MAO-B inhibitor is to elevate brain dopamine concentrations, while causing little or no effect on norepinephrine or 5-HT.

Selegiline has been evaluated as a monotherapy in early-stage PD, and it improves motor function and reduces freezing. Additionally, when combined with levodopa, selegiline can strengthen motor improvements. Selegiline is partly metabolized in the liver to amphetamine and methamphetamine which can result in adverse stimulant effects. Alternative formulations, including a transdermal patch and sublingual disintegrating tablet, are available to reduce hepatic first-pass conversion to the amphetamine metabolites.

Rasagiline is an MAO-B inhibitor that is not metabolized to toxic amphetamine metabolites and is several-fold more potent than selegiline. Rasagiline can provide mild improvement of motor symptoms as monotherapy and adjunct to levodopa.

Adverse effects of selegiline and rasagiline include nausea, dry mouth, confusion, occasional visual hallucinations, dizziness, headache, and insomnia, especially at higher doses. The combined use of these agents at high doses and levodopa results in an increased incidence of dyskinesia and psychoses. For selegiline, the effect may result from the formation of toxic quantities of an amphetamine metabolite. Although MAO-B inhibitors are thought to have fewer drug interactions than MAO-A inhibitors, clinical data have found that when the dose is increased, typical MAO-A drug interactions, such as the "cheese effect," may be seen. The U.S. Food and Drug Administration (FDA) labels warn against combining with most foods that contain elevated tyramine; however, reactions are unlikely unless high amounts of tyramine are consumed. MAO-B inhibitors are contraindicated with meperidine, methadone, propoxyphene, and dextromethorphan. MAO-B inhibitors are relatively contraindicated with most antidepressants due to potential risk of serotonin syndrome and theoretical concerns regarding hypertensive reactions. Caution is advised with any sympathomimetic amines as they could potentiate the noradrenergic effects of these agents.

Direct Dopamine Receptor Agonists

The discovery of dopamine receptor subtypes, recognition of the limits of levodopa therapy, and advances in knowledge of the neurochemistry of normal and parkinsonism-altered synaptic pathways have justified the use of dopamine agonists as a therapeutic option in the treatment of PD. These agents act directly on postsynaptic dopamine receptors; thus they exhibit a separate, but complementary mechanism to levodopa. These drugs offer several advantages over levodopa: (1) they do not require metabolic conversion to an active compound, (2) they do not require the presence of nigrostriatal neurons or nerve impulses for their activity, (3) they have longer durations of action than levodopa with fewer on/off changes, (4) they are more selective than levodopa on specific subpopulations of dopamine receptors, and (5) they are less likely to generate damaging free radicals. Perhaps most importantly, the initiation of treatment with a dopamine agonist delays the need for treatment with levodopa, thus extending the time of treatment without development of dyskinesias seen after long-term levodopa use.

The first dopamine receptor agonist discovered for this purpose was bromocriptine, an ergot alkaloid that contains a dopamine-like substructure (Fig. 13-5). Bromocriptine is a potent D_2 receptor agonist, a weak D_1 antagonist, and also has modest agonist activity at serotonin and glutamate receptors. When combined with levodopa therapy, bromocriptine alleviates the "on/off" phenomenon and reduces the risk of developing dyskinesias. It can also be useful in patients who are unresponsive to levodopa-carbidopa. Although the actions of bromocriptine are similar to levodopa, the adverse effects such as hallucinations, nausea and orthostatic hypotension are more common. In addition, the off-target receptor effects of bromocriptine lead to an increased risk of peripheral vasospasm and pulmonary fibrosis. The use of bromocriptine has declined with the advent of more selective dopamine receptor agonists that do not exhibit these non-dopamine receptor effects.

Ropinirole (Fig. 13-5), pramipexole, and rotigotine are non-ergot-derived dopamine receptor agonists. Their antiparkinsonian effect is thought to be caused by activity at the D_2 or D_3 receptor. These agents can be used as initial monotherapy in patients younger than 60 (delays risk of dyskinesia compared with levodopa) or as an adjunct to levodopa therapy to smooth out its fluctuating propensity (on/off phenomena). Rotigotine is thought to stimulate D_1 dopamine receptors as well.

Pramipexole is cleared primarily by renal excretion (96%); whereas ropinirole is metabolized mainly by the CYP1A2 isoform. Rotigotine has been marketed as a time-release patch to reduce blood level fluctuations and may be helpful when compliance or inability to use an oral dosage form is an issue. It is eliminated primarily by conjugation and renal excretion, but also to a certain extent by oxidative dealkylation.

Several side effects have been noted with direct dopamine receptor agonists. Postural hypotension and peripheral edema can occur. Asthenia (weakness), fatigue, and somnolence are reported. Sleep disturbances (both daytime sleepiness and insomnia), hallucinations, and panic attacks have also been reported. Motor side effects include dyskinesias and extrapyramidal reactions, although less frequently compared with levodopa. Patients can experience increased behavioral drive and have difficulty controlling gambling, sexual activity, and appetite. Gastrointestinal side effects of nausea, constipation, xerostomia, sialorrhea, and dysgeusia have been reported. Rotigotine has a higher incidence of skin reactions associated with the patch adhesives and the drug.

Apomorphine has been recognized as a direct dopamine agonist since 1951. It has been rarely used clinically, however, because of nausea. It has been rediscovered and approved by the FDA as a fast-acting agent to reverse off periods; subcutaneous injection is more efficacious than oral therapy for this indication. The actions of apomorphine are less selective than other approved dopamine agonists in that it stimulates signaling through both D_1 and D_2 dopamine receptors.

Drugs with Antimuscarinic Activity

Before the discovery of levodopa, the standard drugs for the treatment of PD were the antimuscarinic agents. Antimuscarinic drugs such as **benztropine** and **trihexyphenidyl** act to restore the dopaminergic/cholinergic balance by antagonizing the action of acetylcholine; they may also inhibit dopamine uptake. The antimuscarinic drugs are used as adjunct agents because they are not highly effective antiparkinson agents, but tremor often responds better to these drugs than to levodopa-carbidopa.

The antimuscarinic drugs produce sedation and, in high doses, can elicit visual hallucinations and changes in mood. Toxic doses of antimuscarinic drugs can cause severe mental disturbances, including excitement, confusion, hallucinations, delirium, depression, and coma. Because of muscarinic receptor blockade, these drugs produce anticholinergic effects including xerostomia, increased intraocular pressure in closed-angle glaucoma, urinary retention, constipation, and possible cardiac effects (tachycardia, palpitations, and arrhythmias).

Miscellaneous Drugs

Amantadine

The antiparkinson effects of **amantadine**, an antiviral agent, were discovered when the drug was used to treat a viral infection in a patient who had PD. The mechanism of action of amantadine is unknown. It has been proposed that the drug (1) prevents dopamine reuptake and facilitates the release of dopamine; (2) has weak anticholinergic properties; and (3) blocks the glutamate *N*-methyl-D-aspartate (NMDA) receptor, which could contribute to reducing excitation-induced neurotoxicity and dyskinesias. Amantadine offers mild benefit in treating motor symptoms associated with PD in early course of the illness; however, these effects do not last long, and often patients will require more advanced treatment. Amantadine is often used later in the disease course to reduce the severity and extent of dyskinesias induced by levodopa.

Approximately 80% to 90% of amantadine is excreted unchanged in the urine, and accumulation occurs in patients with impaired renal function. This accumulation may lead to the toxic manifestations of confusion, hallucinations, toxic psychosis, and convulsions. Geriatric populations tend to be more sensitive to these adverse effects. Amantadine may cause livedo reticularis of the lower extremities. More common side effects include anorexia, insomnia, nausea, vomiting, dizziness, dry mouth, lightheadedness, lower-extremity edema, and sweating. These side effects are not severe and are limited further by the development of tolerance.

Benzodiazepines

Benzodiazepines can help alleviate anxiety associated with PD and may help alleviate tremor aggravated by anxiety. Additionally, the benzodiazepine **clonazepam** has shown to be useful in patients experiencing REM sleep behavior disorder. Benzodiazepines should be avoided in PD patients with cognitive impairment and those at a higher risk for falls.

Antidepressants

Antidepressants may be useful in PD patients who may exhibit depression. No specific antidepressant is recommended for patients with PD. However, selective-serotonin reuptake inhibitors (SSRIs), tricyclic antidepressants, and selective norepinephrine reuptake inhibitors (SNRIs) are commonly used. Concurrent treatment with selegiline or rasagiline may limit antidepressant selection due to potential drug–drug interactions.

Antipsychotic drugs

As noted earlier, patients with PD may experience psychotic-like signs either from the disease or from the drugs used to treat the disease. The atypical antipsychotics clozapine and quetiapine have been found to be helpful in reducing psychosis in PD patients and have minimal effects on worsening motor symptoms due to their minimal extrapyramidal effects. A serotonin 5-HT_{2A} inverse agonist, pimavanserin, has been shown safe and effective for the treatment of PD psychosis, but it remains investigational.

Acetylcholinesterase inhibitors

Acetylcholinesterase inhibitors initially developed for use in the treatment of Alzheimer disease (e.g., rivastigmine, donepezil, galantamine) have been effective for patients with memory difficulties, behavioral disturbances, and cognitive decline associated with PD.

Adrenergic agents

Adrenergic agents may be helpful in reducing orthostatic hypotension and symptoms associated with orthostatic hypotension. **Midodrine** forms an active metabolite that is an alpha-1 adrenergic receptor agonist. It has been successful in treating orthostatic hypotension associated with PD. Droxidopa, a synthetic amino acid precursor of norepinephrine, is approved for treating neurogenic orthostatic hypotension associated with PD. Other nonadrenergic medications to improve orthostatic hypotension include fludrocortisone and domperidone.

Phosphodiesterase inhibitors

Erectile dysfunction can occur in patients with PD, due to autonomic dysfunction and dopaminergic medication side effect. Inhibitors of phosphodiesterase-5 (e.g., sildenafil, vardenafil) are effective at improving erectile dysfunction and can be used in patients complaining of erectile dysfunction associated with PD. These medications should be used cautiously in patients with uncontrolled orthostatic hypotension due their additive hypotensive effects.

Antiemetics

Due to the nauseating effects of dopaminergic agents, antiemetics are occasionally used adjunctively to treat nausea and vomiting if slower titration or dose reduction of dopaminergic agents is not successful. Many antinausea agents should not be used in patients with PD as they may worsen symptoms due to the blockade of dopamine receptors (e.g., metoclopramide, prochlorperazine). The peripheral dopamine blocker **domperidone** has shown to be effective to reduce nausea and poses low risk of worsening motor symptoms in PD. Trimethobenzamide and ondansetron offer antiemetic effects that are achieved without inhibition of dopamine receptors, and they can be considered for use in PD.

General Therapeutic Uses

Dopaminergic agents continue to represent the mainstay treatment in PD. Treatment strategies vary depending on the severity and predominant symptoms presenting at diagnosis. Some physicians initiate therapy with an MAO-B inhibitor, a dopamine agonist, amantadine, or antimuscarinic agents. When the disease is judged to be moderate, levodopa-carbidopa and a COMT inhibitor can be added, although there is no objective evidence supporting a delay in treatment with levodopa until the disease has progressed. There is still a strong interest in drugs that may provide a neuroprotective effect and reduce progression of the disease. Finally, patients with PD will often present with nonmotor symptoms that may require additional pharmacologic management.

SURGICAL THERAPY

When pharmacologic management is inadequate to control disabling motor symptoms of PD, stereotactic surgical approaches provide an alternative and adjunctive option. Early techniques of lesioning of the globus pallidus (pallidotomy) or thalamus (thalamotomy) have lost favor due to their destructive and irreversible nature. Deep brain stimulation (DBS) has become the standard surgical management for PD. Stimulating electrodes are placed in either the subthalamic nucleus, globus pallidus interna, or less commonly the thalamus. The former two provide control of most of the cardinal features of PD, while thalamic stimulation offers only tremor control. Disabling motor fluctuations (waxing and waning control of symptoms as medications come and go), medically refractory tremor, and disabling levodopa-induced hyperkinetic movements are all common indications for pursuing DBS. The presumed effect of surgery is to reduce excessive excitatory neuronal activity or to increase inhibitory tone by stimulation. Efferent pathways of the subthalamic nucleus seem to be excitatory and mediated by glutamate, as are cortico-subthalamic pathways. Intracranial deep brain electrodes are surgically implanted, and the patient has a battery-powered neurostimulator(s) below the clavicle. There has been longstanding interest in the cellular restorative potential of pluripotent cell (such as fetal and other stem cell lines) implantation for the treatment of PD and other neurodegenerative disorders; however these therapies remain investigational.

DRUGS USED FOR OTHER MOVEMENT DISORDERS

PD is among an extensive list of other disorders that also cause movement disabilities. These diseases include essential tremor, Huntington disease, Tourette/tic disorders, Wilson disease, and dystonic syndromes. Although these movement disorders are more refractory to pharmacotherapy than PD, some drugs are beneficial, and they have furthered our understanding of the role of the basal ganglia in motor control.

Essential tremor is the most prevalent movement disorder, presenting with monosymptomatic tremor of the head, extremities, and voice during activity. Increased incidence and prevalence with age (as common as 1 in 10 over the age of 80) often result in the misconception of this condition being a normal part of aging. Strongly inherited, over 60% have a known family history. Alcohol responsiveness with tremor attenuation is common. Tremor suppression is sought when functional disability or social handicap develops. First-line therapy includes **beta-adrenergic receptor blockers** (e.g., propranolol) and the antiepileptic medication primidone (see Chapters 9 and 12).

Huntington disease is characterized by choreic hyperkinesias, psychiatric/behavioral symptoms of depression, anxiety, irritability, aggression, and cognitive impairment progression to dementia. This inherited neurodegenerative disorder is caused by a mutation in the huntingtin gene and subsequent abnormal synthesis of a huntingtin protein that contains excess polyglutamine repeats. The pathologic change in early Huntington disease includes selective degeneration of GABAergic neurons in the striatum and development of chorea, bradykinesia, and reduced coordination. Reducing dopamine signaling has the most reliable efficacy in attenuating chorea. The **antipsychotic drugs**, which are potent dopamine antagonists, are often used to reduce chorea. A presynaptic dopamine-depleting drug, tetrabenazine, is also useful in controlling chorea.

Tourette and other tic disorders are characterized by phonic and/or motor tics and complex mannerisms. The pathophysiology is not well understood; however, it may share properties with obsessive-compulsive disease that has been associated with orbital frontal cortex disorders and basal ganglia disorder associated with motor program regulation. Symptoms of Tourette disorder are responsive to **clonidine** and **guanfacine** (α_2-adrenergic receptor agonist), first- and second-generation **antipsychotics** (dopamine receptor blockers), **benzodiazepines**, and **topiramate**.

Wilson disease, also known as hepatolenticular degeneration, is an inherited disorder of **copper metabolism** that can be diagnosed by the presence of a brown stain at the edge of the cornea (Kayser–Fleischer rings). Wilson disease can be managed by **chelating excess copper** with penicillamine, zinc supplementation, and a low copper diet. If treatment is begun late in the course of the disease, however, damage to the basal ganglia occurs resulting in motor disorders, including coarse tremor, dysarthria, akinesia, rigidity, and dystonia. At this point, chelating agents are ineffective, and levodopa and the anticholinergic antiparkinson drugs are useful to allay the symptoms.

Primary dystonic disorders may occur in a generalized and focal pattern of involvement. Hallmark clinical features include sustained muscular contractions, abnormal postures, and co-contractions of opposing agonist/antagonist muscle groups. Common adult onset forms of focal dystonia (cervical dystonia, blepharospasm, writer's cramp, oromandibular jaw opening or closing dystonia) are largely refractory to oral pharmacotherapy. An uncommon form of dopa-responsive dystonia shows a robust response to dopaminergic replacement therapies. In most other cases, the underlying pathology and cause of these syndromes remain unknown. Higher doses of antimuscarinic antiparkinson agents can be helpful, though better tolerated in effective doses in young patients. **Botulinum toxin** injections are a common and effective therapeutic option for focal dystonia, by reducing the peripheral neuromuscular junction signaling to produce muscle relaxation (see Chapters 7 and 11). **Antimuscarinic drugs** may also be useful for treating focal dystonias.

IMPLICATIONS FOR DENTISTRY

Physical Barriers

Patients with untreated PD face many potential challenges to maintaining adequate oral health. **Orofacial motor impairments** of PD include disorders of mastication, swallowing, and speech, and they may be different from motor impairments in the extremities and may not respond to pharmacotherapy in the same manner. Jaw muscle function is altered with reduced voluntary and rhythmic activity. Parkinson's patients have difficulty in sustaining repetitive motions, such as those used for toothbrushing or flossing. Electric toothbrushes are recommended and can help circumvent some of the problem, although a patient with motor freezing may still have difficulty and need assistance. Oral tremor or dyskinesias can also make oral health care challenging for the dentist, and prosthetic restoration may pose additional challenges because of the presence of uncontrolled oral movements. Patients with PD who can perform regular dental hygiene procedures do not have an elevated risk for dental disorders, thus extra preventions can be successful.

Patients with PD may have **xerostomia** or **sialorrhea** and experience nausea and vomiting more frequently than other patients, with possible adverse effects on oral health. Reduced gastric acid in elderly patients may prompt caregivers to administer levodopa with acidic juices, with potential impact on enamel and dentin.

PD patients have difficulty maintaining postural stability and normal walking gait and may be more prone to falling; assistance entering and leaving the office should be considered. Orthostatic hypotension can also be present due to dysautonomia in combination with symptomatic PD therapies, so patients should be allowed to change position slowly and stabilize their blood pressure. During a procedure, consideration should be given to the patient's **difficulty with swallowing.** Aggressive saliva control and not tipping the patient too far back in the dental chair can be helpful. PD patients may also react slowly to pain and not provide rapid feedback about progressive tissue damage.

PD is a **motor function disorder**, and so caution should be used with agents that could compromise motor function further. Various agents used in dentistry should be carefully considered and dosed. Drugs that may depress respiratory function need to have their doses adjusted appropriately for the weight, age, and physical condition of the patient. Opioids, barbiturates, skeletal muscle relaxant agents (peripherally and centrally acting), and some antibiotics (clindamycin and aminoglycosides) should be used with caution.

Behavioral Barriers

PD patients report higher levels of anxiety, which may be associated with the disease and possibly some of the treatments. In addition to motor freezing, these patients may have difficulty comprehending or remembering prolonged instructions; written or taped treatment plans and medication instructions should be provided to the patient and responsible accompanying parties.

Patients may be unable to effectively communicate their specific needs because of motor problems or cognitive decline; thus the presence of a caregiver is important to ensure that the treatment plan is clearly understood and approved. In particular, lack of facial muscular control can compromise the patient's ability to express emotion. Patients should be carefully observed during treatment for other signs of pain, such as eye or limb movements, that may indicate pain during a procedure. As a general rule, special care should be taken to reduce the stress of a dental patient with PD by taking the preventive efforts described and by scheduling short appointments with a caregiver present.

Use of Medications and Potential Interactions

Levodopa

It has been recommended that patients be scheduled for treatment within 60 to 90 minutes of the patients' levodopa dosage to reduce their disability during treatment. For some patients this timing may lead to a higher incidence of **dyskinesias** during the visit because of pulsatile exposure of the brain to elevated dopamine at the peak of the absorption curve. Facial movements induced by levodopa may cause numerous dental problems, including inflammation, damage to oral structures, protrusion of anterior teeth (because of tongue thrusting), and difficulty in wearing and retaining dentures. Dyskinesias can become so severe that they interfere with swallowing, speech, and respiration.

Levodopa and other antiparkinsonian agents can cause dysgeusia, or alteration in the sensation of taste, in addition to those changes explained by the loss of olfaction. This reaction is less common when levodopa is combined with a decarboxylase.

Orthostatic hypotension is common in PD, and most commonly provoked with transition to a standing position after prolonged supine and recumbent positioning necessary for dental care. This effect is exacerbated during the peak of levodopa effects. Patients should therefore be transitioned to upright position very slowly. If orthostatic hypotension persists, reducing the levodopa dosage prior to dental visits may be required.

Many **drug interactions** involving levodopa are of potential concern to the dentist. It is believed by some investigators that levodopa sensitizes the heart to epinephrine-induced arrhythmias. The mechanism responsible for this effect is unknown, but the excitatory action of levodopa on the heart may result from an action of dopamine on cardiac beta-adrenergic receptors. Although some practitioners believe that this interaction provides a valid contraindication for the use of local anesthetics with vasoconstrictors in patients taking levodopa, the clinical significance of these interactions is not established. The use of phenothiazines (including promethazine), hydroxyzine, and metoclopramide as antinauseants should be avoided. Such agents can exacerbate motor impairment because of their dopamine receptor–blocking properties. Analgesics may be used with levodopa, but if general anesthesia is required, consultation with the patient's physician is recommended.

Dopaminergic agonists, amantadine, and selegiline

Side effects of dopaminergic agonists, amantadine, and selegiline are generally related to their effect of stimulating (directly or indirectly) dopaminergic receptors. If a patient has recently been started on any of these medications, transient nausea and vomiting may occur. A patient scheduled for dental work at this time is more susceptible to **gagging, nausea, and vomiting.** As with other PD treatments, hypotension is a common side effect with the drug class. Dopamine agonists can cause oral dyskinesia similar to dyskinesias produced by levodopa. The selective dopamine agonists may induce daytime sleepiness in some patients; caution should be used if sedative or opioid therapy is planned. In some cases, ergot-derived dopamine agonists may be used, which can produce possible cardiac valvular damage; this may lead to heart sounds of regurgitation. In some cases, antibiotic prophylactic coverage may be required.

Although MAO-B inhibitors are thought to produce a selective MAO block, package warnings of possible drug interactions with meperidine, other opiates, antidepressants, and many foods suggest that careful screening for potential drug and food interactions is important. Some MAO-B inhibitors are available in buccally dissolving "oral disintegrating tablets." No adverse reports have been associated with this route of administration yet; however, dentists are in a position to evaluate adverse oral effects.

Catechol-O-methyltransferase inhibitors

COMT inhibitors have caused **drug interactions** such as tachycardia, an increase in blood pressure, or arrhythmias with vasoconstrictors (e.g., epinephrine), and increased sedative effects with antianxiety drugs, sedating antihistamines, opioid analgesics, and other drugs with CNS depressant properties.

Anticholinergic agents

A patient taking antimuscarinic agents may have typical antimuscarinic side effects. **Xerostomia** may increase the incidence of caries, impair swallowing, increase the likelihood of soft tissue disease in the oral cavity, and make speech difficult. Drugs with which the antiparkinson anticholinergics might summate include antihistamines, tricyclic antidepressants, and other drugs with antimuscarinic effects. Adverse reactions and drug interactions involving antimuscarinic drugs are discussed further in Chapter 6.

ANTIPARKINSON DRUGS

Nonproprietary (Generic) Name	Proprietary (Trade) Name
Anticholinergics	
Benztropine	Cogentin
Biperiden	Akineton
Procyclidine	Kemadrin
Trihexyphenidyl	Artane
Other Drugs with Anticholinergic Activity	
Diphenhydramine	Benadryl
Orphenadrine	Norflex
Dopamine Precursor and Decarboxylase Inhibitors	
Carbidopa	Lodosyn
Levodopa	Dopar, Larodopa
Levodopa + carbidopa	Sinemet, Duopa, Rytary
Levodopa + carbidopa + entacapone	Stalevo
Dopamine Receptor Agonists	
Apomorphine	Apokyn
Bromocriptine	Parlodel
Pergolide	Permax
Pramipexole	Mirapex
Ropinirole	Requip
Rotigotine	Neupro
Other Antiparkinson Drugs	
Amantadine	Symmetrel
Entacapone	Comtan
Rasagiline	Azilect
Selegiline (L-deprenyl)	Eldepryl, Zelapar
Tolcapone	Tasmar

CASE DISCUSSION

Strategic planning of PD medication timing will ideally serve Mr. WP and minimize the difficulties in providing his dental care. The patient should receive his levodopa or other symptomatic medication approximately 1 hour prior to his planned procedure. This will serve to minimize muscle tone resisting jaw opening or possible uncontrolled tremor. To avoid uncontrolled levodopa-induced dyskinesia, additional consideration may be given to slight dose reduction in levodopa or administration of a short-acting benzodiazepine. For any considered dosing changes, consultation with the treating physician/neurologist is indicated.

GENERAL REFERENCES

1. Connolly BS, Lang AE: Pharmacological treatment of Parkinson disease: a review, *JAMA* 311(16):1670–1683, 2014.
2. Cummings J, Isaacson S, Mills R, et al.: Pimavanserin for patients with Parkinson's disease psychosis: a randomised, placebo-controlled phase 3 trial, *Lancet* 383(9916):533–540, 2014.
3. DiPiro JT, Talbert RL, Yee GC, et al.: *Pharmacotherapy: a pathophysiologic approach*, ed 9, New York, 2014, McGraw-Hill Education.
4. Fahn S, Jankovic J, Hallett M: *Principles and practice of movement disorders*, ed 2, New York, 2011, Elsevier/Saunders.
5. Fukayo S, Nonaka N, Shimizu T, et al.: Oral health of patients with Parkinson's disease: factors related to their better dental status, *Tohoku J Exp Med* 201:171–179, 2003.
6. Goodman LS, Brunton LL, Chabner B, et al.: *Goodman & Gilman's pharmacological basis of therapeutics*, ed 12, New York, 2011, McGraw-Hill.
7. Jost WH, Bruck C: Drug interactions in the treatment of Parkinson's disease, *J Neurol* 249(Suppl 3):III/24–29, 2002.
8. Kaakkola S: Problems with the present inhibitors and a relevance of new and improved COMT inhibitors in Parkinson's disease, *Int Rev Neurobiol* 95:207–225, 2010.
9. Kakkar AK, Dahiya N: Management of Parkinson's disease: current and future pharmacotherapy, *Eur J Pharmacol* 750:74–81, 2015.
10. Lobbezzo F, Naeije M: Dental implications of some common movement disorders: a concise review, *Arch Oral Biol* 52:395–398, 2007.
11. Mhyre TR, Boyd JT, Hamill RW, et al.: Parkinson's disease, *Subcell Biochem* 65:389–455, 2012.
12. Ogawa N: Factors affecting levodopa effects in Parkinson's disease, *Acta Med Okayama* 54:95–101, 2000.
13. Olanow CW, Kieburtz K, Odin P, et al.: Continuous intrajejunal infusion of levodopa-carbidopa intestinal gel for patients with advanced Parkinson's disease: a randomised, controlled, double-blind, double-dummy study, *Lancet Neurol* 13(2):141–149, 2014.
14. Stacy M: Medical treatment of Parkinson disease, *Neurol Clin* 27(3):605–631, 2009.
15. Tomlinson CL, Stowe R, Patel S, et al.: Systematic review of levodopa dose equivalency reporting in Parkinson's disease, *Mov Disord* 25(15):2649–2653, 2010.
16. Verstraeten A, Theuns J, Van Broeckhoven C: Progress in unraveling the genetic etiology of Parkinson disease in a genomic era, *Trends Genet* 31:140–149, 2015.

14

Local Anesthetics*

Daniel A. Haas and Christine L. Quinn

KEY INFORMATION

- Local anesthetics are the most important drug group in dentistry.
- All local anesthetics in use today share similar chemical structures and can be categorized as being either esters or amides.
- Their mechanism of action is by blockade of the propagation of peripheral nerve impulses through binding to their receptor within sodium channels.
- Their duration of anesthetic action is determined by redistribution away from the site of action, not metabolism.
- Most local anesthetics cause vasodilation, necessitating addition of a vasoconstrictor to provide appropriate duration of action for use in dentistry.
- The most common adverse reaction is psychogenic in nature, manifested as syncope.
- Toxicity can occur with excessive doses or by intravascular injection.
- Pediatric patients are most susceptible to overdose.

CASE STUDY

A 36-year-old female patient presented to the dental office for periodontal surgery in the mandibular left quadrant. This procedure would involve raising a mucogingival flap followed by osseous re-contouring. It was estimated that the surgery would take approximately 1 hour. The patient's medical history was noncontributory. She had no known allergies and was not on any medication. Her blood pressure on examination was 122/70 mm Hg. Shortly after the injections of local anesthetic, the patient felt faint, which required management on the part of the dentist. At this stage her blood pressure had fallen to 100/60 mm Hg.

What local anesthetic(s) would be appropriate for this procedure?

Was the patient feeling faint due to a reaction to the local anesthetic?

Local anesthetics are the most important drug group in dentistry. These agents reversibly block nerve conduction when applied to a circumscribed area of the body. Although numerous substances of diverse chemical structure are capable of producing local anesthesia, most drugs of proven clinical usefulness share a fundamental configuration with the first true local anesthetic, cocaine. For centuries, natives of the Peruvian highlands have relied on the leaves of the coca bush to prevent hunger, relieve fatigue, and uplift the spirit. European interest in the psychotropic properties of ***Erythroxylon coca*** led to the isolation of cocaine by Niemann in 1859 and to a study of its pharmacology by von Anrep in 1880. Although Niemann and von Anrep reported on the local anesthetic action of cocaine, credit for its introduction into medicine belongs to Karl Koller, a Viennese physician. In 1884, Koller was familiarized with the physiologic effects of cocaine by Sigmund Freud. Koller recognized the drug's great clinical significance and demonstrated its pain-relieving action in several ophthalmologic procedures. The benefits of cocaine were widely appreciated; within 1 year, local anesthesia had been successfully administered for various medical and dental operations.

Knowledge of cocaine's potential for adverse reactions soon followed its general acceptance as a local anesthetic. Several deaths attributed to acute cocainization testified to the drug's low therapeutic index. The abuse liability of cocaine was dramatically illustrated by the self-addiction of William Halsted, a pioneer in regional nerve blockade. A chemical search for safer, nonaddicting local anesthetics was instituted by Einhorn and associates in 1892, culminating 13 years later in the synthesis of procaine. Since then, numerous improvements in the manufacture of local anesthetic solutions have been made, and many useful agents have been introduced into clinical practice. Because no drug is currently devoid of potentially serious toxicity, however, the search for new and better local anesthetic agents continues.

CHEMISTRY AND CLASSIFICATION

Certain physicochemical characteristics are required of a drug intended for clinical use as a local anesthetic. One prerequisite is that the agent **must depress nerve conduction.** Because an axon whose cytoplasmic contents have been completely removed can still transmit action potentials, a drug must be able to interact directly with the axolemma to exert local anesthetic activity. A second important consideration is that the agent **must have lipophilic and hydrophilic properties** to be effective by parenteral injection. Lipid solubility is essential for penetration of the various anatomic barriers existing between an administered drug and its site of action, including the nerve sheath. Water solubility ensures that the drug can be dissolved in an aqueous medium, and when injected in an effective concentration, the drug does not precipitate on exposure to interstitial fluid. These requirements have placed important structural limitations on the clinically useful local anesthetics.

Structure–Activity Relationships

The typical **local anesthetic molecule can be divided into three parts**: (1) an aromatic group, (2) an intermediate chain, and (3) a secondary or tertiary amino terminus (Fig. 14-1). All three components are important determinants of a drug's local anesthetic activity. The aromatic residue confers lipophilic properties on the molecule, whereas the amino group furnishes water solubility. The intermediate portion is significant in two

* The authors wish to recognize Dr. John Yagiela as the author of this chapter in previous editions.

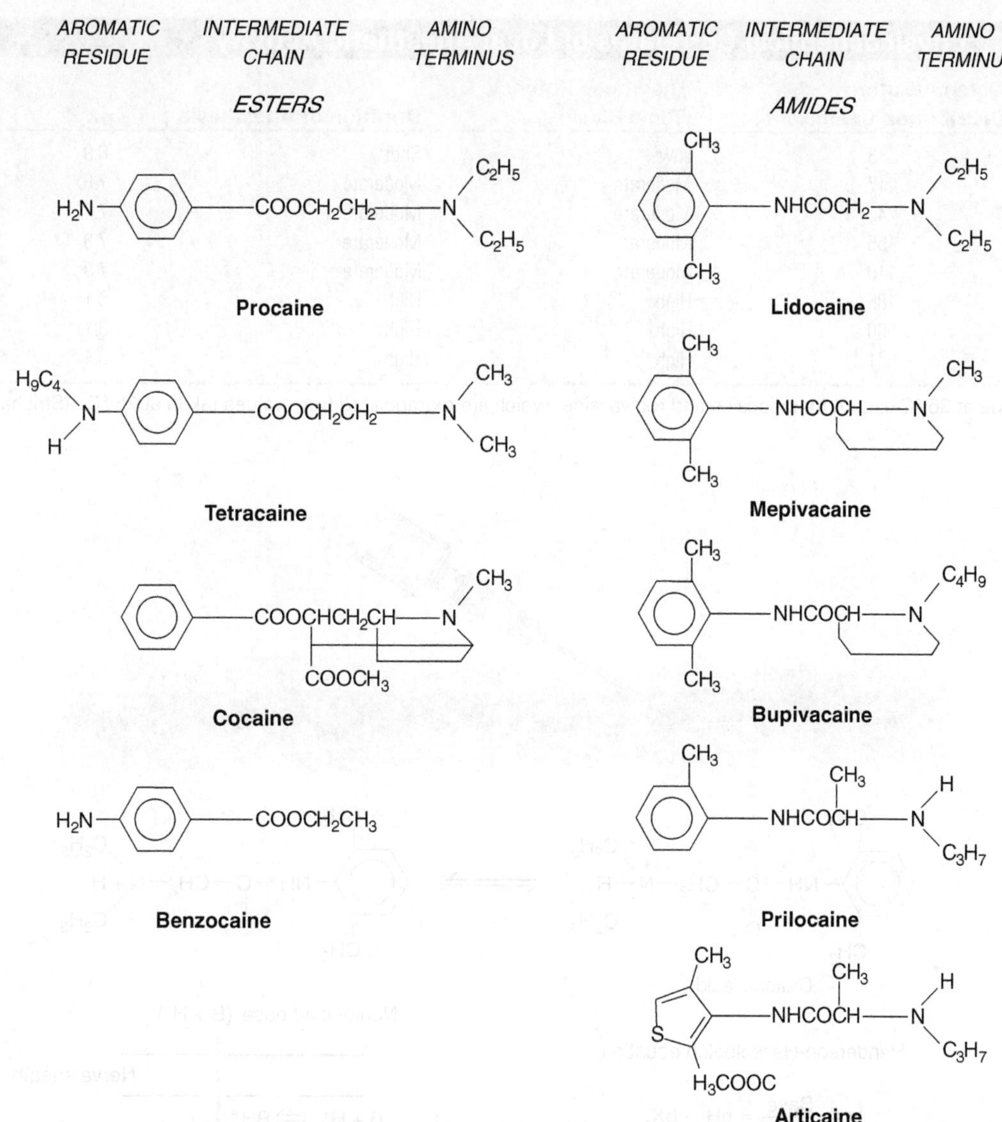

FIG 14-1 Structural formulas of some commonly used local anesthetics.

respects. First, it provides the necessary spatial separation between the lipophilic and hydrophilic ends of the local anesthetic. Second, the chemical link between the central hydrocarbon chain and the aromatic moiety serves as a suitable basis for classification of most local anesthetics into two groups: the esters (—COO—) and the amides (—NHCO—). This distinction is useful because there are marked differences in allergenicity and metabolism between the two drug categories.

Minor modifications of any portion of the local anesthetic molecule can significantly influence drug action. The addition of a chlorine atom to the ortho position on the benzene ring of procaine yields chloroprocaine, a more lipophilic local anesthetic four times as potent as the parent compound yet half as toxic when injected subcutaneously. Table 14-1 lists several important physicochemical properties of local anesthetics and how they correlate with clinical activity.

Influence of pH

By virtue of the substituted amino group, most local anesthetics are weak bases with a negative logarithm of the acid ionization constant (pK_a) ranging from 7.5 to 9.0. A local anesthetic intended for injection is usually prepared in salt form by the addition of hydrochloric acid. Not only is water solubility improved, but also stability in aqueous media is increased. When injected, the acidic local anesthetic solution is quickly neutralized by tissue fluid buffers, and a fraction of the cationic form is converted to the nonionized base. As determined by the Henderson-Hasselbalch equation (Fig. 14-2), the percentage of drug converted depends primarily on the local anesthetic pK_a and the tissue pH. Because only the nonionized base form can diffuse rapidly into the nerve, drugs with a high pK_a tend to be slower in onset than similar agents with more favorable dissociation constants. Tissue acidity may also impede the development of local anesthesia. Products of inflammation can lower the pH of the affected tissue and limit formation of the free base. Ionic entrapment of the local anesthetic in the extracellular space delays the onset of local anesthesia and may render effective nerve blockade impossible.

Numerous attempts have been made to augment local anesthesia by capitalizing on the influence of pH. Theoretically, alkalization should increase local anesthetic activity by promoting tissue penetration and nerve uptake. Many topical agents are marketed in the base form to improve diffusion across epithelial barriers. Although it has been shown experimentally that alkalization of local anesthetic solutions just before use enhances nerve blockade, practical considerations have limited routine clinical application. Even so, extracellular fluid has in most instances sufficient buffering capacity to negate differences

TABLE 14-1 **Physicochemical Correlates of Local Anesthetic Activity**

Drug	Octanol/Buffer Distribution Coefficient*	Anesthetic Potency (Tonic Block)	Duration of Anesthesia	pK_a*	Rate of Onset
Procaine	3	Low	Short	8.9	Moderate
Articaine	17	Moderate	Moderate	7.8	Fast
Mepivacaine	42	Moderate	Moderate	7.7	Fast
Prilocaine	55	Moderate	Moderate	7.8	Fast
Lidocaine	110	Moderate	Moderate	7.8	Fast
Ropivacaine	186	High	High	8.1	Moderate
Bupivacaine	560	High	High	8.1	Moderate
Tetracaine	541	High	High	8.4	Moderate

*Measurements made at 36 °C except for prilocaine and ropivacaine, which are extrapolated from values taken at 25 °C . (Strichartz et al., 1990.)

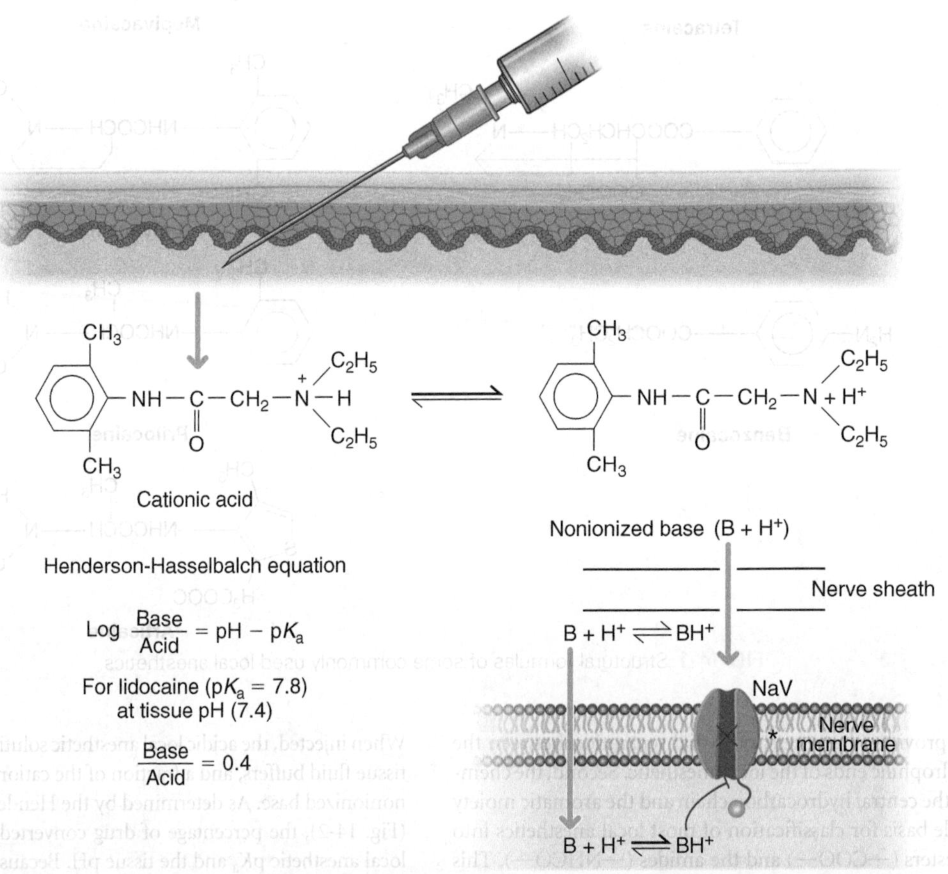

FIG 14-2 Distribution of a local anesthetic during nerve block. On injection of a local anesthetic solution, a portion of the cationic acid is converted to the free base. Calculated for lidocaine is the base-to-acid ratio in the extracellular fluid at equilibrium, favoring the free base form of the local anesthetic ($B + H^+$). The free base form is able to enter the nerve cell. Although the acid form is responsible for most of the blocking activity, the contribution of the nonionized base to blocking the sodium channel must not be overlooked.

in local anesthetic pH soon after injection. There are currently two commercially available systems for buffering dental local anesthetics (OnPharma™, Anutra™).

An alternative approach to modifying drug distribution is through the addition of carbon dioxide. Carbonation of a local anesthetic solution can increase the rate of onset and sometimes the depth of anesthesia. It has been suggested that the hydrocarbonate salt of the local anesthetic penetrates membranes more rapidly than the conventional formulation and that the injected carbon dioxide diffusing into the nerve trunk lowers the internal pH and concentrates local anesthetic molecules by ion trapping. Although promising, carbonated local anesthetic solutions are unavailable in the United States, and a study of carbonated lidocaine used for mandibular anesthesia failed to reveal any significant benefit compared with lidocaine hydrochloride.

MECHANISM OF ACTION

Local anesthetics block the sensation of pain by interfering with the propagation of peripheral nerve impulses. The generation and the conduction of action potentials are inhibited. Electrophysiologic

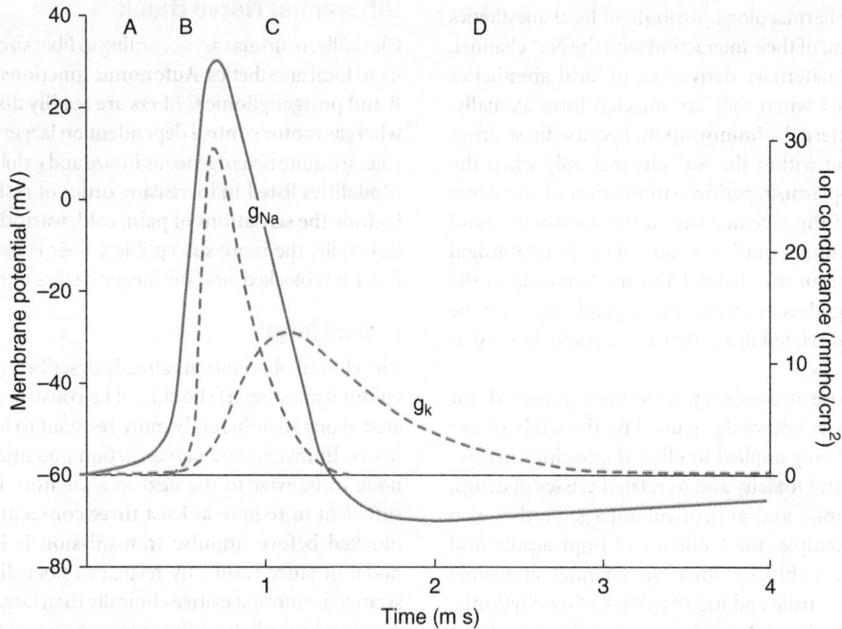

FIG 14-3 The action potential. *Dashed lines* indicate the Na^+ (*gNa*) and K^+ (*gK*) conductance changes responsible for membrane depolarization and recovery. *A*, Resting state; Na^+ channels are in the resting (closed) configuration. *B*, Depolarization phase; Na^+ channels open. *C*, Repolarization phase; Na^+ channels become inactivated, and the nerve becomes refractory to stimulation. *D*, Recovery phase; Na^+ channels convert from the inactivated to the resting state, and the nerve regains the ability to conduct action potentials.

data indicate that local anesthetics do not significantly alter the normal resting potential of the nerve membrane; instead they impair certain dynamic responses to nerve stimulation.

Effects on Ionic Permeability

The quiescent nerve membrane is impermeable to Na^+. Excitation of the neuron by an appropriate stimulus temporarily increases Na^+ conductance and causes the nerve cell to become less electronegative relative to the outside. If the transmembrane potential is sufficiently depressed, a critical threshold is reached at which the depolarization becomes self-generating. Local electrotonic currents induce a rapid influx of Na^+ through activated Na^+-selective channels traversing the nerve membrane. The inward Na^+ current creates an action potential of approximately +40 mV, which is propagated down the nerve. The action potential is quite transient at any given segment of membrane; loss of Na^+ permeability (inactivation of the Na^+ channels) and an outward flow of K^+ (in nonmyelinated axons) quickly repolarize the membrane. These events are reviewed in Figure 14-3.

Local anesthetics interfere with nerve transmission by blocking the influence of stimulation on Na^+ conductance. A developing local anesthetic block is characterized by a progressive reduction in the rate and degree of depolarization and a slowing of conduction. When the depolarization is retarded sufficiently such that repolarization processes develop before the threshold potential can be reached, nerve conduction fails.

Site of Action

Several sites exist within the nerve membrane where drugs could potentially interfere with Na^+ permeability. It was argued that local anesthetics could interact with membrane lipids to impair Na^+ channel function, just as had long been proposed for general anesthetics (see Chapter 15). In recent years, evidence has accumulated that conventional **local anesthetics interact directly with Na+ channels to inhibit nerve conduction.**

The active site for local anesthetics resides within the internal aspect of the Na^+ channel, and thus access becomes an important issue. Local anesthetics gain access to their receptor by traveling up an aqueous route within the Na^+ channel, which must be fully open or at least partially activated to permit their entry from the cytoplasm. Lipophilic molecules, such as benzocaine or the uncharged form of lidocaine, can reach the channel and receptor site by traversing a hydrophobic route, which may include the membrane lipid and hydrophobic portions of the Na^+ channel. The major subunit (α subunit) of the sodium channel comprises the channel through which Na^+ enters and with which local anesthetics interact. The α **subunit is made up of four homologous domains** each **containing 6 helical transmembrane domains.** Segment 4 of each domain is positively charged and rotates outward when the channel opens. These segments are intimately tied to the **"m" or activation gate** (Fig 14-4). Two S4 segments are picture in Figure 14-4 along with the "m" gate and an **"h" gate**, which is the inactivation gate for the channel.

Local anesthetics block nerve conduction by impeding the **gating mechanisms** that underlie cycling of the Na^+ channel. Other actions that could contribute to nerve blockade include a physical occlusion of the channel, an allosterically mediated change in channel conformation, and (at least with local anesthetic cations) a distortion of the local electrical field. Figure 14-4 depicts the Na^+ channel as it cycles through its primary configurations in response to a depolarizing stimulus and postulated interactions with neutral and charged local anesthetic species (See Armstrong, 2006).

Similarities in molecular structure among voltage-gated ion channels provide the basis by which local anesthetics influence the movement of ions other than Na^+. Inhibition of specific K^+ and Ca^{2+} currents may contribute to various local anesthetic effects, including the blockage of nociception.

Use-Dependent Block

Conventional **local anesthetics inhibit high-frequency trains of impulses more readily than they do single action potentials.** This phenomenon, variously referred to as use-dependent or frequency-dependent conduction block, phasic or transitional block, or Wedensky inhibition, is an important pharmacologic attribute of local anesthetics and one vital to the elucidation of their interaction with the Na^+ channel.

It has been stated that quaternary derivatives of local anesthetics retain nerve-blocking activity when they are injected intra-axonally, but they are ineffective by external administration. Because these drugs can reach their site of action within the Na^+ channel only when the channel is open to the cytoplasm, repetitive stimulation of the nerve should increase exposure of the receptor site to the anesthetic—and lead to increasing drug action—until a steady state is established between the bound drug within the channel and the free drug in the axoplasm. A similar, although less extensive, use dependency could be anticipated for lidocaine and related drugs that are partially ionized at physiologic pH.

Marked differences in use dependency have been recorded for various local anesthetics. Basic knowledge gained by the study of use dependency is increasingly being applied to clinical questions involving local anesthetic efficacy and toxicity and to related classes of drugs, such as various antiarrhythmic and anticonvulsant agents that also exhibit phasic block, for example, the tendency of bupivacaine and several other local anesthetics to block cardiac Na^+ channels at normal heart rates, resulting in bradycardia and increased risk of dysrhythmia. Ultimately, new drugs and modes of therapy are expected to arise from the pharmaceutical exploitation of this phenomenon.

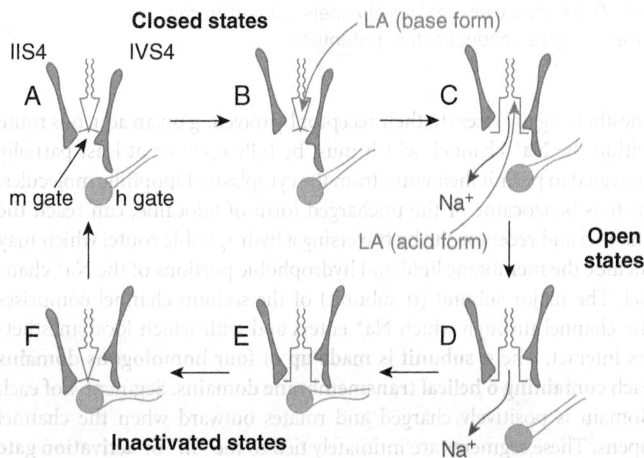

FIG 14-4 Normal Na^+ channel cycling and local anesthetic blockade. **A,** In the basal resting state, the S4 segments of all domains are fully deactivated, forced inward by the negative resting polarity. The m gate is fully closed. **B,** With partial depolarization of the membrane, the S4 segments of domains I, II, and III rotate outward independently. The m gate remains closed. Noncharged local anesthetics can gain access to the channel at any stage of the channel cycle by traversing a hydrophobic pathway. **C,** Conduction begins when the S4 segment of domain IV moves partway out. The steric hindrance on the m gate is relieved, and the gate opens sufficiently for influx of Na^+. Charged local anesthetic molecules can reach the receptor only when the channel is in an open configuration. **D,** Subsequent movement of the S4 domain IV segment allows the channel to open fully. The immediate area assumes a positive polarity as Na^+ rushes inward. This movement also exposes the receptor site for the inactivation, or *h*, gate. **E,** Inactivation of the channel by docking of the h gate to its receptor automatically follows. The influx of Na^+ is terminated. **F,** As the local internal Na^+ concentration dissipates, and the membrane begins to repolarize, the S4 segments of domains I and II return to their resting configurations. At this point, the m and h gates are closed. Return to the normal resting state occurs as the S4 domain returns to its fully resting state, evicting the h gate from its binding site in the process. (Adapted from Armstrong CM: Na channel inactivation from open and closed states, *Proc Natl Acad Sci* 103:17991-17996, 2006. © 2006 National Academy of Sciences, U.S.A.)

Differential Nerve Block

Clinically, neurons vary according to fiber size and type in their susceptibility to local anesthetics. **Autonomic functions subserved by preganglionic B and postganglionic C fibers are readily disrupted by local anesthetics, whereas motor control dependent on larger A fibers is not.** Sensory neurons are quite heterogeneous in size and exhibit a wide range of sensitivity. **Modalities listed in increasing order of resistance to conduction block include the sensations of pain, cold, warmth, touch, and deep pressure.** Generally, the more susceptible a fiber is to a local anesthetic agent, the faster it is blocked, and the longer it takes to recover.

Critical length

The clinical observations already described (and best seen after spinal or epidural anesthesia) should not be construed as proof that large myelinated axons are inherently more resistant to local anesthetics than smaller fibers. In myelinated nerves, action potentials are propagated from one node of Ranvier to the next in a saltatory fashion, with a safety factor sufficient to require **at least three consecutive nodes to be completely blocked before impulse transmission is interrupted.** Because internodal distance is directly related to fiber diameter, small neurons may seem to be more sensitive clinically than large fibers to conduction block. As a local anesthetic diffuses into the nerve trunk, it reaches an effective concentration over a length required to inhibit small axons (i.e., block three nodes) before it spreads sufficiently to block large fibers. Anatomic barriers to diffusion, nonuniform distribution of drug, or the use of a minimal amount of local anesthetic may preclude some large axons from ever being affected. As local anesthesia fades, small neurons are the last to recover because circumscribed areas of drug concentrations adequate for their inhibition remain along the nerve after the more substantial areas required for large axons have broken up.

When the concentration of local anesthetic is insufficient to block three adjacent nodes completely, anesthesia may still occur if a larger train of nodes is partially blocked. As long as more than 70% of the Na^+ channels in a node are inhibited, the resulting action potential at that node is reduced in size. Progressive declines in the action potentials of partially blocked nodes along the axon ultimately result in failure of conduction if a sufficient length of nerve is exposed to the drug. As shown in Figure 14-5, smaller neurons are again more readily blocked because of the shorter length required for exposure of the requisite number of nodes.

The critical length hypothesis may also be applied to unmyelinated axons as a group. Differences in modes of impulse transmission preclude direct comparisons based on fiber size between myelinated and unmyelinated axons. Smaller in diameter, C fibers nevertheless have approximately the same apparent critical length as small myelinated axons.

Peripheral nerve organization

The location of various axons within a nerve trunk has an important bearing on the rate and sometimes the depth of local anesthesia. In major nerve blocks, the epineurium and perineurium limit the spread of anesthetic solution by bulk flow, and the drug must rely more on diffusion to reach the axons within the nerve. Diffusion takes considerable time with nerves that are 1 mm in diameter or greater, and the net result is that the outer, or mantle, fibers are blocked well before the inner core fibers have been exposed to an effective concentration of drug. Removal of the agent by the bloodstream, particularly by intraneuronal blood vessels, may prevent anesthesia of core fibers altogether. Generally, the more proximal tissues supplied by a nerve are more readily affected by local anesthetics because the axons that serve them are located peripherally. The nonuniform distribution of various fiber types within a particular nerve may lead to differential blockade of sensory, motor, and autonomic axons innervating a given structure.

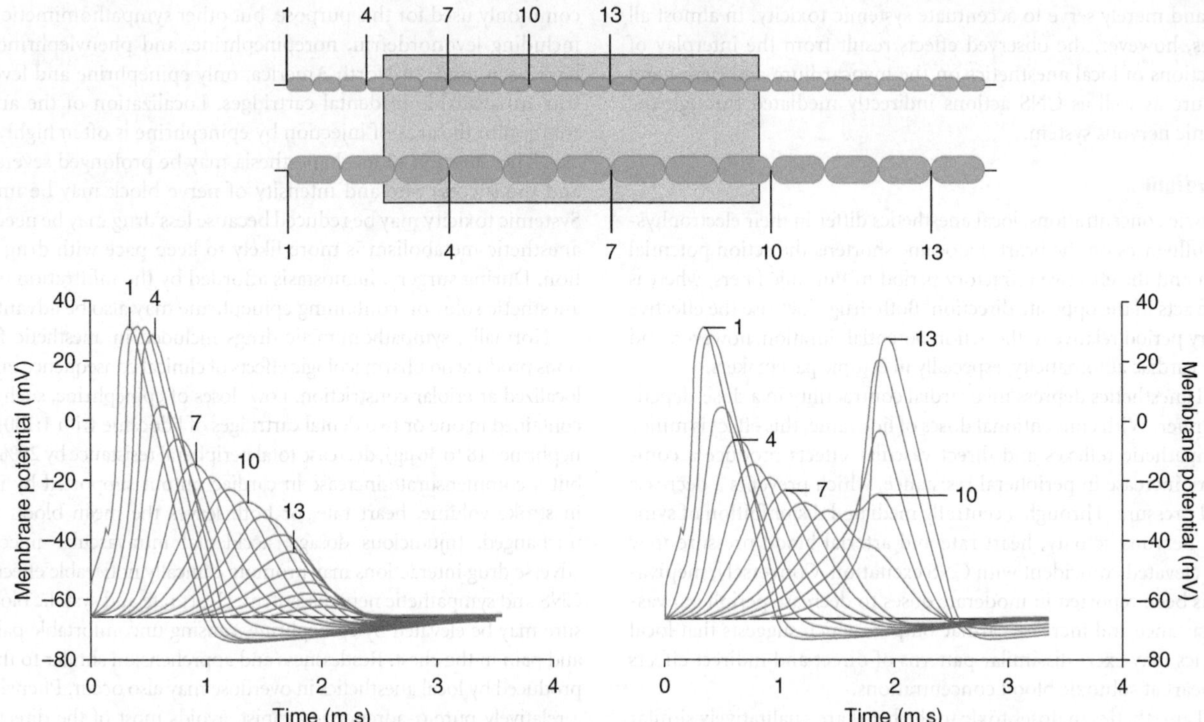

FIG 14-5 Differential nerve block. Two adjacent myelinated axons, differing in diameter and internodal distance by a factor of 2, are exposed to a local anesthetic (*gray zone*). Impulses arising from successive nodes of the small axon are plotted on the left. Exposure of 14 nodes to a specific concentration of local anesthetic causes conduction to fail. Identical exposure of the larger axon (right) results in seven nodes being affected, an insufficient number to prevent conduction at this local anesthetic concentration.

Inflammation

The failure to obtain satisfactory clinical pain relief in inflamed tissues is a well-known and undesirable form of differential nerve block. Clinically, this phenomenon is encountered in a patient who exhibits profound local anesthetic effect except in the specific area requiring treatment. If inflammation lowers the pH at the injection site, diffusion of the drug into the axolemma would be impaired as described previously. There is some evidence, however, that the buffering capacity of inflamed tissues is not always reduced and that other reasons for local anesthetic failure must exist in these conditions.

Increased blood flow and decreased catecholamine effectiveness in inflamed tissues may speed removal of the local anesthetic from the injection site. Alteration of Na^+ channel number, function, or type may offset the ability of local anesthetics to block nerve conduction. Analogous changes in the expression or activity of other ion channels involved in nociception may have a similar effect. Neuromediators and other products released or synthesized during inflammation may increase responsiveness of nociceptors and/or enhance nerve conduction in response to painful stimuli. These include histamine, prostaglandin E_1, kinins, adenine nucleotides, and substance P.

PHARMACOLOGIC EFFECTS

Although primarily used to depress peripheral nerve conduction, **local anesthetics are not selective and may interfere with impulse transmission in any excitable tissue.** Most prominent of the systemic effects of local anesthetics are effects related to the cardiovascular system and the central nervous system (CNS), but virtually any organ with dependence on nervous or muscular activity may be affected. Local anesthetics may also influence various tissues through actions unrelated to specific disturbances in Na^+ conductance.

Central Nervous System

Local anesthetics readily pass from the peripheral circulation into the brain. Because CNS neurons are particularly sensitive to local anesthetics, blood concentrations incapable of altering peripheral nervous activity may profoundly influence CNS function. In general, the concentrations of local anesthetics required to elicit CNS effects are inversely proportional to their anesthetic potencies.

Sensitive psychomotor tests and subjective reports of mild drowsiness indicate that systemic effects caused by local anesthetics can occur with plasma concentrations that are achieved in dental patients. Analgesic and anticonvulsant effects also occur in subtoxic concentrations. Initial signs and symptoms of a toxic effect are often excitatory in nature and consist of a feeling of lightheadedness and dizziness, followed by visual and auditory disturbances, apprehension, disorientation, and localized involuntary muscular activity. Depressant responses, such as slurred speech, drowsiness, and unconsciousness, may also occur and are especially prominent with certain drugs (e.g., lidocaine). As higher blood concentrations of drug are attained, muscular fasciculations and tremors intensify and develop into generalized tonic-clonic convulsions. On termination, seizure activity is often succeeded by a state of CNS depression identical to general anesthesia. With excessively large doses, respiratory impairment becomes manifest; if untreated, death by asphyxiation may ensue.

Cardiovascular System

Local anesthetics can exert various effects on the cardiovascular system. Some influences are beneficial and serve as a basis for the use of selected agents in the treatment of cardiac arrhythmias; others are not helpful and merely serve to accentuate systemic toxicity. In almost all instances, however, the observed effects result from the interplay of direct actions of local anesthetics on the myocardium and peripheral vasculature as well as CNS actions indirectly mediated through the autonomic nervous system.

Myocardium

At nontoxic concentrations, local anesthetics differ in their electrophysiologic influences on the heart. Lidocaine shortens the action potential duration and the effective refractory period in Purkinje fibers, whereas procaine acts in the opposite direction. Both drugs increase the effective refractory period relative to the action potential duration, however, and decrease cardiac automaticity, especially in ectopic pacemakers.

Local anesthetics depress myocardial contractility in a dose-dependent manner. With conventional doses of lidocaine, this effect is minor and sympathetic reflexes and direct vascular effects produce a compensatory increase in peripheral resistance, which prevents a decrease in blood pressure. Through a centrally mediated disinhibition of sympathetic nervous activity, heart rate and arterial blood pressure may become elevated coincident with CNS excitation. Conversely, mepivacaine has been reported in moderate doses to decrease peripheral vascular resistance and increase cardiac output, which suggests that local anesthetics may exert dissimilar patterns of direct and indirect effects on the heart at subtoxic blood concentrations.

Local anesthetics in doses toxic to the heart are qualitatively similar in action. Membrane excitability and conduction velocity are depressed throughout the heart. Sinus bradycardia and impairment of myocardial contractility contribute to a reduction in cardiac output. These effects are magnified by hypoxia, but even if respiration is supported artificially, circulatory collapse occurs after excessively large doses.

Bupivacaine and certain other highly lipophilic local anesthetics are cardiotoxic when compared with less lipophilic congeners. Serious ventricular arrhythmias and cardiovascular collapse are more likely to occur, and resuscitation is more problematic. One explanation for these observations involves use-dependent blockade.

Peripheral vasculature

The effects of local anesthetics on blood vessels are complex and dose dependent. Dilute solutions enhance spontaneous myogenic contractions and peripheral resistance in certain vascular beds, presumably by increasing the cytoplasmic concentration of Ca^{2+} within smooth muscle fibers. Coincidentally, **local anesthetics reduce vascular tone** related to autonomic function by diminishing neurotransmitter release and smooth muscle responsiveness. Subconvulsive doses of local anesthetics exert minor influences on the peripheral vasculature as a whole. Toxic blood concentrations may cause arteriolar dilation and profound hypotension.

The net effect on any vasculature bed depends on the local anesthetic, its concentration, and the existing sympathetic tone in the tissue. A therapeutically relevant estimate of local anesthetics listed in decreasing order of vasodilatory potential includes procaine, bupivacaine, lidocaine, articaine, prilocaine, mepivacaine, ropivacaine, and cocaine. With the possible exception of ropivacaine, local anesthetics administered submucosally inhibit myogenic activity and autonomic tone clinically and cause vasodilation in the area of injection. Cocaine is unique in its ability to decrease local blood flow after topical application to mucosal surfaces. Cocaine potentiates the vasoconstrictive effect of catecholamines by inhibiting their transport into adrenergic nerve terminals.

Vasoconstrictor Effects

Vasoconstrictors are often added to local anesthetic solutions to impede systemic absorption of the anesthetic agent. Epinephrine in concentrations of 5 μg/mL to 20 μg/mL (1:200,000 to 1:50,000) is most commonly used for this purpose, but other sympathomimetic amines, including levonordefrin, norepinephrine, and phenylephrine, are or have been used. In North America, only epinephrine and levonordefrin are available in dental cartridges. Localization of the anesthetic solution in the area of injection by epinephrine is often highly beneficial. The duration of local anesthesia may be prolonged several times, and the success rate and intensity of nerve block may be improved. Systemic toxicity may be reduced because less drug may be needed, and anesthetic metabolism is more likely to keep pace with drug absorption. During surgery, hemostasis afforded by the infiltration of a local anesthetic solution containing epinephrine may also be advantageous.

Normally, sympathomimetic drugs included in anesthetic formulations produce no pharmacologic effects of clinical consequence other than localized arteriolar constriction. Low doses of epinephrine, such as those contained in one or two dental cartridges of lidocaine with 1:100,000 epinephrine (18 to 36 μg), decrease total peripheral resistance by 20% to 30%, but a commensurate increase in cardiac output supported by increases in stroke volume, heart rate, or both leaves the mean blood pressure unchanged. Injudicious dosage, accidental intravascular injection, or adverse drug interactions may promote clinically noticeable effects on the CNS and sympathetic nervous system. Heart rate and systolic blood pressure may be elevated by epinephrine, causing uncomfortable palpitation and pain in the chest. Restlessness and apprehension similar to the effects produced by local anesthetics in overdose may also occur. Phenylephrine, a relatively pure α-adrenergic agonist, avoids most of the direct cardiac stimulation associated with epinephrine, but it may significantly elevate systolic and diastolic pressures and reflexively slow the heart for an extended period. Other sympathomimetics, such as norepinephrine and levonordefrin, are intermediate in their systemic effects.

As a guideline for cardiac patients, current evidence indicates that minimizing epinephrine to a level of less than 40 μg with appropriate vital sign monitoring is appropriate. Several studies have shown that the intraoral injection of 20 μg of epinephrine effectively doubles the preoperative plasma concentration and that higher doses produce proportionately greater elevations. At doses approaching 200 μg, the resulting epinephrine titers can surpass titers associated with heavy exercise, surgery, and pheochromocytoma. Increases in cardiac work become significant, and myocardial ischemia and cardiac arrhythmias are more likely to occur.

ABSORPTION, FATE, AND EXCRETION

Pharmacokinetic considerations regarding local anesthetics are vital because the balance between the uptake of a local anesthetic into the systemic circulation and its removal through redistribution, metabolism, and excretion in large measure determines the drug's toxic potential.

Absorption

The rate of absorption depends on several factors, including the dosage and pharmacologic profile of the drug used, the presence of a vasoconstrictor agent, and the nature of the administration site. The more drug that is injected, the higher its resultant blood concentration. Less obvious are the qualitative influences of the anesthetic solution and how these interact with the site of administration. Drugs with potent vasodilating properties, such as procaine and lidocaine, may significantly enhance their own uptake, particularly when injected into a highly vascular space. Inclusion of epinephrine or another vasoconstrictor is especially important in these instances. Drugs that are not strong vasodilators, such as mepivacaine and prilocaine, do not markedly accentuate their own absorption and do not require as much vasoconstrictor to limit uptake.

Absorption after topical application varies widely. Although intact skin and keratinized mucosa are relatively impermeable, local anesthetics are **readily absorbed from most mucosal surfaces.**

TABLE 14-2 Onset of Action for Select Local Anesthetics

Local Anesthetic	Onset of Action (in minutes)
Articaine	2-3
Bupivacaine	6-10
Lidocaine	2-3
Mepivacaine	1.5-2
Prilocaine	2-4

TABLE 14-3 Elimination Half-Lives of Local Anesthetics (in minutes)

Local Anesthetic	Elimination Half-Time (in minutes)
Articaine	30-146
Bupivacaine	162-210
Lidocaine	80-96
Mepivacaine	114
Prilocaine	93-96

For those local anesthetics used in dentistry, the onset of action is somewhat similar, as shown in Table 14-2.

Distribution

It is important to note that the duration of action of local anesthetics is dependent on its absorption into the bloodstream and distribution away from the site of injection.

On entering the circulation, a local anesthetic is partially (5% to 95%) bound by plasma proteins—α_1-acid glycoprotein in particular and albumin to a much lesser extent—and red blood cells. Because the concentration of α_1-acid glycoprotein is influenced by many factors (see Chapter 2), the fractional binding of local anesthetics differs among individuals and within the same individual at different times.

After distribution throughout the intravascular space, the unbound drug is free to diffuse into the various tissues of the body. So-called barriers to diffusion are ineffective against local anesthetics. In addition to entering the CNS, these drugs readily cross the placenta and occasionally may induce severe cardiac depression in the fetus.

Distribution to peripheral tissues is a major means for the removal of amide and slowly metabolized ester local anesthetics from the bloodstream and for keeping their plasma concentrations below the toxic range. By virtue of the pulmonary circulation, the lung plays a unique role in this process when a local anesthetic is injected intravenously. Initially, 90% of the drug may be taken up by the lung. Although most of the agent diffuses back into the bloodstream within the first minute after injection, the evanescent buffering action of the lung can nevertheless reduce the peak arterial blood concentration by a factor of 3.

Metabolism and Excretion

The metabolic fate of a particular agent largely depends on the chemical linkage between the aromatic residue and the rest of the molecule. Ester drugs are inactivated by hydrolysis. **Derivatives of *p*-aminobenzoic acid (PABA), such as procaine and tetracaine, are preferentially metabolized in the plasma by pseudocholinesterase;** the ratio between plasma and tissue hydrolysis with other esters is variable. Products of hydrolytic cleavage may undergo further biotransformation in the liver before being eliminated in the urine. The half-life for the hydrolysis of procaine is normally less than 1 min and less than 2% of the drug is excreted unchanged by the kidneys.

Metabolism of amide drugs primarily occurs in the liver. The initial reaction is usually N-dealkylation of the tertiary amino terminus, principally by CYP3A4 and CYP1A2. The resultant secondary amine of most amides is susceptible to hydrolysis by hepatic amidase activity, but conjugation, hydroxylation, and further dealkylation may also occur. Hepatic blood flow seems to be the rate-limiting factor governing metabolism of lidocaine and some other amides; elimination half-lives range greatly as can be seen in Table 14-3. Inactivation of prilocaine, a secondary amine, is unusual because dealkylation is not required before hydrolysis can occur, which may explain why almost half of its metabolism is extrahepatic. Articaine is also atypical because it is inactivated in the blood and other tissues by hydrolysis of an ester side chain required for local anesthetic activity. With an initial plasma half-life of approximately 30 min, articaine is removed from the circulation faster than other injected amides, although patient variability can lead to a range of up to 146 min for elimination half-life.

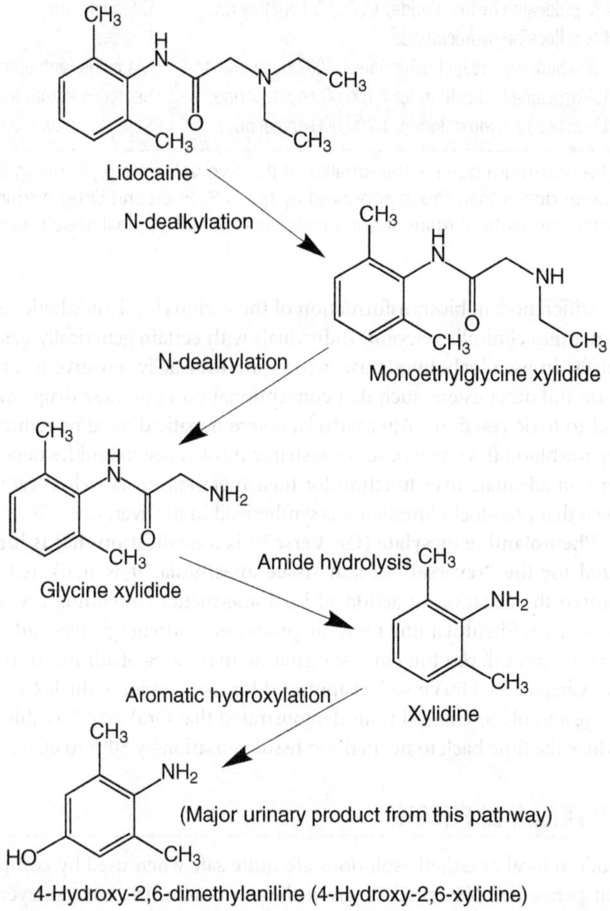

Some local anesthetic metabolites retain significant pharmacologic activity and may contribute to drug toxicity. Much of the sedative effect of lidocaine has been attributed to its de-ethylated metabolites monoethylglycine xylidide and glycine xylidide (Fig. 14-6). As with the ester compounds, minimal amounts (1% to 20%) of administered amides appear in the urine as unmetabolized compounds. 4-Hydroxyxylidine constitutes about 70% of the aniline-containing urinary metabolites of lidocaine (see Fig. 14-6).

FIG 14-6 The major pathway reactions in the metabolism of lidocaine. These reactions occur in the liver. 4-Hydroxyxylidine is the major urinary metabolite of lidocaine. Non-aniline-containing products of the chemical reactions are not pictured.

TABLE 14-4 Comparison of Local Anesthetics Used in Dentistry

		MAXIMUM DOSE*		DURATION OF ANESTHESIA (SOFT TISSUE)	
Preparation Contents	Proprietary (Trade) Name	(mg/kg)	(mg)	Maxillary Infiltration (min)	Inferior Alveolar Block (min)
2% lidocaine hydrochloride; 1:100,000 epinephrine	Xylocaine with epinephrine, 1:100,000	7	500	170	190
2% lidocaine hydrochloride; 1:50,000 epinephrine	Xylocaine with epinephrine, 1:50,000	3.5†	250†	170	190
2% lidocaine	Xylocaine	4.5	300	40‡	100‡
2% mepivacaine hydrochloride; 1:20,000 levonordefrin	Carbocaine 2% with Neo-Cobefrin	6.6	400	150	190
3% mepivacaine hydrochloride	Carbocaine	6.6	400	90	165
4% prilocaine hydrochloride; 1:200,000 epinephrine	Citanest Forte	8	600	140	205
4% prilocaine hydrochloride	Citanest	8	600	105	175
0.5% bupivacaine hydrochloride; 1:200,000 epinephrine	Marcaine with epinephrine	2	90	340	440
4% articaine hydrochloride; 1:100,000 epinephrine	Septocaine with epinephrine, 1:100,000	7		200	230
4% articaine hydrochloride, 1:200,000 epinephrine	Septocaine with epinephrine, 1:200,000	7		180	200

*The maximum dose is the smaller of the two values (e.g., 7 mg/kg lidocaine up to a maximum dose of 500 mg).
†Lower doses than those approved by the U.S. Food and Drug Administration are recommended on the basis of the high epinephrine content.
‡Lidocaine without epinephrine produces unreliable pulpal anesthesia, especially of the maxilla.

Differences in biotransformation of the various local anesthetics are sometimes clinically relevant. Individuals with certain genetically based defects in pseudocholinesterase activity are unusually sensitive to procaine and other esters, such that conventional doses of these drugs may lead to toxic reactions. Alternatively, severe hepatic disease or reduced hepatic blood flow may produce systemic intolerance to amides dependent on adequate liver function for their metabolism, as well as esters, given that pseudocholinesterase is synthesized in the liver.

Phentolamine mesylate (OraVerse™) is a medication that is indicated for the "reversal" of soft tissue anesthesia. It is marketed to shorten the duration of action of local anesthetics containing a vasoconstrictor. Phentolamine mesylate produces α-adrenergic blockade of vascular smooth resulting in vasodilatation in the area of administration (see Chapter 9). OraVerse™ is approved for usage in individuals 6 years of age and older. Clinical trials demonstrated that OraVerse™ is able to reduce the time back to normal soft tissue sensation by 50% to 60%.

ADVERSE EFFECTS

Modern local anesthetic solutions are quite safe when used by competent personnel. Nevertheless, given their common use, adverse events are seen. These can be categorized into four areas: systemic toxicity, local tissue responses, psychogenic/idiosyncratic reactions, and allergic reactions.

Systemic Toxicity

Most serious toxic effects are related to excessive blood concentrations caused by inadvertent intravascular injection or the administration of large quantities of drug. Such reactions can usually be prevented by observing three precautions: (1) **administer the smallest dose that provides effective anesthesia; (2) use proper injection techniques, including aspiration; and (3) use a vasoconstrictor-containing solution when not contraindicated by patient history or operative need.**

In dentistry, intravenous injection of even the small amounts of drug in a single dental cartridge can cause adverse responses in sensitive individuals, particularly if the drug is given rapidly. Aspiration tests with dental syringes indicate that the needle is placed inside a blood vessel in approximately 3% of all injections and much more frequently during blockade of the inferior alveolar and posterior superior alveolar nerves. For any technique where intravascular injection is possible, aspiration should be performed using a 25- or 27-gauge needle, avoiding use of the smaller 30-gauge needle. Negative aspiration does not guarantee that the needle lumen is outside the vessel; using inadequate force or time for aspiration or placing the lumen against a vessel's intimal lining can prevent blood from entering the anesthetic cartridge.

Regarding excessive doses, in general, there is a correlation between potency and toxicity. The rate of injection can be a factor as the rapidity of increased blood level predisposes to toxicity. Increased $PaCO_2$ and decreased pH also tend to increase the likelihood of toxicity. Toxicity manifests primarily in the CNS, with the cardiovascular system the next most susceptible. Initially, sedation can be seen. As blood levels rise, signs and symptoms include lightheadedness, slurred speech, drowsiness, euphoria or dysphoria, diplopia, sensory disturbances, and/or muscle twitching. As blood levels get even higher, disorientation, tremors, respiratory depression, and tonic/clonic seizures can result. When blood levels reach the lethal range, one can find coma, respiratory arrest, and complete cardiovascular collapse.

This has led to recommended maximum doses, as seen in Table 14-4. Calculations should be made on the assumption that each dental cartridge is 1.8 mL. Although variably listed by the manufacturers as either 1.8 or 1.7 mL, all dental cartridges contain approximately 1.76 mL. (See Robertson et al., 2007.) In dental practice, these guidelines should make it apparent that overdose should be a rare event in healthy adult patients. Toxicity has been a more common issue in pediatrics, simply because of the greater likelihood of an inadvertent overdose.

In Table 14-5, the maximum doses recommended earlier are used to calculate the values for the local anesthetics for children weighing 14, 18, and 23 kg. These weights correspond to the 50th percentile weight for a 3-, 5-, and 7-year-old child, respectively. Bupivacaine is not listed, as it is not a preferred agent in the young child.

Methemoglobinemia is a subcategory of toxicity found with certain agents. It is most common with prilocaine or benzocaine overdose, although it can occur with any local anesthetic in susceptible individuals. This is a condition in which cyanosis develops in the absence of cardiac or respiratory abnormalities. It may be congenital or acquired through drugs or chemicals. Methemoglobin is normally less than 1% in humans. Cyanosis and respiratory distress may occur when levels exceed 10%. Pulse oximeter readings are abnormal, usually reading in the mid- to high 80s, and the patient is unresponsive to oxygen administration.

TABLE 14-5 Maximum Number of Dental Anesthetic Cartridges for Children

Child's age-->	3 yr old	5 yr old	7 yr old
Weight at 50th percentile for that age	14 kg	18 kg	23 kg
	MAXIMUM NUMBER OF CARTRIDGES*		
Articaine with epinephrine	1.4	1.8	2.2
Lidocaine with epinephrine	2.7	3.5	4.5
Mepivacaine plain	1.7	2.2	2.8
Mepivacaine with vasoconstrictor	2.6	3.3	4.2
Prilocaine with epinephrine	1.6	2	2.6

*Using the 50th percentile weight for age.
Calculations should be based on the child's body weight and not his or her age.

The blood has a chocolate brown appearance. Prilocaine's metabolite *o*-toluidine can block methemoglobin reductase, leading to increased methemoglobin levels. This appears 3 to 4 hours after administration. In patients with congenital methemoglobinemia, prilocaine and benzocaine must be avoided, but any local anesthetic can be problematic in these patients. Bupivacaine should be considered for administration when a local anesthetic is needed as it should be the least likely to induce a response. When methemoglobinemia occurs, it should be considered a medical emergency, and treatment includes intravenous administration of methylene blue (see Chapter 40).

Local Tissue Responses

Commercially available local anesthetics are relatively nonirritating to tissues. Local anesthetic concentrations necessary to damage peripheral nerves usually far exceed the concentrations required for transmission blockade. Accidental intraneural injection may lead to nerve damage, however, from the combination of undiluted local anesthetic, strong hydrostatic pressure, and direct physical injury. Although the overall incidence is very low, there is evidence that high-concentration agents, such as 4% solutions of prilocaine or articaine, are significantly more likely to cause long-lasting or permanent nerve injury when administered for inferior alveolar nerve block. Exposure of unsheathed neurons to these concentrations results in an irreversible increase in intracellular Ca^{2+} and necrotic cell death.

Conventional anesthetic preparations may induce focal necrosis in skeletal muscle tissue approximating the injection site. The damage occurs rapidly after a single administration and is completely reversed in several weeks. In certain circumstances, local anesthetics may also impede cell motility, depress collagen synthesis, and delay wound healing.

Adverse tissue responses to injected local anesthetic preparations are usually caused or augmented by vasoconstrictor additives. Epinephrine creates tissue hypoxia by reducing local blood flow while increasing oxygen consumption. Although tissue injury may be induced by any of the sympathomimetics currently used, norepinephrine is particularly apt to cause ischemic necrosis. The injection of local anesthetic with a vasoconstrictor has been described historically as especially hazardous in areas supplied by terminal arteries (e.g., nose, digits, and penis). More recent research has shown, however, the safety of epinephrine used with local anesthetics in digital nerve blocks and for injections of the nose and ear.

Psychogenic/Idiosyncratic Reactions

A psychogenic reaction is the most common adverse event from the injection of local anesthetic in dental practice. It must be made clear that these reactions are not due to the local anesthetic drug but to the insertion of the needle. The most common manifestation of this is syncope, very often vasovagal in nature. In this case the patient faints and most commonly has a very low heart rate and blood pressure. The second-most common manifestation of a psychogenic reaction to the injection of local anesthetic is hyperventilation. Various other forms of anxiety attacks may also be seen, including anaphylactoid reactions.

In rare instances, patients have had toxic reactions to small amounts of local anesthetic. Some of these reactions may represent an abnormal susceptibility to the local anesthetic. Most often, these responses are anxiety related, associated with the vasoconstrictor, or the result of inadvertent intravascular injection. Regarding the last possibility, it has been accidentally determined that the convulsant dose of lidocaine in humans is only 10 mg when the drug is injected into the vertebral artery.

Amide local anesthetics were previously thought by some authorities to be causative agents for malignant hyperthermia (MH). This conclusion was based on a few anecdotal cases of supposed MH and on the ability of lidocaine-like drugs to potentiate contracture of skeletal muscle in various experimental situations. Subsequently, direct evidence indicated that no injectable local anesthetic is a triggering agent. Amide local anesthetics are safe for routine dental use in patients susceptible to MH.

Allergic Phenomena

Local anesthetics rarely cause allergic reactions; however, when one does occur, an ester derivative of PABA is usually involved. PABA is a breakdown product of the ester local anesthetics, and it is the most likely antigen when an allergy occurs after its administration. Since all esters produce PABA, an allergy to one ester local anesthetic rules out the use of all esters.

A confirmed allergy in an appropriately tested patient to an amide anesthetic is rare. In the event that this does occur, there is no evidence of cross-reactivity among the amide anesthetics, meaning that it is acceptable to substitute another amide when a local anesthetic is required.

Methylparaben, a preservative used in multidose local anesthetic preparations, has also served as an antigenic stimulant. For this reason, and because it is not required in single-use formulations, methylparaben was removed from dental cartridges in the United States in 1984. Thus, patients having a documented allergic reaction before that date likely reacted to methylparaben, and they would be fine with the formulations in use today.

Certain individuals, mostly asthmatic patients, are intolerant of sulfites, including the bisulfite and metabisulfite preservatives used in local anesthetic solutions with vasoconstrictors. Findings suggest that most affected individuals are hyperreactive to sulfites that are inhaled or ingested but not injected. These reactions are more properly classified as idiosyncratic and do not necessarily contraindicate the use of sulfite-containing local anesthetics, except perhaps in some patients with severe asthma. Isolated case reports of bisulfite allergy occurring after the intraoral administration of local anesthesia constitute the rare absolute contraindication. It should be noted that there is no cross-reactivity with sulfonamide antibacterials.

Despite the low incidence of verifiable allergy to local anesthetic solutions in patients, a high percentage of individuals have medical histories of presumptive local anesthetic hypersensitivity. Many of these cases undoubtedly represent anxiety or toxic reactions misdiagnosed as immunologic in origin. Such mistakes are particularly apparent when amides are involved because most investigations have shown these compounds to be virtually nonallergenic. When a single agent is involved, substitution with another local anesthetic is the simplest method of resolving the problem if consideration is given to the fact that esters may exhibit cross-allergenicity with each other and with methylparaben.

Use During Pregnancy

Local anesthetics are generally regarded as safe for use throughout pregnancy. Studies of women receiving local anesthesia for emergency procedures in the first trimester and/or routine dental procedures in the second trimester have supported this view. The U.S. Food and Drug Administration (FDA) has classified lidocaine and prilocaine in pregnancy risk category B and articaine, mepivacaine, and bupivacaine in category C (Table 3-9). Given these categorizations, clearly the use of lidocaine or prilocaine is a better medicolegal decision in the pregnant patient.

DRUG INTERACTIONS

Because of their influences on excitable membranes, local anesthetics are potentially capable of interacting with a wide spectrum of therapeutic agents. The most important interaction featuring vasoconstrictors is the intended one: inhibition of local anesthetic uptake from the injection site.

The CNS depressant effects of local anesthetics summate with the effects of the general anesthetics, barbiturates, and opioid analgesics, yielding interactions with therapeutic and toxicologic significance. Lidocaine combined with another antiarrhythmic drug may generate profound disturbances in cardiac automaticity and conduction, far in excess of what either compound would have caused if given alone. Although feeble by itself, the neuromuscular blocking activity of local anesthetics has been used to advantage in preventing succinylcholine-induced fasciculations and in reducing the dose of succinylcholine required during surgery for adequate muscle relaxation. Elucidation of the role of CYP3A4 and CYP1A2 enzymes in the metabolism of amide local anesthetics has led to the discovery that inhibitors of these enzymes, such as erythromycin (CYP3A4) and fluvoxamine (CYP1A2), can modestly increase plasma concentrations of lidocaine and related agents.

A unique interaction may occur between certain esters and the sulfonamides. As mentioned earlier, procaine and several other local anesthetics (benzocaine, tetracaine) are metabolized to yield *PABA*. The antibacterial action of sulfonamides is competitively antagonized by this metabolite. This interaction is not relevant for amide dental anesthetics; however, it is a likely interaction with the use of high levels of PABA in certain "health food supplements."

Although the potential for interactions involving local anesthetics is great, clinical manifestations appear infrequently outside the hospital and then only when very large doses are used or when unusual patient factors are present. Much more likely to occur are interactions between various drugs and the vasoconstrictors used during local anesthesia. Epinephrine may generate ventricular arrhythmias during general anesthesia given by some inhaled agents. Similarly, catecholamines can induce undesirable changes in cardiac action and blood pressure in patients taking tricyclic antidepressants and related norepinephrine transporter inhibitors, cocaine, nonselective β-adrenergic blockers, digoxin, inhibitors of catechol-O-methyltransferase, or adrenergic neuron–blocking drugs (e.g., guanethidine). Compounds with prominent α-adrenoceptor–blocking activity, such as the phenothiazine and butyrophenone antipsychotics, may lead to hypotension if coadministered in large doses with epinephrine.

Despite statements to the contrary in local anesthetic product information approved by the FDA, local anesthetics containing epinephrine may be used without special reservation in patients taking monoamine oxidase (MAO) inhibitors. Exogenous catecholamines are mostly degraded by the enzyme catechol-O-methyltransferase; inhibition of MAO has little impact on their respective metabolic fates or cardiovascular actions. Moreover, the effect of injected catecholamines is not appreciably affected by MAO inhibitors because these injected catecholamines do not release endogenous prejunctional catecholamines.

Largely because of the cardiovascular stimulation associated with the sympathomimetic amines, attention has been focused on noncatecholamine alternatives for vasoconstriction. Of these, several analogs of the antidiuretic hormone (vasopressin) have proved suitable, and one, felypressin (2-phenylalanine-8-lysine vasopressin), is used in Europe and elsewhere as a vasoconstrictor for local anesthesia. Although felypressin is not as effective as epinephrine and cannot be relied on for surgical hemostasis, it avoids the drug interaction problems of the catecholamines. Local toxicity is also reduced because felypressin does not stimulate tissue oxygen consumption. Local anesthetics with felypressin are unavailable in the United States.

GENERAL THERAPEUTIC USES

Local anesthetics are widely used for pain relief. By obviating the necessity of general anesthesia, these drugs have been instrumental in reducing the mortality and morbidity associated with various operative procedures. They also render valuable service by obtunding the pain of sunburn, toothache, and other ailments. In addition, local anesthetics are increasingly being used for purposes unrelated to pain control.

Techniques of Anesthesia

The onset, quality, extent, and duration of local anesthesia vary markedly with the technique of administration used. As might be expected, no single agent is capable of performing all the clinical duties local anesthetics are expected to fulfill.

Surface application

Local anesthetics are prepared for topical use in several different forms. Aqueous solutions and sprays are especially suited for coverage of large surfaces; anesthesia of small areas is often best accomplished with an ointment or viscous gel. Although penetration of the intact epidermis is insignificant, uptake by injured skin or by mucous membranes can be rapid. Topical activities are often not related to efficacies determined for other administration sites; tetracaine and lidocaine are useful topically as single agents, whereas mepivacaine, prilocaine, and procaine are not. Benzocaine, ineffective parenterally, is well adapted for surface anesthesia because of its slow systemic absorption and relative safety.

Infiltration, field block, and nerve block

Inhibition of transmission in circumscribed portions of the peripheral nervous system is accomplished by the techniques of infiltration, field block, and nerve block. Infiltration anesthesia is performed by injecting a local anesthetic into the area to be anesthetized. In this manner, the nerve endings exposed to the anesthetic solution are quickly made unresponsive. Field block refers to the subcutaneous or submucosal injection of anesthetic agents where the extent of anesthesia extends distal to the tissues infiltrated with drug. In dentistry, anesthesia of the tooth pulp after supraperiosteal injection is a form of field block because the local anesthetic does not gain access to the pulp but nevertheless renders it insensitive to stimulation. Nerve block is produced by depositing a local anesthetic solution close to the appropriate nerve trunk but proximal to the intended area of anesthesia. After a certain latency period required for penetration of the local anesthetic into the nerve interior, sensations are lost in all tissues innervated by the distal portion of the affected nerve. Although infiltrations, field blocks, and single nerve blocks usually anesthetize discrete areas, compound injections (e.g., brachial plexus or sciatic-femoral blocks) may affect large segments of the body, including whole limbs. All of the many local anesthetics suitable for infiltration are also useful for field and nerve blocks.

Spinal anesthesia

Deposition of a local anesthetic solution in the subarachnoid space can be used to produce surgical anesthesia in all structures of the body below the diaphragm. Injection is ordinarily made inferior to the first lumbar vertebra to avoid possible injury to the spinal cord. When introduced, the drug mixes with the cerebrospinal fluid and begins to spread throughout the subarachnoid space. The extent of cephalad diffusion of the local anesthetic, and the level of anesthesia obtained, is governed by several factors, including the dose, specific gravity (baricity), and volume of local anesthetic solution administered; the size and position of the spinal canal; and the degree of cerebrospinal fluid mixing imposed by the rate of injection and by movements of the patient. Tetracaine, lidocaine, and bupivacaine are most commonly used for spinal anesthesia in the United States, but numerous other agents are also used.

Epidural block

Local anesthetic infusion into the potential space between the dura mater and the connective tissue lining of the vertebral canal provides an effective alternative to subarachnoid anesthesia. Patient resistance to epidural injection is less of a problem, and the neurologic difficulties sometimes encountered after spinal block are avoided. Epidural anesthesia is comparatively slow in onset, however, and requires considerably more total drug than its subarachnoid counterpart. The level of anesthesia is also less predictable and more difficult to control. Bupivacaine, ropivacaine, and lidocaine are especially popular for epidural anesthesia, but virtually any local anesthetic available for nerve blockade may be used.

Intravascular injection

Local anesthetics are sometimes introduced directly into a blood vessel to effect short-term regional analgesia. One popular technique consists of injecting an anesthetic solution (e.g., 0.5% lidocaine) intravenously into a limb previously exsanguinated by elevation or with an Esmarch bandage. Isolation of the local anesthetic solution from the systemic circulation is accomplished by placing a pneumatic tourniquet proximal to the injection site. Egress of the local anesthetic from the vascular compartment to peripheral tissues is so rapid that releasing the tourniquet 5 min after injection does not result in toxic blood concentrations. Other techniques that use intravascular local anesthetics have also occasionally been practiced. Lidocaine may be mixed with some drugs known to be irritating in an attempt to alleviate the pain associated with their intravascular injection.

Other Uses

Local anesthetics are sometimes administered intravenously to produce or to supplement general anesthesia. As an adjunctive agent, lidocaine has been used to prevent postoperative muscle pain caused by succinylcholine and to depress airway reflexes and sympathetic nervous system responses during endotracheal intubation and extubation and other procedures affecting the bronchial tree. Local anesthetics have also been used, with mixed success, to treat protracted cough and laryngospasm and as intravenous analgesic and anticonvulsant medications. An adhesive patch containing 5% lidocaine is approved for relief of postherpetic neuralgia.

USES IN DENTISTRY

It would be difficult to overstate the profound influence of local anesthesia on the practice of dentistry. Most of the complex restorative procedures routinely performed on conscious patients would be inconceivable without effective pain control. By eliminating nociceptive sensations associated with dental care, local anesthetics improve patient acceptance of dental treatment and thereby contribute significantly to oral health. Because local anesthetics are so frequently used and, for many practitioners, represent the only drugs administered parenterally, the toxicity and efficacy of these agents is of particular interest and concern.

Safety in Dentistry

Without question, local anesthesia is often considerably safer in dentistry than in medicine. Statistics related to local anesthetic toxicity in dentistry are meager and subject to error. Mortality figures range from 1 death in 1.4 million local anesthetic administrations to one in 45 million. These values are open to question. It is possible that some deaths from local anesthetics go unreported and that others are mistakenly identified as myocardial infarctions or cerebrovascular accidents. It is also quite likely that some deaths imputed to local anesthetics are caused by procedural stress or are merely accidents of time and place and are not causally related to drug administration at all. Tabulations of nonfatal adverse reactions directly attributable to local anesthetics in clinical practice are limited; however, **Persson (1969) recorded adverse effects in 2.5% of 2960 patients given one to two cartridges of various anesthetic agents.** Because most of the complications observed—pallor, unrest, sweating, fatigue, palpitation, nausea, and fainting—are common manifestations of acute anxiety, it is evident that many adverse effects ascribed to local anesthesia are actually generated by the process of injection and not by the drugs themselves.

Drug Selection

Selection of a local anesthetic for dental application must include considerations of efficiency, safety, and individual patient and operative needs. That such factors are difficult to evaluate is illustrated by the diversity of results obtained in various clinical trials. One of the few areas of agreement is that the introduction of the amide lidocaine in 1948 marked a significant advance over the ester preparations then available. **For routine use, 2% lidocaine hydrochloride with 1:100,000 epinephrine remains a standard dental anesthetic.**

Besides lidocaine, four additional amides are available in dental cartridges that possess similar advantages in stability, nonallergenicity, and efficacy over the ester agents (see Tables 14-2 and 14-4). **Mepivacaine,** introduced in 1957, is generally equivalent to lidocaine in its pharmacologic profile. Two distinctive features of mepivacaine are its topical ineffectiveness and its use as a 3% solution without a vasoconstrictor. **Prilocaine,** used clinically for the first time in 1960, is a less potent alternative to lidocaine. Similar to mepivacaine, it is not used topically as a single agent but is effective for dental application without epinephrine.

Articaine, the only thiophene-based amide local anesthetic, was first tested in humans in 1970 and made available in the United States in 2000. An issue of current interest is whether the marketed formulations of 4% articaine are equivalent or superior to other amide preparations. Properly controlled clinical trials have not generally shown increased efficacy with standard mandibular block injections. Several studies have indicated clinical superiority of articaine over lidocaine (both with epinephrine) when injected supraperiosteally for mandibular anesthesia.

Bupivacaine was used initially in 1963 but not marketed in a dental cartridge until 1983. It exhibits a slightly slower onset time than the other amides but is similarly efficacious after nerve block and has a much longer duration of action, making it well suited for providing postoperative pain relief. Given its slow onset and yet prolonged duration of action, consideration can be given to administering this at the end of the dental procedure before the duration of action of the initial local anesthetic has worn off and to provide more prolonged postoperative pain control. The bupivacaine preparation intended for dental use is a 0.5% solution with 1:200,000 epinephrine.

A significant dissimilarity among the amide preparations concerns the presence or absence of a vasoconstrictor additive. Local anesthetic formulations without epinephrine-like drugs are particularly useful when sympathomimetic amines are contraindicated. Plain solutions are additionally promoted on the basis of a shorter duration of action. Although soft tissue anesthesia is comparatively brief after maxillary injection with 3% mepivacaine or 4% prilocaine (both without vasoconstrictor), differences in duration after mandibular nerve block are trivial (see Table 14-4). Because the period of pulpal anesthesia is often 20% to 25% that of soft tissue anesthesia, the limited maxillary duration of these agents is sometimes disadvantageous.

The use of local anesthetics without vasoconstrictors in pediatric dentistry warrants special comment. It is sometimes said that the shorter duration of soft tissue symptoms with plain local anesthetic solutions should reduce the incidence of self-inflicted tongue, cheek, and lip trauma. Such claims are dubious because blockade of the lingual, inferior alveolar, and buccal nerves that supply most of the tissues at risk is not significantly shortened by these preparations. No studies relating a reduction in traumatic cheilitis to the use of plain solutions have been reported. Consideration of systemic toxicity should limit the pediatric dental use of local anesthetics without vasoconstrictors. **Because the safety margin of local anesthetics is quite low in small children, it is advisable to use a preparation containing a vasoconstrictor if not doing so would result in more total drug being administered.** Injection of phentolamine (OraVerse™) may be a superior alternative strategy to reduce the incidence of accidental soft tissue injury.

PREPARATIONS AND DOSAGE FOR USE IN DENTISTRY

Agents for Parenteral Administration

In dentistry, today only amides are available for injection. As stated earlier, although variably listed by the manufacturers as either 1.8 or 1.7 mL, all dental cartridges contain approximately 1.76 mL. Pyrogen-free distilled water with sodium chloride added for osmotic balance serves as the local anesthetic vehicle. Local anesthetic solutions in cartridges range in pH from less than 3.0 to greater than 6.0; preparations with vasoconstrictors are adjusted to a lower pH than are plain formulations to enhance stability of the sympathomimetic amine constituents. Citric acid and sodium metabisulfite (or an equivalent antioxidant) are also included to help prevent vasoconstrictor breakdown. (Oxidation of the catecholamine compounds produces acids that tend to lower the pH over time.) Currently available local anesthetics marketed for dentistry in the United States and Canada are discussed next.

Lidocaine hydrochloride

Lidocaine is an aminoethylamide derivative of xylidine. It is several times more potent and toxic than procaine and provides local anesthesia that is by comparison more prompt, more extensive, and longer lasting. The administration of 2% lidocaine hydrochloride with 1:100,000 epinephrine is most suitable for routine dental use, but the drug is also available as a plain solution (in multidose vials) and with 1:50,000 epinephrine. Although 2% lidocaine with vasoconstrictor provides satisfactory dental anesthesia in normal circumstances, it has sometimes proved ineffective in rendering extremely sensitive teeth completely pain-free. Lidocaine is the only amide marketed as a single agent for topical anesthesia in dentistry. Formulations of lidocaine hydrochloride include a 2% gel, a 2% viscous solution, a 4% solution, and in Canada a 10% topical spray. Lidocaine base is marketed in a 2.5% and 5% ointment and solution and a 10% aerosol spray. A mucosal adherent patch 2 cm long × 1 cm wide and containing 46.1 mg of lidocaine is also available.

Mepivacaine hydrochloride

Mepivacaine is an amide product of xylidine and N-methylpipecolic acid. Similar in many respects to lidocaine, mepivacaine hydrochloride is marketed in a 2% concentration with 1:20,000 levonordefrin and as a 3% solution without vasoconstrictor.

Prilocaine hydrochloride

In contrast to other amide anesthetics, prilocaine is a secondary amino derivative of toluidine. Less potent than lidocaine, prilocaine hydrochloride is marketed as a 4% solution with and without 1:200,000 epinephrine. As discussed earlier, instances of cyanosis observed after large doses of prilocaine (over 400 mg) result from its metabolic breakdown to *o*-toluidine, an inducer of methemoglobinemia. Prilocaine has also been associated with a greater incidence of nerve damage after inferior alveolar nerve block injections than seen with lidocaine or mepivacaine.

Articaine hydrochloride

Articaine is unique among the amides because it is based on a thiophene ring structure. Marketed in North America in a 4% concentration with 1:100,000 or 1:200,000 epinephrine, articaine has become a popular agent for routine use in dentistry. The rapid hydrolysis of the ester side chain helps reduce toxicity associated with slow absorption from the injection site; conversely, the high concentration of the agent may accentuate the danger of intravascular injection and the risk of nerve damage in the immediate area of injection, especially affecting the lingual and inferior alveolar nerves after inferior alveolar nerve blocks.

Bupivacaine hydrochloride

Bupivacaine is a homologue of mepivacaine rendered highly lipid-soluble by replacement of the N-methyl group with a butyl chain. Bupivacaine is approximately four times as potent and as toxic as mepivacaine; it also has a slightly higher pK_a and a slower onset of action. For dentistry, 0.5% bupivacaine hydrochloride is available with 1:200,000 epinephrine. Bupivacaine with epinephrine given for nerve block produces operative anesthesia several times longer than that afforded by other drugs. Additionally, the formulation provides postoperative analgesia averaging 8 hours in the mandible and 5 hours in the maxilla. Bupivacaine is less effective and shorter acting than lidocaine (both with epinephrine), however, for pulpal anesthesia after maxillary supraperiosteal injection. Bupivacaine is so lipid-soluble that the agent is largely absorbed by the mucosal tissues, leaving little free drug to diffuse into bone.

Tetracaine

A new product just reaching the market is a combination of 3% tetracaine with 0.5% oxymetazoline. The intent is to use this combination drug as a nasal spray to anesthetize the middle superior alveolar and the anterior superior alveolar nerves, effectively giving profound needle-less anesthesia to the maxillary anterior teeth and premolars. It has a tentative brand name of *Kovacaine Mist*, and it is expected to have FDA approval in early 2016. (See Ciancio et al., 2013.)

Agents Limited to Surface Application

Topical anesthetics are used in the oral cavity for various purposes. Formulations marketed as pressurized sprays produce widespread surface anesthesia appropriate for making impressions or intraoral radiographs. Such preparations are potentially hazardous, however, and only products with metered valve dispensers to help prevent inadvertent overdose should be used. Topical liquids, which avoid the possibility of aerosol inspiration, may also be used for anesthetic coverage of large surface areas. Nonaqueous topical preparations are suitable for most other procedures. Common local anesthetic vehicles include lanolin, petrolatum, sodium carboxymethylcellulose, and polyethylene glycol.

Benzocaine

Benzocaine is a derivative of procaine in which the amino terminus is lacking. Poorly soluble in aqueous fluid, benzocaine tends to remain at the site of application and is not readily absorbed into the systemic circulation. Because of its low toxic potential, benzocaine is especially useful for anesthesia of large surface areas within the oral cavity. Benzocaine is not totally innocuous, however; cases of methemoglobinemia have been reported after the administration of very large doses, especially in unmetered spray form. Benzocaine is available in a variety of preparations; a 20% concentration in the form of an aerosol spray, gel, ointment, paste, and solution is most commonly advocated for intraoral use. A mucosal gel patch (containing 36 mg per 2-cm-long × 1-cm-wide patch) is also available.

Tetracaine hydrochloride

Tetracaine is an ester derivative of PABA in which a butyl chain replaces one of the hydrogens on the *p*-amino group. The drug has approximately 10 times the toxicity and potency of procaine. It is no longer available for injection in dentistry; for surface application, it is most commonly marketed as a 2% hydrochloride salt in combination with 14% benzocaine and 2% butamben in an aerosol spray, solution, gel, and ointment under the proprietary name Cetacaine. Tetracaine is one of the most effective topical anesthetics, but the drug's toxic potential after surface application should dictate caution in its use.

Cocaine hydrochloride

Cocaine, the first anesthetic used in dentistry and medicine, is a naturally occurring benzoic acid ester. The pharmacologic characteristics of cocaine are unique among the local anesthetics because, in addition to its action as an anesthetic, the drug inhibits the uptake of catecholamines by adrenergic nerve terminals. Cocaine potentiates the action of endogenously released and exogenously administered sympathomimetic amines. As a result, cocaine may cause pupillary mydriasis, vascular constriction, and other manifestations of sympathetic nervous system activity. Cocaine is also a powerful CNS stimulant and a popular drug of abuse (see Chapter 39). Restricted to therapeutic applications in which its vasoconstricting property is of special benefit (as in intranasal surgery), cocaine has no place in the routine practice of dentistry.

Lidocaine/prilocaine

Marketed under the acronym of EMLA, a eutectic mixture of 2.5% lidocaine and 2.5% prilocaine is available in the form of a cream for topical anesthesia of the skin. When placed under an occlusive dressing for 1 hour, EMLA obtunds the pain of venipuncture and is useful in young children and other patients intolerant of needle insertion. Although this formulation is not intended for topical anesthesia of the oral cavity (it has a poor taste and unfavorable physical characteristics for intraoral use), several investigations have proved its superiority over other topical anesthetics in relieving pain associated with manipulation of oral tissues. EMLA significantly relieved the discomfort of palatal injections after a 5-min application and allowed deeper probing of the gingival sulcus without discomfort than did 5% topical lidocaine.

An intraoral preparation with the same active ingredients of EMLA has been marketed with the trade name of Oraqix™. A low-viscosity fluid at room temperature, the anesthetic mixture becomes an elastic gel after being applied to the gingival sulcus to provide local anesthesia for periodontal scaling and root planing. The packaging of Oraqix™ is intended to avoid the possibility of administering the drug by parenteral injection. The overall effect is a 50% reduction of treatment pain.

It is becoming more common for physicians to prescribe special drug mixtures that are not available through other commercial sources. These are formulated at local compounding pharmacies. An example is a topical cream containing lidocaine + prilocaine + meloxicam (a nonsteroidal antiinflammatory drug) + lamotrigine (an antiepileptic drug) for the treatment of musculoskeletal pain.

CASE STUDY DISCUSSION

There are several possible choices for local anesthetics. The duration of the procedure was estimated to be 1 hour, and therefore a mandibular block by any one of articaine with epinephrine, lidocaine with epinephrine, mepivacaine with levonordefrin, or prilocaine with epinephrine would be appropriate. Periodontal flap surgery sometimes requires strong vasoconstriction, so consideration of infiltration of lidocaine with 1:50,000 epinephrine might be appropriate. If it is determined that prolonged pain control is warranted, then consideration could be given to administering 0.5% bupivacaine with 1:200,000 epinephrine at the end of the procedure.

The finding that the patient felt faint is the common psychogenic reaction that is found with local anesthetic administration leading to syncope. It is not the drug that causes it but the act of injection. Her drop in blood pressure is consistent with this being vasovagal in nature.

A SUMMARY OF THE LOCAL ANESTHETICS AVAILABLE FOR DENTISTRY. THE FIRST FIVE ARE THE ONES PREPARED IN DENTAL CARTRIDGES AND MOST COMMONLY USED

Nonproprietary (Generic) Name	Proprietary (Trade) Name
Agents for Parenteral Administration	
Articaine	Articadent, Orabloc, Posicaine, Septocaine, Zorcaine
Bupivacaine	Marcaine, Sensorcaine, Surgicaine, Vivacaine
Lidocaine	Xylocaine, Lignospan, Lignospan Forte, Octocaine
Mepivacaine	Carbocaine, Isocaine, Polocaine, Scandonest
Prilocaine	Citanest, Citanest Forte
Procaine	Novocain (brand discontinued in United States)
Ropivacaine	Naropin
Tetracaine	Pontocaine
Agents Limited to Surface Application	
Benzocaine	Americaine, Gingicaine, Hurricaine, Topicale, in Cetacaine
Butamben	Butesin Picrate, in Cetacaine
Dibucaine	Nupercainal
Lidocaine/prilocaine	EMLA, Oraqix
Other Related Drugs	
Sodium bicarbonate injection	OnPharma, Anutra
Phentolamine mesylate	OraVerse

GENERAL REFERENCES

1. Armstrong CM: Na channel inactivation from open and closed states, *Proc Natl Acad Sci U S A* 103:17991–17996, 2006.
2. Berde CB, Strichartz GR: Local anesthetics. In Miller RD, editor: *Miller's anesthesia*, ed 6, Philadelphia, 2005, Churchill Livingstone.
3. Catterall WA, Mackie K: Local Anesthetics. In Brunton: *Goodman & Gilman's the pharmacological basis of therapeutics*, 12th Edition, McGraw-Hill Professional Publishing.
4. Ciancio SG, Hutcheson MC, Ayoub F, Pantera Jr EA, Pantera CT, Garlapo DA, Sobieraj BD, Almubarak SA: Safety and efficacy of a novel nasal spray for maxillary dental anesthesia, *JDR* 92(suppl 7):S43–S48, July 2013.
5. Cousins MJ, Bridenbaugh PO, Carr DB, et al.: *Cousins and Bridenbaugh's neural blockade in clinical anesthesia and pain medicine*, ed 4, Philadelphia, 2008, Lippincott Williams & Wilkins.
6. Liu SS, Joseph Jr RS: Local anesthetics. In Barash PG, Cullen BF, Stoelting RK, editors: *Clinical anesthesia*, ed 5, Philadelphia, 2006, Lippincott Williams & Wilkins.
7. Local anesthetics. In Strichartz GR, editor: *Handbook of experimental pharmacology*, vol. 81. Berlin, 1987, Springer-Verlag.
8. Persson G: General side effects of local dental anaesthesia, *Acta Odontol Scand Suppl* 53:1–140, 1969.
9. Robertson D, Nusstein J, Reader A, Beck M, McCartney M: The anesthetic efficacy of articaine in buccal infiltration of mandibular posterior teeth, *JADA* 138:1104–1112, 2007.
10. Strichartz GR, Sanchez V, Arthur GR, et al.: Fundamental properties of local anesthetics, II: measured octanol/buffer partition coefficients and pKa values of clinically used drugs, *Anesth Analg* 71:158–170, 1990.

15

General Anesthesia*

Steven I. Ganzberg and Daniel A. Haas

KEY INFORMATION

- The first public demonstration of anesthesia was carried out by a dentist.
- The mechanism(s) of general anesthesia is not known with certainty, but there are many theories.
- Agents are classified as either inhalational or intravenous.
- Balanced anesthesia, using multiple drugs, is the common technique used today.
- Inhalational anesthetics are now used primarily for maintenance of anesthesia.
- The inhalational anesthetics are nitrous oxide, isoflurane, desflurane, and sevoflurane.
- Intravenous anesthetics are now used primarily for induction of anesthesia.
- Intravenous anesthetics include propofol, methohexital, ketamine, and midazolam.
- A number of adjuncts are used as premedicants or part of the balanced approach.
- Adjuvant drugs include peripheral skeletal neuromuscular blockers, dexmedetomidine, analgesics, sedatives, antihistamines, and antimuscarinic drugs.

CASE STUDY

A 33-year-old male patient, whose medical history includes cognitive impairment and a controlled seizure disorder, was undergoing general anesthesia for general dentistry involving several restorations, endodontic therapy, and a scaling. His medications included valproic acid and, he had no known allergies The patient was administered 100 µg of fentanyl and 2 mg of midazolam, intravenously. This was then followed by an intravenous injection of 2 mg/kg of propofol for induction, which was followed by a drop in blood pressure from a preoperative reading of 120/80 to 80/40 mm Hg. Was this an expected event? How should it be managed? After management of the blood pressure, desflurane was then administered for maintenance of the anesthetia. Later on in the case, blood pressure was found to rise. How should this be managed?

HISTORY

The history of anesthesia is relevant to dentistry, as two dentists, Horace Wells and his one-time pupil and partner, William T.G. Morton, pioneered its use. In the United States in the early 1800s, traveling entertainers who called themselves professors went about delivering lectures on ether and nitrous oxide and demonstrating their effects. Crawford W. Long, a Georgia physician had attended ether frolics while a student, and in 1842, he used ether when he removed two small tumors from the neck of his friend, James Venable. Because Long wanted to include observations of the effects of ether in major surgical procedures, he did not publish reports of his pioneering use of ether until 1849, 3 years after the accounts of Morton's use of ether had appeared.

On December 10, 1844, Horace Wells attended a demonstration, staged by Gardner Quincy Colton in Hartford, Connecticut, of the effects of "laughing gas." One subject who volunteered to take the gas injured himself in the leg. Wells noticed that he was unaware of his injury and apparently had no pain until the effects of the gas wore off. The next day, Wells persuaded John Riggs, a prominent Hartford dentist, to remove one of his own teeth while under nitrous oxide anesthesia administered by "Professor" Colton. Wells claimed that he felt no more than a pinprick. Wells then obtained permission to demonstrate his technique before a class at the Harvard Medical School and administered nitrous oxide to a student, who proceeded to scream loudly while his tooth was being removed. The boy later said he had felt no pain but the demonstration was deemed a failure. Discouraged by the hostile reception that followed, Wells became ill and was unable to practice dentistry on a regular basis. He nevertheless continued to administer nitrous oxide, with mixed success, for dental and medical operations. Wells also experimented with ether in 1845 and with chloroform when its anesthetic effect became known. Wells died in January 1848 when he became deranged by overexposure to chloroform and committed suicide while in jail for having accosted a prostitute.

William Morton of Boston, a former student and partner of Wells, had begun to use ether topically for its local numbing effect on his dental patients. With the help of his chemistry professor at Harvard, Charles T. Jackson, Morton refined his technique and successfully administered anesthesia to a patient for the extraction of a molar tooth. Convinced of the importance of his discovery, he obtained an invitation to demonstrate his technique for John C. Warren, a surgeon at Massachusetts General Hospital. On October 16, 1846, Morton prepared a young patient for the surgical removal of a large mandibular tumor. Morton is credited with the discovery of anesthesia and the custom of saying, "Doctor, your patient is now ready." Morton then went on to become the first professional anesthetist. In 1846, Holmes addressed a letter to Morton suggesting that the term *anesthesia* be given to the state produced by ether and that the agent itself be called an *anesthetic*.

* The authors wish to acknowledge the past contributions of Dr. John A. Yagiela to this chapter.

No new anesthetic agents were added until the 1920s and 1930s, when ethylene, cyclopropane, and divinyl ether were introduced. Since the early 1950s, a series of halogenated agents containing fluorine have been introduced clinically and have essentially replaced other inhalation agents except nitrous oxide. Halothane was the prototype for this group, but its use was discontinued as superior agents, such as isoflurane, sevoflurane, and desflurane, were developed. Similarly, enflurane and methoxyflurane were, at one time, commonly used, but they are no longer available. Intravenous agents became popular in the late 1930s. Initially these were the ultrashort-acting barbiturates, followed in the late 1960s by other agents and adjuncts such as ketamine, etomidate, midazolam, and propofol.

GOALS OF ANESTHESIA

General anesthesia may be defined as a drug-induced reversible depression of the central nervous system (CNS) resulting in a loss of sensation and response to all external stimuli. A complete anesthetic is one that produces unconsciousness, unresponsiveness, amnesia, analgesia, and muscle relaxation by itself without eliciting undue homeostatic disturbances in the patient. An example of such a complete anesthetic is diethyl ether, an anesthetic that was in use for a century. Although there are other complete anesthetics, the tendency in modern anesthesiology is to use a combination of drugs to take advantage of the best properties of each and to minimize unwanted side effects. Combining anesthetics from different drug classes allows for a reduction in the dose of each agent as the majority of such interactions are supra-additive in nature. In fact, ***balanced anesthesia*** is a term used to describe a concept in which combinations of drugs are used to produce general anesthesia, with each drug chosen for a specific effect.

The primary goals of general anesthesia are to preserve the life of the patient, to provide the operator with an adequate surgical field, and to obtund pain and awareness. A general anesthetic ideally should (1) provide a smooth and rapid induction; (2) produce a state of unconsciousness or unresponsiveness; (3) produce a state of amnesia; (4) maintain essential physiologic functions while blocking reflexes that might lead to bronchospasm, salivation, and arrhythmias; (5) produce skeletal muscle relaxation, but preferably not of the respiratory muscles, through the blockade of various efferent impulses; (6) block the conscious perception of sensory stimuli so that there is adequate analgesia to perform the procedure; and (7) provide a smooth, rapid, and uneventful emergence and recovery with no long-lasting adverse effects.

The goals of anesthesia for general surgery also apply to dentistry, but there are some important differences. Dental patients are generally outpatients; in most circumstances, particularly situations not involving extensive oral and maxillofacial surgery, the procedures are not as traumatic as general surgical procedures, and it is often not necessary or desirable to render the patient unconscious. Although general anesthesia for dental and oral surgery is necessary under many circumstances, specific techniques have been developed for producing varying degrees of sedation in dental patients, as are described in Chapter 38.

MECHANISMS OF ANESTHESIA

Since the discovery of general anesthesia, considerable efforts have been directed toward elucidating the mechanism of action of these agents. Numerous theories have been proposed.

Molecular Mechanisms of Action

Many investigators have sought to describe the action of the extremely diverse chemicals known to be general anesthetics by their ability to perturb the molecular structure and function of neurons. Most early anesthetic agents seemed to be indiscriminate in affecting biophysical properties of cellular and subcellular membranes, and for many years, it was generally agreed that there were no specific receptors for general anesthetics, and therefore no direct antagonists, as there are for neurotransmitters. In this setting, a universal mechanism of action of general anesthesia based on the physicochemical properties of anesthetic agents was postulated. More recently, many actions of general anesthetics have been documented, and it is now believed that diverse molecular perturbations may result in unconsciousness and lack of response to external stimuli.

Correlates of anesthetic potency

Various mechanistic theories of general anesthesia began to appear shortly after the landmark demonstration of ether-induced insensibility by Morton, but the first important observation was made independently by Meyer in 1899 and Overton in 1901, who emphasized the correspondence between the lipid solubility of an agent and its anesthetic potency (Fig. 15-1). The **Meyer-Overton correlation** suggested that anesthesia begins when any chemical substance has attained a certain molar concentration in the hydrophobic phase of the cell membrane. When olive oil is used to represent the hydrophobic medium, this concentration is approximately 50 mmol/L. Experiments with different lipid media indicate that the best fit between solubility and anesthetic potency is obtained with lipids that are amphophilic (i.e., they have polar and nonpolar attributes) and can serve as hydrogen bond acceptors. These characteristics are descriptive of membrane phospholipids and cholesterol.

In 1954, Mullins, in his **critical volume hypothesis**, modified the original correlation to include consideration of the volume of the hydrophobic region occupied by the anesthetic agent. He reasoned that large anesthetic molecules would have greater effects on the membrane than would smaller molecules.

Membrane lipid theories

Numerous investigators since Mullins have sought to link the notion of a critical number or volume of anesthetic molecules with plasma membrane disturbances that could result in general anesthesia. Until the early 1980s, most attention was directed at the lipid bilayer of the plasma membrane, specifically the ability of anesthetics to cause membrane expansion, lipid fluidization, or lateral phase separation. With each of these effects, it was postulated that, as a result of the alteration in the lipid bilayer, the neuronal membrane becomes unable to

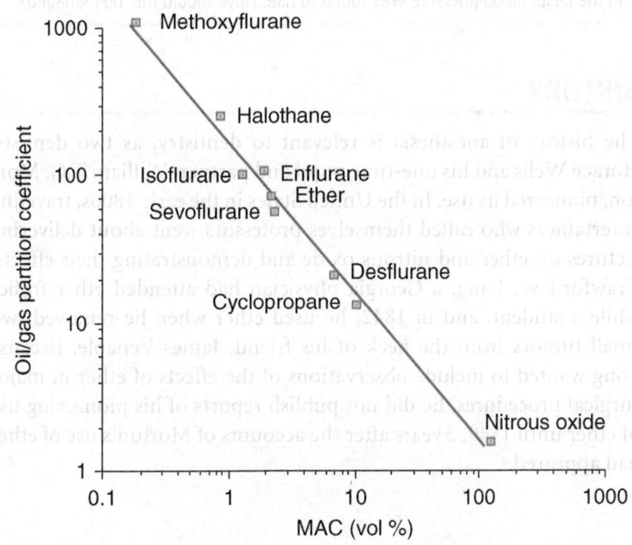

FIG 15-1 Linear correlation between anesthetic potency and lipid solubility. Potency is indicated by the minimum alveolar concentration (*MAC*) and lipid solubility by the olive oil/gas partition coefficient.

facilitate the changes in protein configuration that are required for such essential steps in the transmission of nerve impulses as ion gating, synaptic transmitter release, and binding of the transmitter to the receptor.

The **membrane expansion theory** was a natural outgrowth of the critical volume hypothesis. It holds that the absorption of anesthetic molecules by the lipid phase causes the membrane to expand, preventing important intrinsic membrane constituents from functioning properly. Measurements indicate that the expansion associated with general anesthesia is approximately 0.4%. Fluidization, or disordering, of lipids by anesthetic agents was noted in studies of lipid bilayers prepared with phospholipid and cholesterol to mimic cell membranes. Parallel shifts in measures of lipid fluidization and the activity of membrane-bound enzymes suggested that this perturbation of the normal lipid structure may result in functional changes sufficient to disrupt nerve transmission. The lateral phase separation theory was based on the idea that membrane lipids exist in two states: a high-volume, disordered sol state and a compact, ordered gel state. The ability of lipids to convert from the sol to the gel configuration, or to be compressed laterally within the membrane, was thought to accommodate conformational changes that need to occur for the opening of ion channels.

These lipid perturbation theories were supported by findings that hyperbaric pressures and certain convulsant drugs antagonize anesthesia, presumably by reversing membrane expansion or reestablishing order. It is now understood, however, that pressure or drug reversal of anesthesia arises from a physiologic antagonism of anesthetic action brought on by independent neurologic stimulation. Different anesthetics are affected differently by the same pressure, including chloral hydrate, whose anesthetic effect is immune to pressure reversal. Evidence has also mounted to cast doubt on membrane expansion or lipid perturbation per se as a cause of anesthesia. Direct measurements of the expansion of lipid bilayers and red blood cell membranes in response to anesthetic concentrations of ethanol and halothane yield values that are effectively insignificant, and other measurements have shown non-anesthetic long-chain alcohols to cause membrane expansion similar to that of inhalation anesthetics.

Calculations based on the Meyer-Overton relationship argue in general against a significant effect of anesthetic drugs on membrane lipids. At concentrations sufficient to produce surgical anesthesia, there is only about one molecule of drug in the membrane for every 60 to 80 molecules of the much larger lipid constituents. Unless anesthetic molecules are distributed unevenly in the membrane (e.g., concentrated in lipids adjacent to ion channels) or the lipid phase serves as a barrier to the diffusion of anesthetic agents (i.e., limiting access of anesthetics to their effector site) or as a reservoir for them (i.e., retaining anesthetic molecules where they have direct access to their effector sites), it is unlikely that membrane lipids play a major role in the mechanism of anesthesia.

Mechanisms involving membrane proteins

Membrane proteins constitute a second hydrophobic environment with which anesthetic molecules may interact. The idea that membrane proteins are the targets of anesthetic action is attractive for several reasons. First, it is consistent with the mode of action of most drugs that influence the CNS. Second, allosteric selection (described in Chapter 1) of a protein conformation by the binding of even a single small molecule can have pronounced effects on protein function. Third, it can best explain differences in action among the various anesthetics by assuming that these agents exert different effects on the same protein or influence different proteins altogether.

A close correspondence between the anesthetic potencies of stereoisomers of the agents halothane and isoflurane and their ability to perturb ion channel function provides strong evidence that membrane proteins are the immediate targets for general anesthetic action. It is now firmly established that certain classes of general anesthetics inhibit or activate specific ligand-gated ion channels in clinically relevant concentrations. Binding studies indicate a specific active site for volatile anesthetics on neuronal nicotinic receptors. Inhibition of nicotinic receptors in skeletal muscle probably contributes to the ability of volatile anesthetics to enhance muscle relaxation. Actions at neuronal nicotinic receptors promote effects such as amnesia, hyperalgesia, and excitation observed at subanesthetic concentrations of volatile anesthetics and barbiturates.

The **γ-aminobutyric acid$_A$ (GABA$_A$) receptor** has been implicated in the CNS depressant effect of most anesthetic drugs. Specific binding sites for benzodiazepines, barbiturates, other intravenous anesthetics, and volatile anesthetics have been described. Stimulation of these receptor sites increases the activity of GABA at its own separate site; many agents other than benzodiazepines can also open the GABA$_A$ Cl^- channel in the absence of GABA. Hyperpolarization of the affected neuron inhibits neuronal activity. Glycine receptors constitute another group of inhibitory receptors that are activated by at least some general anesthetics (inhalation anesthetics, alcohols, thiopental, and propofol) in clinically relevant concentrations.

Excitatory receptors blocked by specific anesthetic agents include *N*-methyl-D-aspartate (NMDA), kainate, and α-amino-3-hydroxy-5-methyl-4-isoxazole propionate (AMPA) receptors. Ketamine and nitrous oxide selectively inhibit NMDA receptors, whereas barbiturates and certain inhalation anesthetics block AMPA and kainate receptors.

In addition to the classic ligand-gated ion channels described previously, other ion channels may be involved in the actions of specific general anesthetics. Several types of 2-pore-domain K^+ channels are variably activated by inhalation anesthetics. These channels are responsive to intracellular second messengers and are believed to regulate background neuronal excitability and neurotransmitter release. Several types of **Ca^{2+} and Na^+ channels are inhibited** by clinical concentrations of drugs and may contribute an inhibitory influence on neurotransmitter release.

Several **G protein–coupled receptors (GPCRs)** are influenced by clinical concentrations of general anesthetics. An important example is the α_2-adrenergic receptor effector system. Stimulation of this system by the selective α_2 agonist dexmedetomidine significantly potentiates the anesthetic potency of volatile anesthetics. Similar potentiation can be obtained by drugs that stimulate opioid receptors or block nitric oxide synthase. Demonstration of a blocking action of halothane on the GPCR rhodopsin underscores the possibility that similar interactions with other GPCRs may support the effects of inhalation anesthetics on consciousness, nociception, and various autonomic effects observed during general anesthesia.

Other sites

Several investigators have raised the possibility that proteins other than membrane receptors/ion channels may be involved in the mechanism of anesthesia. Certain anesthetics have been shown to impair the ability of synaptosomes (isolated nerve terminals) to sequester and retain catecholamine neurotransmitters and of mitochondria to produce adenosine triphosphate (ATP) and to take up Ca^{2+}. There is some evidence suggestive that a specific anesthetic effect on mitochondrial function is a possible mechanism of action.

Neurophysiologic Mechanisms of Anesthesia

Molecular influences of general anesthetics may provide a fundamental explanation of their pharmacodynamic properties, but they are not useful in describing the selective changes in consciousness, pain perception, and muscle relaxation observed clinically. Much research has been directed toward determining the neurologic sites and pathways affected by the various anesthetics. Studies of the sympathetic nervous system have conclusively shown that synaptic transmission is much more susceptible to anesthetic block than axonal conduction. Nevertheless, this finding does not rule out an axonal contribution to general anesthesia. Anesthetic agents in clinical concentrations can diminish the amplitude of the action potential, which may impair synaptic transmission prejunctionally by reducing the evoked release of neurotransmitter. Conduction block is strongest at branch points of small-diameter axons and becomes even more prominent as the frequency of nerve transmission increases.

A crucial unknown in the study of general anesthesia is the site at which unconsciousness is produced. Areas in the CNS that have been implicated in this primary anesthetic action include the dorsal lamina of the spinal cord (substantia gelatinosa), the reticular system (including the midbrain reticular formation), sensory relay nuclei of the thalamus, and cortical areas.

Much attention has been directed toward the role of the mesencephalic **reticular activating formation.** This system, which receives various nonspecific sensory inputs, is a major center supporting consciousness and alertness of higher brain centers. As the activity of the system is depressed, the ascending influences on the limbic system and cortical structures are reduced, and unconsciousness ensues. This complex of neurons may also respond quite differently to various anesthetics. Barbiturates and most volatile anesthetics cause depression of spontaneous electrical activity, whereas ketamine alters the pattern of firing. All agents seem to block neuronal responses in the reticular formation to sensory input.

General anesthetics in clinically relevant concentrations may also exert direct effects on various nuclei of the **thalamus, the hippocampus, the olfactory cortex, and various circuits in the cerebral cortex**. Most reactions are consistent with the inhibition of excitatory neuronal pathways or facilitation of inhibitory influences, or both. As with the reticular formation, however, net excitatory reactions also occur depending on the anesthetic administered and region studied. Numerous investigators have argued for a central role of thalamocortical-corticothalamic loop circuits in maintaining consciousness.

Amnesia, which may be present in an awake patient or absent in an apparently unconscious patient, is most closely linked to anesthetic-induced suppression of the limbic system structures (e.g., amygdala, hippocampus). Drugs that potentiate the actions of GABA are likely to have specific amnestic properties.

Because of its role in modulating pain, the spinal cord has been studied as a possible site of anesthetic action. Investigators have shown that the analgesic action of nitrous oxide involves the laminar structures (substantia gelatinosa) of the dorsal horns, often referred to as the gateway for nociceptive impulses into the CNS. The similarity of analgesia produced by opioids, nitrous oxide, and ketamine suggests a common mode of action. Cross-tolerance to the analgesic effect of morphine and nitrous oxide and the ability to partially block nitrous oxide analgesia with the opioid antagonist naloxone indicate that nitrous oxide may release endogenous opioid substances. That the endogenous opioid system cannot be invoked as a mechanism of anesthesia generally is shown by the failure of naloxone to block the analgesic action of several anesthetics and the anesthetic action of nitrous oxide (and other drugs).

The analgesic action of nitrous oxide involves α_1-adrenergic and α_2-adrenergic receptor activation. Blockade of either α_1 receptors by prazosin or α_2 receptors by yohimbine negates the analgesic effect of nitrous oxide in animals. A possible sequence of events underlying nitrous oxide (and ketamine) analgesia is as follows: (1) nitrous oxide inhibition of NMDA receptors, (2) release of endogenous opioid neurotransmitters, (3) activation of descending norepinephrine pathways, (4) activation of α-adrenergic receptors in the spinal cord, and (5) inhibition of the classic nociceptive pathways. The analgesic action of isoflurane and dexmedetomidine may also be explained by their ability to stimulate α_2 receptors.

Behavioral manifestations of anesthesia

Progressive depression. In 1920, **Guedel divided the progression of ether anesthesia** into a sequence of four stages and subdivided the third, or surgical, stage further into four planes (Fig. 15-2). Each of these stages and planes represented a progressive and deepening depression of the CNS. In modern anesthesiology, these observations are no longer used in their entirety because the anesthetic signs are frequently obscured by the presence of other drugs used before and during the anesthetic period, and because different anesthetics create different patterns of responses. Nevertheless, Guedel's scheme is useful in describing some of the effects caused by various anesthetic drugs. The classic stages of anesthesia, as described by Guedel, are stage I, analgesia; stage II, delirium; stage III, surgical anesthesia (planes 1, 2, 3, and 4); and stage IV, medullary paralysis.

Stage I starts with the beginning of anesthetic administration and ends with the loss of consciousness. The patient is unresponsive to mild pain-provoking stimuli and is able to respond to verbal commands. This stage is followed by delirium in *stage II*, during which uncontrolled movements, vomiting, and laryngospasm can occur. It is desirable to traverse this stage rapidly; propofol or another intravenous anesthetic is often given to bypass this stage and induce anesthesia immediately prior to the administration of inhalation agents. *Stage III* has been subdivided, as indicated previously, into four planes in order of increasing depth of anesthesia by using various indices, including the diameter of the pupil; loss of ocular, oropharyngeal, and other reflexes; muscle relaxation; depth and regularity of respiration; and separation of the thoracic and abdominal (diaphragmatic) phases of respiration. *Stage IV* begins with the disappearance of the purely diaphragmatic respiration of stage III plane 4 and ends with complete respiratory and circulatory collapse, culminating in death if the anesthetic is not discontinued and the patient given support for the cardiopulmonary systems.

The recovery from general anesthesia is the reverse of the process of induction. The patient progressively regains reflexes, and a short period of excitement similar to that previously encountered during stage II may occur, followed by emergence to consciousness with residual analgesia.

Although the stages of anesthesia can be useful in a descriptive sense, the further subdivision of the surgical stage into planes is no longer useful. Anesthetic agents currently used do not produce the same pattern of concentration-dependent changes in autonomic, motor, and reflex activity observed with ether, and many adjunctive drugs used during anesthesia tend to obscure these same signs. Muscular relaxation can hardly be used to gage the depth of anesthesia if a neuromuscular blocking agent has been administered, and the arterial blood pressure cannot be useful if an adrenergic amine has been given to prevent hypotension. Nevertheless, measures of autonomic function, such as progressive reduction of blood pressure and alterations in heart rate, can be valuable guides to the patient's status during anesthesia in the absence of medications that specifically obscure these functions.

Selective depression

Generally, volatile anesthetic agents follow Guedel's scheme of progressive anesthesia. Certain discrepancies noted with these agents and experience with injectable drugs (e.g., ketamine), however, make clear

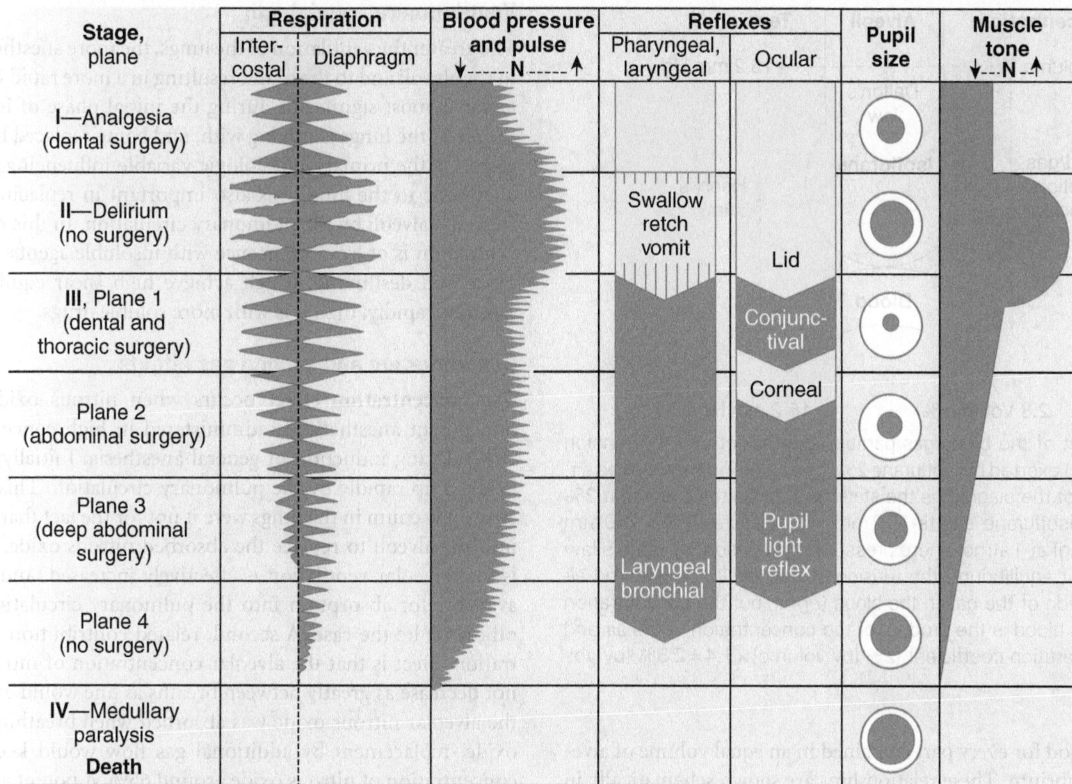

FIG 15-2 Guedel's scheme of progressive central nervous system depression produced by the anesthetic ether. Changes in physiologic functions are shown for the different stages and planes of Guedel's classification. Examples of surgery that can be performed at these anesthetic levels are given in parentheses.

the fact that surgical anesthesia is not synonymous with generalized CNS depression. Neurophysiologic investigations have indicated that amnesia and a loss of responsiveness to painful stimuli can occur with or without comprehensive CNS depression.

AGENTS USED IN GENERAL ANESTHESIA

General anesthesia can be induced by many compounds of diverse chemical structure, including inorganic compounds, halogenated hydrocarbons, simple alcohols, aromatic agents, steroids, and other drugs that affect the CNS. General anesthetics are available as gases and volatile liquids for administration by inhalation, and solutions suitable for intravenous injection.

INHALATION ANESTHETICS

Administration

General anesthetics are administered through delivery systems that incorporate the following features: (1) gases, including oxygen, stored in either local tanks or a central delivery system; (2) regulators to control the pressure of gases delivered; (3) safety systems that warn of dangerous pressures and shut off flow if oxygen delivery is interrupted; (4) mixing valves (adjustable flowmeters) to regulate the percentages of gases; (5) vaporizers to volatilize anesthetic liquids; (6) carbon dioxide absorber system (not required for nonrebreathing systems); (7) reservoir bag, ventilator, or both; (8) assorted tubing and one-way valve systems; (9) face mask, laryngeal mask, or endotracheal tube; and (10) vacuum exhaust line.

Central to the administration of volatile general anesthetics is the temperature-compensated, variable-bypass vaporizer. This device provides the simple selection of anesthetic concentration because it automatically compensates for changes in total gas flow and for changes in the ambient temperature. In the case of desflurane, which boils at 23 °C, the vaporizer must be heated electrically to 39 °C to ensure controlled delivery.

Pharmacokinetics

Uptake and distribution

The depth of anesthesia produced by an inhalation anesthetic depends on the concentration of the anesthetic agent in the brain. The speed of induction and the speed of recovery follow the rate at which the concentration of the agent changes in the brain. During induction, the gas must move from the anesthetic apparatus to the pulmonary alveoli, from the alveoli to the blood, and from the blood to the brain. On termination of anesthesia, the inhaled gas moves in the opposite direction across the same interfaces. The principal force governing this movement of anesthetic gas is the diffusion or concentration gradient, and the behavior of the gases as they move from one compartment to another across biologic interfaces is defined by two gas laws. Dalton's law deals with the partial pressure (or tension) of gases and states that in a gas mixture, the partial pressure of each component gas is directly related to its concentration in the mixture. Henry's law describes the solubility of gases in liquids and states that the quantity that will dissolve in a liquid is proportional to the partial pressure of that gas in direct contact with the liquid.

The partition coefficient is an expression of the relative solubility of a substance in two immiscible phases. When applied to anesthetic gases, it compares the relative amount of gas dissolved in one phase when one part is present in the other phase. The **blood/gas partition coefficient** of 1.4 for isoflurane indicates that 1.4 parts of isoflurane are

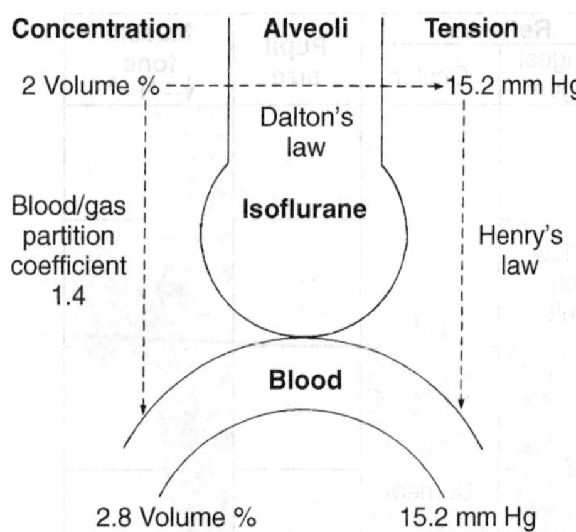

FIG 15-3 Effect of the blood/gas partition coefficient and the tension (partial pressure) exerted by isoflurane 2% (by volume) in the inspired air. Across the top of the diagram is the statement of Dalton's law that 2% (by volume) of isoflurane exerts 15.2 mm Hg pressure (0.02 × 760 mm Hg = 15.2 mm Hg) at 1 atmosphere pressure. Application of Henry's law indicates that, at equilibrium, the tension of the gas in the inspired air equals the tension of the gas in the blood (*right*), but the concentration dissolved in the blood is the product of the concentration in the air and the blood/gas partition coefficient (2% [by volume] × 1.4 = 2.8% [by volume], *left*).

dissolved in blood for every part contained in an equal volume of alveolar air at equilibrium. These relationships are shown schematically in Figure 15-3.

As mentioned earlier, during induction the various compartments of the body are brought into equilibrium regarding the inhaled anesthetic gas. When equilibrium is reached, the tensions of the anesthetic gas in the inspired air, alveolar air, arterial blood, body tissues, and mixed venous blood become equal, but the concentrations vary in concert with the relative solubility of the agent in each compartment. The speed with which equilibrium is achieved is influenced by many variables, and each of these is considered subsequently, particularly regarding how it affects the alveolar concentration.

The **alveolar concentration of an inhalation anesthetic** is of pivotal importance to the onset of anesthesia. Because the brain is extremely well perfused, the tension of an inhaled anesthetic in the brain closely follows that of the arterial blood, which itself is equilibrated with the alveolar tension as the blood passes through the pulmonary microvasculature. Within broad limits, anything that increases delivery of anesthetic to the alveoli, and increases its alveolar partial pressure, would hasten anesthesia onset, and anything that enhances its removal from the lungs—in other words, anything that increases overall alveolar transfer to the pulmonary circulation, and hence systemic uptake—would reduce its alveolar partial pressure and delay anesthesia onset.

Concentration in inspired air

The greater the concentration of the anesthetic gas in the inspired air, the more rapid is the induction of anesthesia. This inspired concentration normally is not held constant during induction. With agents that can be irritating to the airways, such as isoflurane, the concentration is increased slowly. With sevoflurane, which is nonirritating, or in situations in which acceleration of the speed of induction is desired, the concentration at the outset may be two to three times what it would be during the maintenance phase of anesthetic administration. This technique, sometimes referred to as *overpressurization*, is analogous to administering a loading dose of drug (see Chapter 2).

Ventilation rate and depth

The greater the ventilation of the lungs, the more anesthetic is delivered to the alveoli and to the brain, resulting in a more rapid induction. This factor is most significant during the initial phase of induction when the air of the lungs is mixing with, and being replaced by, the inspired gases. As the primary physiologic variable influencing the delivery of anesthetic to the lung, it is also important in replacing gas removed from the alveoli by the pulmonary circulation. In this regard, alveolar ventilation is of less importance with insoluble agents such as nitrous oxide and desflurane, which achieve high (near equilibrium) blood tensions rapidly, than it is with more soluble drugs.

Concentration and second gas effects

The **concentration effect** occurs when nitrous oxide, a relatively non-potent anesthetic, is administered in high concentrations (e.g., 70%) during induction of general anesthesia. Initially, nitrous oxide is taken up rapidly by the pulmonary circulation. This uptake would create a vacuum in the lungs were it not for the fact that fresh gas flows into the alveoli to replace the absorbed nitrous oxide. The net result is that alveolar ventilation is effectively increased, and more agent is available for absorption into the pulmonary circulation than would otherwise be the case. A second, related contribution to the concentration effect is that the alveolar concentration of nitrous oxide does not decrease as greatly between breaths as one would expect. If half of the alveolar nitrous oxide was absorbed when breathing 70% nitrous oxide, replacement by additional gas flow would keep the alveolar concentration of nitrous oxide around 65%. A potent anesthetic given in a concentration of 0.75% with air, for comparison, would yield an alveolar concentration of only 0.38% (only slightly more than half) after removal of half of the drug by the circulation because so little additional gas is included in the inspired gas mixture to offset the loss.

Although the concentration effect is negligible with potent drugs given in low concentrations, if a potent anesthetic is administered along with nitrous oxide, the potent anesthetic will also be delivered to the alveoli in increased amounts as gas rushes inward to replace the nitrous oxide absorbed by pulmonary blood. This phenomenon is called the ***second gas effect.*** Oxygen delivery to the lungs is also enhanced during induction of anesthesia by the second gas effect when nitrous oxide is administered in high concentrations.

Solubility in blood

Inhalation anesthetic solubility in blood is a major factor in the rate of induction of anesthesia. Solubility is generally expressed as the blood/gas partition coefficient, which, as previously mentioned, is the ratio of the concentration of the anesthetic gas in arterial blood to that in the alveolar air at 37 °C when the partial pressures in the two compartments are the same. The anesthetic gases are generally divided into three groups: agents of low solubility in blood (e.g., desflurane, nitrous oxide, and sevoflurane), agents of intermediate solubility (e.g., isoflurane), and agents of high solubility (e.g., older drugs such as halothane, methoxyflurane, and ether). The blood/gas partition coefficients and other related properties of the respective anesthetics are shown in Table 15-1. Physical properties are listed in Table 15-2.

If an agent is poorly soluble in blood, as is true of nitrous oxide and desflurane, only a small percentage of it is removed from the alveolar air before equilibrium is reached between pulmonary blood and alveolar gas. The alveolar concentration of gas increases quickly, the attainment of anesthetic concentrations in the brain is rapid, and the induction phase is short. For instance, nitrous oxide has a blood:gas solubility of approximately 0.5. Therefore, at equilibrium between the alveolar gas and pulmonary venous blood phases, there is a ratio of one molecule of nitrous oxide in the blood for every two molecules in the alveoli

TABLE 15-1 Properties of Inhalation Anesthetics

Anesthetic	Blood/Gas Partition Coefficient*	Brain/Blood Partition Coefficient	Fat/Blood Partition Coefficient	MAC (%)†
Nitrous oxide	0.47	1.1	2.3	104
Isoflurane	1.4	1.6	45	1.15
Desflurane	0.42	1.3	27	6
Sevoflurane	0.65	1.7	48	2.05

*All coefficients are taken at 37 °C.
†MAC is defined as the alveolar concentration (in volume %) of a gas necessary to prevent a skeletal muscle response to a standard surgical stimulus in 50% of patients.

TABLE 15-2 Physical Properties of Anesthetics

Agent	Molecular Weight	Boiling Point (°C [1 atm])	Vapor Pressure (mm Hg [20 °C])
Nitrous oxide	44	−88.5	38,770 (gas)
Desflurane	168	23.5	669
Isoflurane	184.5	48.5	238
Sevoflurane	200	58.6	157

(blood:gas solubility = 0.5 = 0.5:1 or 1:2). With agents of very high blood solubility, such as halothane (B:G solubility ~2.5), large fractions of gas are removed from the alveolar air that are dissolved in the blood, and large amounts have to be delivered over time from the inspired air before the uptake abates significantly. The alveolar tension increases slowly, and induction is similarly slow. At equilibrium, there are five molecules in the blood for every two molecules in the alveoli (blood:gas solubility = 2.5:1 or 5:2). Agents of intermediate solubility have an induction time slower than that of nitrous oxide and faster than that of halothane.

Inasmuch as recovery or emergence is essentially a reversal of the process of induction, anesthetics that are insoluble in blood leave the blood very rapidly after the anesthetic gas is removed from the inspired air, and recovery is very rapid. Conversely, recovery is slow with ether. High solubility is not completely disadvantageous, however, because transient fluctuations of the anesthetic's concentration in the inspired air during maintenance has little effect on the depth of anesthesia.

Cardiac output and blood flow

Cardiac output influences anesthetic uptake and onset of anesthesia in opposite ways. On the one hand, if the cardiac output is very high, it removes large quantities of gas from the alveoli and reduces the alveolar tension, delaying the achievement of equilibrium between inspired air and arterial blood. On the other hand, a high cardiac output delivers a greater amount of anesthetic to the tissues as a whole, hastening the rate at which the body comes to equilibrium with the arterial blood. Because the brain generally autoregulates its own blood flow, keeping flow relatively constant despite changes in cardiac output and arterial partial pressure, increasing total cardiac output generally slows the induction of general anesthesia since alveolar partial pressure, the key determinant in anesthetic uptake, is decreased during high cardiac output states.

The tissue uptake of an anesthetic agent depends on several parameters: the local blood flow, the arterial gas tension, and the blood/tissue coefficient, which varies according to the amount of lipid present. The uptake of anesthetic gases proceeds sequentially into three main compartments of the body, based on differences in vascularity and lipid content of the tissues. Initially, the most active compartment is the vessel-rich group (VRG), consisting of the heart, liver, kidneys, lungs, and brain. As previously stated, equilibration between blood and brain is usually very rapid because the brain receives a large share of the cardiac output and because the brain/blood coefficient is relatively low (see Table 15-1). Nitrous oxide is initially absorbed into the VRG compartment at a rate of 1 L/min for the first 10 to 15 minutes. The uptake decreases to less than 0.5 L/min over the next 1 to 1.5 hours, during which time the anesthetic fills the muscle compartment. If anesthetic administration is continued beyond this time, the uptake rate decreases still further (to <0.1 L/min) until the fat group of tissues is equilibrated. The sequence of isoflurane uptake is similar to that of nitrous oxide except that considerably more time is needed for equilibration of each compartment.

In patients who are mechanically ventilated, high concentrations of anesthetic may hasten anesthesia by inhibiting cardiac output. During induction, this effect increases the danger of overmedication when overpressurization is being used.

Elimination and biotransformation

The same factors that determine the uptake of anesthetic gas and the rate of induction are also important during the elimination phase. This process is initiated by the removal of the gas from the inspired air mixture so that the inspired air tension of anesthetic gas decreases to zero. When this happens, the anesthetic begins to diffuse from the blood through the alveoli, and as the blood tension decreases, there is a decrease in tissue tension. The less soluble the agent, the more completely and quickly the anesthetic is removed from the blood and tissues, and the more rapid is the recovery.

Although recovery might be considered a near mirror image of induction, several important differences do exist. The delivery of anesthetic to the lungs is not under the control of the clinician, but it is a function of the cardiopulmonary status of the patient. Also, many differences arise because anesthesia is normally terminated well before equilibrium with the inspired gas is attained in the various tissue compartments, at least for anesthetics other than nitrous oxide. Often muscle and fat continue to absorb anesthetic from blood and the VRG for some time after administration has ceased. A possible outcome of this redistribution is a rapid recovery from short anesthetic courses.

Nevertheless, the high fat/blood partition coefficients of most agents indicate that anesthetic retention may last for many hours and that recovery from prolonged anesthesia can be delayed. A final disparity between induction and recovery is the influence of metabolism. It was long believed that inhalation anesthetics were eliminated through the lungs without any metabolic transformation. It is now recognized, however, that many agents are biotransformed in the liver, particularly many of the older agents. Newer agents display relatively minimal metabolism, with sevoflurane being the greatest at <5%, while the other currently used agents are fractions of 1%. Table 15-3 lists, for each currently used, the percentage of agent metabolized.

Pharmacologic Effects of Inhalation Anesthetics

The potency of inhalational anesthetic agents is determined by its "**minimum alveolar concentration,**" commonly referred to as MAC. This is defined as the minimal concentration of the inhalational anesthetic agent in the alveolus that prevents movement of 50% of patients following surgical stimulation, specifically a skin incision. Doses of inhaled agents are expressed as percent of total gas mixture, as opposed to milligrams as with oral or parenteral drugs. $MAC_{99\%}$ refers to the anesthetic concentration at which 99% of patients will not move during surgical skin incision and is 1.3 times MAC.

TABLE 15-3 Pharmacologic Properties of Inhalation Anesthetics

Attribute or Effect	Nitrous Oxide	Isoflurane	Desflurane	Sevoflurane
Analgesia	Good	Moderate	Moderate	Moderate
Muscle relaxation	None	Good	Good	Moderate
Heart rate	May increase	Increased	Increased	Unchanged
Myocardial depression	Mild	Moderate	Moderate	Moderate
Cardiac output	Unchanged	Unchanged	Unchanged	Decreased
Vascular resistance	Unchanged	Decreased	Decreased	Decreased
Blood pressure	Unchanged	Decreased	Decreased	Decreased
Arrhythmogenic potential	None	Low	Low	Low
Respiratory depression	Mild	Moderate–marked	Marked	Moderate–marked
Respiratory rate	Slightly increased	Increased	Increased	Increased
Tidal volume	Decreased	Decreased	Decreased	Decreased
Bronchi	No effect	Dilation	Brief constriction	Dilation
Airway irritation	None	Moderate	Marked	Mild
EEG activity	No effect	Depressed	Depressed	Depressed
Renal function	No effect	Decreased	Decreased	Decreased
Biotransformation	0.004%	0.2%	0.02%	2-5%
Hepatotoxicity	None	Rare	Rare	None

EEG, Electroencephalography.

Cardiovascular system

All inhalation agents depress myocardial contractility; the extent is related to the potency of the particular agent used, its concentration, and the duration of anesthesia. As a group, the halogenated anesthetics cause significant changes in cardiovascular parameters. Cardiac rates are variably influenced, and the anesthetic effects may be masked by the preoperative administration of atropine or glycopyrrolate, both of which block activity of the vagus nerve. Some agents may indirectly increase sympathetic tone by depressing respiration or arterial blood pressure. Nevertheless, baroreceptor sensitivity, as measured by a change in heart rate in response to a vasoactive drug, is generally depressed.

All currently used potent inhalation agents cause a dose-dependent decrease in mean arterial pressure due to decreased peripheral vascular resistance, while nitrous oxide may increase it mildly. Heart rate increases occur at lower concentrations of isoflurane (0.25%), at intermediate concentrations with desflurane (1%), and with higher concentrations of sevoflurane (1.5%). Sudden increases in desflurane concentration can increase in heart rate, although this wanes as anesthesia is maintained.

Respiration

The effect of most anesthetics on the respiratory centers in the brain is depression; the amount of respiratory depression is related to the type and concentration of anesthetic used. Respiratory depression with inhalation anesthetics, measured by decreased medullary responsiveness to carbon dioxide tensions, is associated with a progressive decline in tidal volume. This effect is accompanied by a pronounced increase in respiratory rate but not enough to maintain minute ventilation. The most sensitive component of respiration to inhalation anesthetics is the ventilatory response to hypoxemia. Peripheral chemoreceptors that normally respond to low oxygen tensions are strongly inhibited by concentrations of 0.1 MAC and become completely inoperative during general anesthesia. Hypercarbia resulting from depressed ventilatory exchange excites the sympathoadrenal system, causing a release of catecholamines. When breathing is impaired, increased oxygen tensions or mechanical respiratory assistance may be necessary.

Liver

Liver function tests indicate that almost all inhalation anesthetic agents cause some alterations in hepatic function. In most cases, the effects are reversible and not serious. Halothane was associated with serious hepatic necrosis, however, especially if the patient had prior anesthesia with halothane or has preexisting liver disease.

Kidney

General anesthetics depress glomerular filtration and urine output by reducing renal blood flow. These alterations in renal function are generally transitory and readily reversible. Older agents, such as methoxyflurane, caused the release of F^- that occasionally produced serious renal damage, which led to its discontinued use in North America.

Skeletal muscle

Although most general anesthetics produce muscle relaxation by their actions on spinal cord and brainstem motor reflex centers, the volatile anesthetic agents have an additional effect on the neuromuscular junction. Ether is most prominent in this respect and can produce sufficient muscle relaxation by itself for surgical procedures. Even agents with a lesser degree of action, such as isoflurane, can decrease the required dose of neuromuscular blockers by 65%. Cholinesterase inhibition by neostigmine does not antagonize this effect as it does for such nondepolarizing blocking agents as *cis*-atracurium and vecuronium.

SPECIFIC INHALATION AGENTS

Gases and volatile liquids are the oldest known anesthetic agents and have been the most widely used. Today, the only commonly used gas is nitrous oxide. Although general anesthetic agents administered by inhalation are often divided into gases and volatile liquids, there are few differences between these two classes of substances other than boiling point (see Table 15-2) and effects in various tissues (see Table 15-3). Regarding boiling point, which determines the vapor pressure of the gaseous phase, liquids need vaporizers, which produce and maintain an adequate amount of anesthetic in the inspired air. Because tissue solubility (i.e., solubility in brain membranes) is normally greater with the volatile liquids than gases, a smaller concentration of volatile agent is required in the inspired air to produce general anesthesia. An ideal inhalation anesthetic should possess numerous characteristics, as outlined in Box 15-1.

BOX 15-1 Ideal Characteristics of an Inhalation Agent

Stable in light, alkali, and soda lime
Nonflammable
Highly potent, allowing use with high concentrations of oxygen
Low solubility in blood to allow rapid induction and rapid recovery
No or minimal biotransformation
No toxicity
Nonirritating to respiratory mucosa
Minimal cardiovascular and respiratory effects

Ether (diethyl ether) was the most widely used volatile anesthetic in the century that followed the first successful demonstration of general anesthesia in 1846. It is the basis for Guedel's stages of anesthesia. Ether has been superseded by newer inhalation agents and is rarely used as a general anesthetic in North America.

Halothane was one of the most widely used anesthetics after its introduction into clinical anesthesia in the 1950s. Its use in developed countries has greatly declined with the introduction of newer volatile agents, and it is no longer marketed in the United States. Its cardiovascular effects and potential for hepatotoxicity led to its replacement by the newer volatile agents.

Malignant hyperthermia (MH) is a rare adverse effect of general anesthesia involving all volatile inhalation anesthetics (this does not include nitrous oxide) and the neuromuscular blocking drug succinylcholine. In the United States, the incidence of MH is 1:50,000 in adults and 1:15,000 in children. It is a genetic disorder of multifactorial etiology. Most cases are associated with mutations in the ryanodine receptor (type 1), which forms a Ca^{2+} channel in the sarcoplasmic reticulum and is involved in Ca^{2+}-induced Ca^{2+} release. MH has been associated with some inherited muscular disorders, such as the muscular dystrophies, but at least 80 genetic defects have been associated with MH.

An acute crisis of MH is a hypercatabolic reaction that often manifests initially as masseter or generalized muscle rigidity; other early signs include elevation of oxygen use and carbon dioxide production, tachypnea, and tachycardia. Cardiovascular instability, cardiac dysrhythmias, electrolyte disturbances, and elevation in temperature are other classic signs. The body temperature, often unaffected early in an acute attack, progressively increases to alarming and sometimes fatal levels. The elevated heat production, associated with increased Ca^{2+} concentrations in the myoplasm and hypermetabolic activity of skeletal muscle, is responsible for the hyperthermia.

Immediately on recognition, all triggering agents should be discontinued, and hyperventilation with 100% oxygen should be instituted. **Dantrolene**, an inhibitor of Ca^{2+} transport (see Chapter 7), must be administered intravenously as soon as possible because this drug provides lifesaving, definitive treatment. Dantrolene should be administered as a bolus intravenously at a dose of 2 to 3 mg/kg and then titrated in response to the patient's clinical condition. If present, metabolic acidosis and any dysrhythmias or electrolyte disturbances should be treated. Cooling in the form of cold intravenous solutions, packing the patient in ice, and ice water lavage of body cavities should be performed to increase heat loss and reduce body temperature. Effective treatment rendered quickly after prompt recognition of MH has reduced its mortality rate from 70% to less than 10%.

Nitrous Oxide

Nitrous oxide is arguably the oldest general anesthetic agent and the only gaseous anesthetic currently in use. Nitrous oxide is also the only inorganic substance used clinically as an anesthetic. Several features unique to nitrous oxide among available agents include a MAC greater than 100%, strong analgesic properties in subanesthetic concentrations, and minimal relaxation of skeletal muscle.

Physical and chemical properties

Nitrous oxide is a colorless, nonirritating gas with a pleasant, mild odor and taste. The structural formula is shown in Figure 15-4. Its **blood/gas partition coefficient of 0.47** means that it is poorly soluble in blood. It is nonflammable but can support combustion in the absence of oxygen. It is available in pressurized steel cylinders as a liquid in equilibrium with its gas phase. As the nitrous oxide gas is delivered from the cylinder, liquid nitrous oxide spontaneously vaporizes to replace the lost gas phase. Cylinder pressure is maintained unaltered by this process until all the liquid has vaporized, at which point approximately 80% of the contents have been released. This vaporization process requires heat, which is provided from the cylinder and the air around it, causing the tank to become cold with use.

Anesthetic properties

Because of its very low solubility in blood, a state of equilibrium between the alveolar and arterial tensions is quickly reached, allowing induction and awakening to occur very rapidly. The primary disadvantage of nitrous oxide as a general anesthetic is its lack of potency, as reflected by its high MAC of approximately 104%. (A concentration above 100% value is unobtainable at ambient conditions due to hypoxia but is achieved by placing the subject in a hyperbaric chamber.) At normal concentrations and when given with adequate amounts of oxygen, nitrous oxide is incapable of producing full surgical anesthesia by itself, and it is most commonly used as a supplement to volatile anesthetics. To ensure adequate oxygenation of the patient, nitrous oxide is normally not used at a concentration greater than 70%. When it is administered with other anesthetic agents, the maintenance concentration normally used is 50% to 70%.

In dentistry, nitrous oxide is usually administered in subanesthetic concentrations of 20% to 50% via nasal hood to provide minimal to moderate sedation and analgesia. Concentrations above this range may impair the patient's ability to maintain consciousness and lead to a greater incidence of adverse effects, such as nausea or dysphoria. At a 40% concentration, there is good hard and soft tissue analgesia. Awareness of sensory input is reduced, with the exception that sounds may seem louder and qualitatively different.

When nitrous oxide is used with a more potent agent, it is possible to reduce the concentration of the other drug and still achieve a more rapid induction and a shorter recovery period. This phenomenon is a reflection of the fact that the MAC of the rapidly acting nitrous oxide is additive with that of other, slower acting inhalation anesthetics. The addition of 70% nitrous oxide, which is approximately 0.6 MAC, reduces the MAC of isoflurane from 1.15% to 0.5%, a 60% reduction. This additive effect is less pronounced for sevoflurane, particularly in children. In addition, the concentration and second gas effects described earlier can help hasten the onset of anesthesia.

Cardiovascular effects

In contrast to the volatile anesthetics in current use, nitrous oxide does not usually produce any clinically significant cardiovascular effects. It has a weak, dose-dependent myocardial depressant effect and a mild sympathomimetic effect. These opposing influences tend to cancel each other, leading to minimal to no change in cardiac output. Patients at increased risk of the cardiac depressant effects of nitrous oxide include patients with chronic hypertension, left ventricular failure, and advanced atherosclerotic disease.

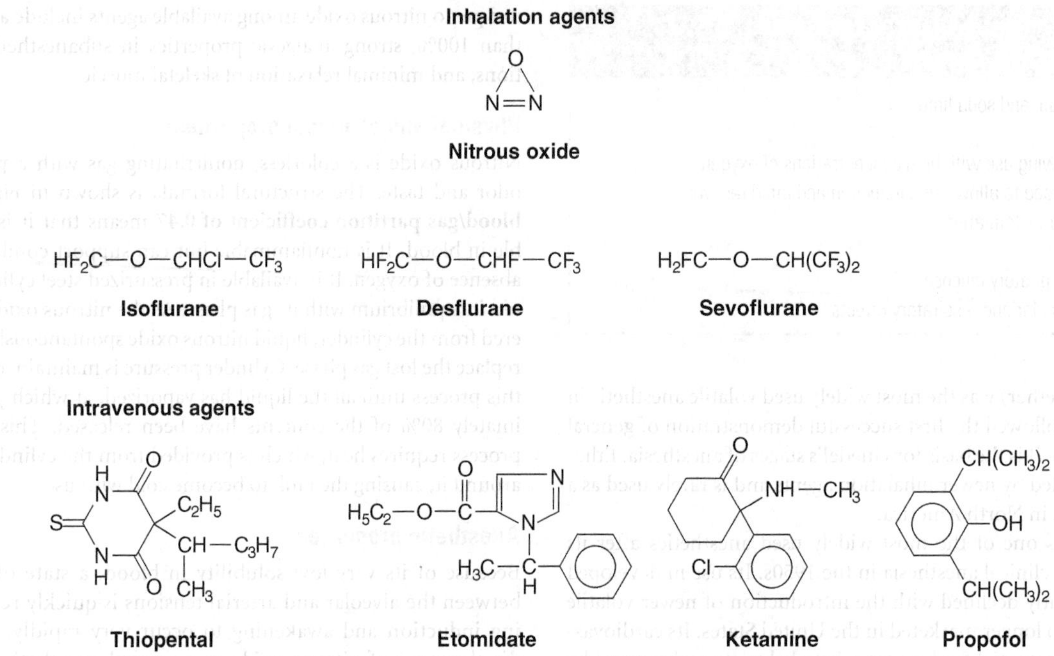

Inhalation agents

Nitrous oxide

$HF_2C—O—CHCl—CF_3$
Isoflurane

$HF_2C—O—CHF—CF_3$
Desflurane

$H_2FC—O—CH(CF_3)_2$
Sevoflurane

Intravenous agents

Thiopental

Etomidate

Ketamine

Propofol

FIG 15-4 Structural formulas of anesthetic drugs.

Respiratory effects

Nitrous oxide is not a strong respiratory depressant, but it decreases tidal volume and increases respiratory rate. Even so, there is likely to be less respiratory depression than would be caused by an equal depth of anesthesia induced by a single potent anesthetic drug. Although nitrous oxide has little effect on respiration in normal individuals, whose ventilation is regulated by the arterial carbon dioxide tension ($PaCO_2$), patients with severe chronic obstructive pulmonary disease whose ventilatory drive depends on the arterial oxygen tension may become severely hypoxic on exposure to even sedative concentrations of anesthetic. Even if hypoxemia is prevented by the high concentration of oxygen that is being coadministered (which by itself blunts the hypoxic drive for respiration), hypoventilation and respiratory acidosis are likely outcomes.

Elimination

Nitrous oxide is eliminated unchanged in the exhaled gas; however, 0.004% undergoes reductive metabolism to nitrogen by bacteria in the gastrointestinal tract.

Adverse effects

When used for sedation, nitrous oxide usually provides a feeling of relaxation, along with the possible symptoms of body warmth, tingling of the hands and feet, circumoral numbness, auditory effects, and euphoria. As the dose increases, the patient is more likely to develop adverse symptoms such as dysphoria and nausea. Some patients may develop acute tolerance to these effects.

For general anesthesia where concentrations of 50% to 70% are used, and because its solubility in blood greatly exceeds that of nitrogen, nitrous oxide increases the volume of any **enclosed air pocket** in the body. This is because nitrous oxide enters a closed space faster than the similar concentration of nitrogen (79%) in ambient air can leave that space. There are several situations in which this property can be problematic: with a pneumothorax or lung bullae as in emphysema, an obstructed bowel, a blocked eustachian tube (with potential damage to the tympanic membrane), or after eye surgery that uses intraocular gases. With respect to **vitreoretinal surgery**, such as the surgical repair of retinal detachments and macular holes, perfluoropropane or sulfur hexafluoride is introduced within the eye to act as a tamponading agent. These gases may persist in the eye for up to 3 months. Administration of general anesthesia during this interval has led to case reports of irreversible loss of vision. These case reports suggest that nitrous oxide should be avoided in patients who have had vitreoretinal surgery with intraocular gas infusion in the past 3 months.

High concentrations of nitrous oxide, particularly when given for long periods of time, may also result in a considerable accumulation of dissolved gas within the body, and when the administration is stopped, large volumes of nitrous oxide diffuse from the blood into the lung alveoli, diluting oxygen. This temporary reduction in the amount of alveolar oxygen is termed ***diffusion hypoxia*** and can be prevented by administering 100% oxygen for 3 to 5 minutes after the cessation of nitrous oxide.

Nitrous oxide is not acutely toxic, but it can **affect DNA synthesis** by inducing changes in folate and amino acid metabolism. Its administration leads to an increase in homocysteine and 5-methyltetrahydrofolate. Nitrous oxide oxidizes the cobalt atom in vitamin B_{12}, which renders inactive the vitamin B_{12}–dependent enzyme methionine synthase. Methionine synthase is required to form the essential amino acid methionine (from homocysteine) and to transform 5-methyltetrahydrofolate into an active form for subsequent reactions. The enzyme is quickly inactivated in vivo by brief exposures to nitrous oxide. This inactivation increases with the nitrous oxide concentration and duration of exposure, is permanent, and requires synthesis of new enzyme for restoration of normal metabolism. Methionine deficiency is believed to be associated with degenerative nervous system changes. It has been suggested that preoperative administration of methionine may counteract some of the adverse effects of nitrous oxide on the hematologic and nervous systems, and methionine has been used in the treatment of nitrous oxide–induced neuropathy.

Continuous inhalation of nitrous oxide can result in **altered hematopoiesis** because of the suppression of DNA synthesis. Patients exposed to 50% nitrous oxide for 6 hours may begin to show evidence of impaired thymidylate metabolism; hematopoietic changes suggestive of pernicious anemia occur after 24 hours of continuous inhalation. Intermittent exposures have a cumulative effect if spaced more frequently than once every 3 to 4 days. These findings have limited the use of nitrous oxide as an analgesic agent for extended use and for procedures that must be repeated often, such as debridement of burned skin.

The inhibition of methionine synthesis by nitrous oxide has been associated with an increased risk of myocardial ischemia in patients undergoing vascular surgery. Patients at special risk include patients with genetic mutations that cause a deficiency in 5,10-methylenetetrahydrofolate reductase activity. This enzyme generates the 5-methyltetrahydrofolate required for methionine synthesis; its deficiency potentiates the pathway block caused by nitrous oxide. This concern, as well as the increased risk of postoperative nausea and vomiting, has prompted many anesthesiologists to abandon the use of nitrous oxide for any patient with known or suspected cardiovascular disease regardless of surgical procedure. Pretreatment with B vitamin supplements for 1 week before anesthesia can prevent the hyperhomocysteinemia believed to cause these adverse effects. More recent studies have not shown a detrimental cardiovascular effect but the use of nitrous oxide for medical surgery has decreased significantly in many parts of the world. There were contradictory data on effects on myocardial infarction, yet no difference in mortality. The proposed mechanism was N_2O effect on homocysteine. Later studies questioned these conclusions (see Leslie et al., 2013 reference) stating that an appropriately designed large randomized control trial is needed to determine exact relationship. More recent studies (see Turan et al., reference) have concluded that intraoperative nitrous oxide was associated with decreased, rather than increased, morbidity and mortality. A well-controlled recent study determined that nitrous oxide had no negative cardiovascular effects for at-risk patients in non-cardiac surgery, did not lead to increased surgical site infection, but did increase the frequency of postoperative nausea and vomiting (see Myles et al., 2014 reference). Therefore the evidence **does not support** the suggestion that nitrous oxide effects are significant on predisposition to **cardiovascular complications**.

Similar to other mood-altering drugs, nitrous oxide may be abused by individuals with access to the drug, including members of the dental profession. This abuse is associated with myeloneuropathic changes indicative of a pernicious anemia–like syndrome: numbness and paresthesia, muscular weakness and incoordination, altered spinal reflexes, impotence, and shooting sensations on flexion of the neck (Lhermitte sign).

Nitrous oxide has been shown to inhibit the release of luteinizing hormone–releasing hormone by the hypothalamus, which theoretically may impair fertility. Potential reproductive toxicity has also been proposed to be caused by the sympathomimetic effects of nitrous oxide leading to vasoconstriction and diminished uterine blood flow. Clinical use in pregnant women carries no apparent increased risk to the fetus, however, over other acceptable forms of pain control. Long-term exposure has been strongly implicated in other reproductive abnormalities, such as spontaneous abortion and impaired fertility, but these effects have not been substantiated by controlled prospective studies.

Retrospective surveys have provided evidence that operating room personnel (surgeons, anesthesiologists, nurses) and dentists and their employees exposed to nitrous oxide may be adversely affected by trace amounts of inhalation anesthetics. Specifically, exposed health care workers reported a higher incidence of hepatic, renal, and neurologic disorders; increased congenital malformations in children born to exposed women; and increased spontaneous abortions in exposed women and wives of exposed men.

Animal studies indicate that nitrous oxide is an agent of major concern and that the threshold concentration of nitrous oxide for producing a biologic response is approximately 500 to 1000 ppm. Although retrospective studies that used examination of public health registries could find no link between working in an operating room (or being exposed to anesthetic gases) and increased risk of miscarriage or congenital malformation. Reproductive toxicity in dental assistants has been linked to nitrous oxide exposure of more than 3 to 5 hours per week (See Rowland et al., reference) Most authorities therefore favor using anesthetic delivery devices in conjunction with **scavenger exhaust systems** and ventilation systems that remove leaked anesthetic gases from the vicinity of the patient. Because many dentists function as sedationist and surgeon, the nonrebreathing flow machine is most commonly used. Its simplicity of operation and compatibility with minimal to moderate sedation is coupled with the major disadvantage of exposing operatory personnel to potentially high concentrations of anesthetic gases (i.e., nitrous oxide) unless a concerted effort is made to minimize pollution, as was outlined in Box 15-2. The National Institute for Occupational Safety and Health has prepared a monograph (see reference) to assist dentists in minimizing exposure to nitrous oxide in the workplace. There is the possibility that long-term exposure to trace concentrations of nitrous oxide may be a health hazard to dental office and operating room personnel. An early report of inhaled concentrations of as little as 50 ppm over a 2-hour span causing impairment in audiovisual performance tasks has not been reproduced (see Bruce and Bach, reference). Nevertheless, this finding prompted the National Institute for Occupational Safety and Health to recommend 25 ppm as a maximum permissible time-weighted exposure limit per anesthetic administration for all health care workers. This level may not be achievable with some existing scavenging systems, so other measures (e.g., using rubber dam, using high-velocity suction, limiting the patient's talking) must be used to minimize the gas escaping into the room.

BOX 15-2 Steps to Reduce Nitrous Oxide Exposure

Facility and Equipment Preparation

- Purchase scavenging nitrous oxide delivery systems with air sweeper capabilities
- Check plumbing for leaks by pressure retention of closed system
- Check all fittings for leaks with disclosing solution or nitrous oxide analyzer
- Ensure exhaust system vents to the outside away from air intake
- Maximize room air circulation
- Consider use of a local exhaust system

Daily Use

- Adjust vacuum setting to manufacturer 's maximum recommended value
- Place hood on nose before administering nitrous oxide
- Adjust flow to patient 's minute respiratory volume
- Instruct patient to exhale through nose
- Instruct patient not to talk
- Use rubber dam whenever possible
- Use high-vacuum suction when mouth is open
- Administer 100% oxygen for 3 to 5 minutes before removing hood

Monitoring

- Inspect delivery apparatus each day of use, particularly the reservoir bag
- Periodically monitor exposure by passive dosimetry or nitrous oxide analyzer
- Record monitoring results

Therapeutic uses

Nitrous oxide is a widely used inhalation anesthetic and continues to play a role in the delivery of medical and dental anesthesia. It is valuable in reducing the concentration of volatile anesthetics during inhalation anesthesia and as a component of "balanced anesthesia." Historically, nitrous oxide was first used for dental surgery, but with the advent of local anesthetics, it was replaced as the drug of choice for providing pain control sufficient for most dental procedures. Since the late 1950s, there has been an upsurge in the use of nitrous oxide, not to provide dental surgical anesthesia, but to provide relief from anxiety in the form of minimal to moderate sedation. In this role, it is often the agent of first choice. Its therapeutic application in dentistry is described in Chapter 38. Conversely, its use for general anesthesia in medicine is declining because of the increasing reliance on intravenous anesthesia coupled with concerns about occupational exposure to the gas and previously reported cardiovascular concerns.

Isoflurane

After its release in the United States in 1981, **isoflurane** became the most widely used volatile anesthetic. It is an isomer of enflurane, which was a halogenated methyl ethyl ether introduced into clinical use in the United States in 1972, but since withdrawn from use. Isoflurane combines the desirable cardiovascular properties of enflurane with a freedom from seizure activity and less respiratory depression and hepatic metabolism. Although the newer, less soluble volatile anesthetics are more frequently used in the United States, isoflurane is less expensive and remains a useful anesthetic for many purposes.

Physical and chemical properties

The **blood/gas partition coefficient of 1.4** for isoflurane results in a slower onset of action compared with sevoflurane and desflurane. Isoflurane is chemically stable, nonflammable, and marketed in brown glass bottles. The vapor is pungent and irritating to breathe.

Anesthetic properties

Isoflurane is the most potent of the currently used volatile anesthetics (MAC of 1.15%). Inhalation induction should theoretically be relatively rapid with isoflurane, but it is limited by its pungent odor, which, if induction is allowed to proceed too rapidly, leads to breath holding, laryngospasm, and coughing. This problem is usually overcome by inducing the patient with an intravenous agent prior to administering isoflurane. Isoflurane is sufficiently potent to provide muscle relaxation adequate for any surgical procedure, but neuromuscular blocking agents are normally used for procedures that require profound muscle relaxation instead of the high concentrations of anesthetic needed to secure muscle relaxation. As with other potent inhalation anesthetics, isoflurane increases the action of the nondepolarizing neuromuscular blocking drugs.

Cardiovascular effects

Similar to all volatile anesthetics, isoflurane produces a dose-dependent depression of myocardial contractility, but it is similar to that of desflurane and sevoflurane. Isoflurane also causes coronary vasodilation, mostly at the distal (resistance) arterioles. Although this effect may be beneficial for heart muscle, it was also proposed to cause "coronary steal" in patients with ischemic heart disease, a situation in which blood flow is redistributed from myocardial tissues supplied by atherosclerotic arteries to areas with healthy coronary vessels. Coronary steal develops only when the coronary perfusion pressure is decreased, is more likely to occur with excessive tachycardia, and is most probably not a special concern with isoflurane. Cardiac output is well maintained with isoflurane, even though stroke volume is decreased, by virtue of an increase in the heart rate, showing isoflurane's relatively good preservation of baroreceptor reflexes. Decreases in arterial blood pressure are similar to the other volatile agents in equal MAC doses. Isoflurane does not significantly sensitize the heart to dysrhythmias; the permissible tissue injected dose of epinephrine during isoflurane anesthesia is at least 7 mcg/kg. Maximum local anesthetic doses would be reached well before this dose of epinephrine in local anesthetic solutions.

Respiratory effects

Respiratory depression manifests as a decreased ventilatory response to hypercapnia with a complete loss of sensitivity to hypoxia. Isoflurane increases respiratory rate only up to 1 MAC. Bronchodilation is similar to other volatile agents.

Other effects

Isoflurane depresses cerebral metabolism and cerebral metabolic requirement for oxygen. It is a cerebral vasodilator, however. Isoflurane causes little change in the cerebrospinal fluid pressure and does not significantly alter cerebrospinal fluid production. All these effects intracranially can be beneficial in neurosurgery.

Metabolism

Biotransformation of isoflurane is quite low (≤0.2%). This finding suggests that it is neither nephrotoxic nor hepatotoxic, a conclusion supported by observations that repeated and prolonged exposures to isoflurane have not caused hepatorenal injury in animals. Although there are a few case reports of hepatic necrosis after isoflurane administration, it is currently believed that isoflurane is highly unlikely to be responsible for postoperative hepatotoxicity.

Therapeutic uses

Isoflurane is a suitable drug whenever a potent inhalation anesthetic is to be administered, except when a mask induction of anesthesia is contemplated. In pediatric patients, induction with isoflurane is more likely to elicit coughing, salivation, and laryngospasm than induction with sevoflurane. These effects can be prevented by prior administration of an intravenous induction agent. Isoflurane has numerous advantages: it is chemically stable, nonflammable, and potent; induction is rapid, and muscle relaxation is adequate; and it is not dysrhythmogenic or toxic to the kidneys or liver. Isoflurane depresses the cardiovascular and respiratory systems. It is also contraindicated in patients with a history of malignant hyperthermia.

Desflurane

Desflurane, approved for clinical use in 1992, is the first volatile anesthetic agent whose **blood/gas partition coefficient (0.42)** compares favorably with that of nitrous oxide (0.47). The theoretic advantages desflurane should have regarding rapid induction and recovery of anesthesia are partially offset by the drug's tendency to irritate the airway during induction. Nevertheless, desflurane is particularly suited for ambulatory anesthesia and is commonly used for other situations in which an inhalation anesthetic is indicated. Also, the increased cost of desflurane is counterbalanced by the faster recovery of the patient.

Physical and chemical properties

Desflurane is chemically very similar to isoflurane, with only a single substitution of fluorine for a chlorine atom (see Fig. 15-4). Desflurane shows marked chemical stability, possibly because of the additional fluorine, which provides resistance to break down in soda lime and to biotransformation. The anesthetic has a high vapor pressure of 664 mm Hg at 20 °C, becomes a gas (vapor pressure 760 mm Hg) at

23 °C, and is not flammable at concentrations less than 17%. The low potency and high volatility of desflurane require the use of a heated vaporizer to enable precise delivery of this agent.

Anesthetic properties

The low solubility of desflurane in blood results in rapid onset, recovery, and adjustment of anesthetic depth, similar to that found with nitrous oxide. A propensity to cause breath holding, coughing, and laryngospasm during mask induction precludes its routine use as a primary induction agent.

With a MAC of 6% (in middle-aged adults), desflurane is less potent than the other volatile agents. Its physiologic effects are similar, however, to those induced by isoflurane. The systemic vascular resistance, mean arterial blood pressure, and stroke volume are reduced, but the cardiac output is maintained by a progressive increase in heart rate. Discernible increases in heart rate occur as the anesthetic concentration exceeds 1.25 MAC. Similar to isoflurane, desflurane theoretically may cause coronary steal in hypotensive cardiac patients. There is no significant sensitization of the myocardium to catecholamines. Desflurane causes a dose-related decrease in tidal volume and, despite an increase in the respiratory rate, a significant depression of minute ventilation. As with other halogenated ethers, respiratory depression is reduced if desflurane is used with nitrous oxide for anesthesia.

Desflurane is contraindicated in patients susceptible to malignant hyperthermia because it can trigger the syndrome in the swine model and has been linked to malignant hyperthermia in the clinical setting. Because desflurane is notable for having minimal biotransformation, it has a very low likelihood for causing serious hepatotoxicity.

Therapeutic uses

Despite its favorable blood/gas partition coefficient, desflurane is not indicated for the inhalation induction of anesthesia. When anesthesia has been achieved with other agents, desflurane may be administered for maintenance purposes. Desflurane then permits a more rapid control over the depth of anesthesia than other inhalation agents and a more rapid recovery, allowing for a more precise duration of general anesthesia.

Sevoflurane

First synthesized in the United States in 1968, sevoflurane became widely used in Japan in 1990 and available for clinical use in the United States in 1995. A relatively pleasant odor, lack of airway irritation, and rapid onset of action make sevoflurane an attractive agent for inhalation induction of anesthesia in pediatrics.

Physical and chemical properties

Sevoflurane is characterized by a low **blood/gas partition coefficient (0.65)** and chemical stability under normal storage conditions. A potential drawback is the agent's reactivity to chemicals (e.g., soda lime) used as carbon dioxide absorbents.

Anesthetic properties

As would be expected, the low solubility of sevoflurane results in rapid onset, recovery, and adjustment of anesthetic depth. The benefit of the low blood:gas solubility in regard to offset of anesthesia is counterbalanced in longer cases (>2 hours) where transfer into fat can occur. Similar to other volatile agents in current use, sevoflurane is relatively potent, with a MAC of 2%. Sevoflurane undergoes oxidative defluorination by the hepatic enzyme CYP2E1. This same enzyme may also be largely responsible for the degradation of isoflurane and desflurane. The degree of **biotransformation** is approximately **2% to 5%**, with plasma inorganic F^- concentrations similar to those previously found in patients with renal dysfunction after methoxyflurane anesthesia. However, plasma F^- declines much more rapidly with sevoflurane, a lack of renal metabolism precludes excessive formation of F^- in kidney cells, and there is no evidence of nephrotoxicity in humans. Sevoflurane is not believed to be hepatotoxic because it is not broken down to yield the trifluoroacetyl halide metabolite.

The cardiovascular effects induced by sevoflurane are somewhat similar to isoflurane. At 1 MAC, sevoflurane causes a decrease in cardiac output, peripheral vascular resistance, and arterial blood pressure. At greater than 1 MAC, further decreases in peripheral vascular resistance and myocardial contractility are partially offset by an increase in heart rate. Sevoflurane does not significantly sensitize the myocardium to catecholamines. There is a decrease in alveolar ventilation similar to that observed with isoflurane.

Therapeutic uses

Sevoflurane has the advantages of a rapid onset, good control over the depth of anesthesia, and a rapid recovery, as previously noted for desflurane. One important advantage of sevoflurane over desflurane is that it is much less irritating to the respiratory tract, which, combined with its rapid induction and maintenance of heart rate, makes it suitable for inhalation induction of anesthesia in children. A potential drawback is that it breaks down in soda lime to compound A, greatly limiting its potential use in low-flow systems with conventional carbon dioxide absorbers. This problem can be circumvented by avoiding low gas flows (<2 L/min) or by using specific carbon dioxide absorbents without this characteristic. One other drawback is the potential for emergence agitation when used in pediatric patients.

INTRAVENOUS AGENTS

Intravenous agents are used widely in anesthesiology. Historically, their primary role was as single-dose induction agents prior to maintenance of general anesthesia with inhalation agents. In recent years, they have also been commonly used for maintenance of general anesthesia in "total intravenous anesthesia" (TIVA) and for various modes of sedation, as described earlier. TIVA has increased in popularity because of **(1)** the introduction of drugs with rapid redistribution and/or shorter elimination half-lives, **(2)** freedom from the risk of malignant hyperthermia associated with volatile anesthetics, and **(3)** continued concern regarding occupational exposure to inhalation agents. For this technique, the drugs are ideally administered by continuous infusion via a computer-controlled pump, with intermittent boluses as needed to adjust the anesthetic depth rapidly.

The primary clinical advantage of intravenous agents is their rapid distribution into the VRG of tissues, which includes the brain. Reduced cardiovascular depression is an additional advantage. The rapid uptake into the CNS due to their high lipid solubility facilitates a rapid onset of action. For most intravenous anesthetics, the termination of effect depends largely on redistribution of the drug out of the brain. Metabolic inactivation generally assumes a more central role when the agent is administered over an extended period. With the exception of the benzodiazepines and dexmedetomidine, these drugs can easily induce anesthesia, at which time maintenance may be carried out by either inhalation agents or continued infusion of the intravenous drug. Suggested ideal properties for an intravenous anesthetic drug are listed in Box 15-3.

Although short-acting and ultrashort-acting barbiturates were previously widely administered to produce all modes of anesthesia and sedation, drugs from other classes are now used more frequently. These

BOX 15-3 Characteristics of an Ideal Intravenous Anesthetic Agent

Physical Properties	Pharmacokinetic Properties	Pharmacodynamic Properties
Soluble in water	Rapid onset of action	Reliable induction of anesthesia
Stable in solution	Ability to titrate	Anxiolytic at subanesthetic doses
Stable to light exposure	Predictable duration of effect	Analgesic at subanesthetic doses
Absence of pain on injection	Short duration of effect	Amnestic at subanesthetic doses
No local irritation	Short elimination half-life	Antinauseant at subanesthetic doses
Long shelf life	Rapid recovery	Minimal respiratory effects
	Rapid biotransformation	Minimal cardiovascular effects
	Inactive metabolites	No effects on other systems
	Nontoxic metabolites	High therapeutic index
		Small interindividual variation
		No allergy

agents include various combinations of antianxiety/sedative drugs, opioids, and anesthetics such as propofol and ketamine. The relatively short action of most of these drugs and their relative freedom from emetic properties (except for opioids and ketamine) make their use especially suited for sedation or general anesthesia in dentistry. The basic pharmacologic features of many intravenous agents are discussed elsewhere in this book, and a more complete review of their use in the control of fear and anxiety for the dental patient is provided in Chapter 38.

Barbiturates

Ultrashort-acting barbiturates were the first drugs widely adopted as intravenous anesthetics. Much of what is known about intravenous anesthesia was developed through their use. Barbiturates available for this purpose included thiopental and methohexital. The use of both drugs has greatly diminished since the introduction of propofol, described subsequently. In fact, thiopental is not available in the United States.

Thiopental

Thiopental, the thiobarbiturate analogue of the oxybarbiturate pentobarbital, was the most commonly used intravenous barbiturate in medicine and is prototypic of the group. Due to its use in executions in the United States, the main manufacturers in the European Union no longer allow export of thiopental to the US. Its molecular structure is depicted in Figure 15-4. Further information on thiopental is available in the 6th edition of this text.

Methohexital

Methohexital, a methylated barbiturate, is rarely used for the induction of general anesthesia in hospital operating rooms, but it has been used more widely for anesthesia in dentistry. The sleep time after a single dose is 5 to 7 minutes, and the mean elimination half-life is 3.9 hours. Methohexital is biotransformed in the liver, with a clearance rate three times greater than that of thiopental. Excitatory phenomena, such as hiccups, spontaneous movements, and seizures, occur more frequently than with other barbiturates used clinically. These excitatory phenomena represent the primary disadvantage of methohexital. Methohexital does not induce histamine release. Although it is more likely than thiopental to cause pain on intravenous injection, methohexital in a 1% concentration is much less damaging after intraarterial injection or extravasation into local tissues. Its primary advantage is the rapid recovery and lower cumulative effect compared with thiopental, making it more suitable for outpatient procedures. Methohexital also is much more stable when reconstituted with sterile water; a 1% solution can be stored at room temperature and used for 6 weeks (versus 1 week for thiopental when refrigerated). Manufacturers state that unused reconstituted drug should be discarded after 24 hours, however, to avoid concerns about loss of sterility.

Propofol

Propofol (2,6-diisopropylphenol) is unrelated to any other general anesthetic. Its structure is illustrated in Figure 15-4. Propofol is formulated in an oil-in-water emulsion containing soybean oil, glycerol, and egg lecithin.

Anesthetic properties

Clinically, the pharmacokinetic properties of propofol include a **rapid onset of action**; an initial distributional half-life of 1 to 8 minutes, which results in an extremely short duration of action; and a terminal elimination half-life reported to be as short as 2 hours. It is extensively conjugated in the liver to inactive glucuronide and sulfate metabolites, with less than 0.3% of an administered dose appearing in the urine as the unchanged drug. Propofol's extensive plasma (98%) and tissue protein binding contributes partly to an enormous steady-state volume of distribution of 2 to 12 L/kg. The clearance of propofol exceeds hepatic blood flow, implying that continued tissue uptake and extrahepatic metabolism are factors in its removal from the blood. After a continuous 10-day infusion of propofol that produces tissue saturation, the volume of distribution approaches 60 L/kg with a metabolic half-life of 1 to 3 days. After bolus administration, the plasma concentrations of propofol and thiopental are similar initially, but propofol subsequently disappears from the bloodstream more rapidly.

Cardiovascular effects

Propofol can depress mean arterial pressures by 20% to 30% without eliciting a reflex increase in heart rate. This finding may be attributed to the drug's ability to decrease myocardial contractility, to dilate the peripheral vasculature, to depress baroreflex activity, and possibly to inhibit the sympathetic nervous system. Effects on cardiac output vary, depending on the $PaCO_2$. Clinically, these hemodynamic effects are transient and rarely require pharmacologic correction. The cardiovascular effects are well tolerated in healthy patients, but significant hypotension may ensue in elderly patients, hypovolemic patients, or patients with limited cardiac reserve.

Respiratory effects

Apnea is the most significant respiratory effect of propofol, with a reported incidence varying from 22% to 45% after an induction dose. Other respiratory effects include decreased sensitivity to carbon dioxide, decreased laryngeal reflexes, and decreased functional residual capacity. Propofol does not release histamine and generally is safe for use in asthmatic patients.

Other effects

Propofol decreases cerebral blood flow, cerebral metabolic rate and oxygen consumption, and intracranial pressure. Although it is believed to have anticonvulsant properties, there are reports of grand mal seizures, opisthotonus (spasm of back muscles inducing an arched back and hyperextension of the neck), and unusual muscle activity with propofol.

The most common adverse reaction is pain on injection, which is noted more frequently when propofol is administered in the small veins on the dorsum of the hand. The incidence of pain may be reduced by using larger veins (e.g., antecubital veins), diluting the drug with a rapidly flowing intravenous line, or mixing the drug with lidocaine. Propofol is associated with less postoperative nausea and vomiting compared with inhalation anesthetics, and it has antiemetic properties in low doses. Propofol may have antipruritic properties. There is no analgesic effect.

Therapeutic uses

Propofol's major advantage is its extremely **rapid and clear awakening** in patients. In addition to induction, propofol can be used for maintenance of general anesthesia or for intravenous sedation. The dose for induction is 2 to 2.5 mg/kg. For TIVA, a maintenance infusion rate of 50 to 300 μg/kg/min is recommended, depending on the age and health of the patient. If used alone, a dose of 25 to 75 μg/kg/min should maintain moderate sedation in healthy adults after an initial infusion of 100 to 150 μg/kg/min for 3 to 5 minutes. Doses must be reduced in elderly patients, debilitated patients, and when propofol is used with other CNS depressants. Due to propofol's low margin for maintaining consciousness, only those with general anesthesia training are approved to use the drug. A history of true type I allergy to any of the emulsion constituents (e.g., soybeans) potentially contraindicates the use of propofol. Because the soybean vehicle is an excellent bacterial culture medium, strict antiseptic technique should be used when administering propofol, and any unused portion should be discarded after 12 hours.

Infusion of propofol is also used long-term in intensive care units to provide sedation. A rare syndrome has been described when propofol is administered in high doses (>4 mg/kg/hr) for long durations (>48 hours). This potentially fatal "propofol infusion syndrome" involves only critically ill patients, primarily children. The main features of this syndrome include acidosis, bradyarrhythmia, and rhabdomyolysis of cardiac and skeletal muscle, signs that mimic mitochondrial myopathies. The use of propofol in lower doses or shorter durations has not been associated with these outcomes.

Etomidate

Etomidate, a carboxylated imidazole derivative, is chemically and pharmacologically unrelated to other intravenous anesthetics. Its pharmacokinetic profile is similar, however, to that of thiopental. Onset of anesthesia is rapid, and the duration of action is brief after conventional doses.

Etomidate is believed to **enhance** the action of the inhibitory neurotransmitter γ-aminobutyric acid (GABA) on $GABA_A$ receptors. The amplitude and duration of inhibitory currents are increased. Etomidate has the advantages over thiopental of causing only mild respiratory depression and little effect on the cardiovascular system. Induction doses of 0.3 mg/kg elicit a mild (15%) decrease in total peripheral resistance, which is mirrored by similar decrements in cardiac output and myocardial oxygen consumption. Coronary blood flow is mildly increased. Nevertheless, this drug is noted for its cardiovascular stability. Several significant liabilities limit the use of etomidate, however. The drug inhibits adrenocorticosteroid synthesis, particularly after prolonged administration; causes severe pain on injection in up to 50% of patients; and is associated with a high incidence of nausea and vomiting, thrombophlebitis, involuntary myoclonic movements, hypertonus, and hiccups. These adverse events have greatly limited the clinical application of etomidate for general anesthesia to the small group of patients who require the cardiovascular stability afforded by it.

Ketamine

Ketamine, a relative of the psychedelic drug phencyclidine (PCP, angel dust), produces a unique state known as dissociative anesthesia, which is characterized by profound analgesia, amnesia, and catalepsy. This excitatory state is quite different from that seen after administration of other general anesthetic agents previously discussed. It has been suggested that this dissociative state is a result of a functional and electrophysiologic dissociation between the thalamoneocortical and limbic systems. In this state, it is believed that the brain fails to correctly transduce afferent impulses because of disruption in normal communications between the sensory cortex and the association areas. The molecular structure of ketamine is shown in Figure 15-4.

Ketamine is an **antagonist of the NMDA class of glutamate receptors**, which is largely responsible for its anesthetic and behavioral effects. NMDA inhibition produces catalepsy, consistent with the effect of ketamine administration. Ketamine also produces profound analgesia, which seems to be at least partially mediated by μ opioid receptors, in addition to its binding to the phencyclidine binding site on the NMDA receptor.

Anesthetic properties

The onset of action and peak plasma concentrations occur within 1 minute after intravenous administration, 5 to 15 minutes after intramuscular injection, and 30 minutes after oral ingestion. The distributional half-life ranges from 11 to 16 minutes, and the elimination half-life is 2 to 3 hours. Ketamine is highly lipid-soluble, with minimal plasma protein binding (12%), which facilitates rapid transfer across the blood–brain barrier. The duration of anesthesia is about 5 to 10 minutes after a bolus intravenous infusion and 10 to 20 minutes after intramuscular injection. The dissociative state resembles catalepsy, in which the eyes may remain open with slow nystagmus and intact corneal and pupillary reflexes. Most protective reflexes are maintained. Varying degrees of skeletal muscle hypertonus may be present, along with non-purposeful skeletal muscle movements that are independent of surgical stimulation.

Cardiovascular effects

Ketamine differs from most anesthetic agents in that, in a healthy patient, it **stimulates the cardiovascular system**, producing increases in heart rate, cardiac output, and blood pressure. Ketamine, however, can directly depress myocardial contractility and enhance vasodilation. Ketamine's induction of central sympathetic stimulation and its ability to inhibit catecholamine uptake usually override the negative inotropism. Its ability to maintain arterial blood pressure is useful in hypovolemic patients and patients in cardiogenic shock.

Caution should be used when ketamine is administered to critically ill patients or patients who have chemical-induced or trauma-induced sympathectomy, in which case the cardiovascular depressant effect of ketamine may be unmasked and lead to myocardial depression and cardiovascular collapse. Ketamine increases pulmonary vascular resistance and may exacerbate pulmonary hypertension or cor pulmonale. The sympathomimetic and cardiovascular stimulating effects contraindicate the use of ketamine in patients in whom an elevation of blood pressure or heart rate should be avoided, such as patients with cerebrovascular accident, significant hypertension, or advanced ischemic heart disease.

Respiratory effects

Compared with other anesthetic agents, ketamine seems to be unique in its ability to maintain functional residual capacity on induction of anesthesia, decreasing the chances of intraoperative hypoxemia. During ketamine anesthesia in spontaneously breathing patients, the minute ventilation may be maintained at the same level as in the awake state. Ventilatory responses to hypercarbia and airway reflexes seem to be preserved. Ketamine has other beneficial effects on the respiratory apparatus, including increased lung compliance and decreased airway resistance. Ketamine is safe for asthmatic patients because it causes bronchodilation and does not induce histamine release. Ketamine is a potent stimulator of salivary and tracheobronchial secretions, however, and antimuscarinics are often administered concurrently.

Other effects

In doses less than those used to induce general anesthesia, ketamine may produce sedation, analgesia, and amnesia. Excitatory activity in the thalamus and limbic systems, without clinical evidence of seizure activity, has been recorded. This electrical activity does not seem to spread to the cortex, and ketamine has been shown to have anticonvulsant properties. Ketamine strongly dilates cerebral blood vessels, increasing cerebral blood flow by 60% to 80%, which increases intracranial pressure in patients with compromised intracranial compliance.

Emergence phenomena have been the most frequently reported adverse effects of ketamine. These reactions, occurring in <5% of patients in some studies and >30% of patients in others, include a feeling of floating, vivid dreams, hallucinations, and/or delirium. The incidence is related to the dose and rate of drug administration and is reduced when benzodiazepines are administered concomitantly. The frequency of emergence delirium is less in children than in adults.

Therapeutic uses

Ketamine may be administered by the intravenous, intramuscular, oral, and rectal routes. Induction of anesthesia may be achieved typically by an intravenous dose of 1 to 2 mg/kg or intramuscularly at a dose of 4 to 6 mg/kg. Intramuscular injection may be necessary when a patient is unable to cooperate with attaining intravenous access. Anesthesia can be maintained by repeated injections or by using a continuous infusion, the latter in a dose of 15 to 90 μg/kg/min. Smaller doses or infusion rates are useful for sedation and analgesia. Ketamine is safe for use in malignant hyperthermia patients, although it may induce some signs (e.g., muscle rigidity, tachycardia) that mimic the early stages of a crisis. Ketamine is usually administered with drugs such as midazolam or propofol to reduce the incidence of untoward excitatory effects.

ADJUNCTS FOR GENERAL ANESTHESIA

Dexmedetomidine

Serendipitous findings that clonidine, an **α_2-adrenoceptor agonist** used to treat hypertension (see Chapter 23), significantly reduces the MAC of inhalation anesthetics and produces significant analgesia independently of the opioid system generated attempts to develop congeners for use as sedatives and anesthetic adjuncts. The first successful outcome of this effort was **dexmedetomidine**, approved by the U.S. Food and Drug Administration (FDA) in 1999 for sedation of initially intubated and mechanically ventilated patients in the intensive care unit. In 2008, dexmedetomidine was approved for preoperative and intraoperative sedation of nonintubated patients. Administration is usually initiated with a loading infusion of 1 μg/kg for the first 10 minutes, followed by a maintenance infusion of 0.2 to 0.7 μg/kg/hr.

Structurally similar to etomidate, dexmedetomidine is approximately seven times more selective than clonidine for the α_2-adrenergic receptor. Stimulation of the α_{2A}-adrenoceptor subtype in the nucleus tractus solitarius and locus coeruleus of the brainstem reduces sympathetic outflow and elicits sedation. Similarly, release of excitatory neurotransmitters by nociceptive afferent axons in the dorsal horn is inhibited, reducing pain. (See Chapter 11.)

Dexmedetomidine has several pharmacokinetic advantages over clonidine. After bolus injection, dexmedetomidine displays a distributional half-life of about 6 minutes (versus 11 minutes for clonidine) and an elimination half-life of 2 hours (versus 9 hours for clonidine). The drug is completely transformed to inactive metabolites in the liver, most of which are excreted in the urine. A significant range in context-sensitive half-times exists, with values ranging from 4 minutes after a 10-minute infusion to 4 hours after an 8-hour infusion.

Clinically, dexmedetomidine is remarkable for its ability to produce a natural sleep from which the patient can be easily aroused. The sedation is characterized by **anxiolysis, analgesia, blunting of cardiovascular responses to stress, and freedom from respiratory depression**. Although intravenous injection initially can cause a transient increase in peripheral vascular resistance and arterial blood pressure by stimulating peripheral vascular α_2 receptors, the subsequent response is a decrease in blood pressure and heart rate in response to the centrally mediated sympatholytic and vagal-stimulating effects. Cardiovascular responses are minimized by slow infusion of low doses. The most common side effects of dexmedetomidine in approved doses are hypotension, bradycardia, and xerostomia. Large, accidental overdoses may produce significant vasoconstriction, profound bradycardia, and decreases in cardiac output possibly leading to cardiovascular collapse. The potential for cardiovascular derangements precludes the use of dexmedetomidine as a sole agent for general anesthesia, and the delayed recovery after prolonged infusions limits its use in outpatient surgery to short procedures. The development of atipamezole, a selective α_2-adrenoceptor antagonist used to reverse the effects of dexmedetomidine in veterinary medicine, suggests that such agents may become available to terminate the effects of dexmedetomidine in humans.

Benzodiazepines

Benzodiazepines have enjoyed widespread use as adjuncts to general anesthesia, as induction agents in patients with serious cardiovascular abnormalities, and as agents for all levels of sedation. Their pharmacologic advantages have given them a major role in the management of fear and anxiety in dentistry (see Chapters 11 and 38). As described in Chapter 11, all benzodiazepines are capable of producing in varying degrees anxiolysis, sedation, anterograde amnesia, skeletal muscle relaxation, and anticonvulsant activity. There is minimal depression of the cardiovascular and respiratory systems when benzodiazepines are administered alone in therapeutic doses, reflecting the fact that benzodiazepines have a wide safety margin in the absence of interacting drugs. These agents are useful for their ability to attenuate the stress response and associated catecholamine release.

Although all benzodiazepines share similar pharmacodynamic effects, they are differentiated by their pharmacokinetic characteristics. Although rarely used alone for general anesthesia because they lack analgesic properties and may be insufficient to induce or maintain general anesthesia in some patients, benzodiazepines are routinely used with other agents in balanced anesthesia for their superior sedative and amnestic effects and relative freedom from cardiovascular depression. The agent most commonly used in anesthesia is midazolam.

Midazolam

Midazolam, the first water-soluble benzodiazepine, is prepared in an aqueous vehicle buffered to a pH of 3.5. Below a pH of 4, the benzodiazepine ring is open, making the molecule highly polar. Above a pH of 4, as is found physiologically, the ring closes, making midazolam very lipid-soluble and leading to a rapid onset of action. This pharmaceutical sleight of hand eliminates the problem of thrombophlebitis on intravenous administration and improves uptake after intramuscular administration, both important advantages over diazepam. Midazolam is biotransformed into metabolites with little significant activity (although they may contribute sedative effects after oral administration), another advantage over diazepam. Midazolam is classified as a **short-acting agent** because its elimination half-life is approximately

1.7 to 2.6 hours in young adults. The usual intravenous dose for induction of general anesthesia is 0.2 mg/kg, but in common practice, midazolam is usually provided as an anxiolytic premedication, or as an adjunctive agent to smooth the overall process and contribute to deep sedation.

Opioids

The opioid analgesics play a major role in facilitating the delivery of general anesthesia and sedation, primarily as adjuncts used in combination with other agents. They also have a role as regional analgesics when administered as part of an epidural or spinal anesthetic. As described in more detail in Chapter 16, all opioids share the properties of analgesia; sedation; mood alteration; and the potential for tolerance, physical dependence, and addiction. Their antitussive effect may be valuable in the immediate postoperative period or for procedures such as bronchoscopy. Nausea and vomiting are common adverse effects and are characteristically exacerbated if the patient is ambulatory. Opioids decrease the MAC of inhalation anesthetics.

An important action is respiratory depression caused by a dose-dependent decrease in the response of the medullary respiratory center to carbon dioxide. High doses can totally block spontaneous respiration, sometimes without inducing unconsciousness. In susceptible patients, this effect may be seen in low to medium doses. Clinically, the respiratory depression manifests as a decrease in the breathing rate, with an overall decrease in minute ventilation and a compensatory increase in tidal volume. The $PaCO_2$ is elevated in a dose-dependent manner. Because of these respiratory effects, opioids must be administered with extreme caution to patients with respiratory disorders, such as chronic obstructive pulmonary disease.

Specific sedation techniques with opioids are discussed in more detail in Chapter 38. Opioid doses should be reduced in elderly patients, in patients with preexisting respiratory disease, and in patients with significant hepatic disease. Several drugs, most notably sufentanil, may be used as primary agents for cardiac anesthesia. Their cardiac stability is attributable to a lack of negative inotropic effects. The anesthetic properties of individual opioids used for anesthesia and sedation are discussed next.

Morphine

Morphine, the **prototypic opioid analgesic**, has been widely used as an adjunct to general anesthesia. It has been administered by numerous techniques, including high doses with oxygen or as a supplement to inhalation agents, to obtain profound analgesia. When used as an adjunct to general anesthesia, the recommended dose of morphine is 0.1 mg/kg intravenously. Because of advantages (discussed subsequently) found in the newer opioids, many centers favor these other medications over morphine when used during general anesthesia. Morphine still has wide acceptance, however, as an inexpensive choice for analgesia during general anesthesia, particularly when postoperative analgesia will be required.

Peak action after intravenous administration takes more than 20 minutes (Table 15-4). This delay reflects morphine's poor lipid solubility and limited ability to cross the blood–brain barrier. Some metabolites of morphine have significant opioid activity.

Cardiovascular effects. Morphine exerts little direct effect on cardiovascular function. This discovery led to the use of morphine for a time as a primary anesthetic for patients with significant cardiovascular disease. High doses, such as 1 mg/Kg, significantly decrease systemic vascular resistance and mean arterial pressure, however, predisposing the patient to orthostatic hypotension. Hypotension may also result from morphine-induced histamine release, bradycardia, or a sympatholytic action. Bradycardia is believed to be caused by stimulation of the vagal nuclei in the brainstem. There may also be a direct depressant effect at the sinoatrial node of the heart. The hypotensive actions of morphine lead to an increased requirement for fluid administration. In combination with nitrous oxide, morphine administration can result in cardiovascular depression, decreased cardiac output, and hypotension.

Respiratory effects. The maximum respiratory depression from morphine occurs approximately 30 minutes after intravenous injection. Increased intracranial pressure may also result because of hypercarbia. Morphine should not be used in patients for whom increased intracranial pressure is a concern, such as patients with an intracranial lesion or traumatic head injury.

Other effects. Emesis is a result of direct stimulation of the chemoreceptor trigger zone. There is also decreased gastrointestinal motility (which contributes to the direct emetic effect). Sphincter tone is increased, which in the case of the sphincter of Oddi (which controls the bile duct flow into the duodenum) can lead to increased bile pressure and epigastric distress that may mimic anginal pain.

For therapeutic use, precautions apply to asthmatic patients because of the histamine release and cough suppression. The same precautions are relevant to patients with a history of chronic obstructive pulmonary disease or other causes of decreased respiratory reserve. As with the administration of all opioids, severely ill or elderly patients are generally more susceptible to the depressant effects of morphine. Chest wall rigidity has been reported and tends to occur when morphine is administered rapidly and in combination with nitrous oxide.

TABLE 15-4 Comparison of Opioids Used for Sedation/Anesthesia

Drug (Proprietary [Trade] Name)	Equipotent Dose (mg)	Time to Peak Analgesic Effect (min)	Duration of Analgesia	Protein Binding (%)	Elimination Half-Life (hr)
Morphine	10	20	4-5 hr	30	2-3
Hydromorphone (Dilaudid)	1.5	15-30	2-3 hr	20	2.6-4
Meperidine (Demerol)	80	5-7	2-4 hr	60	2.4-4
Fentanyl (Sublimaze)	0.1	3-5	30-60 min	85	3-4
Alfentanil (Alfenta)	0.7	1-2	10-15 min	92	1-2
Sufentanil (Sufenta)	0.015	3-5	15-30 min	93	2-3
Remifentanil (Ultiva)	0.05	1-2	5-10 min	70	0.05-0.1
Pentazocine (Talwin)	60	15-30	2-3 hr	65	2-3
Nalbuphine (Nubain)	10	30	3-4 hr	50	2-5
Butorphanol (Stadol)	2	30	2-4 hr	80	2.5-4

Hydromorphone

Hydromorphone is a hydrogenated ketone derivative of morphine. It is 7.5 times more potent than morphine. The change of a single hydroxyl group to the ketone significantly increases lipid solubility such that onset time is only 3 to 5 minutes versus 20 to 30 minutes for morphine. Hydromorphone is minimally bound to plasma proteins. This allows hydromorphone to be more easily titrated to effect than morphine. The duration of action is 2 to 4 hours. There are no clinically significant active metabolites. Hydromorphone weakly releases histamine and is safe for asthmatics. At equianalgesic doses, the cardiovascular and respiratory effects are similar to morphine once peak effect has been reached. Hydromorphone is commonly used for postoperative pain control but can be used intraoperatively as part of a balanced anesthetic technique.

Meperidine

For many years, meperidine was the most widely used opioid for outpatient sedation and anesthesia in dentistry, although its use is has declined significantly. This synthetic opioid has approximately one-tenth the potency of morphine (see Table 15-4), and it has atropine-like properties in addition to its opioid agonist effects. The vagolytic actions may result in a decrease in upper respiratory tract secretions and an increase in heart rate, although these effects are minimal in the usual doses administered for sedation. At equianalgesic doses, meperidine has the same effects as morphine except that it differs from morphine in having a shorter duration of action, more complex biotransformation, and greater lipid solubility. Meperidine has a high hepatic extraction ratio, leading to a major first-pass effect if the drug is administered orally.

Cardiovascular effects of meperidine administration include hypotension caused by a direct negative inotropism, decreased systemic vascular resistance, and decreased venous return. Orthostatic hypotension is commonly seen because of interference with compensatory sympathetic reflexes. As with morphine, meperidine is contraindicated when histamine release or increased intracranial pressure is undesirable and when decreased respiratory reserve exists.

Meperidine is biotransformed into several metabolites. One of them, normeperidine, has a long elimination half-life, can accumulate, and has been associated with CNS toxicity. The adverse reaction manifests as excitation, including agitation, seizures, hallucinations, and disorientation, particularly in patients with hepatic and renal disease and the elderly. Meperidine is therefore not desirable choice for chronic therapy.

Exaggerated toxic responses to meperidine are especially likely in patients concurrently taking monoamine oxidase (MAO) inhibitors or amphetamines. Potential interactions between meperidine and amphetamines include increased risk of hypotension, possibly leading to cardiovascular collapse, severe respiratory depression, and convulsions. Potential interactions between meperidine and MAO inhibitors can be similar but are particularly characterized by unpredictable excitatory effects such as seizures, delirium, rigidity, coma, and hypertension leading to cardiovascular collapse. Meperidine is contraindicated in patients having taken an MAO inhibitor within the past 3 weeks. The ability of meperidine to increase 5-hydroxytryptamine concentrations at serotonergic synapses within the CNS has also led to concerns about interactions regarding serotonin reuptake inhibitors, such as fluoxetine, paroxetine, sertraline, venlafaxine, citalopram, and others.

Fentanyl

The synthetic opioid agonist fentanyl is approximately 100 times as potent as morphine and is characterized by a rapid onset and short duration of action after a single dose (see Table 15-4). It is most commonly administered intravenously but may be given intramuscularly, transmucosally in the oral cavity, and, for chronic pain, transdermally. Fentanyl's high lipid solubility contributes to its **rapid onset** because it readily crosses the blood–brain barrier. It also contributes to rapid redistribution as well as significant accumulation in peripheral tissues with high doses or long continuous infusions. The subsequent slow release of fentanyl from muscle and fat lengthens the terminal half-life to beyond that of morphine. Histamine is not released, which makes it preferable in patients predisposed to bronchospasm.

Cumulative intravenous doses of less than 10 μg/kg can be given as an adjunct to volatile agents in general anesthesia to minimize cardiovascular responses to specific stimuli such as pain, anxiety, or endotracheal intubation. Hemodynamic stability is maintained with fentanyl as a result of its lack of direct myocardial depression, absence of histamine release, and suppression of stress responses to surgery. A typical initial dose for surgery is 1 - 5 μg/kg. In intravenous doses of 25 to 100 μg, fentanyl is commonly used as a sedation adjunct in dentistry. Rapid administration of fentanyl is associated with bradycardia, an event more common in children. It is a potent respiratory depressant, but this lasts only 5 to 15 minutes if doses less than 100 μg are given. Chest wall rigidity has been reported but is unlikely to occur if fentanyl is administered at a rate of 1 μg/kg/min or less. The incidence of nausea is reported to be less than with morphine or meperidine.

Alfentanil

An analog of fentanyl, alfentanil is 5 to 10 times less potent and is characterized by a rapid elimination half-life. This property contributes to a duration of action that is much shorter than that of fentanyl after prolonged infusion. Alfentanil has an especially rapid onset of action because of its low pK_a causing most of the drug to be uncharged at plasma pH. The drug can be used for induction of anesthesia after bolus administration and maintenance by infusion. For bolus administration, recovery is more rapid than with fentanyl or sufentanil, whereas no significant differences occur with short infusions. Because alfentanil is not prone to significant accumulation after continuous infusion, it is commonly used for TIVA in the outpatient setting.

Sufentanil

Sufentanil is 5 to 10 times as potent as fentanyl and has a more rapid recovery after prolonged intravenous infusion. It is more lipid-soluble than fentanyl but has a smaller volume of distribution and a shorter elimination half-life. Cardiovascular effects are similar to effects found with fentanyl; however, sufentanil produces better hemodynamic stability during cardiac anesthesia and exhibits a more favorable ratio of analgesia to respiratory depression. Histamine is not released. High doses of sufentanil may reduce the dose of neuromuscular blocker required. As with fentanyl and alfentanil, sufentanil can be used for induction of anesthesia after bolus administration and maintenance by infusion.

Remifentanil

Remifentanil is also an opioid agonist used as an adjunct in general anesthesia. It is structurally unique because it contains ester linkages, which lead to distinctive pharmacokinetic characteristics. Compared with fentanyl, remifentanil has a more rapid onset and offset of action. Entry into brain tissue is hastened by a comparatively high percentage of drug in the nonionized state. The ultrashort duration of action is not caused by redistribution of the drug but by its unique metabolic inactivation by nonspecific esterases in the blood and tissue. A small volume of distribution also helps to hasten metabolism. One of the most notable characteristics of remifentanil is its invariant context-sensitive half-life, which approximates 3 to 4 minutes regardless of the duration or dose of infusion. The drug is almost always given by intravenous infusion because less controlled administration results in unstable effects and easily leads to chest wall rigidity or respiratory depression or both. Addition of remifentanil to a propofol infusion has been shown to provide a more rapid recovery and reduced use of propofol.

Opioid Agonist-Antagonists

Opioid agonist-antagonists are sometimes used for anesthesia and sedation in lieu of pure opioid agonists. These are compared with pure opioid agonists in Table 15-4. Although the analgesic and respiratory depressant effects of the agonist-antagonists are similar to the effects of morphine and other agonists in conventional doses, a ceiling effect occurs at high doses. These drugs are not indicated as replacements for high-dose opioids as used in open-heart surgery. Pentazocine, butorphanol, and nalbuphine all have been administered for outpatient sedation procedures. All are κ receptor agonists.

Pentazocine depresses myocardial contractility, but myocardial oxygen demand is greater than normal because of increases in peripheral resistance, systolic blood pressure, and plasma catecholamines. Although the antagonist action of pentazocine is weak, it is sufficient to precipitate opioid withdrawal reactions in physically dependent individuals. Adverse reactions include a potential for psychotomimetic effects, such as disorientation, confusion, depression, hallucinations, and dysphoria. Doses that produce sedation have also been associated with diaphoresis and dizziness. Butorphanol shares many of the cardiovascular and psychotomimetic side effects of pentazocine, although it is less likely to precipitate withdrawal in an opioid-dependent individual. Nalbuphine is a strong μ receptor antagonist, but it does not increase blood pressure or heart rate, which makes it the agonist-antagonist of a choice in patients with cardiac disease. The strong ability of nalbuphine to reverse the sedative and analgesic effects of pure opioids can lead to marked and potentially dangerous withdrawal reactions in patients dependent on opioids.

ANESTHETIC ADJUVANTS AND PREMEDICATION

Numerous drugs may be used for premedication or as anesthetic adjuvants. The pharmacologic features of the **neuromuscular blocking agents**, which are frequently used during anesthesia to provide greater muscle relaxation, are discussed in Chapter 7. Many of the **sedatives, analgesics, antihistamines, and antimuscarinics** previously mentioned in this chapter and reviewed elsewhere in the book are administered to the patient minutes to several hours before anesthesia and surgery. Table 15-5 lists commonly used drugs for premedication.

Indications for premedication include relief of anxiety; induction of sedation, analgesia, and amnesia; vagal blockade; reduction of secretions in the upper respiratory tract; and prevention of nausea and vomiting. Premedicants are also used to decrease the acidity and volume of gastric secretions. Finally, they are administered to reduce the dose of the general anesthetic agent needed for a smooth induction.

An effective method of alleviating preoperative anxiety is the preoperative visit by the anesthesiologist, which allows information to be given to the patient and permits questions to be answered. The following classes of drugs, whose pharmacologic features are described elsewhere in this text, are routinely used as adjuncts to the careful psychological preparation of the patient.

Opioid analgesics offer analgesia, euphoria, and sedation. Complicating problems include respiratory depression, nausea and vomiting, gastric retention, and reduced sympathetic tone. Benzodiazepines can relieve anxiety without significant effects on respiration or cardiovascular function. They are also effective in providing amnesia and sedation. The antimuscarinics atropine, glycopyrrolate, and scopolamine may be used as premedicants to block vagal reflexes and inhibit salivation and respiratory tract secretion. They may also oppose the bradyarrhythmias that may accompany the use of other drugs in anesthesia, such as succinylcholine. Scopolamine also has central effects leading to sedation and amnesia as well as being used as an antiemetic in a transdermal patch. Glycopyrrolate does not cross the blood–brain barrier, is a more efficacious antisialagogue than atropine, and is less likely to induce tachycardia. H_1 and H_2 antihistamines may be given for premedication. H_1 antagonists, such as hydroxyzine or promethazine, offer antiemetic effects and some sedation. H_2 antagonists, such as cimetidine or ranitidine, decrease gastric secretion and acidity. These effects are important in certain patients because general anesthesia eliminates the usual protective reflexes that prevent aspiration after regurgitation of stomach contents. The dopaminergic antagonist metoclopramide is also sometimes administered to speed gastric emptying.

Postoperative nausea and vomiting are common adverse events after general anesthesia. To improve comfort and safety, patients who are predisposed to nausea and vomiting may be given one of a wide variety of antiemetics, which include the adrenocorticosteroid dexamethasone; 5-HT_3 antagonists, including ondansetron, granisetron, and dolasetron; anticholinergics/antihistamines, such as scopolamine and hydroxyzine; the substance P/neurokinin (NK1) antagonist, aprepitant; and the

TABLE 15-5 Agents Used for Premedication in General Anesthesia

Drug Name	Adult Dose (mg)	Route of Administration	Indications
Antimuscarinics			
Atropine	0.5	IV, IM	Secretion decrease, vagal blockade
Glycopyrrolate	0.2	IV, IM	Secretion decrease
Scopolamine	0.3	IV	Secretion decrease, sedation, amnesia
Antihistamines			
Hydroxyzine	25-100	Oral	Anxiolysis, sedation, antiemetic effect
Promethazine	25-50	IM	Sedation, antiemetic effect
Ranitidine	150	Oral	Aspiration prophylaxis
Benzodiazepines			
Diazepam	5-20	Oral, IV	Anxiolysis, sedation, amnesia
Lorazepam	0.5-4	Oral, IV	Anxiolysis, sedation, amnesia
Midazolam	2-5	IM, IV*	Anxiolysis, sedation, amnesia
Triazolam	0.125-0.5	Oral	Anxiolysis, sedation, amnesia
Prokinetic			
Metoclopramide (Reglan)	5-15	IV	Aspiration prophylaxis
Opioids			
Fentanyl	0.025-0.1	IV	Sedation, analgesia
Meperidine	50-100	IM	Sedation, analgesia
Morphine	5-10	IM	Sedation, analgesia

*Midazolam is also supplied as a syrup for oral use in pediatric patients.

dopamine antagonists droperidol and prochlorperazine. Although droperidol is an effective antiemetic, its use was greatly limited after the FDA placed restrictions on its use based on reports of its association with a prolonged cardiac QT interval and related arrhythmias (Chapter 19). The applicability of these reports to the small, prophylactic doses of droperidol used in anesthesiology has been widely questioned.

GENERAL ANESTHETICS

Nonproprietary (Generic) Name	Proprietary (Trade) Name
Inhalation Agents	
Nitrous oxide	—
Desflurane	Suprane
Isoflurane	Forane
Sevoflurane	Ultane
Injectable Agents	
Propofol	Diprivan
Methohexital	Brevital
Thiopental	Pentothal
Etomidate	Amidate
Ketamine	Ketalar
Dexmedetomidine	Precedex
Midazolam	Versed
Opioids see Chapter 16.	

CASE DISCUSSION

This case represents a typical general anesthetic regimen with respect to the agents delivered. A drop in blood pressure following induction would be expected since propofol decreases mean arterial blood pressure without a concomitant increase in heart rate due to blunted baroreceptor reflexes. This could be managed in one of two ways. The pharmacokinetic properties of propofol result in a very short duration of action, so blood pressure would be expected to rise without any further pharmacologic intervention. If this is insufficient, then increasing the volume of intravenous fluid or administering an appropriate dose of a sympathomimetic may be needed. The finding of an increase in blood pressure later on in the case could be due to a number of factors. If early after induction, dissipation of the effects of the intravenous agents given at the beginning of the case may be responsible. Later in the case, one would consider an inadequate depth of anesthesia relative to surgical stimulation as the likely cause. Although the patient is unconscious, he may not be adequately anesthetized such that pain can still stimulate the sympathetic nervous system. Its management would be to consider either increasing the administration of the inhalational agent desflurane, readministering fentanyl, or, if appropriate, administering local anesthetic to the site being treated.

GENERAL REFERENCES

1. Barash PG, Cullen BF, Stoelting RK, editors: *Clinical anesthesia*, ed 5, Philadelphia, 2005, Lippincott Williams & Wilkins.
2. Bruce DL, Bach MJ: Effects of trace anaesthetic gases on behavioural performance of volunteers, *Br J Anaesth* 48:871–876, 1976.
3. Leslie K, Leslie P, Devereaux PJ, Forbes A, et al.: Nitrous oxide and serious morbidity and mortality in the POISE trial, *Anes Analg* 116:1034–1040, 2013.
4. Miller RD, editor: *Miller's anesthesia*, ed 6, Philadelphia, 2005, Elsevier.
5. Myles PS, Leslie K, Chan MTV, Forbes A, et al.: The safety of addition of nitrous oxide to general anaesthesia in at-risk patients having major non-cardiac surgery (ENIGMA-II): a randomised, single-blind trial, *Lancet* 384:1446–1454, 2014.
6. Patel PM, Patel HH, Roth DM: General anesthetics and therapeutic gases. In Brunton L, Chabner B, Knollman B, editors: *Goodman and Gilman's the pharmacological basis of therapeutics*, ed 12, New York, 2011, McGraw-Hill.
7. Rowland AS, Baird DD, Weinberg CR, et al.: Reduced fertility among women employed as dental assistants exposed to high levels of nitrous oxide, *N Engl J Med* 327:993–997, 1992.
8. Turan A, Mascha EJ, You J, Kurz A, et al.: The association between nitrous oxide and postoperative mortality and morbidity after noncardiac surgery, *Anes Analg* 116:1026–1033, 2013.

WEBSITE

http://www.cdc.gov/niosh/docs/hazardcontrol/pdfs/hc3.pdf (accessed March 2016).

16

Opioid Analgesics and Antagonists

Robert B. Raffa, Michael H. Ossipov, and Frank Porreca

KEY INFORMATION

- Pain is a common symptom in dentistry: it either prompts a visit to a dentist or may result from a dental procedure.
- Morphine and codeine are prototypic naturally occurring opiates.
- Opioids (opiate-like drugs such as hydrocodone, codeine, and oxycodone) are efficacious analgesics; consequently, they find widespread application in dentistry.
- Treatment of dental pain associated with inflammation may be accomplished with antiinflammatory drugs, either alone or in combinations with opioids. Opioids do not have antiinflammatory properties.
- The mechanism of action of opioids is the binding to ("affinity" for) and activation of ("efficacy") 7-transmembrane G protein–coupled opioid receptors located on neurons located primarily within the central nervous system (CNS).
- The target receptor for most commonly used opioid analgesics is termed μ, mu, or MOR.
- Opioids also produce undesirable effects, including sedation and somnolence, constipation, nausea and vomiting, respiratory depression, and urinary retention.
- Repeated use of opioids can lead to analgesic tolerance, physical dependence, and in some patients, addiction.
- Opioids that are agonists are used principally for relief of pain; antagonists prevent or reverse the effects of agonists and are used principally to reverse opioid intoxication.

CASE STUDY

Your patient is a 50-year-old male complaining of severe pain in an upper left molar (tooth #14). He reports that the tooth has been sensitive to cold temperatures in the past, but in the last two days the pain has become persistent, with a dull, aching, and throbbing quality. Examination reveals a deep filling and a periapical radiolucency on the MB root. The tooth is exquisitely tender to percussion. You have numbed the tooth with 4% articaine as buccal infiltration and Greater Palatine injections so you can begin endodontic therapy. After initial treatment of the canals, you prescribe clindamycin (300 mg). What, if anything, would you prescribe for postoperative pain?

INTRODUCTION: GENERAL THERAPEUTIC USES OF OPIOIDS

Pain is a common symptom that initiates a visit to a dentist or physician. Pain is almost always present after invasive procedures or surgery. Morphine and other opioid analgesics are the most efficacious analgesic (i.e., pain-relieving) drugs known and are without peer in their ability to control pain. These drugs provide symptomatic relief of pain without influencing its underlying cause. When administered at therapeutic doses to produce analgesia, opioids also produce drowsiness, from which the patient is generally easily aroused, and tranquilization. There is a significant antianxiety or sedating component in the analgesic effect of opioids. Opioids can also produce nausea and initial vomiting, depress respiration, suppress cough, and elicit constipation, as well as tolerance, and can induce physical dependence. Though some of these undesirable effects can be drawbacks to their use, opioids produce an important combination of desirable effects (e.g., analgesia and sedation) in patients with pain.

Aside from their application for pain relief, opioids can be useful in inducing sleep, provided that sleeplessness is caused by pain or coughing. Opioid analgesics should not be used for nighttime sedation in the absence of coughing or pain and should be used with caution in patients with sleep apnea. Morphine is also effective in the treatment of pulmonary edema. Opioids are not used for anesthesia, but they are often used in perioperative procedures. Opioids are also used therapeutically as antidiarrheal and antitussive agents.

OPIOIDS

Morphine and **codeine**, the prototypic opioid analgesics, are natural phenanthrene alkaloids contained in opium, which is derived from the poppy plant *Papaver somniferum*. The unripe seed capsules of the plant are incised, and the milky exudate is collected, dried, and powdered. Opium powder contains 5% to 20% morphine and 0.5% to 2.5% codeine, depending on the source.

Descriptions of the pharmacologic properties of extracts from *P. somniferum* appeared by 1550 BC. Sertürner first isolated morphine from opium and linked its properties to that of *P. somniferum* in 1806. Besides morphine and codeine, all current opioid analgesics are either semisynthetic congeners of morphine (e.g., **hydromorphone, oxymorphone, hydrocodone,** and **oxycodone**) or entirely synthetic (e.g., **meperidine, fentanyl,** and **methadone**). Morphine and codeine can also now be produced for commercial use through modern synthetic methods.

Basis of Opioid Action

Opioids act at specific CNS and peripheral sites to produce their analgesic and side effects through mechanisms that are fairly well understood. In the early 1970s, it was discovered that opioids stereospecifically, saturably, and reversibly activate specific receptors in

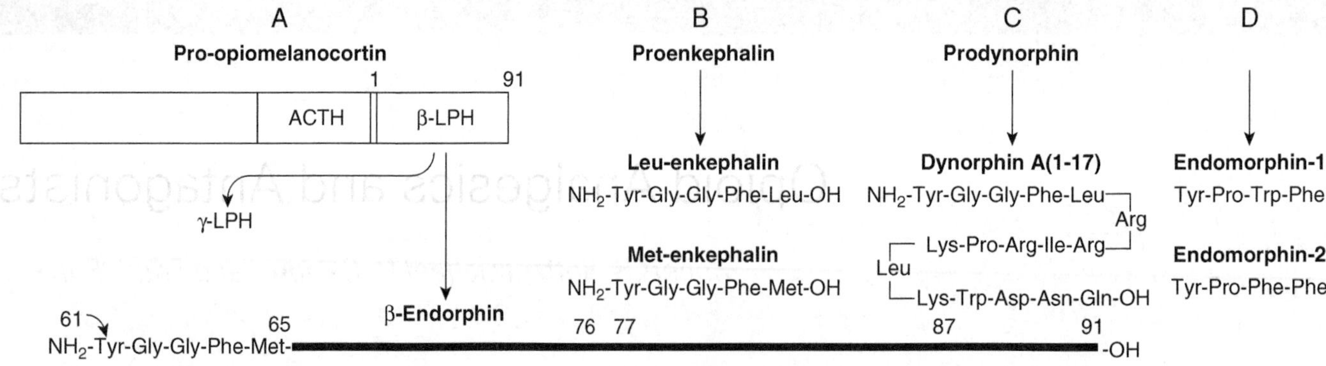

FIG 16-1 Derivations and structures of endogenous opioids. **A,** Endorphins. Proteolysis products of the pituitary hormone β-lipotropin (*β-LPH*), endorphins are ultimately derived from the precursor molecule pro-opiomelanocortin. Other peptides of biologic importance obtained from pro-opiomelanocortin include adrenocorticotropin (*ACTH*), γ-lipotropin (*γ-LPH*), and several melanotropins (not shown). The initial amino acid sequence of β-endorphin is shown (*at bottom left*) to illustrate its structural relationship to the enkephalins and dynorphins; the numbers refer to amino acid residues of β-LPH. **B,** Enkephalins. In addition to met-enkephalins and leu-enkephalins, proenkephalin may give rise to at least two other biologically active molecules, a heptapeptide and an octapeptide, both of which contain met-enkephalin as part of their structure. **C,** Dynorphins. A common precursor, prodynorphin, yields several dynorphins, including dynorphin α(1-17) (shown here), dynorphin A(1-8), dynorphin B(1-13), and at least two other peptides, α-neoendorphin and β-neoendorphin. **D,** Endomorphins. The precursor for these two endogenous opioid peptides is unknown.

the brain. These "opioid" receptors were later shown to be the natural effectors of opioid action; that is, specific pharmacologic effects were produced by binding of opioid agonists to opioid receptors, resulting in transduction through a cascade of intracellular mechanisms that influence ion channels and the excitability of the cell. The discovery of opioid receptors naturally raised questions about their biologic significance, spurring research that led to the discovery of endogenous circuits of opioid receptors and ligands. Subsequently, several families of endogenous opioid peptides and opioid receptors have been characterized.

Endogenous opioid peptides

There are four families of endogenous opioid peptides: **enkephalins, endorphins, dynorphins,** and **endomorphins.** Figure 16-1 illustrates their biologic derivations and structural relationships. The pentapeptide enkephalins—met-enkephalin (Tyr-Gly-Gly-Phe-Met) and leu-enkephalin (Tyr-Gly-Gly-Phe-Leu)—were the first endogenous opioids discovered. They were subsequently shown to be potent opioid receptor agonists in the same biologic systems in which morphine is active.

Proenkephalin, the peptide precursor of the enkephalins, is present in the CNS and the adrenal medulla. In the brain, cleavage of proenkephalin results in free enkephalins including four copies of met-enkephalin and one copy of leu-enkephalin. Prodynorphin is the common precursor for several larger opioid peptides, three dynorphins and two neoendorphins, all of which share with the enkephalins the same N-terminal amino acid sequence: NH_2-Tyr-Gly-Gly-Phe-Met/Leu. The products of prodynorphin are often localized with the enkephalins within the CNS. Differential processing of proenkephalin and prodynorphin (i.e., enzymatic cleavage at different sites in the precursor peptide sequence) in various brain areas leads to multiple products having a diversity of functions in different brain circuits.

The endorphins are a group of endogenous peptides that are larger in size and distributed differently in the CNS than are the endomorphins, enkephalins, or dynorphins. The precursor for the endorphins, pro-opiomelanocortin, gives rise to several important hormones, including adrenocorticotropic hormone (ACTH) and β-lipotropin, which are further processed to form additional biologically active products. The most important opioid derived from β-lipotropin is β-endorphin, a 31-amino acid carboxy terminal sequence of β-lipotropin. Shorter cleavage products of β-endorphin, such as α-endorphin and γ-endorphin, have been isolated from the pituitary.

Endomorphin-1 and endomorphin-2 are more newly discovered endogenous opioid peptides. Both are short tetrapeptides (NH_2-Tyr-Pro-Trp/Phe-Phe-$CONH_2$) and are structurally distinct from the other opioid peptides (see later). Although the genes for the endorphins, enkephalins, and dynorphins are known, the gene for the endomorphins has yet to be identified. The endomorphins, enkephalins, and dynorphins are stored in nerve terminals, and after receptor activation, they are quickly destroyed by peptidases (aminopeptidase N [EC 3.4.11.2] and neutral endopeptidase [EC 3.4.24.11]). β-Endorphin is present in high concentrations in the intermediate lobe of the pituitary and in neurons in the mediobasal hypothalamus, whose axons terminate in the amygdala, periaqueductal gray matter, and brainstem. β-Endorphin coexists with adrenocorticotropic hormone in pituitary secretory granules, and both peptides can be released simultaneously. β-Endorphin is believed to function more as a neurohormone than as a neurotransmitter, mediating diverse autonomic and psychological responses to pain and stress.

Endogenous opioid peptides have been localized to areas in the CNS associated with opioid receptors and pain processing (e.g., spinal dorsal horn, trigeminal nucleus, midbrain periaqueductal gray, and cortex) (Fig. 16-2) and in the endings of sensory neurons that terminate in the spinal dorsal horn.

Opioid receptors

Three opioid receptors have been pharmacologically characterized and cloned: MOR (μ, mμ, and other designations), KOR (κ, kappa, and other designations), and DOR (δ, delta, and other designations). They share 60% to 65% structural homology (Fig. 16-3), contain seven membrane-spanning α-helical segments, and are coupled to transducing G proteins (Fig. 16-4). G proteins couple opioid receptors to

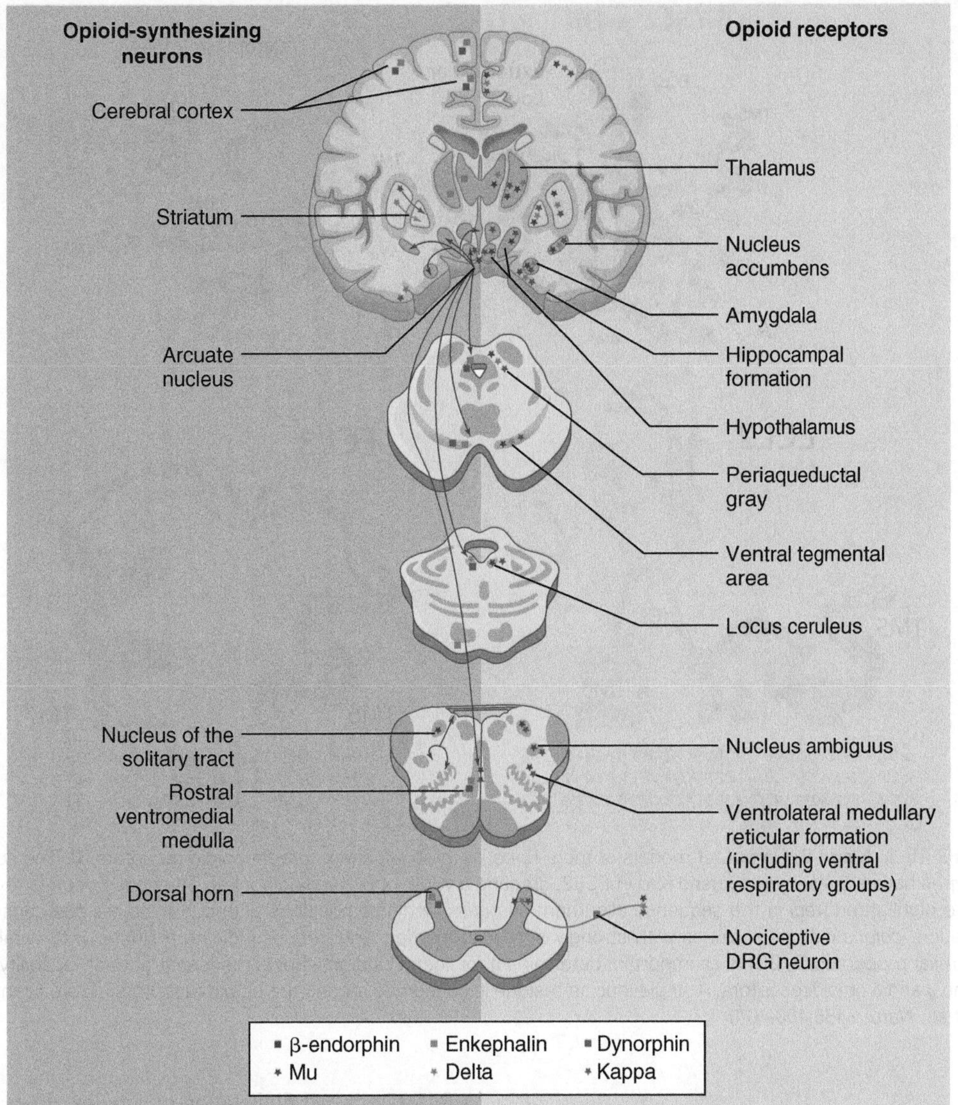

FIG 16-2 Overlapping distribution of opioid peptides and opioid receptors in the central nervous system. For clarity, opioid pathways are shown on the left and opioid receptors are shown on the right.

intracellular effectors and exist as heterotrimers. There is structural and functional diversity in the three G protein subunits: each heterotrimer consists of an α subunit isoform (of which there are at least 18) and a dimer of β-γ subunits (which also exist in multiple isoforms) that link with specific (and potentially diverse, given the numbers of isoform combinations that are possible) effector systems. Opioid receptors couple in this way with adenylyl cyclase and with ion channels to reduce neurotransmitter release and inhibit action potentials in nerves that promote pain (see later).

A receptor with high sequence homology to the three cloned opioid receptors, termed *ORL-1* (for opioid receptor–like, an "orphan" receptor), has been discovered. Despite its structural similarity to opioid receptors, opioids do not bind to ORL-1 with high affinity (Box 16-1). The μ opioid receptor is the site at which all the currently available agonists primarily act to produce analgesia. Morphine and other agonists have greatest affinity for μ receptors and lower affinity for δ and κ receptors (Box 16-2). The δ receptor is also involved in analgesia, mainly through spinal mechanisms, and in opioid reinforcement (see Chapter 39). Although morphine and other agonists preferentially bind at μ receptors, they can produce effects at δ and κ opioid receptors as well, particularly as the dosage is increased. Activation of δ and κ opioid receptors can result in modulation of μ-induced analgesic action and/or elicit adverse actions (e.g., activation of CNS κ opioid receptors has been associated with dysphoric effects).

Receptor isoforms may be produced by alternative splicing in the coding regions of the three cloned opioid receptors. Variant mRNAs have been reported for all three opioid receptors, although their expression is typically very low, and it is not clear that splice variants can be distinguished pharmacologically or to the degree to which they participate in clinical effects. Other mechanisms (e.g., posttranslational regulation, variable activation of receptors by different ligands, receptor dimerization, intracellular interactions with proteins associated with different effectors) could also explain the diverse pharmacologic actions linked to opioid receptor subtypes. Interestingly, opioid receptors can exist as dimers (two receptors linked), and heterodimerization could result in a complex pharmacologic profile.

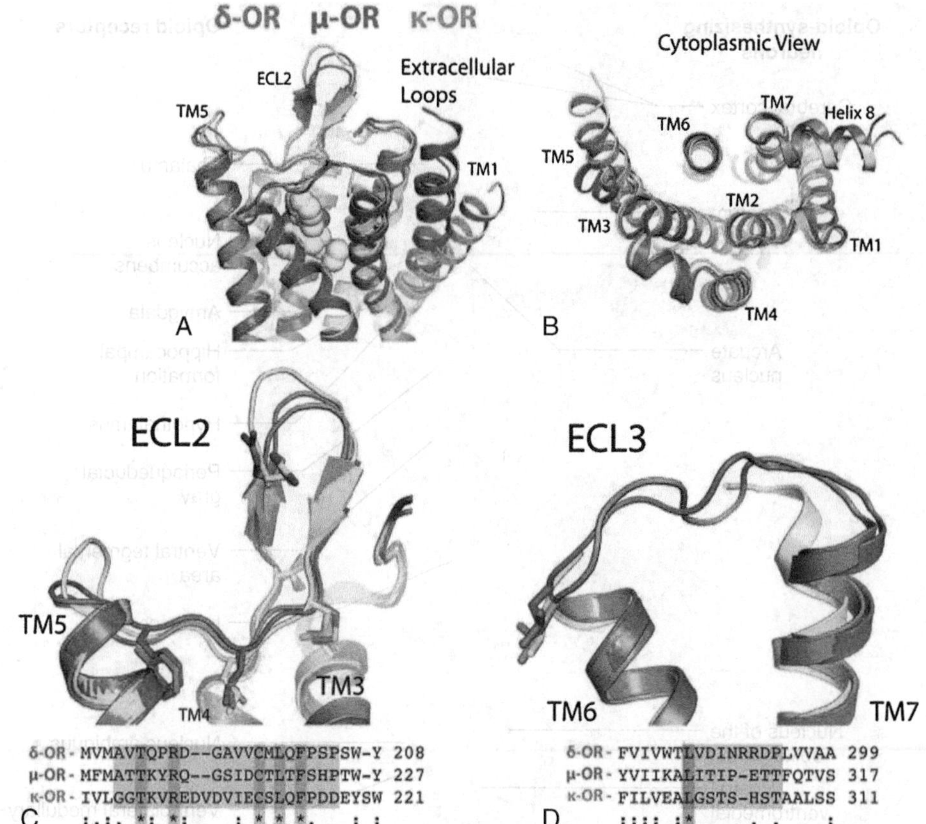

FIG 16-3 A and B, Computer models of the μ (*blue*), δ (*orange*), and κ (*green*) opioid receptors. **C,** The subtypes have a conserved β-strand fold in ECL2, creating a wide, open binding pocket. The conserved residues are highlighted (*red*) in the sequence alignment. *Asterisks* indicate positions with complete residue conservation, *colons* indicate residues with strongly similar properties, and *periods* indicate residues with weakly similar properties. **D,** ECL3, an important determinant for ligand binding, shows modest structural variability in the μ and δ opioid receptors. A single leucine residue is conserved among the opioid receptors. (From Granier et al.: *Nature* 485:400-404)

Physiologic roles

Enkephalins are present principally in local circuits or interneurons in the CNS, and following their release, they have an inhibitory effect on other cells expressing opioid receptors. Endogenous opioids also tonically modulate the secretion of gonadotropins from the pituitary. When naloxone, an opioid receptor antagonist (see below), is administered to normal subjects, the plasma concentrations of luteinizing hormone and follicle-stimulating hormone are increased (this is because naloxone releases hypothalamic neurons from tonic endogenous opioid inhibition). One might also expect naloxone to lower the response threshold for pain if endogenous opioids tonically modulated nociception, but administration of naloxone to normal human volunteers does not affect their resting pain thresholds or responses to experimental pain stimuli. Nevertheless, naloxone has been reported to attenuate the analgesic effects of placebo administration after minor oral surgery and to be hyperalgesic in humans after major surgery. From these and other findings, two clinically important physiologic roles of endogenous opioids are revealed. Endogenous antinociceptive opioid systems are normally quiescent, but they are engaged to diminish pain when significant injury or stress is present. Endogenous opioid activity also underlies the naloxone-reversible placebo response that diminishes the perception of pain (i.e., elicits analgesia).

Sites and mechanism of action

Opioids act at opioid receptors at **spinal** and **supraspinal** sites to produce clinically effective analgesia. Emerging evidence suggests that opioids may also act in the **periphery** to contribute to analgesic actions; for example, administration of very low doses of morphine directly into the knee joint after arthroscopic knee surgery has been reported to diminish postoperative pain (Box 16-3).

Early studies attempted to determine the central locus of opioid analgesic action by administering morphine directly into selected brain sites of animals. These studies succeeded in identifying an area of the brainstem surrounding the midbrain cerebral aqueduct (i.e., **periaqueductal gray** or **PAG**) as a site important to morphine analgesia. Corollary studies found that electrical stimulation of this same area in the midbrain in animals and humans produced a potent, long-lasting analgesia largely mediated by endogenous opioids. Exogenous opioid agonists, including morphine, act in part by activating the opioid receptors in the PAG to produce analgesia in part by engaging an endogenous pain modulatory circuit that involves descending neuronal pathways from the brain to the spinal cord (see below).

However, the most important mechanism by which morphine and other opioid agonists modulate pain is by acting at opioid receptors in the brain (e.g., the cortex). Critically, actions of opioids at cortical brain sites do not affect the response threshold to a painful stimulus but rather influence the interpretation of—and emotional reaction to—the stimulus. This is termed the "motivational-affective dimension" of pain that is the most important aspect of pain clinically and is discussed later in this chapter.

Nociceptors are specialized peripheral nerves that respond preferentially to high intensity stimuli that have the potential to produce tissue injury. Afferent information resulting from activation of nociceptors

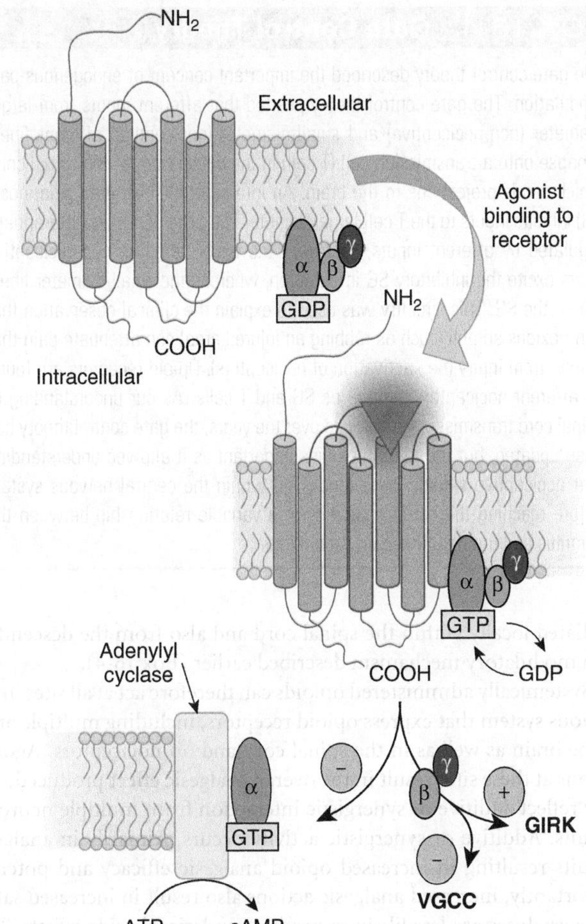

FIG 16-4 Diagram of a G protein–coupled opioid receptor. Opioids bind within the hydrophobic membrane-spanning domains of the receptor. Opioid agonist effects at the receptor are mediated by G proteins, an α_i subunit associated with guanosine diphosphate (*GDP*), and a β-γ dimer. When an opioid agonist binds, the conformation of the receptor is changed as the membrane-associated G proteins assemble with the receptor. GDP is exchanged with guanosine triphosphate, and this activated G_α complex negatively regulates adenylyl cyclase. The β-γ dimer activates conductance in a G protein inwardly rectifying K^+ (*GIRK*) channel and inhibits voltage-gated Ca^{2+} channels (*VGCC*) in the cell membrane. (See Chapters 1 and 5 for more details on signal transduction.) *ATP*, Adenosine triphosphate; *cAMP*, cyclic 3′,5′-adenosine monophosphate.

that innervate the skin, muscle, joints, viscera, and dental pulp (i.e., noxious stimuli) can be influenced at the first central synapse (spinal or medullary dorsal horn) by the descending system of endogenous pain modulation arising from supraspinal sites including the cortex (Fig. 16-5). It is important to appreciate two features of this pain-modulating system: the descending pathway from the midbrain is indirect, arising from a synaptic relay in the medulla (there is also a synaptic relay in the dorsolateral pons), and although engaged by an opioid acting at opioid receptors in the midbrain, the neurotransmitters in the spinal cord or medullary dorsal horn that ultimately inhibit pain transmission are nonopioids such as 5-hydroxytryptamine (5-HT, serotonin) and norepinephrine. Engagement of the descending pain inhibitory circuit is also partly responsible for placebo-induced analgesia.

Another means by which morphine and other opioid agonists produce analgesia is by acting at opioid receptors located on the central (spinal) terminals of nociceptors. Opioid receptors are located on both the central and peripheral terminals of these specialized nerve fibers,

BOX 16-1 Nociceptin and Nocistatin

A heptadecapeptide termed *orphanin FQ* (or nociceptin), which is structurally similar to the endogenous opioid peptide dynorphin, seems to be the endogenous ligand for an opioid-related receptor termed ORL-1 (which has been renamed the *N/OFQ receptor* [NOP]). Nociceptin does not act at any of the three cloned μ, δ, or κ opioid receptors, but the nociceptin–NOP ligand–receptor complex may function to inhibit, or facilitate, pain at some sites. Another heptadecapeptide, termed *nocistatin*, is derived from the same gene that gives rise to nociceptin. Nocistatin is reported to "block" the effects of nociceptin, but nocistatin does not displace nociceptin from its receptor (ORL-1), and it is believed to exert its effect through a presynaptic G_i/G_o-coupled receptor not related to either the opioid receptors or the NOP receptor.

BOX 16-2 Opioid Receptor Subtypes

- Two subtypes of mu (μ) opioid receptors have been characterized: μ_1, associated with supraspinal analgesia, and μ_2, associated with spinal analgesia, respiratory depression, and gastrointestinal actions.
- Pharmacologic studies also suggest the existence of two subtypes of delta (δ) opioid receptor, at which the endogenous enkephalins are considered to be the prototypic agonists.
- Three subtypes of kappa (κ) opioid receptor have been characterized pharmacologically. Two mediate spinal (κ_1 and κ_2) and supraspinal (κ_3) analgesia.
- The sigma (σ) receptor, initially thought to be an opioid receptor, is now known to mediate the dysphoric and psychotomimetic effects of opioids and those of phencyclidine, a nonopioid hallucinogen. This receptor has now been recognized as an inhibitory component of the *N*-methyl-D-aspartate receptor complex, which modulates opioid tolerance and dependence.

BOX 16-3 Peripheral Opioid Analgesia

An increasingly important peripheral analgesic action of opioids is now appreciated. Opioid receptors are located on the central and peripheral terminals of nociceptors. When tissue is inflamed, peripheral opioid receptors upregulate (increase in number or are inserted into peripheral nociceptor terminals in greater number). This event is presumably part of the normal response to tissue insult where endogenous opioid peptides contained in monocytic cells or lymphocytes, attracted to the site of injury, are released to modulate pain associated with the tissue insult. Therapeutically, the upregulation of opioid receptors can be taken advantage of by application of exogenous opioid agonists directly to the site of insult (e.g., intraarticular injection of morphine or topical application of μ opioid receptor agonists).

typically Aδ and C fibers, which connect the periphery directly with the CNS. Therefore, analgesic effects of opioids can be produced by direct administration of an opioid into the epidural or intrathecal space. The impetus for exploring spinal administration of opioids for pain relief arose from the discovery of opioid receptors in the spinal dorsal horn. Epidural or intrathecal administration of opioids is now frequently used in multiple clinical situations for pain control.

An important advance in pain research was the realization that excitatory and inhibitory transmitters within the spinal dorsal horn allowed for the "processing" of nociceptive information before ascending to the brain (i.e., the "gate control" theory). These mechanisms allow for either amplification or inhibition of nociceptive signaling depending on the context in which an injury may occur and interpretation and memories of the individual. Modulation of nociception is

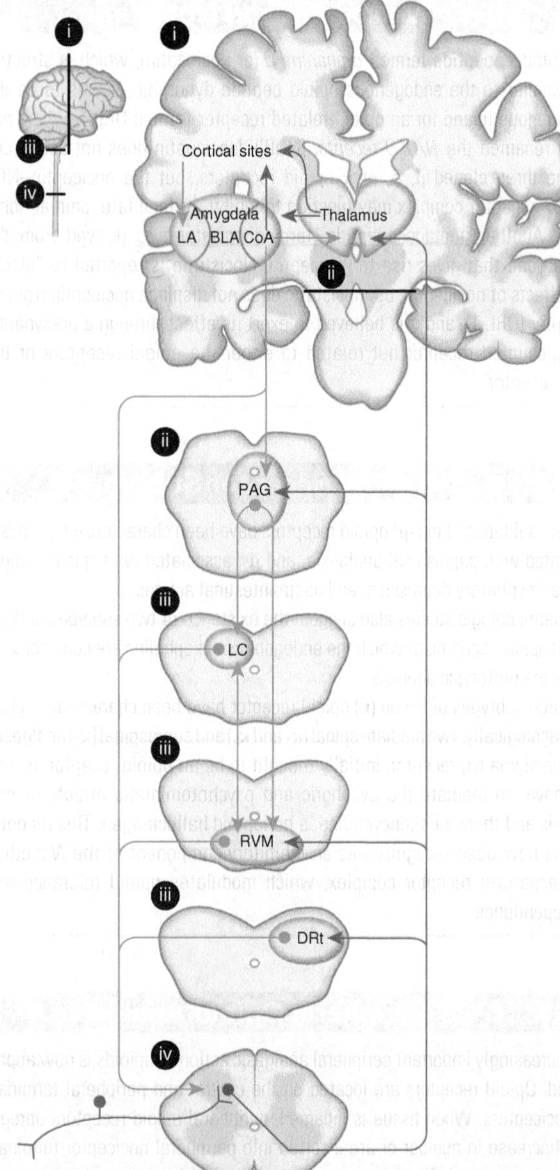

FIG 16-5 Schematic representation of pain transmitting (ascending, *red*) and pain-modulating (descending, *green*) pathways. Nociceptive signals are transmitted to the dorsal horn of the spinal cord via primary afferent neurons. Projection neurons ascend through the contralateral spinothalamic tract (and other pathways). Ascending pathways involve the thalamus, mesencephalic nuclei, and the midbrain periaqueductal gray (PAG). Rostral projections from the thalamus target areas that include the cortex and amygdala. Descending pain modulation is mediated through projections to the PAG, which also receives inputs from other sites (including the hypothalamus) and communicates with the rostral ventral medulla (RVM) and other medullary nuclei that send descending projections to the dorsal horn of the spinal cord and to the medullary dorsal horn for cephalic pain. The locus coeruleus (*LC*), which contains a high density of noradrenergic nuclei, receives input from the PAG, communicates with the RVM, and sends descending noradrenergic inhibitory projections to the level of the spinal and medullary dorsal horns. Anti- and pro-nociceptive spinopetal projections from the RVM inhibit and enhance, respectively, nociceptive inputs and constitute an endogenous pain regulatory system. Areas labeled "*i–iv*" in the inset correspond to the same labels in the larger diagram. *DRt*, Dorsal reticular nucleus. (From Ossipov et al.: *Journal Clin Invest*, 120:3779-3787, 2010.)

BOX 16-4 Gate Control Theory

The gate control theory described the important concept of endogenous pain modulation. The gate control theory posited that afferent inputs from large-diameter (non-nociceptive) and small-diameter (nociceptive) afferent fibers synapse onto a transmission cell (T cell) in the dorsal horn of the spinal cord, which sends projections to the brain. An interneuron (substantia gelatinosa; SG) inhibits inputs to the T cell large-diameter fiber. The SG cell is differentially regulated by afferent inputs, such that the large-diameter, non-nociceptive fibers excite the inhibitory SG interneuron, whereas the small-diameter fibers inhibit the SG. This circuitry was used to explain the clinical observation that non-noxious stimuli (such as rubbing an injured area) can attenuate pain that results from injury (i.e., activation of nociceptors). Opioid receptors are found on afferent nociceptors as well as SG and T cells. As our understanding of spinal cord transmission developed over the years, the gate control theory has been updated, but the theory remains important as it allowed understanding that nociceptive signals were processed within the central nervous system before reaching the cortex, resulting in a variable relationship between the stimulus and the resulting pain experience.

mediated locally within the spinal cord and also from the descending pain modulatory mechanism described earlier (Box 16-4).

Systemically administered opioids can therefore act at all sites in the nervous system that express opioid receptors, including multiple areas in the brain as well as in the spinal cord and on nociceptors. Agonist actions at these sites result in the overall analgesic effect produced, and they reflect additive or synergistic interaction from multiple neuronal circuits. Additive or synergistic activity occurs primarily in analgesic circuits resulting in increased opioid analgesic efficacy and potency. Importantly, increased analgesic actions also result in increased safety as lower doses are less likely to produce undesirable side effects. This knowledge can be used to improve pain control and limit the incidence or severity of undesirable opioid effects. Because pain modulation descending from the brainstem is mediated in the spinal cord by norepinephrine and 5-HT, the direct effects of an opioid given into the epidural space can be enhanced by epidural administration of an α-adrenoceptor agonist such as clonidine; this procedure is only used in specialized settings for specific patients. Likewise, tricyclic antidepressants that block the reuptake of norepinephrine are also effective adjuvants that are used for the treatment of chronic, but not acute, pain. This strategy allows reduction of the dose of opioid without compromising the analgesia produced (an "opioid-sparing" effect). Two drugs in particular, tramadol and tapentadol, produce analgesic actions by agonist activity at opioid receptors plus inhibition of neuronal reuptake of norepinephrine (tapentadol) and serotonin (tramadol). By requiring less opioid for adequate pain control, undesirable opioid effects, such as urinary retention, respiratory depression, sedation, and development of analgesic tolerance, can be reduced.

The cellular mechanisms by which opioids produce their effects are best established for direct actions at opioid receptors located on neurons. Actions commonly produced at all three opioid receptors include inhibition of adenylyl cyclase, inhibition of Ca^{2+} conductance, activation of K^+ conductance, and inhibition of neurotransmitter release (Fig. 16-6). Acute inhibition of adenylyl cyclase by an opioid results in a decrease in intracellular cyclic 3′,5′-adenosine monophosphate (cAMP); a decrease in inward nonselective cation current; and decreased cell excitability. All three opioid receptors also activate a G protein, inwardly rectifying K^+ conductance, and inhibit voltage-activated Ca^{2+} currents, both events mediated by G protein β-γ subunits. Because Ca^{2+} influx is required for the stimulus-secretion coupling of neurotransmitter release, opioids decrease the release of excitatory neurotransmitters

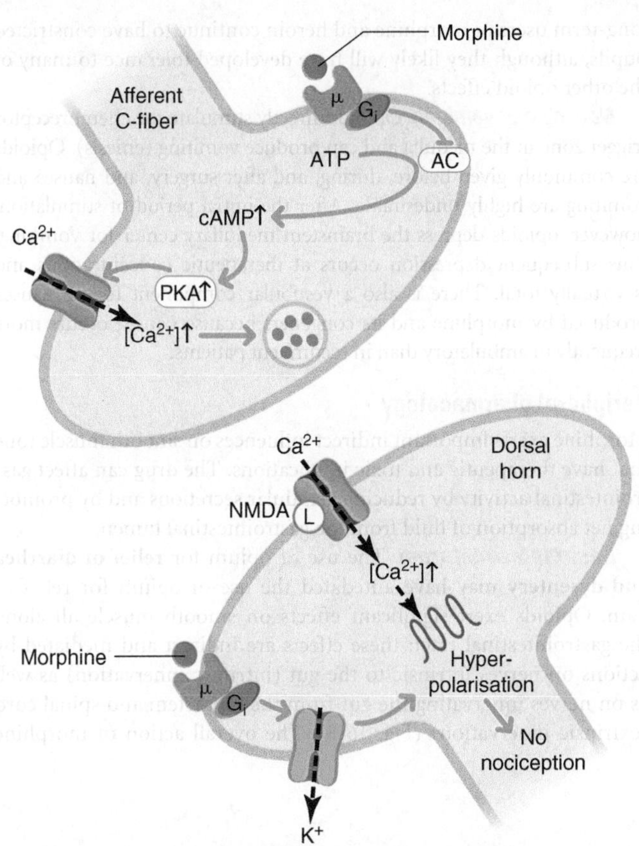

FIG 16-6 Opioids act both presynaptically and postsynaptically on neurons in pain circuits. Activation of presynaptic opioid receptors leads to a reduced intracellular cAMP concentration and decreased Ca^{2+} influx (and thus inhibition of release of excitatory neurotransmitters such as glutamate and substance P). Opioid receptor binding postsynaptically hyperpolarizes the neuronal membrane, which decreases the probability of the generation of an action potential in response to excitatory input at "L" (such as during pain transmission).

(such as glutamate, substance P, and calcitonin gene–related peptide) from nociceptor terminals and attenuate the transmission of nociceptive information at the first central synapse in the spinal dorsal horn (or medullary dorsal horn for cephalic pain). Activation of the rectifying K^+ conductance produces a relative hyperpolarization of neurons, making them more resistant to excitation (i.e., a higher pain threshold).

Morphine as the Prototype Opioid Analgesic

Morphine (Fig. 16-7) is the prototypic opioid analgesic agonist and the one about which most is known. It can be given by virtually any route of administration. All opioid analgesics share with morphine the ability to produce analgesia, respiratory depression, constipation, gastrointestinal spasm, antitussive actions, and physical dependence. The incidence of untoward effects (e.g., respiratory depression) differ little among the opioid agonists when they are compared at doses that produce equivalent analgesia. Consequently, morphine is discussed in greater detail, and what is stated for morphine applies in general to other opioid agonists. Significant differences are mentioned for individual agents.

Central pharmacologic effects

The CNS effects of morphine include **analgesia, drowsiness, euphoria, respiratory depression, suppression of the cough reflex, pupillary constriction, suppression of the secretion of some (e.g., luteinizing)**

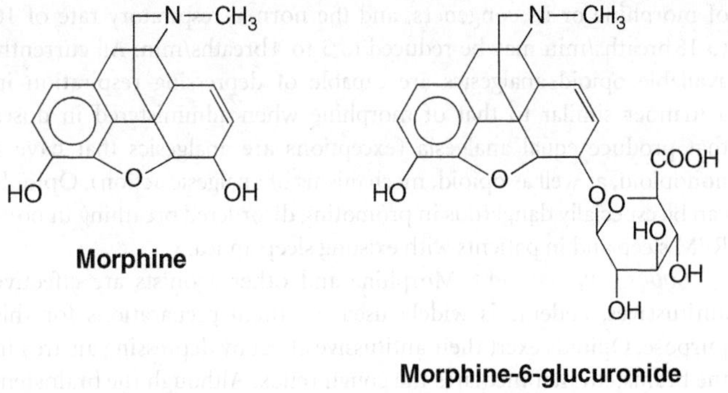

Morphine

Morphine-6-glucuronide

FIG 16-7 Structural formulas of morphine and its active metabolite morphine-6-glucuronide.

hormones and enhancement of other (e.g., prolactin) hormones, and initial stimulation of the medullary chemoreceptor trigger zone (to produce vomiting) followed by depression of vomiting through actions in medullary centers. Dysphoria occurs in a small percentage of opioid-naïve individuals.

Analgesia. The **analgesia** produced by morphine and other agonists occurs without loss of consciousness; thus opioids are not suitable for anesthesia. When opioids are administered for relief of pain (or for cough or diarrhea), they provide only symptomatic relief without alleviation of the cause of the pain (or cough or diarrhea). The analgesia produced by opioid analgesics is dose-dependent and selective in that other sensory modalities (e.g., vision, audition, touch) are unaffected at therapeutic doses. Likewise, systemic opioids do not impede the physiologic role of pain (i.e., withdrawal and protective responses to noxious stimuli). The standard parenteral (oral) analgesic dose of morphine, 10mg (30mg)/70kg of body weight, is considered a therapeutic dose for relief of moderate to severe pain. Pain is a highly subjective and personal experience that is influenced by many factors. Adequate pain relief is best achieved by titrating the dose to a patient's individual (and perhaps changing) requirement.

It is generally accepted that opioid-induced analgesia involves both sensory-discriminative and motivational-affective components of pain. However, opioids preferentially modulate the **motivational-affective (aversive) qualities of pain.** The **sensory-discriminative component** of pain is associated with identification and localization of the source and intensity of pain, whereas the motivational-affective component of pain is related to the perception of unpleasantness of the pain. Pain is not a simple sensation associated with a single neuronal circuit, but rather, it is a complex experience that can be influenced by the context in which the pain arises; prior experience and expectation; attention, anxiety, mood, and stress levels; and other societal, emotional, and cognitive contributions. As noted earlier, the nociceptive component (sensation) of pain is generally unaffected by systemically delivered opioid analgesics, a feature that allows these drugs to be used relatively safely. Clinical impressions and patients' reports suggest a prominent action by opioid analgesics on the motivational-affective component of pain, presumably resulting from opioid actions at opioid receptors within the cortical and limbic system of the brain. A common report from patients after receiving an opioid for relief of pain is that the pain is still present but that it is not discomforting.

Respiratory depression. Morphine and its congeners **depress respiration** (tidal volume and rate) in a dose-related fashion. Respiratory depression represents the principal potentially life-threatening effect of opioids. In humans, morphine decreases the response of brainstem respiratory centers to carbon dioxide tension of the blood and depresses pontine and medullary centers that regulate respiratory frequency. Irregular rhythms and periodic breathing are common after toxic doses of morphine or its congeners, and the normal respiratory rate of 16 to 18 breaths/min may be reduced to 3 to 4 breaths/min. All currently available opioid analgesics are capable of depressing respiration in a manner similar to that of morphine when administered in doses that produce equal analgesia (exceptions are analgesics that have a nonopioid, as well as opioid, mechanisms of analgesic action). Opioids can be especially dangerous in promoting disordered breathing in non-REM sleep and in patients with existing sleep apnea.

Cough suppression. Morphine and other agonists are effective antitussives; codeine is widely used in cough preparations for this purpose. Opioids exert their antitussive effect by depressing an area in the brainstem that mediates the cough reflex. Although the brainstem sites for the respiratory depressant and antitussive effects of opioids are anatomically close, there is no apparent relationship between opioid depression of one or the other because suppression of the cough reflex occurs at opioid doses lower than those required to produce an analgesic effect or to depress respiration.

Pupillary reaction. At therapeutic doses, morphine and most of its congeners produce pupillary constriction (miosis) in humans. The miosis produced by opioids results from a central effect mediated by the oculomotor nerve and not from a direct action on the circular or radial muscles of the iris of the eye. Although tolerance to opioids has not yet been discussed, it is appropriate to indicate here that tolerance to the pupillary-constricting effect of morphine and some other opioids does not develop to any appreciable extent. Consequently, long-term users of morphine and heroin continue to have constricted pupils, although they likely will have developed tolerance to many of the other opioid effects.

Nausea and vomiting. Opioids directly stimulate the chemoreceptor trigger zone in the medulla and can produce vomiting (emesis). Opioids are commonly given before, during, and after surgery, and nausea and vomiting are highly undesirable. After the initial period of stimulation, however, opioids depress the brainstem medullary center for vomiting. This subsequent depression occurs at therapeutic concentrations and is virtually total. There is also a vestibular component to the nausea produced by morphine and its congeners because nausea occurs more frequently in ambulatory than in recumbent patients.

Peripheral pharmacology

Morphine exerts important indirect influences on smooth muscle tone that have therapeutic and toxic implications. The drug can affect gastrointestinal activity by reducing glandular secretions and by promoting net absorption of fluid from the gastrointestinal lumen.

Gastrointestinal tract. The use of opium for **relief of diarrhea and dysentery** may have antedated the use of opium for relief of pain. Opioids exert significant effects on smooth muscle all along the gastrointestinal tract; these effects are indirect and mediated by actions on nerves intrinsic to the gut (intrinsic innervation) as well as on nerves innervating the gut from the brainstem and spinal cord (extrinsic innervation) (Fig. 16-8). The overall action of morphine

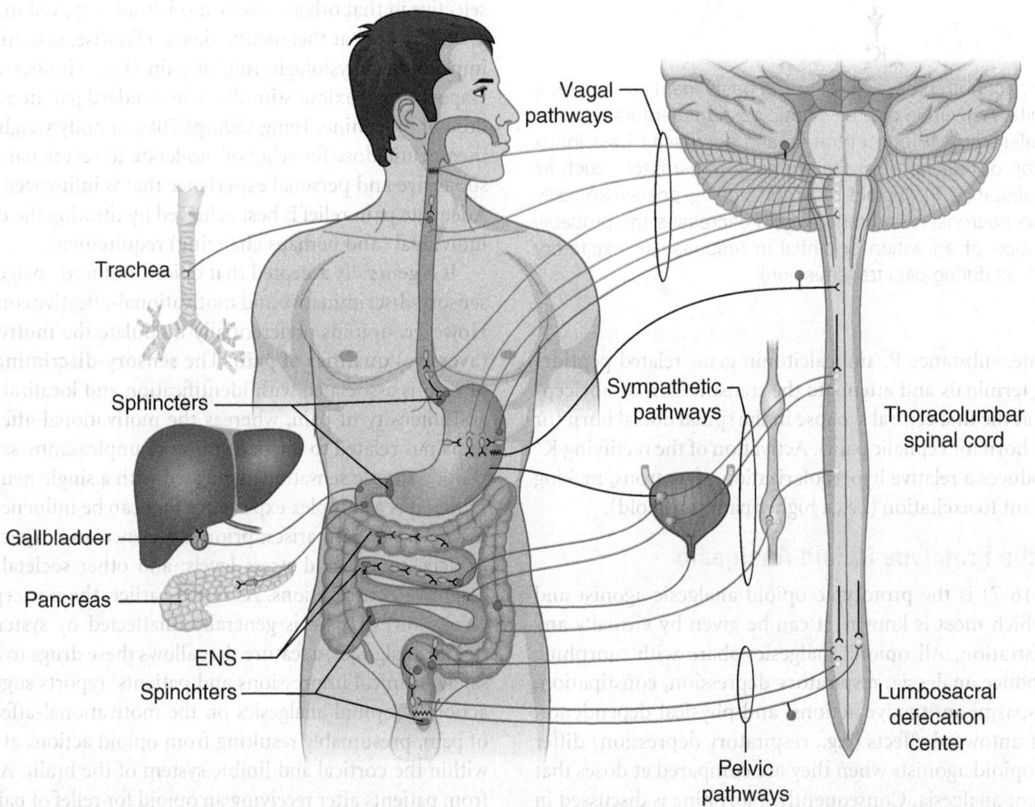

FIG 16-8 Opioids exert effects on the gastrointestinal tract (*GIT*) through interaction with both intrinsic and extrinsic innervation by the central nervous system (*CNS*) and within the enteric nervous system (*ENS*) (motor neurons and interneurons indicated in *blue*, sensory neurons indicated in *purple*). (Colors refer to cell bodies.) Control of function is reciprocal: signals from the CNS are transmitted to the ENS and GIT via vagal (10th cranial nerve), sympathetic, and pelvic pathways; signals from the GIT are transmitted via intestinofugal neurons (*red*) to the CNS (neurons in *yellow*), sympathetic ganglia, and organs (e.g., gallbladder and pancreas). Neurons within sympathetic prevertebral ganglia (indicated in *green*) receive input from both the CNS and the ENS. Sensory information is transmitted to both the ENS, via intrinsic primary afferent (sensory) neurons (indicated in *purple*), and to the CNS, via extrinsic primary afferent neurons (also indicated in *purple*) that follow spinal and vagal afferent pathways.

and its congeners is constipating, an effect that is either a desired therapeutic effect (antidiarrheal) or an unintended adverse effect (constipation). Constipation elicited by long-term opiate exposure can reach such a point as to be intolerable by patients who discontinue the use of opioids in spite of adequate analgesic efficacy. Opioid analgesics can act at opioid receptors on the intrinsic neuronal network in the gastrointestinal tract to inhibit motility. Endogenous opiate peptides have been identified in myenteric neurons and opiate receptors have been localized at presynaptic and postsynaptic sites of the enteric neuronal (myenteric and submucosal) plexus. Thus opiates can inhibit the firing of secretomotor and submucosal neurons as well as inhibit the release of transmitter from these neurons. In addition, opioids can also influence gastrointestinal activity by actions at opioid receptors in the CNS; opioids can decrease autonomic (parasympathetic) excitation of gastrointestinal smooth muscle and decrease propulsive motility throughout the gastrointestinal tract. In addition, opioids also suppress gastrointestinal motility by increasing sympathetic activity, which enhances the release of NE acting on presynaptic α2-adrenergic receptors of enteric neurons. Opioids may also exert a direct effect via opiate receptors expressed on smooth muscle cells (Fig. 16-9).

In the large intestine, muscle spasms can result from the marked increase in muscle tone and nonpropulsive muscle contractions. Spasm of the smooth muscle of the biliary tract can occur after the administration of therapeutic doses of morphine and related drugs, which can be very painful. Morphine and other opioids inhibit relaxation of the sphincter of Oddi in part by enhancing sympathetic tone, which suppresses the activity of inhibitory neurons that mediate relaxation of the sphincter.

Morphine and other agonists delay gastric emptying. In addition, gastric acid secretion is usually depressed, and pancreatic, biliary, and intestinal secretions are routinely depressed by opioid administration. Combined inhibition of intestinal fluid secretion and enhancement of absorption are important contributors to the beneficial effect of morphine in the treatment of diarrhea.

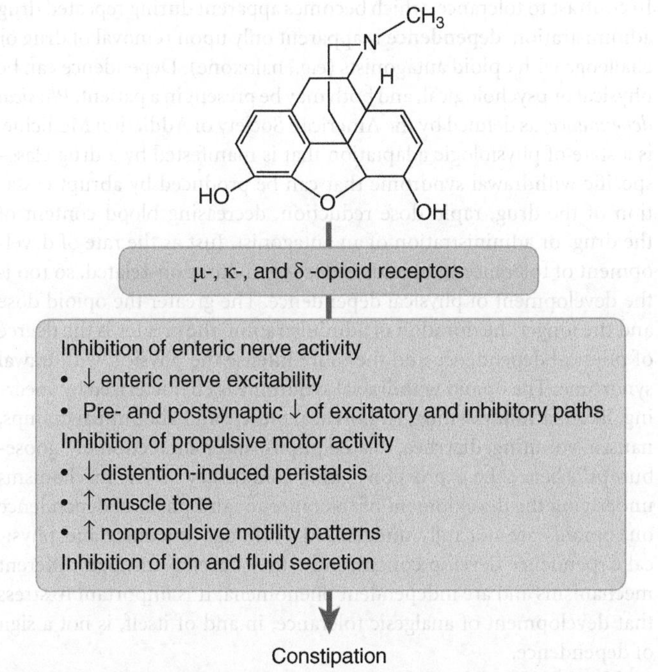

CH_3 N H HO O OH

μ-, κ-, and δ -opioid receptors

Inhibition of enteric nerve activity
- ↓ enteric nerve excitability
- Pre- and postsynaptic ↓ of excitatory and inhibitory paths

Inhibition of propulsive motor activity
- ↓ distention-induced peristalsis
- ↑ muscle tone
- ↑ nonpropulsive motility patterns

Inhibition of ion and fluid secretion

Constipation

FIG 16-9 Opioid agonists (morphine is pictured) produce constipation (or inhibit diarrhea) through a combination of multivariate mechanisms involving decrease in enteric nervous system excitability, inhibition of propulsive motor activity, and inhibition of ion and fluid secretion.

Other smooth muscle. Morphine and other opioid agonists also increase muscle tone in smooth muscle of the ureters, urinary bladder, uterus, and bronchioles, but at therapeutic doses the effect of opioids on these muscles is generally unremarkable. Urinary retention, characterized by urgency and increased tone of the bladder sphincter, is common after all routes of opioid administration. In addition to effects on tone and contractility of smooth muscle, opioids also possess antidiuretic effects. Although opioids increase uterine tone, they do not generally influence the duration of labor. Likewise in the bronchial musculature, opioids administered at usual therapeutic doses do not produce significant bronchoconstriction, even though they may aggravate an asthmatic condition or precipitate an asthmatic attack resulting in part from stimulation of **histamine release**.

In large doses, opioid effects on smooth muscles may be significant. For example, contraction of the ureter contributes to cessation of urine flow.

Cardiovascular system. The effects of morphine and other opioid agonists on blood pressure, heart rate, and cardiac work are generally minor at analgesic doses. The vasomotor center of the medulla is relatively unaffected by opioid analgesics, and blood pressure is maintained near normal even after intoxicating doses of opioids. A decrease in blood pressure observed during acute opioid intoxication is primarily caused by hypoxia that results from opioid-induced respiratory depression.

Morphine and several other opioid analgesics release histamine and produce some vasodilation of the peripheral vasculature, often resulting in an overall sensation of warmth accompanied occasionally by itching on the face and nose. Mast cell degranulation and histamine release does not appear to be mediated by opioid receptors, but rather, it may be influenced by the chemical properties of individual compounds. For example, morphine produces significant histamine release, whereas fentanyl does not. There also seems to be a poorly understood contribution by the CNS to peripheral vasodilation. The resultant decrease in peripheral resistance is the primary cause of the orthostatic hypotension and fainting that occur occasionally in some recumbent patients when the head-up position is suddenly assumed. Opioids have no direct effect on the vasculature and circulation of the brain, but cerebral vasodilation is a common consequence of opioid administration. Cerebral vasodilation is considered to be a consequence of the respiratory depression produced by morphine and its congeners and the subsequent retention of carbon dioxide in the blood. The result is an increase in cerebrospinal fluid pressure, which requires that opioids be used cautiously in cases of cranial trauma and head injury, where cerebrospinal fluid pressure may already be elevated. Morphine is also occasionally used in the treatment of pulmonary edema, where it is quite effective. The mechanism by which morphine exerts this beneficial action is unclear, but morphine seems to inhibit adrenergic tone centrally, promoting redistribution of blood to the periphery and reducing pressure in the pulmonary veins and capillaries without causing concomitant reduction of systemic arterial pressure.

Acute opioid intoxication

Death from acute intoxication by an opioid analgesic is the result of direct respiratory depression. The cardinal signs of acute opioid intoxication (overdose) represent an extension of the pharmacologic features of these drugs: **stupor, constricted pupils, and depressed respiration**. As the severity of intoxication increases, coma ensues, and the blood pressure, initially maintained close to normal, steadily decreases if the hypoxia associated with the respiratory depression is unaltered. Measures must be instituted to support respiration in cases of intoxication; pupillary dilation and shock, both caused by persistent hypoxia. Hypoxia precedes death in the absence of alteration in the respiratory status of an intoxicated individual.

Restoration of ventilation is most rapidly and dramatically achieved by administration of an opioid receptor antagonist (e.g., naloxone), but in the absence of immediately effective opioid receptor antagonism, a patent airway must be established, and efficient pulmonary gas exchange must be restored (by artificial respiration if necessary). Restoration of adequate pulmonary ventilation prevents the hypoxic cardiovascular sequelae of opioid intoxication. Although the details of opioid antagonists have not yet been discussed, it is important to interject two notes of caution regarding their use in cases of opioid intoxication. First, the duration of action of naloxone, the standard opioid receptor antagonist, is shorter than that of most opioid analgesics. Consequently, an opioid-intoxicated individual typically requires continued monitoring and readministration of additional naloxone as necessary. Second, administration of an opioid receptor antagonist to an acutely intoxicated, opioid-dependent individual can precipitate a withdrawal syndrome that cannot readily be attenuated during the period of action of the antagonist.

Tolerance

Tolerance is an observed decrease in effect of a drug as a consequence of prior administration of that drug. Hence, increasingly greater doses of drug must be administered over time to maintain an effect equivalent to the effect produced on initial administration. Interestingly, tolerance does not develop uniformly to all opioid effects. Generally, tolerance develops to the depressant effects of opioids but not to the same extent to the stimulant effects. Tolerance develops to opioid-induced analgesia, euphoria, drowsiness, and respiratory depression but not to any appreciable extent to opioid effects on the gastrointestinal tract or the pupil.

In the therapeutic setting, the initial indication that tolerance has developed is generally reflected in a shortened duration or reduced analgesic effect. The rate at which tolerance develops is a function of the dose and the frequency of administration. Although some patients remain normally sensitive, most patients treated for 5 to 7 or more days exhibit tolerance to the analgesic (and other) effects of opioids. Generally, the greater the opioid dose and the shorter the interval between doses, the more rapidly tolerance develops. Tolerance can develop to such an extent that the lethal dose of the opioid is increased significantly. For any individual, however, there always exists an opioid dose capable of producing death by respiratory depression, regardless of the extent to which tolerance has developed.

The mechanisms by which tolerance develops to opioids are not fully known, and many different hypotheses have been proposed. One hypothesis points to a role of internalization of G protein–coupled receptors, which include opioid receptors, after being bound by an agonist. Internalization is a multistep process in which opioid receptors are uncoupled from their heterotrimeric G proteins, phosphorylated by a receptor kinase, and targeted for endocytosis by clathrin-coated pits. When in the intracellular endosomal compartment, opioid receptors can be recycled for reinsertion into the cell membrane, sustaining agonist activity (i.e., diminishing tolerance), or degraded, which can result in receptor downregulation (a reduction in the number of receptors) and enhancement of opioid tolerance. Although acute desensitization is common to virtually all G protein–coupled receptors and occurs rapidly (seconds to minutes) after occupation of a receptor by its agonist, the time course of these cellular effects does not seem to match loss of agonist activity observed in humans. Tolerance may represent longer term desensitization and downregulation of receptor–effector coupling by mechanisms not yet fully understood.

More recent studies point to neuroplastic changes in the neuraxis as underlying the tolerance to the analgesic action of opioids. Clinical studies have shown that patients with persistent exposure to opiates show enhanced sensitivity to painful stimuli, even while the opiate is still present in the body. This condition of opiate-induced hyperalgesia (OIH) results from multiple neuroadaptive changes elicited by the opioid exposure. Persistent exposure to opioids may cause an increase in release of excitatory neurotransmitters from primary afferent terminals in the spinal cord and trigeminal ganglion, thus enhancing nociceptive inputs. This increased nociceptive input is associated with additional adaptations in the pain-processing centers of the CNS, resulting in an increase in activity of descending pain facilitation, as well as activation of microglia that can signal to nerves. Collectively, these mechanisms amplify the transmission of nociceptive inputs to the brain. This increase in "gain" contributes to the requirement for increased doses of opioids to produce inhibition and to offset the augmented pain. The consequence is a requirement for increased doses of opioids, resulting in a rightward displacement of the dose–response function and the manifestation of analgesic tolerance. Importantly, this state of amplified signaling can persist so that later insults, such as surgical incision, produce an exaggerated painful response. These amplification mechanisms may also contribute to findings that preoperative loading doses of opioids fail to reduce the postoperative requirement for analgesics, and they can actually increase the need for pain relief. The development of OIH is likely not due to nonselective effects of the drug used, since it has occurred with different structural classes of opioids and is stereospecific (i.e., receptor-mediated). Activation of the mechanisms driving hyperalgesia might be "buried" within the analgesic activity of the opioid, but it is unmasked once the analgesic effect has terminated. In addition, manipulations that block OIH often also enhance analgesia and the expression of analgesic tolerance.

Dependence

In contrast to tolerance, which becomes apparent during repeated drug administration, **dependence** is apparent only upon removal of drug or challenge with opioid antagonists (e.g., naloxone). Dependence can be physical or psychological, and both may be present in a patient. *Physical dependence*, as defined by the American Society of Addiction Medicine, is a state of physiologic adaptation that is manifested by a drug class–specific withdrawal syndrome that can be produced by abrupt cessation of the drug, rapid dose reduction, decreasing blood content of the drug, or administration of an antagonist. Just as the rate of development of tolerance to opioids is dose- and duration-related, so too is the development of physical dependence. The greater the opioid dose and the longer the duration of administration, the greater is the degree of physical dependence and the more intense the physical withdrawal syndrome. The opioid withdrawal syndrome is characterized by sneezing, lacrimation, yawning, rhinorrhea, muscle and abdominal cramps, nausea, vomiting, diarrhea, dilated pupils, and piloerection or "goosebumps" (hence the expression "going cold turkey"). The mechanisms underlying the development of tolerance to, and physical dependence on, opioids are not fully understood. Although tolerance and physical dependence develop concurrently, they develop through different mechanisms and are independent phenomena. It is important to stress that development of analgesic tolerance, in and of itself, is not a sign of dependence.

Physical dependence results from adaptations at cellular, synaptic, and systemic levels that in some ways are analogous to adaptive processes better understood as nervous system plasticity in the context of learning and memory (i.e., **long-term potentiation**). The underlying cellular and synaptic mechanisms that contribute to the development of opioid physical dependence are unknown.

Psychological dependence is more difficult to define and measure. Psychological dependence may contribute more to drug-seeking behavior than does physical dependence and contributes more significantly to addiction. As defined by the American Society of Addiction Medicine, *addiction* is the extreme of compulsive drug use and is characterized by continued use, and most importantly, loss of control over drug use and craving despite harm. Physical dependence can exist in the absence of psychological dependence, and it is inappropriate to identify as "addicted" an individual who becomes physically dependent after repeated opioid administration. All three phenomena—tolerance, physical dependence, and psychological dependence—are reversible, although psychological dependence provides a strong drive to continue the use of opioids.

It is now well documented that opioids activate endogenous reward pathways in the brain and that this mechanism contributes to their abuse. Opioids release or prolong the actions of the monoamine neurotransmitter dopamine in the mesocortical or mesolimbic systems, likely through actions on neurons in the midbrain ventral tegmental area, resulting in rewarding effects and promoting repeated use. Although the commonly abused drugs are structurally and pharmacologically heterogeneous (e.g., nicotine, alcohol, opioids, cannabinoids, cocaine), they all possess the ability to activate dopaminergic transmission in the mesocorticolimbic system to promote and maintain drug craving.

Opioid analgesics are sometimes ranked in terms of "abuse potential." However, it is unclear how significant the differences are among opioid analgesics when compared at equianalgesic doses given by the same route of administration and adjusted for relative availability.

Health professionals and patients are justifiably concerned about the repeated use of opioids for pain control, particularly in cases of chronic non-cancer pain (see later). This concern reflects the fear of dose escalation and unintended overdose that can lead to opioid poisoning and death in some individuals. Additionally, whether use of opioids for chronic pain provides significant benefit to the patient is not firmly established.

Absorption, fate, and excretion

Morphine is approximately one-third to one-sixth as potent when administered orally for relief of pain as the same dose given parenterally. Much of the difference is due to metabolic inactivation during morphine's first pass through the liver (first-pass effect). The primary pathway for the metabolism of morphine is conjugation with glucuronic acid, and the principal metabolite is morphine-3-glucuronide (approximately 55% of the administered dose). Morphine is also glucuronidated at the 6 position (approximately 10% of the administered dose) (see Fig. 16-7). **Morphine-6-glucuronide has a high affinity for the μ receptor** and is a potent and efficacious analgesic, especially when injected. Because it accumulates in the bloodstream, morphine-6-glucuronide may make a major contribution to the analgesic effects of morphine administered on a long-term basis.

Most of conjugated morphine is eliminated by the kidney; only small amounts of free morphine appear in the urine. Some morphine glucuronide appears in the bile, and a small percentage is excreted in the feces. Morphine does not generally accumulate in tissues; the total excretion of an administered dose is usually approximately 90% complete within the first 24 hours.

Although morphine is subject to significant first-pass metabolism after oral administration, it is widely used orally for the management of chronic pain (e.g., cancer pain). The oral dose of morphine in liquid form can range from less than 10 mg every 4 hours to 2500 mg every 4 hours (the latter in a highly opioid tolerant patient); most patients require no more than 200 mg/day. Morphine is also available for oral use in controlled-release tablets or capsules to produce longer lasting analgesia (e.g., 12 hours).

Regarding the wide dose ranges reported necessary for pain control in cases of chronic pain, it first must be appreciated that chronic pain is controlled by titration of the dose in individual patients to achieve a desired effect and, second, that analgesic tolerance is likely present or will develop. A common phenomenon in the treatment of chronic pain is "breakthrough" pain. Breakthrough pain is sharp, intense pain that "breaks through" the doses of opioid that are effectively controlling pain. Breakthrough pain can occur from movement (incident pain) or for unknown reasons and requires very fast-acting opioids such as fentanyl. Fentanyl is often given as a "lollipop" specifically for the treatment of breakthrough pain allowing the patient to titrate the effect as needed. In general, dosages of morphine required to manage chronic pain can be quite high. In terminally ill patients, concern that the development of physical dependence is an indication of "addiction"—which it is not—should not be dose-limiting.

OTHER COMMON OPIOIDS

Analgesics that act through opioid receptors display similar pharmacologic properties to morphine. The properties of some specific agents are highlighted in Table 16-1. In general, they offer little or no theoretical advantage over morphine or codeine and for the most part are less widely used. New opioid analgesics continue to be developed, and it is likely that some of these will find clinical application.

Mixed Agonist-Antagonists and Opioid Receptor Antagonists

Mixed agonist-antagonists

Some opioids possess both agonist and antagonist effects and are therefore referred to as "mixed" agonist-antagonists. Drugs possessing agonist and antagonist properties were first synthesized 100 years ago. It was hoped that such drugs would be potent analgesics devoid of dependence and abuse liability. It was quickly learned, however, that drugs having agonist and antagonist properties are often unsuitable for clinical use as analgesics because of undesirable dysphoric side effects. The dysphoric actions of opioids are most prominent if the κ opioid receptor is engaged. The opioid receptor–blocking aspect of their pharmacologic profile does not prevent their abuse or free these drugs from tolerance and dependence. The properties of specific agents are summarized in Table 16-1.

In carefully controlled studies in animals, mixed agonist-antagonists have been shown to possess reinforcing properties that lead to self-administration. In this respect, the mixed agonist-antagonists are similar to agonists, although they have less reinforcing efficacy. Tolerance develops to the agonist, but not antagonist, effects of these drugs. Subjects who repeatedly use mixed agonist-antagonists may become physically dependent, just as can occur with repeated use of morphine and other opioid agonists. However, the withdrawal symptoms differ from those of morphine-like agonists.

Opioid receptor antagonists for treatment of opioid toxicity

Naloxone (Fig. 16-10), **naltrexone,** and nalmefene are opioid receptor antagonists currently available that are essentially devoid of

TABLE 16-1 Characteristic Features of Some Opioid Agonists and Agonist-Antagonists

Drug	Features
Codeine See Fig. 16-12	• A naturally occurring alkaloid present in opium powder. • Differs from morphine only in that a methoxy substitution (—OCH_3) replaces the hydroxyl group at position 3 of the molecule. • This subtle structural change provides codeine with significant oral effectiveness. • Primarily used as an orally administered analgesic and antitussive. • Is metabolized primarily by the liver and is excreted chiefly in the urine, largely in inactive forms. • Demethylated at position 3 to form morphine, and free and conjugated morphine are found in small quantities in the urine after therapeutic doses of codeine. This conversion, plus the fact that codeine itself binds poorly to the μ opioid receptor, has led to classification of codeine as a prodrug insofar as its analgesic action is concerned. • The analgesic and antitussive actions of codeine (and its respiratory depressant and sedative effects) are central in origin. • That codeine is a mild analgesic incapable of providing an analgesic effect equivalent to morphine is an erroneous, but widely held, impression. At present, however, doses of codeine greater than 60mg (orally) are not commonly used and are not officially recognized as generally safe and effective by the U.S. Food and Drug Administration. • The recommended analgesic dose of codeine is 30-60mg orally. • The most common adverse effects are nausea, constipation, dizziness, and sedation. At greater doses, the incidence of nausea and vomiting is increased, a particularly undesirable effect in individuals who have undergone dental surgery. • Codeine is especially suitable for relief of pain in ambulatory individuals because it is orally effective; can provide significant analgesia and relief of dull, continuous pain; and can be taken for relatively long periods with little or no risk of physical dependence. A dose of 60mg of codeine taken 3-4 times daily over 6-8 weeks is not associated with the development of significant physical dependence. Tolerance develops to the analgesic effect of codeine over time. • The demonstrated analgesic usefulness of codeine in some situations that show little or limited response to nonopioid analgesics makes codeine a useful drug for certain pain states.
Dihydrocodeine, oxycodone, and hydrocodone	• Opioids similar in structure to morphine and codeine. • Similar to codeine, they have a methoxy substitution (—OCH_3) for the hydroxy group at position 3 of the morphine molecule. • Have good oral efficacy. • Do not differ significantly from morphine in terms of their pharmacology. • Oxycodone is approximately equipotent with morphine when given parenterally. • An oral dose of 5mg of oxycodone is approximately equivalent to 30-60mg of codeine. • A controlled-release preparation of oxycodone (OxyContin) was the subject of controversy because of abuse potential and toxicity. The abuse potential for this form of oxycodone seems to be due, at least in part, by the higher quantity of the drug present in the controlled-release formulation. • Hydrocodone is slightly less potent than oxycodone (the usual analgesic dose of dihydrocodeine is half that of codeine).
Meperidine (pethidine)	• A synthetic phenylpiperidine structurally dissimilar to morphine. • Initially developed as an atropine-like drug, but subsequently discovered to possess analgesic efficacy. • In therapeutic doses (80-100mg parenterally), it produces analgesia, sedation, respiratory depression, and the other CNS actions common to opioids as a class. • Approximately one-eighth to one-tenth as potent as morphine. • Given parenterally; at equianalgesic doses, the degree of sedation and respiratory depression is the same for both drugs. • Because it has some atropine-like action, pupillary constriction is less, as is the incidence of spasm of the biliary tract. • Similar to other opioid analgesics, meperidine can be spasmogenic to the smooth muscle of the gastrointestinal tract, but it differs from other opioids in that it is generally not considered to be valuable in the treatment of diarrhea. A congener, diphenoxylate (contained in Lomotil®), is widely used for that purpose. • Peak analgesic effect occurs soon after parenteral administration; duration of action is short (3-4 hours). • Acute intoxication differs from morphine: CNS excitation produced by the normeperidine metabolite, manifested as tremors and convulsions. • Commonly abused by health professionals who mistakenly believe that it has a lower dependence liability and is easier to stop using than morphine.
Methadone	• A synthetic pure agonist opioid. • The diphenylheptane structure, although it does not resemble morphine, is induced by steric factors to assume the configuration that apparently is required for agonist interaction with MOR. Might also have other relevant pharmacologic actions. • Approximately equipotent to morphine. • Aside from greater oral efficacy, differs little from morphine. • Produces analgesia, sedation, respiratory depression, miosis, antitussive effects, and subjective effects similar to those of morphine. • Is constipating and can cause biliary tract spasm. • Well absorbed from the gastrointestinal tract, eventually becomes localized in the lung, kidney, and liver, where it undergoes extensive biotransformation. • The major metabolites are excreted in the urine and in the bile, along with small quantities of unchanged drug. • Because methadone is a potent, orally effective analgesic agent, it was initially restricted by law for use in the treatment of opioid addiction. • Possesses a combination of properties that makes it useful in opioid addiction treatment (e.g., oral delivery and duration of action). • The term *blockade* of the effects of opioids and a disappearance of "drug hunger" is misleading because methadone is an opioid receptor agonist not antagonist. • Use of methadone (or any other opioid agonist) in maintenance programs relates to cross-tolerance and cross-dependence and not to some unique ability of methadone to "block" heroin's effects. • As used in maintenance programs, methadone simply represents the substitution of one opioid for another, and methadone is used rather than other opioids primarily because it can be given orally and has an extended duration of action.

TABLE 16-1 Characteristic Features of Some Opioid Agonists and Agonist-Antagonists—cont'd

Fentanyl and congeners	• Fentanyl, alfentanil, sufentanil, and remifentanil are 4-anilopiperidines that have relatively short durations of action and thus are often used as intravenous supplements during general anesthesia with inhalation or intravenous anesthetic drugs or as the principal component of balanced anesthesia (e.g., with nitrous oxide and a neuromuscular blocking drug), especially for cardiac surgery. • The primary advantage of these more potent opioids is the cardiovascular stability they provide during surgery. Also, they are more effective than morphine in reducing the endocrine and metabolic responses to surgery. • Opioids are not anesthetics, and such use is associated with a high incidence of signs of inadequate anesthesia (e.g., sweating, pupillary dilation, or opening of the eyes during surgery). • Awareness during surgery and inadequate amnesia after surgery can occur. Other disadvantages include bradycardia (which can be prevented by pretreatment with atropine); respiratory depression; and muscle rigidity, particularly of the abdominal and thoracic cavities. • Fentanyl is about 80-100 times more potent than morphine. • Sufentanil is 5-10 times more potent than fentanyl; alfentanil is less potent than fentanyl. • Because of its rapid onset and short duration of action even after repeated administrations, alfentanil has become a popular choice for outpatient anesthesia. • Remifentanil is quickly broken down in bloodstream and tissues by esterases, so it has the shortest duration of action and can be beneficial in brief procedures. • Available as an adherent skin patch for transdermal delivery of drug. This formulation, used principally for treatment of chronic pain (e.g., cancer pain), provides continuous drug delivery in therapeutic concentrations with reduced incidence of constipation and nausea. • Available for rapid onset (sublingual absorption) to control episodes of breakthrough pain.
Buprenorphine	• Multimechanistic. • Partial agonist at MOR, KOR partial antagonist, plus some nonopioid receptor activity. • Agonistic effects qualitatively similar to the effects of morphine in comparative clinical trials. • Produces less respiratory depression than does morphine at equianalgesic doses; may be more difficult to reverse using naloxone. • Causes less euphoria than many other opioids and opiates. • Useful in chronic addiction control.
Pentazocine	• Agonist-antagonist. • Used parenterally • Benzomorphan derivative structurally related to morphine, but it has an allyl-like substitution on the nitrogen of the piperidine ring, as do many opioid receptor antagonists. • Agonist at KOR and a partial agonist or weak antagonist at MOR. • Produces its major agonist effects on the CNS and gastrointestinal tract and induces morphine-like subjective effects and euphoria. • In contrast to pure agonists, pentazocine does not suppress withdrawal symptoms in individuals dependent on other opioids, but it also does not antagonize morphine-induced respiratory depression. • Can precipitate signs of withdrawal in an opioid-dependent individual (due to antagonist activity at MOR). • Approximately one-third as potent an analgesic as morphine when given intramuscularly. Generally, the maximal analgesic effect of mixed agonist-antagonist analgesics is less than that of morphine or other pure opioid agonists. • At therapeutic doses, pentazocine exhibits adverse effects on the CNS and gastrointestinal tract that are qualitatively similar to effects of other opioids (e.g., dizziness, nausea, and sedation and analgesia). • In contrast to most other opioids, pentazocine can increase heart rate and blood pressure. In toxic doses, it produces dysphoric effects and opioid-like respiratory depression, although the respiratory depression does not increase proportionately with increasing doses as it does for pure opioid agonists.
Butorphanol	• Agonist-antagonist. • A morphinan derivative approximately 4-6 times more potent than morphine as an analgesic. • An agonist at KOR and a weak partial agonist at MOR. • Shows no cross-dependence, unlikely to precipitate withdrawal symptoms in opioid-dependent individuals. • Has a low abuse potential, and respiratory depression tends to plateau beyond therapeutic doses. Has been tested as an analgesic anesthetic, but because it has a tendency, similar to pentazocine, to increase cardiac work, it is not well suited for this application. Another limitation of butorphanol is the possibility of dysphoric side effects. • Subject to significant first-pass metabolism; bioavailability after oral administration is low. Available in an injectable form for obstetric use and as a nasal spray formulation (used for migraine headache).
Nalbuphine	• Agonist-antagonist. • Structurally related to naloxone. • Agonist at KOR (but produces few dysphoric reactions) equipotent with regular analgesic doses of morphine. • Pronounced antagonist action at MOR, which distinguishes it from other available mixed agonist-antagonists. • Has been used to reverse respiratory depression produced by other opioids without causing a loss of analgesia and in debilitated surgical patients for whom the abrupt loss of pain relief caused by naloxone reversal can be life-threatening (also beneficial in this setting since it produces minimal myocardial depression). Nevertheless, opioid reversal even with nalbuphine is potentially dangerous in a patient at risk of heart attack. • Should not be considered a replacement for naloxone for treatment of drug overdose, except in special settings. • Marketed only as an injectable solution in the United States; rarely used outside the hospital setting; rarely found in forensic analyses; the only opioid analgesic not scheduled under the Controlled Substances Act.

Continued

TABLE 16-1 Characteristic Features of Some Opioid Agonists and Agonist-Antagonists—cont'd	
Tramadol	• Multimechanistic. • Aminocyclohexanol derivative, marketed as the racemic mixture. • The (+) enantiomer is a weak MOR agonist and inhibits the reuptake of 5-HT; the (–) enantiomer is a norepinephrine reuptake inhibitor. • The *O*-demethylated (M1) metabolite is a potent MOR agonist. • All of these properties contribute synergistically to the analgesic action. • Only partially reversed by naloxone. • The most common adverse effects include nausea, vomiting, and drowsiness; effects on respiratory or cardiovascular parameters are not clinically relevant at recommended doses; seizures and serotonin syndrome have been reported. • Has abuse potential, but generally less than equianalgesic doses of other opioid agonists.
Tapentadol	• Multimechanistic. • Opioid plus neuronal NE reuptake inhibition. • In contrast to tramadol, does not have relevant serotonin reuptake inhibition. • Opioid and norepinephrine reuptake inhibition mechanisms contribute (synergistically) to analgesia. • Does not have an analgesically active metabolite. • Efficacy greater than tramadol and similar to morphine. • The dual mechanism of action contributes to an improved gastrointestinal side-effect profile.

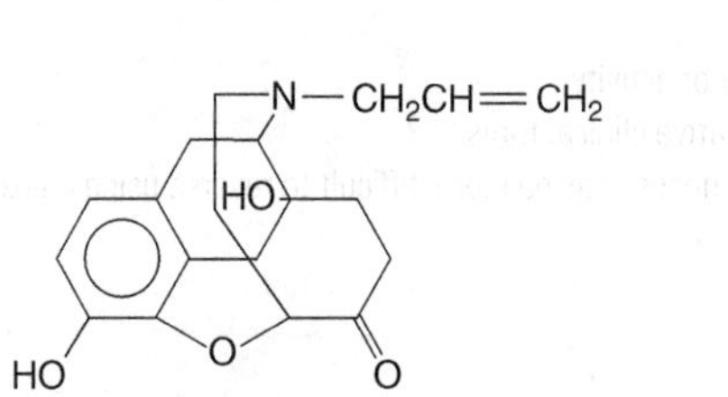

FIG 16-10 Structural formula of naloxone.

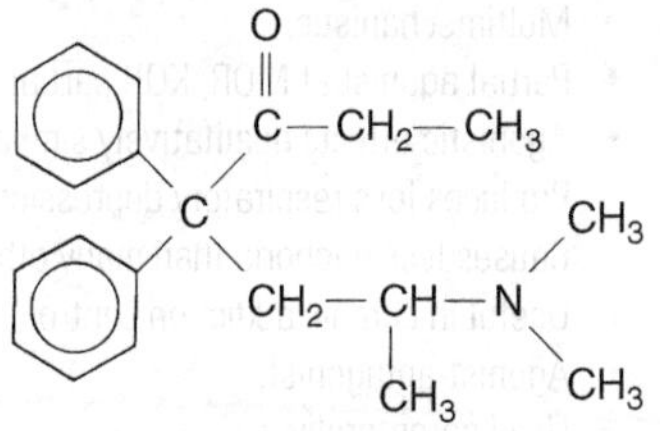

FIG 16-11 Structural formula of methadone.

opioid agonist effects. The principal use of opioid receptor antagonists is in the treatment of acute opioid intoxication. They rapidly improve ventilation. The antagonists are not general respiratory stimulants, however. Conversely, they do not diminish respiration further if administered to individuals with respiratory depression produced by other drugs (e.g., barbiturates or alcohol). The lack of response to naloxone, naltrexone, or nalmefene in a case of respiratory depression of unknown cause can be highly suggestive of nonopioid drug intoxication.

Naloxone, which is not very effective when given orally, has an almost immediate onset and a short duration of action (1 to 4 hours) when given parenterally. Additional doses may be required at 20- to 60-minute intervals, especially if naloxone is being used to reverse intoxication by a long-acting opioid agonist. Naltrexone differs from naloxone in that it is more effective orally and has a remarkably longer duration of action. A single oral dose can suppress the effects of opioid agonists for 48 to 72 hours. These attributes suggest that naltrexone may be useful in the maintenance of an opioid-free state in detoxified, formerly opioid-dependent, individuals. A single daily administration of the drug can effectively block the action of 25 mg of heroin injected intravenously 24 hours after the last dose of naltrexone. Naltrexone may also prove useful in treating morphine overdose because it might obviate the need to monitor the patient for a relapse of respiratory depression. Nalmefene is an orally active drug that has an even longer duration of action than does naltrexone, but it is not as commonly used.

Opioid receptor antagonists for treatment of constipation as a result of opioids or bowel surgery

Alvimopan and methylnaltrexone are antagonists of MOR. They do not pass the blood–brain barrier and therefore do not affect the actions of opioids in the CNS, making them useful in treating one adverse effect of MOR stimulation in the GI tract without compromising the central analgesic effects of opioids. Alvimopan is an oral drug given in the hospital setting before and after bowel surgery. Methylnaltrexone is given subcutaneously to treat constipation due to opioids.

USE OF OPIOIDS FOR THE CONTROL OF CHRONIC NON-CANCER PAIN

A full discussion of the differentiating types of pain is beyond the scope of this chapter, but discussion of some general principles will aid in a better understanding of the use of opioids in the clinical management of pain. Opioids can be used satisfactorily as analgesics for the relief of acute pain and are appropriate for the treatment of cancer pain. Whether opioids should be used for the treatment of chronic non-cancer pain is controversial. Meta-analysis data suggest that opioids used for the treatment of chronic non-cancer pain are not very effective and may decrease the patient's quality of life. Care should be taken before embarking on opioid therapy for chronic nonmalignant pain.

The long-term use of opioids requires taking into account the choice of opioid, the route of administration, and the role that will be played by the development of tolerance and physical dependence in therapy. Although the bioavailability of oral morphine is limited because of first-pass metabolism, the dose can be adjusted for successful pain control by administration in liquid or sustained-release tablet form. Methadone (Fig. 16-11) is a useful alternative to morphine, but because its plasma half-life averages 24 hours, methadone accumulates with repeated dosing, and greater care is required with its use. Oral administration is generally considered optimal for the treatment of chronic pain, but epidural, intrathecal, and intravenous routes of administration are also used, more recently in situations of patient-controlled analgesia (PCA). Studies indicate that the total amount of opioid that is self-administered by PCA is usually no more than, and often less than, that given conventionally by health care professionals. The use of PCA is important because it gives patients control over when they treat their pain, thereby diminishing fear and providing psychological benefit.

The use of mixed agonist-antagonists in chronic pain management is limited. For example, escalating doses of pentazocine and related drugs can lead to psychotomimetic effects. More importantly, the antagonistic properties of mixed agonist-antagonists at the μ opioid receptor restrict the ability to switch between pure agonists and mixed agonist-antagonists.

USE IN DENTISTRY

Pain of dental origin frequently arises from, or is accompanied by, inflammation. Because opioids are not antiinflammatory, nonopioid analgesic drugs with antiinflammatory efficacy (e.g., aspirin, ibuprofen) are often the first choice for relief of pain. Opioids are particularly useful when additional pain control is required. The opioids used in dentistry are primarily those available for oral administration, including codeine, hydrocodone, and oxycodone. Morphine, meperidine, and fentanyl are used parenterally. Combinations of **opioids with acetaminophen, aspirin, or ibuprofen are commonly used and are rational** because different, complementary central and peripheral mechanisms of pain relief are invoked. Although aspirin and ibuprofen have antiinflammatory efficacy, acetaminophen is not antiinflammatory and is not a good choice, used singly, when it is desired to reduce inflammation. Acetaminophen does, however, have analgesic activity.

Cautions

The opioid analgesics are subject to misuse and abuse. The pharmacologic and sociologic aspects of opioids are discussed in Chapter 39. Additional implications for dentistry relate to the possible interactions of opioids with other medications that may be prescribed or substances (prescription and nonprescription drugs, herbals, nutritional supplements, etc.) that patients may take for other reasons. Drug interactions with orally administered opioids are uncommon or not usually of great clinical importance when they do occur. There are recognized interactions, however, between opioids and CNS depressants, neuroleptics, tricyclic antidepressants, monoamine oxidase inhibitors, local anesthetics, and oral anticoagulants that can be clinically significant, particularly if opioids are given parenterally.

Generally, the coadministration of **CNS depressants** produces summation of effects and occasionally a greater than anticipated depression (i.e., supra-additive effect). Opioids and phenothiazines (e.g., chlorpromazine) are known to produce at least additive CNS depression, including respiratory depression. This combination may also produce a greater incidence of orthostatic hypotension than either drug administered alone. Increased hypotension has also been reported with combinations of opioids and tricyclic antidepressants. The clinical significance of these interactions, particularly at the doses of opioids used orally in dentistry, is uncertain. When combinations of opioids with other CNS depressants are given by intravenous infusion, the effects can be titrated to the desired level. When opioids are used orally, doses should have a sufficient margin of safety to avoid dose-dependent toxicity.

The coadministration of local anesthetics and parenteral opioid analgesics is a common and generally safe practice. Large doses of these classes of drugs display supra-additive toxicity, however. It is likely that

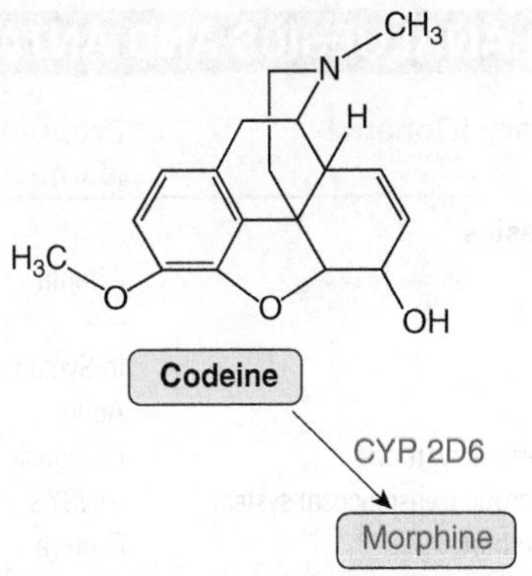

CH_3 N H H_3C O O OH

Codeine

CYP 2D6

Morphine

FIG 16-12 Codeine undergoes metabolism and activation (demethylation) to morphine accounting for most of its analgesic effect. Cytochrome P450 2D6 is the enzyme system responsible. Genetic variation in this enzyme accounts for differences in analgesic or toxic effects of codeine. For simplicity, other routes of metabolism of codeine (to inactive metabolites) are not shown.

respiratory acidosis caused by an opioid can increase the entry of a local anesthetic into the CNS.

Interaction of opioids with oral anticoagulants has been reported to result in an enhanced response to the latter, but the clinical significance has not been established, and it is unlikely that short-term opioid administration has an appreciable effect on the patient's response to oral anticoagulants.

A well-documented interaction between **meperidine** and **monoamine oxidase inhibitors** results in severe and immediate reactions that include excitation, rigidity, hypertension, and sometimes death. Chemically unrelated opioids are unlikely to cause a similarly violent reaction.

Dentists are often confronted with the report by patients that they are allergic to codeine. The nature of these adverse effects needs to be explored with the patients. Nausea and vomiting, without hives and itching, is most like due to stimulation of the chemoreceptor trigger zone (CTZ) during the initial period of therapy. This is not a hypersensitivity reaction. If on the other hand, the previous adverse reaction had the appearance of a hypersensitivity reaction with hives, itching, and perhaps difficulty in breathing, codeine and other phenanthrenes such as morphine, hydrocodone, dihydrocodeine, and oxycodone should be avoided. The CTZ mechanism is more likely to occur than the hypersensitivity reaction.

Genetic Variation in Response to Codeine

Figure 16-12 shows the pathway of **codeine metabolism** by which it is activated to morphine. Variations in the activity of cytochrome P450 2D6 range from poor metabolizers, to intermediate metabolizers, to extensive metabolizers (the most common genetic type), to ultra-rapid metabolizers. Therefore, depending on the patient's genetic profile, the rate and degree of conversion of codeine to morphine can range from low to high. Codeine, at typical doses, would be ineffective in the patient who is a poor metabolizer but potentially toxic in the patient who is an ultra-rapid metabolizer. Codeine is more affected than other opioids by variations in enzyme makeup, although **tramadol and hydrocodone** are also somewhat affected by variations in activity of cytochrome P450 2D6. (See case study for chapter 4.) Future medicine and dentistry will take into account these variations using the benefits of genetic testing. Dentists should be aware that a higher percentage of some Asian groups have slower metabolism involving cytochrome P450 2D6 (intermediate metabolizers) and therefore are likely to have a lower analgesic response to codeine than most Caucasians.

OPIOID ANALGESICS AND ANTAGONISTS

Nonproprietary (Generic) Name	Proprietary (Trade) Name
Agonist Analgesics	
Alfentanil	Alfenta
Codeine	—
Dihydrocodeine	In Synalgos DC
Fentanyl	Actiq
Fentanyl transdermal system	Duragesic
Fentanyl iontophoretic transmucosal system	IONSYS
Fentanyl buccal tablet	Fentora
Fentanyl sublingual	Abstral
Hydrocodone	In Hycodan
Hydromorphone	Dilaudid
Levomethadyl	ORLAAM
Levorphanol	Levo-Dromoran
Meperidine	Demerol
Methadone	Dolophine
Morphine	—
Oxycodone	Oxycontin; in Percodan
Oxymorphone	Numorphan
Remifentanil	Ultiva
Sufentanil	Sufenta
Mixed Agonist-Antagonist Analgesics	
Buprenorphine	With naloxone in Suboxone; Belbuca
Butorphanol	Stadol
Nalbuphine	Nubain
Pentazocine	Talwin
Antagonists	
Alvimopan	Entereg
Methylnaltrexone	Relistor
Nalmefene	Revex
Naloxone	Narcan
Naltrexone	Revia, Vivitrol
Others	
Tramadol	Ultram
Tapentadol	Nucynta

CASE DISCUSSION

Given the bone and soft tissue involvement, an analgesic would be indicated. You decide on hydrocodone (5mg)+acetaminophen (325mg), with instructions to take one "pain pill" every 6hours as needed for pain. The patient left the dentist's office with the intention of going home before having the prescriptions filled. Unfortunately, before getting his prescription filled, the effect of the local anesthetic began to wear off, and the patient became aware of a gradually intensifying persistent throbbing type of pain on the left side of his mouth that became increasingly unbearable. He immediately had the prescriptions filled and took one hydrocodone/acetaminophen tablet. Within 45minutes, the pain had largely subsided. The patient estimated that on a 10-point pain scale the pain fell from a high score of 8 to a low score of 2. The patient then took two ibuprofen tablets (200mg each), and he was pain-free within 15minutes. At this point the patient should have been instructed to take ibuprofen and, if that was sufficient, to continue with ibuprofen until the pain subsided. The hydrocodone/acetaminophen combination can be added if needed for pain.

GENERAL REFERENCES

1. Dickenson AH, Besson J-MR, editors: *The pharmacology of pain*, handbook of experimental pharmacology (vol. 130). Berlin, 1997, Springer.
2. Dostrovsky J, Carr DB, Koltzenburg M, editors: *Proceedings of the 10th World Congress on Pain*, Seattle, 2003, IASP Press.
3. Gebhart GF, Proudfit HK: Descending modulation of pain processing. In Hunt S, Koltzenburg M, editors: *The neurobiology of pain*, Oxford, 2004, Oxford University Press.
4. Kieffer BL: Molecular aspects of opioid receptors. In Dickenson AH, Besson J-MR, editors: *The pharmacology of pain*, handbook of experimental pharmacology, vol. 130. Berlin, 1997, Springer.
5. Moore PA: JADA Continuing Education: pain management in dental practice: tramadol vs codeine combinations, *J Am Dent Assoc* 130: 1075–1079, 1999.
6. Raynor K, Kong H, Chen Y, et al.: Pharmacological characterization of the cloned kappa-, delta-, and mu-opioid receptors, *Mol Pharmacol* 45:330–334, 1994.
7. Reisine T: Opiate receptors, *Neuropharmacology* 34:463–472, 1995.
8. Stein C, Cabot PJ, Schafer M: Peripheral opioid analgesia: mechanisms and clinical implications. In Stein C, editor: *Opioids in pain control*, Cambridge, 1999, Cambridge University Press.
9. Stein C, editor: *Opioids in pain control*, Cambridge, 1999, Cambridge University Press.
10. Taylor DA, Fleming WA: Unifying perspectives of the mechanisms underlying the development of tolerance and physical dependence to opioids, *J Pharmacol Exp Ther* 297:11–18, 2001.
11. Williams JT, Christie MJ, Manzoni O: Cellular and synaptic adaptations mediating opioid dependence, *Physiol Rev* 81:299–343, 2001.
12. Wynn RL: Non-traditional analgesics for dental pain, *Gen Dent* 56: 122–124, 2008.
13. Zakrezewska JM, Harrison SD, editors: *Assessment and management of orofacial pain*, pain research and clinical management (vol. 14). Amsterdam, 2002, Elsevier.

17

Nonopioid Analgesics

Elliot V. Hersh and Raymond A. Dionne

KEY INFORMATION

- Inflammatory mediators include histamine, prostaglandins, leukotrienes, platelet-activating factor, cytokines, bradykinin, and nitric oxide.
- The nonsteroidal antiinflammatory drugs (NSAIDs) block the production of prostaglandins by inhibiting cyclooxygenase (COX).
- The two major COX enzymes are the constitutive COX-1 and the inducible COX-2.
- Aspirin is the only enzyme that irreversibly inhibits COX.
- Inhibition of the synthesis of thromboxane A2 by aspirin accounts for its antiplatelet effect.
- Aspirin and other NSAIDs have analgesic, antipyretic, and antiinflammatory effects.
- NSAIDs that inhibit both COX-1 and COX-2 include aspirin, ibuprofen, naproxen, ketorolac, and several others.
- Celecoxib is a selective COX-2 inhibitor, and therefore it is associated with less GI toxicity compared to aspirin and the other nonselective COX inhibitors.
- Acetaminophen has analgesic and antipyretic properties, but it is not an effective antiinflammatory drug.
- Hepatotoxicity is a manifestation of acute toxicity of acetaminophen.
- NSAIDs, chiefly aspirin and ibuprofen, as well as acetaminophen are often used in combination with opioids to treat dental pain.
- Disease-modifying agents for rheumatic diseases (DMARDs) include antineoplastic drugs, antimalarial and immunosuppressant drugs, and the newer protein biopharmaceuticals.
- Antigout drugs are drugs that reduce uric acid or its inflammatory effects.

CASE STUDY

Your patient, Ms. K, has rampant caries in her remaining dentition. You previously diagnosed that she needs to have her remaining 16 teeth removed, three quadrants of alveoloplasty, and two mandibular tori removed to prepare her for upper and lower dentures. She is 55 years old, admits to being a "pain wimp," and has been avoiding your recommended care out of phobia and reluctance to convert to dentures. She now presents with acute pulpitis in #19 and wants to get "lots of narcotics" to blunt the pain. How will you manage her acute pain needs and then (hopefully soon) her postoperative pain management when she does submit to having the rest of her teeth removed?

Nonopioid analgesics, including the NSAIDs, represent a diverse group of chemical compounds whose mechanism of action typically involves the inhibition of one or more components of the inflammatory response. Acute pain, which typically accompanies tissue injury and subsequent inflammation, results from a variety of dental procedures and can often be controlled by the use of the nonopioid analgesics such as acetaminophen or ibuprofen. In addition, the NSAIDs play an important role in the symptomatic relief of the inflammation and pain that accompany chronic orofacial pain and generalized arthritic pain. However, they do not eliminate or reduce the underlying causes of the chronic disorder, and joint damage can continue to progress despite the long-term use of these drugs.

CAUSES OF INFLAMMATION

Inflammation typically represents the response to tissue injury and includes products of activated mast cells, leukocytes, and platelets; prostaglandins (PGs); leukotrienes; and complement-derived products. The clinical features of inflammation include edema (tumor), redness (rubor), heat (calor), pain (dolor), plus loss of function. Inflammation is often thought of as a pathologic event, but it actually serves a normal repair function. In the case of tissue injury from minor trauma or a surgical procedure, the inflammatory process results in a series of well-regulated humoral and cellular events leading to localization of injury, removal of noxious agents, repair of physical damage, and restitution of function in the injured tissue. In patients unable to mount a competent inflammatory response, such as those with neutropenia induced by some cancer chemotherapeutic drug regimens, the results may lead to fulminant infection and death.

The inflammatory response is, of course, not always beneficial to the host. If it becomes excessive or chronic, as is the case with rheumatoid arthritis, it may result in the progressive destruction of joint tissue and untoward systemic effects. In the dental setting, acute inflammation can result in moderate to severe pain, edema, limited mouth opening, and diminished quality of life for four or six days following oral surgical procedures. Pharmacologic intervention may be desired to minimize symptoms.

Inflammation can be divided into three phases: acute inflammation, subacute inflammation, and chronic inflammation. In acute inflammation, inflammatory mediators such as histamine are released, causing vasodilation and increased capillary permeability. In the subacute stage, inflammatory cells migrate and invade the site. PGs, leukotrienes, platelet-activating factor (PAF), and cytokines also play major roles. The third, or chronic, stage of inflammation involves the lymphocytic phase of injury cleansing and repair. Cytokines, especially interleukins and tumor necrosis factor-alpha (TNF-α), are prominent in this stage. In reality, these phases are not distinct entities. For example, components of the subacute phase participate in the acute inflammatory process and acute inflammatory mediators are present in chronic inflammatory disorders such as arthritis. Even so, this classification offers a useful way to categorize this highly complex process. The following section briefly reviews some of the key mediators of the inflammatory process. A more complete list of inflammatory mediators is provided in Table 17-1.

Tissue Mediators

Histamine is a vasoactive amine that is widely distributed in the body, mostly stored in mast cells and basophil granules in a physiologically inactive form. A variety of physical and chemical stimuli, such as antigens, complement fragments, or simple mechanical trauma, can cause extrusion of the granules and release of active histamine into the extracellular fluid. One of the most characteristic actions of histamine is dilation of vessels of the microcirculation and a marked, but transient, increase in the permeability of capillaries and postcapillary venules reflecting an activation of histamine-1 (H_1) receptors in these tissues. The histamine content of tissue fluid at the site of injury rises within minutes after the insult and then falls. Prior depletion of tissue histamine stores by various means or pretreatment with classic antihistamines (H_1 receptor blockers) will reduce the initial vascular response to injury (Chapter 18). The role played by histamine in inflammation is early, transient, yet nonessential for subsequent events that may lead to lasting tissue alterations.

Pharmaceutical antihistamines have little use as general antiinflammatory agents. In certain situations, such as immediate allergic reactions, large amounts of histamine are released locally or systemically from sensitized mast cells and basophils as a consequence of antigen–antibody reactions. In these instances, antihistamines that block the H_1 receptor are useful in reducing symptoms attributable to histamine. Antihistamines that block the action of histamine at the H_2 receptor have a supporting role in the management of anaphylaxis and a major role in the treatment of gastric hyperacidity conditions.

The **prostaglandins** (PGs) are a unique family of closely related lipids found in all tissues. The basic structure of all PGs is a prostanoic acid skeleton composed of a 20-carbon polyunsaturated fatty acid with a five-member ring at C8 through C12. Like the leukotrienes described later, PGs are derived from arachidonic acid and similar other 20-carbon polyunsaturated fatty acids that are liberated from damaged cell membranes of local tissues. Inflammatory cells, including human monocytes and mast cells, also have the ability to generate PGs.

One of the key events in the acute inflammatory process is the liberation of arachidonic acid from damaged cell membranes upon exposure to phospholipase A_2 (Fig. 17-1). This step can be inhibited indirectly by a powerful group of antiinflammatory steroid agents known as **glucocorticoids**, which are described in detail in Chapter 30. From this point, the oxidative metabolism of arachidonic acid can proceed along two divergent pathways. One pathway uses the enzyme **cyclooxygenase (COX)**, whereas the second uses the enzyme **lipoxygenase**. Virtually all cells in the body, with the exception of red blood cells, contain the COX enzyme, whereas lipoxygenase appears to be limited to inflammatory cells (neutrophils, mast cells, eosinophils, and macrophages). COX catalyzes the transformation of arachidonic acid to the short-lived cyclic endoperoxide PGG_2. PGG_2 is then converted to PGH_2 by peroxidation, which is an additional function of COX. From this point, PGH_2 is converted to the stable PGE_2 and $PGF_{2\alpha}$, thromboxanes, or prostacyclin (PGI_2) by appropriate enzymes.

It is now well established that COX exists in three isoforms. The two most common are 72-kd proteins but differ in terms of their sequence homology (approximately 60%) and their genomic regulation. COX-1 is regarded as the constitutive or "housekeeping" isoform and is the major isoform found in healthy tissues. It is always present in a number of tissues, including the central nervous system (CNS), gastric mucosa, platelets, and kidneys. In the gastric mucosa, COX-1 plays a major role in the synthesis of PGs involved in the formation of the mucous protective barrier against stomach acid. In platelets, COX-1 is the key enzyme involved in thromboxane production and its subsequent platelet activation properties necessary for proper hemostasis. COX-2 is an inducible isoform upregulated by such products as cytokines, growth factors, and mitogens in human monocytes, macrophages, endothelial cells, chondrocytes, synoviocytes, and osteoblasts. It is associated with elevated concentrations of PGs during inflammation, pain, and fever. Although initially it was hoped the COX-2 products only participated in inflammatory and other pathologic processes, it is now known that oxidation products of the COX-2 isoform help regulate some normal physiologic processes, including the maintenance of adequate water and Na^+ excretion by the kidneys, the inhibition of excessive platelet aggregation and dilation of certain vascular beds. Finally, COX-3 is an elongated isoform of COX-1 (it has an extra intron that is alternately

TABLE 17-1 Classification of Some Endogenous Mediators of Inflammation

Major Groups	Major Mediators
Tissue	
Lymphocyte products	MCP-1
	GM-CSF
	Other chemoactive factors
	Interferon γ
	Interleukins
	Skin reactive factor
Macrophage products	Interleukin-1
	Interferon γ
	TNF-α
	PAF
Mast cell products	Histamine
	Cytokines
	TNF-α
	Leukotrienes
	Prostaglandin D_2
	PAF
Eosinophil products	Lysosomal enzymes
	Major basic protein
	Other cationic proteins
	Leukotrienes
	PAF
Others	Reactive metabolites of oxygen
	Endogenous pyrogens from leukocytes
	Leukocytosis factors
	Nitric oxide
Plasma	
Kinin system	Bradykinin
Complement system	C3 fragments
	C5 fragments
	C5b67 complex
	Membrane attack complex
Clotting system	Fibrinopeptides
	Fibrin degradation products

GM-CSF, Granulocyte-macrophage colony-stimulating factor; *MCP-1*, monocyte chemoattractive protein-1; *PAF*, platelet-activating factor.

spliced), and in the animal model, it has properties that are mainly found in the transmission of pain in the spinal cord. There is debate if this isoform exists in humans.

PGs and the other active metabolites of the intermediate endoperoxides (e.g., PGI_2 and thromboxane A_2 [TXA_2]) exert a multitude of effects in almost every biologic process examined so far. There is abundant evidence that PGs and the intermediate endoperoxides are mediators of inflammation. In acute inflammatory reactions, PGs appear in fluids and exudates later (2 to 12 hours after injury) than some other mediators, such as histamine and bradykinin. PGs are being formed, then, at a time when tissue damage is more prominent. It is possible that some of the PG content found in sites of inflammation is derived from infiltrating neutrophils and macrophages because these cells are capable of PG synthesis. The precise roles of PGs in the inflammatory process are still evolving, but these unique compounds clearly occupy a central regulatory position as mediators, modulators, or both.

Slow-reacting substance of anaphylaxis (SRS-A) is an important mediator of anaphylactic and other immediate allergic reactions. SRS-A can be found in most tissues, especially in the lung, after appropriate antigenic challenge. It is released along with histamine and other active products from mast cells. SRS-A belongs to a class of compounds known as **leukotrienes**. The leukotrienes are formed by the conversion of arachidonic acid by the combined actions of 5-lipoxygenase and leukotriene A synthase to generate leukotriene A_4. Leukotriene A_4 may be converted to leukotriene B_4 by a hydrolase enzyme or, alternatively, to leukotriene C_4 by the addition of glutathione. Removal of glutamate from leukotriene C_4 generates leukotriene D_4. These lipid-peptide derivatives appear to account for all the biologic activity of SRS-A in immediate allergic reactions. Leukotrienes C_4 and D_4 constitute SRS-A. However, asthmatic reactions may also involve other leukotrienes. The ability of cells to produce leukotrienes appears to be limited to the lung, leukocytes, blood vessels, and epicardium. In contrast, all cells except erythrocytes can convert arachidonic acid to PGs and related compounds by the action of COX.

Leukotrienes C_4 and D_4 are potent constrictors of bronchial smooth muscle with 1000 times more potency than histamine. Because these leukotrienes also increase vascular permeability, it seems likely that either one or both play a role in the bronchial constriction and mucosal edema of asthma. Leukotriene B_4 can enhance chemotactic and chemokinetic responses in human neutrophils, monocytes, and eosinophils. These findings suggest that leukotrienes are involved

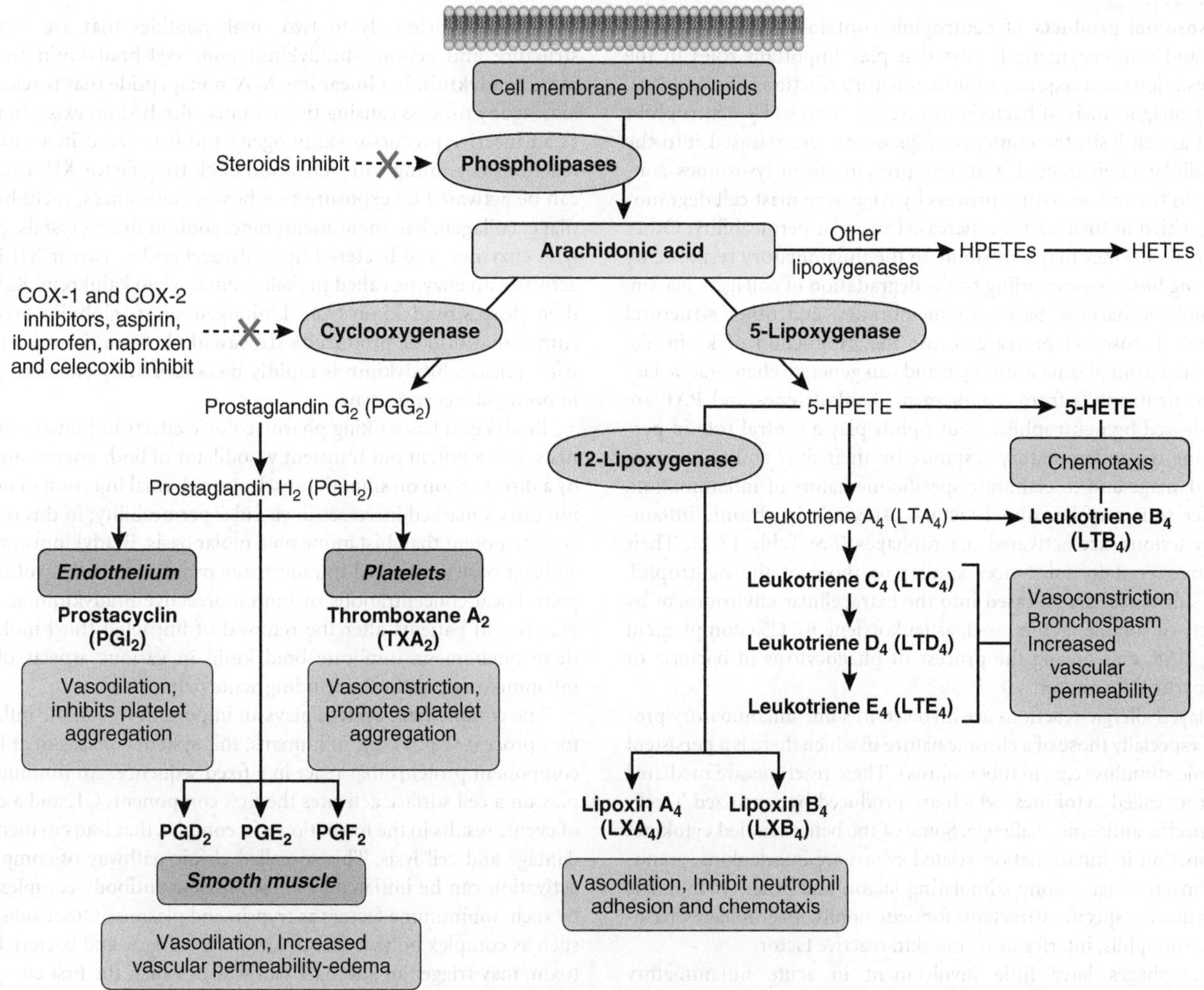

FIG 17-1 Pathways of arachidonic acid metabolism to prostaglandins and leukotrienes and their subsequent effects on the endothelium, platelets, and smooth muscle. Areas where NSAIDs and steroids inhibit the pathway are illustrated. (Modified from Kumar V et al.: *Robbins and Cotran Pathologic Basis of Disease*, ed 8, Philadelphia, 2010, Saunders and from Batmanian L, Ridge J, Worrall, S: *Biochemistry for Health Professionals*, Sydney, 2011, Mosby.)

TABLE 17-2 Factors in the Neutrophil with Inflammatory Potential

Tissue-damaging enzymes	Elastase
	Cathepsins B and G
	Collagenase
	Other proteases
Microbicidal enzymes	Myeloperoxidase
	Lysozyme
Permeability factors	Leukotrienes
	PAF
	Leukokinin-forming enzyme
	Basic peptides
Leukotactic factors	Leukotrienes
	PAF
	C5-cleaving enzyme
	Basic peptides (chemotactic for monocytes)

in localized inflammatory processes as well as in asthma. Drugs that block leukotriene receptors or inhibit leukotriene synthesis by blocking the enzyme lipoxygenase are used in the treatment of asthma (see Chapter 27).

Lysosomal products of neutrophils contain a variety of enzymatic and non-enzymatic factors that play important roles in the manifestations and sequelae of inflammatory reactions (Table 17-2). During phagocytosis of bacteria or foreign material by neutrophils, as well as cell lysis, the contents of lysosomes are released into the extracellular environment. Cationic proteins from lysosomes contribute to the inflammatory process by triggering mast cell degranulation, which in turn leads to increased vascular permeability. Other lysosomal enzymes may contribute to the inflammatory response by damaging host tissues leading to the degradation of collagen, elastin, mucopolysaccharides, basement membranes, and other structural elements. Lysosomal proteases cause the production of kinin-like substances from plasma kininogen and can generate chemotactic factors for neutrophils from complement. **Leukotrienes** and **PAF** are also released by neutrophils. Neutrophils play a central role in perpetuating the inflammatory response by their dual ability to cause tissue damage and to elaborate specific mediators of inflammation. Another source of lysosomal factors, especially in chronic inflammatory lesions, are activated macrophages (See Table 17-2). Their lysosomes contain substances similar to those of the neutrophil. These substances are released into the extracellular environment by a variety of soluble factors, such as leukotriene B_4, C5a complement factor, PAF, and during the process of phagocytosis of bacteria or other particulate matter.

Delayed allergic reactions are involved in some inflammatory processes, especially those of a chronic nature in which there is a persistent antigenic stimulus (e.g., in tuberculosis). These reactions are mediated by factors called **cytokines**, which are produced by sensitized T cells after specific antigenic challenge. Some of the better studied cytokines that function in inflammation-related events are interleukins, granulocyte/macrophage colony-stimulating factor, and other chemotactic factors that are specific attractants for neutrophils, macrophages, basophils, eosinophils, interferon-α, and skin reactive factor.

Macrophages have little involvement in acute inflammatory responses but do play a very prominent role in chronic inflammation and are crucial to the immune response. In addition to their phagocytic activity, **macrophage secretory products** have a major function in established inflammatory lesions. Secretory products include the constituents of lysosomes (described earlier), reactive metabolites of oxygen, interferon-α, interleukin-1 (IL-1), and TNF-α. The latter two substances are crucial mediators of the complex interplay between macrophages and lymphocytes, which in large measure determines the course and eventual outcome of an inflammatory process. IL-1 is produced by macrophages exposed to bacterial, viral, and fungal products; antigens; or macrophage activation factor. It may have several roles, but chief among these seems to be the stimulation of differentiation of a pre–T-lymphocyte population to mature T cells capable of responding to an antigen processed and presented by macrophages. Another mediator of inflammation produced by macrophages and other cells is PAF. PAF initiates a variety of actions, including platelet activation, vasodilation, vascular permeability, neutrophil chemotaxis, and discharge of lysosomal enzymes.

Mast cells release a number of inflammatory mediators in addition to histamine, including cytokines (e.g., TNF-α), leukotrienes, PGD_2, and PAF. Mast cells are activated by immunoglobulin (Ig) E antibodies that are bound to their plasma membrane that sensitize them to specific allergens. Several allergic reactions, including allergic asthma, involve this mechanism. Basophils have many of the same characteristics as mast cells. Eosinophils release a number of enzymes and toxins that can lead to tissue destruction. as well as leukotrienes and PAF.

Plasma Mediators

Kinins refer primarily to two small peptides that are similar in structure and actions: bradykinin and lysyl-bradykinin (or kallidin). **Bradykinin** is a linear low MW nonapeptide that is released by almost any process causing tissue injury. Bradykinin exists in plasma as an inactive precursor (kininogen) and is released in a cascade of reactions beginning with activation of clotting factor XII. Factor XII can be activated by exposure to a host of substances, including cartilage, collagen, basement membrane, sodium urate crystals, proteolytic enzymes, and bacterial lipopolysaccharides. Factor XII in turn activates an enzyme called prekallikrein to yield kallikrein. Kallikrein then cleaves bradykinin from kininogen, an α_2-globulin precursor. Kinins may also be produced extravascularly from tissue kininogen. After release, bradykinin is rapidly metabolized by enzymes present in both plasma and tissues.

Bradykinin has striking pharmacologic effects in humans and animals. It is a potent but transient vasodilator of both arteries and veins by a direct action on smooth muscle. Intradermal injection of bradykinin causes marked increases in vascular permeability; in this regard, it is more potent than histamine on a molar basis. Bradykinin applied to a blister base or injected intradermally or intraarterially evokes sharp pain. Local concentrations of immunoreactive bradykinin as well as PGs rise in patients after the removal of impacted third molars. All these phenomena implicate bradykinin in various aspects of acute inflammatory reactions, including acute pain.

The **complement system** plays an important role in the inflammatory process (Fig. 17-2). In humans, this system consists of at least 20 component proteins that react in a fixed sequence. An immune complex on a cell surface activates the first component, C1, and a cascade of events results in the formation of a complex that leads to membrane damage and cell lysis. This so-called classic pathway of complement activation can be initiated by most antigen–antibody complexes and by such nonimmune factors as trypsin and plasmin. Other substances, such as complex polysaccharides, aggregated IgA, and bacterial endotoxin, may trigger an alternate pathway in which the first component to be activated is C3, followed then by the usual components in the activation scheme.

In addition to the direct cellular damage cited earlier, certain fragments produced during the cascade of complement activation have biologic properties of importance. Two of them (C3a and C5a) cause

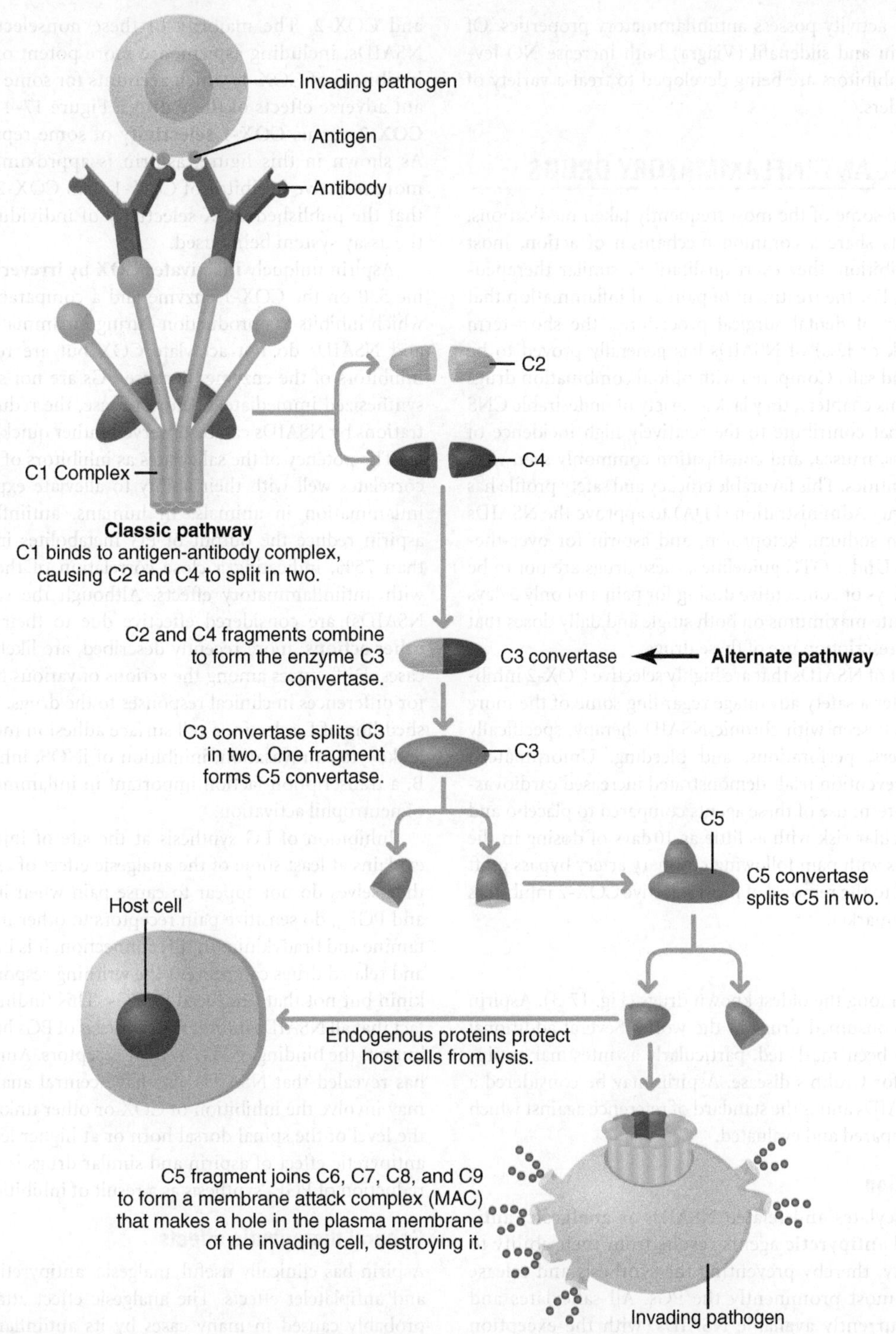
Invading pathogen
Antigen
Antibody
C2
C4
C1 Complex
Classic pathway
C1 binds to antigen-antibody complex, causing C2 and C4 to split in two.
C2 and C4 fragments combine to form the enzyme C3 convertase.
C3 convertase
Alternate pathway
C3 convertase splits C3 in two. One fragment forms C5 convertase.
C3
C5
C5 convertase splits C5 in two.
Host cell
Endogenous proteins protect host cells from lysis.
C5 fragment joins C6, C7, C8, and C9 to form a membrane attack complex (MAC) that makes a hole in the plasma membrane of the invading cell, destroying it.
Invading pathogen

FIG 17-2 The complement cascade. The classic and alternate pathways are shown. The steps by which bacterial polysaccharides interact with several plasma proteins (B, D, and properdin) to generate the C3 convertase of the alternate pathway, C3bBb, are not shown.

increased vascular permeability by inducing the release of histamine from mast cells. These substances have been implicated in anaphylaxis and other allergic reactions. Complement fragments can be produced by other mechanisms extrinsic to the complement system, which suggests that complement fragments may participate in tissue injury and in the subsequent inflammatory response without classic or alternative complement activation.

The small gaseous molecule **nitric oxide** (NO) plays a regulatory and a proinflammatory role in various inflammatory conditions including arthritis, asthma, and inflammatory bowel disease. In mammalian cells (and somewhat similar to COX), two isoforms of the NO-producing enzyme nitric oxide synthetase are constitutively expressed, while a third inducible isoform (iNOS) is upregulated in response to bacterial products and proinflammatory cytokines. Compounds that inhibit iNOS expression or activity possess antiinflammatory properties. Of interest, nitroglycerin and sildenafil (Viagra) both increase NO levels. Specific iNOS inhibitors are being developed to treat a variety of inflammatory disorders.

NONSTEROIDAL ANTIINFLAMMATORY DRUGS

The NSAIDs include some of the most frequently taken medications. Because these agents share a common mechanism of action, most notably COX-1 inhibition, they exert qualitatively similar therapeutic and toxic effects. For the treatment of pain and inflammation that accompany a variety of dental surgical procedures, the short-term use (typically 1 week or less) of NSAIDs has generally proved to be highly efficacious and safe. Compared with opioid combination drugs (described later in this chapter), they lack a variety of undesirable CNS depressant effects that contribute to the relatively high incidence of drowsiness, dizziness, nausea, and constipation commonly seen with opioid-containing entities. This favorable efficacy and safety profile has led the Food and Drug Administration (FDA) to approve the NSAIDs ibuprofen, naproxen sodium, ketoprofen, and aspirin for over-the-counter (OTC) use. Under OTC guidelines, these drugs are not to be used more than 10 days of consecutive dosing for pain and only 3 days for fever, plus absolute maximums on both single and daily doses that are lower than the prescription use of these drugs.

The development of NSAIDs that are highly selective COX-2 inhibitors appeared to offer a safety advantage regarding some of the more serious adverse effects seen with chronic NSAID therapy, specifically gastrointestinal ulcers, perforations, and bleeding. Unfortunately, large colon polyp prevention trials demonstrated increased cardiovascular risk with long-term use of these agents compared to placebo and increased cardiovascular risk with as little as 10 days of dosing in the treatment of patients with pain following coronary artery bypass graft surgery. This has led to the removal of most selective COX-2 inhibitors from the worldwide market.

Salicylates

The salicylates are among the oldest known drugs (Fig. 17-3). Aspirin is one of the most consumed drugs in the world. Several additional salicylates have also been marketed, particularly as intestinal antiinflammatory agents for Crohn's disease. Aspirin may be considered a prototype of the NSAIDs and is the standard of reference against which these agents are compared and evaluated.

Mechanism of action

The efficacy of salicylates and related NSAIDs as **analgesic, antiinflammatory, and antipyretic** agents results from their ability to inhibit COX activity, thereby preventing the synthesis and release of COX products, most prominently the PGs. All salicylates and almost all of the currently available NSAIDs, with the exception of the highly selective COX-2 inhibitors, inhibit both COX-1 and COX-2. The majority of these nonselective COX-inhibiting NSAIDs, including aspirin, are more potent or at least equipotent inhibitors of COX-1, which accounts for some of the more important adverse effects of these drugs. Figure 17-4 displays the relative **COX-2** versus **COX-1 selectivity** of some representative NSAIDs. As shown in this figure, aspirin is approximately a hundredfold more selective inhibitor of COX-1 than COX-2. It should be noted that the published COX selectivity of individual drugs varies with the assay system being used.

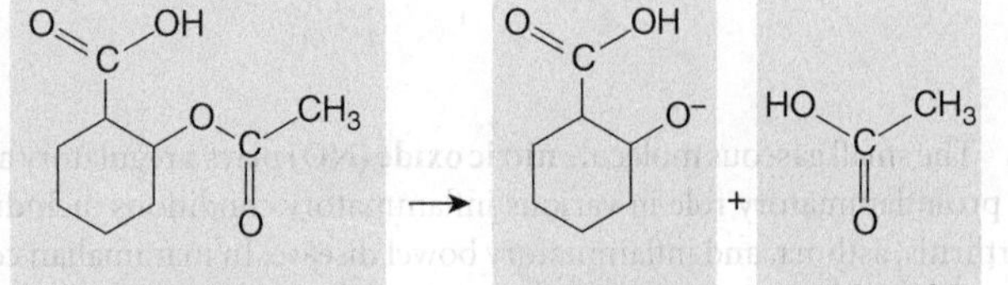

FIG 17-3 The structure of aspirin and how it is broken down to salicylate and acetic acid.

Aspirin uniquely **inactivates COX by irreversibly acetylating** serine 530 on the COX-1 enzyme and a comparable serine on COX-2, which inhibits PG production during inflammation. Other salicylates and NSAIDs do not acetylate COX but are reversible competitive inhibitors of the enzyme. Because PGs are not stored, but rather are synthesized immediately before release, the reduction of PG concentrations by NSAIDs can be observed rather quickly.

The potency of the salicylates as inhibitors of PG synthesis in vitro correlates well with their ability to alleviate experimentally induced inflammation in animals. In humans, antiinflammatory doses of aspirin reduce the output of PG metabolites in the urine by more than 75%, indicating a close correlation of the inhibition of COX with antiinflammatory effects. Although the salicylates (and other NSAIDs) are considered effective due to their inhibition of COX, **other actions**, more recently described, are likely important in some cases. Differences among the actions of various NSAIDs may account for differences in clinical responses to the drugs. Salicylates may cause shedding of L-selectin, a cell surface adhesion molecule, important in leukocyte extravasation; inhibition of iNOS; inhibition of NF-Kappa B, a transcription faction important in inflammation; and inhibition of neutrophil activation.

Inhibition of PG synthesis at the site of injury or inflammation explains at least some of the analgesic effect of aspirin. Although PGs themselves do not appear to cause pain when injected locally, PGE_2 and $PGF_{2\alpha}$ do sensitize pain receptors to other mediators such as histamine and bradykinin. In this connection, it is interesting that aspirin and related drugs can prevent the writhing response elicited by bradykinin but not that produced by PGs. This finding is explained by the fact that all NSAIDs inhibit the synthesis of PGs induced by bradykinin but not the binding of PGs to their receptors. Animal experimentation has revealed that NSAIDs also have central analgesic actions, which may involve the inhibition of COX or other unknown mechanisms at the level of the spinal dorsal horn or at higher levels of the CNS. The antipyretic effect of aspirin and similar drugs is also mediated by the reduction of PGE_2 synthesis as a result of inhibition of COX.

General therapeutic effects

Aspirin has clinically useful analgesic, antipyretic, antiinflammatory, and antiplatelet effects. The analgesic effect attained with aspirin is probably caused in many cases by its antiinflammatory actions. In addition to their widespread use for the symptomatic relief of acute pain and fever, salicylates (most commonly aspirin) are drugs of major importance in the treatment of numerous chronic inflammatory diseases.

Acute pain. It is difficult to separate the analgesic and antiinflammatory effects of NSAIDs because the majority of painful conditions have an inflammatory component. There is little doubt that the cascade of reactions leading to the formation of PGs is integrally involved with the inflammatory response and that aspirin's efficacy in treating inflammation and pain is closely related to its inhibition of PG synthesis. By using microdialysis techniques, it has been demonstrated that after dental surgery the analgesic effects of NSAIDs correlate with a local reduction in PG synthesis. Nevertheless, several observations suggest that the analgesic and antiinflammatory effects of NSAIDs may occur by different mechanisms. First, there is a different time course for the onset of analgesic and antiinflammatory effects. Clinically significant analgesia usually occurs within 1 hour of drug administration, whereas antiinflammatory effects sometimes take several days or weeks to reach maximum levels because chronic inflammatory processes may be occurring that cannot be quickly reversed by inhibiting PG production. Also, the maximum human **analgesic effect usually occurs at lower doses than do the antirheumatic** and other antiinflammatory effects.

Aspirin is an effective analgesic for almost any type of acute dental pain. Double-blind, controlled studies of the relief of pain after the surgical extraction of third molars have demonstrated that 650 mg of aspirin is substantially more effective than 60 mg of codeine in relieving postoperative pain. Aspirin, as well as other NSAIDs and acetaminophen, has a ceiling or plateau effect in the treatment of acute pain at 650 to 1000 mg. Increasing the dose beyond these amounts does not further enhance the analgesic effect but does increase the likelihood for toxic effects.

Rheumatic fever. Now considered a rare condition, aspirin markedly reduces the acute inflammatory components of rheumatic fever, such as fever, joint pain, swelling, and immobility. However, the salicylates do not affect other aspects of the disease, such as the proliferative reaction in the myocardium leading to scarring, and they do not alter the progression of the disease. While antiinflammatory drugs, including corticosteroids, may be used to reduce inflammation, antibiotic therapy is the major therapeutic strategy.

Rheumatoid arthritis. Rheumatoid arthritis is a chronic systemic disease of unknown origin, but in most patients the chief clinical and pathologic features result from chronic inflammation of synovial membranes. Irreversible joint injury (subluxation, loss of motion, or ankylosis) results from formation of chronic granulation tissue that causes erosions of articular cartilage, subchondral bone, ligaments, and tendons. Extraarticular manifestations such as subcutaneous or subperiosteal nodules of granulation tissue, peripheral neuropathy, and chronic skin ulcers occur to a variable extent and appear to result from generalized focal vasculitis. Patients with rheumatoid arthritis are at increased risk of developing cardiovascular disease including myocardial infarction.

Rheumatoid arthritis is considered an autoimmune disease with many contributing factors, including lymphocytes that have become activated and produce TNF-α and IL-1. These cytokines lead to the release of other inflammatory mediators, such as the PGs and autoantibody immunoglobulins that attach to the Fc component of IgG (referred to as the **rheumatoid factor**). These dual-antibody complexes may activate complement, which in turn triggers a number of inflammatory phenomena in the joint tissues, including histamine release, production of factors chemotactic for neutrophils and mononuclear cells, cell membrane damage, and PG synthesis. The dual-antibody complexes also activate antigen-presenting cells, which in turn stimulate T cells, leading to further release of cytokines. Both neutrophils and macrophages accumulate in the synovial fluid and are found to contain aggregated IgG, rheumatoid factor, complement fragments, and fibrin. These substances are acquired by phagocytosis with subsequent release of lysosomal materials that amplify the inflammatory reaction and may directly damage tissues. Cytokines produced by the lymphocytic cell infiltrate may also help propagate the reaction and participate in tissue destruction.

Salicylates (usually aspirin) are still widely used in the clinical management of rheumatoid arthritis. Salicylates produce a measurable reduction of inflammation in the joints and associated tissues, a lessening of pain symptoms, and improved mobility. Salicylates may also reduce neutrophil activity in addition to inhibiting PG synthesis.

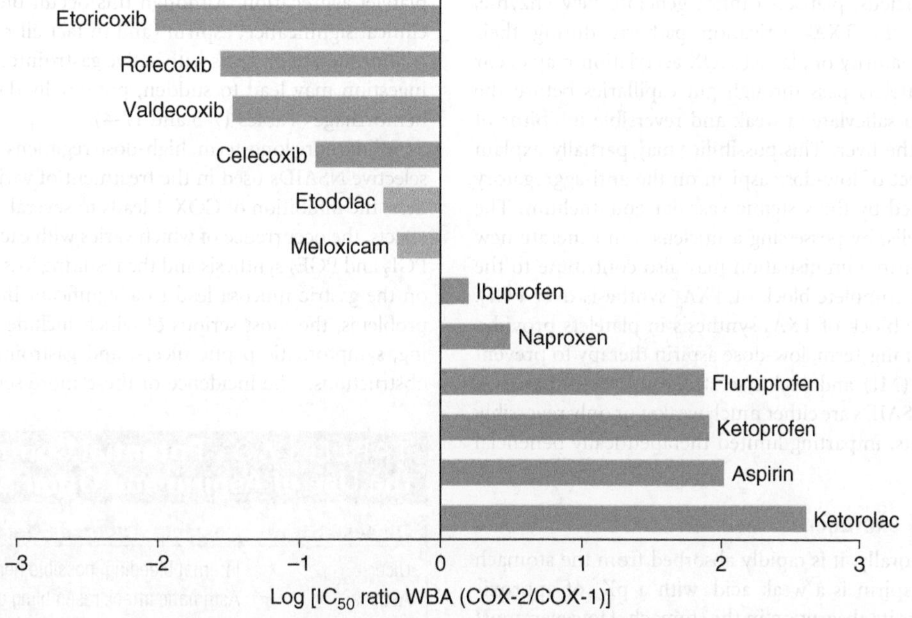

FIG 17-4 The ratio of the log of inhibitory concentrations (*IC*) of various NSAIDs needed to block 50% of COX-2 activity versus 50% of COX-1 activity in the whole-blood assay (*WBA*). The *zero line* indicates equipotency. Bars on the *right* represent drugs with greater selectivity for COX-1, whereas those on the *left* represent drugs with greater selectivity for COX-2. (Adapted from Riendau D, Percival MD, Brideau C et al.: Etoricoxib (MK-0663): preclinical profile and comparison with other agents that selectively inhibit cyclooxygenase-2, *J Pharmacol Exp Ther* 296:558–566, 2001; Warner TD, Guiliano F, Vojnovic I et al.: Nonsteroid drug selectivities for cyclooxygenase-1 rather than cyclooxygenase-2 are associated with human gastrointestinal toxicity: a full in vitro analysis, *Proc Natl Acad Sci* 96:7563–7568, 1999.)

Salicylates are given in doses sufficient to control the symptoms, often 3 to 6 g/day. The degree of suppression of inflammation increases with the plasma salicylate concentration even beyond the point of toxicity. When salicylate therapy is not effective or is not well tolerated, other drugs can be used such as ibuprofen, naproxen, or corticosteroids.

Other inflammatory diseases. Aspirin is a commonly used antiinflammatory agent in various other inflammatory diseases, including juvenile rheumatoid arthritis, ankylosing spondylitis, psoriatic arthritis, Reiter syndrome, and degenerative joint disease (osteoarthritis). The arthralgia and fever of mild lupus erythematosus may also be alleviated by aspirin. Acute episodes of inflammation in isolated joints, tendons, or bursae caused by trauma are also best treated with aspirin given in full doses immediately after the injury.

Fever. Fever is typically a symptom of a disease process, usually a viral or bacterial infection brought about by both exogenous (microbial products) and endogenous pyrogens. It is believed that exogenous proteins stimulate host cells to produce endogenous pyrogens, of which IL-1 has been the best characterized. IL-1 is thought to act on the anterior hypothalamus, generating the local release of PGs. Injection of PGs into the brain of various animal species is known to raise body temperature. The PGs and possibly other **non-PG endogenous pyrogens** elevate the thermal set point of the body so that it retains the ability to closely regulate its temperature but at a higher temperature than normal. In mild–moderate fevers, this allows better migration and activity by the immune cells.

By inhibiting the synthesis of PGs in the hypothalamus, aspirin, other NSAIDs, and acetaminophen are thought to reduce the thermal set point back toward normal. This is particularly important when the fever is very high. Because of its association with Reye's syndrome, aspirin is no longer recommended to treat most febrile episodes in children.

Prophylaxis against platelet aggregation. Aspirin inhibits the synthesis of $\mathbf{TXA_2}$ by irreversible acetylation of the COX enzyme in platelets. Lacking a nucleus, platelets cannot generate new enzyme, permanently blunting the TXA_2 activation pathway during their 10-day lifetimes. The majority of platelet COX acetylation may occur pre-systemically as platelets pass through gut capillaries before the hydrolysis of aspirin to salicylate (a weak and reversible inhibitor of COX) in the gut and the liver. This possibility may partially explain the relative lack of effect of low-dose aspirin on the anti-aggregatory $\mathbf{PGI_2}$ molecule produced by the systemic vascular endothelium. The fact that endothelial cells, by possessing a nucleus, can generate new COX enzyme after aspirin administration may also contribute to the relatively selective and complete block of TXA_2 synthesis over PGI_2. This relatively selective block of TXA_2 synthesis in platelets provides the rationale for using long-term, low-dose aspirin therapy to prevent myocardial infarction (MI) and occlusive stroke in at-risk patients. Other salicylates and NSAIDs are either much weaker or only reversibly inhibit COX in platelets, imparting limited therapeutically beneficial antiplatelet effects.

Absorption, fate, and excretion

When aspirin is taken orally, it is rapidly absorbed from the stomach and small intestine. Aspirin is a weak acid, with a pK_a of approximately 3.5, which favors its absorption in the stomach. However, most absorption takes place in the small intestine because of its much larger surface area. The rate-limiting steps in the absorption of aspirin are the disintegration and dissolution of the tablet. Aspirin has a very short **15-minute half-life.** However, since its binding to COX in the platelet is irreversible, the full extent of its antiplatelet action is dependent on the **life span of the platelet (10 days)** and not its short half-life. Aspirin is quickly metabolized by gastric and plasma esterases to salicylate ion. Although some aspirin becomes bound to plasma proteins, 80% to 90% of the salicylate ion is bound for only a short time, principally to albumin. Salicylate is distributed throughout most body fluids and tissues and crosses the placenta from mother to fetus.

The **elimination half-life of salicylate is 2 to 3 hours** after a single analgesic dose. The liver is the main site of biotransformation, and conjugation is the primary route. Because the metabolism of salicylate is capacity limited, large repeated doses or single toxic ingestions result in plasma half-lives of 5 to 30 hours. In fact, when describing the duration of analgesic and antiinflammatory action of aspirin, its ultimate dosing interval reflects the summed half-lives of the parent molecule and the salicylate metabolite. Free salicylate and the salicylate metabolites are excreted both by glomerular filtration and by active proximal tubular secretion in the kidney. In normal humans, approximately 10% of ingested salicylate appears unchanged in the urine; however, this fraction may fall to 2% or rise to 30% with urinary acidosis or alkalosis, respectively. Furthermore, a higher percentage of free salicylate is excreted at higher doses because the liver is not able to maintain the same percentage of metabolism at higher doses of salicylates.

Adverse effects

The severity of side effects that can accompany aspirin ingestion depends on the overall health of the patient, the length of dosing, and the total daily intake of drug. When used under OTC package insert guidelines (for no more than 10 days and no more than 4 g/day), the majority of reported side effects are more annoying than serious, with **dyspepsia and nausea** occurring in up to 10% of patients. In addition, occult bleeding (hidden amounts of blood in the stool), which is usually less than 10 ml/day, develops in more than 70% of patients ingesting the drug (Table 17-3). The **bleeding** is thought to originate from both direct capillary and mucosal damage as aspirin disintegrates in contact with gastric tissues and from the ability of aspirin to inhibit COX-1, which interferes with cytoprotective mechanisms and platelet aggregation. Although this occult bleeding is usually of little clinical significance, aspirin (and in fact all related NSAIDs) are contraindicated in patients with active gastrointestinal ulcers because their ingestion may lead to sudden, potentially dangerous gastrointestinal hemorrhage (Tables 17-3 and 17-4).

With more long-term, high-dose regimens of aspirin and other nonselective NSAIDs used in the treatment of various inflammatory disorders, the inhibition of COX-1 leads to several common and predictable effects, the occurrence of which varies with each drug. The inhibition of PGI_2 and PGE_2 synthesis and the resulting loss of their protective effects on the gastric mucosa lead to a significant increase in gastrointestinal problems, the most serious of which include significant gastric bleeding, symptomatic peptic ulcers, and gastrointestinal perforations and obstructions. The incidence of these more serious events ranges from

TABLE 17-3 Potential Contraindications to the Use of Aspirin and Other Salicylates

Disease State	Possible Adverse Effect of Aspirin
Ulcer	Internal bleeding, possible hemorrhaging
Asthma	Asthmatic attack resembling an allergic reaction
Diabetes	High doses may cause hyperglycemia or hypoglycemia
Gout	Low doses increase plasma urate; high doses lower plasma urate
Influenza, varicella, and other viral conditions	Reye's syndrome in children
Hypocoagulation	Excessive bleeding states

1% to 5% of patients per year. Even long-term, low-dose (81 mg/day) aspirin therapy is associated with an increased risk of serious gastrointestinal events, at a rate of 0.1% to 0.2% of patients per year. This increase in gastrointestinal complications has led experts to question the widespread use of low-dose aspirin therapy in patients without significant cardiovascular or cerebrovascular risks. The non-aspirin salicylates generally elicit fewer adverse effects in the gastrointestinal tract but cannot be used for platelet anti-aggregatory therapy. Most other NSAIDs have some reversible antiplatelet effect based on inhibition of the production of TXA_2, but the effects are not as pronounced as with aspirin because aspirin is an irreversible inhibitor of COX.

The antiplatelet effects of aspirin, particularly at higher doses, can theoretically lead to pronounced increases in intraoperative and postoperative hemorrhage in dental surgical patients, but in clinical practice this is rare. **Accepted practice is to not stop low-dose aspirin therapy for dental procedures but to consider local control measures (suturing, collagen in the socket, etc.) if necessary.** If the patient has been ingesting higher doses of aspirin prior to surgery, a medical consultation and platelet function assay is recommended.

The adverse effects of aspirin and other NSAIDs on the kidney are well known. Normal **renal function** is partly dependent on PG synthesis. It is believed that both COX-1 and COX-2 are important in producing PGs that reduce water and Na^+ reabsorption at the ascending loop of Henle and maintain proper dilation of the renal vasculature. With NSAID therapy, dose-dependent water and Na^+ retention manifested by peripheral edema, elevation in blood pressure, and rarely congestive heart failure are thought to follow the inhibition of PGE_2 synthesis. Acute renal failure is more likely to develop in patients with preexisting renal insufficiency, congestive heart failure, or dehydration because the renal arterioles are more dependent on PGs to maintain normal perfusion of the glomeruli. Acute renal failure is also more likely when NSAIDs are given concurrently with an angiotensin-converting enzyme (ACE) inhibitor because the lack of angiotensin II weakens reactive constriction of the efferent arteriole, a normal protective response for maintaining glomerular filtration in patients with reduced renal blood flow.

The NSAIDs are likewise responsible for chronic renal toxicity, commonly known as **analgesic-associated nephropathy**. This disorder sometimes occurs with long-term use of high doses of NSAIDs and is characterized by papillary necrosis and chronic interstitial nephritis.

TABLE 17-4 Some Drug Interactions Involving Aspirin

Drug	Possible Interaction with Aspirin
Warfarin	Internal bleeding, possible hemorrhaging
Heparin	Internal bleeding, possible hemorrhaging
Insulin	Aspirin may cause hyperglycemia or enhancement of hypoglycemic effect
Sulfonylureas (oral hypoglycemic agents)	Enhancement of hypoglycemic effect
Phenytoin/valproic acid	Increased free plasma concentration of phenytoin, valproic acid
Methotrexate	Increased free plasma concentration of methotrexate
Ethanol	Internal bleeding, possible hemorrhaging
Probenecid, sulfinpyrazone	Decreased uricosuric effect, reappearance of gout
ACE inhibitors, β-adrenergic blockers, diuretics	Loss of antihypertensive effect with high doses of aspirin

The mechanism may be related to the acute ischemic response described previously, but the cause has not been definitely established. It is estimated that serious renal problems requiring hospitalization occur in 0.5% to 1.0% of long-term NSAID users.

The use of aspirin in **children with viral infections** has been associated with **Reye's syndrome.** First described in 1963, Reye's syndrome is an acute childhood illness that produces metabolic encephalopathy and liver disease. Typically, the children are recovering from influenza or varicella when the acute encephalopathic symptoms of lethargy, agitation, delirium, and seizures appear. Without aggressive supportive treatment, the disease progresses to deep coma, brainstem dysfunction, and in 80% to 90% of cases, death. Even with heroic treatment, the mortality rate can exceed 30%, and survivors can be left with permanent brain damage. Clinical reviews and case-controlled studies performed in the 1970s and 1980s reported a strong association between the development of Reye's syndrome and the ingestion of aspirin in children and teenagers with viral infections. Aspirin and related salicylates are thus contraindicated for the treatment of flulike symptoms, chicken pox, gastroenteritis, and in the opinion of most pediatricians, any febrile respiratory condition in children or teenagers. It is of note that both acetaminophen and ibuprofen have not been associated with the development of Reye's syndrome.

Toxicity caused by aspirin overdose is common. Its symptoms and severity depend on the dose. Chronic toxicity caused by salicylates results in a syndrome termed **salicylism**, which is characterized by tinnitus, nausea, vomiting, headache, hyperventilation, and mental confusion. Aspirin holds the dubious distinction of being one of the more frequently used drugs for attempted suicide. The drug is commonly involved in accidental poisoning, especially in children, because many households do not follow proper precautions for its storage. Serious clinical manifestations of acute aspirin overdose typically occur at doses greater than 6 to 10 g in adults or when intake exceeds 150 to 200 mg/kg of body weight. The cardinal signs and symptoms of acute aspirin overdose include nausea, vomiting, tinnitus, hyperthermia, and hyperventilation. Hyperventilation arises in part from a direct stimulation of respiratory centers in the brain and from a compensatory increase in respiration in response to excessive carbon dioxide produced by large doses of aspirin partially uncoupling oxidative phosphorylation. This uncoupling also accounts for a paradoxical (because therapeutic doses of aspirin are used for antipyresis) increase in body temperature. The hyperventilation eventually can lead to respiratory alkalosis, which may be followed by a combined respiratory and metabolic acidosis accompanied by dehydration. Acidosis is more prominent as the level of overdose increases. Acidosis is also more likely to occur in children and infants. Impaired vision, hallucinations, delirium, and other CNS effects may be evident, and the situation is considered life-threatening.

The treatment of aspirin overdose is primarily palliative and supportive. Chronic toxicity usually is treated simply by withholding the drug temporarily and then reinstituting therapy at lower doses. Acute toxicity often requires respiratory support, gastric lavage, maintenance of electrolyte balance (e.g., K^+ replacement if necessary), maintenance of plasma pH, and alkalinization of the urine with intravenous bicarbonate. Alkalinization of the urine increases the percentage of ionized salicylate in the glomerular filtrate. Salicylate reabsorption is reduced, and renal clearance is increased up to fourfold. The carbonic anhydrase inhibitor acetazolamide may also be used to promote urinary alkalinization.

Allergic reactions to aspirin can also occur. Many patients, however, confuse side effects such as nausea or tinnitus with true allergic responses manifested by skin rashes, hives, angioedema, or anaphylaxis. Patients with a history of skin eruptions caused by aspirin ingestion should be cautioned to avoid all proprietary compounds containing aspirin or any other salicylate to avoid more serious anaphylactic reactions.

Intolerance to salicylates can occur, with symptoms ranging from rhinitis to severe asthma. This reaction does not appear to be immune mediated, even though it resembles drug allergy in clinical presentation. Aspirin intolerance is more common in patients with preexisting asthma or nasal polyps. The incidence of this reaction in asthmatic patients has been reported to be as high as 20%. Patients with a history of asthma, allergic disorders, or nasal polyps should be questioned to be sure that they can tolerate aspirin and other NSAIDs. The bronchoconstriction may be caused by a shift in the arachidonic acid cascade when the COX enzyme is blocked. This inhibition prevents arachidonate metabolism from producing bronchodilating PGs, primarily PGE_2. The lipoxygenase pathway then predominates and produces leukotrienes that constrict bronchioles in sensitive persons, mimicking an asthmatic attack. Other manifestations of aspirin intolerance include urticaria (hives) and angioedema. Switching from aspirin to another salicylate or even another NSAID does not prevent the reaction; acetaminophen is the only antipyretic analgesic that may be used safely in patients with aspirin intolerance. The clinician should be aware that while relatively rare, there are reports of aspirin-intolerant asthmatic patients also displaying severe respiratory symptoms when ingesting therapeutic doses of acetaminophen.

Contraindications and precautions

Aspirin is contraindicated or at least must be used with caution in a number of medical conditions (See Table 17-3). Serious internal bleeding can result from the ingestion of aspirin by a patient with an ulcer. Patients with compromised liver function should use aspirin cautiously because, when used on a long-term basis, aspirin raises the prothrombin time, which could aggravate bleeding problems. Low doses of aspirin can increase plasma urate concentrations and exacerbate gouty arthritis as a result of competition between salicylate and uric acid at the active secretion sites in the proximal tubule of the kidney or by an increase in uric acid reabsorption. High doses of aspirin may either raise or lower plasma glucose concentrations by stimulating epinephrine and glucocorticoid release or by depleting liver glycogen, respectively. Salicylates may also increase insulin secretion because PGE_2 inhibits insulin secretion. Asthma patients, patients with nasal polyps, and those with chronic allergic disorders (e.g., urticaria) should use aspirin cautiously because, as previously mentioned, as many as 20% of these patients have reported intolerance to aspirin, other salicylate drugs, and other NSAIDs. Of course, aspirin (and other NSAIDs) is contraindicated in patients with aspirin intolerance or true salicylate allergy.

Aspirin is not absolutely contraindicated in pregnancy, but it should be used with caution. In the third trimester, aspirin tends to prolong labor by inhibiting the synthesis of PGs involved in initiating uterine contractions. Aspirin has also been reported to increase blood loss at the time of delivery and may cause premature closure of the ductus arteriosus in the fetus. Some evidence also suggests that, in very high doses, aspirin can have teratogenic effects.

A number of **drug interactions** may involve **aspirin** (see Table 17-4). Because of its effects on blood glucose, aspirin can interact adversely with insulin or oral hypoglycemic agents, causing unpredictable changes in blood glucose concentrations. Furthermore, aspirin and other salicylates compete with oral hypoglycemic drugs for binding sites on plasma proteins. This interaction theoretically leads to higher amounts of unbound oral hypoglycemic in the plasma and an enhanced hypoglycemic effect. Internal bleeding may occur if aspirin, which causes gastrointestinal irritation and inhibition of platelet aggregation, is used in conjunction with anticoagulants such as warfarin and heparin. In addition, warfarin can be displaced from plasma proteins by aspirin. As with the oral hypoglycemic drugs, this competition for binding is more of a theoretical concern than a practical issue. Another potentially dangerous drug combination is aspirin and alcohol because alcohol sensitizes the gastric mucosa to aspirin. Aspirin and other NSAIDs also increase the toxicity of methotrexate and valproic acid and can decrease the effect of certain antihypertensive drugs (e.g., β-adrenoreceptor blockers, diuretics, and ACE inhibitors). However, long-term low doses of aspirin used for antiplatelet therapy appear not to interact with antihypertensive drugs.

Diflunisal

Diflunisal is a difluorophenyl derivative of salicylic acid with antiinflammatory, analgesic, and antipyretic activity. Although structurally related to salicylates, diflunisal is not hydrolyzed in vivo to salicylate and therefore is unique among the salicylates. Like other salicylates, diflunisal blocks the synthesis of PGs by inhibiting COX. Diflunisal is approximately tenfold more potent than aspirin in suppressing PG formation in rats.

The drug is well absorbed after oral administration, with peak blood concentrations occurring in 2 to 3 hours. It is highly bound to plasma protein. Diflunisal has a long plasma half-life (8 to 12 hours versus 2.5 hours for salicylate), which permits dosing intervals of up to 12 hours. The drug is excreted in the urine, with two soluble glucuronide conjugates accounting for approximately 90% of the administered dose.

Diflunisal is indicated for the treatment of mild to moderate pain and for osteoarthritis and rheumatoid arthritis. In postoperative dental pain, 500 to 1000 mg of diflunisal produces greater analgesia than does aspirin or acetaminophen (both 650 mg), and peak analgesic effects are comparable to those obtainable with fixed combinations containing optimal doses of opioids. Because diflunisal has an extended duration of action and a relatively slow onset of action in acute pain models, the recommended dosage regimen is a 1000-mg loading dose followed by 500 mg every 8 to 12 hours. The effectiveness of diflunisal in osteoarthritis appears to be comparable to that of aspirin.

In terms of adverse effects, diflunisal qualitatively resembles aspirin. Effects on the gastrointestinal tract range from nausea and epigastric pain to peptic ulcer and gastrointestinal bleeding. However, diflunisal is less problematic in this respect than aspirin. Platelet function and bleeding time are affected in a dose-related fashion but to a lesser degree than with aspirin because diflunisal is a competitive, reversible inhibitor of COX. Like aspirin, diflunisal prolongs the prothrombin time in patients receiving oral anticoagulants, perhaps by competitive displacement of coumarins from protein binding sites. Diflunisal does not penetrate the blood–brain barrier as well as does aspirin, and diflunisal therefore causes fewer CNS effects, including tinnitus. For this same reason, it is not used as an antipyretic.

Other NSAIDs

Many NSAIDs unrelated to the salicylates are available that inhibit COX, but they vary in their relative potencies against COX-1 and COX-2. A number of these NSAIDs have been evaluated in postoperative dental pain and have been found to be superior to optimal doses of either aspirin or acetaminophen in terms of peak analgesic effect and duration of effect. For more long-term use, the choice of an NSAID for therapy is largely empiric and often based on what drug is best tolerated and best relieves symptoms in the individual patient.

Propionic acid derivatives

Among the NSAIDs, the substituted phenylpropionic acid derivatives constitute the largest group of aspirin alternatives (Fig. 17-5, ibuprofen, naproxen, and ketoprofen). In addition to their antiinflammatory indications in treating the symptoms of rheumatoid arthritis, osteoarthritis, and degenerative joint disease, ibuprofen, naproxen, ketoprofen, and fenoprofen are also approved as analgesic agents. The short-term use of ibuprofen, naproxen, and ketoprofen is available without a prescription for relief of **headache, fever, dysmenorrhea,**

and mild to moderate musculoskeletal and postoperative pain. In patients with rheumatoid and osteoarthritis, the propionic acid derivatives and other NSAIDs reduce joint swelling, pain, and morning stiffness, and they improve mobility as measured by an increase in walking time. When used in patients treated with corticosteroids, these agents may permit reduction of the steroid dose.

Like aspirin and other NSAIDs, these drugs inhibit PG synthesis by nonselective inhibition of COX. Their ability to inhibit COX, and thereby prevent the effect of PGs on uterine smooth muscle, makes them useful in the treatment of dysmenorrhea. Although they share a common pharmacologic profile, some unique characteristics exist among individual drugs. Naproxen, for example, appears to be especially effective in reducing leukocyte activity in inflammation, and ketoprofen appears to prevent lysosomal enzyme release by stabilizing the membranes of lysosomes.

Because the propionic acid derivatives as a group are less likely than usual doses of aspirin to cause gastrointestinal or bleeding disturbances, they have increasingly been used in place of aspirin. The propionic acid NSAIDs are almost completely absorbed from the gastrointestinal tract. The rate of absorption is generally rapid but can be altered for some drugs by the presence of food in the stomach. Peak blood concentrations are reached in 1 to 4 hours. All these agents are highly bound (>90%) to plasma proteins; they are theoretically capable of interfering with the binding of other drugs such as phenytoin, warfarin, or the sulfonamides. The drugs are variably metabolized and conjugated, and they are then largely excreted in the urine. Ibuprofen, fenoprofen, and ketoprofen have short plasma half-lives (1 to 4 hours), whereas naproxen has a plasma half-life of approximately 15 hours, which allows less frequent dosing.

Ibuprofen. Ibuprofen was the first single-entity oral analgesic to be approved by the FDA that showed a greater peak analgesic effect than 650 mg of aspirin. It is also available as a nonprescription drug. The recommended prescription analgesic dose of ibuprofen is 400 to 600 mg every 4 to 6 hours with a maximum daily dose of 3200 mg. When used OTC without a health professional's guidance, the maximum daily dose should not exceed 1200 mg. Doses of ibuprofen larger than 400 mg have not consistently demonstrated enhanced analgesic efficacy in nonrheumatic pain, although a recent meta-analysis of various analgesic interventions in postsurgical dental pain studies reported a modest increase in pain relief (at least with the first dose of drug) with ibuprofen 600 mg compared to ibuprofen 400 mg. Preoperative or immediately postoperative ibuprofen can delay the onset and lessen the severity of postoperative pain. Such treatment may be particularly useful when there is a high likelihood of moderate to severe postoperative discomfort. Ibuprofen is widely used as an antipyretic and is second to acetaminophen as the most used antipyretic in the pediatric population. Dosages for antipyresis are based on the child's age and body weight.

Ibuprofen is a weak organic acid and is highly (approximately 99%) bound to plasma albumin. It is extensively metabolized and then excreted as the metabolites or their conjugates in the urine, with an elimination half-life of approximately 2 hours.

Naproxen. Naproxen is approved for a variety of inflammatory conditions and for the relief of pain. It is the only NSAID manufactured as the pure active (S) enantiomer. It is available as both the free acid and as the sodium salt, the latter of which is more rapidly absorbed from the gastrointestinal tract and is the preferred form for analgesic use. The sodium salt of naproxen at a 220-mg dose is available OTC

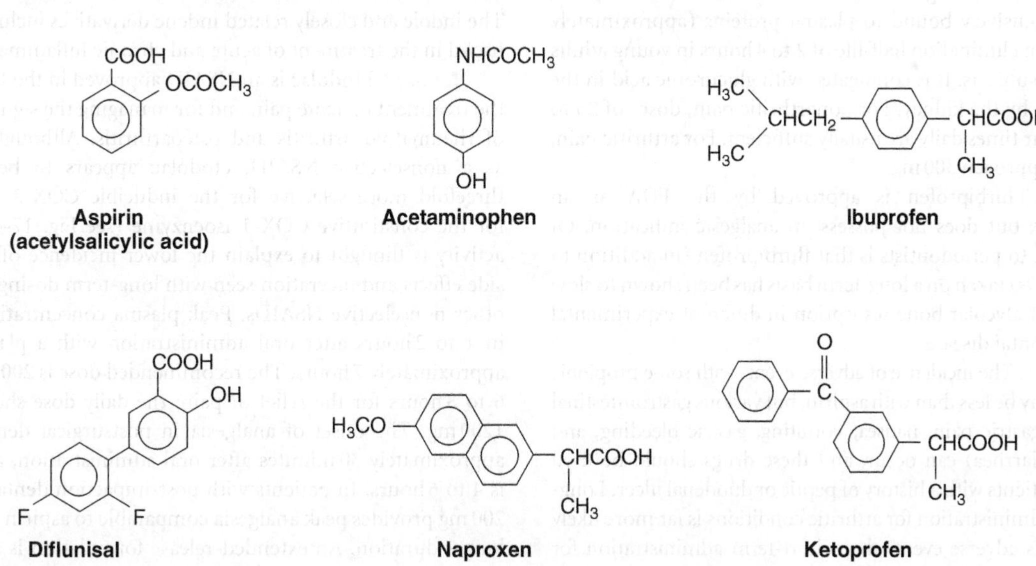

COOH OCOCH$_3$ — **Aspirin (acetylsalicylic acid)**

NHCOCH$_3$ OH — **Acetaminophen**

H$_3$C, H$_3$C CHCH$_2$ CHCOOH CH$_3$ — **Ibuprofen**

COOH OH F F — **Diflunisal**

H$_3$CO CHCOOH CH$_3$ — **Naproxen**

O C CHCOOH CH$_3$ — **Ketoprofen**

O C N COOH — **Ketorolac**

SO$_2$NH$_2$ N N F$_3$C CH$_3$ — **Celecoxib**

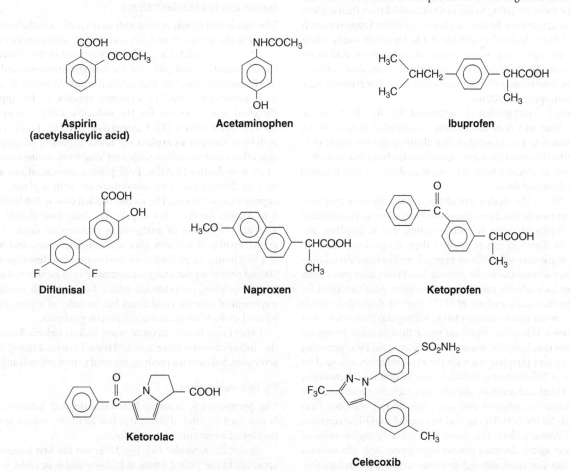

FIG 17-5 The structures of common NSAID analgesics and acetaminophen used in the practice of dentistry.

with a maximum recommended daily dose of 660 mg (440 mg if greater than 65 years old). Naproxen sodium at 220 mg is approximately equivalent in analgesic efficacy and duration to 200 mg ibuprofen. A dose of 440 mg of naproxen sodium appears to be superior to 1000-mg acetaminophen in peak analgesia and duration and equivalent in efficacy to 400-mg ibuprofen. At a dose of 440 mg, naproxen sodium displays a **duration of action of between 8 and 12 hours,** which is the recommended dosing interval. This extended duration of action is explained by its relatively long half-life of approximately 15 hours. Naproxen is somewhat more irritating to the gastrointestinal tract than ibuprofen, possibly due to its greater selectivity for blocking COX-1. The drug is partially metabolized, and its clearance is almost entirely renal. Like ibuprofen, naproxen is highly bound to plasma albumin.

Fenoprofen. Fenoprofen is marketed with both analgesic and antiinflammatory indications. The recommended dose of 200 mg every 4 to 6 hours is likely to be superior to 650 mg of aspirin. As with the other propionic acid derivatives, fenoprofen is extensively (approximately 99%) and reversibly protein bound. It has a mean plasma half-life of approximately 2.5 hours in healthy adults. Most of the drug is excreted by the kidney as hydroxylated and conjugated metabolites.

Ketoprofen. Ketoprofen is an FDA-approved analgesic that is also effective for the symptomatic management of rheumatoid arthritis, osteoarthritis, and dysmenorrhea. Like the other propionic acid derivatives, it inhibits PG synthesis. However, ketoprofen has also been shown to inhibit leukotriene synthesis in at least two in vitro cell culture systems. In addition, ketoprofen stabilizes lysosomal membranes and has an antibradykinin effect. A dose of 25 to 50 mg of ketoprofen is about equally effective for mild to moderate pain as 400 mg of ibuprofen.

Although approved OTC at a 12.5-mg dose, ketoprofen has been reported to be more irritating to the gastrointestinal tract than aspirin. Ketoprofen is extensively bound to plasma proteins (approximately 99%), and it has an elimination half-life of 2 to 4 hours in young adults and middle-aged subjects. It is conjugated with glucuronic acid in the liver and excreted by the kidney. For nonarthritic pain, doses of 25 to 50 mg three or four times daily are usually sufficient. For arthritic pain, daily doses may approach 300 mg.

Flurbiprofen. Flurbiprofen is approved by the FDA as an antiarthritic drug, but does not possess an analgesic indication. Of particular interest to periodontists is that flurbiprofen (in addition to some other NSAIDs) taken on a long-term basis has been shown to slow the progression of alveolar bone resorption in different experimental models of periodontal disease.

Adverse effects. The incidence of adverse events with some propionic acid derivatives may be less than with aspirin, but various gastrointestinal disturbances (epigastric pain, nausea, vomiting, gastric bleeding, and constipation or diarrhea) can occur, and these drugs should be used with caution in patients with a history of peptic or duodenal ulcer. Long-term, high-dose administration for arthritic conditions is far more likely to produce serious adverse events than short-term administration for acute pain. In fact, meta-analyses of OTC doses of ibuprofen (800 to 1200 mg/day) or naproxen sodium (440 to 880 mg/day) taken for 10 or fewer days have a side-effect profile no worse than placebo. Propionic acid derivatives can, however, injure the gastric mucosa by suppressing COX-1 activity and therefore decrease the cytoprotection afforded by PGI_2 and PGE_2. CNS effects may include headache, dizziness, drowsiness, vertigo, and visual and auditory disturbances including tinnitus. Skin rashes are somewhat common, and immediate allergic reactions have been reported. All the NSAIDs can lead to anaphylactoid-like reactions in aspirin-intolerant patients (i.e., those susceptible to aspirin-induced asthma). These agents decrease platelet aggregation and adhesiveness and increase bleeding time, although to a lesser degree than aspirin; they should be avoided in patients with bleeding disorders and used with caution in patients receiving anticoagulants. These drugs may promote Na^+ retention, and their use may lead to the formation of edema in susceptible persons. They can interfere with the antihypertensive effects of β-adrenergic blockers, ACE inhibitors, and diuretics if they are administered for more than 1 week. In elderly patients, especially during long-term therapy, the dosage of the propionic acid NSAIDs may have to be reduced by up to 50%.

Of recent concern are epidemiologic reports indicating an increased risk of gastrointestinal bleeding when these drugs and other NSAIDs are taken concomitantly with antidepressants of the selective serotonin reuptake inhibitor (SSRI) class such as fluoxetine (Prozac) and paroxetine (Paxil). It appears that SSRIs block the reuptake of serotonin in the platelet as they do in neurons in the CNS. Like the COX-1 arachidonic acid product thromboxane A_2, serotonin stimulates platelet aggregation. Thus the combined intake of SSRIs and NSAIDs can result in an additive or supra-additive antiplatelet effect. Another recent concern has been the reported ability of NSAIDs like ibuprofen to inhibit the antiplatelet and cardioprotective effects of low-dose aspirin. Because NSAIDs such as ibuprofen and naproxen can compete with aspirin for COX-1 binding sites in the platelet, less aspirin will be bound. Unlike aspirin, the antiplatelet effects of the bound NSAIDs would only be temporary plus a large proportion of unbound aspirin would then be converted to salicylic acid. Warnings of this potential interaction now appear on both OTC and prescription formulations of NSAIDs.

Because all NSAIDS reduce prostaglandins in the kidney, they present a risk of renal toxicity as explained above. This is due in part to decreased perfusion of glomeruli. This risk is especially pertinent for those with pre-existing kidney disease.

Indole and indene derivatives

The indole and closely related indene derivatives include several drugs useful in the treatment of acute and chronic inflammatory diseases.

Etodolac. Etodolac is an NSAID approved in the United States for the treatment of acute pain and for managing the signs and symptoms of rheumatoid arthritis and osteoarthritis. Although it is classified as a nonselective NSAID, etodolac appears to be approximately threefold more selective for the inducible COX-2 isoenzyme than for the constitutive COX-1 isoenzyme (see Fig. 17-4). This relative activity is thought to explain the lower incidence of gastrointestinal side effects and ulceration seen with long-term dosing compared with other nonselective NSAIDs. Peak plasma concentrations are reached in 1 to 2 hours after oral administration with a plasma half-life of approximately 7 hours. The recommended dose is 200 to 400 mg every 6 to 8 hours for the relief of pain; the daily dose should not exceed 1200 mg. The onset of analgesia in postsurgical dental pain occurs approximately 30 minutes after oral administration, and its duration is 4 to 6 hours. In patients with post-impaction dental pain, etodolac 200 mg provides peak analgesia comparable to aspirin 650 mg but with longer duration. An extended-release formulation is available for the treatment of arthritic conditions, but its onset of action is too slow to be used in the treatment of acute postsurgical pain.

Other drugs in this chemical group include indomethacin and sulindac. Indomethacin is more toxic and is used to treat forms of arthritis and acute gout. Sulindac is a prodrug also used to treat arthritis and acute gout.

Pyrrole derivatives

The pyrrole acetic acids include tolmetin and ketorolac. Tolmetin is not used in clinical dentistry, but ketorolac enjoys special status because of its parenteral dosage form.

Ketorolac. Ketorolac (see Fig. 17-5) was the **first injectable NSAID** approved in the United States. It is also available in tablet form for oral use but only after initial intramuscular or intravenous injection. It is recommended that the total course of therapy with ketorolac not exceed 5 days. These limitations follow the drug's relatively high incidence of nephrotoxicity, gastrointestinal ulceration, and bleeding complications if used chronically, compared with other NSAIDs. The more than 400-fold selectivity for inhibiting COX-1 over COX-2 (see Fig. 17-4) probably accounts for ketorolac's enhanced toxicity. Although ketorolac is marketed as a racemic mixture, only the S-enantiomer is an active analgesic.

Injectable ketorolac has an important application in postoperative pain management in patients who are unable to consume oral analgesics or when the pain is severe and injectable opioids are contraindicated. Clinical trials have shown that in some circumstances, parenteral ketorolac is as effective as standard doses of intramuscular morphine or meperidine, longer lasting, and with fewer adverse effects. In patients with moderate to severe postoperative pain, 30 mg of intramuscular ketorolac is comparable to 12 mg of morphine and equal or superior to 100 mg of meperidine.

Both the oral and the intramuscular forms are well absorbed. Like other NSAIDs, ketorolac is highly bound (approximately 99%) to plasma proteins. Plasma concentrations of 0.3 µg/mL are estimated to be required for effective analgesia; when plasma concentrations exceed 5.0 µg/mL, side effects are frequent. Onset of analgesia after parenteral ketorolac is similar to that after injectable opioids. The S- and R-isomers have half-lives of about 2.5 and 5 hours, respectively, and they are metabolized largely to oxidized and conjugated products.

An initial intramuscular dose of 15 to 30 mg ketorolac is recommended, followed by 10- to 20-mg doses every 6 hours with a maximum daily dose not to exceed 120 mg. The initial intravenous dose is 15 to 30 mg. Oral doses are recommended at 4- to 6-hour intervals. Oral ketorolac (10-mg) has also been evaluated in postoperative dental pain and found to be superior to 650 mg of aspirin, 600 mg of acetaminophen, and combinations of 600-mg acetaminophen/60-mg codeine or 1000-mg acetaminophen/10-mg hydrocodone; it is at least as effective as 400 mg of ibuprofen. However, FDA recommendations clearly state that the oral ketorolac should only be employed if a patient was started on the parenteral formulation. A relatively new intranasal spray formulation has also shown efficacy in postsurgical dental pain and an opioid-sparing effect in other postsurgical pain models.

Clinical studies have shown that ketorolac does not produce several of the common adverse effects associated with opioid analgesics. It does not depress respiration or cardiovascular function and causes less constipation and drowsiness than equivalent doses of opioids. As with other NSAIDs, physical dependence and tolerance do not develop. The most common adverse effects after ketorolac are drowsiness, dyspepsia, gastrointestinal pain, and nausea. Peptic ulcers and gastrointestinal bleeding have occurred after oral ketorolac. Renal toxicity has also been associated with ketorolac. The drug is contraindicated before surgery because its intense antiplatelet effect is likely to result in increased intraoperative bleeding, which reflects its potent COX-1 blocking activity.

Selective Cyclooxygenase-2 Inhibitors

The introduction of drugs that are highly **selective for inhibiting** the inducible **COX-2 isoform** while sparing the constitutive COX-1 isoform was initially thought to be a major advance in NSAID therapy. Unlike preferential or semi-selective COX-2 inhibitors such as etodolac, diclofenac, and meloxicam, whose COX-2 selectivity does not exceed twofold to threefold, COX-2 selective drugs display selectivity in the range of eightfold to 35-fold in whole-blood assay systems (see Fig. 17-4). The selectivity of these so-called "coxibs" leads to roughly a 50% to 60% reduction in serious gastrointestinal complications—including symptomatic ulcers and gastrointestinal bleeds, perforations, and obstructions—compared with standard NSAIDs (e.g., ibuprofen and naproxen) in long-term safety studies in arthritic patients. This reduction represented a major potential health cost savings because clinically important gastroduodenal ulceration occurs in up to 6% of patients on long-term NSAID therapy and results in more than 100,000 hospitalizations and 16,000 deaths annually. It is stressed, however, that short-term NSAID use for treating acute postsurgical dental pain is typically measured in a few days, and it is rarely associated with serious gastrointestinal side effects, thus the safety advantage of these drugs in the dental patient population was dubious at best.

Celecoxib

With the removal of rofecoxib and valdecoxib from the market, celecoxib presently is the only FDA-approved highly selective COX-2 inhibitor available for use in the United States. Celecoxib's COX-2 selectivity in whole-blood assays approaches eightfold (see Fig. 17-4). It is highly protein bound (approximately 97%) and has a plasma elimination half-life of 10 to 12 hours. Its metabolism is mediated primarily by CYP2C9, yielding three inactive metabolites: a primary alcohol, the corresponding carboxylic acid, and its glucuronide metabolite. In randomized trials in patients with rheumatoid arthritis and osteoarthritis, the therapeutic responses seen with celecoxib are equal to that of nonselective and COX-2 preferential NSAIDs, including naproxen and ibuprofen. Celecoxib 200 mg is inferior to ibuprofen 400 mg in terms of both analgesic onset and peak effects in patients with acute postsurgical dental pain. Therefore, an initial loading dose of 400 mg (followed by 200 mg every 12 hours) provides a somewhat quicker onset and greater peak effects, and it is considered the recommended dosing regimen for acute postsurgical pain. At the 400-mg dose, celecoxib's duration of action is longer than an equal dose of ibuprofen, but its analgesic onset is still somewhat slower.

An additional FDA indication for celecoxib is to reduce the number of adenomatous colorectal polyps in patients with familial adenomatous polyposis. This is a genetic condition in which more than 90% of affected individuals develop colorectal cancer. Celecoxib at 400 mg twice per day, which is the recommended dose for this indication, reduced the number of polyps by roughly 25% after 6 months of therapy. COX-2 is overexpressed in human colorectal adenomas and adenocarcinomas, and the ability of celecoxib to inhibit COX-2 probably explains its usefulness in this condition. However, in a large trial of subjects who were high polyp formers, with an average age of 60 years and almost half with cardiovascular disease or related risk factors (angina, previous MI, hypertension, and/or poor lipid profile), celecoxib at 200 mg and 400 mg taken twice per day increased the risk of a **serious cardiovascular event** (MI, stroke, or heart failure) by 2.5- to 3.4-fold, respectively, compared to placebo after 36 months of treatment.

Despite celecoxib's COX-2 selectivity, patients still must be warned of the potential for the drug to cause serious gastrointestinal toxicity. Because COX-2 plays a normal constitutive role in the kidney, celecoxib and other COX-2s can cause renal toxicity, including Na^+ and water retention, hypertension, and acute renal failure. Like other NSAIDs, celecoxib may interfere with the antihypertensive effects of ACE inhibitors, diuretics, and β-adrenergic blockers. In patients with aspirin intolerance, the use of COX-2 inhibitors may precipitate potentially life-threatening asthmatic or allergic-type reactions. Because celecoxib is a sulfonamide, patients with documented allergies to other sulfonamides (including the thiazide diuretics) should avoid celecoxib. Drug interactions involving celecoxib resemble those of aspirin and other NSAIDs. As with other NSAIDs, reports of significant bleeding episodes have occurred in patients taking warfarin who subsequently received celecoxib. Drugs that are inhibitors of CYP2C9, such as fluconazole and metronidazole, may significantly increase celecoxib blood concentrations.

Implications for Dentistry

The major use of aspirin and other NSAIDs in dentistry is to relieve acute pain associated with pathologic processes (e.g., pulpitis, dentoalveolar abscesses) or after surgical procedures. In both situations, the antiinflammatory actions of the NSAID may contribute significantly to the therapeutic effect sought. Aspirin at doses between 650 and 1000 mg is an acceptable drug for mild to moderate dental pain. However, for more traumatic surgical procedures such as the removal of impacted third molars, the newer NSAIDs at dosages that approach their analgesic ceiling are more efficacious and sometimes better tolerated than aspirin. In fact, postsurgical dental pain studies that have used ceiling analgesic doses of NSAIDs, such as ibuprofen at 400 mg and naproxen sodium at 440 mg, have displayed efficacy at

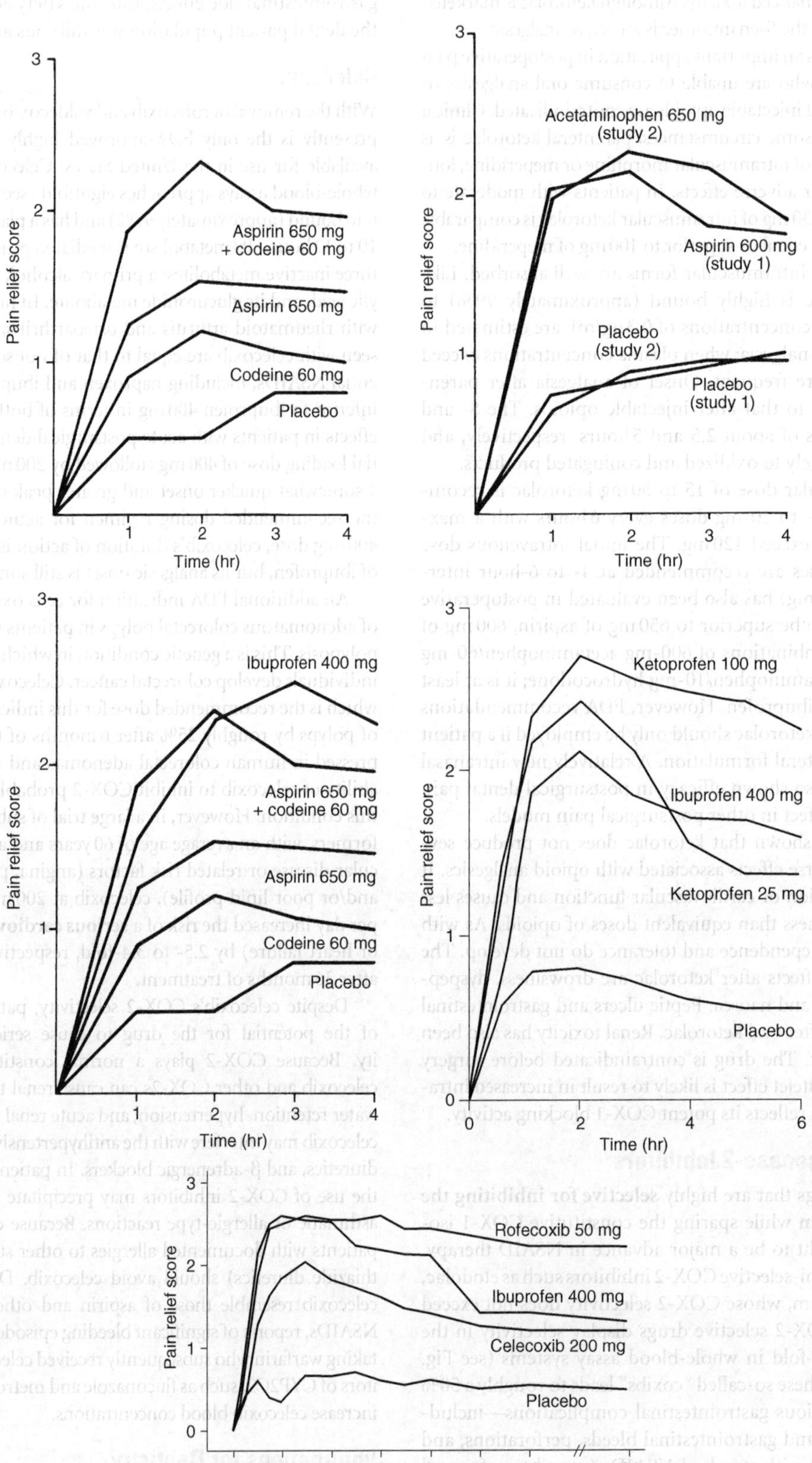

FIG 17-6 Various curves showing pain relief versus time for various drugs and drug combinations compared to placebo.

least equal to that obtained with opioid combination drugs (Fig. 17-6). In addition, the NSAIDs produce far fewer side effects of drowsiness, dizziness, nausea, and vomiting than do opioid-containing analgesics. The recommended dosing schedules of NSAIDs for acute pain of dental origin are shown in Table 17-5.

There are very few instances where the use of the highly selective COX-2 inhibitor celecoxib can be recommended, considering that in most instances NSAIDs are only used for a few days in the dental setting, thus negating any gastrointestinal benefit with the long-term use of the drug, the relatively high cost of the drug compared to traditional prescription and OTC NSAIDs, and concerns about cardiovascular risk of highly selective COX-2 inhibitors as a whole. One possible exception would be in the treatment of temporomandibular joint (TMJ) pain where the duration of NSAID therapy is measured in weeks and significant GI toxicity of NSAIDs becomes a greater concern. Still, it would behoove the clinician not to prescribe celecoxib to patients with cardiovascular risk factors including previous MI or stroke, unstable angina, or poorly controlled hypertension. Finally, naproxen has demonstrated better efficacy in TMJ pain overall than celecoxib.

Contraindications to the NSAIDs must be heeded. For instance, salicylates must be avoided in children or teenagers with viral or suspected viral infections. The antiplatelet effect of NSAIDs, especially aspirin and ketorolac, must be considered if the patient is at risk from a bleeding abnormality or anticoagulant therapy. Hypersensitivity to aspirin may indicate a risk to NSAIDs in general, including COX-2 inhibitors. The elimination of methotrexate and lithium is reduced with NSAIDs; other drug interactions may occur because of the ability of NSAIDs to displace drugs from plasma albumin and otherwise alter their pharmacokinetic properties. The common adverse effects for NSAIDs on the gastrointestinal tract and CNS should be considered, especially when the patient is taking drugs with overlapping toxicity. The NSAIDs can reduce the therapeutic effects of several antihypertensive drugs, most prominently β-adrenoreceptor blockers, ACE inhibitors, and diuretics (see Table 17-4).

ACETAMINOPHEN

Acetaminophen (N-acetyl-*p*-aminophenol) is widely promoted as the antipyretic analgesic of choice when aspirin cannot be used because of gastric problems or other contraindications.

Chemistry and Classification

The history of acetaminophen dates back to the late 1800s, when the antipyretic activity of aniline derivatives was discovered and several congeners, including acetaminophen, were synthesized. For some reason, two other aniline derivatives, acetanilid and phenacetin, became popular, and acetaminophen was not used. Chemists eventually realized that acetaminophen was an active metabolite of both of these drugs, but it was not until the mid-1900s that acetaminophen became commercially successful.

Mechanism of Action

Acetaminophen has both **analgesic and antipyretic** activity that is essentially equivalent to that of aspirin. The drug's mechanism of action also appears to stem from an inhibition of PG synthesis, although there may be some differences in the spectrum of COX enzymes that are inhibited. It has been suggested that acetaminophen may be more active than aspirin as an inhibitor of CNS COX and less active in the periphery, based largely on the differences in the therapeutic and toxic effects of aspirin and acetaminophen rather than on direct experimental evidence. For example, acetaminophen has **very weak antiinflammatory** effects compared with aspirin, but it may be a more selective inhibitor of neuronal PG synthesis. More recent evidence suggests that a peripheral mechanism of acetaminophen may indeed be partially responsible for its analgesic effects. However, the presence of peroxides from leukocytes in inflamed tissues leads to inhibition of acetaminophen, which may severely limit any effect of acetaminophen on inflammation. Other proposed mechanisms of action for acetaminophen do not involve PGs and include the activation of spinal serotonergic pathways and the inhibition of nitric oxide synthase.

Pharmacologic Effects

Compared with aspirin, acetaminophen exerts relatively few important effects on specific organs or systems. The potency and efficacy of acetaminophen as an antipyretic are similar to those of aspirin. At therapeutic doses, acetaminophen has little if any effect on the cardiovascular or respiratory systems. Acetaminophen does not inhibit platelet aggregation, cause occult bleeding or gastric irritation, affect uric acid excretion, or have as many drug interactions as aspirin. **In overdose, the organ most affected is the liver.** Acute renal toxicity may also occur. With long-term use, analgesic nephropathy is a possibility, but the risk is low.

Absorption, Fate, and Excretion

Acetaminophen is well absorbed in the small intestine after oral administration. The drug is evenly distributed throughout the body fluids and tissues, and it freely crosses the placenta. The half-life is approximately 2 to 4 hours, and the primary site of biotransformation (by glucuronide

TABLE 17-5 Some Nonopioid Analgesics Approved for Acute Pain

Nonproprietary (Generic) Name	Proprietary (Trade) Name	Analgesic Dosage*	Maximum Daily Dose*
Aspirin (OTC)	ASA, others	650-1000 mg every 4-6 hours	4000 mg
Diflunisal	Dolobid	1000 mg to start, then 500 mg every 8-12 hours	1500 mg
Acetaminophen (OTC)	Tylenol, others	650-1000 mg every 4-6 hours	3000 mg
Ibuprofen (OTC)	Motrin, Advil, Nuprin, others	400-600 mg every 4-6 hours	3200 mg
Naproxen sodium (OTC)	Aleve	220-440 mg every 8 hours	660 mg
Fenoprofen	Nalfon	200 mg every 4-6 hours	1200 mg
Ketoprofen (OTC)	Orudis KT, Actron	12.5-25 mg every 4-6 hours	75 mg
Diclofenac	Cataflam	50 mg every 8 hours	150 mg
Etodolac	Lodine	200-400 mg every 6-8 hours	1200 mg
Ketorolac	Toradol	15-30 mg IV/IM to start, then 10-20 mg PO/IV/IM every 6 hours; no more than 5 days of therapy	60-120 mg

*Doses are for acute pain only. Higher doses are sometimes used for control of inflammatory disorders.
IM, Intramuscularly; *IV*, intravenously; *PO*, orally.

conjugation) is the liver. A highly reactive and **hepatotoxic intermediate metabolite,** N-acetyl-*p*-benzoquinoneimine (NAPQI), is usually of little significance. However, in the case of acetaminophen overdose, the accumulation of this metabolite can be disastrous and result in acute liver failure due to swelling of the hepatocytes to the point of lysis. The binding of acetaminophen to plasma proteins is variable but rarely exceeds 40% of the total drug. Elimination is through the kidneys by glomerular filtration and active proximal tubular secretion.

General Therapeutic Uses

Although acetaminophen is approximately equipotent to aspirin as both an analgesic and an antipyretic, it is not a true antiinflammatory drug, and thus aspirin and other NSAIDs are far superior for conditions such as dental pericoronitis and rheumatoid arthritis. For patients in whom aspirin and other NSAIDs are contraindicated, acetaminophen is usually the drug of choice. Tables 17-3 and 17-4 list some of the disease states and potentials for drug interactions that make acetaminophen a more acceptable antipyretic analgesic than aspirin or related NSAIDs. Even though acetaminophen is not used to reduce inflammation, it can be effective in treating pain resulting from inflammation. Because of its low toxicity at therapeutic dosages (up to 3 g per day), acetaminophen is still considered first-line therapy for osteoarthritis, despite the fact that NSAIDs are generally more efficacious. Acetaminophen remains the antipyretic of choice in children and teenagers because, unlike aspirin, it is not associated with the development of Reye's syndrome.

Therapeutic Uses in Dentistry

The wide attention given to the adverse effects of aspirin has caused increasing numbers of dentists to substitute acetaminophen for aspirin in the treatment of postoperative dental pain, even though the antiinflammatory effects of acetaminophen are poor. In clinical studies, aspirin and acetaminophen are similar in their effectiveness in relieving pain after the extraction of third molars (see Fig. 17-6).

Acetaminophen has a positive dose–effect curve for analgesia up to 1000 mg. On the basis of this finding, some clinicians recommend the use of 1000 mg of acetaminophen rather than the customary 650-mg dose, but that pushes the limit for staying under the 3 g daily limit of the drug. For postsurgical dental pain, acetaminophen is most often used in combination with an opioid analgesic agent (see later).

Adverse Effects

The potential for adverse effects from acetaminophen seems to be confined to situations in which there is an acute or chronic overdose with the drug. At therapeutic doses, acetaminophen has very few side effects. Allergy to acetaminophen is rare and is generally manifested as skin eruptions. In rare cases, acetaminophen has been associated with neutropenia, thrombocytopenia, and pancytopenia.

Acute overdose from acetaminophen has become a problem because of the extent of its use. In 1992, acetaminophen-containing products accounted for more than 40% of all OTC analgesic drugs sold in the United States, and they remain popular today by still accounting for approximately a third of the market share. Acetaminophen is frequently used in suicide attempts because of its availability in sizable quantities. The therapeutic index for acetaminophen is high; it is estimated that 6 g or more must be ingested within a relatively short time for hepatotoxicity to occur. In children younger than 10 years, a therapeutic overdose, which typically involves multiple dose miscalculations on the part of the parent administering the drug, has also led to severe hepatotoxicity. The degree of liver damage is directly related to the amount of drug ingested, and people with preexisting liver disease are most susceptible.

Hepatotoxicity appears to result from the formation of the highly reactive metabolite NAPQI, which normally reacts rapidly with glutathione and, as a result, is quickly neutralized. In acetaminophen overdose, this metabolite depletes glutathione and accumulates, resulting in the alkylation of liver proteins and cellular injury. When enough liver cells are damaged, clinical signs of toxicity, such as nausea and jaundice, appear. Clinicians should also be aware that in patients who have consumed supratherapeutic doses of acetaminophen alone or combined with an opioid for a number of days, as sometimes happens with untreated toothache pain, an early sign of liver injury may in fact be intraoral bleeding, since the blood coagulation factors are synthesized in the liver. In contrast to the rapid onset of toxic signs seen after an overdose with aspirin or related NSAIDs, clinical manifestations of acetaminophen poisoning may not appear until several days after ingestion of the drug, thus making diagnosis and treatment much more difficult than with aspirin overdose. Severe **hepatotoxicity** after acetaminophen overdose is a life-threatening situation. Fortunately, there is a satisfactory treatment for acetaminophen overdose if initiated in sufficient time. Gastric lavage may be of some benefit if started within a few hours of drug ingestion, even before clinical signs of toxicity appear. N-Acetylcysteine is an effective treatment in many cases of toxicity. It enables the formation of new glutathione and dramatically reduces mortality rates. However, to be effective, N-acetylcysteine must be administered as soon as possible and ideally within 10 h. At present, acetaminophen overdose presents a more dangerous and difficult management problem than does aspirin overdose. The clinician should not be lured into a false sense of security because of acetaminophen's relative freedom from adverse effects at therapeutic doses. To some extent, the dramatic rise in reported cases of acetaminophen toxicity results from a reluctance of the health professions to realize the potential hazards of this drug and to warn their patients of the consequences of misuse.

Warning labels now appear on all acetaminophen products concerning the potential adverse drug interaction between it and alcohol. As with acetaminophen overdosage, chronic alcohol use is associated with hepatotoxicity. The theoretical basis of the interaction is that in patients who consume alcohol, CYP2E1 is highly induced. More CYP2E1 would then be available to promote the conversion of acetaminophen to NAPQI. In addition, hepatic glutathione, usually available to bind and inactivate NAPQI, tends to be depleted in chronic alcoholics. Interestingly, when patients are actively consuming alcohol, CYP2E1 is preferentially occupied by alcohol and not acetaminophen, which may limit the production of NAPQI. This protective effect of alcohol has been demonstrated in suicidal patients showing little hepatotoxicity after ingesting acute overdoses of acetaminophen in combination with large quantities of alcohol.

In theory, patients may in fact be at greatest risk of hepatotoxicity when, after acute **alcohol consumption** (which may be as little as a few drinks every day), they stop drinking and begin taking acetaminophen for fever, pain, or a hangover. In this scenario, CYP2E1 is induced, alcohol is no longer present, and the enzyme is free to convert a large portion of the acetaminophen to NAPQI. Whether chronic alcohol consumption (3 or more drinks per day for an extended period) followed by a period of abstinence and the ingestion of high therapeutic doses of acetaminophen challenge could produce toxic levels of NAPQI is open to debate. In reality, cases of acetaminophen toxicity in alcoholics invariably involve an overdose of the analgesic.

COMBINATION ANALGESICS

Nonopioids

Aspirin and acetaminophen are sometimes combined in proprietary compounds (Table 17-6). The rationale for combining an NSAID with

TABLE 17-6 Common Analgesic Combinations Used in Dentistry

NSAID	Opioid	Brand Name	Usual Adult Dose (mg)
ASA	Codeine		300/30
ASA	Oxycodone	Percodan	325/5
Acetaminophen	Codeine	Tylenol #3	300/30
Acetaminophen	Hydrocodone	Vicodin, Lortab, Norco	325/5 325/7.5 325/10
Acetaminophen	Oxycodone	Percocet	325/5 325/10
Acetaminophen	Tramadol	Ultracet	325/37.5
Ibuprofen	Hydrocodone	Vicoprofen	200/7.5
Ibuprofen	Oxycodone	Combunox	400/5

Note: No attempt has been made to present a complete listing of drug combinations or proprietary preparations (which are available in a dazzling variety of dosage forms). Such listings can be found in a variety of sources. It should be noted that a number of the combinations provide less than optimal amounts of aspirin or acetaminophen. In such cases, taking two tablets instead of one can remedy this problem, but it may result in administration of an excessive amount of the opioid analgesic, and unwanted side effects may occur.

acetaminophen appears to have some justification based on the fact that acetaminophen has some actions that are distinct from those of the NSAIDs. Studies have demonstrated an additive analgesic effect of when acetaminophen is combined with ibuprofen. Recently published flexible analgesic guidelines recommend employing 500 mg of acetaminophen with an optimal dose of an NSAID (i.e., ibuprofen 400 mg), especially when the postoperative dental pain is more severe, because the combination produces an additive analgesic and opioid-sparing effect.

Many OTC combinations of aspirin plus acetaminophen also contain caffeine. Caffeine is considered to be an analgesic adjuvant. Caffeine does not appear to have analgesic effects when used alone. However, when 65 to 100 mg of caffeine is combined with traditional analgesics (aspirin, acetaminophen, or ibuprofen), it improves their analgesic efficacy. The mechanism for this adjuvant effect is not known but may include the ability of caffeine to block adenosine receptors at free nerve endings or in mast cells, to enhance central catecholamine effects, or to increase the absorption of weak acids such as aspirin. The central vasoconstrictive effects of caffeine probably help alleviate migraine headaches.

Opioid and Nonopioid Analgesics

There is a sound scientific basis for combining NSAIDs or acetaminophen with opioids. The former drugs combat pain principally by interfering with production of biochemical mediators that cause sensitization of nerve endings at the site of injury or spinal cord, whereas the opioids alter CNS perception and reaction to pain. These complementary actions support the use of the drugs in combination; abundant clinical data exist to support the validity of their combined use. However, there is a common misconception that such combinations produce a synergistic phenomenon, that is, a total effect greater than the sum of individual effects expected from both drugs. No evidence currently supports this belief, and, at best, there is a purely additive effect when drugs from these two classes of analgesics are combined.

Another misconception is that the opioid component in an oral analgesic combination is the major contributor to the preparation's overall effectiveness. Clinical studies indicate quite the opposite, showing that the **non-opioid component is an equal or, more often, greater contributor to the overall efficacy** of the combination for most types of pain. When comparisons are limited to studies evaluating dental pain, there is no question that the aspirin-like drugs provide most of the pain relief, whereas the opioids cause most of the side effects.

The clinical significance of the opioids is that they provide additional analgesia beyond the ceiling effect of the NSAID or acetaminophen alone, and they also contribute a centrally mediated sedative effect. Therefore, the most effective combinations are those that use the optimal amount of an aspirin-like drug combined with the appropriate dose of an opioid analgesic. The clinician must be aware of the epidemic of prescription opioid abuse in the United States, and the number of tablets prescribed must be kept at a minimum. Acetaminophen plus hydrocodone was reported to be the most frequently diverted immediate-release opioid formulation among 19 to 44 year olds in the United States, which is a major reason why this combination was moved from a DEA Schedule III to DEA Schedule II drug. In addition, because of acetaminophen-induced hepatoxicity concerns, all currently marketed opioid combination tablets contain a maximum of 325 mg of acetaminophen.

Oral Analgesic Combinations Used in Dentistry

Although the pharmacologic features of the opioids are discussed in Chapter 16, combinations of opioids and peripherally acting analgesics that are widely used in dentistry are described here. The highest oral potency for the commonly used centrally acting analgesics includes **codeine, hydrocodone, and oxycodone**. A general problem with the opioid analgesics is their relatively high incidence of undesirable side effects. They all cause nausea, constipation, and CNS depression, which become more intense as the dosage is increased. Mild CNS depression manifested as drowsiness may sometimes be useful, but ambulatory dental patients generally want to be able to function normally after they leave the dental office.

Codeine is a commonly used opioid in combination analgesics. Its effective oral dose range is 30 to 90 mg, with 30 mg providing only minimal analgesia, 60 mg providing a little more analgesia with considerably more nausea and sedation, and 90 mg approaching the dose at which intolerable side effects appear. Codeine is available in combination with aspirin or acetaminophen. For most patients, 600 to 650 mg of either drug combined with 60 mg of codeine should provide adequate pain relief for most acute dental pain situations. However, codeine is a prodrug requiring demethylation by CYP2C9 to its active metabolite morphine. It is thought that up to 10% of the population possesses relatively low concentrations of CYP2C9, and in this population, codeine is unlikely to possess analgesic activity. Of more recent concern is that there appears to also be a subset of patients that are "high" metabolizers of codeine to morphine (See chapter 4). Cases of significant respiratory depression (because of **excessive morphine blood levels) have been reported in pediatric patients when codeine-containing analgesics were employed for postoperative pain control.** Serious adverse effects and some deaths have occurred in children after taking codeine for pain relief following tonsillectomy and/or adenoidectomy for obstructive sleep apnea syndrome. Today, there is a trend away from using codeine in children.

Hydrocodone and oxycodone are close analogues of codeine but are approximately 6 and 12 times more potent, respectively. Hydrocodone/acetaminophen combinations (Table 17-6) are now

TABLE 17-7 Drug Treatments for Gout

Drug	Mechanism	Adverse Effects	Indications
Colchicine	Inhibits leukocyte phagocytosis by binding to tubulin	GI, liver necrosis, renal toxicity, coagulation disorders	Acute gout (reduces inflammation and pain)
NSAIDs*, e.g., Indomethacin	Antiinflammatory	GI, dizziness, renal toxicity	Acute gout (reduces inflammation and pain)
Allopurinol	Inhibits xanthine oxidase (reduces uric acid production)	GI, peripheral neuritis, hepatic and renal toxicity, vasculitis	Chronic treatment of gout
Febuxostat	Inhibits xanthine oxidase	GI, headache, rash, liver function abnormalities	Chronic treatment of gout
Probenecid	Increases uric acid excretion (uricosuric)	GI, renal toxicity, blood dyscrasias	Chronic treatment of gout
Sulfinpyrazone	Uricosuric	GI, rash, blood dyscrasias	Chronic treatment of gout
Pegloticase	An enzyme that catalyzes conversion of uric acid to allantoin	Immune response, GI, confusion, pharyngitis, chest pain	Chronic treatment of gout for patients who have failed other therapy

*Salicylates are contraindicated because they reduce uric acid excretion at lower doses.

the most widely prescribed analgesics in the United States. A formulation combining ibuprofen 200 mg with hydrocodone 7.5 mg is also being marketed, but in reality the 200-mg ibuprofen dose is suboptimal, while the 7.5-mg dose of hydrocodone may be too much for most patients. In patients with severe pain, 5 to 10 mg of oxycodone combined with either aspirin or acetaminophen is an effective oral analgesic combination, although side effects such as nausea, dizziness, and sedation should be expected. A formulation of ibuprofen 400 mg with oxycodone 5 mg possesses optimal concentrations of both components. These combinations are categorized as Schedule II narcotics by the United States Drug Enforcement Agency (See Table 17-6).

Hydromorphone is another potent narcotic that occasionally has merit in the dental arena, particularly with narcotic-experienced patients. It is not available as a combination medication, but the dental professional can consider adding OTC ibuprofen, aspirin, or acetaminophen to create an equivalent effect. Normal dosing is 1- to 2-mg hydromorphone every 4 to 6 hours.

The majority of drug combinations on the market include codeine, hydrocodone, and oxycodone combined with either aspirin or acetaminophen (see Table 17-6). Opioids such as morphine, meperidine, and oxymorphone have such low oral absorption that they are of little use in routine dental analgesic therapy. In general, single-entity opioid analgesics are not the drugs of choice for the management of acute dental pain in ambulatory patients.

Implications for Dentistry

Abundant evidence suggests that **dental pain is most amenable to treatment by NSAID analgesics and acetaminophen,** and these drugs have become the mainstay for the management of acute dental pain. Their use, however, is associated with some risks that are readily reduced by understanding the pharmacologic characteristics of these drugs, including the contraindications and precautions to be followed in selected populations. Opioid combination drugs are most useful in patients with a strong emotional component to their pain, in which the mood-altering and sedative effects of the opioid may be desirable. Side effects of drowsiness, impaired psychomotor function, and nausea are common with these drugs and should be expected. In addition, the practicing dentist must be aware of the drug-seeking patient who will often request a prescription including a specific opioid, most often oxycodone or hydrocodone.

OTHER INFLAMMATORY MEDIATORS

Miscellaneous Drugs Used to Treat Inflammation

Diclofenac, meclofenamate, piroxicam, meloxicam, sulindac, tolmetin, oxaprozin, and nabumetone are NSAIDs used to treat inflammatory conditions. Adverse effects and other factors tend to limit the use of these drugs to inflammatory indications such as arthritis, although diclofenac is also used to treat dysmenorrhea and migraine. Salsalate is a salicylate use to treat arthritis and other rheumatoid disorders.

Disease-Modifying Agents for Rheumatic Diseases

These drugs reduce inflammation but also slow the progression of the disease. They include several classes of drugs, including antineoplastic drugs (azathioprine, cyclophosphamide, and methotrexate); hydroxychloroquine, an anti-malarial drug; cyclosporine, an immunosuppressant drug; sulfasalazine, an antimicrobial drug; and miscellaneous drugs such as leflunomide. A number of protein biopharmaceutical DMARDs are available to treat rheumatic diseases. These include monoclonal antibodies and fusion proteins. They are summarized in Appendix 1, including their compositions, mechanisms, and indications. These agents inhibit inflammatory immune responses by a variety of mechanisms, often inhibiting T-cell and B-cell function.

Drugs Used to Treat Gout

Gout is an inflammatory disease that stems from elevated concentrations of uric acid in blood and other body fluids. Treatment of gout is either acute or chronic. Table 17-7 summarizes the drugs that are used in treatment.

NSAIDS, ANALGESIC COMBINATIONS, AND ANTIRHEUMATIC AND ANTIGOUT DRUGS

Nonproprietary (Generic) Name	Proprietary (Trade) Name
Salicylates*	
Aspirin	(many)
Salsalate	Amigesic, Disalcid
Other NSAIDs Used for Analgesia*	
Ibuprofen	Motrin
Ketoprofen	Orudis
Etodolac	Lodine
Flurbiprofen	Ansaid
Celecoxib	Celebrex
Naproxen	Aleve
Other NSAIDs Used for Inflammation	
Diclofenac	Voltaren
Indomethacin	Indocin
Meclofenamate	—
Meloxicam	Mobic

Continued

NSAIDS, ANALGESIC COMBINATIONS, AND ANTIRHEUMATIC AND ANTIGOUT DRUGS—cont'd

Nonproprietary (Generic) Name	Proprietary (Trade) Name
Nabumetone	Relafen
Oxaprozin	Daypro
Piroxicam	Feldene
Sulindac	Clinoril
Tolmetin	Tolectin
Analgesic Combinations‡	
Other Antirheumatic Drugs	
Azathioprine	Imuran
Chloroquine	Aralen
Cyclophosphamide	Cytoxan
Cyclosporine	Neoral
Hydroxychloroquine	Plaquenil
Leflunomide	Arava
Methotrexate	Rheumatrex
Sulfasalazine	Azulfidine
Antigout Drugs	
Allopurinol	Zyloprim
Colchicine	—
Febuxostat	Uloric
Indomethacin	Indocin
Pegloticase	Krystexxa
Probenecid	Benemid
Sulfinpyrazone	Anturane

*See also Table 17-6.
‡See Table 17-5.

CASE DISCUSSION

Although Ms. K wants a narcotic pain reliever for her acute pulpitis, there are better therapies you can offer. First and foremost, addressing the crisis with local anesthesia followed by either pulpectomy/endodontic irrigation or extraction would be best. If she is unwilling to consent to this care today, your next best option is to use one of the antiinflammatory medications discussed in this chapter. Ibuprofen 400 to 600 mg every 4 to 6 hours or aspirin 650 mg every 4 hours is an ideal choice. You can explain to Ms. K that these drugs will be more efficacious than opioids for most dental pain. Then, if you feel she needs it, you can prescribe a narcotic for breakthrough pain, such as oxycodone 5 mg.

In the future, when she consents to surgery and there is less active inflammation, a combination drug such as hydrocodone/acetaminophen 5/325 may be ideal. She can supplement it with the same ibuprofen or aspirin to get additional NSAID pain relief.

Be sure that she understands that her pain will be reduced from about 7 or 8 (out of 10 on the pain scale), for instance, down to a tolerable 2 or 3. Guiding her expectations away from complete pain relief will likely improve her response to therapy because she will know what to expect.

Also let her know that the opioids may cause nausea/vomiting, dry mouth, and constipation. Use these facts as more reasons to support the NSAIDs as your primary pain control method and the narcotics as backup for breakthrough pain.

Finally, tell her that you will manage her pain for 4 to 10 days depending on the number of surgery appointments. Likely in a few days after the last surgery, she should be off her narcotic pain medications. Knowing this, she will be less likely to seek additional prescriptions of narcotic pain relievers.

GENERAL REFERENCES

1. Aoki T, Narumiya S: Prostaglandins and chronic inflammation, *Trends Pharmacol Sci* 33:304–311, 2012.
2. Bello AE, Holt RJ: Cardiovascular risk with non-steroidal anti-inflammatory drugs: clinical implications, *Drug Saf* 37:897–902, 2014.
3. Borchers AT, Keen CL, Cheema GS, Gershwin ME: The use of methotrexate in rheumatoid arthritis, *Semin Arthritis Rheum* 34:465–483, 2004.
4. Dale MM, Foreman JC, Fan T-PD, editors: *Textbook of immunopharmacology*, ed 3, Boston, 1994, Blackwell Scientific.
5. Dart RC, Kuffner EK, Rumack BH: Treatment of pain of fever with paracetamol (acetaminophen) in the alcoholic patient: a systemic review, *Am J Ther* 7:123–134, 2000.
6. Diaz-Gonzales F, Sanchez-Madrid F: NSAIDs: learning new tricks from old drugs, *Eur J Immunol* 45:679–686, 2015.
7. Drugs for pain, *Med Lett* 128(April 11):31–42, 2013. http://www.uspreventiveservicestaskforce.org/Page/Document/draft-recommendation-statement/aspirin-to-prevent-cardiovascular-disease-and-cancer (website on aspirin prophylaxis, to prevent cardiovascular disease and cancer, accessed January, 2016).
8. Famaey JP, Paulus HE, editors: *Therapeutic applications of NSAIDs: subpopulations and new formulations*, New York, 1992, Marcel Dekker.
9. Glaser KB, Vadas P: *Phospholipase A_2 in clinical inflammation. Molecular approaches to pathophysiology*, Boca Raton, FL, 1995, CRC Press.
10. Graves DT, Jiang Y: Chemokines, a family of chemotactic cytokines, *Crit Rev Oral Biol Med* 6:109–118, 1995.
11. Jackson JL, Roszkowski MT, Moore PA: Management of acute postoperative pain. In Fonseca RJ, Frost D, Hersh EV, Levin LM, volume editors: *Oral and maxillofacial surgery, vol. 1: anesthesia/dentoalveolar surgery/office management*, Philadelphia, 2000, WB Saunders.
12. Prescott LF: *Paracetamol (acetaminophen). A critical biographical review*, Bristol, PA, 1996, Taylor & Francis.
13. Rainsford KD, Powanda MC, editors: *Safety and efficacy of non-prescription (OTC) analgesics and NSAIDs*, Hingham, MA, 1998, Kluwer Academic Publishers.
14. Ruddy S, Harris ED, Sledge CB, et al.: *Kelley's textbook of rheumatology*, ed 6, Philadelphia, 2001, WB Saunders.
15. Stockley IH: *Stockley's drug interactions*, ed 6, London, UK, 2002, Pharmaceutical Press.

18

Histamine and Histamine Antagonists*

Matthew R. Cooke and Joseph A. Giovannitti Jr.

KEY INFORMATION

- Autacoids are potent endogenous substances with complex physiologic and pathophysiologic functions with non-autonomic pharmacologic effects. They include histamine, serotonin, prostaglandin, vasoactive peptides, and nitric oxide.
- Histamine, formed from the amino acid histidine, is a ubiquitous amine, that modulates local immune responses and regulates physiologic function including gastric secretion, neurotransmission in the central nervous system, and local control of the microcirculation.
- Most histamine is produced and stored within granules in mast cells, leukocytes (basophils and eosinophils), and enterochromaffin cells of the stomach.
- Physical or chemical agents that nonspecifically cause injury to tissue can cause the immediate release of histamine from mast cells in the affected area.
- Histamine release can occur as a consequence of the binding of specific antigens to allergen-specific antibodies via reaginic (IgE) antibodies. These are attached to the plasma membranes of mast cells and basophils.
- Histamine exerts its effects by binding G protein–coupled histamine receptors, (see chapter 1), designated H_1 through H_4.
- Histamine antagonists do not alter the formation, release, or degradation of histamine but competitively antagonize it at the receptor sites.
- H_1 blockers are clinically used for allergies of the immediate type (e.g., hay fever, allergic rhinitis, urticaria), such as those caused by antigens, which act on IgE antibody-sensitized mast cells.
- Older H_1 antihistamines, first generation, are highly sedating agents with significant autonomic receptor blockade.
- Second-generation H_1 blockers, typified by cetirizine, fexofenadine, and loratidine, have less lipid solubility than first-generation agents and do not cross the blood–brain barrier, therefore greatly reducing their sedative and autonomic effects.
- Side effects of first-generation H_1 blockers may be the desired therapeutic (sedation and dry mouth) outcome.
- Four H_2 blockers are available: cimetidine, ranitidine, famotidine, and nizatidine. They are potent competitive antagonists of the H_2 receptors, therapeutically reducing gastric acid secretion.
- Cimetidine is a competitive inhibitor of the hepatic mixed-function oxidase enzymes responsible for the metabolism of some drugs.
- Cimetidine has been shown to increase blood concentrations of numerous drugs, including anticoagulants of the warfarin type, tricyclic antidepressants, various benzodiazepines, phenobarbital, theophylline, propranolol and other β-adrenoceptor blockers, Ca^{2+} channel blockers, lidocaine, estradiol, and phenytoin.
- Ranitidine, famotidine, and nizatidine have fewer adverse effects than cimetidine because binding of these agents to cytochrome P450 enzymes is much less firm than that of cimetidine.

CASE STUDY

Mr. H. is your 67-year-old dental patient. He needs to have tooth #19 extracted and an immediate implant placed. He tells you he is extremely anxious and would like moderate sedation for the procedure. You review his medical history and find a past medical history significant for benign prostatic hyperplasia (BPH) and hypertension (HTN). His HTN is well controlled with lisinopril, and he takes no medicines for his BPH. His surgical history is significant for a hernia repair 3 years ago. He does note a history of severe postoperative nausea and vomiting in recovery. You evaluate the patient, discuss risks versus benefits, and decide to use moderate IV sedation for treatment. Would you include a first-generation antihistamine, promethazine, in your sedation regimen to help with the patient's sedation and possible postoperative nausea and vomiting?

*The authors wish to recognize Clarence L. Trummel for his past contributions to this chapter.

AUTACOIDS

Autacoids from the Greek *autos* ("self") and *akos* ("cure") are endogenous organic molecules with potent pharmacologic effects, that are not part of traditional immune or autonomic groups. Histamine and serotonin (5-hydroxytryptamine) are two important amine autacoids. Other autacoids, which produce paracrine type effects, include polypeptides (angiotensin, bradykinin, and kallidin), lipid-derived substances (prostaglandins, leukotrienes, and platelet-activating factor), and nitric oxide. This chapter will focus on histamine and histamine antagonists.

HISTAMINE

Histamine, formed from the amino acid histidine (Fig. 18-1), is a ubiquitous amine that modulates local immune responses and regulates physiologic function including gastric secretion, neurotransmission in the central nervous system (CNS), and local control of the microcirculation. Pharmacologic properties of histamine suggest that this substance is involved in **inflammatory and anaphylactic reactions.**

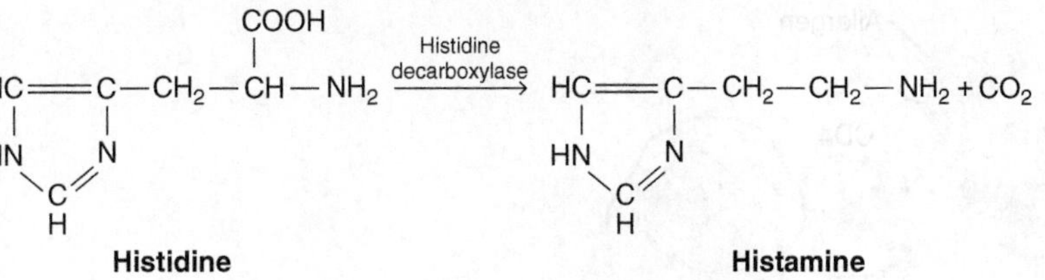

$$\text{Histidine (imidazole–}CH_2\text{–}CH(COOH)\text{–}NH_2) \xrightarrow{\text{Histidine decarboxylase}} \text{Histamine (imidazole–}CH_2\text{–}CH_2\text{–}NH_2) + CO_2$$

Histidine **Histamine**

FIG 18-1 Conversion of histidine to histamine.

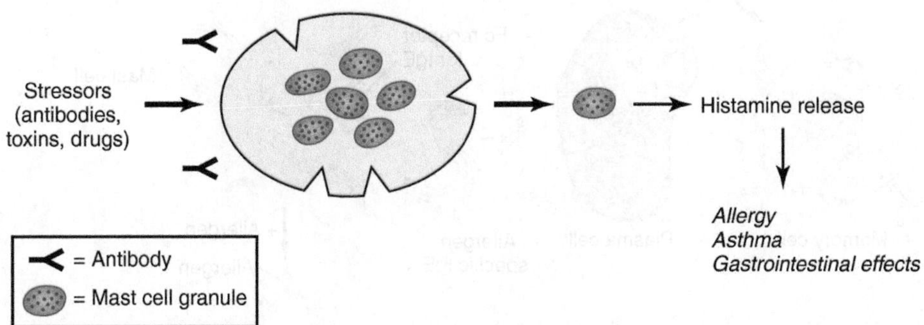

FIG 18-2 Summary of mast cell release of histamine. Some stimuli act through receptors for immunoglobulins (indentations in the membrane), whereas others act directly by causing an increase in intracellular Ca^{2+}, which triggers the release of histamine from mast cells. (From Wecker L, Crespo L, et al: *Brody's human pharmacology*, ed 5, Philadelphia, 2010, Mosby.)

Local application of histamine causes redness, swelling, and edema, mimicking a mild inflammatory reaction. Large doses of systemically administered histamine have the potential to produce profound vascular changes similar to those seen in shock of traumatic or anaphylactic origin.

Formation, Distribution, and Release

The histamine content of different tissues varies greatly. The highest concentrations are found in lung, skin, and intestinal mucosa. Organs such as the pancreas, spleen, liver, and kidney have low histamine content. The physiologic significance of this pattern of distribution is unknown. Histamine may be derived from dietary sources or synthesized by bacteria in the gastrointestinal tract. However, most is formed in situ.

High concentrations of histamine are found in vesicles within mast cells, leukocytes (basophils and eosinophils), enterochromaffin cells of the gastrointestinal tract, some neurons, and other cells. **Mast cells synthesize histamine** and store it as a proteinaceous complex with heparin or chondroitin sulfate in membrane-bound secretory granules where it can be discharged from the cell by a process called **exocytosis,** or **degranulation** (Fig. 18-2).

Histamine outside the mast cell or basophil is found within neurons of the hypothalamus. The function of these histaminergic neurons is unknown. Another site of non–mast cell histamine is the enterochromaffin cell in the gastric mucosa. Here histamine stimulates gastric acid secretion by mucosal parietal cells. Certain neoplasms, collectively known as **carcinoids,** also secrete various autacoids, including histamine, which likely contribute to the so-called carcinoid syndrome.

Various conditions (or stimuli) trigger the release of histamine:

Tissue injury

Physical or chemical agents that nonspecifically cause injury to tissue, particularly skin or mucosa, cause the immediate release of histamine from mast cells in the affected area. Depending on the severity of injury, histamine continues to be released for several minutes and seems to be largely responsible for the initial sharp increase in vascular permeability that is characteristic of acute inflammation. This histamine-dependent change in permeability is transient (≤30 minutes) but is followed in 2 to 4 hours by a more prolonged increase in permeability lasting up to 4 hours. Although inhibitors of histamine release, or inhibitors of the subsequent action of histamine, can block the initial phase of vascular permeability after injury, they have little effect on the secondary or delayed phase, suggesting that autacoids or factors other than histamine mediate the secondary phase. The mechanism by which a nonspecific injury triggers mast cell degranulation is unclear. Proposed mechanisms include direct physical damage to mast cells or alternatively via initial production of factors such as activated complement components or vasoactive polypeptides, which stimulate histamine release.

Allergic reactions

Presentation of a specific antigen to a previously sensitized subject can trigger immediate allergic reactions, ranging in intensity from mild (localized edema, erythema, and itching) to severe (marked decrease in blood pressure and bronchospasm). The pathophysiologic manifestations of such reactions are caused largely by the release of histamine (Fig. 18-3). Release occurs as a consequence of the binding of specific antigens to allergen-specific reaginic (IgE) antibodies that are attached to the plasma membranes of mast cells and basophils; these are transmembrane high-affinity receptors termed *FcεRI*. Antigen–antibody interaction is an appropriate stimulus for the series of events leading to degranulation of these cells (see Fig. 18-3).

Drugs and other foreign compounds

Large groups of drugs and other chemicals can trigger histamine release directly without a requirement for previous sensitization through an immune response. For convenience, these agents can be classified as basic histamine releasers, macromolecular compounds, and enzymes. The basic histamine releasers include aliphatic and arylalkyl amines, amides, amidines, diamidines, quaternary ammonium compounds,

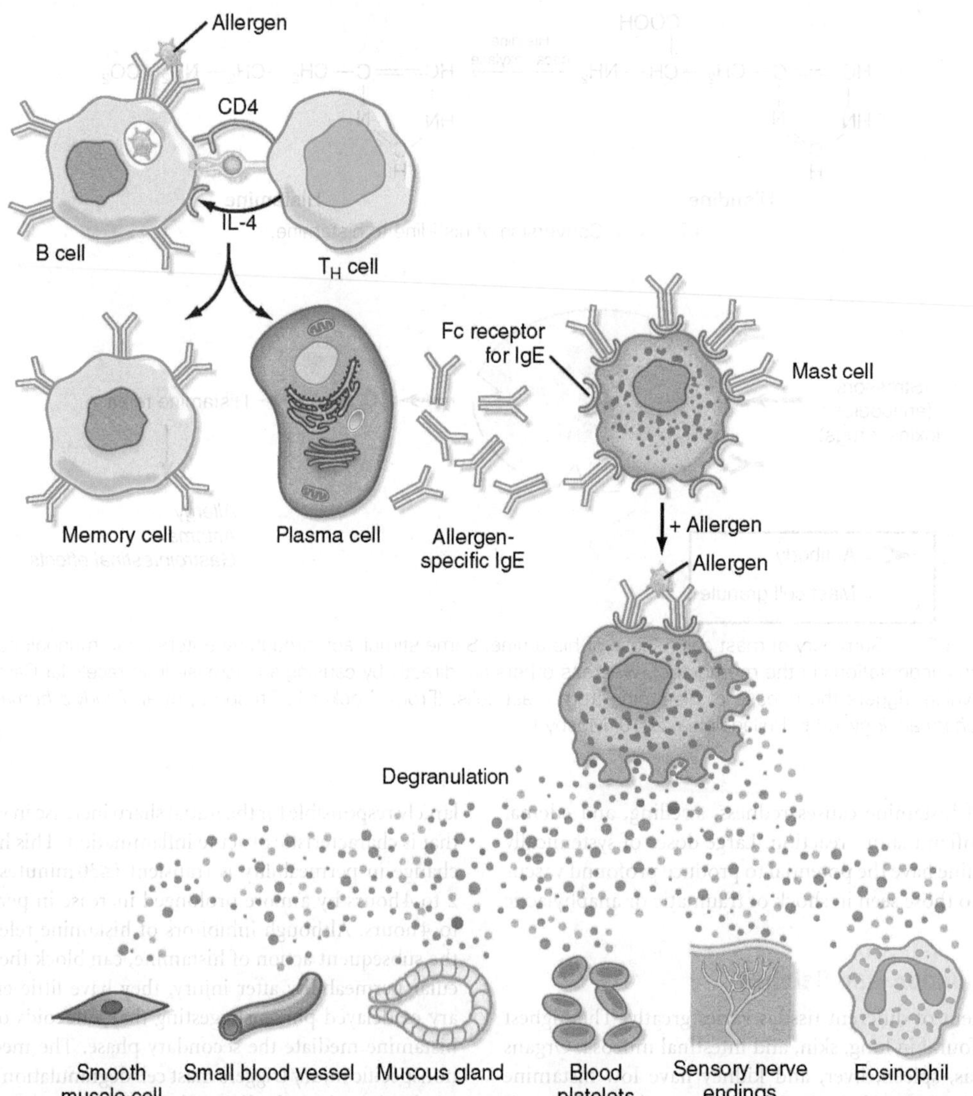

FIG 18-3 General mechanism underlying an allergic reaction. Exposure to an antigen activates B cells to form IgE-secreting plasma cells. The secreted IgE molecules bind to IgE-specific Fc receptors on mast cells. After a second exposure to the allergen, the bound IgE is cross-linked, which triggers the release of active mediators (e.g., histamine) from mast cells. The mediators cause smooth muscle contraction, increased vascular permeability, and vasodilation. (From Koeppen B, Stanton B: *Berne and Levy physiology*, ed 6, Philadelphia, 2010, Mosby.)

alkaloids, piperidine derivatives, pyridinium compounds, **opioids**, antimalarial drugs, dyes, and basic polypeptides.

Metabolism

Histamine of either exogenous or endogenous origin is rapidly inactivated by two routes. The more important of these is methylation of the imidazole ring by the enzyme histamine-N-methyltransferase, which is widely distributed throughout the body. The other route involves the oxidative deamination of histamine by diamine oxidase to produce imidazole acetic acid, much of which is subsequently conjugated with ribose. All metabolites are inactive and, along with a small amount of free histamine, are excreted by the kidney.

Mechanism of Action

Histamine exerts its effects by binding to G protein–coupled histamine receptors, (Chapter 1) designated H_1 through H_4 (Table 18-1). Most of the important effects of histamine can be attributed to its actions on smooth muscle and glands. The existence of compounds that can selectively block the actions of histamine strongly supports the existence of four histamine receptors: H_1, H_2, H_3, and H_4. Although the first two seem to be unique (i.e., have selective agonists and antagonists), the H_3 and H_4 receptors share a degree of homology and are more difficult to distinguish pharmacologically from one another (see Table 18-1).

General Therapeutic Uses

Although no valid therapeutic applications exist for histamine, it is of limited use as a diagnostic tool in the assessment of gastric acid production and in testing for nonallergic bronchial hyperreactivity in asthmatics.

Adverse Effects

The toxic effects of histamine are predictable based on its pharmacologic actions and include cutaneous flushing, hypotension, headache, visual disturbances, dyspnea, and gastrointestinal disturbances such

TABLE 18-1 G Protein–Coupled Histamine Receptors

Type	Location	Post-Receptor Mechanism	Function
Histamine H_1 receptor	• CNS: Produced in the tuberomammillary nucleus, projecting to the dorsal raphe, locus coeruleus, and either to and/or through the hippocampal formation, amygdala, basal ganglia, thalamus, superior colliculus, cerebellum, and additional structures. • PNS: Smooth muscle and endothelium	Gq ↑ IP3 DAG	• CNS: Sleep–wake cycle, body temperature, nociception, endocrine homeostasis, appetite, mood, learning, and memory • PNS: Causes bronchoconstriction, bronchial smooth muscle contraction, vasodilation, separation of endothelial cells (responsible for hives), and pain and itching due to insect stings; the primary receptors involved in allergic rhinitis symptoms and motion sickness
Histamine H_2 receptor	Located on parietal cells and vascular smooth muscle cells	Gs ↑ CAMP	Primarily stimulates gastric acid secretion; also involved in vasodilation
Histamine H_3 receptor	Central nervous system and to a lesser extent peripheral nervous system tissue/nerve endings	Gi ↓ CAMP	Decreased neurotransmitter release: histamine, acetylcholine, norepinephrine, serotonin
Histamine H_4 receptor	Leukocytes, primarily in the basophils; also found on thymus, small intestine, spleen, and colon	Gi ↓ CAMP	Plays a role in mast cell chemotaxis

CAMP, Cyclic adenosine phosphate; *CNS*, central nervous system; *DAG*, diacylglycerol; *IP3*, inositol triphosphate; *PNS*, peripheral nervous system.

as nausea, vomiting, and diarrhea. Massive doses may lead to shock and circulatory failure. Histamine, even in low doses, may have serious adverse consequences in elderly individuals or patients with cardiovascular disease, asthma, or recent gastrointestinal bleeding.

HISTAMINE ANTAGONISTS

Histamine antagonists, or antihistamines, encompass a group of compounds with the characteristic ability to block the actions of histamine. These compounds do not alter the formation, release, or degradation of histamine but competitively antagonize it at receptor sites. Four groups of antihistamines are now known by their ability to selectively block effects of histamine mediated by the various receptors. These groups of antihistamines are appropriately termed ***H_1, H_2, H_3, and H_4 receptor antagonists***. The generic term ***antihistamine*** is often used to refer to the "classic" antihistamines, or **H_1 antagonists.**

H_1 Receptor Antagonists

Most antihistamines with the ability to block H_1 receptors contain a side chain that resembles the ethylamino group in histamine. These H_1 receptor antagonists, or H_1 antihistamines, can be represented by the following general formula:

$$\begin{matrix} \text{Aryl}_1 & & & & R_1 \\ & \searrow & | & | & \nearrow \\ & X- & C- & C- & N \\ & \nearrow & | & | & \searrow \\ \text{Aryl}_2 & & & & R_2 \end{matrix}$$

A general conclusion from examination of structure–activity relationships is that a basic nitrogen atom is essential, whether it exists in an aliphatic side chain, as in diphenhydramine, or in a ring structure, as in meclizine (Table 18-2).

By using the general formula just presented, most H_1 antihistamines can be grouped according to the substitution made at the X position (see earlier). Levocabastine is a piperidine, but it does not fit the structural chemistry in the six aforementioned categories. Azelastine, used only topically on the nasal mucosa, is a phthalazinone and is structurally unrelated to these other categories.

The chemical structures of representative compounds of each of the major classes of H_1 antihistamines are shown in Table 18-2. Despite their structural heterogeneity, the older antihistamines have only minor differences in pharmacologic properties, and these are mainly in potency, duration of action, and intensity of effects on other systems. In the last few decades, several H_1 antihistamines have been developed that differ from older antihistamines in that they are largely devoid of effects on the CNS. Because of this difference, this group of agents, which are predominantly **piperidine** derivatives and include **fexofenadine, levocabastine, and loratadine,** is often termed ***second-generation antihistamines*** to distinguish them from the older, or **first-generation, antihistamines**. Other second-generation H_1 antihistamines include **acrivastine (an alkylamine), cetirizine (a piperazine),** and azelastine (a phthalazinone).

Pharmacologic effects

H_1 antihistamines exert various effects. Although the basis of some of these effects is obscure, many clearly result from histamine antagonism. **These agents inhibit the contraction of gastrointestinal and bronchial smooth muscle and decrease capillary permeability and the flare and itch components of the "triple response."** H_1 antihistamines do not block histamine-induced gastric secretion. However, they do antagonize the increased secretions of the salivary and lacrimal glands and the increased release of epinephrine from the adrenal medulla stimulated by histamine. **Xerostomia** is a common side effect of H_1 antihistamines. As with many other pharmacologic inhibitors, the basic mechanism of action can be explained in terms of a competitive blockade of receptors. Antihistamines interact with the **H_1 receptors** on the target cell, resulting in a decreased availability of these receptors for histamine. This interaction is reversible, or competitive, because the inhibition produced by a given concentration of antihistamine can be overcome by increasing the concentration of histamine.

No evidence indicates that antihistamines interfere with the synthesis, release, or biotransformation of histamine. Cetirizine seems to be unique among antihistamines because it has been reported to have antieosinophilic activity, so it inhibits the late phase of inflammation in addition to the more immediate histaminic effects.

The action of H_1 antihistamines in antagonizing histamine is specific. H_1 antihistamines "reverse" the effects of histamine by inhibiting further action, but they have no directly opposing actions of their own. **In contrast, epinephrine** nonspecifically antagonizes histamine by exerting its own distinct effects, such as vasoconstriction, bronchodilation, and decreased gastrointestinal motility. The distinction is important in

TABLE 18-2 Chemical Classification, Representative Structures, and Dosages of Major H_1 Antihistamines

Class	Representative Compound* (Proprietary Name)	Usual Adult Dose (Oral)	Duration of Action	Some Other Compounds in the Same Class
Alkylamines	Chlorpheniramine maleate (Chlor-Trimeton, others)	4 mg	4-6 hr	Acrivastine (in Semprex-D): 8 mg, 6-8 hr Brompheniramine maleate (Dimetane): 4 mg, 4-6 hr Dexchlorpheniramine maleate (Polaramine): 2 mg, 4-6 hr Triprolidine hydrochloride (Actidil): 2.5 mg, 4-6 hr
Ethanolamines	Diphenhydramine hydrochloride (Benadryl, others)	25-50 mg	6-8 hr	Carbinoxamine maleate (in Carbiset): 4-8 mg, 6-8 hr Clemastine fumarate (Tavist): 1.34-2.68 mg, 8-12 hr Dimenhydrinate (Dramamine): 50-100 mg, 4-6 hr Doxylamine succinate (Unisom): 12.5-25 mg, 4-6 hr
Ethylenediamines	Tripelennamine citrate (PBZ, others)	25-50 mg	4-6 hr	Pyrilamine maleate (Nisaval): 25-50 mg, 6-8 hr
Piperazines	Meclizine hydrochloride (Bonine, others)	25-50 mg	24 hr	Buclizine hydrochloride (Bucladin-S): 50 mg, 4-12 hr Cetirizine hydrochloride (Zyrtec): 5-10 mg, 24 hr Cyclizine hydrochloride (Marezine): 50 mg, 4-6 hr Hydroxyzine hydrochloride (Atarax, others): 50-100 mg, 6-24 hr Hydroxyzine pamoate (Vistaril): 50-100 mg, 6-24 hr
Phenothiazines	Promethazine hydrochloride (Phenergan)	12.5-25 mg	4-12 hr	Methdilazine hydrochloride (Tacaryl): 8 mg, 6-12 hr Trimeprazine tartrate (Temaril): 2.5 mg, 6 hr
Piperidines	Loratadine hydrochloride (Claritin)	10 mg	24 hr	Azatadine maleate (Optimine): 1-2 mg, 8-12 hr Cyproheptadine hydrochloride (Periactin)[†]: 4 mg, 6-8 hr Fexofenadine hydrochloride (Allegra): 60 mg, 12 hr Levocabastine hydrochloride (Livostin): topical Phenindamine tartrate (Nolahist): 25 mg, 4-6 hr

TABLE 18-2 Chemical Classification, Representative Structures, and Dosages of Major H_1 Antihistamines—cont'd

Class	Representative Compound* (Proprietary Name)	Usual Adult Dose (Oral)	Duration of Action	Some Other Compounds in the Same Class
Phthalazinones	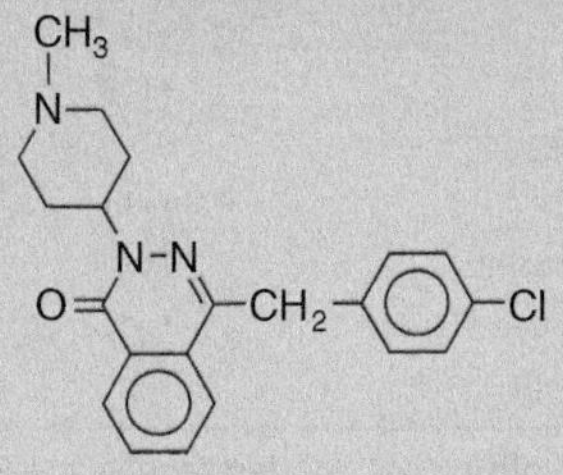 Azelastine hydrochloride (Astelin)	274 μg (topical nasal application; per nostril)	8-12 hr	

Second-generation H_1 antihistamines are acrivastine, azelastine, cetirizine, desloratadine, fexofenadine, levocabastine, levocetirizine, and loratadine.
H_1 histamine receptor blockers used in ophthalmology are emedastine, epinastine, ketotifen, and olopatadine.
*Each structural formula is of the free base form.
†Also a serotonin-receptor antagonist.

understanding why a physiologic antagonist such as epinephrine is a more effective agent than an antihistamine for relieving bronchospasm associated with asthma, anaphylaxis, and other allergic reactions. The ineffectiveness of H_1 antihistamines in relieving these physiologic effects is partly the result of involvement of autacoids other than histamine in mediating allergic bronchospasm in humans. These substances include leukotrienes and kinins, against which classic antihistamines show little antagonism.

The older H_1 antihistamines, typified by diphenhydramine, are sedative agents with significant autonomic receptor blockade (Table 18-2). **Second-generation H_1 blockers**, typified by **cetirizine, fexofenadine, and loratidine**, have less lipid solubility than first-generation agents and **do not cross the blood–brain barrier**, therefore greatly reducing their sedative and autonomic effects. Sedation is mediated by the inhibition of H_1 receptors in the brain. The ability to cause sedation varies widely among the available first-generation H_1 antihistamines. The agents with the most sedation are the ethanolamines and phenothiazines, whereas the alkylamines have a low incidence of drowsiness. Tolerance to the sedative effects of H_1 antihistamines may develop with long-term use. However, concomitant decreases in peripheral antihistaminic effects have not been observed.

Another clinically useful CNS effect of first-generation H_1 antihistamines is **inhibition of nausea and vomiting**, associated with motion sickness. These agents also possess mild anti-Parkinson activity. They work via a central cholinergic receptor–blocking action. Because H_1 agents possess antimuscarinic activity, there is a decrease in salivary secretion. Second-generation H_1 antihistamines have little or no antimuscarinic activity.

Antihistamines have some **degree of local anesthetic activity**. This property is most notable in **diphenhydramine**, promethazine, pyrilamine, and tripelennamine. Antihistamines have occasionally been used clinically in dentistry when conventional local anesthetics are contraindicated.

Large doses of first-generation H_1 antihistamines can cause CNS stimulation that may result in convulsions. Paradoxical excitement, restlessness, or insomnia may occasionally be encountered even at therapeutic doses.

Absorption, rate, and excretion

H_1 antihistamines are well absorbed after either oral or parenteral administration. The onset of action occurs 15 to 60 minutes after an oral dose. Effects are typically maximal in 1 to 2 hours, with a duration of 4 to 6 hours, although the duration is longer for some agents (see Table 18-2). In contrast, most second-generation H_1 antihistamines have a considerably longer duration of action. Loratadine is transformed to an active metabolite with an average elimination half-time of greater than 24 hours, which allows once-daily dosing.

TABLE 18-3 Classification of H_1 Receptor Blockers

H_1 Receptor Class	X Substitution on Antihistamine Molecule
Alkylamines	Carbon
Ethanolamines	Oxygen
Ethylenediamines	Nitrogen
Piperazines	Piperazine ring
Phenothiazines	Phenothiazine nucleus
Piperidines	Piperidine ring

Biotransformation of first-generation H_1 antihistamines is terminated by conversion to inactive metabolites through hydroxylation in the liver. Second-generation antihistamines are extensively metabolized in the liver by the CYP3A4 microsomal enzyme. In some cases, such as with loratadine, these result in active metabolites. Concurrent administration of other agents metabolized by this same enzyme can reduce the biotransformation of these particular antihistamines. Other second-generation H_1 antihistamines (e.g., acrivastine and cetirizine) are not metabolized to an active form and are largely excreted unchanged in the urine. Cetirizine is a metabolite of the first-generation agent hydroxyzine.

General therapeutic uses

The introduction of antihistamines into clinical medicine stimulated great interest regarding application in histamine-mediated pathologic states. The early enthusiasm for antihistamines often led to their irrational use in various clinical situations. Although subsequent experience has brought about a better appreciation of the therapeutic indications and limitations of antihistamines, they are often still used when their clinical efficacy is doubtful or when other agents might be more appropriate.

The most prominent use of H_1 antihistamines is in countering the manifestations of various allergic conditions, that is, reactions resulting from antigen–antibody combination in which histamine release occurs. Remember, antihistamines have no effect on the interaction of antigens and antibodies or on the release of histamine that may be triggered by this interaction. Antihistamines act by competitively antagonizing the binding of liberated histamine to its receptor. They cannot alter the allergic basis of a given disease, but they may only provide relief from some of the symptoms. Antihistamines are most effective when given before the release of histamine. After histamine release has occurred, an antihistamine can only reduce further undesirable effects.

The clinical applications and efficacy of H_1 antihistamines (Table 18-4) can be summarized as follows:

1. H_1 antihistamines are generally useful in the treatment of nasal allergies of either a seasonal (e.g., hay fever) or perennial (nonseasonal) nature because they relieve rhinorrhea, sneezing, lacrimation, and itching of the eyes and nasal mucosa. Azelastine is effective for 12 hours when applied topically to the nasal mucosa. This route of administration minimizes unwanted systemic effects such as drowsiness. Antihistamines are often combined with decongestants such as pseudoephedrine for the management of allergic symptoms in the upper respiratory tract. H_1 antihistamines are less effective in treating chronic or vasomotor (nonallergic) rhinitis.
2. Allergic dermatoses are treated with H_1 antihistamines. Acute and chronic urticarias respond favorably to these agents. Angioedema also responds to antihistamine therapy; however, a severe attack involving the larynx almost certainly requires epinephrine for proper management of this serious complication. H_1 antihistamines may, also, be useful in controlling the itching associated with eczematous pruritus, atopic or contact dermatitis, and insect bites. In some situations (e.g., atopic dermatitis), topical corticosteroids are usually more effective. Although antihistamines are topically effective in treating pruritus and urticaria, topical application can also cause an allergic dermatitis.
3. H_1 antihistamines have minimal effect on the acute manifestations of bronchial asthma. The pathogenesis of bronchial asthma is complex, and mediators of bronchial muscle constriction other than histamine are involved. β-Adrenergic receptor agonists and corticosteroids are the primary drugs used to alleviate an acute asthmatic episode. Antihistamines have been used in an attempt to decrease pre-asthmatic cough in children, although the efficacy of this therapy is not established.
4. H_1 antihistamines, particularly chlorpheniramine, combined with nasal decongestants and analgesics, are widely used for symptomatic relief of the common cold. There are dozens of such preparations on the market, which indicates the popularity of these nostrums. Unless the cold is superimposed on an allergic rhinitis, any relief obtained from this combination stems largely from the drying of the mucosa caused by the anticholinergic action of the antihistamine and the actions of the vasoconstrictor and analgesic. Antihistamines alone are of no proven value in either preventing or shortening the duration of the common cold.
5. A CNS action of first-generation H_1 antihistamines can be used to prevent or treat nausea and vomiting induced by motion. In general, these agents exert less anti–motion sickness activity than do anticholinergics such as scopolamine. H_1 antihistamines may also be useful in counteracting nausea and vomiting in vestibular disturbances such as Meniere disease and other forms of vertigo. The effectiveness of individual antihistamines varies widely; promethazine, diphenhydramine, dimenhydrinate, and cyclizine are probably the most effective of all. The more effective agents also tend to have greater sedative effects.

TABLE 18-4 Efficacy of H_1 Antihistamines

Clinical Applications of H_1 Antihistamines	Efficacy
Nasal allergies	+++
Allergic dermatitis	+++
Bronchial asthma	++
Severe anaphylactic reaction*	0
Symptom relief of colds	+++
Prevent and/or treat nausea	+++
Hypnotics	+
Local anesthetics	+

0, No effect; +, modest effect; ++, moderate effect; +++, significant effect.
*H_1 antihistamines have no primary therapeutic role because they cannot control either the marked hypotension or the bronchospasm associated with a severe anaphylactic reaction.

6. Various over-the-counter (OTC) preparations sold as **hypnotics** include H_1 antihistamines, especially **diphenhydramine**. These agents are added because of their ability to cross the blood–brain barrier and induce sleep. Antihistamines are less effective sedatives than benzodiazepines and sedative-hypnotics, even at higher doses.
7. Some miscellaneous uses of H_1 antihistamines include reduction of tremors and muscle rigidity in Parkinson disease, treatment of headaches of unknown cause, and control of nonhemolytic, nonpyrogenic reactions to blood transfusion. They are also useful in relieving acute dystonias caused by phenothiazines and other neuroleptics. Promethazine is used as an adjunct to general anesthesia to produce drowsiness and to prevent or control nausea and vomiting induced by anesthetic agents and opioid analgesics.

Adverse effects

At therapeutic doses, H_1 antihistamines are relatively free of serious adverse reactions. The most common side effects result from CNS depression, which is generally manifested as drowsiness, diminished alertness, lethargy, and decreased motor coordination. The incidence of sedation varies with individual agents, but in general the ethanolamines and the phenothiazines are the most sedating, the ethylenediamines are intermediate, and the alkylamines and piperazines are the least sedating. As previously mentioned, loratadine and other second-generation H_1 antihistamines are essentially devoid of sedative or other CNS effects. Sedation caused by antihistamines may be a serious liability in a patient whose daily activities require mental alertness and coordination. In such cases, a reduction of dosage or substitution of agents may be necessary. If antihistamines are to be used as part of balanced sedation/anesthesia (i.e., preop promethazine), the patient should be monitored closely.

The anticholinergic properties of antihistamines occasionally cause insomnia, tremors, nervousness and irritability, palpitations, tachycardia, dry mouth, blurred vision, urinary retention, and constipation. Gastrointestinal disturbances—nausea, vomiting, and epigastric distress—also occur but are uncommon. The incidence of these effects is dose-related.

Serious disturbances of cardiac rhythm have occurred in patients receiving astemizole or terfenadine, second-generation H_1 antihistamines of the piperidine class. These drugs have been off the market for several years. Newer second-generation H_1 antihistamines are not associated with these adverse effects.

Large doses of a first-generation H_1 antihistamine can cause **marked stimulation of the CNS** manifested by hallucinations, excitement, and motor disturbances such as tremors and convulsions. Deaths from overdosage almost invariably occur outside a therapeutic setting (e.g., accidental poisoning in the home).

TABLE 18-5 Comparison of First and Second-Generation Antihistamines (H_1 Blockers)

	First Generation	Second Generation
Useful against allergies	Yes	Yes
Pass the blood–brain barrier	Yes	No
Cause sedation	Yes	No
Antimuscarinic effect	Yes	Little
Local anesthetic effect	Yes	No
Useful vs Parkinsonism*	Yes	No
Useful vs nausea	Yes	No

*As an adjunct.

Allergic reactions to H_1 antihistamines can occur; they are more frequent after topical application than after oral administration and can complicate the treatment of allergic lesions of the skin or oral mucosa. Allergic reactions can take the form of urticarial, eczematous, bullous, or petechial rashes; fixed drug eruptions; or, more rarely, anaphylaxis.

As with most drugs, various blood dyscrasias (hemolytic anemia, agranulocytosis, pancytopenia, and thrombocytopenia) have been reported after the use of antihistamines. Patients receiving long-term antihistamine therapy should be periodically monitored. Although certain piperazine H_1 antihistamines have been shown to be teratogenic in some laboratory animal models, there is no clinical evidence to indicate that antihistamines cause birth defects in humans. More specifically, meta-analysis of human pregnancy outcomes following first semester exposure to antihistamines has shown no increase in birth defects.

Antihistamines are variably excreted in breast milk. Because infants, especially newborns and premature infants, are at higher risk of adverse effects, the use of antihistamines in nursing women should be avoided. Antihistamines, similar to other anticholinergic drugs, may inhibit lactation.

Table 18-5 shows a comparison between the two generations of H_1 antihistamines.

Uses in dentistry

H_1 antihistamines are used in dentistry primarily for their CNS actions, rather than for their specific antihistaminic effects. Promethazine, hydroxyzine, and diphenhydramine may be used in **minimal–moderate sedation** procedures and as premedication for deep sedation and general anesthesia. The sedative effect is increased by the concomitant administration of an opioid analgesic and a benzodiazepine; fentanyl and midazolam are commonly used for this purpose. The preoperative administration of these agents may also cause some inhibition of salivary and bronchial secretions, although more effective anticholinergic drugs should be used if control of secretions is essential. Another particular benefit of antihistamines is their ability **to reduce postoperative nausea and vomiting** in the outpatient setting.

H_1 antihistamines have **some local anesthetic activity**, and their feasibility as local anesthetic agents for dental procedures has been shown. They have not been used much for this purpose because far more effective agents (e.g., lidocaine) are available. However, the local anesthetic activity of antihistamines may be useful in the exceedingly rare case of allergy to conventional amide local anesthetics.

H_1 antihistamines can be used as secondary agents in the management of systemic anaphylactic reactions that may occur in the course of dental therapy. They can also be valuable in the **treatment of allergic lesions** of the oral mucosa and as adjuncts in treating angioneurotic edema of the orofacial region.

H_2 Receptor Antagonists

Chemistry and classification

H_2 receptor antagonists, or H_2 antihistamines, are basically structural analogues of histamine (Fig. 18-4). Two changes in the histamine molecule are necessary to achieve H_2 receptor–blocking activity. One is modification of the imidazole ring or its substitution by a furan or thiazole ring. A second modification is the presence of a flexible connecting chain linked to a polar substituent capable of hydrogen binding.

The four available drugs in this group are **cimetidine, ranitidine, famotidine, and nizatidine**. Ranitidine is a modification of cimetidine, in that it does not contain an imidazole ring but rather contains a furan ring. Famotidine and nizatidine are based on a thiazole ring structure (see Fig. 18-4).

Pharmacologic effects

The H_2 blockers are relatively selective and potent competitive antagonists of the H_2 receptors, with the main therapeutic effect being reduction of gastric acid secretion. H_2 antagonists cause a marked reduction in H^+ output, pepsin activity, and the total volume of gastric secretions (Fig. 18-5). Blockade of cardiovascular and mast cell H_2 receptor–mediated effects have been demonstrated but with minimal clinical significance.

Absorption, fate, and excretion

H_2 antihistamines are rapidly and completely absorbed after oral administration, except for famotidine. All undergo a variable degree of first-pass metabolic degradation in the liver, resulting in an oral bioavailability of approximately 50% for cimetidine, ranitidine, and famotidine and more than 90% for nizatidine. Therapeutic concentrations are reached in approximately 1 to 2 hours. The elimination half-life is 2 to 3.5 hours, except for nizatidine, which has a half-life of 1 to 1.5 hours. Urinary excretion of the parent compound accounts for 60% to 70% of the dose of each drug. The remainder is oxidized with sulfoxide being a major metabolite excreted in the urine and feces. Cimetidine (300 mg), the least potent agent, reduces basal gastric acid secretion by at least 80% for 4 to 5 hours, whereas famotidine (20 mg), the most potent, lasts for 10 to 12 hours. Because of the relative safety of these drugs, increased doses can be used to extend the duration of effect.

General therapeutic uses

H_2 antihistamines are used clinically for their marked ability to **inhibit basal and stimulated secretion of gastric acid.** They are approved for use in a wide variety of gastrointestinal disorders in which reduction of acid secretion may relieve symptoms, lead to healing, and prevent recurrence of previously resolved disease. Specifically approved indications include **duodenal ulcer disease (active or in maintenance), active gastric ulcer disease, gastroesophageal reflux disease** (GERD), and pathologic hypersecretory conditions (e.g., systemic mast cell disease and Zollinger-Ellison disease). H_2 antihistamines are generally given orally, but parenteral forms for famotidine and ranitidine are also available for acute suppression of gastric acid secretion. Oral dosage may be divided into once- or twice-daily administration; if once daily, the dose is best given at bedtime to block nocturnal gastric acid secretion.

A major use of H_2 antihistamines is treatment of active benign gastric ulcers and prophylaxis or treatment of active duodenal ulcers. All the currently available agents (cimetidine, ranitidine, famotidine,

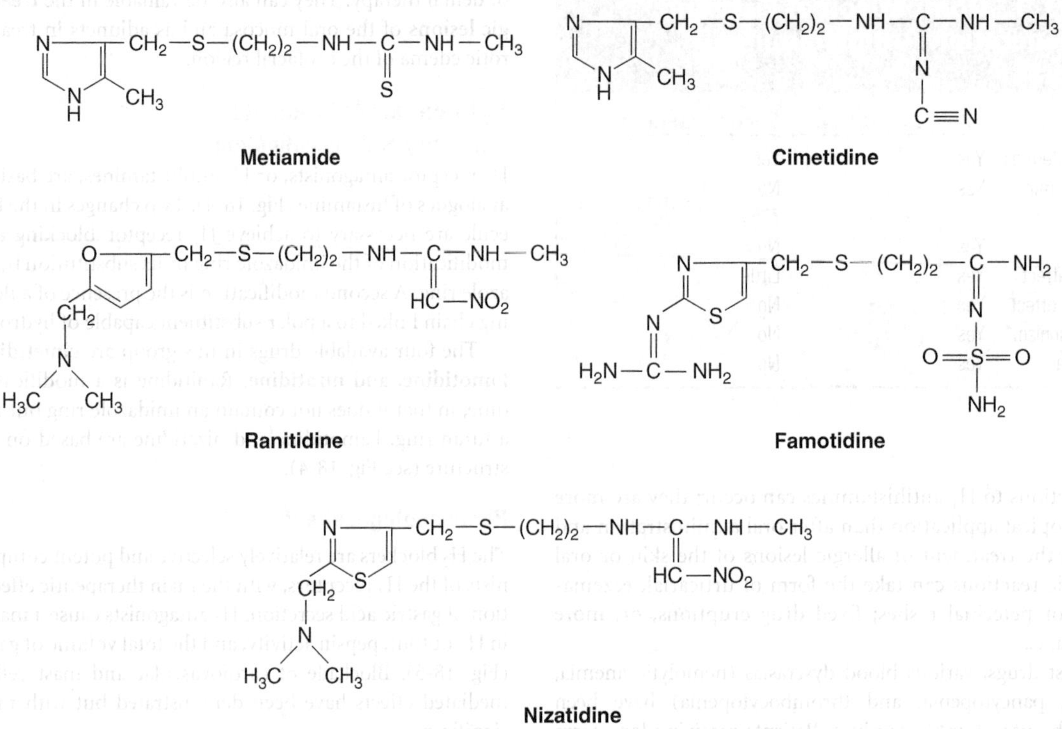

Metiamide

Cimetidine

Ranitidine

Famotidine

Nizatidine

FIG 18-4 Structural formulas of four H_2 receptor antagonists.

and nizatidine) have been shown to be equally effective in appropriate doses in suppressing gastric acid secretion (by up to 90%) and accelerating the healing of duodenal and, to a lesser extent, gastric ulcers. Healing of ulcers generally occurs within 2 to 4 months of therapy; if healing is not achieved in this period, further therapy is unlikely to be successful. Although cimetidine and other H_2 antihistamines have been used to treat upper gastrointestinal bleeding caused by liver disease, such as cirrhosis, little evidence supports their effectiveness in these conditions. Finally, H_2 antihistamines may be used before general anesthesia, particularly in patients with gastrointestinal obstruction, to elevate gastric pH and reduce the danger of aseptic pneumonia if gastric contents are aspirated during induction.

After their introduction, H_2 receptor antagonists became one of the most widely prescribed groups of drugs in the world. Their use has declined considerably in recent years because of the introduction of proton pump inhibitors. The U.S. Food and Drug Administration now allows OTC marketing of all four currently available H_2 antihistamines for symptomatic relief of occasional heartburn, GERD, acid indigestion (hyperchlorhydria), or "sour" stomach. This decision reflected the extensive use of H_2 antihistamines previously dispensed by prescription for unapproved conditions, while acknowledging the relative safety of these agents in unsupervised use. Such OTC use may risk delaying diagnosis of more serious disease, such as peptic ulcer or gastric cancer.

Adverse effects

The initial impression that H_2 antagonists are generally free of serious adverse effects has been validated by the passage of time and extensive clinical use. However, cimetidine and, to a lesser extent, other H_2 antihistamines can cause various toxic reactions and side effects. Perhaps untoward responses are a result of an incomplete understanding of the presence and function of H_2 receptors in tissues other than the gastric mucosa.

Adverse effects of cimetidine are manifested in the CNS. These are highly variable and range from minor symptoms (dizziness, lethargy, and fatigue) to more serious disturbances (mental confusion, delirium, focal twitching, hallucinations, and seizures). The CNS effects often seem to be dose-related and are most commonly seen in elderly patients or patients with impaired liver or kidney function.

Cimetidine exerts many effects on **endocrine function** that are generally minor and reversible on cessation of therapy. The most notable of these is gynecomastia. Other complications include elevation of serum prolactin concentrations, galactorrhea, loss of libido, impotence, and reduction in sperm counts. Small but definite increases in serum creatinine concentrations occur in most patients treated with cimetidine. This effect is not associated with other changes in renal function and ceases when the drug is withdrawn. With cimetidine there is a transient leukopenia, granulocytopenia, and thrombocytopenia reported. It is difficult to implicate cimetidine as a direct bone marrow suppressant because the cases reported almost always involve the concomitant use of other drugs or the existence of other serious systemic diseases. Although cimetidine enhances cell-mediated immune reactions, no evidence suggests that this phenomenon is related to any of the observed clinical responses.

Although cimetidine initially seemed to have no significant drug interactions, subsequent clinical reports and laboratory studies indicate that this is not the case. Cimetidine has been shown to increase blood concentrations of numerous drugs, including anticoagulants of the warfarin type, tricyclic antidepressants, various benzodiazepines, phenobarbital, theophylline, propranolol and other β-adrenoceptor blockers, Ca^{2+} channel blockers, lidocaine, estradiol, and phenytoin, creating a risk of toxicity. The **basis of these interactions** is competitive inhibition by cimetidine of the hepatic mixed-function oxidase enzymes responsible for the metabolism of these drugs. **Several cytochrome enzymes are inhibited.** Also, a cimetidine-induced decrease in hepatic blood flow may depress the entry of drugs into the liver and slow metabolism. Patients receiving cimetidine together with any from a long list of drugs should be carefully monitored; if appropriate, reduction of dosages or use of alternative agents should be considered.

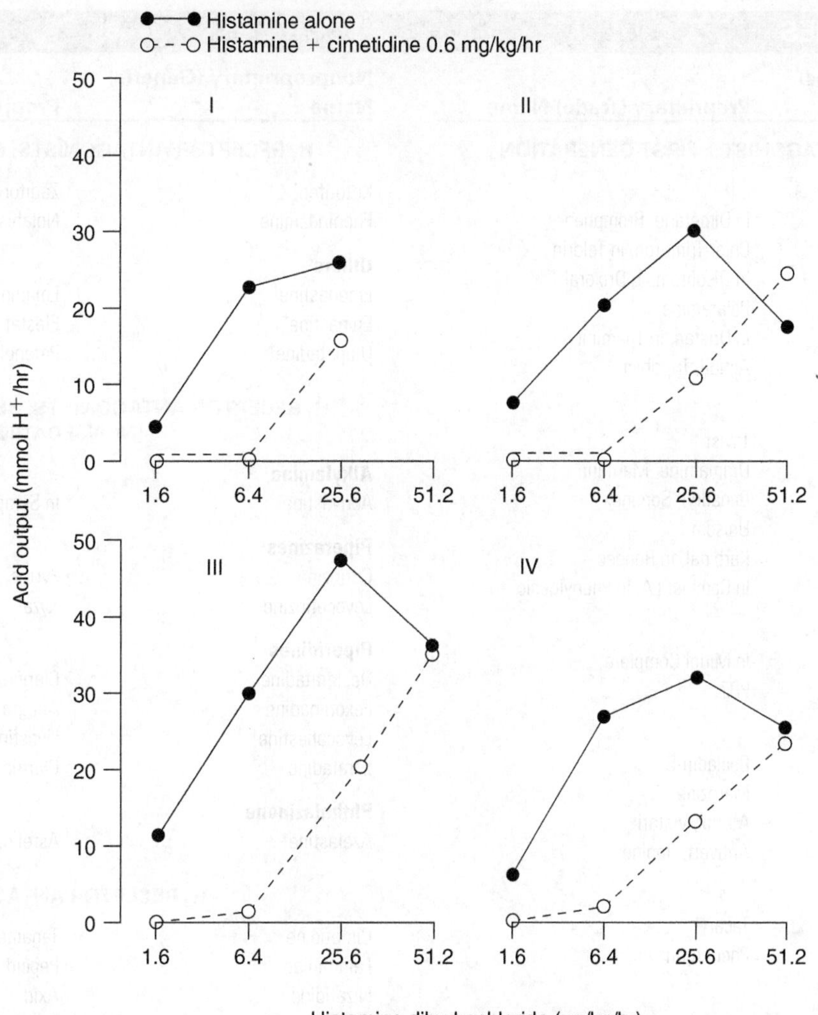

FIG 18-5 Inhibition of histamine-stimulated gastric acid production by cimetidine in humans. Histamine dihydrochloride in doses of 1.6 to 51.2 μg/kg/hr was infused intravenously with or without cimetidine at a dose of 0.6 mg/kg/hr for 105 minutes. When cimetidine was given, its administration was begun 15 minutes before the histamine infusion was started. Gastric juice was collected at 15-minute intervals and analyzed for acid concentration; the last four 15-minute intervals were used to establish the dose–response curves. Data shown are individual results from four normal adult subjects (*I-IV*). (From Aadland E, Berstad A: Inhibition of histamine- and pentagastrin-stimulated gastric secretion by cimetidine in man. In Creutzfeldt W, editor: *Cimetidine,* Amsterdam, 1978, Excerpta Medica Foundation.)

Ranitidine, famotidine, and nizatidine have fewer adverse effects than cimetidine. These drugs have little if any antiandrogenic effects. Serum prolactin concentrations, impotence, and gynecomastia are of minimal concern. Mental disturbances are less likely with these drugs, and they have not been reported to elevate serum creatinine concentrations. Because the binding of these agents to cytochrome P450 enzymes is much less firm than that of cimetidine, they do not significantly inhibit the microsomal metabolism of other drugs.

H_3 and H_4 Receptor Antagonists

Discovery of the histamine H_3 and H_4 receptor some years ago has opened the door to potential new therapeutic agents. H_3 receptors are located mainly in the CNS, while H_4 receptors are primarily expressed on leukocytes. Structural similarities and differences between H_3 and H_4 receptors and species differences are causes of limitations in the evaluation of their biologic profile. Drugs that target the H_3 receptor will likely focus on neurotransmission, improving neuronal diseases, such as cognitive impairment, schizophrenia, sleep/wake disorders, epilepsy, and neuropathic pain. The H_4 receptor, the newest identified members of the histamine receptor family, will likely target immunomodulation. Research suggests it may have therapeutic indications in allergy, inflammation, autoimmune disorders, and possibly cancer.

ANTIHISTAMINES

Nonproprietary (Generic) Name	Proprietary (Trade) Name
H_1 RECEPTOR ANTAGONISTS: FIRST-GENERATION	
Alkylamines	
Brompheniramine	In Dimetane, Bromphen
Chlorpheniramine	Chlor-Trimeton, in Teldrin
Dexbrompheniramine	In Disobrom, in Drixoral
Dexchlorpheniramine	Polaramine
Pheniramine	In Dristan, in Triaminic
Triprolidine	Actidil, Tripohist
Ethanolamines	
Clemastine	Tavist
Dimenhydrinate*	Dramamine, Marmine
Diphenhydramine	Benadryl, Sominex
Doxylamine	Unisom
Carbinoxamine	Karbinal, in Rondec
Phenyltoloxamine	In Comhist LA, in Phenylgesic
Ethylenediamines	
Pyrilamine	In Midol Complete
Tripelennamine	PBZ
Piperazines	
Buclizine	Bucladin-S
Cyclizine	Marezine
Hydroxyzine	Atarax, Vistaril
Meclizine	Antivert, Bonine
Phenothiazines	
Methdilazine	Tacaryl
Promethazine	Phenergan
Piperidines	
Azatadine	Optimine
Cyproheptadine	Periactin

Nonproprietary (Generic) Name	Proprietary (Trade) Name
H_1 RECEPTOR ANTAGONISTS: FIRST-GENERATION	
Ketotifen†	Zaditor
Phenindamine	Nolahist
Others	
Emedastine†	Emadine
Epinastine†	Elestat
Olopatadine†	Patanol
H_1 RECEPTOR ANTAGONISTS: SECOND-GENERATION (NONSEDATING)	
Alkylamine	
Acrivastine	In Semprex-D
Piperazines	
Cetirizine	Zyrtec
Levocetirizine	Xyzal
Piperidines	
Desloratadine	Clarinex
Fexofenadine	Allegra
Levocabastine†	Livostin
Loratadine	Claritin
Phthalazinone	
Azelastine‡	Astelin, Azelex
H_2 RECEPTOR ANTAGONISTS	
Cimetidine	Tagamet
Famotidine	Pepcid
Nizatidine	Axid
Ranitidine	Zantac

*The chlorotheophylline salt of diphenhydramine.
†For topical ophthalmic use.
‡For topical use.

CASE DISCUSSION

Promethazine may effectively alleviate anxiety, facilitating the surgery and preventing postoperative nausea and vomiting. Older antihistamines readily enter the CNS causing sedation and preventing motion sickness. However, promethazine and several other first-generation H_1 antihistamines are also effective alpha blockers. Thus, when the patient attempts to get out of the dental chair after the procedure, he may experience severe orthostatic hypotension and faint. When sudden changes are made (supine to standing) the blood pressure may rapidly drop, causing syncope. Replacing the patient in the horizontal position will allow him to regain consciousness. Also, patients with BPH may have difficulty with micturition due to increased urinary retention, a possible side effect of promethazine. If this patient had narrow-angle glaucoma, he could be at risk for increased ocular pressure due to the anticholinergic properties of the older first-generation antihistamine.

GENERAL REFERENCES

1. Church MK, Church DS: Pharmacology of antihistamines, *Indian J Dermatol* 58(3):219–224, May 2013, http://dx.doi.org/10.4103/0019-5154.110832. http://www.ncbi.nlm.nih.gov/pubmed/23831018-comments.
2. Monczor F, Fernandez N, Fitzsimons CP, Shayo C, Davio C: Antihistaminergics and inverse agonism: potential therapeutic applications, *Eur J Pharmacol* 715(1–3):26–32, September 5, 2013. http://dx.doi.org/10.1016/j.ejphar.2013.06.027. Epub July 4, 2013.
3. Tabarean IV: Histamine receptor signaling in energy homeostasis, *Neuropharmacology*, June 21, 2015. http://dx.doi.org/10.1016/j.neuropharm.2015.04.011. pii:S0028-3908(15)00140-9; Epub ahead of print.
4. Thurmond RL: The histamine H_4 receptor: from orphan to the clinic, *Front Pharmacol* 6:65, March 31, 2015. http://dx.doi.org/10.3389/fphar.2015.00065.

19

Antiarrhythmic Drugs

Frank J. Dowd

KEY INFORMATION

- Automaticity, refractoriness, and conduction velocity of the heart are affected by antiarrhythmic drugs.
- Sodium, potassium, and calcium channels, as well as β-adrenergic receptors and adenosine receptors, are targets for antiarrhythmic drugs.
- Cardiac arrhythmias arise as a result of errors in impulse generation, a conduction defect, or both.
- Arrhythmias may arise in the atria; atrial fibrillation is the most common.
- Other arrhythmias may arise in the ventricles.
- Antiarrhythmic drugs are classified according to their action, a modification of the original classification scheme of Vaughan-Williams:
  - Class I sodium channel blockers
  - Class II β-adrenergic receptor blockers
  - Class III potassium channel blockers
  - Class IV calcium channel blockers
  - Misc. e.g., adenosine receptor agonists
- Drugs affect automaticity, conduction velocity, or refractoriness in different structures of the heart, depending on their effects on channels and other receptors.
- Antiarrhythmic drugs can paradoxically be proarrhythmic, and these drugs have typical and often unique adverse effects, both cardiac and non-cardiac.
- Drug–drug interactions are an important consideration for several antiarrhythmic drugs, including interactions at cytochrome P450 enzymes.
- These drug–drug interactions include drugs used in dentistry such as the opioids and sedatives.

CASE STUDY

Your 60-year-old dental patient has recently been diagnosed with atrial fibrillation and has been placed on amiodarone for the arrhythmia. After a loading dose period of about 3 weeks, a maintenance dose is established at 400 mg once a day. The patient needs the extraction of impacted tooth #17, and you wish to prescribe an analgesic for postsurgical pain. In the oral cavity, you notice some diffuse patches of a bluish-gray discoloration. Would this information influence your treatment or choice of analgesic?

Antiarrhythmic drugs are used to correct or reduce the risk of cardiac arrhythmias (technically dysrhythmias; true arrhythmia is synonymous with asystole). They are classified into several categories on the basis of their mechanisms of action and resulting cardiac effects. All antiarrhythmic agents influence impulse generation or impulse conduction in the heart and impart definable electrophysiologic effects.

BASIC CARDIAC ELECTROPHYSIOLOGY

Under normal conditions, the chambers of the heart contract as synchronized rhythmic units driven by electrical impulses generated and conducted in the heart. The normal pacemaker impulse is generated in the sinoatrial (SA) node and travels through the atria to stimulate contraction and then to the atrioventricular (AV) node. After a brief pause, the impulse will move through specialized conduction pathways in the common bundle of His, bundle branches, and Purkinje network to reach the ventricular muscle cells (Fig. 19-1).

Automaticity

Automaticity describes the unique ability of cells of the SA node, AV node, and specialized other conducting system cells to exhibit spontaneous impulse generation. An increase in automaticity refers to an increase in the rate of impulse generation, and conversely, a decrease in automaticity refers to a decrease in the rate of impulse generation. Under normal conditions, the pacemaker cells of the SA node exhibit "leaky" ionic flows in the resting part of the cycle. As the ions leak into the cells, a threshold is released, and the cells spontaneously depolarize. Because the SA nodal cells normally have the most rapid leakiness, the SA node is the controlling pacemaker of the heart. The rate at which pacemaker cells initiate impulses is a function of the rate of phase 4 "leaky" depolarization and the magnitude of the **threshold potential**. An increase in the rate of phase 4 depolarization in the SA node increases heart rate, whereas a change in the threshold voltage to a more positive value decreases the heart rate. These functions are under nervous and hormonal control and can be altered by injury or drugs (Fig. 19-2).

Refractoriness

The period after the initiation of an action potential during which another action potential cannot be initiated and propagated regardless of stimulus is known as the **effective refractory period** (**ERP**). Many drugs with antiarrhythmic effects prolong the duration of the ERP, and some decrease it.

Conduction Velocity

Conduction velocity in cardiac fibers is altered by several factors, including anatomic characteristics, the electrophysiologic state, pathologic conditions, and many antiarrhythmic drugs. The rate of phase 0 depolarization strongly influences the conduction velocity. The rate (or slope) of phase 0 depolarization (measured as the change in voltage per unit of time [dV/dt]) depends on the membrane potential during phase 4. The more negative the membrane potential at the beginning

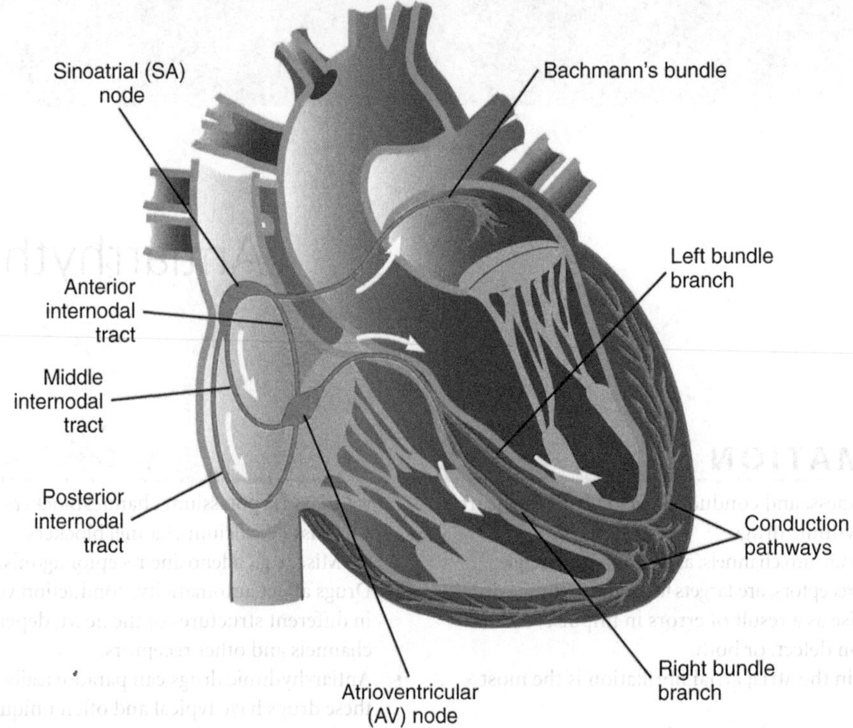

FIG 19-1 The basic electrical system of the heart. In normal health the impulses originate in the sinoatrial (SA) node, then travel through three basic intermodal pathways to trigger atrial contraction. They arrive at the atrioventricular (AV) node where there is a brief pause to allow filling of the ventricles. From there, they travel down the common bundle of His, which is a neural bundle that splits into the left and right bundle branches. Once at the apex, the neural bundles separate to feed the various areas of the ventricular muscle; these nerve endings are called the Purkinje fibers. (From Workman ML, LaCharity LA: *Understanding pharmacology: essentials for medication safety*, St. Louis, ed. 2, 2016, Elsevier.)

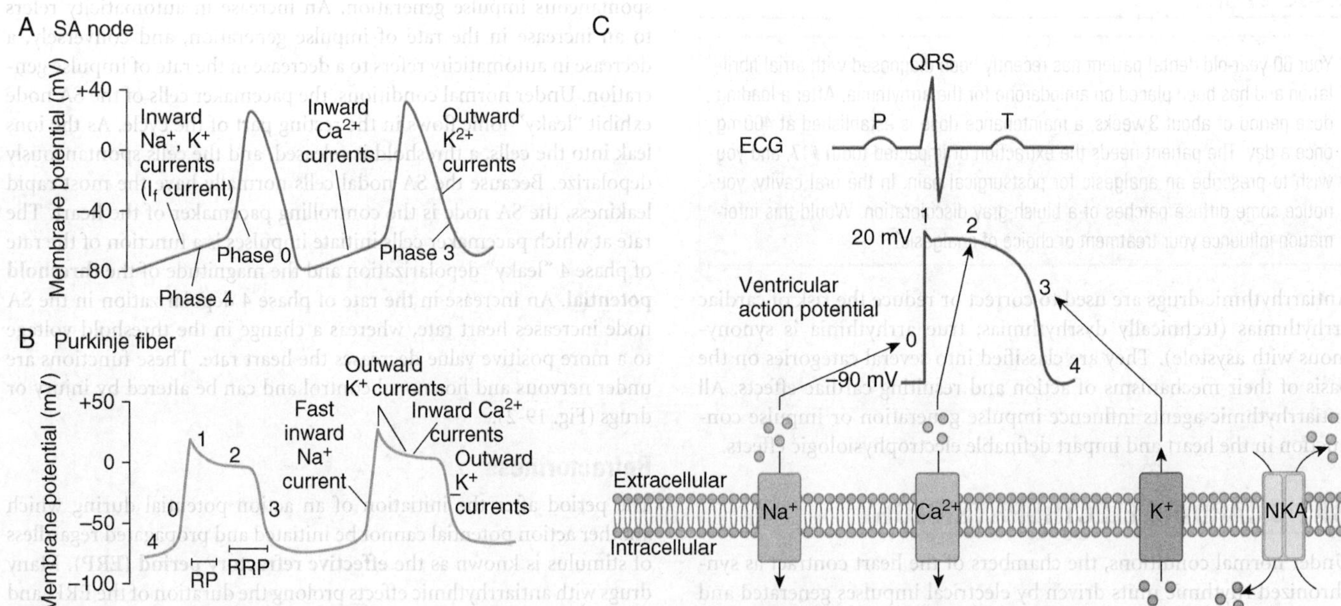

FIG 19-2 A comparison of the "leaky" sinoatrial (SA) node **(A)** and the action potential of a ventricular myocyte. In the SA node, phase 4 is leaky and allows slow depolarization until the firing threshold is reached. There is then a more rapid depolarization (phase 0) and a nebulous phase 1 and 2. Phase 3 is repolarization. In comparison, these phases are much more defined in the Purkinje fiber **(B)** and ventricular myocardium **(C)** and demonstrate a clear refractory period (phases 1 and 2 and part of 3). Conduction velocity is directly related to the slope of phase 0, and the refractory period is directly related to the duration of the action potential. Note that in the SA (and atrioventricular (AV)) node, phase 0 is slower than in the Purkinje fibers and ventricular myocardium because phase 0 in the SA and AV nodes primarily depends on Ca^{2+} influx. In **C**, the temporal relationship between the ECG tracing and the ventricular action potential is shown, as well as important ion conductances for the ventricular action potential. NKA, Na^+, K^+-ATPase pump. (**A and B**, Modified from Waller DG, Sampson, AP, et al.: *Medical pharmacology and therapeutics*, ed 4, St. Louis, 2014, Saunders; **C** from Goldman L, Schafer AI, et al.: *Goldman-Cecil medicine*, ed 25, Philadelphia, 2016, Elsevier.)

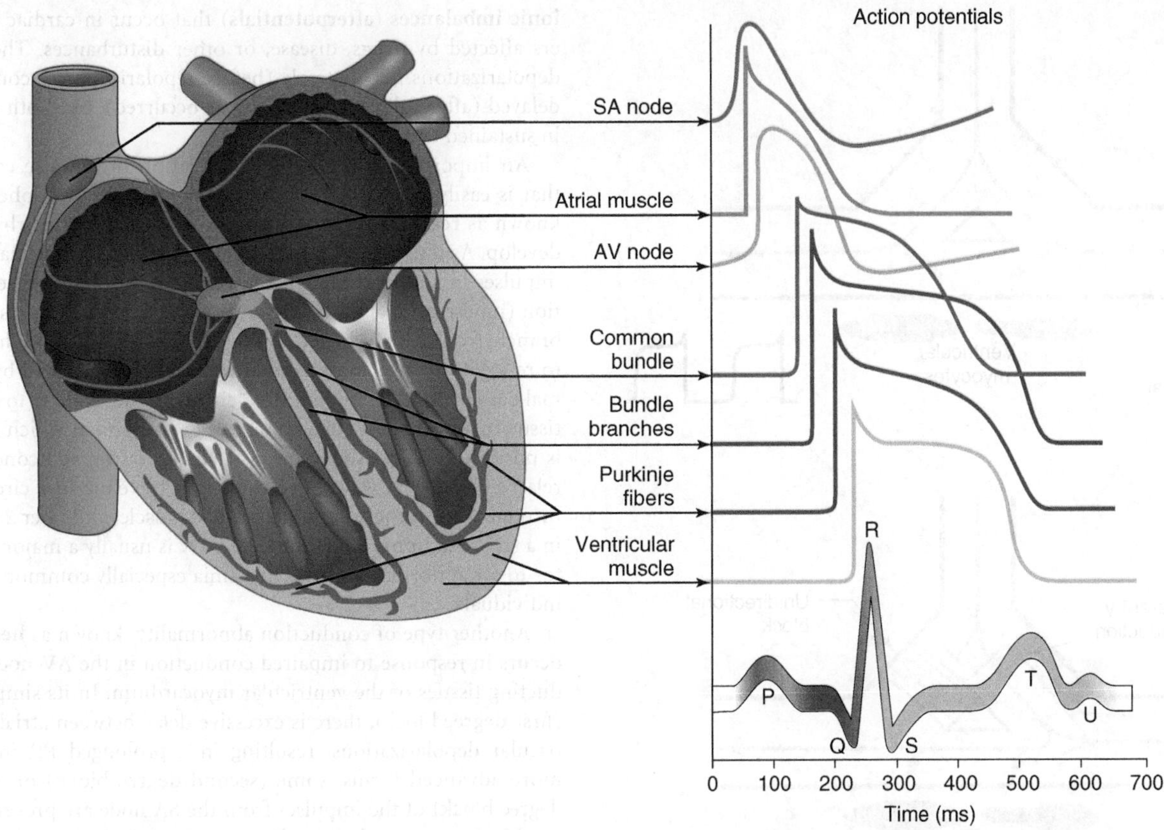

FIG 19-3 Characteristic membrane action potentials from a sinoatrial (SA) nodal cell (*top*) down to ventricular myocardium (*bottom*). The differences between leaky phase 4s and rapid versus slower phase 0s can easily be seen. Note that the atrioventricular node resembles the SA node because it can assume the pacemaking functions of the heart should the SA node become damaged. All of the action potentials are related to the various phases of the ECG in the lower part of the figure.

of phase 0 depolarization, the greater is the maximal dV/dt for phase 0. In this sense, what happens in phase 4 influences what happens in phase 0.

Ion Channels

Ions and the channels that control their movements play major roles in the various phases of cardiac depolarization and repolarization. Figures 19-2A and 2B; and 19-3 illustrates the membrane action potential in an SA nodal cell and a Purkinje fiber—two characteristically different action potentials—and the flow of ions through specific channels in the Purkinje fiber.

In Purkinje fibers and in atrial and ventricular myocardium, depolarization in phase 0 results from an initial, "fast channel" current of Na^+ in the inward direction. Na^+ channels also contribute to the pacemaker current in phase 4 of pacemaker cells. The **hyperpolarization-activated cyclic nucleotide-gated K^+ channels (HCN)** participate in this pacemaker activity. These channels are permeable to both Na^+ and K^+. The various HCN channels generate the I_f current that is important in initiating and maintaining diastolic depolarization (Fig.19-2A). Another major inward current, carried by Ca^{2+} and conducted through "slow channels," contributes to the plateau phase (phase 2) of the action potential. **Ca^{2+} channels are of two main types: T (transient) and L (long-lasting)**. These channels remain open for different periods during the action potential and respond differently to antiarrhythmic drugs.

Outward K^+ currents are responsible for repolarizing the muscle fiber in phase 3 and, by slowly deactivating in phase 4, contribute to spontaneous depolarization in pacemaker cells. As K^+ conductance through inwardly rectifying K^+ (**Kir**) channels decreases, and Na^+ and Ca^{2+} conductance increases, spontaneous depolarization during phase 4 occurs. Another major difference between pacemaker cells (e.g., cells of the SA and AV nodes) and non-pacemaker cells (e.g., cardiac muscle cells) is the slope of phase 0. Phase 0 has a much lower slope in pacemaker cells, where the major membrane event governing depolarization in phase 0 is Ca^{2+} influx through slow channels. As indicated, the faster phase 0 depolarization of the myocardium and Purkinje fibers is caused primarily by the Na^+ influx through fast channels. Differential effects on these ion fluxes help explain variations in the therapeutic uses and adverse effects of the antiarrhythmic drugs.

The K^+ current that is responsible for repolarization of the action potential is termed the delayed outwardly rectifying K^+ current (I_K). I_K is composed of several distinct currents carried through separate channels. Each current and its corresponding channel are defined by the rapidity with which they activate. The **K^+ currents, I_{Ks}, I_{Kr}, and I_{Kur}**, referring to slow-, rapid-, and ultrarapid-activating currents, are conducted through Ks, Kr, and Kur channels, respectively.

The complex interplay of ionic currents that constitute the cardiac action potential is based on the ability of ion channels to sense and respond to variations in the membrane potential. Channels that are in a closed resting state open when a particular threshold potential is reached. Ions capable of diffusing through these activated channels immediately begin flowing in response to

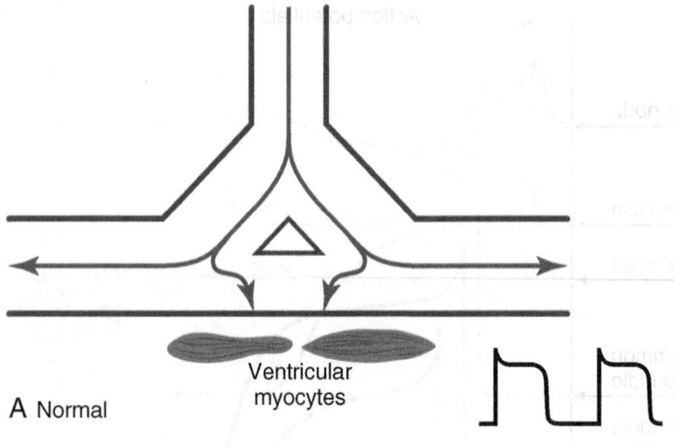

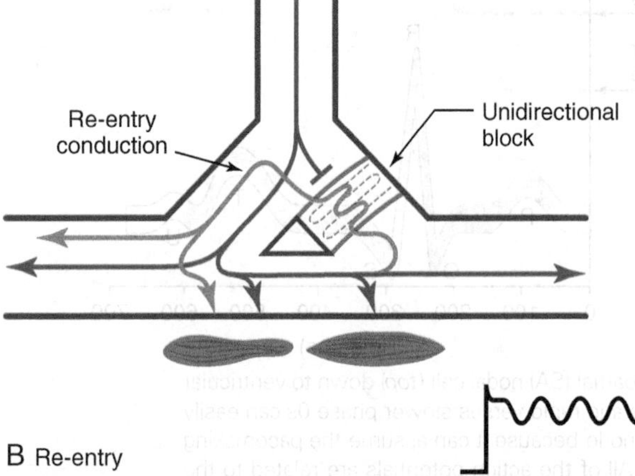

FIG 19-4 Reentry in the presence of unidirectional block. In **B**, "unidirectional block" indicates an area of damage that blocks normal electrical flow but allows the impulse to find its way back against the flow where it can trigger another unintended cycle. Reentry is commonly associated with supraventricular tachycardias.

their electrochemical gradients across the cell membrane. Most ion channels spontaneously close, or become inactivated, over a characteristic time frame, and the ion flux abruptly decreases. Channels in the inactivated state are unresponsive, or refractory, to the original stimulus and remain so until the membrane potential returns to a value that permits the channels to assume again a ready-to-open conformation. As discussed in subsequent sections of this chapter, many antiarrhythmic drugs bind preferentially to specific conformations of ion channels and exert differing effects on the action potential.

ORIGINS OF ARRHYTHMIAS

Rhythm disturbances, often occurring as a result of myocardial infarction, are the most common cause of death from heart disease. Arrhythmias are thought to originate from abnormal impulse generation, impulse conduction, or both in combination. Some arrhythmias caused by abnormal impulse generation result from increased automaticity. These **tachyarrhythmias** are usually in response to an increase in the rate of diastolic depolarization (increased slope of phase 4) in pacemaker cells. Phase 4 depolarization can be altered by autonomic nervous system activity, by hormones, or by drugs. Changes in the threshold potential voltage can also affect automaticity. Abnormal impulse generation may also be triggered by **ionic imbalances (afterpotentials)** that occur in cardiac pacemakers affected by drugs, disease, or other disturbances. The induced depolarizations may be early (before repolarization is complete) or delayed (after full repolarization has occurred), but both can result in sustained tachyarrhythmias.

An important example of an alteration in impulse conduction that is easily induced in experimental animals is the phenomenon known as **reentry**. Figure 19-4 shows how a reentrant rhythm may develop. As illustrated, conduction in one branch is normal, whereas impulses in a second branch can proceed in only the reverse direction (unidirectional block). A normally conducted impulse through branch *1* can be conducted in retrograde fashion through branch *2* to re-excite an area of tissue that was previously excited by the normal path of conduction. For this "circadian movement" to occur, the tissue in path 1 must have repolarized to a point at which excitation is possible (which usually means that the retrograde conduction is relatively slow). A wave of re-excitation traveling in a circular path through fiber *1*, the contractile cardiac muscle, and fiber *2* can result in a self-sustaining arrhythmia. Reentry is usually a major contributor to atrial fibrillation, an arrhythmia especially common in elderly individuals.

Another type of conduction abnormality, known as **heart block,** occurs in response to impaired conduction in the AV node or conducting tissues of the ventricular myocardium. In its simplest form (first-degree block), there is excessive delay between atrial and ventricular depolarizations, resulting in a prolonged PR interval. In more advanced forms, some (second-degree block) or all (third-degree block) of the impulses from the SA node are prevented from reaching the ventricles, resulting in a ventricular rate that is lower than the atrial rate.

Disturbances in the relationship of the fast and slow electrical responses of certain cardiac cells may play an important role in the genesis of arrhythmias. The **fast response** refers to the rapid phase 0 depolarization caused by rapid Na^+ influx (see Figs. 19-2 and 19-3). This kind of activity is seen in atrial and ventricular muscle fibers and specialized conducting fibers. In addition to the rapid inward current carried by Na^+, the fast fibers exhibit a second, slower inward current carried by Ca^{2+}. The slower current does not normally constitute a major factor in phase 0 depolarization of the atrial and ventricular myocardium and Purkinje fibers, but it persists after rapid depolarization and is responsible for the prolonged plateau phase characteristic of these fibers. However, fibers located in the SA and AV nodes, the AV ring fibers, and the mitral and tricuspid valve leaflets show the **slow response** in phase 0, during which the depolarization is carried largely by the inward Ca^{2+} current.

ELECTROCARDIOGRAPHY AND COMMON ARRHYTHMIAS

Arrhythmias are generally classified as supraventricular (originating in the atria or conducting system not in the ventricle) or ventricular. A few of the most common arrhythmias are described here. For comparison, a diagram of a normal electrocardiogram (ECG) is provided in Figure 19-5. In Figure 19-5, also note the **PR, QT, and ST** intervals and the duration of the **QRS** complex.

The arrhythmias in general fall into several classifications. Aberrancies that have their origin above or in the AV node are considered supraventricular. Dysrhythmias originating in the ventricles are obviously ventricular. Next, the rate is considered. Is it faster than normal (tachydysrhythmia), normal, or slower (bradydysrhythmia)? Does it have some kind of repeating rhythm, or is it chaotic? Is there

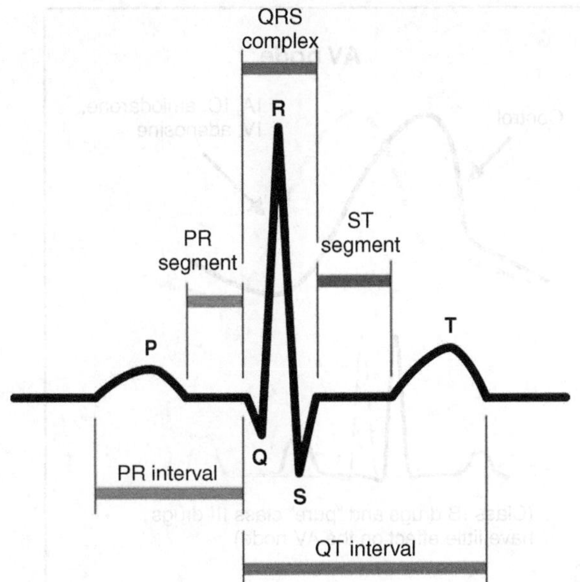

FIG 19-5 Normal ECG. The *P wave corresponds with* atrial depolarization; the *QRS complex corresponds with* ventricular depolarization; the *T wave corresponds with* ventricular repolarization. The atrial repolarization is "lost" in the QRS complex. The PR segment is the pause at the atrioventricular node to allow ventricular filling with blood. The ST segment corresponds to phase 1 and 2 (refractory period) of the ventricular myocardium. (From Workman ML, LaCharity LA: *Understanding pharmacology: essentials for medication safety*, ed. 2, 2016, Saunders.)

some kind of block in the normal conduction system leading to the unusual pattern, or are there hyperresponsive areas in the myocardium that are firing without control? Are there only a few abnormal beats, or is it truly an abnormal rhythm that is sustained or recurrent? And most of all, is the dysrhythmia able to sustain cardiac output sufficient to keep the patient from needing emergency CPR and medical intervention?

The role of the cardiologist is to determine the cause and effect of the various dysrhythmias and then try to find medications suitable to correct or manage the clinical outcomes. In recent years, a remarkable number of cardiac medications have been introduced to the market that have truly allowed better survival and quality of life for those who are diagnosed in time. In this chapter, we will discuss the antiarrhythmic drugs. In Chapter 20, the drugs used in heart failure are covered, and in Chapter 21 the drugs used for angina are discussed. Of course, proper cardiac care often involves other classifications of drugs such as anticoagulants, diuretics, pulmonary medications, and others.

ANTIARRHYTHMIC DRUGS

Antiarrhythmic drugs are used to modify or restore to normal, aberrant electrophysiologic properties of cardiac muscle. Arrhythmias may result from various disease conditions or drug treatments. In all arrhythmias, some facet of the normal electrophysiologic system that governs cardiac contraction is behaving abnormally. Several methods of treating arrhythmias are used today. Nonpharmacologic interventions for cardiac arrhythmias include electrical cardioversion, automatic implantable cardioversion/defibrillation devices, ablation therapy, and pacemakers.

The type of arrhythmia that presents is a major factor in the selection of an antiarrhythmic drug. Enhanced impulse generation can be reduced by drugs that slow phase 4 depolarization by reducing the inward Na^+ current or the inward Ca^{2+} current. The treatment of reentry includes drugs that reduce Na^+ channel and Ca^{2+} channel activity, which in turn slows conduction velocity. Drugs that block K^+ channels, prolonging repolarization and the refractory period, may also be useful.

Drugs used in the treatment of cardiac arrhythmias are not easily classified because they often have more than one action. Drugs within each class vary in their magnitudes of action or types of effects produced. The most common scheme classifies drugs according to certain specific properties. Type I drugs, such as quinidine, lidocaine, and flecainide, depress Na^+ current. The type I agents are subdivided further according to their relative effects on phase 0 depolarization, conduction velocity, and action potential duration. Na^+ channels exist in at least three states: closed, open, and inactivated. At resting membrane potentials, the Na^+ channels are closed except for a Na^+ "leak" associated with phase 4 depolarization in the cells that display automaticity. During rapid depolarization (phase 0, especially in Purkinje fibers and ventricular muscle), the Na^+ channels are open. The Na^+ channels then convert to the inactivated state before returning to the resting, closed state. The inactivated state occurs mostly in phases 2 and 3 of the action potential.

Class IA and IC drugs bind more selectively to the open state of the channel. Class IB drugs bind more selectively to the inactivated state of the channel. Because the Purkinje fibers and ventricular myocardial cells have longer plateau phases (phase 2), class IB drugs are able to block Na^+ channels more effectively in these tissues since the Na^+ channels remain in an inactivated state longer during systole. Inasmuch as ischemic ventricular tissue is more depolarized, it, too, is especially sensitive to Na^+ channel blockade by class IB drugs.

Quinidine-like, or class IA, drugs depress phase 0 depolarization at all heart rates. They prolong the action potential duration of the ventricle because they also inhibit K^+ (chiefly Kr) channels (Fig. 19-6). Class IB agents, such as lidocaine, block Na^+ channels more selectively, but the rapid onset and recovery of Na^+ channel blockade results in little accumulated lidocaine effect on phase 0 and conduction velocity in healthy tissue at normal heart rates. In damaged or rapidly firing cells, lidocaine causes a frequency-dependent or use-dependent block to reduce the slope of phase 0 and lowers the slope of phase 4 in ectopic pacemakers and in Purkinje fibers under high sympathetic tone. The faster the heart rate, the greater is the effect of lidocaine. (Use-dependent block is discussed in Chapter 14.) In contrast to other class I agents, lidocaine and related class IB antiarrhythmics may actually shorten the action potential duration. Flecainide and other class IC antiarrhythmics are characterized by their profound depression of phase 0 depolarization and slowing of conduction in the atria, AV node, and ventricles at normal heart rates. This pronounced effect results from their slow dissociation from Na^+ channels and accumulation of the channel-blocking effect over several contraction cycles. There is little or no prolongation of the action potential duration.

Metoprolol and related β-adrenergic–blocking agents constitute class II drugs and inhibit cardiac stimulation brought on by β-adrenergic agonists. They depress the slope of phase 4 depolarization (see Fig. 19-6). The class III group drugs, including amiodarone and sotalol, block K^+ channels (chiefly Kr channels) and prolong the action potential duration by delaying phase 3 repolarization.

Diltiazem and Amlodipine and other class IV drugs selectively block Ca^{2+} channels (L type) and depress slow fiber conduction (phase 0 of the SA and AV nodes) and depress the slope of phase 4

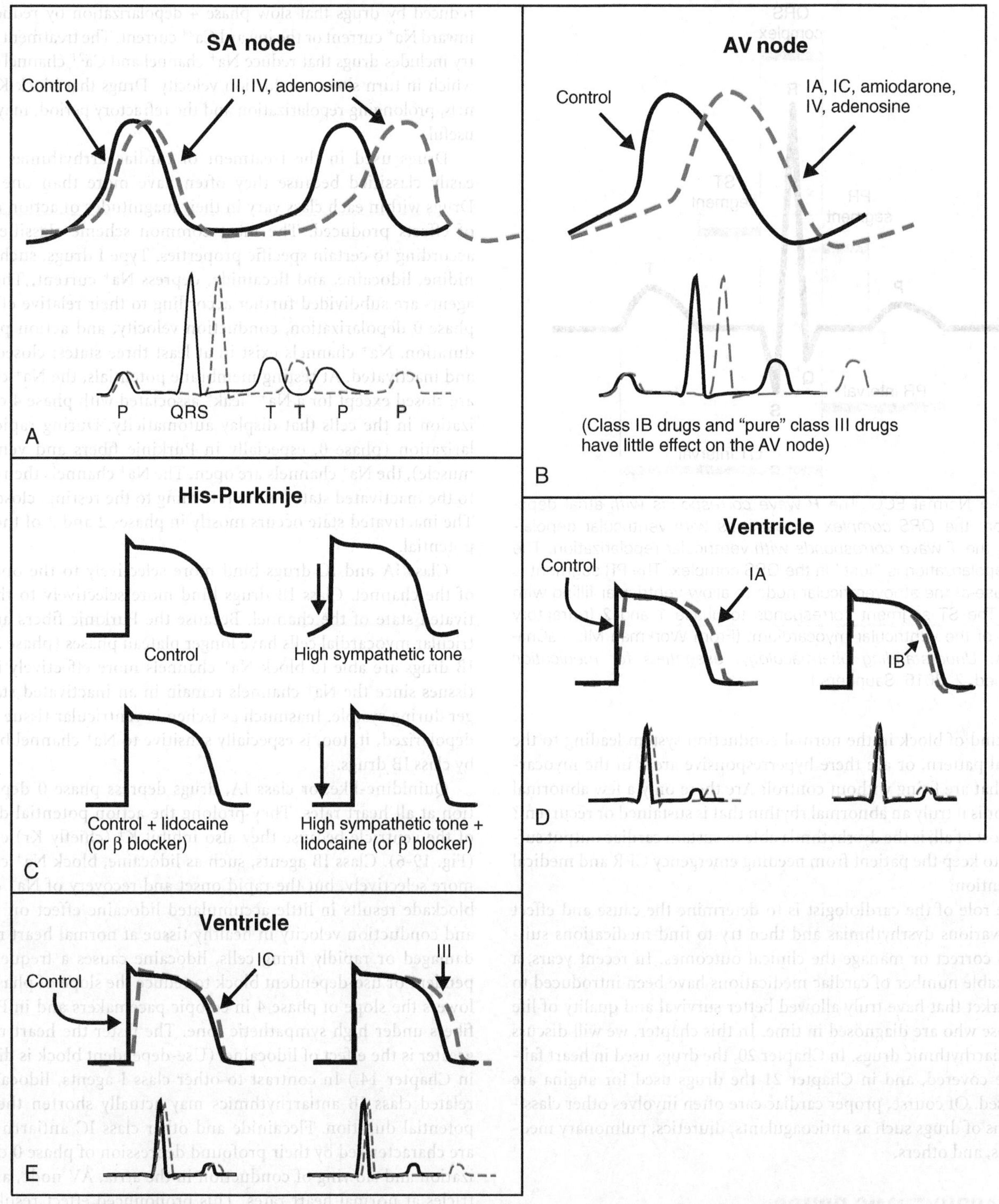

FIG 19-6 Effect of the various antiarrhythmic drug classes on the action potentials in the heart. Where relevant, the corresponding ECG pattern is also shown. Omitted drug classes have little effect on the action potentials depicted. The changes shown do not imply the same magnitude of change for each drug class. Amiodarone is specifically identified because, although it is classified as a class III drug, it has additional actions. **A,** Sinoatrial node. Note the delay in appearance of the QRS complex, T wave, and subsequent P wave caused by the identified drugs. **B,** Atrioventricular node. Various drugs delay conduction through the node. **C,** His-Purkinje system. Active drugs reduce phase 4 depolarization (*arrows*). **D and E,** Ventricular muscle. In **D,** class IB drugs minimally alter the ECG pattern in normal cardiac rhythms.

depolarization (see Fig. 19-6). Drugs that cannot be classified by the Vaughan-Williams scheme include digitalis and adenosine.

Table 19-1 outlines the various categories of antiarrhythmic agents. The drugs vary widely in their clinical usefulness. Class IA drugs are almost never used today, partly because of the **introduction of class IC and class III drugs**. In Table 19-1, the action responsible for the classification of each drug, which is usually its major action, is enclosed in a box. In the discussion of individual agents that follows, reference should also be made to Table 19-2 for the electrophysiologic actions of representative antiarrhythmic drugs. The net effects of the relevant

TABLE 19-1 Actions of Antiarrhythmic Drugs

	Block Na^+ Channels						
Drug*	**Slow**	**Medium**	**Fast**	**Block β Receptors**	**Block K^+ Channels**	**Block Ca^{2+} Channels**	**Other Actions**
Class IA							
Quinidine		[X]			X	X	α-Adrenergic blockade, vagolytic action
Procainamide		[X]			X		Ganglionic blockade
Disopyramide		[X]			X		Muscarinic blockade
Class IB							
Lidocaine			[X]				
Mexiletine			[X]				
Class IC							
Flecainide	[X]				X		
Propafenone	[X]			X		X	Vagolytic action
Class II							
Metoprolol			X	[X]			
Esmolol				[X]			
Class III							
Amiodarone			[X]	X	[X]	X	α-Adrenergic blockade, muscarinic blockade
Ibutilide					[X]		
Dofetilide					[X]		
Dronedarone			[X]	X	[X]	X	α-Adrenergic blockade, blocks effect of acetylcholine on K/ACh channels
Sotalol				X	[X]		
Class IV							
Verapamil			X			[X]	α-Adrenergic blockade
Diltiazem						[X]	
Amlodipine						[X]	
Miscellaneous							
Adenosine							A_1-receptor stimulation

*The distinguishing characteristics for the main classes of antiarrhythmic drugs are the following: class I drugs block Na^+ channels. The subclassification is based on the characteristics of the block. The terms *slow, medium,* and *fast* refer to the rates of onset of, and recovery from, Na^+ channel blockade. Class II drugs block β-adrenergic receptors. Class III drugs block K^+ channels. Class IV drugs block Ca^{2+} channels. The major action responsible for the classification of each drug is enclosed in a box.
Ibutilide is exceptional because a major action, not shown, is to increase conductance through a slow Na^+ channel.

drug classes and various action potentials in the heart are shown in Figure 19-6. Pharmacokinetic data for specific drugs are given in Table 19-3. The use of digoxin for certain kinds of arrhythmias is discussed in Chapter 20.

Quinidine

Although rarely used today, **Quinidine** is a useful drug to discuss as an example of class IA antiarrhythmic drugs. Historically, quinidine has been effective in the treatment of some atrial and (to a lesser extent) ventricular tachyarrhythmias. It was discovered that during treatment of patients with malaria, the reversal of atrial fibrillation was noted in some of them. Quinidine, the *d* isomer of quinine, is found in the bark of the cinchona tree, which is indigenous to certain regions of South America.

Pharmacologic effects

Quinidine reduces automaticity and conduction velocity and increases refractoriness. Quinidine tends to inhibit reentrant pathways. Automaticity is depressed through a more positive threshold potential and a decrease in the slope of spontaneous diastolic

TABLE 19-2 Effects of Antiarrhythmic Drug Classes

Drug Class	Sinoatrial Automaticity	Atrioventricular Conduction Velocity	ECG Changes: PR	ECG Changes: QRS	ECG Changes: QT	Affinity for Na^+ Channels in Ischemic Tissues	Antiarrhythmic Use: Supraventricular	Antiarrhythmic Use: Ventricular
IA	↓	↑*, ↓	↓*, ↑	↑↑	↑↑	+	Yes	Yes
IB	0	0	0	0	0	+++†	No	Yes
IC	0	↓	↑	↑↑↑	0	+	Yes	Yes
II	↓↓	↓↓	↑↑	0	0	+‡, 0	Yes	Yes
III	↓↓	↓	↑↑	0	↑↑↑	+§, 0	Yes	Yes
IV	↓↓‖	↓↓	↑↑‖	0	0	+¶, 0	Yes	No
Adenosine	↓↓	↓↓↓	↑↑	0	0	0	Yes	No

This table does not include unique qualities of individual drugs that may contrast with the qualities of other drugs within the same class. *ECG changes* refer to an increase or decrease in the respective intervals. The number of *plus signs* or *arrows* indicates the relative magnitude of effect or relative affinity for Na^+ channels in ischemic tissue; *zero* indicates no or little effect.

*From antimuscarinic and anti-vagal effects.

†Ischemic tissue is more depolarized and has a higher percentage of inactivated Na^+ channels. Class IB drugs bind most selectively to inactivated Na^+ channels.

‡Propranolol and esmolol can block Na^+ channels in depolarized cells.

§Amiodarone has more blocking effects on Na^+ channels than other class III drugs.

‖Direct cardiac effect of the drug; it does not include reflex effects from vasodilation.

¶Verapamil can block Na^+ channels in the depolarized state, whereas diltiazem has little effect.

TABLE 19-3 Pharmacokinetic Properties of Antiarrhythmic Drugs

Drug Class	Drug	Elimination Half-Life (hr)	Plasma Protein Binding (%)	Urinary Excretion (%)
IA	Quinidine	4-10	85	20
	Procainamide	3-4	20	60
	Disopyramide	4-10	20 to 60	50
IB	Lidocaine	1.5-2	65	<2
	Mexiletine	10-12	55	10
IC	Flecainide	12-27	40	25
	Propafenone	6-30	90	<2
II	Esmolol	0.2	55	<2
	Propranolol	4-6	90	<2
III	Amiodarone	25-100 days	>90	<1
	Dronedarone	24-30	>99	<5
	Sotalol	7-15	0	>90
	Ibutilide	2-12	40	<5
	Dofetilide	8-10	65	80
IV	Verapamil	3-7	90	<5
	Diltiazem	4-8	75	<5
Miscellaneous	Adenosine	<10 s	0	0

depolarization (phase 4) in pacemaker fibers, particularly at sites other than the SA node. Quinidine has the potential to slow or abolish tachyarrhythmias. Quinidine decreases the slope of phase 0 depolarization and decreases conduction velocity in cells such as those of the AV node and ventricular myocardium (see Fig. 19-6). Quinidine influences automaticity and conduction velocity by blocking Na^+ channels, particularly channels in the open state. The rate of recovery from quinidine block is intermediate between class IB and IC antiarrhythmic drugs (see Table 19-1).

Lidocaine

Lidocaine has been used as a local anesthetic for more than half a century. In contrast to procaine, however, lidocaine has also long been a primary drug for arresting and preventing certain ventricular arrhythmias in emergency situations. For additional discussion of its pharmacologic characteristics, see Chapter 14.

Pharmacologic effects

Lidocaine decreases automaticity but is devoid of antimuscarinic activity. Lidocaine preferentially influences ventricular function. Lidocaine acts by blocking Na^+ channels, particularly inactivated Na^+ channels. This effect on Na^+ channels is rapidly reversed, which restricts its use-dependent blocking effect to patients with rapid heart rates. Because lidocaine has a preferential effect on Na^+ channels in the inactivated state, it selectively inhibits automaticity in ischemic tissue where membrane depolarization or an enhanced frequency of excitation occurs, such as in the His-Purkinje system (see Table 19-2). Lidocaine also reduces delayed afterdepolarizations seen with digoxin

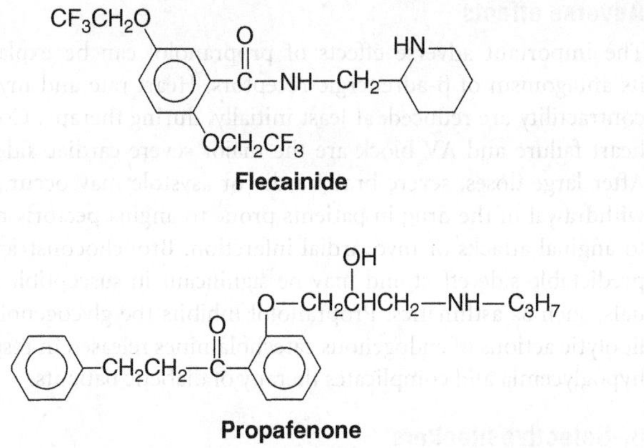

FIG 19-7 Structural formulas of flecainide and propafenone.

toxicity. Lidocaine does not slow repolarization but instead may hasten it. The drug has little effect on conduction velocity and phase 0.

Lidocaine is usually administered intravenously for the treatment of ventricular ectopic rhythms. Because lidocaine must be administered parenterally, it is largely restricted to emergency situations and hospital settings. Its use is contraindicated in supraventricular arrhythmias because it is largely ineffective against these arrhythmias and excessive ventricular rates may result.

Absorption, fate, and excretion

After intravenous administration, the plasma concentration initially decreases rapidly, followed by a slower decline. For this reason, various loading regimens are used to achieve therapeutic plasma concentrations quickly. Lower constant perfusion rates are subsequently used. Lidocaine is broken down in the liver to various metabolites.

Adverse effects

Lidocaine exhibits only minor effects on the autonomic nervous system. Arterial pressure is not depressed. After acutely high dosages or prolonged infusion, lidocaine may cause convulsions and respiratory depression. Note that these reactions rarely occur with the dosages and routes of administration used in dentistry, especially if proper precautions are taken to avoid intravenous administration. Cardiac arrest may occur if lidocaine is administered to a patient with higher degrees of heart block.

Flecainide

A third category of type I antiarrhythmics (class IC) is represented by drugs that are newer to clinical use than the drugs in classes IA and IB. **Flecainide** (Fig. 19-7) belongs to this class (see Table 19-1). Flecainide is indicated for the prevention of supraventricular arrhythmias including atrial fibrillation and for sustained life-threatening ventricular arrhythmias unresponsive to other medications.

Pharmacologic effects

Although possessing some similarity to lidocaine, flecainide and related class IC drugs significantly depress conduction velocity by strongly reducing Na^+ conductance during phase 0 of the action potential. This effect is felt throughout the heart but is especially strong in the atrium and His-Purkinje system. It results from the slow association of drug with, and dissociation from, Na^+ channels, especially channels in the open configuration. Recovery from Na^+ channel blockade is protracted.

Flecainide does not selectively reduce phase 0 in diseased tissues. Rather, it inhibits phase 0 more or less uniformly in diseased and healthy tissues and tends to be effective on reentry mechanisms. Flecainide widens the QRS complex. Flecainide also reduces conduction velocity in the AV node but to a lesser degree than in ventricular muscle (see Fig. 19-6 and Table 19-2).

Absorption, fate, and excretion

Flecainide is not significantly metabolized on its first pass through the liver and has good bioavailability after oral administration. Approximately 75% of a flecainide dose is eventually metabolized to inactive products. The large range in reported half-lives for the drug stems partly from genetically determined variations in the rate of hepatic metabolism by cytochrome CYP2D6. As discussed in Chapter 4, some individuals lack this enzyme or have a CYP2D6 variant that is less able to metabolize the drug. The resulting potential differences in patient response necessitate careful monitoring of drug effects.

Adverse effects

Central nervous system toxicity is the most common adverse effect. Dizziness, blurred vision, tremor, paresthesia, and headache may occur. Nausea and a metallic taste have been reported for flecainide. Flecainide administration to patients with recent myocardial infarction shows twofold to threefold increase in mortality. An arrhythmogenic effect of these drugs is suspected despite the fact that they suppressed premature ventricular depolarizations in these patients. These data have led to cautions concerning the use of flecainide after myocardial infarction. Similar concern exists for the other class IC drugs.

Propafenone

Propafenone is classified as a class IC antiarrhythmic because of its strong tendency to depress the maximum rate of depolarization and conduction velocity. The drug is indicated for life-threatening ventricular arrhythmias and is prescribed for atrial fibrillation and other types of supraventricular arrhythmias. The structure of propafenone is depicted in Figure 19-7.

Pharmacologic effects

Propafenone exerts several actions on the heart. In addition to blocking Na^+ channels, it blocks Ca^{2+} channels and exerts β-adrenergic receptor–blocking effects (see Table 19-1). The drug reduces the slope of phase 0, prolongs the PR and QRS intervals, and suppresses ectopic pacemakers (see Table 19-2). Negative inotropic effects are possible but usually occur only with high doses.

Absorption, fate, and excretion

Propafenone is well absorbed orally, but approximately 80% of a given dose is destroyed in the first pass through the liver. The same genetic predisposition for inefficient or slow metabolism by CYP2D6 of the drug exists as for flecainide, and the half-life may be prolonged in patients who are slow metabolizers. At least one major metabolite is pharmacologically active.

Adverse effects

Adverse effects include dizziness, blurred vision, dysgeusia, and gastrointestinal symptoms. CNS toxicity seems to be more likely with slow metabolizers. Asthma may be exacerbated in susceptible individuals. Untoward cardiac signs include SA nodal dysfunction, AV nodal block, and worsening of heart failure. The arrhythmogenic potential of the drug must be considered in light of the problems documented for other class IC agents. Competition for metabolism by CYP2D6 is the basis for interactions involving propafenone and other drugs. Propafenone may increase the anticoagulant effect of warfarin given concurrently.

β-Adrenergic Receptor–Blocking Drugs

Since the introduction of **propranolol** in 1968 for clinical use in the United States, a number of β-adrenergic receptor–blocking agents have been approved. (The β-adrenergic antagonists are discussed in Chapters 9, 21, and 23.) Two β-adrenergic blockers—propranolol and **esmolol**—are the primary class II antiarrhythmic drugs discussed here (see Table 19-1). Sotalol, a third drug with ability to block the β-adrenergic receptor, is discussed under class III drugs. Propranolol is reviewed here as the prototypic agent; special features of the other β blockers are also noted.

Pharmacologic effects

Propranolol, the prototypic type II antiarrhythmic, has two types of effects on the heart: indirect effects as a consequence of blockade of β-adrenergic receptors and "membrane-stabilizing" effects similar to those of quinidine. The membrane-stabilizing effects of propranolol have antiarrhythmic effects in addition to those due to β-adrenergic receptor blockade. Propranolol decreases automaticity and conduction velocity and increases refractoriness. The drug's greatest effects are on SA nodal automaticity, AV node refractoriness, and (if it exists) His-Purkinje automaticity (see Fig. 19-6 and Table 19-2).

Activation of the sympathetic nervous system leading to β receptor stimulation enhances automaticity by increasing the slope of phase 4 depolarization, speeds conduction velocity, and shortens the ERP (especially in the AV node). By blocking β receptors, propranolol can produce opposite effects proportional to the sympathetic input to the heart at the time of administration. In addition to decreasing automaticity in the SA node (and decreasing the heart rate), propranolol variably reduces automaticity and conduction velocity in the atria, AV node, His-Purkinje system, and ventricles. Increased refractoriness in the AV node is an especially important manifestation of blockade. The direct actions of propranolol include decreasing the slope of phase 0 and phase 4 depolarization and prolonging the ERP. The β-adrenergic blockers, with the exception of sotalol, do not appreciably affect repolarization.

The major antiarrhythmic indication for propranolol is in the management of supraventricular tachyarrhythmias in which protection of the ventricles (by interfering with AV transmission) is the major clinical objective. Propranolol is also useful in suppressing paroxysmal supraventricular tachycardia and in treating afterdepolarizations and other ventricular arrhythmias in which catecholamine stimulation is involved. Because propranolol reduces the ratio of oxygen demand to oxygen supply, arrhythmias caused by myocardial ischemia may also be relieved. β Blockers have been shown to reduce the incidence of heart attack and death in patients with previous myocardial infarction. The mechanism is not established, but it may relate to an antiarrhythmic mechanism.

Absorption, fate, and excretion

Propranolol is readily absorbed after oral administration, but more than two-thirds of the drug is destroyed in its first pass through the liver. Peak plasma concentrations are reached in 1 to 2 hours. The rate of metabolism of propranolol, which involves CYP2D6, varies considerably among individuals, so plasma titers may differ markedly with long-term therapy. Propranolol is metabolized by hydroxylation, deamination, and glucuronide conjugation.

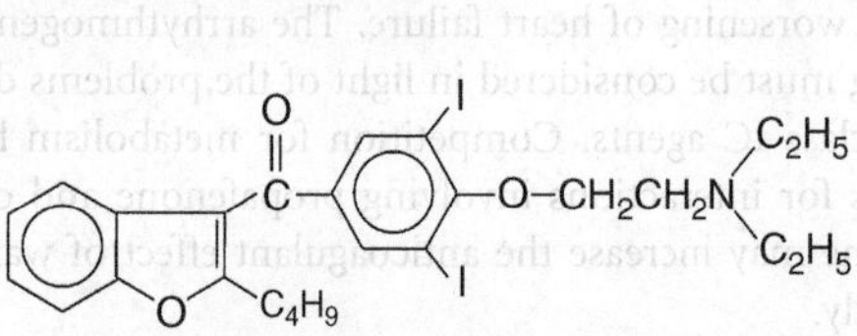

FIG 19-8 Structural formula of amiodarone.

Adverse effects

The important adverse effects of propranolol can be explained by its antagonism of β-adrenergic receptors. Heart rate and myocardial contractility are reduced, at least initially, during therapy. Congestive heart failure and AV block are the major severe cardiac side effects. After large doses, severe bradycardia or asystole may occur. Sudden withdrawal of the drug in patients prone to angina pectoris may lead to anginal attacks or myocardial infarction. Bronchoconstriction is a predictable side effect and may be significant in susceptible individuals, such as asthmatics. Propranolol inhibits the glycogenolytic and lipolytic actions of endogenous catecholamines released in response to hypoglycemia and complicates therapy of diabetic patients.

β_1-Selective blockers

Metoprolol is used in chronic therapy for the same indications as propranolol. Esmolol is a very short-acting selective β_1-adrenergic receptor blocker that is metabolized by plasma esterases. It is used intravenously for short-term β-adrenergic receptor blockade. The adverse effects of these drugs resemble the adverse effects of propranolol. Despite their selectivity for β_1-adrenergic receptors, these drugs as well as other β blockers should be avoided if possible in asthmatic patients. This drug is primarily used by anesthesiologists to give short-acting beta blockade in patients undergoing general anesthesia.

Sotalol

Sotalol, a β-adrenergic–blocking drug, also has properties of and is classified as a class III drug. It increases the ERP in addition to its β-adrenergic–blocking activity. The relative importance of its β-blocking properties and its class III antiarrhythmic effects has yet to be determined. Sotalol is well absorbed when taken orally, with a bioavailability of nearly 100%. Sotalol is useful in supraventricular arrhythmias such as atrial fibrillation and in certain cases of ventricular tachycardia. It has been shown to be effective in preventing recurrences of ventricular tachyarrhythmias.

Amiodarone

Amiodarone, a benzofuran derivative resembling thyroid hormone (Fig. 19-8), was originally introduced in Europe as a coronary vasodilator for the treatment of angina pectoris. It is now widely used for various acute and chronic arrhythmias. It has an interesting mix of blocking several ion channels, including sodium, potassium, and calcium.

Pharmacologic effects

Amiodarone's major action is to increase the ERP by slowing the rate of repolarization. Blockade of K^+ channels is a major mechanism of action (see Table 19-1). Repolarization is slowed in the His-Purkinje system and in ventricular and atrial myocardium. The Q-T interval is increased (see Fig. 19-6). In addition to blocking K^+ channels, amiodarone blocks Na^+ and Ca^{2+} channels. Inhibition of these latter channels probably prevents much of the inward depolarizing current that can trigger early afterdepolarizations.

Amiodarone decreases automaticity in the SA node and in ectopic pacemakers, but it has little effect on automaticity elsewhere in the heart. Conduction velocity is slowed in the AV node by Na^+ and Ca^{2+} channel blockade (see Table 19-1), and the ERP in the AV node is lengthened. Conduction velocity in the His-Purkinje system and ventricular muscle is also slowed. The ventricular fibrillation threshold is increased.

Amiodarone has an active metabolite, desethylamiodarone, which also contributes to the antiarrhythmic effect. Desethylamiodarone binds to cellular thyroid hormone receptors, inhibiting thyroid hormone–induced gene expression. Of the numerous genes normally induced by thyroid hormone, several support the synthesis of certain K^+ channels. This finding is consistent with the fact that amiodarone's effects on K^+ channels are generally delayed compared with its effects on Na^+ and Ca^{2+} channels. Long-term therapy with amiodarone is more likely to generate a class III antiarrhythmic effect (K^+ channel block), largely because of reduction in the number of Kr channels. Short-term therapy is more likely to limit effects to Na^+ channels, Ca^{2+} channels, and β-adrenergic receptors. The resulting cardiac effects with short-term use seem to be different from the effects of long-term therapy and avoid many of the adverse effects seen with long-term administration, such as pulmonary fibrosis and hypothyroidism. Amiodarone is a vasodilator, noncompetitively inhibiting the vascular effect of catecholamines. The cardiac effects of catecholamines are likewise inhibited, and coronary arterial resistance is decreased, resulting in increased coronary blood flow.

Amiodarone is used for various arrhythmias, including ventricular extrasystoles, tachycardia, and fibrillation. It is also efficacious in some atrial arrhythmias, including atrial fibrillation and flutter, in which it may have unique effects on the adverse remodeling changes in the atria, which are thought to be partly responsible for the genesis of atrial fibrillation.

Absorption, fate, and excretion

When administered orally, amiodarone's bioavailability is low (20% to 50%). Amiodarone is also administered intravenously. A highly lipophilic drug, amiodarone is sequestered in tissues, yielding an apparent volume of distribution of approximately 60 L/kg. It is highly bound to protein in plasma. Because the drug would normally take weeks to reach a steady-state concentration after the initiation of therapy, loading doses are routinely used. Amiodarone is extensively metabolized by the liver; a desethyl derivative, which has antiarrhythmic properties as indicated previously, has been identified. When the drug is withdrawn, the tissue concentrations decrease only gradually as the drug is eliminated. Plasma determinations of amiodarone may not reflect tissue concentrations.

Adverse effects

Sinus arrest may occur if amiodarone is given with β-adrenergic–blocking drugs or other antiarrhythmics, and AV nodal conduction abnormalities may be exacerbated. Because amiodarone has negative inotropic properties, its use may be associated with a decrease in cardiac function. Some preexisting arrhythmias may be worsened by the drug.

Non-cardiac adverse reactions are common and occasionally life-threatening. The primary concerns are **pulmonary fibrosis and pneumonitis**, which may become clinically evident in a significant percentage of patients with long-term use, and can be lethal. Amiodarone also commonly causes CNS disturbances (ataxia, dizziness), photosensitivity, and hepatic dysfunction as indicated by an increase of liver enzymes in the blood. The skin may take on a unique blue-gray hue. Corneal microdeposits occur routinely but usually do not interfere with vision and disappear after withdrawal of the drug. Changes in **thyroid function** (hyperthyroidism and especially hypothyroidism) have been reported, and these may be related to the aforementioned facts that amiodarone resembles thyroid hormone and influences thyroid hormone actions. Amiodarone can reduce the action of thyroid hormone by binding to the thyroid hormone receptor and blocking its cellular effects. It has also been shown that amiodarone can inhibit the action of thyroid-stimulating hormone, which could also contribute to a hypothyroid effect by amiodarone. The drug inhibits the conversion of thyroxine to triiodothyronine in peripheral tissues and causes the buildup of reverse triiodothyronine (see Chapter 29). Finally, amiodarone inhibits several cytochrome P450 enzymes and can cause a number of drug–drug interactions.

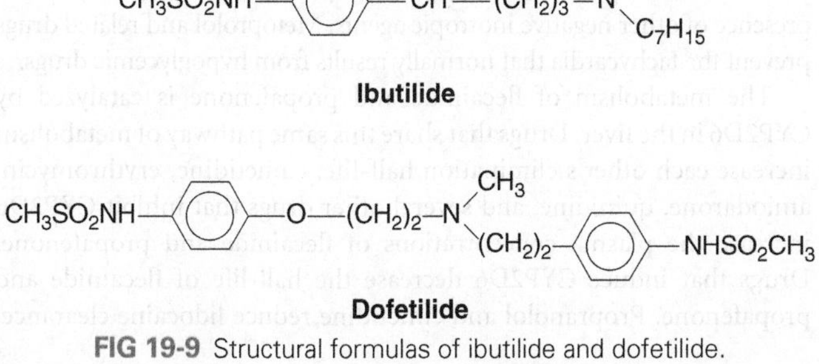

Dronedarone

Dronedarone is structurally similar to amiodarone, but it lacks the iodine atoms and is more water-soluble, giving it a half-life of about 20 hours. It is similar in its pharmacodynamics to amiodarone and is considered to be a class III antiarrhythmic, although, like amiodarone, it has effects on several ion channels. Lacking the iodine atoms, it does not have the thyroid-related adverse effects associated with amiodarone. Pulmonary fibrosis and pneumonitis are also not associated with dronedarone. Dronedarone can cause bradycardia, an increase in the Q-T interval, and GI symptoms. It also can interact with other drugs because of its ability to inhibit and be metabolized by CYP3A4.

Ibutilide and Dofetilide

Ibutilide is classified as a class III drug because it delays repolarization. It blocks Kr channels and causes the opening of Ca^{2+} channels, which promote Na^+ influx through slow channels, extending phase 2 of the action potential. The drug is administered intravenously for atrial fibrillation and atrial flutter. It can be used to convert these arrhythmias, especially of recent onset, to normal sinus rhythm. Hypotension and arrhythmias are adverse effects.

Dofetilide is considered a "pure" class III drug, blocking the Kr channel selectively. It is used for acute conversion of atrial fibrillation and atrial flutter and for short-term maintenance of normal sinus rhythm. Dofetilide is available for intravenous and oral use. The structures for ibutilide and dofetilide are shown in Figure 19-9.

Ca^{2+} Channel Blockers

Ca^{2+} channel blockers, represented by **verapamil, diltiazem,** and **amlodipine,** are used for the treatment of certain cardiovascular diseases. Verapamil and diltiazem are prescribed primarily for their antianginal (see Chapter 21) and antiarrhythmic effects. Amlodipine, which has a greater effect on vascular smooth muscle, is a major antihypertensive drug (see Chapter 23) and is used as an antiarrhythmic

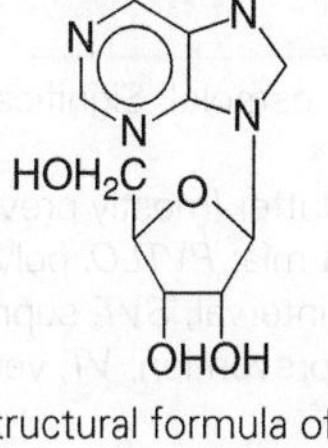

Ibutilide

Dofetilide

FIG 19-9 Structural formulas of ibutilide and dofetilide.

FIG 19-10 Structural formula of adenosine.

drug. In each case, the drugs are selective for potential-dependent Ca^{2+} channels rather than receptor-operated channels. The potential-dependent Ca^{2+} channels are of at least three types: L, N, and T. These channels are distinguished by their electrical properties and anatomic location. The L (long-lasting) channels are selectively inhibited by these drugs. The fact that they are the predominant Ca^{2+} channels in the heart and vascular smooth muscle is consistent with the major effects of Ca^{2+} channel blockers on these organs. The N (neuronal) and T (transient) channels are not affected by these channel blockers to a major degree, although the T-type channels play a role in phase 2 of action potentials in the heart (see Fig. 19-2).

By interfering with the slow inward current in pacemaker cells, these drugs depress the rate of phase 4 depolarization; automaticity in the SA node and the AV node is decreased. The major direct cardiac effect is to reduce conduction velocity and to increase the refractory period of the AV node (see Fig. 19-6). Verapamil and diltiazem are useful in treating supraventricular arrhythmias such as atrial fibrillation and flutter. This helps indirectly to control ventricular rate, which can be affected by the aberrant supraventricular activity. Both drugs have also been used successfully in preventing attacks of atrial tachycardia. Verapamil and diltiazem have a negative inotropic effect. Other aspects of the pharmacologic features of the Ca^{2+} channel blockers are discussed in Chapters 21 and 23.

Adenosine

The endogenous purine nucleoside, **adenosine,** is approved for terminating attacks of supraventricular tachycardia. It does not match the profile of any other antiarrhythmic. The structure of adenosine is shown in Figure 19-10.

Pharmacologic effects

Adenosine stimulates the A_1 adenosine receptor in the heart. This receptor is linked to the G protein G_i, which, when activated, increases K^+ conductance and decreases Ca^{2+} channel activity, leading to hyperpolarization. Adenosine also reduces the release of norepinephrine from nerve endings. The net effect on the heart is to reduce automaticity in the SA node and Purkinje fibers and reduce the AV nodal conduction rate (see Fig. 19-6 and Table 19-2). The drug is useful for short-term treatment of supraventricular tachycardia involving reentry with rapid ventricular response. Adenosine also dilates coronary vessels and reduces contractility. Selective adenosine receptor agonists offer promise for future drug development.

Adverse effects

Adenosine must be injected intravenously as a rapid bolus with a saline flush behind it because of its extremely short plasma half-life, due to its rapid transport into tissues. This is followed by incorporation into purine biosynthetic pathways. Many patients have transient flushing and dyspnea with the drug. Arrhythmias, including heart block and transient asystole, may also occur immediately after injection. Patients are warned they may feel a metallic taste and may become dizzy or black out as the drug is injected. Because of the drug's rapid uptake into tissues, however, therapeutic and adverse responses are normally short-lived.

TABLE 19-4 Major Antiarrhythmic Indications of Antiarrhythmic Drugs

		INDICATIONS	
Class	Drug	Supraventricular	Ventricular
Ia	Procainamide		VT, life-threatening
	Disopyramide	AF/F	VT, life-threatening
Ib	Lidocaine		Acute VT, DVA
Ic	Flecainide	AF/F, SVT	VT, life-threatening
	Propafenone	AF/F, SVT	VT, life-threatening
II	β-Blockers*	AF/F, SVT	
III	Amiodarone	AF/F	VT, VF
	Sotalol	AF/F	Sustained VT, life-threatening
	Dronedarone	AF/F	
	Dofetilide	AF/F	
	Ibutilide	AF/F	
IV	Diltiazem	AF/F, SVT	
	Verapamil	AF/F, SVT	
Misc.	Adenosine	SVT	
	Magnesium		PVTLQ

*Includes metoprolol and esmolol. Significant differences exist among the β-blockers.
AF/F, Atrial fibrillation or flutter (mostly prevention); *DVA,* digitalis-induced ventricular arrhythmia; *PVTLQ,* polymorphic ventricular tachycardia with long QT interval; *SVT,* supraventricular tachycardia; *VF,* ventricular fibrillation prevention; *VT,* ventricular tachycardia.

Digoxin

Digoxin is used in treating certain supraventricular arrhythmias. Its use is discussed in Chapter 20.

Magnesium

Magnesium sulfate is used intravenously to overcome drug-induced *torsades de pointes*. It may be effective even in the absence of hypomagnesemia.

Indications for Antiarrhythmic Drugs

Table 19-4 presents the general indications of the various agents discussed in this chapter in treating some of the most commonly encountered arrhythmias. It is not intended to be a comprehensive listing of applications of these drugs. Drugs administered orally are largely used to prevent the recurrence of arrhythmias, whereas drugs administered parenterally are usually given to treat acute disorders.

Drug Interactions

Antiarrhythmic drugs can participate in a wide variety of drug interactions. Because the margin of safety with these drugs as a group is narrow, clinically significant interactions may develop whenever the activity or plasma concentration of an antiarrhythmic agent is altered. The following discussion provides an illustrative but not exhaustive list of interactions involving these drugs.

Drugs that slow AV conduction, such as the β-adrenergic–blocking drugs and amiodarone, can exaggerate the AV conduction effects of drugs with similar actions, possibly leading to bradycardia and heart block. Drugs that have negative inotropic effects (e.g., class IA drugs, Ca^{2+} channel blockers, and β blockers) may precipitate heart failure, especially in the presence of other negative inotropic agents. Metoprolol and related drugs prevent the tachycardia that normally results from hypoglycemic drugs.

The metabolism of flecainide and propafenone is catalyzed by CYP2D6 in the liver. Drugs that share this same pathway of metabolism increase each other's elimination half-life. Cimetidine, erythromycin, amiodarone, quinidine, and several other drugs that inhibit CYP2D6 increase the plasma concentrations of flecainide and propafenone. Drugs that induce CYP2D6 decrease the half-life of flecainide and propafenone. Propranolol and cimetidine reduce lidocaine clearance,

TABLE 19-5 Unique or Typical Adverse Effects of Representative Antiarrhythmic Drugs

Drug	Adverse Effect(s)
Adenosine	Flushing, asthma, dyspnea, SA nodal arrest, AV nodal block
Amiodarone	Pulmonary fibrosis, thyroid abnormalities, skin discoloration, corneal deposits, peripheral neuropathy
Calcium channel blockers	Flushing, AV nodal conduction defects, reduced contractility of the heart, bradycardia
Flecainide	Cardiac risk with recent myocardial infarction
Lidocaine	Convulsions
Procainamide	Mental changes, *torsades de pointes*, lupus
Propranolol	AV nodal conduction defects, bronchoconstriction in asthmatics, bradycardia

AV, Atrioventricular; *SA,* sinoatrial.

whereas induction of hepatic microsomal enzymes by drugs such as phenobarbital increases lidocaine clearance.

Amiodarone increases the effect of warfarin and procainamide. There may be more than one mechanism accounting for these interactions. In addition to its effects on metabolism, amiodarone may reduce renal clearance of these drugs by inhibiting the transport function of P-glycoprotein in the kidney. Verapamil, propafenone, amiodarone, flecainide and quinidine have been reported to increase plasma digoxin concentrations. These interactions may also involve the P-glycoprotein.

IMPLICATIONS FOR DENTISTRY

Patients who are being treated on a long-term basis with antiarrhythmic drugs, if under adequate control, are usually not a management problem for the dentist. Because some antiarrhythmic agents may depress cardiovascular function, the potential for an increased incidence of orthostatic hypotension and hypotensive syncope exists. There is also a greater probability that arrhythmias will develop in a patient with a previous history of arrhythmias who is undergoing stressful treatment. The fact that these medications "normalize" a patient should not lull dentists into believing their patients do not have significant cardiac disease; their disease is still quite present but managed. The dentist should therefore consider consulting with the patient's cardiologist regarding the patient's overall constitution and his or her ability to withstand stress and undergo routine dentistry in a private practice setting. If the cardiologist has concerns, referral to a dentist who can provide the care in a hospital environment with a cardiac anesthesiologist monitoring the patient at all times may be warranted.

Many dentists fear the use of epinephrine in cardiac patients. While usually not a problem in the doses used in standard dental practice, it may be necessary to also discuss with the cardiologist the use of epinephrine or other adrenergic vasoconstrictors in patients with a significant arrhythmia history. Most cardiac patients can easily handle 40 mcg of epinephrine per hour (the approximate equivalent of two standard dental cartridges with 1:100,000 epi) without adverse effects if injected slowly after negative aspiration to be sure the medication is not given intravascularly.

As described in Chapter 9, the combination of epinephrine and propranolol may lead to hypertensive reactions. Amiodarone, quinidine, and to a lesser extent propafenone inhibit **dealkylation reactions by CYP2D6** and may therefore limit the effectiveness of certain oral opioid analgesics (e.g., **codeine, hydrocodone, and tramadol**) that are converted in the liver to highly active metabolites (e.g., codeine metabolized to morphine). In most cases these interactions are more of a theoretic concern than a clinically relevant problem.

The dentist should be aware of the manifestations of adverse drug reactions that occur in the oral cavity. Amiodarone therapy can cause pigmentation of the skin and mucous membranes such as in the oral cavity. Calcium channel blockers can cause significant gingival hyperplasia, either generally across the gingiva or as localized lesions. Blockade of β-adrenergic receptors is associated with a change in the profile of salivary proteins. The implications of this effect on oral health have not been fully determined. Table 19-5 lists some unique or typical adverse effects of representative antiarrhythmic drugs.

CASE DISCUSSION

The bluish-gray discoloration in the oral cavity as described is similar to the bluish-gray discoloration on the skin caused by amiodarone. Although there may be other causes, the diffuse nature of the discoloration is highly suggestive of the effects of amiodarone, especially if given chronically. The presence of similar-looking bluish-gray areas on the skin should confirm amiodarone as the cause. These discolorations should not affect the tooth extraction or choice of drugs. More importantly for the choice of an analgesic drug is the fact that amiodarone is an inhibitor of cytochrome P450 2D6 (CYP2D6), an enzyme that catalyzes the conversion of codeine to morphine, thereby allowing codeine to have significant clinical efficacy. Amiodarone is likely to inhibit this conversion and to delay or reduce the analgesic effect of codeine. Therefore if a combination of an opioid and a nonnarcotic analgesic is considered for this patient, codeine should be avoided. Unfortunately, hydrocodone is also activated by this same pathway and would not be a good alternative. Oxycodone can be considered, even though it goes through the same metabolic pathway. Oxycodone is absorbed at a much higher rate and is not as dependent on conversion by CYP2D6 for an analgesic effect. Of course, using NSAIDs such as Ibuprofen or naproxen often will be sufficient for most dental pain and therefore should be considered as the primary analgesic of choice.

ANTIARRHYTHMIC DRUGS

Nonproprietary (Generic) Name	Proprietary (Trade) Name
Adenosine	Adenocard
Amiodarone	Cordarone
Acebutolol	Sectral
Diltiazem	Cardizem
Disopyramide	Norpace
Dofetilide	Tikosyn
Dronedarone	Multaq
Esmolol	Brevibloc
Flecainide	Tambocor
Ibutilide	Corvert
Lidocaine	Xylocaine
Magnesium sulfate	—
Mexiletine	Mexitil
Procainamide	Pronestyl, Procanbid
Propafenone	Rythmol
Propranolol	Inderal
Quinidine*	Quinidex
Sotalol	Betapace
Verapamil	Calan, Isoptin

*Quinidine is available as a gluconate, sulfate, or polygalacturonate salt.

GENERAL REFERENCES

1. Bigger JT, Breithardt G, Brown AM, et al.: The Sicilian gambit: a new approach to the classification of antiarrhythmic drugs based on their actions on arrhythmogenic mechanisms, Task Force of the Working Group on Arrhythmias of the European Society of Cardiology, *Circulation* 84:1831–1851, 1991.
2. Breithardt G, Borggrefe M, Camm JA, Shenasa M, editors: *Antiarrhythmic drugs: mechanisms of arrhythmic and proarrhythmic actions*, New York, 2012, Springer.
3. Drugs for cardiac arrhythmias, Treatment guidelines, *Med Lett Drugs Ther* 5:51–58, 2007.
4. Pamukcu B, Lip GY: Dronedarone as a new treatment option for atrial fibrillation patients: pharmacokinetics, pharmacodynamics and clinical practice, *Expert Opin Pharmacother* 12:131–140, 2011.
5. Roden DM: Pharmacology and toxicology of Na_V 1.5-class 1 antiarrhythmic drugs, *Card Electrophysiol Clin* 6:695–704, 2014.
6. Roden DM: Personalized medicine to treat arrhythmias, *Curr Opin Pharmacol* 15:61–67, 2014.
7. Saeed W, Kowey PR: Antiarrhythmic drug therapy for atrial fibrillation, *Amer Coll Cardiol* 32:533–549, 2014.
8. Shu J, Zhou J, Patel C, Yan GX: Pharmacotherapy of cardiac arrhythmias—basic science for clinicians, *Pacing Clin Electrophysiol* 32: 1456–1465, 2009.
9. Treatment of atrial fibrillation, *Med Lett Drugs Ther* 56:1446, 2014.
10. Vaughan EM, Williams DM: Classification of antidysrhythmic drugs, *Pharmacol Ther [B]* 1:115–138, 1975.

Drugs Used in Treating Heart Failure

Frank J. Dowd

KEY POINTS

- Heart failure involves a loss in the efficiency of contraction in the heart.
- Heart failure reduces cardiac output for any given end-diastolic pressure.
- The usual approach to treating heart failure is to reduce afterload and preload, treat any underlying valvular abnormalities (such as aortic stenosis), reduce remodeling of the heart, and if possible, increase cardiac output via better myocardial function.
- The choices of drugs for treating heart failure include the following: ACE inhibitors, angiotensin II receptor blockers (ARBs), β-adrenergic receptor blockers, aldosterone antagonists, diuretics, hydralazine/isosorbide dinitrate, digoxin, tolvaptan, and ivabradine, roughly in that order of preference.
- The two newest drugs from this list are tolvaptan and ivabradine.
- Digoxin has classically been the mainstay of treating CHF.
  - Digoxin has a positive inotropic effect on the heart by inhibiting Na^+,K^+-ATPase and indirectly increasing intracellular calcium.
  - Digoxin also has a negative chronotropic (direct and vagal) effect on the heart, as well as other electrical effects.
  - Digoxin has a very low therapeutic index and is being used less and less as a result.
- Other drugs are available for the acute management of heart failure.
- Important considerations for dental patients with heart failure include these:
  - Determine the suitability of treating the patient in a private practice/outpatient clinical setting.
  - Use strategies to reduce stress, e.g., shorter appointments, sedation.
  - If necessary, adjust chair position to reduce dyspnea.
  - Make O_2 available to patient if necessary.
  - Be aware of drug–drug interactions, especially involving digoxin if the patient is taking the drug.

CASE STUDY

Mr. B has been a dental patient for several years. He is 60 years old, and recently he was diagnosed with congestive heart failure (CHF). He was prescribed an angiotensin-converting enzyme (ACE) inhibitor, a β-adrenergic receptor blocker, and furosemide. Mr. B has done well on the medications, and his vital signs have reflected this. You have treated him successfully over two dental appointments since he started taking his medications. Today the patient is scheduled to have a full crown preparation on tooth #30. Before starting the procedure, you take his blood pressure and record a reading of 95/60 with a pulse of 65 bpm. (At his previous appointment one month ago, his blood pressure was 110/65, and the pulse was 80 bpm). When you place the patient in the dental chair in a supine position, you observe that the patient is having labored breathing, when this was not the case during the two previous appointments. What would be an appropriate response on your part?

Heart failure is characterized by a decreased ability of the heart to pump blood in adequate amounts. The disorder is common especially as one ages and is associated with considerable morbidity and mortality. Diseases contributing to heart failure include hypertension, valvular abnormalities, and myocardial infarction. In addition to changes in the heart, multiple adaptive mechanisms occur in heart failure; these provide targets for drug therapy. The severity of heart failure is often rated according to the New York Heart Association classification, ranging from class I, in which signs of heart failure occur only at higher exercise levels, to class IV, in which signs of heart failure occur at rest. Another classification incorporates measurable evidence of heart failure: Stage A, only risk factors for heart failure and no symptoms of heart failure; Stage B, some evidence of heart disease but no symptoms; Stage C, heart failure symptoms with clear evidence of heart disease; and Stage D, heart failure with severe symptoms requiring aggressive therapy.

Initial therapy for heart failure involves control of underlying causes such as hypertension and coronary artery disease, eliminating smoking, restricting sodium intake, improving diet, and appropriate exercise. In addition to drug therapy, other strategies for treating heart failure include auxiliary mechanical pumps (ventricular assist devices), ventricular pacing (resynchronization), and surgical procedures including valve repairs, valve replacements, and even heart transplantation.

CARDIAC MUSCLE CONTRACTION AND HEART FAILURE

In addition to its role in the electrical action potential, Ca^{2+} is intimately involved in the mechanical contractile process. The contraction of cardiac muscle is initiated by extracellular Ca^{2+} entering the cell with the slow inward current. However, the immediate source of contractile Ca^{2+} in the heart comes largely from intracellular stores. Ca^{2+} entering the cell during an action potential must first traverse the plasma membrane through voltage-sensitive Ca^{2+} channels. This initial "spark" influx of Ca^{2+} during the slow inward current triggers the release of much larger amounts of intracellular Ca^{2+} from the sarcoplasmic reticulum (SR) via the ryanodine-2 calcium channels. Upon binding calcium, these channels open up to "flood" the cell with additional Ca^{2+}

stored in the SR. The sudden increase in cytoplasmic Ca^{2+} stimulates contraction.

Tropomyosin and troponin, which are associated with actin, regulate the interaction between actin and myosin. The binding of Ca^{2+} to troponin C initiates a series of conformational changes in troponin and tropomyosin that alter the interaction of tropomyosin and troponin I with actin, favoring the coupling of actin with myosin. Adenosine triphosphate (ATP) is hydrolyzed by myosin-bound adenosine triphosphatase (ATPase) when the actomyosin complex is formed, and chemical energy is converted into mechanical work. The contraction cycle is completed by the active reuptake of Ca^{2+} by the SR (and mitochondria) and extrusion of Ca^{2+} from the cell by Na^+-Ca^{2+} exchange.

Drugs such as the β-adrenergic receptor agonists increase cardiac contractility by increasing intracellular cyclic 3′,5′-adenosine monophosphate (cyclic AMP), which enhances Ca^{2+} influx into the cell, accelerates uptake of Ca^{2+} into the SR by increasing sarcoplasmic endoplasmic reticulum Ca^{2+}-ATPase (SERCA), and increases Ca^{2+} release from the SR through the ryanodine-sensitive channels, ultimately making more Ca^{2+} available for contraction (Fig. 20-1). Increasing cyclic AMP also stimulates the phosphorylation of troponin I, thus increasing the effect of Ca^{2+} on contraction.

In heart failure, the heart is unable to maintain the requisite cardiac output. The mechanics underlying this failure are incompletely understood. The ability of the SR to participate in the trafficking of Ca^{2+} seems to be hindered. The Na^+-Ca^{2+} exchange sites seem to be increased in heart failure, leading to spilling the Ca^{2+} out of the cell and a subsequent decrease in intracellular Ca^{2+}. There are likely to be multiple biochemical defects in heart failure, however.

According to Starling's law of the heart, cardiac output, or more precisely, the ventricular stroke volume, increases as ventricular filling pressure increases. Stated simply, the heart pumps whatever is supplied to it by way of venous return, maintaining a near-optimal heart size. As ventricular end-diastolic pressure increases, ventricular stroke work and stroke volume increase. Normal heart function is within well-defined limits and is described by a single curve (Fig. 20-2).

When cardiac contractility is reduced in heart failure, three mechanisms are available by which the heart can compensate for the defect: (1) an increase in ventricular end-diastolic pressure, which enhances cardiac output (Frank-Starling preload mechanism); (2) an increase in number of contractile units (cardiac hypertrophy); and (3) use of chronotropic and inotropic reserves of the heart through reflex mechanisms (sympathetic activity). If these mechanisms are sufficient to produce normal cardiac output, the heart failure is said to be compensated. In this condition, a new ventricular function curve is generated (see Fig. 20-2). For any given ventricular end-diastolic pressure, however, ventricular stroke work, stroke volume, and cardiac output are lower in the failing heart than in the normal heart. Consequently, the heart typically enlarges to maintain cardiac output, and heart rate increases to help compensate for poor cardiac function. This is known as a dilated cardiomyopathy.

If the ventricular end-diastolic pressure becomes too elevated (i.e., the heart is working to the far right along the Frank-Starling curve), venous pressure upstream also increases excessively, leading to symptoms of "backward" heart failure. Signs and symptoms include pulmonary congestion and dyspnea (left-sided failure) and systemic venous distention and peripheral edema (right-sided failure). If compensatory mechanisms are unable to maintain cardiac output sufficient for the needs of the peripheral tissues and organs, "forward" heart failure ensues. Adverse effects from impaired tissue perfusion include weakness, lassitude, and acute renal failure. In chronic heart failure, aspects of backward and forward failure interact to produce clinical manifestations. Salt and water retention caused by forward failure contributes to the venous hypertension and edema associated with backward failure. Conversely, impaired gas exchange in the congested lungs augments muscle weakness and fatigue associated with reduced cardiac output and delivery of oxygen to skeletal muscle.

An increase in total peripheral vascular resistance, as seen in hypertension or as a reflex reaction in CHF, can contribute to heart failure because of increased outflow resistance on cardiac contraction. Reducing preload and afterload by reducing peripheral resistance is an important strategy in treating heart failure.

Figure 20-3 shows some important adaptive mechanisms that result from heart failure. These changes, including an increase in sympathetic discharge, can temporally compensate for the heart failure. If these and other responses are insufficient, however, the heart failure becomes uncompensated. Adaptive mechanisms also include an increase in production of angiotensin II, leading to remodeling of the heart over time. Remodeling results in cardiac hypertrophy and several cellular changes, which although they tend to compensate for heart failure in the short term may unfortunately also hasten the course of the disease. This cardiac remodeling in heart failure has a parallel in hypertension in which vascular smooth muscle slowly undergoes hypertrophy and hyperplasia.

As a result of the complexity of changes in heart failure, there are numerous processes that can be targeted by drugs: neurohumoral events, vascular dynamics, fluid volume, the sympathetic nervous system, and contractility of the heart. The detailed pharmacologic features of ACE inhibitors and other vasodilators, diuretics, β blockers, and catecholamines are discussed elsewhere in this book. They are discussed in this chapter in relation to the clinical treatment of heart failure. The basic pharmacology of the cardiac glycoside, digoxin, is discussed in this chapter, even though its use has declined in recent years due to advances in both surgical and pharmacologic approaches to CHF.

DRUGS USED IN THE TREATMENT OF CHRONIC HEART FAILURE

Table 20-1 lists the drugs used to treat heart failure and their mechanisms of action. The drugs are often used in combination. Heart failure can be classified as diastolic or systolic failure. In diastolic failure, the heart has inadequate distention and inadequate filling capabilities. Contraction as measured by the ejection fraction may be normal. This type of heart failure is often seen in patients with hypertension. Systolic heart failure is a deficiency in contractility with a low ejection fraction.

The primary drugs used to treat chronic heart failure are ACE inhibitors, ARBs, β-adrenergic receptor blockers, loop and thiazide diuretics, aldosterone antagonists, digoxin, and directly acting vasodilators. For short-term acute treatment, certain catecholamines, nesiritide, other vasodilators, and the phosphodiesterase III inhibitors have special application.

Angiotensin-Converting Enzyme Inhibitors and Angiotensin II Receptor Blockers

A major effect of **ACE inhibitors** is to reduce afterload and preload. These drugs improve symptoms in patients with heart failure as well as slowing the progressive deterioration of the heart. ACE inhibitors control remodeling that occurs with chronic heart failure. Remodeling results from growth of the myocardial cell and myocardial fibrosis. This probable cardioprotective effect provides added support for the use of ACE inhibitors in heart failure. Inhibiting the production of angiotensin II or blocking its receptor reduces aldosterone secretion, which reduces Na^+ and water retention. Reduction of aldosterone release by ACE inhibitors also reduces sympathetic discharge, as described in Chapter 23 (see Fig. 20-4).

Evidence also suggests that ACE inhibitors stimulate the proliferation of capillaries in the coronary circulation, increasing blood flow. It is unknown whether this action of ACE inhibitors occurs as a result of the decrease in angiotensin II, an increase in bradykinin, or both.

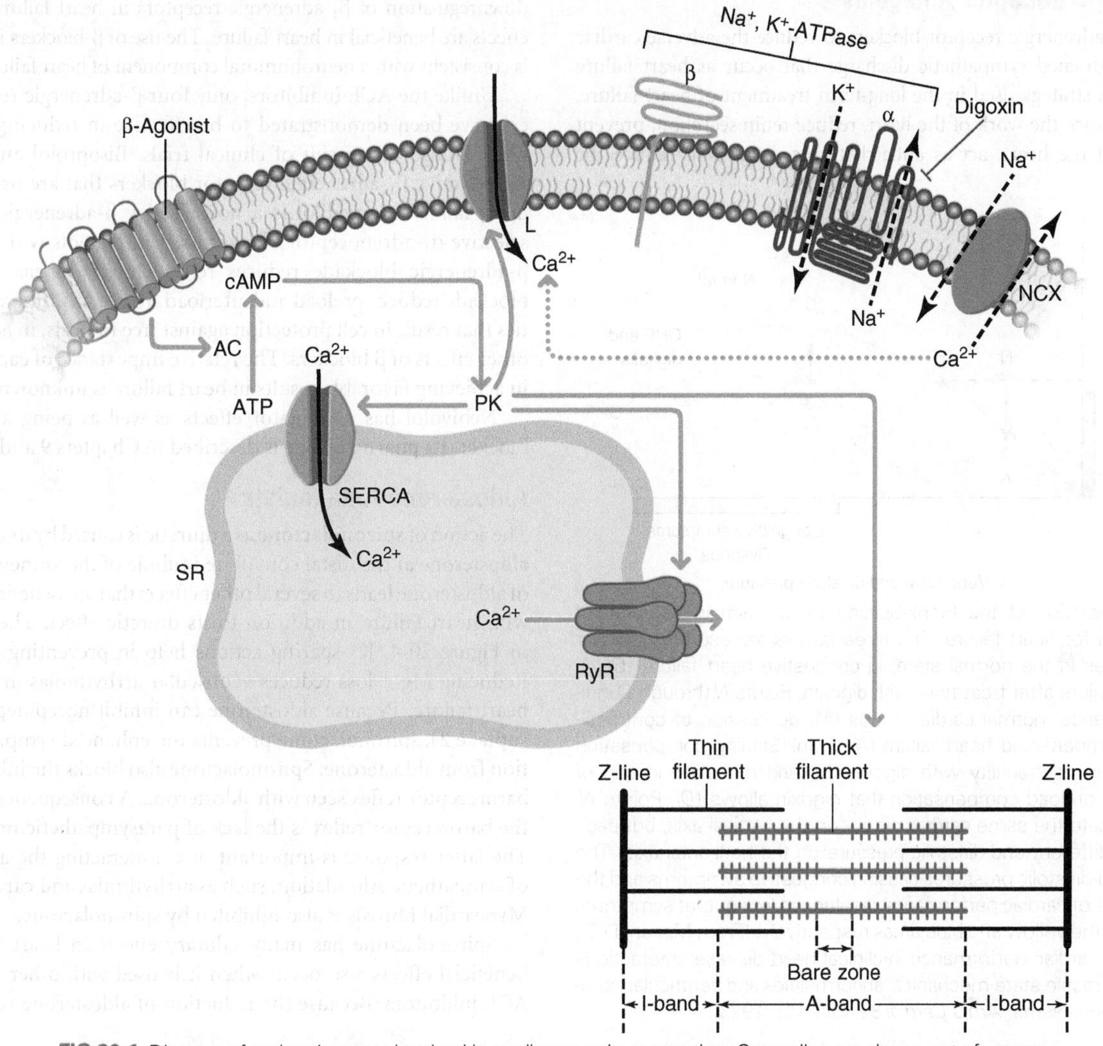

FIG 20-1 Diagram of major elements involved in cardiac muscle contraction. Organelles are shown out of proportion. Calcium, in proportion to its concentration released into the cytosol mostly through the ryanodine receptor (*RyR*), enhances the interaction between actin (thin filament) and myosin (thick filament), leading to contraction. The amount of calcium released at systole depends on its concentration within the sarcoplasmic reticulum (*SR*) and on the concentration of "trigger" calcium in the cytosol. The amount of calcium in the SR is dependent on the level of activity of the sarcoplasmic endoplasmic reticulum Ca^{2+}-ATPase (*SERCA*) pump, which transports calcium into the SR. The level of "trigger" calcium in the cytosol depends on the net effect of the sarcolemma L-type calcium channel (*L*) activity during each depolarization (influx), the high capacity Na^+-Ca^{2+} exchanger (*NCX*), (usually efflux), and the plasma membrane Ca^{2+}-ATPase pump (efflux) (not pictured). (SERCA also removes calcium from the cytosol.) The action of calcium on the contractile apparatus is described in the text. The action of β-receptor agonists is primarily through the production of cyclic AMP (*cAMP*), which stimulates cyclic AMP-dependent protein kinase (PK). The effect of PK is an increase in SERCA activity, an increase in calcium influx through the L-type calcium channel, a greater release of calcium by the RyR receptor, and an enhanced sensitivity of the contractile apparatus due to inhibition of troponin I on actin. These actions lead to a positive inotropic effect. Phosphodiesterase inhibitors inhibit the breakdown of cAMP (not shown) and therefore have effects through PK. Digoxin inhibits Na^+,K^+-ATPase by binding to its α-subunit, leading to a small but significant rise in intracellular sodium, in the vicinity of the plasma membrane. The effect is to reduce the rate, or even to reverse the action of NCX, resulting in an increase in intracellular calcium. This provides more "trigger" calcium and more calcium for contraction, resulting in a positive inotropic effect. The *dotted arrow* indicates the added availability of calcium as a result of the effect on NCX from digoxin. The signal transduction of the β-adrenergic receptor pathway is discussed further in Chapter 1.

Most likely, the ability of ACE inhibitors to reduce blood pressure in hypertensive patients also contributes to a cardioprotective effect. Early treatment of congestive heart disease with an ACE inhibitor could be a major factor in slowing the progress of the disease, relieving symptoms, and extending life. Enalapril is one of the first drugs whose administration was associated with an increased survival time in patients with heart failure. Drugs in this family (most commonly enalapril, lisinopril, benazepril, ramipril, and captopril) also are useful in combination with other drugs, including digoxin and loop diuretics, in treating heart failure.

Angiotensin II antagonists, such as losartan, valsartan, and candesartan, are additional candidates for treating heart failure. As receptor blockers, they share the benefits of ACE inhibitors, while reducing the risk of such side effects as angioedema and persistent coughing. The pharmacologic features of angiotensin II antagonists and ACE inhibitors are discussed in detail in Chapter 23.

β-Adrenergic Receptor Antagonists

The use of β-adrenergic receptor blockers to reduce the adverse cardiac effects of heightened sympathetic discharge that occur as heart failure progresses is a strategy used in the long-term treatment of heart failure. β-Blockers reduce the work of the heart, reduce renin secretion, prevent remodeling of the heart, act as antiarrhythmic drugs, and reduce the downregulation of β_1-adrenergic receptors in heart failure. All of these effects are beneficial in heart failure. The use of β-blockers in heart failure is consistent with a neurohumoral component of heart failure.

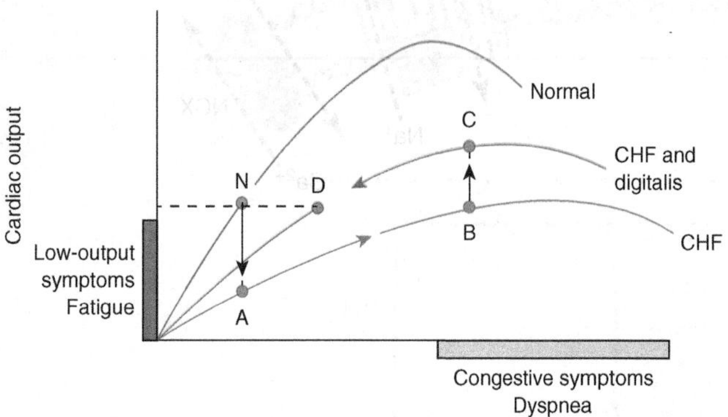

FIG 20-2 Operation of the Frank-Starling mechanism in the preload compensation for heart failure. The three *curves* represent ventricular function curves in the normal state, in congestive heart failure (*CHF*), and in heart failure after treatment with digoxin. Points *N* through *D* indicate, in sequence, normal cardiac status (*N*), depression of contractility with decompensated heart failure (*A*), Frank-Starling compensation (*B*), increase in contractility with digoxin (*C*), and reduction in use of Frank-Starling preload compensation that digoxin allows (*D*). Points *N*, *D*, and *B* indicate the same cardiac output on the vertical axis, but each point is at a different end-diastolic pressure on the horizontal axis. The excessive end-diastolic pressures causing congestive symptoms and the lowered levels of cardiac performance resulting in low-output symptoms are shown by the yellow and blue areas respectively. (From Mason, D.T., Regulation of cardiac performance in clinical heart disease: interactions between contractile state mechanical abnormalities and ventricular compensatory mechanisms, *Am J Cardiol* 32:437–448, 1973.)

Unlike the ACE inhibitors, only four β-adrenergic receptor blockers have been demonstrated to be effective in reducing mortality in heart failure as a result of clinical trials. Bisoprolol and metoprolol are selective β_1-adrenergic receptor blockers that are used in treating heart failure. Carvedilol is a nonselective β-adrenergic blocker and selective α_1-adrenoceptor blocker used in patients with heart failure. β-adrenergic blockade reduces remodeling, whereas α_1-adrenergic blockade reduces preload and afterload. It also has antioxidant properties that result in cell protection against free radicals, in addition to the other effects of β blockers. The relative importance of each mechanism in achieving favorable results in heart failure is unknown.

Nebivolol has vasodilator effects as well as being a β-adrenergic blocker. Its pharmacology is described in Chapters 9 and 23.

Aldosterone Antagonists

The action of **spironolactone** as a diuretic is caused by its antagonism of aldosterone at the distal convoluted tubule of the kidney. Antagonism of aldosterone leads to several other effects that are beneficial in patients with heart failure in addition to its diuretic effect. These are shown in Figure 20-4. K^+-sparing actions help in preventing hypokalemia. Reducing Mg^{++} loss reduces ventricular arrhythmias in patients with heart failure. Because aldosterone can inhibit norepinephrine uptake (uptake 2), spironolactone prevents the enhanced sympathetic activation from aldosterone. Spironolactone also blocks the inhibition of the baroreceptor reflex seen with aldosterone. A consequence of inhibiting the baroreceptor reflex is the lack of parasympathetic nerve response. The latter response is important in counteracting the adverse effects of sympathetic stimulation, such as arrhythmias and cardiac ischemia. Myocardial fibrosis is also inhibited by spironolactone.

Spironolactone has many salutary effects in heart failure. These beneficial effects also occur when it is used with other drugs such as ACE inhibitors. Because the reduction of aldosterone release by ACE

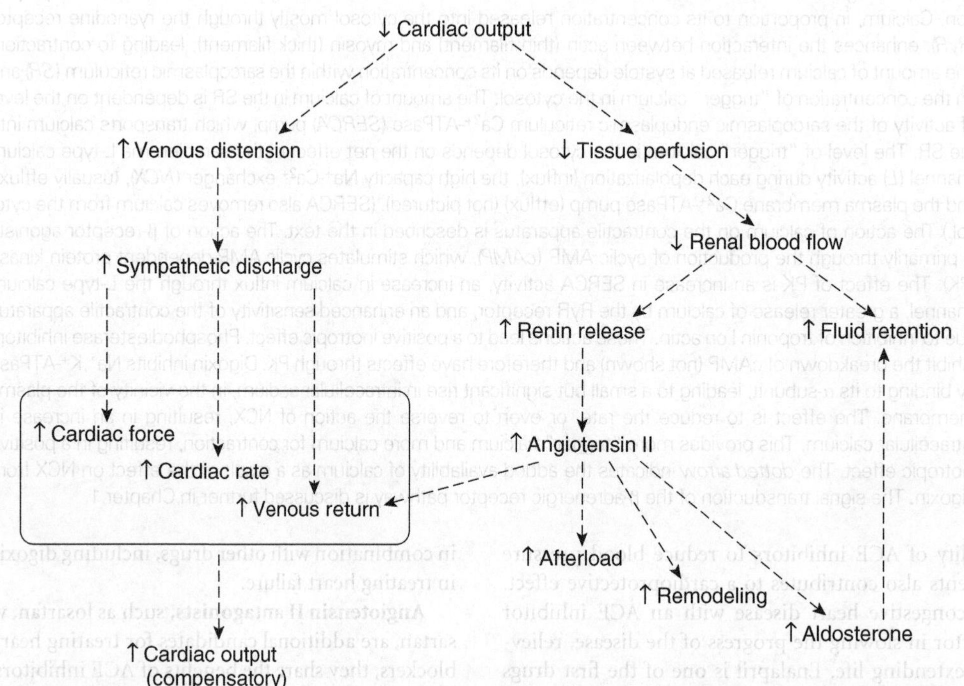

FIG 20-3 Adaptive mechanisms in heart failure. A decrease in cardiac output leads to a cascade of events that results in a compensatory increase in cardiac output (*box*). In addition, activation of the renin-angiotensin system leads to changes that put further burden on the failing heart.

inhibitors is only partial, an added benefit is gained from the use of an aldosterone antagonist synergistically.

Eplerenone is another aldosterone receptor antagonist for the treatment of heart failure. Compared with spironolactone, it has a lower affinity for the androgen receptor and has a lower incidence of related side effects including gynecomastia.

The net effect of aldosterone antagonists in heart failure is to reduce mortality as well as to improve symptoms.

Diuretics

Diuretics reduce edema, which is common with heart failure. Their mechanisms of action are discussed in Chapter 22. A loop diuretic is usually the first choice of this type of drug because a loop diuretic is usually more effective in heart failure than the thiazides. Diuresis results in a reduction in the preload, or diastolic filling pressure. This helps decrease wall tension in the heart and lessens myocardial oxygen demand. Diuresis also aids in reducing afterload, or the arterial pressure against which the heart has to pump in moving blood. Although diuretics other than aldosterone antagonists have not been shown to reduce mortality from heart failure, they do improve symptoms and exercise tolerance.

TABLE 20-1 Treatment of Heart Failure

Drug or Drug Class	Mechanism(s)
Long-Term Treatment (Chronic Therapy)	
ACE inhibitors	Reduce effect of angiotensin II, prevent remodeling
Angiotensin II receptor blockers	Reduce effect of angiotensin II, prevent remodeling
β Blockers*	Reduce sympathetic effect, prevent remodeling, prevent arrhythmias
Aldosterone antagonists	Inhibit effect of aldosterone
Loop and thiazide diuretics	Reduce fluid volume (reduce preload and afterload)
Hydralazine/isosorbide dinitrate	Reduce afterload and preload
Digoxin	Direct cardiotonic effect
Ivabradine	Reduces heart rate, reduces heart rate variability
Sacubitril	Inhibits neprilysin
Short-Term Treatment†	
Dobutamine	Direct cardiotonic effect
Dopamine	Direct cardiotonic effect
Nesiritide	Reduces preload and afterload
Phosphodiesterase III inhibitors	Reduce preload and afterload; direct cardiotonic effect
Nitroglycerin	Reduces preload and afterload
Nitroprusside	Reduces preload and afterload
Diuretics (especially loop)	Reduce edema
Tolvaptan	Reduces edema that is refractory to other drugs

*Carvedilol is a β blocker that also blocks α_1-adrenergic receptors.
†Usually only for a few days.
ACE, Angiotensin-converting enzyme.

Directly Acting Vasodilators

Vasodilators such as nitrates and hydralazine reduce the load on the heart, improve tissue perfusion in heart failure, and increase survival rates in these patients. Their pharmacologic effects are discussed in Chapters 21 and 23. Vasodilators are usually administered in combination with other drugs, such as inotropic agents or ACE inhibitors. Disadvantages of nitrates and hydralazine include the indirect enhancement of sympathetic discharge and activation of the renin-angiotensin pathway. Added interest in vasodilator therapy resulted from evidence supporting the clinical efficacy of two vasodilators in combination: **hydralazine and isosorbide dinitrate.** This fixed-dose therapy was found to be effective in patients of African descent with class III and class IV heart failure. This drug combination may be particularly effective in this group of patients, who may be less responsive to drugs such as ACE inhibitors. The hydralazine/isosorbide dinitrate combination may also be useful as added therapy in resistant cases or in patients who cannot tolerate other heart failure medications.

DIGOXIN

Digoxin is a cardiac glycoside that is often called **digitalis**, referring to the plant from which it is derived. Digoxin is currently indicated for the treatment of CHF and the management of atrial flutter and fibrillation.

The history of the use of digitalis since it was first used has been characterized by a realization of its potential therapeutic benefits on the one hand and its low margin of safety on the other.

Chemistry and Classification

The term **digitalis** is often used interchangeably with the term **cardiac glycoside.** Both terms refer to compounds, naturally occurring or semisynthetic, that have similar cardiotonic effects. Only one such compound, **digoxin**, is commonly used clinically in the United States today. The structure of digoxin is shown in Figure 20-5. The molecule is composed of a steroid ring structure. Other distinguishing molecular

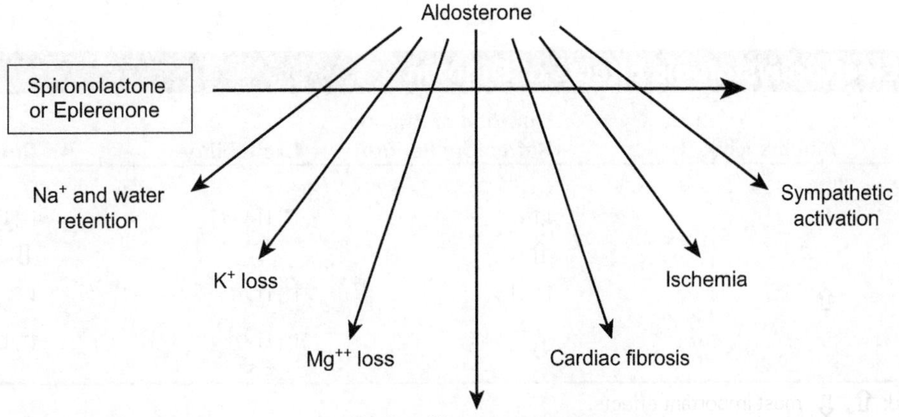

FIG 20-4 Effects of spironolactone or eplerenone in treating congestive heart failure. The beneficial effects of spironolactone and eplerenone are the result of inhibiting the several effects of aldosterone at its receptors.

characteristics include an α,β-unsaturated lactone ring and a carbohydrate moiety in glycosidic linkage at C_3.

Mechanism of Action

Digoxin has a direct inotropic effect on the heart; it increases the force of contraction. The inotropic action of digoxin does not depend on release of endogenous catecholamines. Digoxin is known to be a specific inhibitor of the Na^+-K^+ pump (Na^+,K^+-ATPase). The α subunit of Na^+,K^+-ATPase is responsible for pumping sodium and potassium and contains the binding site for digoxin (see Fig. 20-1). Inhibition of Na^+,K^+-ATPase leads to a small but significant increase in intracellular Na^+ near the plasma membrane. This increase in Na^+, amounting to approximately 2 mmol/L, reduces the rate of Na^+-Ca^{2+} exchange (three Na^+ exchanged into the cell for one Ca^{2+} transported out of the cell) because the increase in Na^+ reduces the net binding of Ca^{2+} to its binding sites on the Na^+-Ca^{2+} exchange system (NCX) (see Fig. 20-1). This alteration results in a reduced efflux of Ca^{2+} and an increase in intracellular Ca^{2+} resulting in enhanced contraction.

The added intracellular Ca^{2+} also increases the amount of Ca^{2+} taken up into the SR during diastole. After several contractions, the amount of Ca^{2+} released from the SR is also increased. The positive inotropic effect results from the increased Ca^{2+} available for contraction during the systolic phase. The inhibition of Na^+,K^+-ATPase resulting in increased intracellular Na^+ and a reduced diastolic membrane potential has important implications for other ion movements and electrical properties of heart cells. Some of these are described subsequently. The relationship between Na^+,K^+-ATPase inhibition by digoxin and its inotropic effect is shown in Figure 20-1.

Pharmacologic Effects

The most important actions of the digitalis glycosides are those exerted on the cardiovascular system. Resulting changes in hemodynamics may indirectly influence other systems, yielding beneficial or adverse responses. Some therapeutic effects may be exerted through the nervous system. Direct actions on the central nervous system (CNS), gastrointestinal tract, and cardiovascular system also contribute to the toxic profile of digoxin.

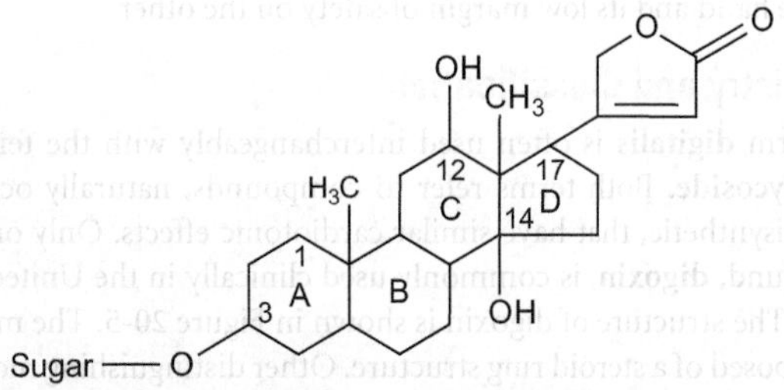

FIG 20-5 Structural formula of digoxin.

Cardiac effects

Digoxin has two powerful influences on the heart: it increases myocardial contractility, and it alters electrical activity throughout the heart. A complex interplay of direct actions and indirect actions through the autonomic nervous system contributes to effects clinically observed.

Contractility. The overall cardiodynamic effect of digoxin on the isolated heart can be summarized as an increased force of contraction caused by an increased rate of force development by the myocardium, resulting in a systolic phase of shorter duration but greater effectiveness.

Digoxin increases cardiac output, reducing the need for compensatory responses by the sympathetic and renin-angiotensin systems during heart failure. Digoxin enhances baroreceptor sensitivity and corrects an impaired baroreceptor response in patients with heart failure. The net result is to further reduce sympathetic activity.

In compensated and decompensated heart failure, digoxin can improve cardiac function so that a greater cardiac output can be achieved without as much reliance on compensatory mechanisms. Figure 20-2 shows that a new ventricular function curve is generated as a result of digoxin. This curve more closely approximates the normal situation.

In the clinical management of CHF, the administration of digoxin is most often associated with a reduction in heart rate. This reduction results from both a vagal and a direct effect on the heart by digoxin. The cardiac glycosides stimulate the vagus nerve—probably indirectly by an effect on baroreceptors, afferent nerve pathways, and central vagal nuclei—and at therapeutic doses reduce the sympathetic tone of the heart indirectly by improving cardiac function and sensitizing the baroreceptor mechanism. Both effects account for a reduction in heart rate. The effect of digitalis on heart rate during the treatment of certain cardiac arrhythmias is discussed subsequently.

Electrophysiology. The effects of digitalis on the electrical properties of the heart can be divided into at least four interrelated categories: **automaticity, refractoriness, excitability, and conduction velocity**. Because digoxin has vagal and nonvagal effects on the heart and because the areas of the heart affected by the vagus include the sinoatrial (SA) node, the atrial myocardium, and the upper portions of the atrioventricular (AV) node, a discussion of discrete regions of the heart is necessary. The direct effects of digoxin on the electrophysiology of the heart are as follows (Table 20-2): reduced conduction velocity and increased duration of the **effective refractory period** in the AV node, increased automaticity of subsidiary pacemaker activity

TABLE 20-2 Electrophysiologic Effects of Digoxin

Site	Automaticity	Duration of Effective Refractory Period	Excitability	Conduction Velocity
SA node	↓,↑A			
Atrial myocardium		↓,↑A	↑*, ↓T	↑*, ↓T
AV node		⇧		⇩
Purkinje fibers	⇧	↑*, ↓T	↑*, ↓T	↓
Ventricular myocardium		⇩	↑*, ↓T	↑*, ↓T

↑, Increased; ↓, decreased; ⇧, ⇩, most important effects.
A, After atropine; *AV*, atrioventricular; *SA*, sinoatrial; *T*, at toxic doses.
*Lower therapeutic doses only.

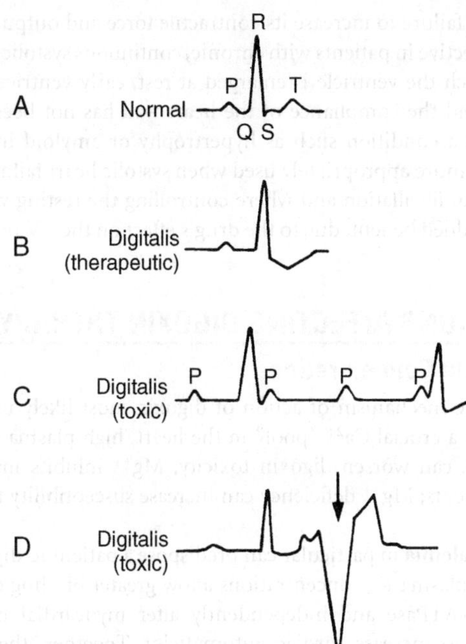

FIG 20-6 Some effects of digoxin on the ECG (lead II). **A,** Normal ECG. **B,** Typical changes at therapeutic concentrations include depression of the ST segment and lengthening of the PR interval. **C,** Toxic effect of digoxin on atrioventricular (AV) conduction promotes AV dissociation, such as complete AV block. Notice the lack of relationship between the P waves and QRS complexes. **D,** Toxic effect of digoxin on ventricular impulse generation results in ectopic ventricular beats. An example of an ectopic beat is marked by the *arrow.*

in the conductive tissues of the ventricle (e.g., Purkinje fibers), and decreased duration of the effective refractory period of the ventricular myocardium. Cardiac vagal effects of digoxin are limited to effects on the atria, the SA node, and the AV node. They consist of a decrease in the duration of the effective refractory period of the atrial myocardium, a decrease in the automaticity of the SA node, and an increase in the duration of the effective refractory period along with a decrease in the conduction velocity of the AV node.

Electrocardiogram. Therapeutic and toxic effects of digoxin are associated with changes on the electrocardiogram (ECG) that reflect the electrophysiologic effects listed in Table 20-2. They include alterations in the shape of the T wave, the configuration of the ST segment, the lengths of the QT and PR intervals, AV dissociation, and the presence of ectopic ventricular beats (Fig. 20-6).

At therapeutic doses, changes often occur in the T wave and the ST segment configuration. The T wave may be inverted or distorted, whereas the ST segment may appear depressed (lead II of the ECG). These changes are caused by alterations in the sequence of repolarization of various ventricular myocardial cells. Also at therapeutic doses, the PR interval is lengthened by digitalis as a result of decreased conduction velocity in the AV node. The QT interval is shortened because of the shortened ventricular action potential.

Although several **cardiac effects of digoxin** are observed at toxic doses, **two effects are typical.** The first is heart block caused by excessive reduction in AV nodal conduction; the second is any of several ventricular arrhythmias caused by ectopic pacemaker activity.

Absorption, Fate, and Excretion

Digoxin is usually given by the oral route. Dose schedules are extremely important for digoxin because attaining a therapeutic effect without toxicity requires precise regulation of the amount of drug administered. Digoxin dosages depend on individual patient variations and disease states and concurrent drug therapy. In all cases, patients must be continually monitored, and final judgment on optimal dosages depends on clinical observations.

Digoxin is **excreted by the kidney** largely in the active form. The mechanism involves glomerular filtration and tubular secretion and accounts for almost all the elimination of the drug. Because digoxin is largely eliminated in the kidney, patients with kidney hypofunction may require downward dosage adjustments of the drug. It has an elimination **half-life** of approximately **36 hours.**

BOX 20-1 Common Signs and Symptoms of Digoxin Toxicity

Gastrointestinal
Salivation
Anorexia
Nausea
Vomiting
Diarrhea

Central Nervous System
Headache
Visual disturbances
Fatigue
Drowsiness

Cardiac
Atrioventricular block
Excessive slowing of the heart
Ventricular extrasystoles
Other arrhythmias

Miscellaneous
Excessive urination

Adverse Effects

Signs and symptoms

Although allergic reactions to digoxin are rare, toxic reactions are not. The drug has a very **low therapeutic index.**

Digoxin toxicity is a significant clinical problem and is one of the reasons the drug is not as commonly used today as in the past. Toxic signs are often seen at roughly twice the minimum effective dose. In practice, adverse reactions usually result from accumulation of the drug or from K^+ depletion caused by diuretic coadministration, or both. Individual differences in patient response exist and may account for unexpected clinical results; dosages have to be tailored for each patient. Common toxic effects of digoxin are listed in Box 20-1.

Extracardiac toxic effects include anorexia, nausea, diarrhea, and vomiting. Gastrointestinal symptoms may also occur at nontoxic concentrations. The mechanism involves stimulation of the chemoreceptor trigger zone of the medulla. Excessive salivation, headache, fatigue, drowsiness, and abdominal pain often accompany these toxic signs and symptoms. Visual disturbances, such as the appearance of halos and distortions in color perception, can also occur, perhaps because of a direct effect of digoxin on the visual cortex. Objects often appear yellow or green. Giddiness and trigeminal neuralgia are sometimes observed; excessive urination often occurs with digoxin intoxication.

Cardiac toxicity is the most serious consequence of digoxin therapy. Although it is difficult to characterize specifically cardiac toxicity caused by digoxin, two effects stand out as the most typical: AV nodal block and ventricular tachyarrhythmias. Complete AV dissociation can occur at toxic concentrations of digoxin. This effect is an extension of a therapeutic effect of the drug and is mediated by a reduction in AV nodal conduction. Dropped ventricular beats caused by partial heart block are also a sign of toxicity. The effect on AV conduction accounts in great measure for the excessive slowing of the heart seen in some toxic situations. Excessive cardiac slowing may be an important sign of toxicity in many patients.

Digoxin also produces tachyarrhythmias in toxic situations. Increased electrical activity can result in premature beats and extrasystoles of ventricular origin, which may progress to ventricular fibrillation. Tachyarrhythmias may be caused by one of several mechanisms. Some may be caused by increased automaticity of Purkinje fibers, others may be due to a reentry process, and still others may be due to delayed afterpotentials whose depolarizations follow quickly on the action potential and in some cases generate a new action potential (Chapter 19). Afterdepolarizations are most likely caused by release of intracellular Ca^{2+} from overloading of the intracellular Ca^{2+} stores. Afterpotentials may also interfere with conduction by reducing the phase 4 resting potential. Other arrhythmias of atrial and of ventricular origin may also occur. Examples of toxic effects on AV conduction and ventricular impulse generation are shown in Figure 20-6.

The arrhythmic effects of digoxin result largely from inhibition of cardiac Na^+,K^+-ATPase. Vagal effects of digoxin can contribute to certain cardiac effects, such as heart block. In addition, at toxic concentrations, digoxin may exert significant stimulatory effects on the sympathetic nervous system, and these actions may account for some arrhythmias. Enhanced sympathetic activity is most likely caused by inhibition of Na^+,K^+-ATPase in the CNS and inhibition of active reuptake of norepinephrine at adrenergic nerve endings.

Drug monitoring

Attempts have been made to correlate blood concentrations of cardiac glycosides with signs of toxicity. These attempts create a technical problem because serum digoxin at therapeutic doses is only 0.7 to 1.2 ng/mL, and toxic effects may start to appear at approximately 2.3 ng/mL or lower.

Treatment of digoxin toxicity

When digoxin toxicity is diagnosed, the drug and any diuretics that may have exacerbated the problem are temporarily discontinued. If digoxin must be readministered before signs of toxicity have abated, small doses are given with constant monitoring. Potassium chloride can be administered intravenously in cases of hypokalemia. In general, it is not used if AV conduction is significantly impaired because K^+ can worsen this condition. Atropine can be helpful in controlling AV block, sinus bradycardia, and SA nodal arrest.

Lidocaine may be useful in treating digoxin toxicity. It is given intravenously in these situations. Lidocaine is useful in suppressing ectopic ventricular pacemaker activity; however, it has little effect on slowing of AV nodal conduction by digoxin. Phenytoin may also be useful in treating ventricular arrhythmias caused by digoxin.

In severe digoxin toxicity, an antidigoxin drug designated digoxin immune Fab (Digibind) may be administered. Digoxin immune Fab consists of antigen-binding fragments derived from sheep antibodies to digoxin.

Therapeutic Use of Digoxin

The primary use for digoxin is in the treatment of **CHF**. The direct effect of digoxin on the myocardium in most cases enables the heart in congestive failure to increase its contractile force and output. Digoxin is most effective in patients with chronic, continuous systolic heart failure in which the ventricle is enlarged at rest, early ventricular filling is rapid, and the compliance of the heart wall has not been reduced because of a condition such as hypertrophy or amyloid infiltration. Digoxin is more appropriately used when systolic heart failure accompanies atrial fibrillation and where controlling the resting ventricular rate is an added benefit, due to the drug's effect on the AV node (Table 20-2).

CONDITIONS AFFECTING DIGOXIN THERAPY

Electrolyte Concentrations

Because the mechanism of action of digoxin most likely involves an increase in a crucial Ca^{2+} "pool" in the heart, high plasma Ca^{2+} concentrations can worsen digoxin toxicity. Mg^{++} inhibits many Ca^{2+}-induced events; Mg^{++} deficiency can increase susceptibility to digoxin toxicity.

Hypokalemia in particular can predispose a patient to digoxin toxicity. Low plasma K^+ concentrations allow greater binding of digoxin to Na^+,K^+-ATPase and independently alter myocardial membrane properties to increase cardiac automaticity. Together, these factors may account for increased digoxin toxicity at low plasma K^+ concentrations. (For drugs that reduce plasma K^+, see the subsequent section on drug interactions.) The effects of major electrolyte changes on digoxin toxicity are summarized in Table 20-3.

Sympathomimetic amines interact with digoxin because both classes of drugs increase the possibility of ectopic cardiac pacemaker activity. Cardiac arrhythmias are more likely to occur when β-adrenergic receptor agonists are used concurrently with digoxin. On the other hand, β-adrenergic receptor antagonists increase the risk of bradycardia and AV nodal block when given with digoxin, even though β blockers and digoxin are both used to treat heart failure.

Cholinergic and anticholinergic drugs alter responses to digoxin. The cholinergic agents enhance and the anticholinergic drugs antagonize the atrial, SA nodal, and AV nodal effects of digoxin. Succinylcholine, by increasing vagal tone and altering the K^+ distribution, may acutely increase digoxin toxicity.

Spironolactone reduces digoxin clearance. This reduction in digoxin clearance may necessitate a lower digoxin dose when these drugs are used concurrently. Spironolactone may also interfere with serum digoxin assays.

In approximately 10% of patients, enteric bacteria, especially *Eubacterium lentum*, metabolize a significant portion of ingested digoxin. In these patients, antibiotics, by inhibiting these bacteria, can increase the amount of digoxin absorbed and increase the potential for digoxin toxicity. Erythromycin, other macrolides, and tetracyclines may increase digoxin plasma concentrations. In some cases, the interaction between antibiotics and digoxin has resulted in a twofold increase in serum digoxin concentrations.

TABLE 20-3 Effects of Plasma Electrolyte Concentrations on Digoxin Toxicity

	Normal Total Plasma Concentration (mmol/L)	Digoxin Toxicity More Likely if Plasma Electrolyte Concentration Is
K^+	3.8-5.4	Decreased
Ca^{2+}	2.2-2.8	Increased
Mg^{++}	0.8-1.1	Decreased

Some important drug–drug interactions involving digoxin are shown in Table 20-4.

Ivabradine

Ivabradine was approved for use in heart failure in the United States in 2015. It blocks the hyperpolarization-activated nucleotide-gated (HCN) channel that conducts the cardiac pacemaker I_f current (see Chapter 19). This current regulates heart rate by controlling the rate of phase 4 depolarization in cardiac pacemaker cells. Lowering the rate of phase 4 depolarization reduces the heart rate, which is useful in controlling heart rates in stable heart failure patients whose heart rate is ≥70 bpm and when β-blockers and other therapy are insufficient. Ivabradine reduces the heart rate variability and therefore the numbers of hospitalizations in these patients.

Ivabradine is given orally and metabolized in the liver. It has a half-life of approximately 6 hours, which includes the half-life of the principal active metabolite. Adverse effects include bradycardia, fetal toxicity, and bright visual flashes (luminous effects or phosphenes). Phosphenes are due to the effects of the drug on photoreceptor signaling.

A priority listing of drugs used in treating chronic heart failure is shown in Table 20-5.

Sacubitril

Sacubitril is a neprilysin (neutral endopeptidase) inhibitor. It is used to treat chronic heart failure with reduced ejection fraction, in combination with an angiotensin II receptor blocker (ARB). The effect of inhibition of neprilysin is to increase the level of peptides such as atrial natriuretic peptide and C-type natriuretic peptide. The result is vasodilation, increased renal blood flow and natriuresis. Sacubitril therapy targets the decrease in sensitivity to natriuretic peptides seen in heart failure, whereas the ARB targets the renin angiotensin system.

DRUGS USED FOR ACUTE THERAPY OF HEART FAILURE

Catecholamines

Drugs that stimulate β_1 adrenoceptors, such as **dobutamine** and **dopamine**, are cardiotonic. An undesirable chronotropic response may occur, but it is less likely than with other catecholamines, such as epinephrine. Dobutamine and dopamine are used to treat heart failure in the acute setting. Dobutamine is a selective β_1-adrenergic agonist, which accounts for the positive cardiac inotropic response. A lesser β_2-adrenergic effect seems to account for its effect of reducing vascular resistance. The effect of dobutamine on α-adrenergic receptors is complex. The negative isomer is an α_1-adrenergic agonist, whereas the positive isomer is an α_1-adrenergic antagonist. The self-negating combination of both isomers in the clinically available preparations ensures primarily a β_1-adrenergic effect of the drug.

At low doses, dopamine stimulates peripheral D_1-dopaminergic receptors selectively. This effect accounts for vasodilation of coronary, renal, and mesenteric blood vessels. At increasingly higher doses, dopamine has a greater net effect in stimulating β_1-adrenergic receptors, leading to an inotropic effect. Finally, at still higher doses, dopamine significantly stimulates α_1-adrenergic receptors and increases vascular resistance. The choice of which catecholamine will be used depends largely on the vascular state of the patient. The pharmacologic features of the catecholamines are discussed in Chapter 8.

Nesiritide

Nesiritide is a human B-type natriuretic peptide that is produced using recombinant DNA methods. The drug binds to and stimulates membrane-bound guanylyl cyclase, causing an increase in cyclic 3′,5′-guanosine monophosphate (cGMP) in blood vessels. This increase in cGMP leads to relaxation of vascular smooth muscle. The half-life of the drug is about 18 minutes; however, the effect of the drug may last several hours. It is used in the acute management of heart failure to reduce preload and afterload.

Diuretics

Diuretics, especially **loop diuretics**, are useful in reducing edema in acute heart failure. Volume reduction is critical to keep both pulmonary and systemic edema under control, which helps tremendously to lessen many of the symptoms of CHF. These drugs are discussed in detail in Chapter 22.

TABLE 20-4 Some Drug–Drug Interactions Involving Digoxin (D)

Mechanism	Drug Examples
Increase D toxicity by decreasing plasma [K+]	Loop and thiazide diuretics, amphotericin B, corticosteroids
Reduce the GI absorption and effect of D	Metoclopramide, cholestyramine, colestipol, kaolin-pectin, oral antacids
Increase D toxicity by decreasing renal clearance of D and/or displacement of D from tissue stores	Quinidine, quinine, amiodarone, diltiazem, flecainide, verapamil, spironolactone
Increase arrhythmogenic effect of D	Sympathomimetic amines
Enhance the bradycardia effect of D	Muscarinic receptor agonists
Increase absorption of D	Macrolide and tetracycline antibiotics
Augment the slowing of the heart from digoxin	β-Blockers and calcium channel blockers

TABLE 20-5 Prioritization of Drugs for Treating Chronic Heart Failure with Reduced Ejection Fraction (Systolic Heart Failure)

Drug	Comments
ACEI	All patients should receive an ACEI except if contraindicated (reduces mortality)
ARB	Substitute for ACEI if patient is unable to take an ACEI (ARB reduces mortality)
β-Blocker	All patients should receive a β-blocker except if it is contraindicated (reduces mortality)
Aldosterone antagonist	It can be added to improve cardiac function (reduces mortality)
Loop or thiazide diuretic	They are useful to reduce edema and volume overload; a loop diuretic is preferred (they reduce symptoms but reduced mortality is not established)
Hydralazine/isosorbide dinitrate	Can be used to add to the effect of other drugs Especially effective in African American patients (reduces mortality)
Digoxin	A positive inotropic drug (reduces symptoms but not mortality)
Ivabradine	Used as add-on therapy for patients whose heart rates are ≥70 bpm (reduces symptoms)

ACEI, Angiotensin-converting enzyme inhibitor; *ARB*, angiotensin II receptor blocker; *β-blocker*, β-adrenergic receptor blocker. Wording in parentheses refers to established outcomes.

Tolvaptan

Tolvaptan is a vasopressin antagonist that is used to treat hyponatremia. It is useful in treating conditions of diuretic-resistant volume overload in heart failure. The drug is selective for the V_2 vasopressin receptor, thus antagonizing the action of vasopressin in the kidney and making it useful in correcting volume overload and hyponatremia.

Milrinone

Milrinone is a bipyridine drug that has a positive inotropic action on the heart. The bipyridines act by inhibiting **phosphodiesterase III**, also termed **cGMP-inhibited phosphodiesterase.** As a result of this inhibition, cardiac concentrations of cAMP are elevated, and a sympathomimetic effect on the heart is achieved. (See effect of cAMP in Fig. 20-1.) Milrinone also reduces arterial and venous pressures because of the increase in vascular smooth muscle relaxation, which aids in relieving heart failure. The latter effect is the major mechanism operable in heart failure patients.

Milrinone is given intravenously. The half-life of milrinone is approximately 3 hours. Arrhythmias have been associated with milrinone. It is for short-term use, especially in cases in which the heart is refractory to other cardiotonic agents and vascular resistance is elevated. Studies have failed to show long-term benefits, however, and evidence indicates that survival is worsened with long-term administration because of an arrhythmogenic effect of the drug.

Directly Acting Vasodilators

Nitroprusside and nitroglycerin are sometimes used for acute treatment of heart failure. These drugs are discussed in Chapters 23 (nitroprusside) and 21 (nitroglycerin).

IMPLICATIONS FOR DENTISTRY

A history of the patient should be obtained to assess the relative severity of the patient's cardiac condition. The dentist should reinforce the need for the patient to keep all medical appointments and be compliant with taking medications. The dentists should also reinforce the physician's advice to the patient about diet, lifestyle, and smoking cessation, if necessary. Dental procedures should not be performed unless the patient is current with medications and considered stable for the private practice/outpatient clinical setting.

TABLE 20-6 Dental Implications for Patients Taking Digoxin

Dental Condition or Drug	Decision
Stress	Use shorter appointments, sedatives as needed to lessen stress
Vasoconstrictors	Consider avoiding vasoconstrictors, especially epinephrine, due to possible arrhythmias
Muscarinic drugs	Avoid use: enhanced bradycardia may result due to mutual effects on SA and AV nodes
Antimuscarinic drugs	Avoid use: antagonism of some effects of digoxin may result
Antibiotic use	Avoid macrolides and tetracyclines and possibly other antibiotics that have broad or extended spectra; these drugs may lead to an increase in GI absorption of digoxin

Blood pressure and pulse readings should be taken before dental treatment to establish baseline values. These should be monitored during and after the dental procedure and before discharging the patient. The practitioner should strive to eliminate needless stress for cardiac patients, especially anxiety or pain associated with dental procedures. Patients being treated for heart failure possess limited cardiac function. These patients are at special risk in stressful situations because stress puts a greater workload on the heart and stimulates the release of endogenous catecholamines. Sedatives may be required to reduce anxiety, and the level of fatigue of the patient may dictate shorter appointments.

Patients with heart failure often experience dyspnea, and the severity of dyspnea is one measure of severity of the disease. This may require that the patient be placed in an upright position for the dental procedure. Supplemental oxygen may also be useful. Suffice it to say that if a patient has evidence of severe heart failure, treatment in a hospital setting with cardiac anesthesiology providing support and monitoring is safest for the patient and represents "best practices."

Dental precautions involving digoxin are summarized in Table 20-6. Dental implications of ACE inhibitors, ARBs, and β-adrenergic receptor blockers are discussed in Chapter 23.

CASE DISCUSSION

Dyspnea is a common finding in patients with heart failure, and recent experience has indicated that this patient usually can breathe normally in a supine position. Yet at this appointment, the blood pressure and pulse pressure have significantly dropped from the previous appointments, which indicates a relatively low ejection fraction and suggests systolic dysfunction. The course of the disease could be getting worse, but probably not this quickly.

With this data in mind, it is best to query the patient about any changes that may have occurred since he was last in. Has he changed medications? Has he been taking them as prescribed? Have there been any other changes in his health status that may have affected his cardiac status?

Given the clearly unstable nature of the patient, at this point the crown preparation should be postponed and his cardiologist consulted. Transport to the cardiologist or (if decompensating quickly) to an emergency department may be warranted.

Further dental care should be postponed if possible until the patient has reestablished compliance and stability with his drug regimen. Cases like this demonstrate how important it is to ask the patient prior to the procedure if he/she has taken all medications as prescribed and is current with all medications. Vital signs and simple observation/recognition of a deteriorating situation are critical. Proper therapy for heart failure can be very complex, but it does extend life in most cases, indicating how important it is to have a quality drug regimen.

DRUGS USED IN TREATING HEART FAILURE

Nonproprietary (Generic) Name	Proprietary (Trade) Name
Diuretics (See Loop and Thiazide-Type and Thiazide-Like Diuretics*)	
ACE Inhibitors	
Benazepril	Lotensin
Captopril	Capoten
Enalapril	Vasotec
Fosinopril	Monopril
Lisinopril	Zestril
Moexipril	Univasc
Perindopril	Aceon
Quinapril	Accupril
Ramipril	Altace
Trandolapril	Mavik
Angiotensin II Receptor Blockers	
Candesartan	Atacand
Eprosartan	Teveten
Irbesartan	Avapro
Losartan	Cozaar
Olmesartan	Benicar
Telmisartan	Micardis
Valsartan	Diovan
Aldosterone Antagonists	
Eplerenone	Inspra
Spironolactone	Aldactone
β Blockers	
Bisoprolol	Zebeta
Carvedilol	Coreg
Metoprolol	Lopressor
Nebivolol†	Bystolic
Directly Acting Vasodilators	
Hydralazine + isosorbide dinitrate	BiDil
Cardiac Glycosides	
Digoxin	Lanoxin
Miscellaneous	
Ivabradine	Corlanor
Sacubitril	Entresto (combined with valsartan)
Drugs for Acute Treatment	
Dobutamine	Dobutrex
Dopamine	Intropin
Milrinone	Primacor
Nesiritide	Natrecor
Nitroglycerin	—
Nitroprusside	Nitropress
Tolvaptan	Samsca

ACE, Angiotensin-converting enzyme.
*Diuretics are discussed in Chapter 22.
†Added vasodilator effect.

GENERAL REFERENCES

1. Adigopula S, DePasquale EC, Deng MC: Management of ACCF/AHA stage C heart failure, *Cardiol Clin* 32:73–93, 2014.
2. Albert NM, Boehmer JP, Collins SP, et al.: Executive summary: HFSA 2010 comprehensive heart failure practice guideline, *J Cardiac Fail* 16:475–539, 2010.
3. Collins S, Storrow AB, Albert NM, et al.: Early management of patients with acute heart failure: State of the art and future directions. A consensus document from the Society for Academic Emergency Medicine/Heart Failure Society of America Acute Heart Failure Working Group, *J Cardiac Fail* 21:27–43, 2015.
4. Drugs for chronic heart failure, *Med Lett Drugs Therap* 57(1460):9–13, 2015.
5. Emdin CA, Callendar T, Cao J, et al.: Meta-analysis of large-scale randomized trials to determine the effectiveness of inhibition of the renin-angiotensin aldosterone system in heart failure, *Am J Cardiol* 116:155–161, 2015.
6. Herman WW, Ferguson HW: Dental update for patients with heart failure, *J Am Dent Assoc* 141:845–853, 2010.
7. Klapholz M: β-blocker use for the stages of heart failure, *Mayo Clin Proc* 84:718–729, 2009.
8. Ramani GV, Uber PA, Mehra MR: Chronic heart failure: contemporary diagnosis and management, *Mayo Clin Proc* 85:180–195, 2010.

21

Antianginal Drugs

*Frank J. Dowd**

KEY POINTS

- The various types of angina pectoris occur when the oxygen demand of the heart exceeds the supply of oxygen supplied through the coronary blood vessels.
- The first-line drugs for treating angina are these:
  - Organic nitrates and nitrites (nitroglycerin being the major drug for treating acute episodes)
  - Calcium channel blockers
  - β-Adrenergic receptor blockers
- Second-line drugs are as follows:
  - Ranolazine
  - Ivabradine
- Other supportive drugs:
  - Angiotensin converting enzyme (ACE) inhibitors
  - Statins
  - Antiplatelet drugs
  - Anticoagulants
- First- and second-line drugs reduce the oxygen demand of the heart or, in some cases, increase the oxygen supply to the heart.
- Supportive drugs tend to prevent the deterioration of vascular dynamics.
- Dentists should make every attempt to reduce stress in the patient and to have available emergency oxygen and nitroglycerin in case they are needed.

CASE STUDY

Mr. G has been your dental patient for several years. He is 60 years old and is seeing a cardiologist for occasional chest pain. His history reveals he has been diagnosed with angina pectoris. Several months ago in your office, he presented with "pain in the lower jaw" on the left side. He had only minor symptoms other than that, and the mandibular pain was intermittent. At that time, the oral examination revealed no oral or hard tissue abnormality and neither did the full mouth radiographs. Subsequent substernal pain brought him to the cardiologist.

Since seeing the cardiologist, the patient was prescribed metoprolol, a β-adrenergic receptor blocker, which has alleviated the chest pain and the pain in the jaw. Nitroglycerin tablets were also prescribed for acute attacks of angina.

Fast forward to today: you plan to do a full crown preparation on #18. You take his blood pressure (130/80) and pulse (63) readings after the patient is seated. Both are typical of past values for this patient. As you begin the injection of anesthesia, the patient experiences intense chest pain that radiates to the left shoulder, arm, and mandible. At this point what would be the best course of action?

Angina pectoris (from the Latin, literally meaning "pain in the chest") is usually manifested as a severe, transient, retrosternal pain that sometimes radiates to the arms, back, or jaw. It is frequently accompanied by fear, anxiety, feelings of suffocation, and a sensation of tightening of the chest. There is a wide variation among individuals in the intensity and quality of the pain, and some ischemic episodes may occur without prominent symptoms. In such cases the patient may only report pressure or "heartburn." The pain and associated changes in the electrocardiogram (e.g., depressed ST segment) **result from ischemia** (hypoxia) of some area of the myocardium, usually a subendocardial area. The most frequent pathologic cause of angina is epicardial coronary artery atherosclerosis leading to compromised blood flow and reduced oxygen delivery to a region of the myocardium. Angina may also result from vasospasm; the coronary vasoconstriction frequently occurs at an atherosclerotic site on the artery.

As shown in Figure 21-1, the normal response to increased myocardial oxygen demand is satisfied by vasodilation of the small coronary resistance vessels, increased blood flow, and increased oxygen supply. In contrast, in the classic anginal patient with exertional (exercise-induced) episodes, significant sclerosis (>70% narrowing of the luminal diameter) of the large conductance arteries precludes increased vasodilation in response to increased myocardial work because the poststenotic resistance vessels are already dilated, and the resultant demand for oxygen cannot be met. Cardiac determinants of oxygen consumption and factors that can precipitate changes in these determinants are also shown in Figure 21-1.

The intraventricular pressure is important in determining flow in subendocardial regions because of compression of blood vessels in the involved area. Coronary blood flow occurs primarily during diastole, when the intraventricular pressure is minimized. Increased heart rate decreases the diastolic time more than the systolic and requires increased oxygen supply in concert with the increased rate of metabolism. Increases in ventricular size, due to increases in chamber volume, such as found in congestive failure, also cause an increase in ventricular work and oxygen demand. Finally, the inotropic state of the myocardium is also a factor in determining oxygen consumption. Sympathetic nervous activity from sources of stress additionally increase oxygen demand by the heart.

Any factor that compromises the balance between oxygen demand and oxygen supply may cause an attack of angina. Anginal pain may follow exercise, emotional upset, exposure to cold, or may occur after meals or smoking. Certain individuals have nocturnal attacks of angina, probably because recumbent posture can increase venous

*The author thanks Dr. Eileen L. Watson for her contributions to this chapter in previous editions.

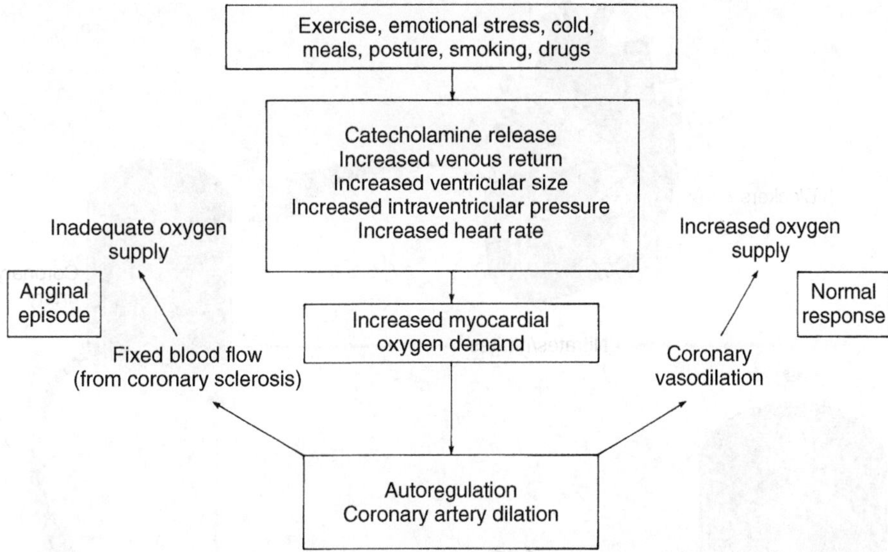

FIG 21-1 Pathophysiologic characteristics and precipitating causes of classic angina pectoris.

TABLE 21-1 Clinical Types of Angina Pectoris

Type	Characteristics
Classic (chronic stable, exertional)	Pain during stress or exertion, due to atherosclerotic coronary disease
Vasospastic (variant or Prinzmetal)	Pain at rest and often during sleep
Unstable (acute coronary syndrome, preinfarction angina)	New onset of severity, different from the normal presentation of angina. Often due to sudden platelet aggregation or plaque emboli in coronary vessels
Cardiac syndrome X	Coronary microvascular dysfunction, angina with normal angiography, abnormal coronary vasodilation, or contraction

return to the heart and increase cardiac work. Anginal attacks in susceptible patients may also result from self-medication with various drugs, such as cocaine and cold remedies that contain sympathomimetic agents.

The **types of angina pectoris** are listed in Table 21-1. Pain in classic angina occurs when the myocardial oxygen requirement reaches a value that cannot be supplied due to ischemia. Patients with vasospastic angina are at a higher risk of near future myocardial infarction. Cardiac syndrome X (rare) often requires the use of additional therapies in addition to first-line drugs.

Drugs that are used to treat angina pectoris have mechanisms aimed at reducing cardiac work and oxygen demand or improving blood supply and delivery of oxygen to the myocardium, or both. The sites of action of three major classes of antianginal drugs are depicted in Figure 21-2.

NITRITES AND NITRATES

Nitroglycerin is the drug of choice for the relief of acute symptoms of angina pectoris. Nitroglycerin is administered sublingually as a tablet or aerosol spray and has a quick onset and short duration of action. Amyl nitrite was used by inhalation for angina pectoris, although its use has waned because of its short duration and unpredictability. Various organic nitrates and sustained-release forms of nitroglycerin have been developed in attempts to find a suitable, long-lasting preparation for the control and prevention of anginal pain. The use of nitrites in the treatment of cyanide poisoning is discussed in Chapter 40.

Chemistry

Nitroglycerin is chemically a simple compound. Figure 21-3 shows its structure and, for comparison, the structures of some of the other organic nitrates marketed for oral, topical, sublingual, buccal, inhalant, or intravenous administration. All nitrites and nitrates with antianginal activity are esters of nitrous or nitric acid. Organic nitrites and nitrates are capable of being metabolized to yield the free radical **nitric oxide (NO)**. These drugs are referred to collectively as *nitrovasodilators*. (See Chapter 6 for further information on NO.)

Pharmacologic Effects

The pharmacologic effects of all the members of this class are similar and result from actions of NO released by denitration reactions of the parent drugs in the tissues (Fig. 21-4). Although more than one pathway for generation of NO from nitroglycerin likely exists, mitochondrial aldehyde dehydrogenase plays the most important role in the synthesis of NO from nitroglycerin. Generation of NO results in dilation of blood vessels. NO has been shown to stimulate the synthesis of **cyclic 3′,5′-guanosine monophosphate (cGMP)**. cGMP initiates a cascade of reactions involving cGMP-dependent protein kinases leading to the various cellular responses that relax vascular smooth muscle (Fig. 21-4).

NO causes **vasodilation** first in veins at low doses and then in arteries at higher doses. Nitroglycerin has been shown to cause varying degrees of change in coronary flow in normal and diseased mammalian hearts. Its efficacy in the various types of angina is attributed in part to a preferentially increased oxygen supply to ischemic areas, with variable actions on total coronary blood flow. More importantly, through a reduction in venous tone, there is a reduction in venous pressure, pulmonary arterial pressure, and end-diastolic filling pressure. These actions lead to a decrease in ventricular volume, producing a decrease in intramyocardial tension and a decline in myocardial oxygen demand. Nitrovasodilators tend to cause **redistribution of coronary blood flow** to the more ischemic areas. As implied earlier,

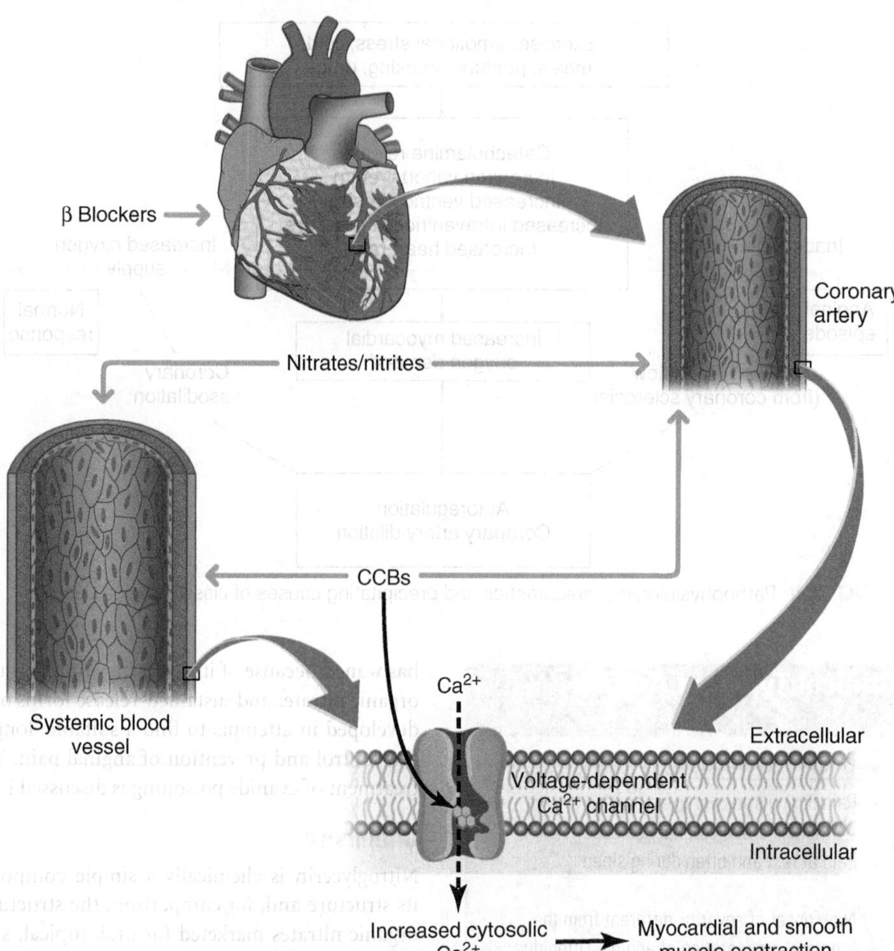

FIG 21-2 Sites of action of β-adrenergic receptor blockers, Ca^{2+} channel blockers (*CCBs*), and nitrates/nitrites. β Blockers reduce the rate and contractility of the heart, reducing energy and oxygen demand of the heart. CCBs reduce vasoconstriction in coronary and noncoronary vessels, increasing coronary blood flow and reducing cardiac load. The nitrates/nitrites act primarily on systemic blood vessels to reduce cardiac load. The effect on coronary arteries is less a factor in alleviating classic angina but plays a major role in variant angina. Three anatomic levels are shown: cardiac anatomy, cell layers of the blood vessel walls, and a blood vessel smooth muscle cell membrane showing a Ca^{2+} channel and the effect of CCBs in preventing Ca^{2+} entry.

arterial smooth muscle is relaxed by these drugs, although to a lesser degree than venous smooth muscle. The efficacy of nitrates and nitrites in relieving variant angina probably stems from a direct alleviation of coronary artery spasm.

Absorption, Fate, and Excretion

Nitroglycerin is rapidly absorbed after **sublingual** administration (onset 1 to 3 minutes, duration 30 to 60 minutes). Nitroglycerin has a much slower onset when applied topically to the skin in a patch or ointment, but it has a comparably longer duration of action. Although nitroglycerin administered orally is readily absorbed, it is extensively metabolized during the first pass through the liver. Sublingual nitroglycerin is highly effective for the treatment of acute anginal episodes; however, its short duration of action makes it unsuitable for long-term prophylaxis.

To avoid the first-pass phenomenon that plagues orally administered nitrates, nitroglycerin has been prepared in several forms. The sublingual tablet is a commonly used preparation. Nitroglycerin ointment is effective prophylactically, but it must be administered every 3 to 4 hours. A further development is the nitroglycerin transdermal system, which comes in the form of an adhesive patch. When applied to the skin, the transdermal patch slowly releases nitroglycerin over a 24-hour period. This system minimizes the potential for toxicity inherent in large-dose oral administration, and it overcomes the inconvenience and frequency of application associated with the ointment. Nitroglycerin is also marketed in a transmucosal preparation. Supplied in a matrix, the drug is made available in a sustained-release fashion when placed between the upper lip and teeth. Swallowing or chewing increases the rate of absorption and could lead to toxicity. The advantages of this preparation are its rapid onset and extended action.

In addition to undergoing denitration activation reactions in tissues, nitroglycerin is metabolized in the liver by glutathione–organic nitrate reductase. The products of hepatic biotransformation, including the released nitrite ions, are much less effective against angina pectoris than the parent compound; they are subsequently excreted in the urine, at least in part, in the form of glucuronide conjugates.

Isosorbide dinitrate is converted to its principal metabolite, **isosorbide-5-mononitrate**, which is responsible for most of the vasodilator action and is also available clinically. When administered sublingually, both are effective against angina pectoris, and each is available for oral administration. The clinical efficacy of a single

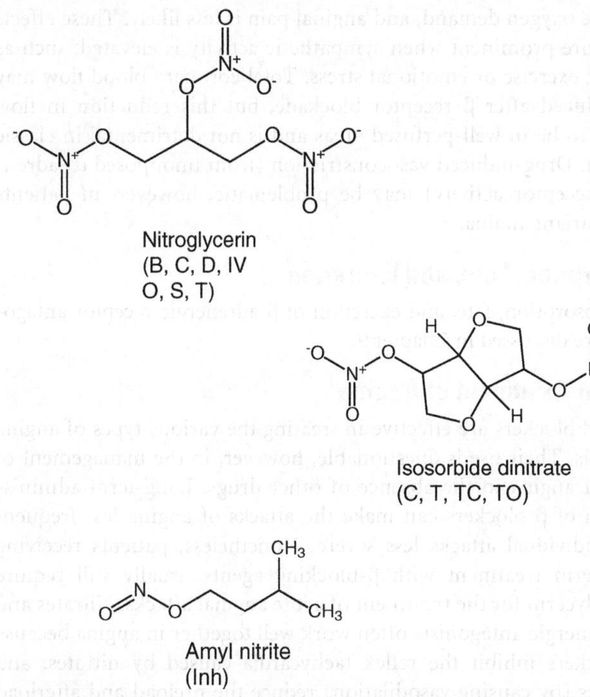

Nitroglycerin
(B, C, D, IV
O, S, T)

Isosorbide dinitrate
(C, T, TC, TO)

Amyl nitrite
(Inh)

FIG 21-3 Structural formulas and methods of administration of selected organic nitrates and amyl nitrite. *B*, Buccal (transmucosal) tablet; *C*, sustained-release capsule or tablet; *D*, transdermal disk; *Inh*, inhalant; *IV*, intravenous injection; *O*, ointment; *S*, lingual spray; *T*, sublingual tablet; *TC*, chewable tablet; *TO*, oral tablet or capsule.

dose of isosorbide-5-mononitrate formulated as a 30% immediate-release/70% sustained-release formulation is observed within a few minutes to increase work and exercise capacity.

Nitrates, by generating NO, also reduce platelet aggregation and adhesion in patients with acute myocardial infarction. This indicates an added benefit of long-acting nitrates. Nitrates have a place in the prophylactic treatment of patients with angina pectoris because their efficacy is not in doubt.

One problem shared by all the long-acting preparations is the development of tolerance. In vitro studies suggest that the causes include volume expansion and tissue tolerance resulting partly from enzyme changes. Such tolerance is not observed with the intermittent administration of sublingual nitroglycerin.

Other problems associated with their use are the following: unreliable absorption, short duration of action, treatment-induced vasodilatory headache, and a rebound phenomenon observed during intermittent dosing. Patient convenience regarding the treatment schedule should also be considered. Controlled-release formulations that produce sufficiently high nitrate concentrations during part of the day, followed by nitrate-poor rather than nitrate-free intervals, have the potential to prevent tolerance and rebound phenomena and to produce a sufficiently long duration of action with a convenient once-daily regimen. The combination of immediate and sustained-release formulations, used once daily, produces a fast onset of action and a longer period during which nitrate concentrations are sufficient to prevent ischemia during the active part of the day. During the night, nitrate levels decrease but offer some protection with low risk of tolerance.

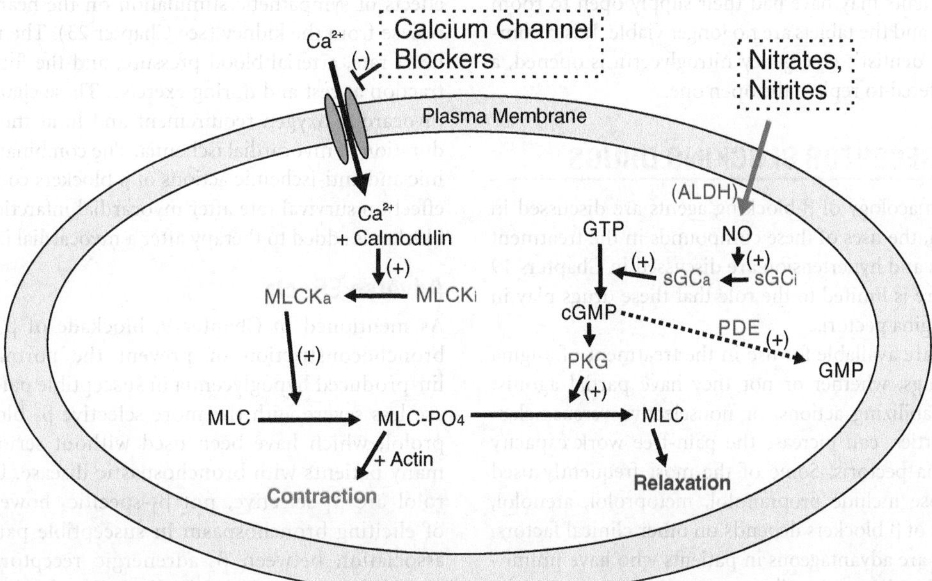

FIG 21-4 Action of calcium channel blockers (*CCBs*) and organic nitrates and nitrites on a vascular smooth muscle cell. CCBs block the influx of calcium through the L-type calcium channel in the plasma membrane. This leads eventually to reduced phosphorylation of myosin light chain (*MLC*) and reduced contraction. Nitrates and nitrites generate nitric oxide (*NO*). NO activates soluble guanylyl cyclase (*sGC*), which catalyzes the synthesis of cyclic GMP (*cGMP*). This leads to activation of cyclic GMP-dependent protein kinase (*PKG*), which results indirectly in the dephosphorylation of the phosphorylated form of myosin light chain and leads to relaxation. The dotted arrow indicates the metabolism of cyclic GMP by phosphodiesterase (*PDE*). This reaction is inhibited by phosphodiesterase-5 inhibitors such as sildenafil (Viagra), which leads to an increase in cyclic GMP and greater relaxation of vascular smooth muscle. This is the reason that nitrates and nitrites are contraindicated when the patient is taking a drug such as sildenafil. The combination can lead to severe hypotension. *ALDH*, Aldehyde dehydrogenase; *GMP*, guanosine monophosphate; *GTP*, guanosine triphosphate; *MLC-PO$_4$*, phosphorylated myosin light chain; *MLCKa*, activated myosin light chain kinase; *MLCKi*, inactive myosin light chain kinase; *sGCa*, activated soluble guanylyl cyclase; *sGCi*, inactive soluble guanylyl cyclase; (+), stimulation.

Adverse Effects

Almost all side effects of these drugs are direct results of their effects on the cardiovascular system. **Headache**, due to dilation of meningeal arteries, is the most common untoward response and can be very severe. Tolerance to this effect may develop in some patients before tolerance to other cardiovascular effects occurs. **Orthostatic hypotension** resulting in **reflex tachycardia**, cerebral ischemia, weakness, dizziness, **flushing**, and **syncope** may follow drug administration. Syncope is likely to occur if the patient is standing and immobile while taking medication or has ingested alcoholic beverages. Because it dramatically reduces placental blood flow, **amyl nitrite** is **contraindicated** for use in pregnant women (**pregnancy risk** category X).

Nitrite ions and high doses of nitrates readily convert hemoglobin to **methemoglobin**; large amounts of methemoglobin can seriously impair the oxygen-carrying capacity of the blood, resulting in anemic hypoxia. Infants are especially sensitive to this effect of nitrates because of their relative inability to reduce methemoglobin back to hemoglobin. Drug rash occasionally may occur, most frequently with topical nitroglycerin.

Nitrates and nitrites should not be taken concurrently with phosphodiesterase-5 inhibitors such as sildenafil. The combination can lead to excessive hypotension. This interaction is depicted in Figure 21-4.

On a clinical note, nitroglycerin tablets are manufactured and packaged in vials filled with pure nitrogen gas to avoid oxidation. Once the vial is opened for the first time and oxygen is introduced to the tablets, they all begin a slow oxidation process that eventually leads to them being ineffective. This takes around 3 months to occur. This is why dentists should always have a fresh supply of nitroglycerin in his or her emergency kit; the patients may have had their supply open to room air for several months, and the tablets are no longer viable. It is recommended that once the dentist's emergency nitroglycerin is opened, a new vial should be ordered to replace the open one.

β-ADRENERGIC RECEPTOR BLOCKING DRUGS

The history and pharmacology of β-blocking agents are discussed in Chapter 9. In addition, the uses of these compounds in the treatment of cardiac arrhythmias and hypertension are discussed in Chapters 19 and 23. Discussion here is limited to the role that these drugs play in the management of angina pectoris.

Several β blockers are available for use in the treatment of angina pectoris. All these drugs, whether or not they have partial agonist activity, membrane-stabilizing actions, or nonselective versus selective β-blocking properties, can increase the pain-free work capacity of patients with angina pectoris. Some of the most frequently used agents for this purpose include propranolol, metoprolol, atenolol, and nadolol. Selection of β blockers depends on other clinical factors. Cardioselective agents are advantageous in patients who have pulmonary disease or peripheral vascular disease. Consideration must be given to the dosage used, however, because all β-blocking drugs have nonselective effects at higher dosages (see Chapter 9).

Pharmacologic Effects

Because exercise and emotional stress are possible precipitating factors in angina (see Fig. 21-1), increases in sympathetic nervous system activity can bring on attacks of angina in susceptible individuals. The blockade of adrenergic responses can be beneficial in the treatment of this condition. Effects of β blockers that are helpful in treating angina include decreased heart rate and protection from reflex tachycardia, depressed myocardial contractility, decreased cardiac output, and reduced blood pressure. Therefore there is a reduction in cardiac oxygen demand, and anginal pain is less likely. These effects are more prominent when sympathetic activity is elevated, such as during exercise or emotional stress. Total coronary blood flow may be reduced after β receptor blockade, but this reduction in flow seems to be in well-perfused areas and is not detrimental in classic angina. Drug-induced vasoconstriction (from unopposed α-adrenergic receptor activity) may be problematic, however, in patients with variant angina.

Absorption, Fate, and Excretion

The absorption, fate, and excretion of β-adrenergic receptor antagonists are discussed in Chapter 9.

Use in Treatment of Angina

Most β blockers are effective in treating the various types of angina pectoris. Their use is questionable, however, in the management of variant angina in the absence of other drugs. Long-term administration of β blockers can make the attacks of angina less frequent and individual attacks less severe. Nonetheless, patients receiving long-term treatment with β-blocking agents usually still require nitroglycerin for the treatment of acute anginal attacks. Nitrates and β-adrenergic antagonists often work well together in angina because β blockers inhibit the reflex tachycardia caused by nitrates, and nitrates (by causing vasodilation) reduce the preload and afterload of the heart and therefore reduce the impact of a negative inotropic effect from β receptor blockade.

Use in Preventing Future Myocardial Infarctions

The primary cardiovascular actions of β blockers are to inhibit the effects of sympathetic stimulation on the heart and to reduce renin release from the kidney (see Chapter 23). The result is a reduction in heart rate, arterial blood pressure, and the force of myocardial contraction at rest and during exercise. These changes reduce the overall myocardial oxygen requirement and limit the intensity, extent, and duration of myocardial ischemia. The combination of the antiarrhythmic and anti-ischemic actions of β blockers contributes to a favorable effect on survival rate after myocardial infarction. For this reason a β blocker is added to therapy after a myocardial infarction.

Adverse Effects

As mentioned in Chapter 9, blockade of β receptors may cause bronchoconstriction or prevent the normal response to insulin-produced hypoglycemia in susceptible patients. These problems are less severe with the more selective $β_1$ blockers, such as metoprolol, which have been used without serious adverse effects in many patients with bronchospastic disease. Drugs such as metoprolol are $β_1$-selective, not $β_1$-specific, however, and are capable of eliciting bronchospasm in susceptible patients. Because of the association between $β_2$-adrenergic receptors and glycogenolysis and gluconeogenesis in the liver, $β_1$-selective blockers are associated with less risk of hypoglycemic reactions in diabetics than the nonselective β receptor blockers.

A problem encountered with both selective and nonselective blockers, because they block cardiac β receptors, is myocardial depression and heart failure if initial dosages are too high or if there is concomitant myocardial incompetence (see Chapter 20 for a discussion of the use of β blockers in the treatment of heart failure). For this reason, dosages should be gradually increased until concentrations offering therapeutic effects in the management of angina are reached. The sudden discontinuance of β blockers has been implicated in rebound overstimulation of the heart, worsening of angina, and myocardial infarction.

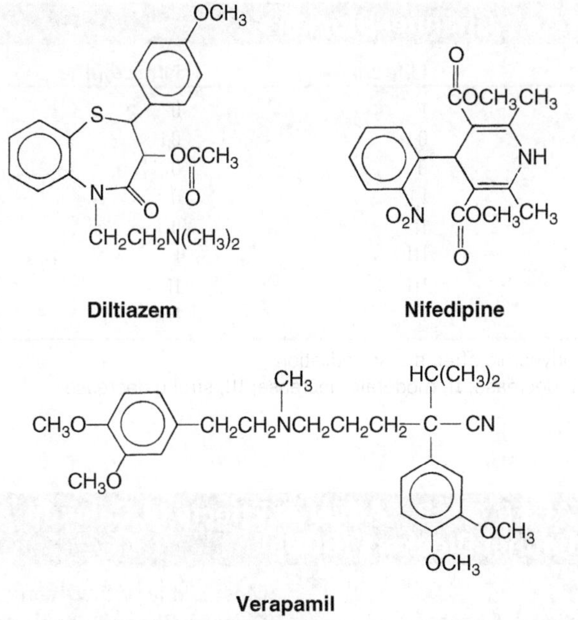

Diltiazem

Nifedipine

Verapamil

FIG 21-5 Structural formulas of three Ca^{2+} channel blockers. The structures of other dihydropyridine calcium channel blockers (most commonly amlodipine) resemble the structure of nifedipine.

CA^{2+} CHANNEL BLOCKERS

Calcium channel blockers (CCBs) include **verapamil** and **diltiazem,** as well as several dihydropyridines represented by **nifedipine.** Many of these compounds are effective in the prophylactic treatment of chronic stable exertional angina, variant angina, and unstable angina. They have also proved to be useful in the treatment of other cardiovascular disorders, such as supraventricular tachyarrhythmias and hypertension (see Chapters 19 and 23). Additional indications for certain CCBs include peripheral vascular disease, pulmonary hypertension, hypertrophic cardiomyopathy, and cerebral vasospasm after subarachnoid hemorrhage.

Chemistry and Classification

Verapamil is a diphenylalkylamine derivative and the only member of its type clinically available. It is closest in pharmacologic profile to diltiazem, a benzothiazepine. The largest category of CCBs consists of dihydropyridines, of which nifedipine is the prototype. Dihydropyridines are characterized by their prominent arterial vasodilatory properties, reduced direct effects, and greater indirect effects on the heart. The structures of the CCBs are shown in Figure 21-5.

Pharmacologic Effects

CCBs relax peripheral and coronary blood vessels (see Fig. 21-2). CCBs exert their primary action on Ca^{2+} channels that carry the slow inward Ca^{2+} current. This and subsequent effects on smooth muscle cells are shown in Figure 21-4. CCBs differ from local anesthetics, which are primarily fast channel blockers inhibiting the rapid inward influx of Na^+. Although the primary action of CCBs is on the slow current, they may also act through other mechanisms. Diltiazem, especially at higher doses, has been shown to depress the Na^+, or fast, channels.

Some of the diverse effects of CCBs can be explained by the roles that Ca^{2+} and slow channels have in different cardiovascular cell types (Box 21-1). In the sinus and atrioventricular (AV) nodes, slow channels are the primary conduit for the generation and propagation of action potentials. They may additionally be involved in regulating sinus node automaticity by altering diastolic depolarization. Ca^{2+} channels also govern conduction velocity in the AV node. The actions of CCBs as antiarrhythmics are discussed in Chapter 19.

BOX 21-1 Cardiovascular Responses to Inhibition of Transmembrane Ca^{2+} Influx by Ca^{2+} Channel Blockers

Myocardium
Excitation-contraction uncoupling
Prevention of Ca^{2+} overload

Specialized Pacemaker and Conducting Tissues
Reduction of automaticity
Damping of ectopic pacemakers
Inhibition of reentrant pathways

Vasculature
Vasodilation
Protection against Ca^{2+} deposition in vessel walls

CCBs directly and preferentially block voltage-dependent Ca^{2+} channels as opposed to receptor-operated channels. By this mechanism, they reduce intracellular Ca^{2+} activity and interfere with the replenishment of Ca^{2+} stores in vascular smooth muscle. Tonic and phasic muscle contractions are depressed in a dose-dependent manner. The various types of voltage-dependent Ca^{2+} channels include *L, N, T, P/Q,* and *R*. Only the L (large, long-lasting current) channel is inhibited by CCBs. Verapamil and diltiazem on the one hand and the nifedipine-like CCBs on the other bind to different receptor sites on the L-type calcium channel. The degree of binding is influenced by the functional state of the channel (resting, open, or inactivated) in a manner similar to the use dependency described for local anesthetics and Na^+ channels (see Chapter 14).

CCBs induce coronary and peripheral arterial dilation. Their action on coronary vessels is especially prominent in vessels that undergo transient vasospasm in variant angina. The vasodilator action in large measure explains their use as antianginals and antihypertensives.

Although all CCBs directly depress the myocardium and slow conduction velocity in the heart, the overall response in vivo depends on the relative mix of direct and indirect effects of each drug on the cardiovascular system. For verapamil and diltiazem, the direct cardiac effects usually predominate (Table 21-2). Nifedipine and other dihydropyridine CCBs typically elicit prominent vasodilation at doses that do not greatly affect Ca^{2+} channels in the heart. Reflex sympathetic activity causes an increase in heart rate and conduction through the AV node and may result in a net positive inotropic effect. Factors that contribute variety to the pharmacologic profile of the different CCBs include the drugs' binding dependence on the frequency of stimulation of the tissue, their binding characteristics to L channels in different tissues, and at least with some agents, their ability to influence other voltage-gated ion channels.

CCBs are important drugs in the treatment of all forms of angina pectoris. They inhibit Ca^{2+} flux in cardiac and smooth muscle and are effective in the treatment of stable angina because of their coronary vasodilator effect, negative inotropic and chronotropic effects (for verapamil and diltiazem), enhancement of diastolic relaxation of the left ventricle (primarily verapamil and diltiazem), and hypotensive effect mediated through peripheral arterial dilation. These effects lead to an increase in coronary blood flow and myocardial perfusion with a decrease in myocardial oxygen demand.

TABLE 21-2 Comparative Pharmacologic Effects of Ca^{2+} Channel Blockers

Parameter	Verapamil	Diltiazem	Nifedipine	Nimodipine
Heart rate	↑,↓	0,↓	↑	0
Sinoatrial node automaticity	↓↓	↓↓	0,↓	0,↓
AV conduction	↓↓↓	↓↓	0	0
Myocardial contractility	↓↓	↓	↓,↑*	0
Cardiac output	↑,↓	0,↑	↑↑	0
Peripheral vascular resistance	↓↓	↓	↓↓↓	↓
Coronary vasodilation	↑↑	↑↑	↑↑↑	↑↑
Cerebral vasodilation	↑	↑	↑	↑↑↑

*The direct myocardial depression of nifedipine is reversed clinically by the hemodynamic effects of vasodilation.
0, No effect; ↑, slight increase; ↑↑, moderate increase; ↑↑↑, strong increase; ↓, slight decrease; ↓↓, moderate decrease; ↓↓↓, strong decrease.
AV, Atrioventricular.

Absorption, Fate, and Excretion

All CCBs are rapidly and almost completely absorbed after oral administration. Bioavailability is reduced, however, by extensive first-pass hepatic metabolism. To extend their duration of action, many CCBs are marketed in sustained-release formulations. Verapamil and diltiazem are converted in part to active metabolites; biotransformation of nifedipine causes complete inactivation. Most CCBs are highly protein bound, especially to plasma albumin. Excretion of the metabolites is primarily by the kidney.

Use in the Treatment of Angina

CCBs as a class have been shown to be effective in the treatment of **all types of angina** regardless of whether coronary spasm is involved. They seem to be especially effective in preventing coronary vasospasm. In chronic stable exertional angina, CCBs may afford relief of pain through one or more mechanisms: coronary and peripheral vasodilation, attenuation of increased heart rate caused by exercise, or a negative inotropic effect on the heart. The latter two characteristics pertain mostly to verapamil and diltiazem.

Adverse Effects

Adverse effects of CCBs may vary with the individual drug; however, many adverse effects are common to all. Typical effects of all include those due to vasodilation. Adverse effects are listed in Table 21-3.

TABLE 21-3 Adverse Effects of Calcium Channel Blockers (CCBs)

Adverse Effect	Most Likely with Which Calcium Channel Blockers
Nausea	All
Dizziness, headache	All
Reduced heart rate and reduced AV node conduction rate*	Verapamil, diltiazem
Tachycardia	Dihydropyridines
Coronary steal caused by abrupt vasodilation from immediate-release CCB therapy†	Dihydropyridines
Gingival hypertrophy‡	All
Peripheral edema	All
Facial flushing	All

*Coadministration with a β-adrenergic receptor blocker poses an added risk.
†Long-acting CCBs are indicated.
‡Clinically and histologically resembles that seen with phenytoin, but it occurs less often and usually less severely than with phenytoin.

SECOND-LINE DRUGS

Ranolazine

Ranolazine is an antianginal agent approved for the treatment of chronic stable angina pectoris for use as combination therapy when angina is not adequately controlled with other antianginal agents.

Chemistry and pharmacologic effects

Ranolazine is a piperazine derivative that inhibits the late Na+ current of the plasma membrane (see Chapter 19). This current may result from ischemia. Inhibition of the late sodium current reduces sodium–calcium exchange, thereby reducing intracellular calcium and diastolic wall tension. This drug exerts its antianginal and anti-ischemic effects without reducing heart rate or blood pressure. The drug can be used in combination with other antianginal drugs or sometimes as monotherapy.

Absorption, fate, and excretion

Ranolazine is administered twice a day by mouth in an extended-release preparation. It undergoes extensive metabolism, some in the intestine and most in the liver. The metabolites are excreted chiefly in the kidney. The terminal half-life of ranolazine is about 7 hours. Ranolazine tends to increase the plasma levels of digoxin and some other drugs. Itraconazole, clarithromycin, and some antivirals increase plasma levels of ranolazine and should not be administered with it. The dosage of ranolazine should be limited when given with verapamil or diltiazem because these drugs tend to inhibit the metabolism of ranolazine.

Adverse effects

Constipation, nausea, dizziness, and headache are the most common adverse effects. Tinnitus, vertigo, and dry mouth may also occur. Some cardiac disorders have been reported. Ranolazine increases the QT interval of the heart. The drug should be avoided in patients with congenital long QT syndromes, patients with tachycardia, and patients taking other medications that increase the QT interval.

Ivabradine

Ivabradine is discussed in Chapter 20 in relation to its use in heart failure. It controls pacemaker activity in the heart and reduces heart rate. The reduction in heart rate results in less cardiac work and enhanced time spent in diastole with longer profusion time for the myocardium.

OTHER SUPPORTIVE DRUGS

ACE inhibitors, by virtue of several of their effects, tend to improve angina pectoris. They reduced the response of the sympathetic nervous system, cause vasodilation of blood vessels including the microvasculature, and improve conditions in heart failure. The pharmacology of heart failure is discussed in Chapter 20.

The HMG-CoA reductase inhibitors (statins) are the most commonly used drugs to control plasma lipids (see Chapter 24). The reduction in cholesterol reduces the risk of atherosclerosis. This has the beneficial effect of reducing coronary artery disease and angina pectoris.

Antiplatelet agents are a heterogeneous group of drugs. Their action is to prevent platelet aggregation and adhesion, thus reducing the risk of platelet clots. The pharmacology of the antiplatelet drugs is discussed in Chapter 26. Aspirin is also discussed in Chapter 17.

Anticoagulant drugs are also discussed in Chapter 26. Certain anticoagulants such as low-molecular-weight heparins are used prophylactically to reduce coronary ischemia.

OTHER DRUGS USED EXTENSIVELY OUTSIDE THE UNITED STATES

Nicorandil is a drug with a dual action. It generates nitric oxide, and it also opens potassium channels in the sarcolemma (ATP-dependent potassium channel). The latter action causes the smooth muscle cell to hyperpolarize and relax, leading to vasodilation of blood vessels.

Trimetazidine has the unique action of inhibiting beta-oxidation and metabolism of fatty acids. Fatty acids are the preferred energy source of the cardiac cells; however, this energy source requires considerable oxygen. A shift to glucose metabolism in the heart reduces oxygen demand and preserves intracellular ATP.

IMPLICATIONS FOR DENTISTRY

Anginal attacks can be precipitated by physical or emotional stress. Because these situations often arise in the dental operatory, dentists must be aware of the symptoms and treatment of angina. A complete medical history reveals whether a patient is being treated for angina. If so, the dentist should ensure that the patient has medication (e.g., nitroglycerin) available before a procedure is performed. The patient will know when an attack is imminent; the patient's medication should be in an easily accessible location such as on a nearby tray or counter. Also, nitroglycerin should be included in the dentist's emergency kit. Although nitroglycerin tablets are now stabilized against breakdown, unused tablets should be discarded 3 months after the original bottle has been opened because of oxidation, volatilization, and adsorption of the drug to the wall of the container.

If a patient experiences angina pain in the dental office, stop the procedure. The patient should be placed in a semireclined position and oxygen administered. Continually monitor vital signs, particularly blood pressure. A nitroglycerin tablet (0.4 mg) should be placed under the tongue. If pain does not subside after approximately 3 to 5 minutes, readminister nitroglycerin. Repeat this procedure again if necessary. If pain is not relieved after three administrations, the patient should be taken to the hospital because the patient may be experiencing a myocardial infarction. Nitroglycerin should be avoided in patients who are hypotensive or may have taken **phosphodiesterase-5 (PDE-5) inhibitors** in the last 24 hours. If such drugs were taken and the

TABLE 21-4 Elimination Half-Lives of Phosphodiesterase-5 Inhibitors

Drug	Half-Life (hr)
Sildenafil (Viagra)	4-5
Tadalafil (Cialis)	17
Vardenafil (Levitra)	4-5
Avanafil (Stendra)	5

blood pressure is normal or high, it is reasonable to treat the angina with nitroglycerin. If the blood pressure is marginal or low, do not give the nitroglycerin, but instead move the patient to a hospital emergency department. The combination of the vasodilatory effects of the PDE-5s and nitroglycerin can lead to hypotension with potentially serious effects. Table 21-4 lists the elimination half-lives of the PDE-5 inhibitors.

In most cases, anginal pain subsides rapidly (2 to 3 minutes), and the patient may have a headache or a stinging sensation under the tongue or both. As a precaution, patients should be treated carefully, be fully informed about the procedure, and if they feel it necessary, be given prophylactic medication. Preoperative sedation may be helpful and is not contraindicated if significant cardiovascular depression is avoided.

The use of epinephrine in gingival retraction cord is contraindicated in patients with angina pectoris because of the potential for an excessive workload on the heart. Similar considerations dictate prudence with, although not avoidance of, adrenergic vasoconstrictors injected with local anesthetics. Orthostatic hypotension might be a problem in patients receiving CCBs, but cardiac depression is not usually clinically significant. Sensations of heat or facial flushing may be evident in these patients.

As previously mentioned, **gingival overgrowth** and inflammation occasionally develop in patients as a result of therapy with CCBs, especially when taken concurrently with other agents that promote gingival enlargement (e.g., phenytoin, cyclosporine). Strict oral hygiene measures, including regular dental prophylaxis, reduce this problem.

CASE DISCUSSION

Mr. G's pain is most likely due to angina pectoris, and the acute symptoms that he is experiencing are typical of anginal pain. The patient should be placed in a semireclined position and oxygen 2 to 4 L/min started via nasal cannula or nitrous mask. Nitroglycerin (0.4-mg tablet) should next be administered sublingually. Ideally the patient will have his supply of nitroglycerin that has been provided to him by his cardiologist; if so, use a tablet from his supply. If he has none, or if his medication is likely to be oxidized and inefficacious, use a tablet from your emergency kit. Wait approximately 3 to 5 minutes, and if the pain has not abated, give another 0.4-mg dose of the nitroglycerin. Repeat a 0.4-mg dose a third time if pain is still present. After the third dose and about 12 to 15 minutes after the first dose, if the pain has not remitted, arrangements should be made to immediately transport the patient to a hospital for evaluation and treatment. The patient may be experiencing myocardial infarction and should be assessed immediately. Of course, at any time if the patient is decompensating and becoming worrisome to the dentist, emergency services should be called regardless of the status of the nitroglycerin doses.

The earlier initial pain in the jaw was most likely due to angina pectoris even though its presentation was somewhat atypical since little substernal pain accompanied the initial jaw pain.

DRUGS USED IN THE TREATMENT OF ANGINA PECTORIS

Nonproprietary (Generic) Name	Proprietary (Trade) Name
Nitrates and Nitrites	
Amyl nitrite	—
Isosorbide dinitrate	Isordil, Sorbitrate, Isochron, Dilatrate SR, ISDN, Isordil Titradose
Isosorbide mononitrate	ISMO, Imdur, Monoket
Nitroglycerin	Nitro-Bid, Nitro-time, Nitro-Dur, Nitrek, NitroQuick, Nitrostat, Nitroglyn E-R, NitroMist, Rectiv, Transderm-Nitro, Nitrolingual pump spray
β-Adrenergic Blocking Drugs	
Atenolol	Tenormin
Betaxolol	Kerlone
Bisoprolol	Zebeta
Carvedilol	Coreg
Labetalol	Normodyne
Metoprolol	Lopressor, Toprol XL
Nadolol	Corgard
Propranolol	Inderal
See other β-adrenergic blocking drugs in Chapter 9.	
Ca^{2+} Channel Blockers	
Amlodipine	Norvasc
Diltiazem	Cardizem, Dilacor XR
Felodipine	Plendil
Isradipine	DynaCirc
Nicardipine	Cardene
Nifedipine	Adalat, Procardia
Nimodipine	Nimotop
Nisoldipine	Sular
Verapamil	Calan, Isoptin, Verelan
Other Drugs	
Ranolazine	Ranexa
Ivabradine	Corlanor
Nicorandil*	Ikorel
Trimetazidine*	Vastarel
Antiplatelet Agents	
See Chapter 26	
Cholesterol-Lowering Drugs	
See Chapter 24	
Anticoagulants	
See Chapter 26	

*Not available in the United States.

GENERAL REFERENCES

1. Angiolillo DJ, Ferreiro JL: Antiplatelet and anticoagulant therapy for atherothrombotic disease: the role of current and emerging agents, *Am J Cardiovasc Drugs* 13:233–250, 2013.
2. Cattaneo M, Porretta P, Gallino A: Ranolazine: drug overview and possible role in primary microvascular angina management, *Int J Cardiol* 181:376–381, 2015.
3. Chen Z, Foster MW, Zhang J, et al.: An essential role for mitochondrial aldehyde dehydrogenase in nitroglycerin bioactivation, *Proc Natl Acad Sci USA* 102:12159–12164, 2005.
4. Cooper-DeHoff RM, Chang SW, Peping CJ: Calcium antagonists in the treatment of coronary artery disease, *Curr Opin Pharmacol* 13:301–308, 2013.
5. Fox K, Ford I, Steg PG, et al.: On behalf of the BEAUTIFUL investigators: Ivabradine for patients with stable coronary artery disease and left ventricular systolic dysfunction (BEAUTIFUL): a randomized, double blind, placebo-controlled trial, *Lancet* 372:807–816, 2008.
6. Frishman WH: β-Adrenergic blockade in cardiovascular disease, *J Cardiovasc Pharmacol Ther* 18:310–319, 2013.
7. Lanza GA, Parrinello R, Figliozzi S: Management of microvascular angina pectoris, *Am J Cardiovascular Drugs* 14:31–40, 2014.
8. Petersen JW, Pepine CJ: Microvascular coronary dysfunction and ischemic heart disease: where are we in 2014? *Trends Cardiovasc Med* 25:98–103, 2015.
9. Tarkin JM, Kaski JC: Pharmacological treatment of chronic stable angina pectoris, *Clin Med* 13:63–70, 2013.
10. Thadani U, Rodgers T: Side effects of nitrates to treat angina, *Expert Opin Drug Saf* 5:667–674, 2006.

22

Diuretic Drugs

William B. Jeffries and Dennis W. Wolff

KEY INFORMATION

- Diuretics increase urine flow, typically by blocking reabsorption of filtered Na^+ in the kidney (i.e., they are natriuretics).
- Natriuretic diuretics are broadly divided into K^+-sparing and K^+-losing agents and can be combined to achieve greater natriuresis with lesser kaliuresis.
- K^+-sparing diuretics used alone produce a small natriuresis by blocking Na^+/K^+ exchange in the cortical collecting tubule, either by antagonizing the actions of the mineralocorticoid hormone aldosterone (e.g., spironolactone) or by blocking apical Na^+ channels in the principal cells (e.g., amiloride, triamterene).
- Diuretics that block Na^+ reabsorption upstream from the Na^+/K^+ exchanger cause K^+ loss as some of that tubular fluid Na^+ is now reabsorbed via this mechanism.
- Thiazide diuretics (e.g., hydrochlorothiazide, chlorthalidone, metolazone) are K^+-losing diuretics that block the Na^+-Cl^- cotransporter in the distal convoluted tubule to cause a moderate diuresis; Ca^{2+} is not lost.
- Thiazide or thiazide-type diuretics are most commonly used alone or in combination with other drugs to treat hypertension, but they also have an adjunct role in the treatment of edema.
- Loop diuretics (e.g., furosemide, bumetanide, torsemide, ethacrynic acid) are K^+-losing (and Ca^{2+}- and Mg^{++}-losing) diuretics that block the Na^+, K^+, $2Cl^-$ cotransporter in the thick ascending limb of Henle to cause a potentially maximal diuresis.
- Loop diuretics impair the formation of the dilute tubular fluid needed for a dilute urine while also disrupting the medullary osmotic gradient needed to excrete concentrated urine, thereby causing urine osmolality to become closer to plasma osmolality irrespective of plasma ADH levels.
- Loop diuretics are used primarily to mobilize the edematous fluid associated with heart, liver, or kidney failure and are also useful for treating hypertension in patients with poor kidney function.
- Aquaretics (e.g., conivaptan, tolvaptan) exert their effects by blocking ADH-regulated water reabsorption by the collecting duct and can be used to help correct the hyponatremia associated with congestive heart failure and the syndrome of inappropriate antidiuretic hormone.
- Most adverse effects associated with diuretic use are related to plasma volume contraction and/or the abnormal plasma electrolyte concentrations (e.g., K^+, Na^+, HCO_3^-, and Ca^{2+}) caused by the elimination of body fluid volume and electrolytes in the urine.
- Nonsteroidal antiinflammatory drugs (NSAIDs) can interfere with diuretic effects in compromised kidneys.
- The use of digoxin and diuretics together to treat congestive heart failure requires careful monitoring since digoxin efficacy/toxicity varies inversely with the plasma K^+ concentration.

CASE STUDY

A 73-year-old man crossing the street at an intersection collided with a bicyclist weaving between cars. His mouth was struck by the bicycle handlebar and teeth #12, 13, 14, 19, and 20 were broken. He is to be scheduled for sedation dentistry to begin the process of repairing this damage. His past medical history includes a myocardial infarction for which he now takes doses of atorvastatin, lisinopril, carvedilol, furosemide, digoxin, and spironolactone at approximately 7 am and additional doses of furosemide and carvedilol at approximately 7 pm. Comment on the potential problems associated with sedation dentistry in this patient and when during the day he might tolerate this procedure best. Which class of analgesics should not be used to treat dental pain in this patient? Family members caring for this patient ask if he should brush his teeth with Sensodyne® (active ingredients: 5% potassium nitrate, 0.15% sodium fluoride). Why is that a potential cause for concern?

The kidney serves the vital function of maintaining fluid and electrolyte homeostasis. Through the processes of glomerular filtration and selective tubular reabsorption and secretion, the kidney maintains plasma volume and the plasma concentration of electrolytes, glucose, amino acids, and other substances within tight physiologic limits, while eliminating metabolic waste products and toxins. The kidneys filter approximately 180 L of plasma each day, one-fifth of the cardiac out, producing approximately 1.5 L of urine.

The kidney selectively reabsorbs approximately 99% of the filtered load of water and solute. Many of the filtered solutes are reabsorbed by specific transport proteins located on the luminal membrane of the nephron. When inside of a nephron cell, solute movement back into the plasma is often directly or indirectly coupled to the actions of Na^+-K^+-activated adenosine triphosphatase (Na^+, K^+-ATPase) located on the basolateral surfaces of the nephron cells. Transepithelial electrochemical potential differences can also drive the reabsorption of various ions by paracellular pathways.

The reabsorption of water in the kidney is passive, following osmotic gradients created by the movement of solutes along the nephrons to the extent permitted by the water permeability of the various segments of the nephron. Water rapidly equilibrates across the nephron as solute is reabsorbed from the tubular fluid or in response to the medullary osmotic gradient as it descends toward the tip of the loop of Henle. The ascending portion of the nephron is relatively impermeable to water, however.

The selective reabsorption of solute while trapping water in the lumen in these regions creates the dilute tubular fluid that could ultimately become maximally diluted urine. The solute selectively reabsorbed during the passage of tubular fluid through the ascending loop of Henle creates the medullary osmotic gradient that pulls water from the tubular fluid of the descending loop of Henle and the collecting duct. With the exception of the terminal portions of the collecting duct, where urea is recycled from concentrated urine, relatively little net solute reabsorption occurs in this nephron segment. Instead, this is the portion of the nephron that governs water reabsorption.

Antidiuretic hormone (ADH), also known as *vasopressin*, determines the extent to which this segment is permeable to water. If ADH is absent, the tubular fluid that reaches the collecting duct becomes, after some solute exchange, the maximally diluted excreted urine. If the collecting duct is responding maximally to ADH, the most concentrated urine that the kidney can generate is excreted; ADH makes collecting duct cells permeable to water, which permits passive water extraction from the tubular fluid as it passes through the progressively more concentrated osmotic gradient of the medullary interstitium. The more solute that reaches the collecting duct, the greater is the volume of urine for any amount of ADH.

Renal function can become disturbed in many clinical conditions, producing metabolic abnormalities such as edema. There is a therapeutic need for drugs that modulate renal function.

All of the drugs discussed in this chapter affect renal function by inhibiting the reabsorptive capacity of the renal nephrons. This action produces an increase in the rate of urine production. Substances that increase the quantity of urine are called **diuretics**. Many substances produce this effect, including caffeine, alcohol, and water itself; however, most clinically useful diuretics produce their effects by inhibiting Na^+ reabsorption by the nephrons. Such drugs are properly called **natriuretics**; even so, in most circumstances, all these drugs are referred to as *diuretics*. All clinically useful diuretics produce their effects by acting at specific segments of the nephron. Common conditions for which diuretics are used include primary hypertension and congestive heart failure.

CLASSES OF DIURETICS

This discussion of diuretics proceeds up the nephron in a retrograde direction. As shown in Figure 22-1, this order of consideration moves from diuretics with a low maximal effect to diuretics with a high maximal effect. The effects of blockade of Na^+ upstream on tubular fluid composition are acted on by downstream mechanisms—mechanisms that act to limit or offset these effects. The effects of the various classes of diuretics on urine volume, urine pH, and urine electrolytes are summarized in Table 22-1.

K^+-Sparing Diuretics

The pathway by which Na^+ is reabsorbed in the late distal tubule/cortical collecting duct is shown in Figure 22-2. The apical membrane of these cells contains Na^+ channels. The primary purpose of these channels is to recover filtered Na^+. The entry of Na^+ through these channels carries a net positive charge along with it (i.e., Na^+ entry is electrogenic), leaving the lumen with a net negative charge. This negative charge in the lumen acts as a driving force for movement in the opposite direction of other cytosolic cations such as K^+ and H^+ from

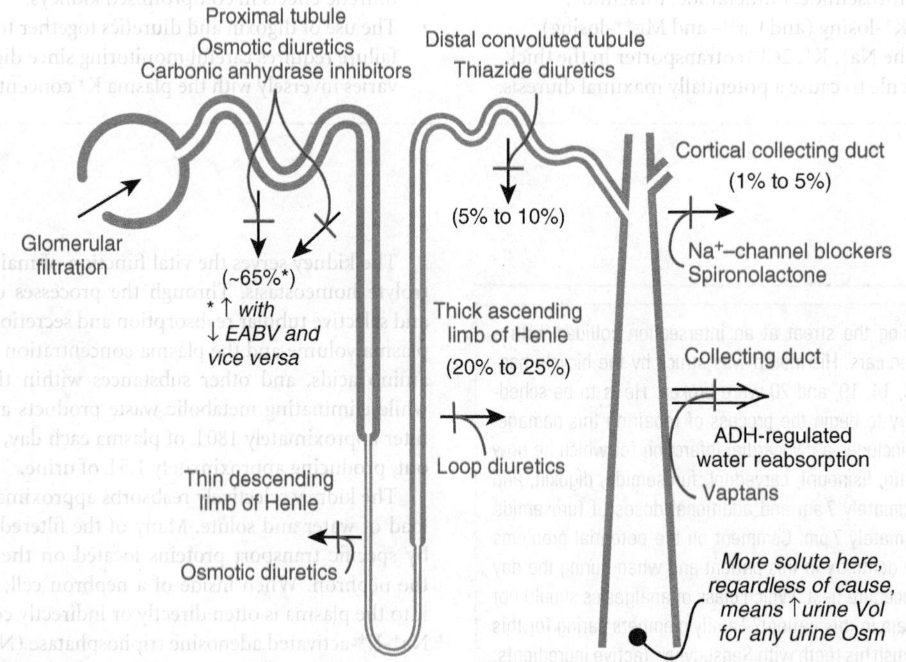

FIG 22-1 Sites of action of diuretics along the nephron. The percentages shown illustrate the approximate amount of the filtered load of Na^+ that is reabsorbed by each nephron segment. Spironolactone exerts its effects by blocking the intracellular aldosterone receptor and the vaptans block ADH receptors on the basolateral membrane. The remaining diuretics exert their effects at the tubular lumen to prevent reabsorption of solute and water. *EABV*, Effective arterial blood volume; *Osm*, osmolality.

TABLE 22-1 Summary of Urinary Effects and Mechanisms of Action of Diuretic Drugs

	Volume (mL/min)	pH	Na^+	$U_{Na}V$	K^+	U_KV	Cl^-	HCO_3^-	$U_{HCO3}V$	Mechanism of Action
Control	1	6	50	50	15	15	60	1	1	—
Thiazides (e.g., hydrochlorothiazide)	3	7.4	150	450	25	75	150	25	75	Decreases Na^+ and Cl^- cotransport in distal tubule*
Loop diuretics (e.g., furosemide)	8	6	140	1120	10	80	155	1	8	Decreases Na^+, K^+, $2Cl^-$ cotransport in medullary ascending loop of Henle
Amiloride, triamterene	2	7.2	130	260	5	10	120	15	30	Decreases Na^+ reabsorption in late distal tubule and collecting ducts; less K^+ secretion and Na^+-H^+ exchange
Spironolactone	2	7.2	125	250	5	10	120	15	30	Inhibits aldosterone receptor activation; net effects similar to effects of amiloride
Carbonic anhydrase inhibitors (e.g., acetazolamide)	3	8.2	70	210	60	180	15	120	360	Inhibits carbonic anhydrase and H^+ production in proximal tubules; less Na^+ and HCO_3^- reabsorption
Osmotic diuretics (e.g., mannitol)	10	6.5	90	900	15	150	110	4	40	Osmotically retains water in proximal tubule and loop of Henle

Values are average peak diuretic responses in humans with a normal water and electrolyte balance. Electrolyte concentrations are given in mEq/L. $U_{Na}V$, U_KV and $U_{HCO3}V$ are rates of excretion of Na^+, K^+, and HCO_3^-, respectively, and given in μEq/minute.
*Thiazide diuretics also variably inhibit carbonic anhydrase.

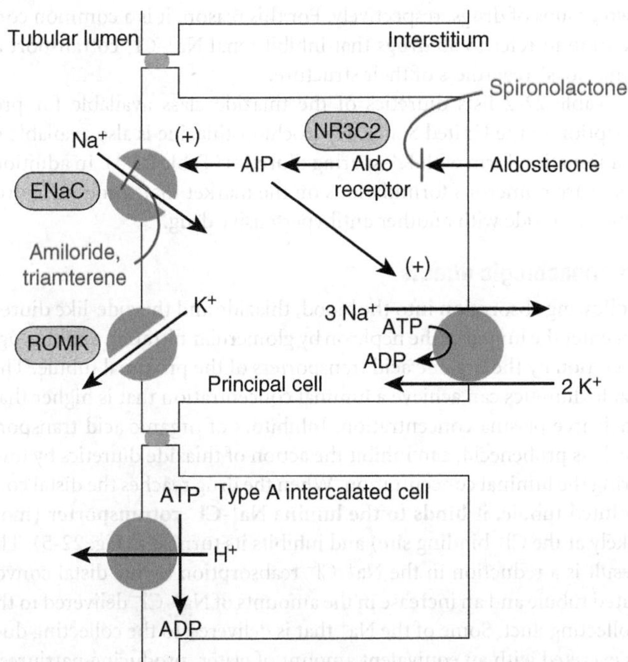

FIG 22-2 Actions of K^+-sparing diuretics in the cortical collecting duct. In this segment, Na^+ is transported passively into the principal cells through ENaC Na^+ channels located on the apical membrane. The conductance of this channel is enhanced by an aldosterone-induced protein (*AIP*). The apical entry of Na^+ (removal of positive charges) creates a negative electrostatic driving force in the lumen that enhances the secretion of K^+ via ROMK K^+ channels from principal cells and H^+ from type A intercalated cells. Amiloride and triamterene are antagonists of apical membrane Na^+ channels. Spironolactone, by antagonizing the action of aldosterone at its nuclear hormone receptor (NR3C2 receptor), prevents AIP activation of Na^+ conductance. Either of these mechanisms can produce a mild natriuresis with a K^+-sparing effect. *ADP*, Adenosine diphosphate; *ATP*, adenosine triphosphate; *ENaC*, epithelial sodium channel.

the collecting duct cells (see Fig. 22-2), resulting in net Na^+ retention and K^+ excretion. This latter process is referred to as **Na^+/K^+ exchange.** Aldosterone, acting through nuclear receptors in the principal cells of the cortical collecting duct, enhances the conductance of these apical Na^+ channels, increasing Na^+/K^+ exchange. Diuretics that act further upstream to block Na^+ reabsorption and increase distal Na^+ delivery to the collecting duct promote Na^+/K^+ exchange, resulting in enhanced urinary excretion of K^+.

Pharmacologic effects

K^+-sparing diuretics are so named because, by blocking Na^+ reabsorption in the cortical collecting duct region of the nephron, they do not produce the hypokalemic effects of the other natriuretic drugs. The three drugs of this class—**spironolactone, triamterene, and amiloride**—are structurally dissimilar (Fig. 22-3), but each produces similar effects (mild natriuresis with a decrease in K^+ excretion) because of the **blockade of Na^+ reabsorption** by this segment. Spironolactone is a 17-spirolactone steroid that is structurally similar to aldosterone and functions as an aldosterone antagonist. Triamterene, a pteridine derivative with structural similarities to folic acid, and amiloride, a pyrazine derivative, exert similar effects by directly blocking the apical membrane Na^+ channels of the principal cells of the collecting duct. By preventing Na^+ entry into these cells, these diuretics reduce the electrogenic driving force for K^+ or H^+, or both, in this segment. The net effect is a mild diuresis with a K^+-sparing effect.

The amount of additional Na^+ excretion and K^+ retention is small when drugs of this class are administered alone. When natriuresis from other drugs is present, the capacity of K^+-sparing diuretic to inhibit K^+ excretion is significantly increased. This characteristic provides the rationale for combining loop and thiazide diuretics with a K^+-sparing diuretic to prevent hypokalemia.

Absorption, fate, and excretion

Spironolactone is administered orally and is rapidly absorbed. The onset of action takes 2 to 4 days, however, and full clinical efficacy is

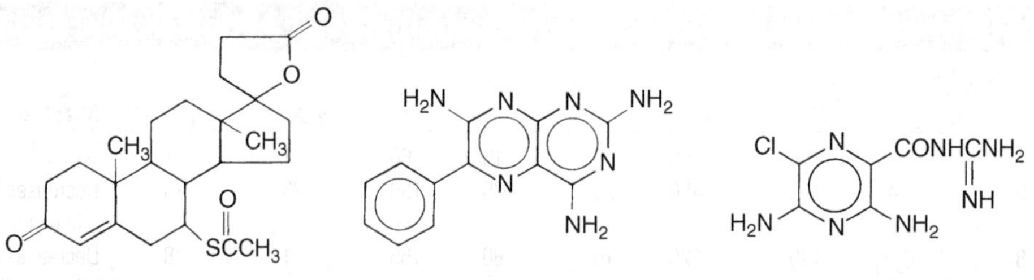

Spironolactone Triamterene Amiloride

FIG 22-3 Structural formulas of K^+-sparing diuretics.

not seen for several weeks. Spironolactone is metabolized by the liver and has two active metabolites, canrenone and canrenoate. Canrenone is prescribed as a K^+-sparing diuretic in Europe.

Amiloride is given orally, despite its poor gastrointestinal absorption. Diuresis begins within 2 hours, and its duration of action is approximately 24 hours. Amiloride does not undergo metabolism and is excreted unchanged in the urine and feces. Triamterene is better absorbed by the gastrointestinal tract and produces a response within 2 hours of administration. Triamterene has a short plasma half-life and is extensively metabolized to products that are excreted in the urine and feces. The duration of diuresis is longer (approximately 14 hours), however, because the hydroxylated metabolites are also active Na^+ channel blockers.

Therapeutic uses

K^+-sparing diuretics are most often used to **prevent hypokalemia** caused by thiazide and loop diuretics. Spironolactone, triamterene, and amiloride are each **available in combination with thiazide diuretics to facilitate this use. Spironolactone is also sometimes used in the treatment of hyperaldosteronism.** Spironolactone and **eplerenone** also have been found to be useful in the treatment of **congestive heart failure** (see Chapter 20). Plasma aldosterone concentration is inappropriately elevated in patients with congestive heart failure, and it contributes to the development of edema, direct hypertrophic effects on the myocardium, and other adverse effects in heart failure. Spironolactone effectively antagonizes these effects and has been shown to reduce the mortality rate of patients with congestive heart failure, but the increased risk for hyperkalemia necessitates careful monitoring of the plasma K^+ concentration.

Adverse effects

The primary toxic effect of K^+-sparing diuretics is **hyperkalemia.** This effect is most common when these drugs are given without another diuretic or concomitantly with other inhibitors of K^+ excretion, such as angiotensin-converting enzyme inhibitors or angiotensin II receptor antagonists. Dietary K^+ supplementation can also precipitate hyperkalemia in patients taking these drugs. Hyperkalemia is infrequent when these drugs are administered in the presence of loop or thiazide diuretics, but using multiple drugs simultaneously as happens during the treatment of congestive heart failure creates challenges. Spironolactone, because of its steroid structure, can also produce gynecomastia and/or decreased libido in men. Menstrual irregularities have been reported for women. Eplerenone is an aldosterone antagonist similar to spironolactone with fewer undesirable effects at sex hormone receptors. Triamterene and amiloride infrequently cause other effects, such as nausea and vomiting, muscle cramping, and dizziness. Triamterene can sometimes accumulate in the renal pelvis and produce renal stones.

Thiazide Diuretics

Benzthiazide diuretics (commonly referred to as **thiazides**) are derived from 1,2,4-benzothiadiazine-7-sulfonamide 1,1 dioxide (Fig. 22-4). Chlorothiazide **inhibits Na^+-Cl^- cotransport in the distal nephron,**

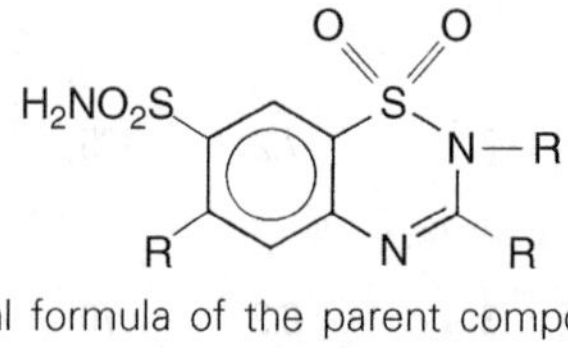

FIG 22-4 Structural formula of the parent compound of the thiazide diuretics.

which produces a large increase in the excretion of NaCl and reduction of extracellular fluid volume. Structural congeners of chlorothiazide, including hydrochlorothiazide, hydroflumethiazide, and methyclothiazide, also share this mechanism. Several other compounds (chlorthalidone, indapamide, metolazone, and quinethazone) that are not structurally related to thiazides also inhibit renal Na^+-Cl^- cotransport and produce natriuresis and diuresis that are indistinguishable from thiazides. Thiazide-type and thiazide-like are designations for these two groups of drugs, respectively. For this reason, it is a common convention to refer to all drugs that inhibit renal Na^+-Cl^- cotransport as "thiazides" regardless of their structure.

Table 22-2 lists diuretics of the thiazide class available for prescription in the United States. Hydrochlorothiazide is also available in combination form with K^+-sparing diuretics (Table 22-3). In addition, there are numerous formulations on the market that combine hydrochlorothiazide with another antihypertensive drug.

Pharmacologic effects

Following absorption into the blood, thiazide and thiazide-like diuretics enter the lumen of the nephron by glomerular filtration and through secretion by the organic acid transporters of the proximal tubule. Thiazide diuretics can achieve a luminal concentration that is higher than their free plasma concentration. Inhibitors of organic acid transport, such as probenecid, can inhibit the action of thiazide diuretics by lowering the luminal concentration. When the drug reaches the distal convoluted tubule, it **binds to the lumina Na^+-Cl^- cotransporter** (most likely at the Cl^- binding site) and inhibits its turnover (Fig. 22-5). The result is a reduction in the Na^+-Cl^- reabsorption by the distal convoluted tubule and an increase in the amounts of Na^+-Cl^- delivered to the collecting duct. Some of the Na^+ that is delivered to the collecting duct is excreted with an equivalent amount of water, producing natriuresis and diuresis, and some is reabsorbed in the cortical collecting duct as it is **exchanged for K^+ or H^+.** The increased excretion of K^+ (kaliuresis) can result in clinically significant reductions in circulating K^+ (hypokalemia). Increased H^+ excretion can lead to metabolic alkalosis.

In addition to increasing the excretion of Na^+, Cl^-, and K^+, thiazide diuretics **increase the reabsorption of filtered Ca^{2+}.** This action distinguishes thiazides from loop diuretics, which promote Ca^{2+} excretion. The mechanism for this action is not completely understood, but Ca^{2+} reabsorption apparently is increased at the proximal tubule as a result of decreased glomerular filtration (because of reduced plasma volume) and at the distal convoluted tubule as a direct result of

TABLE 22-2 **Thiazide and Thiazide-Like Drugs Currently Available in the United States**

Drug	Proprietary (Trade) Name	Daily Dose (mg)	Half-Life (hr)	Duration of Diuretic Action (hr)
Bendroflumethiazide	Naturetin	2.5-10	8.5	6-12
Chlorothiazide	Diuril	500-1000	1-2	6-12
Chlorthalidone	Hygroton	50-100	35-50	48-72
Hydrochlorothiazide	HydroDIURIL, Microzide, Esidrix, Oretic	12.5-100	5.6-14.8	6-12
Indapamide	Lozol	1.25-5	14-18	12-24
Methyclothiazide	Aquatensen, Enduron	2.5-10	NA	>24
Metolazone	Diulo, Zaroxolyn	2.5-10	14	12-24

TABLE 22-3 **Thiazide and K^+-Sparing Combination Drugs**

Proprietary (Trade) Name	Thiazide	Additional Drug
Moduretic	Hydrochlorothiazide 50 mg	Amiloride 5 mg
Aldactazide, Spirozide	Hydrochlorothiazide 25 mg	Spironolactone 25 mg
Aldactazide	Hydrochlorothiazide 50 mg	Spironolactone 50 mg
Maxzide	Hydrochlorothiazide 25 mg	Triamterene 37.5 mg
	Hydrochlorothiazide 50 mg	Triamterene 75 mg

Na^+-Cl^- cotransport inhibition. Ca^{2+} influx into the distal convoluted cells is governed in part by hormones such as parathyroid hormone, and its efflux is powered by a basolateral Na^+/Ca^{2+} exchanger (see Fig. 22-5). Less Na^+ inside the cell from blockade of apical Na^+-Cl^- cotransport creates a larger gradient for the influx of extracellular Na^+ through the basolateral Na^+/Ca^{2+} exchanger, resulting in increased Ca^{2+} reabsorption. Mg^{++} reabsorption is also initially increased by thiazides, likely in a similar manner, but thiazides **ultimately cause Mg^{++} loss** that is perhaps secondary to the effects of the associated K^+ loss on Mg^{++} reabsorption in the thick ascending limb. Depending on their structure, some thiazides are also weak inhibitors of carbonic anhydrase; this may result in alkalinization of the urine from increased HCO_3^- excretion.

At the level of the whole organism, long-term administration of a thiazide diuretic produces a reduction in the extracellular fluid volume. The decrease in blood volume activates the renin-angiotensin system, causing angiotensin II-mediated aldosterone release from the adrenal gland. Aldosterone acts on the cortical collecting duct to increase the conductance of the principal cell Na^+ channels. Blood volume reduction leads to aldosterone-induced increases in the recovery of Na^+ in the cortical collecting duct, which increases the excretion of K^+ in this segment further. Thiazides also lead to a **long-term decrease in blood pressure**. The mechanism for this effect is controversial. A reduction in blood volume would be expected to decrease arterial blood pressure. Blood volume returns to near-normal values, however, after several weeks of thiazide administration, but the antihypertensive action persists. A direct vascular effect—vasodilation caused by reductions in vascular Na^+ content—has been proposed to explain the continued reduction in total peripheral resistance that persists during thiazide administration.

Absorption, fate, and excretion

Absorption of thiazides from the gastrointestinal tract varies with the particular agent. The plasma elimination half-life and duration of diuretic effect for each of the thiazide diuretics are listed in Table 22-2. Plasma protein binding varies considerably among this class of drugs. The parent compounds or metabolites or both are primarily excreted through renal elimination after glomerular filtration and secretion in the proximal tubule.

Therapeutic uses

Thiazide diuretics are primarily used to treat primary hypertension. The Joint National Commission 8 and the World Health Organization recommend thiazide diuretics as a first-line treatment for primary **hypertension** because of their demonstrated efficacy and low cost (see also Chapter 23). The antihypertensive dosage of thiazide diuretics should normally not exceed the equivalent of 25 mg/day of hydrochlorothiazide because clinical studies have shown that doses greater than this produce equivalent antihypertensive effects but greater toxicity. Thiazide diuretics can be given as monotherapy for primary hypertension or as an adjunct agent. Thiazide diuretics enhance the effectiveness of most other antihypertensive agents, especially vasodilators such as hydralazine and minoxidil, which by themselves promote volume expansion. Thiazide diuretics can also mobilize mild edema and are sometimes used for this purpose, but loop diuretics are generally used to treat edema.

In some individuals, excessive Ca^{2+} excretion promotes the formation of calcium oxalate kidney stones. Thiazide diuretics can be used to **lower the concentration of Ca^{2+} in the excreted urine**, an effect that can help prevent the formation of renal stones.

Thiazides are also sometimes (paradoxically) used in the treatment of polyuria of **nephrogenic diabetes insipidus**, which is caused by a loss in renal responsiveness to antidiuretic hormone. Patients with this condition have a high flow rate of dilute urine. The plasma volume contraction that occurs from thiazide diuretic use leads to a decreased glomerular filtration rate and other compensatory changes that increase Na^+-Cl^- reabsorption in the proximal nephron. Less delivery of water to the collecting duct in nephrogenic diabetes insipidus produces a lower urine volume.

Adverse effects

Thiazide diuretics are generally safe and effective drugs. Toxicity usually is a result of plasma electrolyte disturbances, which can result in extracellular volume depletion, hyponatremia, and hypokalemia. Most prevalent among these is hypokalemia, which results from the combined effects of volume depletion–induced aldosterone release and increased delivery of Na^+ and Cl^- to the collecting duct. Both of these effects increase reabsorption of Na^+ through apical channels in the cortical collecting duct, which increases the driving force for the secretion of K^+.

Hypokalemia reduces the resting membrane potential, decreasing the likelihood of action potentials in nerves and muscles. Predictable symptoms occur, such as flaccid muscles; paralytic ileus; confusion and lethargy; and various cardiac arrhythmias such as sinus bradycardia, atrioventricular block, and paroxysmal atrial tachycardia. Hypokalemia also causes hyperglycemia by decreasing insulin production in the pancreatic β cells. **Hyperglycemia** can occur in nondiabetic patients

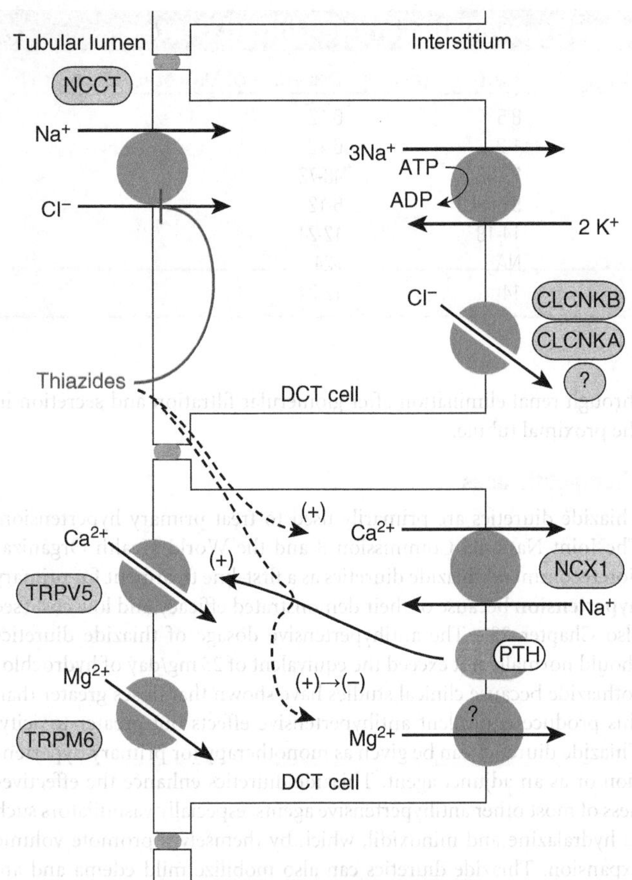

FIG 22-5 The action of the thiazide diuretics on the distal convoluted tubule. Na^+ and Cl^- enter the cell from the tubular fluid by the electroneutral Na^+-Cl^- cotransporter (NCCT) while Ca^{2+} and Mg^{2+} enter via TRPV5 and TRPM6 channels, respectively. Intracellular Na^+ is removed by the action of basolateral Na^+, K^+-ATPase, and Cl^- exits through various basolateral Cl^- channels including CLCNKB and CLCNKA. Thiazides bind to the Cl^--binding site of the Na^+-Cl^- cotransporter, causing an increase in Na^+ and Cl^- delivery to more distal segments, and ultimately increasing Na^+-Cl^- excretion. The increased delivery of Na^+ to the downstream Na^+/K^+ exchange mechanism causes this to be a K^+-losing diuretic. TRPV5 channels reabsorb Ca^{2+} in response to hormonal signals such as that from PTH. A thiazide diuretic-induced decrease in apical Na^+ influx augments the driving force for the basolateral Na^+-Ca^{2+} exchanger (NCX1); while this mechanism potentially contributes to the decreased urinary excretion of Ca^{2+} with thiazides, increased reabsorption of Ca^{2+} in the proximal tubule due to thiazide-induced volume contraction appears to be the primary mechanism. TRPM6 channels reabsorb Mg^{2+} from the tubular fluid, but details related to the regulation of Mg^{2+} reabsorption and its exit from the DCT cells remain to be elucidated. Over the short term, thiazides increase Mg^{2+} reabsorption in a manner presumably somewhat comparable to that for Ca^{2+}. However, longer term thiazide administration leads to decreased Mg^{2+} reabsorption and a potential for hypomagnesemia due to increased excretion. The cause of this is uncertain but may be secondary to the effects of thiazide-induced hypokalemia on Mg^{2+} reabsorption in the thick ascending limb of the loop of Henle (see Fig. 22-6). Unlike Ca^{2+}, which is also reabsorbed in the proximal tubule, Mg^{2+} is only reabsorbed in the more distal portions of the nephron. *DCT*, Distal convoluted tubule; *PTH*, parathyroid hormone.

treated with thiazide diuretics, and glucose control can be destabilized in diabetic patients. Because insulin-dependent glucose uptake promotes cellular uptake of K^+, this hyperglycemia blunts the full effects of diuretic-induced hypokalemia. Severe, sometimes fatal, hypokalemia could result if insulin is administered under these circumstances. Hypokalemia can be avoided by eating foods rich in K^+, especially fruits such as bananas, or by taking K^+ supplements. The concomitant use of K^+-sparing diuretics is an alternative strategy for avoiding hypokalemia, and several combination drugs with hydrochlorothiazide are available for this purpose (see Table 22-3).

Because thiazide diuretics can cause a Na^+ loss in excess of water loss, they can cause **volume depletion and hyponatremia.** Hyponatremia causes systemic **cellular edema and brain swelling,** leading to symptoms such as irritability, depression, and confusion; whereas plasma volume depletion adds symptoms such as postural hypotension, tachycardia, weak pulse, dry mouth, thirst, and oliguria. Other adverse effects of thiazide diuretics include hypercalcemia and hypophosphatemia, simulating hyperparathyroidism. Thiazide diuretics produce **hyperuricemia.** Urate is freely filtered by the glomerulus, reabsorbed in the proximal tubule, secreted by more downstream portions of the proximal tubule, and later largely reabsorbed again. Urate is poorly soluble, and its concentration is normally close to that at which crystals form. Thiazide diuretics interfere with urate transport in a manner that promotes urate retention. This effect combined with thiazide diuretic–induced water loss can increase the plasma urate concentration beyond its solubility limits, leading to the formation of urate crystals that can trigger the inflammatory response known as **gout.** Hyperlipidemia was seen in the past when higher doses of thiazide diuretics (e.g., >25 mg/day of hydrochlorothiazide) were routinely administered to treat hypertension.

Allergic reactions are uncommon with thiazide diuretics, but can lead to fever, skin rash, interstitial nephritis, and renal failure. Patients allergic to sulfonamides should not receive thiazide diuretics.

Loop Diuretics

Loop diuretics are so named for their site of action on the thick ascending limb of the loop of Henle (TALH), where they inhibit Na^+ and Cl^- reabsorption (Fig. 22-6). Because 20% to 25% of filtered Na^+ is reabsorbed in this segment, the resulting natriuresis can be of a much larger magnitude compared with other diuretics. Thus these drugs are sometimes referred to as high ceiling or high efficacy diuretics. Diuretics that act at segments distal to the TALH have a much smaller maximum effect on Na^+ reabsorption. Available loop diuretics are structurally dissimilar (Fig. 22-7). **Furosemide and bumetanide** are sulfonamide derivatives of aminobenzoic acid, **torsemide** is a pyridine sulfonylurea, and **ethacrynic acid** is an unsaturated ketonic derivative of aryloxyacetic acid.

Pharmacologic effects

Na^+ and Cl^- are reabsorbed in the medullary and cortical TALH by the **Na^+, K^+, $2Cl^-$ cotransporter**, as described in Figure 22-6. Evidence obtained with radiolabeled bumetanide suggests that loop diuretics bind to one of the Cl^- binding sites on the cotransporter because bumetanide binding is enhanced by Na^+ and K^+ but inhibited by Cl^-. Loop diuretic binding to the Na^+, K^+, $2Cl^-$ cotransporter effectively arrests ion transport, preventing the reabsorption of Na^+ and Cl^-. K^+ reabsorption is also inhibited, which reduces the intraluminal positive electrical potential normally present in the TALH; this reduces the driving force for the paracellular reabsorption of cations in this segment, further enhancing their excretion (see Fig. 22-6). Additional K^+ excretion occurs in the collecting duct in response to increased Na^+

delivery to the collecting duct and increased aldosterone secretion, as described for the thiazide diuretics. The amount of H^+ secreted by the collecting duct is also enhanced by loop diuretics by the same mechanism. Loop diuretics **increase the excretion of Na^+, K^+, Ca^{2+}, Cl^-, H^+, and Mg^{++}**. The effect on Ca^{2+} is particularly noteworthy because the hypercalciuric effect of loop diuretics is the opposite of the hypocalciuric effect seen with thiazides.

At the level of the whole kidney, inhibition of Na^+ and Cl^- reabsorption in the TALH reduces the medullary interstitial osmotic gradient, which is the driving force for water reabsorption by the adjacent descending loops of Henle and collecting ducts. By blocking the NaCl reabsorption in the TALH, a more isotonic tubular fluid is delivered to the collecting duct, impairing the ability of the kidney to excrete a dilute urine. The associated reduction in the interstitial medullary gradient also means that less water can be extracted from the tubular fluid, impairing the ability of the kidney to excrete a concentrated urine. Thus the urine excreted in the presence of loop diuretics does not differ much from that of plasma, regardless of ADH levels (i.e., free water clearance approaches zero).

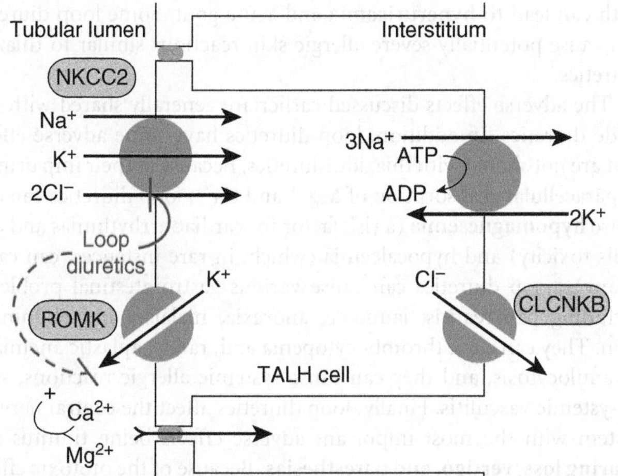

FIG 22-6 The action of the loop diuretics on the thick ascending limb of the loop of Henle. Na^+, K^+, and Cl^- enter the TALH cell from the tubular fluid by the Na^+, K^+, $2Cl^-$ cotransporter (NKCC2). Intracellular Na^+ is removed by the action of basolateral Na^+, K^+-ATPase, and Cl^- exits through basolateral CLCNKB Cl^- channels. K^+ is partially recycled as there is back-leak through an apical ROMK channel. This action creates a net positive potential in the tubular lumen, which acts as an electrostatic driving force for the paracellular reabsorption of cations such as Na^+, Mg^{2+}, and Ca^{2+}. Loop diuretics bind to one of the Cl^--binding sites of the Na^+, K^+, $2Cl^-$ cotransporter, causing an increase in Na^+ and Cl^- delivery to more distal tubule segments, and resulting in increased Na^+ and Cl^- excretion. The increased delivery of Na^+ to the downstream Na^+/K^+ exchange mechanism causes this to be a K^+-losing diuretic. Disruption of the K^+ back-leak in TALH cells, due to inhibition of the cotransporter, decreases reabsorption of Mg^{2+} and Ca^{2+}, thereby also increasing the urinary excretion of these cations.

At the level of the whole body, loop diuretics reduce the extracellular fluid volume and reduce blood pressure as described for thiazides except that these effects are typically of greater magnitude for loop diuretics. Furosemide also increases venous capacitance, which reduces left ventricular filling pressure. This effect seems to be mediated by prostaglandins and occurs before diuresis. This effect is especially useful with intravenous furosemide to treat acute pulmonary edema.

Absorption, fate, and excretion

Although structurally dissimilar, there is substantial similarity among loop diuretics regarding absorption, fate, and excretion. Furosemide is available in oral and injectable forms, with approximately 65% absorption of the oral form. Diuresis begins within 5 minutes of intravenous administration with a duration of 2 hours, and it begins approximately 30 minutes after oral or intramuscular administration and lasts from 6 to 8 hours. Furosemide is highly protein bound, metabolized by the liver, and excreted in the urine and feces. With normal renal function, it has a half-life of 30 to 70 minutes, but this increases to approximately 9 hours in patients with end-stage renal disease.

Torsemide is available in oral and intravenous forms and is rapidly absorbed after oral administration with 80% to 90% bioavailability. Diuresis begins in 30 to 60 minutes after an oral dose and lasts approximately 6 hours. Torsemide is highly protein bound and is 80% metabolized by the hepatic cytochrome P450 system before excretion in the urine. The half-time for elimination is typically 2 to 4 hours but is increased to 7 to 8 hours by cirrhosis of the liver.

Bumetanide is available in oral and injectable forms. Diuresis begins within 2 to 3 minutes of intravenous administration and 30 to 60 minutes after oral or intramuscular administration and has a duration of approximately 6 hours. Bumetanide is highly protein bound, metabolized by the liver, and excreted in the urine.

Ethacrynic acid is available in oral and intravenous forms. Diuresis begins within 5 minutes of intravenous administration and lasts 2 hours, whereas the onset of the diuretic effect after oral administration requires 30 to 60 minutes and has a duration of approximately 12 hours. Ethacrynic acid is highly protein bound, metabolized by the liver, and excreted in the urine and bile. With

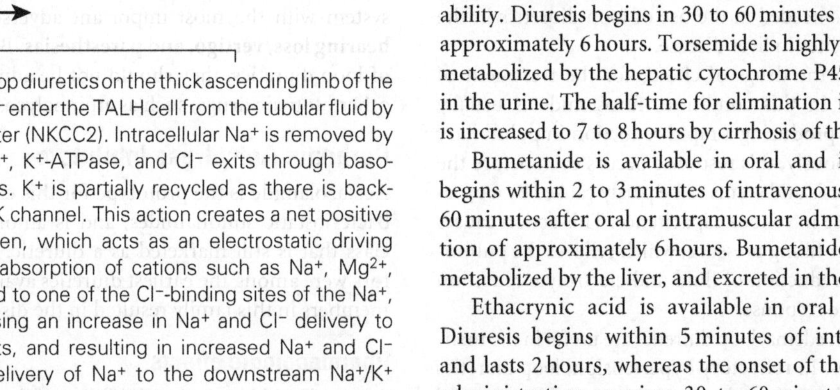

Furosemide

Torsemide

Bumetanide

Ethacrynic acid

FIG 22-7 Structural formulas of loop diuretics.

normal renal function, ethacrynic acid has a half-life of 2 to 4 hours. Ethacrynic acid is not based on a sulfonamide or sulfonylurea backbone like many other diuretics and is therefore especially useful for patients who cannot tolerate other diuretics due to hypersensitivity reactions.

Therapeutic uses

Loop diuretics are predominantly used to treat **edema**. In cardiac failure, low cardiac output results in poor renal perfusion, which causes volume retention. If cardiac dysfunction is severe, this volume retention results in edema and cardiac dilation, which further worsen cardiac failure. Fluid retention in the lungs can also produce grave consequences in heart failure. Loop diuretics reduce plasma volume to cause migration of edema fluid from the tissue back into the circulation, from where it can be excreted.

Many primary and secondary kidney diseases are characterized by salt and water retention and hyperkalemia. Thiazide diuretics can be used in some of these patients, but they become ineffective when the glomerular filtration rate decreases to less than 30 mL/min. Loop diuretics are the primary drugs of choice for **volume management in renal failure.**

Edema can originate from a **primary liver disease.** Edema in this setting is the result of low plasma oncotic pressure from hypoalbuminemia, ascites formation, low renal perfusion, and increased aldosterone release. Loop diuretics have a place in the management of this complex syndrome by reducing fluid and electrolyte retention by the kidney. Some patients with liver disease can be resistant to loop diuretics, however, and these drugs can produce dangerous hypovolemia in others. Great care is needed in the use of loop diuretics in the treatment of edema and ascites in liver disease.

Loop diuretics are also the drugs of choice for the treatment of **acute pulmonary edema.** In this condition, furosemide is usually administered parenterally, producing a rapid reduction in pulmonary congestion. As stated previously, this response occurs even before the onset of significant natriuresis and seems to be partly caused by a prostaglandin-mediated increase in venous capacitance. This action causes a decrease in left ventricular filling pressure, which relieves the pulmonary edema. Longer term reduction of fluid and electrolyte retention by furosemide maintain the response.

In addition to their use in edema, loop diuretics are useful in the management of other conditions. In **refractory hypertension,** loop diuretics are used to combat the fluid and electrolyte retention caused by powerful vasodilators such as minoxidil and hydralazine. In such cases, a K^+-sparing diuretic is also included in the regimen to prevent hypokalemia. Loop diuretics are also used to **treat hypercalcemia.** As discussed earlier (see Fig. 22-6), loop diuretics decrease Ca^{2+} reabsorption in the TALH. In patients with hypercalcemia, furosemide is given intravenously, which produces a prompt reduction in plasma Ca^{2+} concentration. To maintain plasma volume and prevent Na^+ and K^+ wasting, normal saline must be infused simultaneously at a rate that matches urine flow.

Adverse effects

Similar to thiazide diuretics, toxicity from loop diuretics is usually the result of plasma electrolyte disturbances such as **hyponatremia and hypokalemia and extracellular volume depletion**. The magnitude of these effects can be greater than the effects produced by thiazides because of the more prominent natriuresis produced by loop diuretics. The hypokalemia produced by loop diuretics occurs by a mechanism similar to that described for thiazide diuretics (increased exchange of K^+ for Na^+ in the collecting duct) and can be associated with metabolic alkalosis. Also similar to thiazide diuretics, hypokalemia is the most prevalent among these electrolyte disturbances and exerts various neuromuscular and metabolic effects. Inasmuch as loop diuretics are routinely used to help regulate plasma volume in patients with congestive heart failure, this is the appropriate place to draw attention to an important drug interaction. Digoxin and other digitalis-like cardiac glycosides are used to increase myocardial contractility in the failing heart. Various toxic effects are associated with the use of cardiac glycosides (see Chapter 20). Digitalis toxicity increases under conditions of hypokalemia. Thiazide and loop diuretics increase the likelihood and severity of digitalis toxicity.

Hyponatremia causes systemic cellular edema and brain swelling, leading to symptoms such as irritability, depression, and confusion. Plasma volume depletion adds symptoms such as postural hypotension, tachycardia, weak pulse, dry mouth, thirst, and oliguria. Similar to thiazide diuretics, disruption of urate excretion or dehydration or both can lead to **hyperuricemia** and acute gout. Some loop diuretics can cause potentially severe allergic skin reactions similar to thiazide diuretics.

The adverse effects discussed earlier are generally shared with thiazide diuretics. In addition, loop diuretics have some adverse effects that are not shared with thiazide diuretics. Because of their impairment of paracellular reabsorption of Mg^{++} and Ca^{2+}, loop diuretics can also cause **hypomagnesemia** (a risk factor for cardiac arrhythmias and digitalis toxicity) and hypocalcemia (which, in rare instances, can cause tetany). Loop diuretics can cause various gastrointestinal problems, including pancreatitis, jaundice, anorexia, malaise, and abdominal pain. They can elicit thrombocytopenia and, rarely, aplastic anemia or agranulocytosis, and they can cause systemic allergic reactions, such as systemic vasculitis. Finally, loop diuretics affect the central nervous system with the most important adverse effects being tinnitus and **hearing loss, vertigo, and paresthesias.** Because of the ototoxic effects of loop diuretics, they should not be administered concurrently with other ototoxic drugs, such as aminoglycosides.

Carbonic Anhydrase Inhibitors

Acetazolamide is the prototype for this class of drugs, which are nonbacteriostatic sulfonamides, and is among the few members of this class that is still marketed as a diuretic. Carbonic anhydrase inhibitors were among the earliest diuretics available, and the search for new members in this family resulted in the discovery of thiazide diuretics.

Pharmacologic effects

Acetazolamide is a potent inhibitor of the enzyme carbonic anhydrase, the enzyme that catalyzes the reversible reaction of carbonic acid to form either water and carbon dioxide or HCO_3^- and H^+. By blocking this enzyme, reabsorption of HCO_3^- is impaired in the proximal tubule, which leads to increased delivery of Na^+, K^+ and HCO_3^- to the distal nephron and ultimately an alkaline diuresis.

Absorption, fate and excretion

Acetazolamide is readily absorbed from the gastrointestinal tract, with peak concentrations reached in 2 hours. Extended-release capsules are available. Acetazolamide is not metabolized. It is tightly bound to carbonic anhydrase and concentrates in cells with high amounts of this enzyme, such as erythrocytes and the renal cortex. It is excreted unchanged in the urine as a result of active secretion and some passive reabsorption and has a half-life of 2.5 to 6 hours.

Therapeutic uses

Carbonic anhydrase inhibitors can be used to treat the edema of congestive heart failure but are no longer widely used for this purpose. When used to treat edema, best results are obtained when the drug is skipped every other day or every 2 days, giving the kidneys an opportunity to recover lost HCO_3^-. Carbonic anhydrase inhibitors also suppress aqueous humor formation in the eyes and can be used to **reduce intraocular pressure** in open-angle glaucoma and before surgery in cases of angle-closure glaucoma. Treatment of glaucoma is the therapeutic indication for most carbonic anhydrase inhibitors that are now on the market. For reasons that are not well established, but perhaps because of the tendency toward acidosis with these drugs, carbonic anhydrase inhibitors are also useful for treating epilepsy (especially absence seizures in children). A final use for these drugs is the **treatment of altitude sickness** when taken before the ascent and, if necessary, to suppress symptoms for a few days afterward.

Adverse effects

Common side effects with carbonic anhydrase inhibitors include a tingling sensation in the extremities, tinnitus, alterations of taste, loss of appetite, nausea, and vomiting. These side effects are especially common early during therapy. The alkaline diuresis caused by carbonic anhydrase inhibitors can also alter the elimination of other drugs; excretion of weak acids is increased (an effect sometimes harnessed during treatment for drug toxicities), whereas the excretion of weak bases is decreased. In addition, because these drugs are sulfonamide derivatives, some individuals do have allergic reactions typical of these kinds of drugs. These usually manifest as rashes and are rarely fatal, but severe reactions such as anaphylaxis and Stevens-Johnson syndrome have occurred.

Osmotic Diuretics

Mannitol is the prototypic osmotic diuretic, a class of drugs that differs from the drugs previously discussed in two important respects: the amount needed to exert their effects and the site at which they cause diuresis.

Pharmacologic effects

In contrast to the other drugs, which are administered in small amounts to block transporters, mannitol is administered intravenously in **gram quantities** (typically 50 to 200 g over a 24-hour period) and functions as an impermeable solute in the extracellular space. By selectively increasing the osmolality of the extracellular space, water is extracted from the intracellular space to equilibrate the osmotic differences. Mannitol is freely filtered at the glomerulus, is poorly reabsorbed (<10%), and is not secreted. Mannitol carries water extracted from cells with it into the urine. In contrast to the other diuretics discussed here, mannitol selectively decreases intracellular volume (Na^+ and Cl^- excretion are also increased, however).

Absorption, fate, and excretion

Mannitol must be administered intravenously to exert its diuretic effects. When administered to treat cerebral edema, decreases in intracerebral volume are seen within 15 minutes, and diuresis is evident within 1 to 3 hours. There is little metabolism of mannitol, and it is excreted in the urine with a half-time for elimination of 70 to 100 minutes.

Therapeutic uses

There are three major indications for mannitol administration. The first indication is to increase or **maintain urine flow**. Maintaining the flow of urine during the oliguric phase of acute renal failure can block the progression of acute renal failure to irreversible chronic renal failure. This effect can also be harnessed to hasten the elimination of toxins from the body that can be trapped in the urine. Second, by extracting intracellular water, mannitol can be administered to **decrease brain edema and intracranial pressure.** Finally, mannitol is administered preoperatively to **reduce intraocular pressure** before surgery for glaucoma.

Adverse effects

Adverse effects are common during and after the infusion of mannitol. The redistribution of fluid from the intracellular to the extracellular compartment causes various problems, such as pulmonary congestion, electrolyte imbalances, dryness of the mouth, thirst, blurred vision, convulsions, nausea and vomiting, and fever, along with pain, thrombophlebitis, and infection at the injection site. The cardiovascular status of patients must be carefully assessed before administering mannitol because it can cause severe congestive heart failure.

Antidiuretic Hormone Antagonists

In contrast to natriuretics, this class of drugs primarily prevents water reabsorption, producing a selective increase in free water clearance. Several available drugs produce this effect, such as lithium and the antibiotic demeclocycline, but these drugs are rarely used for this purpose in practice. **Conivaptan** and an orally active congener, **tolvaptan**, have been approved more recently for the treatment of acute hyponatremia.

Pharmacologic effects

Conivaptan and tolvaptan are nonpeptide competitive antagonists at vasopressin V_2 receptors (Figures 22-8 and 22-9). These **drugs prevent ADH (vasopressin)-induced insertion of water channels (aquaporins)** into the apical membranes of principal cells in the collecting duct (Fig. 22-8). This prevents the absorption of water by the collecting

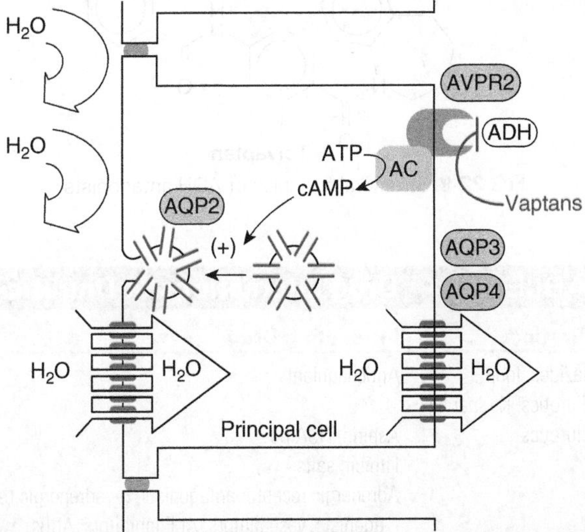

FIG 22-8 The action of the vaptans, ADH antagonists, in the collecting duct. Antidiuretic hormone (*ADH*), also known as arginine vasopressin (*AVP*), maintains plasma osmolality within its normal range by regulating water reabsorption by the principal cells of the collecting duct. ADH binds to G protein-coupled AVPR2 receptors on the basolateral membrane. This results in stimulation of adenylyl cyclase (*AC*) causing formation of the intracellular second messenger cyclic adenosine monophosphate (*cAMP*) from adenosine triphosphate (*ATP*). cAMP facilitates the fusion of aquaporin 2 (*AQP2*)-containing vesicles with the apical membrane of the principal cells. Without AQP2 in the apical membrane of these cells, neither the apical membrane nor the tight junctions between the cells are permeable to water. Reabsorbed water exits across the basolateral membrane by constitutively present aquaporin 3 (AQP3) and aquaporin 4 (AQP4) water channels. By blocking the AVPR2 receptors that regulate this water reabsorption pathway, vaptans selectively increase water excretion, which leads to an increase in plasma osmolality.

ducts, causing increased water excretion. The increase in free water clearance increases urine volume, decreases urine osmolality, reduces plasma volume, and increases plasma osmolality, primarily because of an increase in Na^+ concentration. These actions make conivaptan and tolvaptan particularly suited for the treatment of hyponatremia (Fig. 22-8).

Absorption, fate, and excretion

Conivaptan is available only for intravenous administration. It is extensively bound to plasma proteins with an elimination half-life of approximately 8 hours. Tolvaptan is administered orally, has an onset of action in 2 to 4 hours, and has peak effects in 4 to 8 hours and a half-life of 5 to 12 hours. Conivaptan and tolvaptan are metabolized by cytochrome P450 enzymes in the liver, and their metabolites are primarily excreted in the feces.

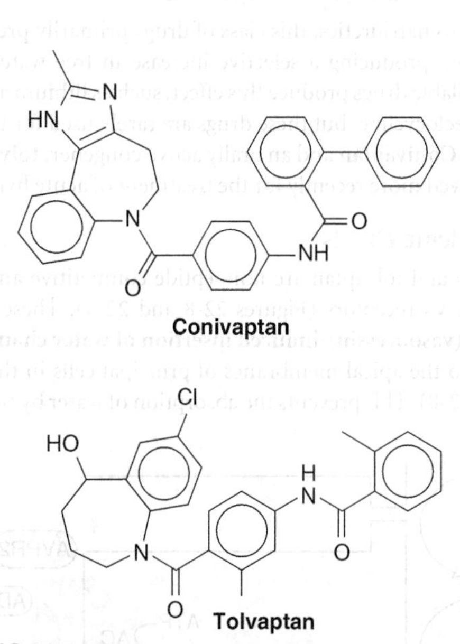

Conivaptan

Tolvaptan

FIG 22-9 Structural formulas of ADH antagonists.

Therapeutic uses

Conivaptan was originally approved for the treatment of euvolemic hyponatremia in hospitalized patients. In 2007, this approval was extended to patients with hypervolemic **hyponatremia**. Tolvaptan now has similar indications. These drugs are useful primarily in the treatment of the **syndrome of inappropriate antidiuresis and the hyponatremia of congestive heart failure that is resistant to water restriction.** Conivaptan can be used only in hospitalized patients because it is administered intravenously, and tolvaptan also must always be started (or re-started) in the hospital because careful monitoring of the plasma sodium concentration is imperative during therapy. Conivaptan is administered for a few days while tolvaptan can be administered for up to 30 days.

Adverse effects

Conivaptan and tolvaptan are generally well tolerated, with few significant adverse effects reported when administered according to protocol. Common adverse effects due to V_2 receptor blockade include thirst, headache, hypokalemia, and vomiting. Conivaptan also blocks vascular vasopressin V_{1A} receptors at therapeutic concentrations, which can lead to vasodilatation and hypotension. Skin reactions at the conivaptan infusion site are common. Care should be taken not to reverse hyponatremia too rapidly because this can lead to osmotic demyelination. Caution should be exercised in patients with renal impairment, which reduces drug elimination. Conivaptan and tolvaptan are **metabolized by cytochrome P450 isozyme CYP3A4** similar to many other drugs, and this creates the opportunity for many potentially dangerous drug interactions. Tolvaptan should not be used for > 30 days because of an increased risk for hepatotoxicity, presumably due in part to its interaction with CYP3A4. Conivaptan has been shown to be teratogenic in laboratory animals and should not be used in pregnant women.

TABLE 22-4 Drug Interactions of Diuretic Agents

Diuretic	Interacting Drug	Effect
Thiazides, loop diuretics, K^+-sparing diuretics	Anticoagulants	Increased concentration of clotting factors from reduction of plasma volume, decreasing anticoagulant effect
	Aspirin, NSAIDs	Natriuresis and hypotensive effect blocked by cyclooxygenase inhibition
	Lithium salts	Decreased Li^+ excretion, leading to increased Li^+ toxicity
	Adrenergic receptor antagonists, α_2-adrenergic receptor agonists, vasodilators, ACE inhibitors, ARBs	Increased antihypertensive response
	Uricosurics	Enhancement of uric acid reabsorption, reducing efficacy of uricosuric agent
Thiazides, loop diuretics	Oral hypoglycemic, insulin	Hypokalemia-induced hyperglycemia
	Nondepolarizing neuromuscular blockers	Hypokalemia-induced potentiation of paralysis
	Adrenergic receptor agonists	Hypokalemia-induced arrhythmias
	Digoxin	Hypokalemia-induced potentiation of digitalis toxicity
	Corticotropin, adrenal steroids	Decreased diuresis, increased hypokalemia
Thiazides	Cholestyramine, colestipol	Decreased thiazide reabsorption
Loop diuretics	Aminoglycosides, cisplatin	Ototoxicity
	Clofibrate, warfarin	Competition for binding to plasma proteins by furosemide increases the free concentration of clofibrate and warfarin.
	Cephalosporin antibiotics	Increased renal toxicity
K^+-sparing diuretics	ACE inhibitors, ARBs, K^+ supplements, cyclosporine	Hyperkalemia
Vaptans	Other drugs metabolized by, or acting on, CYP3A4	Reduced effect or increased potential for toxicity depending on interaction

ACE, Angiotensin-converting enzyme; *ARBs*, angiotensin II receptor blockers; *NSAIDs*, nonsteroidal antiinflammatory drugs.

IMPLICATIONS FOR DENTISTRY

The major drug interactions of diuretics are summarized in Table 22-4, and some additional concerns related to herbal remedies are presented at the end of this section. Diuretic therapy does not usually influence dental practice. Nonetheless, epinephrine, sedatives, opioid analgesics, adrenocorticosteroids, and NSAIDs used in dentistry can interact with patients receiving diuretic agents to cause clinically important adverse effects. Most patients taking diuretics are doing so because of primary hypertension, and the implication of hypertension and its treatment to dental practice are discussed in Chapter 23. Extra caution is especially warranted when dental patients have congestive heart failure, cardiac arrhythmias, and any other conditions in which subtle worsening of plasma K^+ abnormalities could have an adverse effect.

As previously discussed, thiazide and loop diuretics are K^+-losing diuretics that can cause **hypokalemia.** Strategies used to compensate for this K^+ loss include increasing the dietary intake of K^+ or prescribing K^+ supplements or a simultaneous K^+-sparing diuretic. Nonetheless, these patients may still have low plasma K^+ concentrations. Under these circumstances, the epinephrine present in gingival retraction cords and local anesthetic solutions can produce a transient hypokalemia, which increases the propensity of **epinephrine** to **trigger cardiac arrhythmias.**

The use of antiinflammatory dosages of **adrenocorticosteroids** with even modest mineralocorticoid activity, such as hydrocortisone, can also promote **hypokalemia** by exaggerating the hypokalemic effect of thiazide and loop diuretics. In contrast to the rapid-onset transient effects of epinephrine on plasma K^+ concentrations, the hypokalemic effects of adrenocorticosteroids are slow in onset and slow in termination. They may not be of clinical significance until after the patient has left the dental office. Anything that can cause hypokalemia is of greatest concern in patients with congestive heart failure who are receiving digitalis therapy because hypokalemia is a well-known cause of fatal cardiac arrhythmias in these patients.

Conversely, **hyperkalemia** can occur if patients taking a K^+-sparing diuretic or K^+ supplements are placed on a "soft diet" for dental pain since many of the recommended fruits and vegetables are also good dietary sources of K^+.

There is an increased likelihood of **syncope** in dental patients taking diuretics because of a depletion of intravascular volume. Sedative-hypnotics and opioid analgesics are among the drugs that more readily cause orthostatic hypotension in the presence of diuretics.

Renal prostaglandin synthesis plays an increasingly important role in facilitating salt and water excretion when kidney function is compromised due to, for example, suboptimal perfusion or intrinsic renal disease. **NSAIDs** used for dental pain may antagonize these prostaglandin effects, thereby **making the diuretics less effective.** This is of greatest concern when the diuretics are needed to control edema (e.g., for congestive heart failure). Short-term use of NSAIDs in patients taking diuretics for hypertension is unlikely to be clinically significant, but can become relevant if NSAIDs are prescribed to treat chronic dental pain.

Most diuretics are in pregnancy class D, meaning that there is a proven risk of fetal harm. Similarly, breastfeeding is generally contraindicated because most of these drugs enter breast milk.

Because various herbal remedies are touted for their diuretic properties, some patients may be taking diuretic therapy without proper medical supervision, and others may choose to combine the use of herbal remedies with contemporary diuretic pharmacotherapy in the potentially erroneous belief that all diuretics work well together. Herbs used as diuretics include dandelion, horsetail, stone root, cleavers, gravel root, hydrangea, pipsissewa, goldenrod, lovage, and parsley. The mechanism of action for these herbs has generally not been established. Claims that dandelion is a rich source of K^+ while functioning as a K^+-depleting diuretic could be of concern, however, if taken by patients who are also taking a K^+-sparing diuretic. Lastly, the glycyrrhizic acid of "real" (e.g., European) licorice used in candy and for various medicinal purposes has mineralocorticoid properties. Overindulgence in this type of licorice candy has caused hypertension and, if consumed with diuretics, could exacerbate the **K^+-depleting** effects of thiazide and loop diuretics or inhibit the activities of spironolactone. The possibility of drug interaction between diuretics and alternative therapies should not be overlooked.

ADH antagonists are only administered for a short duration and are therefore unlikely to be encountered in a typical dental practice. Nonetheless, these drugs and the water restriction that is sustained once the drugs are discontinued cause thirst, and a significant fraction of these patients experience xerostomia. There are multiple problems associated with this dry mouth including increased dental caries, halitosis, difficulty swallowing, taste alterations, and oral yeast infections.

DIURETIC DRUGS

Nonproprietary (Generic) Name	Proprietary (Trade) Name
Thiazides and Related Derivatives	
Bendroflumethiazide	Naturetin
Chlorothiazide	Diuril
Chlorthalidone	Hygroton, Thalitone
Hydrochlorothiazide	Esidrix, HydroDIURIL, Hydro-Par
Indapamide	Lozol
Methyclothiazide	Aquatensen, Enduron
Metolazone	Zaroxolyn, Mykrox
Loop Diuretics	
Bumetanide	Bumex
Ethacrynic acid	Edecrin
Furosemide	Lasix
Torsemide	Demadex
K^+-Sparing Agents	
Amiloride	Midamor
Eplerenone	Inspra
Spironolactone	Aldactone
Triamterene	Dyrenium
Osmotic Nonelectrolytes	
Mannitol	Osmitrol
Carbonic Anhydrase Inhibitors	
Acetazolamide	Dazamide, Diamox
Antidiuretic Hormone Receptor Antagonist	
Conivaptan	Vaprisol
Tolvaptan	Samsca

CASE DISCUSSION

The best time for scheduling these dental procedures is likely mid- to late-afternoon as this would allow time for the furosemide-induced diuresis after the morning dosage to subside. The diuretic-induced volume contraction makes postural hypotension/syncope more likely, and having carvedilol levels at post-peak in the afternoon should also ensure that the sympathetic nervous system is better able to respond when the sedatives wear off and the patient tries to move. Heart failure also impacts on both hepatic and renal function, which means sedatives likely will not be eliminated as rapidly. This could lead to prolonged sedation with a possible accumulation of sedatives administered by constant infusion [e.g., midazolam (although restricted to those with advanced training)] to concentrations used for deeper sedation than desired. Renal prostaglandins are important for maintaining salt and water excretion in poorly perfused kidneys, and NSAIDs are therefore contraindicated in patients with heart failure because they interfere with diuretic actions. Potassium levels are a concern in this patient given their impact on digoxin toxicity/efficacy. The actions of lisinopril and spironolactone offset the K^+-losing effects of furosemide. The degree to which potassium nitrate from the Sensodyne® enters the body is not readily available but will presumably depend on the number of tooth brushings per day and the extent to which the toothpaste is swallowed. Thus, although unlikely, K^+ from this toothpaste might boost the plasma K^+ concentration into a range in which digoxin becomes less effective and/or the hyperkalemia causes an arrhythmia.

GENERAL REFERENCES

1. Spironolactone from Drugs.com; c2000–15 [Updated: February 2015; Cited: August 5, 2015]. Available from: http://www.drugs.com/pro/spironolactone.html.
2. Amiloride from Drugs.com; c2000–15 [Updated: September 2014; Cited: August 5, 2015]. Available from: http://www.drugs.com/pro/amiloride.html.
3. Triamterene from Drugs.com; c2000–15 [2009 Wolters Kluwer Health; Cited: August 5, 2015]. Available from: http://www.drugs.com/ppa/triamterene.html.
4. Hydrochlorothiazide from Drugs.com; c2000–15 [Updated: May 2015; Cited: August 5, 2015]. Available from: http://www.drugs.com/pro/hydrochlorothiazide.html.
5. Chlorthalidone from Drugs.com; c2000–15 [Updated: March 2014; Cited: August 5, 2015]. Available from: http://www.drugs.com/pro/chlorthalidone.html.
6. Metolazone from Drugs.com; c2000–15 [Updated: June 2015; Cited: August 5, 2015]. Available from: http://www.drugs.com/pro/metolazone.html.
7. Aldactazide from Drugs.com; c2000–15 [Updated: November 2014; Cited: August 5, 2015]. Available from: http://www.drugs.com/pro/aldactazide.html.
8. Furosemide from Drugs.com; c2000–15 [Updated: October 2014; Cited: August 5, 2015]. Available from: http://www.drugs.com/pro/furosemide.html.
9. Torsemide from Drugs.com; c2000–15 [Updated: January 2015; Cited: August 5, 2015]. Available from: http://www.drugs.com/pro/torsemide.html.
10. Ethacrynic acid from Drugs.com; c2000–15 [2009 Wolters Kluwer Health; Cited: August 5, 2015]. Available from: http://www.drugs.com/ppa/ethacrynic-acid-ethacrynate.html.
11. Conivaptan from Drugs.com; c2000–15 [2009 Wolters Kluwer Health; Cited: August 5, 2015]. Available from: http://www.drugs.com/ppa/conivaptan-hydrochloride.html.
12. Tolvaptan from Drugs.com; c2000–15 [2009 Wolters Kluwer Health; Cited: August 5, 2015]. Available from: http://www.drugs.com/ppa/tolvaptan.html.
13. Samsca (Tolvaptan): Drug Safety Communication—FDA Limits Duration and Usage Due to Possible Liver Injury Leading to Organ Transplant or Death from Drugs.com; c2000–15 [2009 Wolters Kluwer Health; Cited: August 5, 2015]. Available from: http://www.drugs.com/fda/samsca-tolvaptan-safety-communication-fda-limits-duration-usage-due-possible-liver-injury-leading-13286.html.
14. Acetazolamide from Drugs.com; c2000–15 [Updated: December 2014; Cited: August 5, 2015]. Available from: http://www.drugs.com/pro/acetazolamide.html
15. Mannitol from Drugs.com; c2000–15 [Updated: March 2014; Cited: August 5, 2015]. Available from: http://www.drugs.com/pro/mannitol-injection.html.
16. Ellison DH: Physiology and pathophysiology of diuretic action. In Alpern RJ, Moe OW, Caplan MC, editors: *Seldin and Giebisch's the kidney: physiology and pathophysiology*, 5th ed, Amsterdam, 2013, Elsevier.
17. Ellison DH, Hoorn EJ, Wilcox CS: Diuretics. In Taal MW, Chertow GM, Marsden PA, Skorecki K, Yu ASL, Brenner BM, editors: *Brenner and Rector's the kidney*, 9th ed, Amsterdam, 2012, Elsevier.
18. Houston BA, Kalathiya RJ, Kim DA, Zakaria S: Volume overload in heart failure: An evidence-based review of strategies for treatment and prevention, *Mayo Clin Proc*, 2015. Available from: http://dx.doi.org/10.1016/j.mayocp.2015.05.002. [Epub ahead of print, 2015].
19. James PA, Oparil S, Carter BL, et al.: 2014 Evidence-Based Guideline for the Management of High Blood Pressure in Adults: Report From the Panel Members Appointed to the Eighth Joint National Committee (JNC 8), *JAMA* 311(5):507–520, 2014.
20. Opie LH, Victor RG, Kaplan NM: Diuretics. In Opie LH, Gersh BJ, editors: *Drugs for the heart*, 8th ed, Philadelphia, 2013, Saunders Elsevier.
21. Verbalis JG, Grossman A, Höybye C, Runkle I: Review and analysis of differing regulatory indications and expert panel guidelines for the treatment of hyponatremia, *Curr Med Res Opin* 30(7):1201–1207, 2014.
22. Yancy CW, Jessup M, Bozkurt B, et al.: 2013 ACCF/AHA guideline for the management of heart failure: a report of the American College of Cardiology Foundation/American Heart Association Task Force on Practice Guidelines, *J Am Coll Cardiol* 62:e147–e239, 2013.

Antihypertensive Drugs

Frank J. Dowd and William B. Jeffries

KEY INFORMATION

- Hypertension is a common disorder that poses significant risk to several end organs.
- Race, gender, and concomitant disorders have important implications as to the choice of therapy.
- Lifestyle and dietary changes have a role in controlling high blood pressure.
- The most commonly used antihypertensive drugs for chronic therapy are diuretics, e.g., hydrochlorothiazide, chlorthalidone, drugs that inhibit the renin-angiotensin system, and some calcium channel blockers.
- Drugs that inhibit the renin-angiotensin system are the angiotensin-converting enzyme (ACE) inhibitors, e.g., lisinopril and enalapril; the angiotensin II receptor (AT_1) blockers (ARBs), e.g., losartan and valsartan; and the renin inhibitor, aliskiren.
- Adrenergic receptor–blocking drugs also have important uses in treating hypertension. These drugs are the β blockers, e.g., propranolol and metoprolol; the α_1 blockers, e.g., prazosin and terazosin; and drugs that block β receptors as well as having a vasodilator effect, e.g., carvedilol and nebivolol.
- Additional drugs, referred to as vasodilators, are useful in certain cases of hypertension. For chronic therapy, these drugs are not as often used as those listed above but include hydralazine and minoxidil.
- Centrally acting α_2-adrenergic receptor agonists, α methyl dopa, clonidine, guanabenz, and guanfacine, reduce sympathetic outflow from the brain and can be used as add-on drug therapy.
- Hypertensive emergencies are treated with drugs that reduce peripheral vascular resistance.
- Drug treatment of pulmonary hypertension primarily involves vasodilator drugs.
- Chronic NSAID therapy may inhibit the antihypertensive effect of certain drugs.
- Postural hypotension is a potential adverse effect of certain antihypertensive drugs.
- Centrally acting antihypertensive drugs often cause sedation and xerostomia.

CASE STUDY

Mr. J is a 45-year-old office worker who has been a dental patient of yours for several years. Monitoring of his blood pressure in your office as well as his physician's has indicated that his blood pressure has risen to 160/95 and has remained at this level. Mr. J's physician has instituted antihypertensive drug therapy. Chlorthalidone, 15 mg once a day, was given as initial monotherapy with potassium supplementation. The chlorthalidone was later increased to 30 mg once a day. This was found to be only partially effective in lowering his blood pressure. Recently, lisinopril, 10 mg once a day, was added to Mr. J's drug regimen, and the potassium supplementation stopped. Ten days after the lisinopril was started, Mr. J arrives for his scheduled dental appointment. The patient has one dental complaint: tightness in the throat. Upon oral examination, you observe that the oral pharynx is swollen, and the airway is partially restricted.

You ask Mr. J how long he has noticed the tightness. He said it started yesterday. Oral examination reveals no other soft tissue abnormality and normal hard tissue. The exam of the teeth indicates no pathology. What would be your best course of action?

Careful examination of the prevalence of hypertension reveals that it is distributed disproportionately among subgroups in the U.S. population (Fig. 23-1).

Hypertension increases with advancing age, but its prevalence is lower in women before menopause than in men of comparable age. This trend reverses in elderly individuals. There also is a racial component to hypertension. In the United States, for those 20 years of age and older, the prevalence of hypertension is shown in Table 23-1.

Because of the asymptomatic nature of this disease, approximately one-third of affected individuals are unaware of their condition. Screening programs are essential to detect the disease early so that treatment can be instituted before major complications ensue. Education of patients is essential to ensure compliance with recommended therapy because of the insidious nature of the disease and because unpleasant side effects of the drugs used to treat it may cause the patient to feel better when not receiving medication. An individual is considered hypertensive if his or her systolic or diastolic arterial blood pressure (or both) is elevated above normal (i.e., **systolic arterial pressure >140 mm Hg or diastolic arterial pressure >90 mm Hg**).

CLINICAL ASPECTS OF HYPERTENSION

Classification

The severity of hypertension is classified as shown in Table 23-2. Hypertension can arise as a primary disease or as a result of an underlying illness. **Primary** or essential **hypertension** is a term used to describe the presence of sustained, elevated blood pressure for which no underlying

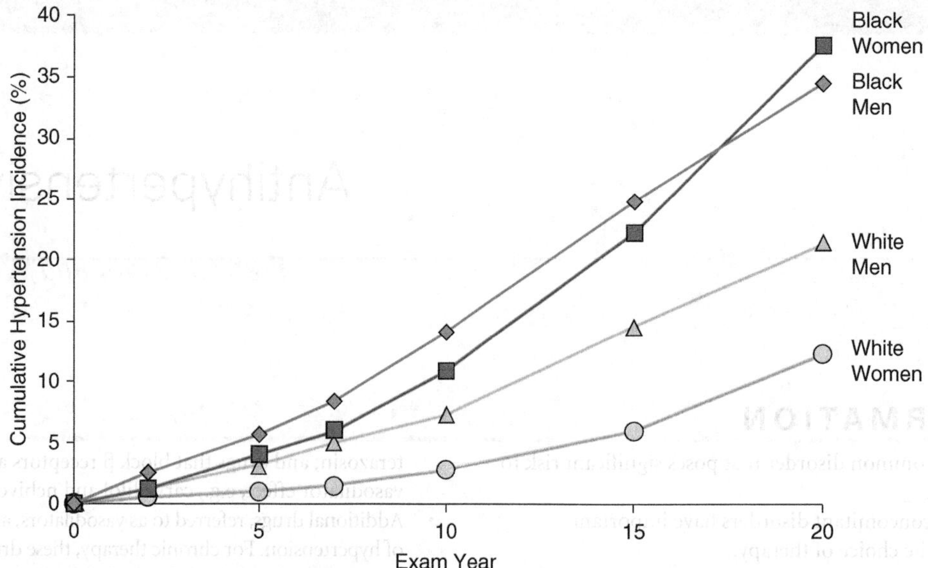

FIG 23-1 Cumulative 20-year hypertension incidence by race/sex, among adults 18 to 30 years of age at baseline: the CARDIA study, 1985 to 2005. (From Levine DA, et al: Geographic and demographic variability in 20-year hypertension incidence, the CARDIA study. *Hypertension* 57:39-47, 2011.)

TABLE 23-1 Percent of Individuals with Systolic Blood Pressure ≥140 mm Hg or Diastolic Blood Pressure ≥90 mm Hg or Both, for Adults 20 years or Older*

	Males	Females
Non-Hispanic whites	33.4	30.7
Non-Hispanic blacks	42.6	47.0
Mexican Americans	30.1	28.8

*Data from the National Health and Nutrition Examination Survey 2007-2010 as reported in Go AS et al., on behalf of the American Heart Association Statistics Committee and Stroke Statistics Committee. Heart disease and stroke statistics 2014 update: a report from the American Heart Association. *Circulation* 129:e28-e292, 2014.

TABLE 23-2 Classification of Severity of Hypertension by Blood Pressure

Stage	Systolic (mm Hg)		Diastolic (mm Hg)
Normal	<120	and	<80
Prehypertension	120-139	or	80-89
Stage 1	140-159	or	90-99
Stage 2	>160	or	>100

Hypertension staging corresponds to the higher of the systolic or diastolic blood pressure values.
From the Seventh Report of the Joint National Committee on the prevention, detection, and treatment of high blood pressure. *JAMA* 289:2534-2573, 2003.

cause can be discovered. Primary hypertension represents 80% to 90% of all cases of hypertension.

Secondary hypertension results from a known disorder, such as renal, vascular, endocrine or parenchymal disease. Treatment of secondary hypertension usually consists of therapy for the underlying disease process. Hypertension may be systolic or diastolic, or both. Until more recently, less emphasis had been placed on the importance of systolic hypertension. More recent evidence indicates, however, its close association with untoward outcomes. Treatment of isolated systolic hypertension in elderly patients with an antihypertensive drug has been shown to reduce mortality rates, especially from stroke. The results are independent of mean arterial pressure. The risk of heart failure is also decreased with reduction in systolic hypertension. It has been suggested that the incidence of dementia is reduced as systolic pressure is reduced in elderly patients.

In metabolic syndrome, hypertension is accompanied by abdominal obesity, hyperlipidemia with atherosclerosis, and hyperglycemia or insulin resistance or both. In this syndrome, hypertension is only one target of therapy. Questions that are still being explored are to what extent each sign of the syndrome is related and how.

Regulation of Blood Pressure

Pressure in a hydraulic system is the product of flow through the system and the resistance to such flow. The relationships between mean arterial blood pressure (MAP), cardiac output (CO), and total peripheral resistance (TPR) can be described in the following equation:

$$MAP = CO \times TPR$$

CO is determined by the load presented to the heart (venous return or preload) and the inotropic and chronotropic state of the myocardium. TPR depends on the diameter and compliance (stiffness) of the arterioles. These factors are regulated by the resting vascular smooth muscle tone, intrinsic reactivity of the vasculature, vasoactive substances in the blood, and sympathetic nervous system activity. Another important factor in the governance of blood pressure is the blood volume, which is regulated by the kidneys. The interrelationships among all these factors are illustrated in Figure 23-2.

Blood pressure tends to remain at a constant value, and there are many physiologic control mechanisms to protect the organism from harmful perturbations in blood pressure. Two of the most important regulatory mechanisms are short-term control afforded by the sympathetic nervous system and long-term control, which is a function of the renal system.

Moment-to-moment control of blood pressure largely depends on baroreflexes, in which sympathetic nervous system output to the heart, resistance vessels, and capacitance vessels is adjusted in response to

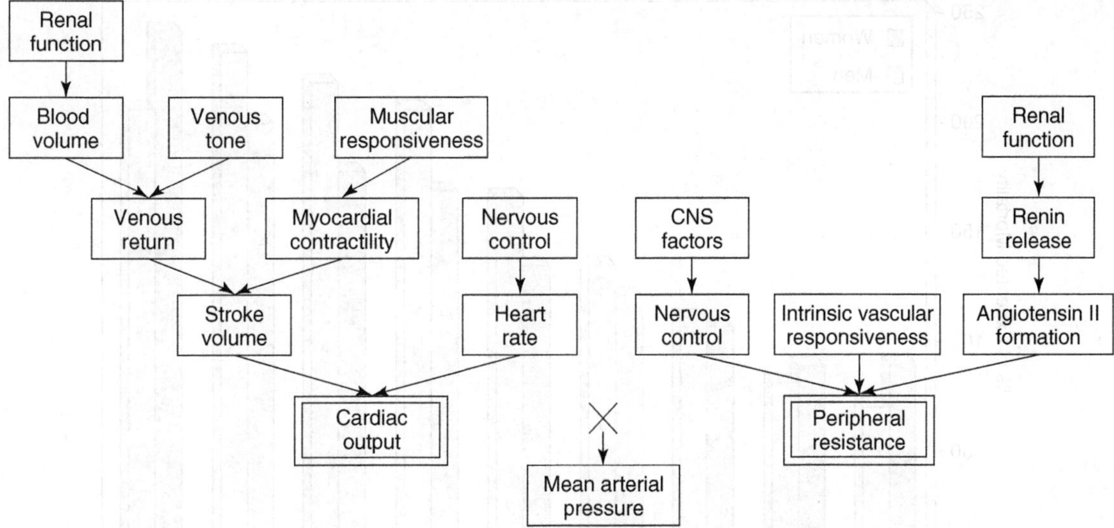

FIG 23-2 Factors that govern mean arterial blood pressure. *CNS*, Central nervous system.

feedback from baroreceptors in the carotid sinus and aortic arch. These baroreceptors respond to mechanical stretch (increased pressure) by increasing the firing rate of sensory neurons that innervate blood pressure control areas of the central nervous system (CNS). If blood pressure increases, the resultant increased activity of these sensory neurons inhibits efferent sympathetic nervous system activity, reducing heart rate, vascular tone, and blood pressure. Conversely, if blood pressure suddenly decreases, baroreceptor output is reduced, allowing increased peripheral sympathetic discharge. This reflex is responsible for the maintenance of blood pressure during rapid stresses to cardiovascular homeostasis, as induced by a change in posture.

Long-term stresses on the maintenance of blood pressure (e.g., alterations in water and salt intake) are handled by the kidneys. A change in blood pressure is sensed by the kidneys as a corresponding change in renal perfusion pressure. This disturbance invokes two compensatory mechanisms. First, the tubular reabsorption of Na^+ and water either decreases (in high perfusion pressure) or increases (in low perfusion pressure). This alteration adjusts blood volume and secondarily changes CO to bring blood pressure back to normal. The kidneys also influence resistance vessel tone more directly by releasing renin (activating the renin-angiotensin system) when renal perfusion is diminished. The resultant increase in vasoactive angiotensin peptides increases peripheral vascular resistance by causing vasoconstriction. Angiotensin peptides also promote volume retention by increasing the release of aldosterone and contribute to muscular hypertrophy and other structural changes in the heart and vasculature (collectively referred to as **remodeling**).

The physiologic mechanisms that control blood pressure are important in the treatment of hypertension in two respects. First, each of these mechanisms represents a potential therapeutic target for reducing blood pressure in a hypertensive patient. Second, because these mechanisms are in place to prevent changes in blood pressure, they become activated in an attempt to restore blood pressure to its former (high) level when steps are taken to reduce the hypertension.

Pathophysiologic Characteristics of Primary Hypertension

The physical findings of a patient with essential hypertension usually reveal that CO is normal and TPR is elevated. In a hypertensive patient, the baroreceptor reflexes function normally, but have been "reset" to maintain MAP at a higher than normal value. The reasons for this shift are not well understood. It is evident that there is a genetic component to primary hypertension and that certain risk factors lead to a worsening of blood pressure elevation (Box 23-1). In many patients, long-term cardiovascular complications of hypertension can be lessened by making appropriate lifestyle changes.

BOX 23-1 Risk Factors for Development or Worsening of Essential Hypertension

Unavoidable Risks

Family history
Age
Male sex
African American race
Diabetes

Lifestyle Risks

Na^+ intake
Obesity
Alcohol consumption
Cigarette smoking
Lack of exercise

Although the cause of primary hypertension is unknown, it is well established that high blood pressure leads to cardiovascular and renal disease. Elevated blood pressure is directly correlated with overall mortality (Fig. 23-3). It is accepted that reducing the blood pressure in hypertensive patients reduces the risk of cardiovascular events including myocardial infarction and stroke, and kidney failure. The damage caused by decades of elevated arterial pressure can be seen in the form of left ventricular hypertrophy, medial thickening of arteries, and nephropathy. These changes contribute to the development of diseases such as congestive heart failure, coronary artery disease, stroke, aneurysm, and renal failure (Box 23-2). Numerous clinical trials have shown a reduction in morbidity and mortality rates after pharmacologic reduction in blood pressure in hypertensive patients.

Diabetic patients are particularly vulnerable to targeted organ damage resulting from hypertension. The current standard of care dictates that antihypertensive therapy be prescribed in diabetics whose blood pressure is in the high-normal range or above (see Table 23-2).

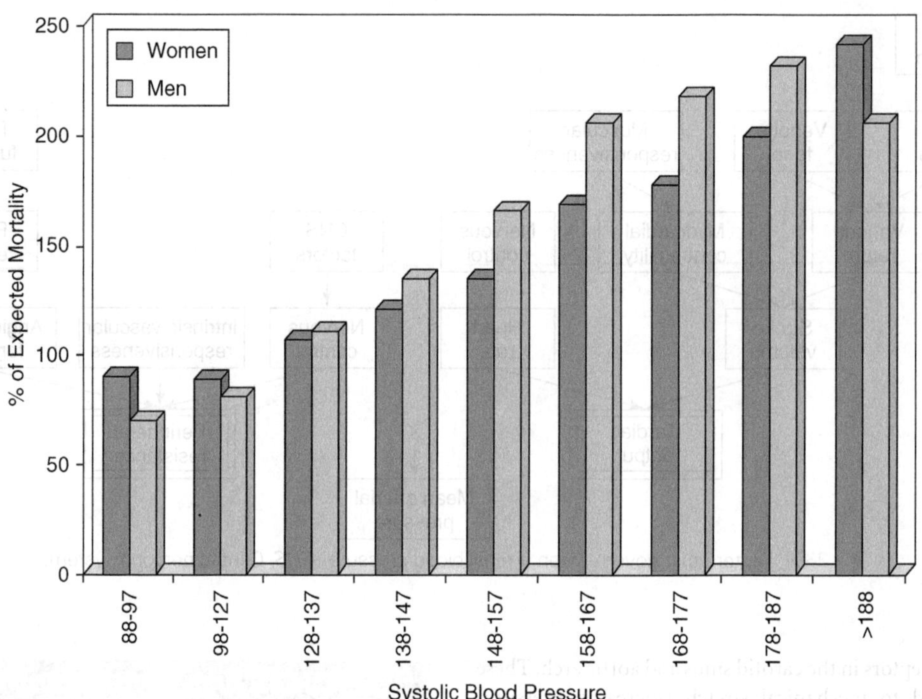

FIG 23-3 Expected mortality as a function of systolic blood pressure at all ages without regard to treatment. (Adapted from *The Society of Actuaries and the Association of Life Insurance Medical Directors of America: Blood pressure study 1979*, Boston, 1980, The Society.)

BOX 23-2 Clinical Disorders Resulting from Hypertension and Atherosclerosis

Hypertension
- Congestive heart failure
- Cerebral hemorrhage or stroke
- Renal failure
- Retinopathy
- Dissecting aneurysm
- Hypertensive crisis

Atherosclerosis
- Coronary artery disease
- Angina pectoris
- Myocardial infarction
- Secondary renovascular hypertension
- Peripheral vascular insufficiency
- Cerebral thrombosis, stroke

ACE inhibitors are most commonly used for this purpose because of their well-documented protective effects in diabetic patients.

General Aims of Antihypertensive Drug Therapy

Treatment of essential hypertension consists of therapy aimed at reducing the blood pressure into the normal range. As shown in Figure 23-2, many factors play a role in the determination of blood pressure, and consequently pharmacologic agents with diverse mechanisms of action can be used singly or in combination to treat essential hypertension. Antihypertensive agents can be categorized according to their mechanism of action and therapeutic use: diuretics, drugs affecting angiotensin or its function, Ca^{2+} channel blockers (CCBs), drugs affecting sympathetic function, directly acting vasodilators, and miscellaneous drugs. Because the basic pharmacologic properties of many drugs useful in treating hypertension are discussed elsewhere, only pharmacologic features not covered elsewhere or those pertinent to the treatment of hypertension are discussed in detail in this chapter. Figure 23-4 shows the major sites of action of antihypertensive agents.

DIURETICS

Thiazide or thiazide-like diuretics are currently among the most widely used drugs for the initial management of essential hypertension. K^+-sparing diuretics are commonly used together with thiazides for their additive effect and to prevent thiazide-induced hypokalemia. Thiazide diuretics may be used alone or in combination with other antihypertensive drugs. Loop diuretics such as furosemide are sometimes used as adjunctive agents in refractory hypertension.

Diuretics reduce plasma volume by increasing Na^+ and water excretion. Initially, this effect reduces blood pressure by decreasing CO. With time, CO and extracellular fluid volume return toward normal values, but the hypotensive effect persists because of a reduction in peripheral resistance. It is probable that electrolyte changes in vascular smooth muscle account for the vasodilation. The use of longer acting thiazide-type or thiazide-like diuretics, such as **chlorthalidone**, appears to be superior to the shorter acting hydrochlorothiazide in preventing some renal and cardiovascular consequences of hypertension. The reasons for this may include better blood pressure control during the nighttime hours with the longer acting diuretic. For a complete discussion of diuretics used in the treatment of hypertension, see Chapter 22.

DRUGS AFFECTING ANGIOTENSIN

The role played by the **renin-angiotensin system** in hypertension has received much attention in recent years. Renin catalyzes the conversion of angiotensinogen, a glycoprotein found in the blood, to angiotensin I, a decapeptide with little cardiovascular activity (see Fig. 23-4). Angiotensin I is activated by conversion to

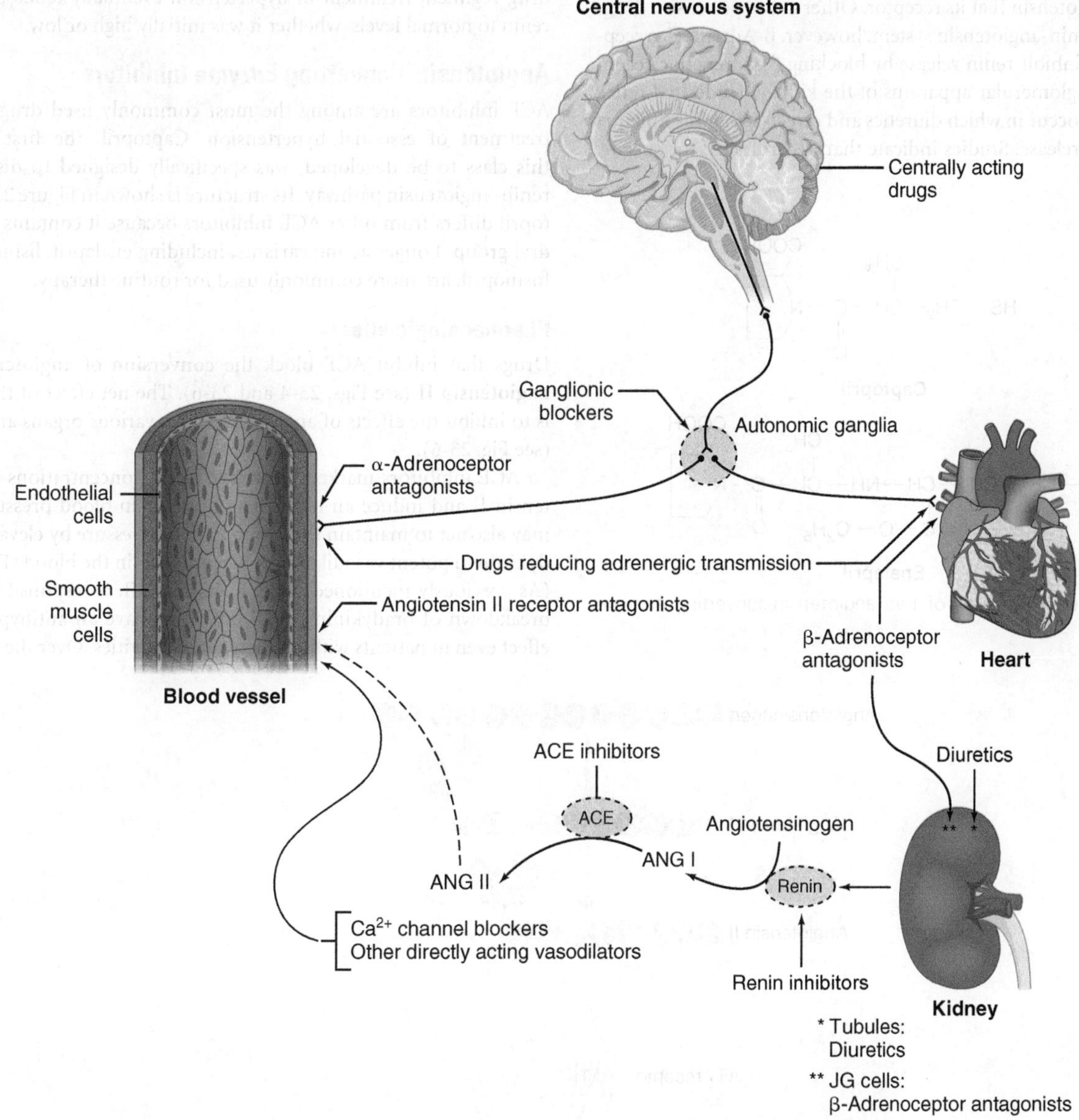

FIG 23-4 Sites of action of antihypertensive drugs. The diagram indicates by drug class the targets for antihypertensive action. *ACE*, Angiotensin-converting enzyme; *ANG*, angiotensin; *JG*, juxtaglomerular.

the octapeptide angiotensin II. This reaction is catalyzed by **angiotensin converting enzyme** (**ACE**), otherwise known as *dipeptidyl carboxypeptidase* or *peptidyl dipeptidase*. Under its designation as *kininase II*, ACE is also the enzyme that inactivates the endogenous vasodilator bradykinin.

Angiotensin II is metabolized by aminopeptidase enzymes to yield the less active and shorter lived heptapeptide angiotensin III. Increased renin activity leads to heightened production of angiotensin II and angiotensin III, vasoconstriction of peripheral arterioles, and elevation of blood pressure. Angiotensin peptides stimulate thirst and the secretion of aldosterone and antidiuretic hormone; the resultant increase in extracellular fluid and electrolytes augments the direct pressor effects. Angiotensin II also influences sympathetic nervous system function centrally and peripherally to increase cardiac activity and peripheral vascular resistance.

Patients with essential hypertension can be divided into three groups according to their renin-Na^+ index (i.e., plasma renin activity relative to Na^+ excretion). Approximately 15% of patients have renin concentrations higher than normal, 25% have renin concentrations lower than normal, and the remaining 60% exhibit normal renin titers. Renin titers tend to decrease with age. African American and elderly individuals tend to have a higher incidence of low-renin hypertension.

The percentage of hypertensive patients with normal renin activity may be misleading because renin release is ordinarily depressed as the result of increased blood pressure. Renin release may still be inappropriately high even in the "normal" group. Although angiotensin II may be the main causative agent in high-renin hypertension and may be a factor in the normal-renin hypertension group, other influences are implicated in low-renin hypertension, and these may contribute to normal-renin hypertension as well.

Pharmacologic intervention to reduce blood pressure theoretically can be anywhere along the angiotensin system—from the release of renin by the kidney juxtaglomerular cells, to the inhibition of renin, to the formation of angiotensin peptides, to the binding of angiotensin II and angiotensin III to receptors in vascular smooth muscle and other effector sites. In the following discussion, attention is limited to drugs whose primary mechanism of action is interference with renin synthesis, renin activity, conversion of angiotensin I to angiotensin II, or action of angiotensin II at its receptor. Other antihypertensive drugs also affect the renin-angiotensin system, however. β-Adrenergic receptor antagonists inhibit renin release by blocking β_1-adrenergic receptors in the juxtaglomerular apparatus of the kidney. Undesired reflex actions can also occur in which diuretics and direct-acting vasodilators stimulate renin release. Studies indicate that, regardless of the specific drug regimen, treatment of hypertension eventually tends to restore renin to normal levels, whether it was initially high or low.

$HS-CH_2-CH(CH_3)-C(=O)-N$ (pyrrolidine ring with COOH)

Captopril

$C_6H_5-CH_2-CH_2-CH(C(=O)-O-C_2H_5)-NH-CH(CH_3)-C(=O)-N$ (pyrrolidine ring with COOH)

Enalapril

FIG 23-5 Structural formulas of two angiotensin-converting enzyme inhibitors.

Angiotensin-Converting Enzyme Inhibitors

ACE inhibitors are among the most commonly used drugs for the treatment of essential hypertension. Captopril, the first drug of this class to be developed, was specifically designed to disrupt the renin-angiotensin pathway. Its structure is shown in Figure 23-5. Captopril differs from other ACE inhibitors because it contains a sulfhydryl group. Longer acting variants, including enalapril, lisinopril and fosinopril, are more commonly used for routine therapy.

Pharmacologic effects

Drugs that inhibit ACE block the **conversion of angiotensin I to angiotensin II** (see Figs. 23-4 and 23-6). The net effect of this action is to inhibit the effects of angiotensin II on various organs and tissues (see Fig. 23-6).

ACE inhibitors markedly decrease blood concentrations of angiotensin II and induce an immediate decrease in blood pressure. They may also act to maintain the lowered blood pressure by elevating **bradykinin** (a potent vasodilator) concentrations in the blood (Fig. 23-7). (As previously mentioned, ACE, as kininase II, is responsible for the breakdown of bradykinin.) ACE inhibitors have an antihypertensive effect even in patients without high-renin activities. Over the course of

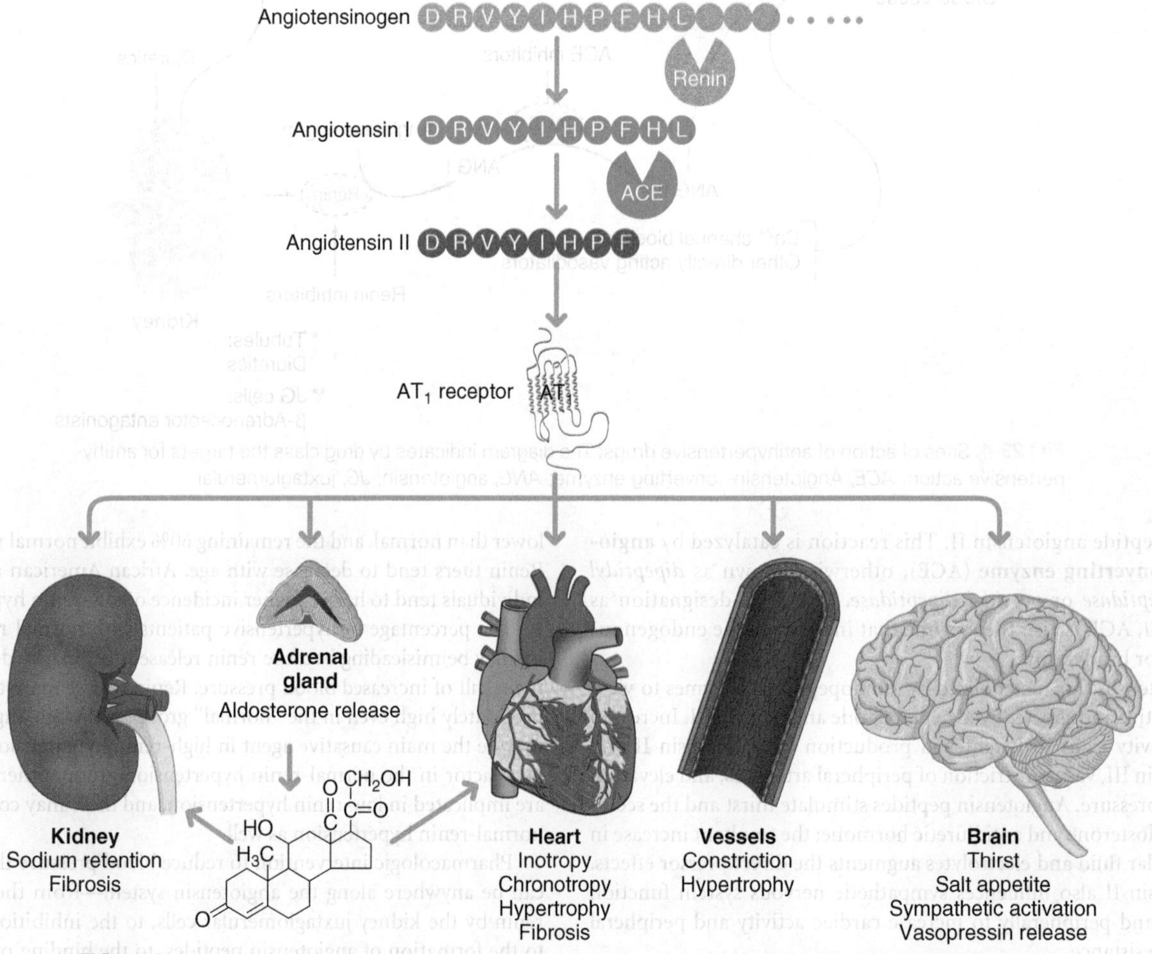

FIG 23-6 Classical renin-angiotensin-aldosterone system. Angiotensin expressed in the liver is cleaved by renin from the kidney to release angiotensin I in plasma. ACE on endothelial cells catalyzes the conversion of angiotensin I to angiotensin II. Angiotensin II binds to angiotensin II receptors (AT_1) in the organs and tissue shown, leading to the effects listed. (From Bader M: Tissue renin-angiotensin-aldosterone systems: targets for pharmacology therapy. *Annu Rev Pharmacol Toxicol* 50:439-465, 2010.)

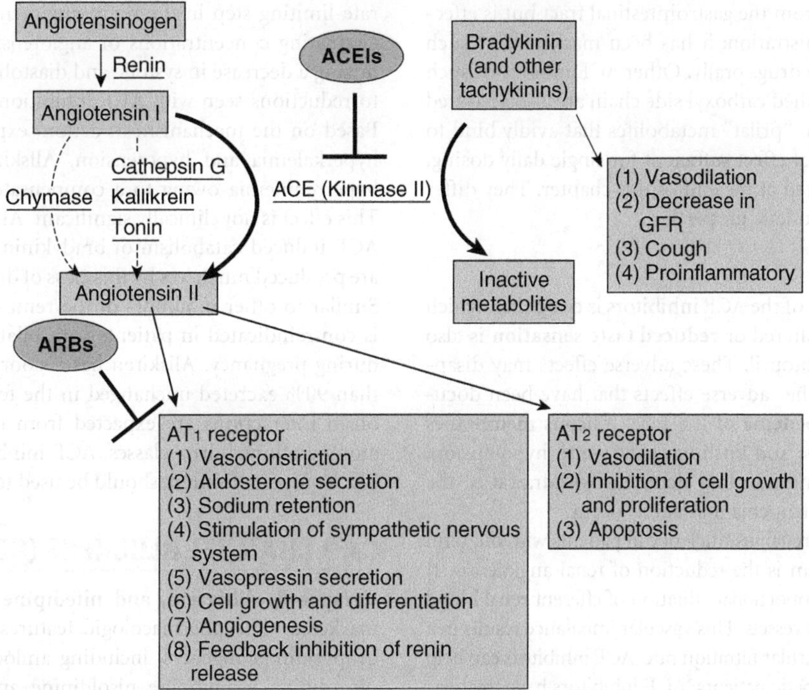

FIG 23-7 The role of angiotensin-converting enzyme inhibitors (*ACEIs*) and angiotensin II receptor blockers (*ARBs*) in treating hypertension. ACEIs block the major, but not the only, synthetic pathway to angiotensin II. ACEIs also increase the concentration of bradykinin and other tachykinins, leading to vasodilation and some undesirable effects. ARBs block the effect of angiotensin II by whatever synthetic pathway because they block the AT_1 receptor and the response to AT_1 receptor stimulation. The ARBs do not block the AT_2 receptor. This is considered a benefit of ARBs because the AT_2 receptor mediates vasodilation, inhibition of growth and proliferation, and apoptosis. ACE located in tissues is less affected by ACEIs. Enzymes are underlined. *GFR*, Glomerular filtration rate.

several weeks, blood pressure is progressively reduced, mainly through decreased peripheral resistance, with little effect on CO or renal blood flow in patients with otherwise normal cardiac function. Salt and water retention is not induced, and orthostatic hypotension and tachycardia are not problems.

The reduction in angiotensin II concentrations as a result of ACE inhibition also leads to a decrease in aldosterone secretion from the adrenal gland, which results in an increase in Na^+ and water excretion and a corresponding increase in the tubular reabsorption of K^+. Thus K^+ supplements and K^+-sparing diuretics should not be used concurrently with ACE inhibitors. With long-term ACE inhibitor therapy, deleterious cardiovascular remodeling may be reduced or even reversed. ACE inhibitors have also been shown to **reduce** long-term hypertension-induced **renal damage** and because of this are useful drugs in patients with chronic renal disease and diabetes. The presence of high-normal (or above normal) blood pressure and diabetes is a clear indication for the use of an ACE inhibitor.

Absorption, fate, and excretion

The onset of action of captopril is rapid, and the duration of effect is short, requiring administration two to three times daily. Because food in the gastrointestinal tract significantly reduces the absorption of captopril, the drug should be taken 1 hour before meals. Approximately 40% of captopril is metabolized in the liver, and most of the metabolites and the parent drug are excreted by the kidney. The elimination half-lives of the ACE inhibitors and angiotensin II receptor blockers are listed in Table 23-3.

TABLE 23-3 Elimination Half-Lives of Some ACE Inhibitors, Angiotensin II Receptor Blockers (ARBs), and Calcium Channel Blockers

ACE INHIBITORS AND ARBS		CALCIUM CHANNEL BLOCKERS	
Drug	**Elimination $t_{½}$ (h)**	**Drug**	**Elimination $t_{½}$ (h)**
Captopril	2	Verapamil	5
Enalapril	11*	Diltiazem	4
Lisinopril	12	Nifedipine	2
Trandolapril	20†	Nimodipine	1.5
Losartan	4‡	Felodipine	13
Valsartan	6	Nitrendipine	15
Eprosartan	6	Nisoldipine	10
Telmisartan	24	Amlodipine	40

*Due to enalaprilat, the active metabolite.
†Due to trandolaprilat, the active metabolite.
‡Includes the longer half-life metabolite.

Lisinopril is less well absorbed than **captopril**, resulting in peak plasma concentrations after approximately 7 hours. Lisinopril is excreted unchanged in the urine.

Enalapril (see Fig. 23-5 and Table 23-3) is a prodrug that must be hydrolyzed in the liver to become fully active. Its absorption is not influenced by food, and it has a longer duration of effect than captopril.

Enalaprilat is not absorbed from the gastrointestinal tract but is effective after intravenous administration; it has been marketed for such use in patients unable to take drugs orally. Other ACE inhibitors, such as trandolapril, with an esterified carboxyl side chain are also activated (by hydrolysis) in the liver to "prilat" metabolites that avidly bind to ACE and provide durations of effect sufficient for single daily dosing. Other ACE inhibitors are listed at the end of this chapter. They differ primarily in their pharmacokinetic properties.

Adverse effects

The most frequent side effect of the ACE inhibitors is **coughing**, which occurs in 20% of patients. Altered or **reduced taste sensation** is also common, especially with captopril. These adverse effects may disappear after continued use. Other adverse effects that have been documented are skin rash; **angioedema** of the face, mucous membranes of the mouth, or extremities; and flushing, pallor, and hypotension. Angioedema is a serious condition that demands withdrawal of the drug. Hyperkalemia and neutropenia may rarely occur.

ACE inhibitors may cause renal insufficiency in patients with **bilateral renal stenosis.** The mechanism is the reduction of renal angiotensin II production, leading to a disproportionate dilation of efferent renal blood vessels compared with afferent vessels. This vascular imbalance results in a significant decline in the glomerular filtration rate. ACE inhibitors can help preserve renal function in diabetic patients. ACE inhibitors have the beneficial effect of reducing proteinuria in patients with some renal diseases.

Although ACE inhibitors are not known to be teratogenic during the first trimester of pregnancy, they can cause significant **developmental defects** and fetal death later on. After pregnancy has been established, discontinuance or substitution with another antihypertensive agent is mandatory.

Angiotensin Receptor Antagonists

Losartan was the first orally active **angiotensin II receptor antagonist** to be introduced (Fig. 23-8). Other angiotensin II antagonists include **candesartan**, eprosartan, irbesartan, telmisartan, and **valsartan**. These nonpeptide analogues of angiotensin bind to the angiotensin II receptor and competitively inhibit the action of angiotensin II and angiotensin III. They are selective inhibitors of the AT_1 receptor, the angiotensin receptor subtype that accounts for the major physiologic effects of angiotensin II. The effect is to inhibit the consequences of AT_1 receptor stimulation without affecting potentially beneficial effects mediated by the AT_2 receptor (see Fig. 23-7). As is the case with ACE inhibitors, AT_1 receptor blockers reduce the blood pressure and the tissue remodeling seen in hypertension and reduce organ damage resulting from hypertension.

The half-lives for the angiotensin II blockers range from 4 to 24 hours (see Table 23-3). The selectivity of angiotensin II antagonists avoids some of the side effects of ACE inhibitors, such as coughing and angioedema, because the bradykinin pathway is not affected by the angiotensin II antagonists (see Fig. 23-7). Orally effective angiotensin II receptor antagonists now constitute a major drug group for treating hypertension.

Renin Inhibitors

Aliskiren is a **renin inhibitor** that binds with high specificity to the proteolytically active site of human renin (see Fig. 23-4). Renin is the rate-limiting step in the renin-angiotensin system. Aliskiren reduces circulating concentrations of angiotensin I and angiotensin II, producing a decrease in systolic and diastolic blood pressure, comparable to reductions seen with ACE inhibition or AT receptor antagonism. Based on the mechanism of action, expected adverse events include hyperkalemia and hypotension. Aliskiren administration produces hyperreninemia owing to a compensatory increase in renin release. This effect is not clinically significant. Aliskiren does not interfere with ACE-induced catabolism of bradykinin, and cough and angioedema are produced much less by this class of drugs than with ACE inhibitors. Similar to other inhibitors of the renin-angiotensin system, aliskiren is contraindicated in patients with bilateral renal artery stenosis and during pregnancy. Aliskiren has a poor bioavailability and is greater than 90% excreted unchanged in the feces, so minimal drug metabolism interactions are expected from this drug. None of the three aforementioned drug classes, ACE inhibitors, angiotensin II receptor blockers, and aliskiren, should be used together.

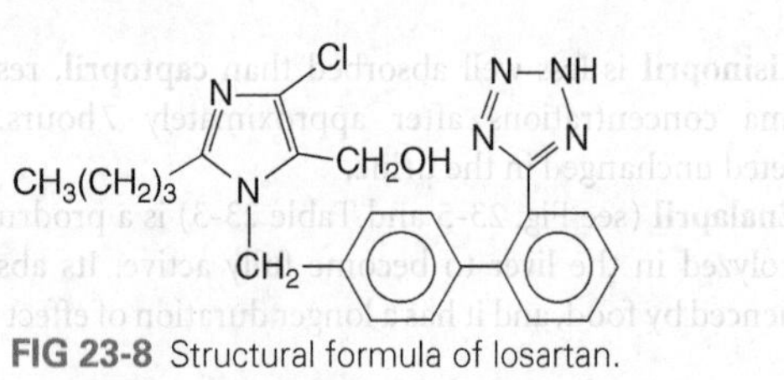

Cl
N—NH
N
N
N
CH₂OH
$CH_3(CH_2)_3$
N
CH_2

FIG 23-8 Structural formula of losartan.

CA^{2+} CHANNEL BLOCKERS (CCBs)

Verapamil, diltiazem, and nifedipine were the first CCBs to be marketed. The pharmacologic features of nifedipine and its dihydropyridine congeners, including amlodipine, felodipine, isradipine, nicardipine, nimodipine, nisoldipine, and nitrendipine, are addressed in this chapter. Other CCBs are discussed in Chapters 19 and 21.

Pharmacologic Effects

All CCBs prevent Ca^{2+} influx into smooth and cardiac muscle cells. The potency of these drugs for each of these actions varies, however, producing some important clinical distinctions between the dihydropyridines and verapamil and diltiazem. These latter two drugs inhibit Ca^{2+} influx into vascular smooth muscle and the heart with roughly the same potency. The effect of verapamil and diltiazem is to reduce blood pressure by vasodilation and reduced CO. Dihydropyridines such as nifedipine are much more potent at inhibiting Ca^{2+} influx at vascular smooth muscle than in the heart. At clinically relevant plasma concentrations, nifedipine produces a pronounced vasodilation with little direct effect on cardiac function. Reflex tachycardia is a common side effect with dihydropyridines but is almost never seen with verapamil and diltiazem. CCBs are contraindicated in patients with cardiac conduction defects and in heart failure. CCBs are useful drugs for treating low-renin hypertension, and are a major drug class for treating hypertension, especially in black patients (Table 23-4).

Dihydropyridines enhance the glomerular filtration rate and renal blood flow. Some patients taking dihydropyridines develop pedal edema. This condition does not result from fluid retention but rather from precapillary dilation. Renal Na^+ excretion may be enhanced.

TABLE 23-4 Initial Monotherapy for Hypertension

Patient	Non-blacks	Blacks
General population	THZD, ACE inhibitor, ARB or CCB	THZD or CCB
+CKD	ACE inhibitor or ARB	ACE inhibitor or ARB
+Diabetes	ACE inhibitor or ARB	THZD or CCB
+Diabetes and CKD	ACE inhibitor or ARB	ACE inhibitor or ARB

THZD, Thiazide-type or thiazide-like diuretic; *ACE*, angiotensin-converting enzyme; *ARB*, angiotensin receptor blocker; *CCB*, calcium channel blocker; *CKD*, chronic kidney disease.
Summary adapted from Drugs for hypertension. *Med Letter*, issue 141, May, Vol 12, 2014, pp. 31-39.

The antihypertensive effect and an apparent direct renoprotective effect of these drugs may make them useful in treating chronic renal failure.

Absorption, Fate, and Excretion

The elimination half-life and duration of action influence the clinical use of these agents (see Table 23-3). Long-term therapy may be associated with some increase in half-lives for some CCBs. The short time course of nimodipine, along with its relative ability to cross the blood–brain barrier, limits the drug's suitability for the treatment of chronic disease but permits its use to prevent vasospasm subsequent to subarachnoid hemorrhage. Short-acting nifedipine has been associated with an increased cardiovascular mortality rate during long-term use, and this rapidly absorbed preparation is no longer used for treating hypertension. The drug's short duration of action causes the blood pressure to wax and wane with each dose. The extended release version of the drug stabilizes blood concentrations and now is the recommended formulation. CCBs with long half-lives and slow-release preparations are recommended for this reason.

Adverse Effects

Toxic reactions and side effects of CCBs are described in Chapter 21.

DRUGS REDUCING SYMPATHETIC FUNCTION

A major homeostatic role of the autonomic nervous system is control of cardiovascular function. Drugs affecting autonomic activity are useful in controlling blood pressure in primary hypertension. This section describes drugs that exert their antihypertensive action on the sympathetic division of the autonomic nervous system. These drugs can conveniently be divided into four groups according to their site of action: (1) α-adrenergic receptor–blocking drugs, (2) β-adrenergic receptor–blocking drugs, (3) drugs altering peripheral adrenergic transmission, and (4) drugs acting on the CNS. Only actions and side effects pertinent to antihypertensive use of agents affecting adrenergic function are described here. For discussion of other uses and actions as well as pharmacokinetics of adrenergic receptor–blocking drugs, see Chapter 9.

β-Adrenergic Receptor–Blocking Drugs

The structures of representative **β-adrenergic receptor–blocking drugs** are shown in Figure 23-9. A more complete list of structures is shown in Chapter 9. **Propranolol**, the prototype for this class of drugs, and its congeners are not only used as antihypertensives, but they also are used in many other disorders, including cardiac arrhythmias, angina pectoris, and migraine headache. As indicated in Chapter 9, some of these agents, including propranolol, block β_1 and β_2 receptors, whereas others, such as **metoprolol,** have a selective effect on β_1 receptors of the heart. Some drugs classified as β-adrenergic blocking drugs are actually partial agonists, and some exert a membrane-stabilizing effect analogous to that of the local anesthetics. Because the local anesthetic action of β-blocking drugs occurs at doses higher than those used clinically, it may not be clinically relevant.

Pharmacologic effects

The various β-adrenergic receptor–blocking drugs are about equally effective in the management of hypertension, regardless of subtype selectivity. They can be used alone or in combination with diuretics and other antihypertensive medications. Their effects have been attributed to the following actions: blockade of β_1 receptors resulting in **decreased CO, decreased renin secretion**, decreased central sympathetic outflow, blockade of prejunctional β receptors on adrenergic nerve endings, and resetting of baroreceptors. Of these mechanisms, the first two are probably the most important for blood pressure control. Some investigators believe that hypertension characterized by high CO or high plasma renin activities represents a specific indication for β receptor antagonist therapy. Partial β receptor agonists produce less bradycardia than β receptor antagonists without partial β receptor agonist effects. Cardioselective β-adrenergic receptor antagonists (β_1-selective), having less affinity for bronchial β_2 receptors, are less likely to precipitate asthmatic attacks in susceptible individuals.

Adverse effects

The adverse effects of β-adrenergic receptor antagonists on the heart, smooth muscle, the CNS, and their adverse metabolic effects are discussed in Chapter 9. Abrupt withdrawal of β-adrenergic receptor antagonists in patients with coronary heart disease increases the likelihood of severe ischemic events and may lead to anginal pain, myocardial infarction, or life-threatening arrhythmia. Abrupt withdrawal in hypertensive patients may result in increased blood pressure and heart rate, palpitation, tremors, and sweating. It is important that dosages be gradually decreased when drug treatment with β blockers is terminated.

Salt and water retention, which is a problem with some antihypertensive medications, has not been reported with the β-adrenergic receptor–blocking drugs. Postural hypotension is also not generally encountered.

Selective α_1-Adrenergic Receptor–Blocking Drugs

Prazosin is the first of a group of selective **α_1-adrenergic receptor–blocking agents** used for the treatment of hypertension. **Terazosin** and **doxazosin** have a similar action. The chemical structure of prazosin is shown in Figure 23-9. The general pharmacologic characteristics of α_1-adrenergic receptor–blocking drugs are discussed in Chapter 9.

Pharmacologic effects

The hypotensive effect of these drugs is ascribed to vasodilation of arterioles and capacitance veins. The action is a result of blockade of α_1 receptors on vascular smooth muscle. In contrast to older, nonselective α blockers such as phenoxybenzamine, these drugs have a low affinity for α_2 receptors. They can be used in hypertension ranging from mild to severe, alone, with diuretics, or with other antihypertensive drugs.

Nonselective α-adrenergic receptor blockers are used only occasionally in therapy. Their ability to block α_1 and α_2 receptors is useful in treating hypertension resulting from pheochromocytoma. With this disease, α_1 and α_2 receptors play a major role in the hypertensive response to the elevated circulating catecholamine concentrations. Phentolamine is a competitive antagonist, whereas phenoxybenzamine is a noncompetitive antagonist.

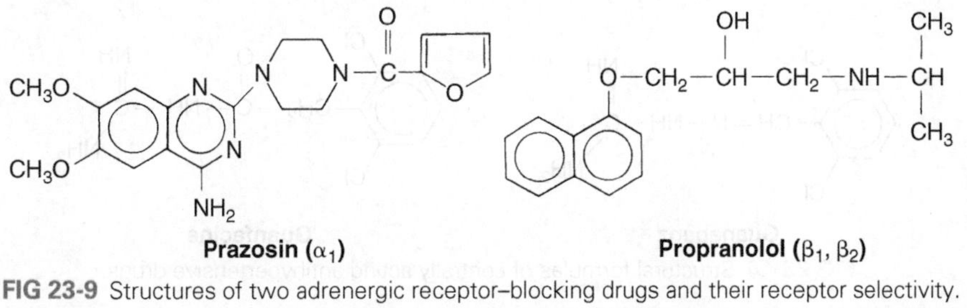

FIG 23-9 Structures of two adrenergic receptor–blocking drugs and their receptor selectivity.

The adverse effects of nonselective α-adrenergic receptor antagonists are more notable than the adverse effects of selective α_1-adrenergic receptor blockers. Inhibition of prejunctional α_2 receptors accounts for the greater reflex tachycardia seen with nonselective blockers. There is a higher incidence of orthostatic hypotension and fluid retention compared with selective α_1-adrenergic receptor antagonists.

Adverse effects

Prazosin and other α_1-adrenergic receptor blockers produce less reflex tachycardia than direct vasodilators or nonselective α-adrenergic receptor blockers. Nevertheless, reflex tachycardia may be significant. Syncope from orthostatic hypotension may occur with the initiation of therapy. This heightened response early in therapy has been termed the **first-dose effect**. This usually requires starting therapy at a low dose. Postural hypotension usually abates with continued therapy. These drugs share an array of other side effects, including gastrointestinal upset, palpitation, tinnitus, headache, rash, edema, and urinary incontinence. Inhibition of ejaculation may also occur.

α_1-Adrenergic and β-Adrenergic Receptor Blockers

Labetalol is a competitive blocker of **α_1, β_1, and β_2** receptors, with a greater affinity for β receptors. It also exerts some β_2-agonistic activity and inhibits norepinephrine uptake by the presynaptic nerve terminal. This extensive pharmacologic profile results from the fact that the drug is composed of four different diastereoisomers, each of which has distinct effects. Labetalol has been used singly and in combination with other antihypertensive agents. Used orally and intravenously, labetalol undergoes significant first-pass metabolism in the liver, accounting for approximately 75% of an oral dose. It has a half-life of approximately 8 hours and is metabolized to the glucuronide conjugate. Labetalol is especially useful in treating pheochromocytoma and hypertensive emergencies. Its adverse effects include gastrointestinal disturbances, dry mouth, fatigue, nervousness, paresthesias, orthostatic hypotension, and bradycardia. Patients with asthma are at risk of bronchospasm.

Carvedilol is the second drug with mixed α_1-adrenergic and β-adrenergic receptor–blocking activity to be marketed for the treatment of hypertension and heart failure. As with labetalol, several stereoisomers contribute to the drug's complex pharmacologic characteristics. The pharmacokinetic profile is similar to that of labetalol; however, one of the isomers of carvedilol, which contributes roughly half of the drug's α-blocking activity, accumulates up to threefold in patients genetically deficient in cytochrome P450 2D6 activity. Carvedilol is available only for oral use.

Although **nebivolol** does not block α-adrenergic receptors, it is a vasodilator because it **releases nitric oxide** in blood vessels, in addition to being a selective β_1-adrenergic receptor blocker. It is indicated for hypertension, but its ability to release nitric oxide appears to give it fewer adverse effects compared to traditional β-adrenergic receptor blockers.

Drugs That Affect Adrenergic Transmission

Guanethidine and guanadrel exert their primary antihypertensive action on peripheral postganglionic adrenergic nerve endings and are classified as adrenergic neuron–blocking drugs. The ultimate effect of guanethidine and guanadrel is depletion of norepinephrine from adrenergic nerve endings. Since these drugs are rarely used today for the treatment of hypertension, they will not be discussed further.

Centrally Acting Antihypertensive Drugs

Methyldopa, clonidine, guanabenz, and guanfacine are drugs that exert their antihypertensive effect by **stimulating α_2-adrenergic receptors** in the **brainstem**. As a result, these drugs reduce sympathetic outflow from the brain. The structures of methyldopa, clonidine, guanabenz, and guanfacine are shown in Figure 23-10. The structural similarity of methyldopa to the catecholamine transmitter norepinephrine is obvious. Clonidine, guanabenz, and guanfacine are not chemically related to norepinephrine.

Pharmacologic effects

Methyldopa, a prodrug, is biotransformed in the brain to α-methyldopamine and then to α-methylnorepinephrine. The latter metabolite probably stimulates important α_2-adrenergic receptor sites in the medulla, resulting in inhibition of central sympathetic outflow. In addition, there is evidence that vagal activity to the heart is increased. Clonidine, guanabenz, and guanfacine seem to act directly as central α_2-adrenergic receptor agonists. With all four drugs, the reduction in central sympathetic outflow and increased vagal activity lead to reduced peripheral vascular resistance and CO. It is uncertain whether presynaptic or postsynaptic medullary α_2 receptors play the predominant role in mediating the antihypertensive response.

Absorption, fate, and excretion

Methyldopa can be given orally or intravenously (as methyldopate hydrochloride). Approximately 25% to 50% of an orally administered dose of methyldopa is absorbed from the gastrointestinal tract. Although methyldopa and its metabolites appear rapidly in the urine, significant concentrations remain in the body for longer periods. It has a long duration of action (up to 24 hours), probably because α-methylnorepinephrine is not metabolized by monoamine oxidase, but is stored in synaptic vesicles in central adrenergic nerve terminals.

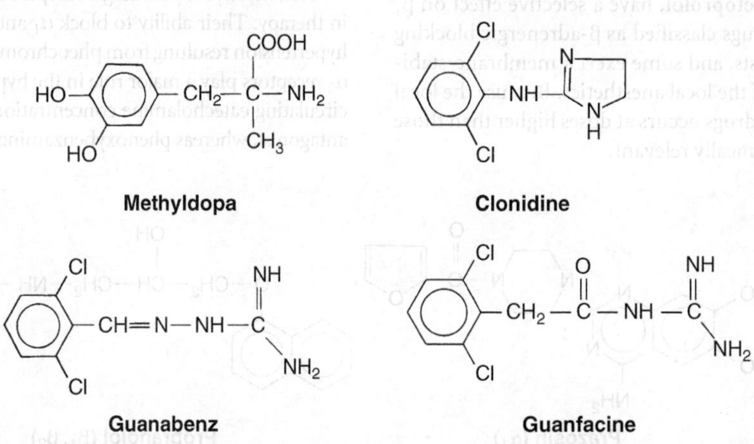

Methyldopa

Clonidine

Guanabenz

Guanfacine

FIG 23-10 Structural formulas of centrally acting antihypertensive drugs.

Clonidine is available for oral and parenteral use and is well absorbed after oral administration. Peak plasma concentrations are achieved in 3 to 5 hours; its half-life is approximately 10 hours. Approximately 50% is metabolized in the liver. The remaining clonidine and its metabolites are primarily excreted in the urine.

Approximately 75% of an oral dose of guanabenz is absorbed, but hepatic metabolism decreases bioavailability. Peak plasma concentrations appear 2 to 5 hours after administration. The plasma half-life is approximately 6 hours. A large percentage of guanabenz is metabolized in the liver and excreted by the kidney. Guanfacine is rapidly and nearly completely absorbed from the gastrointestinal tract. It has a half-life of 14 to 17 hours. The drug is partly hydroxylated, and parent drug and metabolites are excreted in the urine.

Adverse effects

Untoward effects of methyldopa include drowsiness, depression, nightmares, dry mouth, and nasal stuffiness. The drowsiness caused by this drug, although usually transient, may be particularly bothersome. Orthostatic hypotension is not frequent because the baroreceptor reflex is not greatly affected by centrally acting drugs. Extrapyramidal reactions, prolactin release, and impotence may also occur. Hepatitis, a lupus-like syndrome, drug fever, and blood dyscrasias are rare adverse manifestations.

The most common side effects of clonidine are dry mouth and sedation. The incidence of these effects is high, but some tolerance may develop during long-term therapy. Other side effects include parotid gland pain, nightmares, and insomnia. Constipation and impotence occur in a small percentage of patients treated with clonidine. Rebound hypertension has been observed on abrupt withdrawal of clonidine therapy. The sudden withdrawal of clonidine is also associated with tachycardia, anxiety, and insomnia. When withdrawal is necessary, the dosage should be reduced gradually.

Guanabenz has not been found to cause postural hypotension. Adverse side effects, listed in order of decreasing frequency, are drowsiness, dry mouth, dizziness, weakness, and headache. Side effects of guanfacine are mild and dose related. The side effects include fatigue, dizziness, dry mouth, insomnia, and impotence, but they tend to be less disturbing than with clonidine or guanabenz. Abrupt withdrawal of guanabenz and guanfacine has been associated with rebound hypertension.

Directly Acting Vasodilators

Hydralazine, **minoxidil**, **diazoxide**, **nitroprusside**, and **nitroglycerin** exert their primary antihypertensive effect through a direct action on vascular smooth muscle. Figure 23-11 summarizes the site of action of the directly acting vasodilators and other drugs that

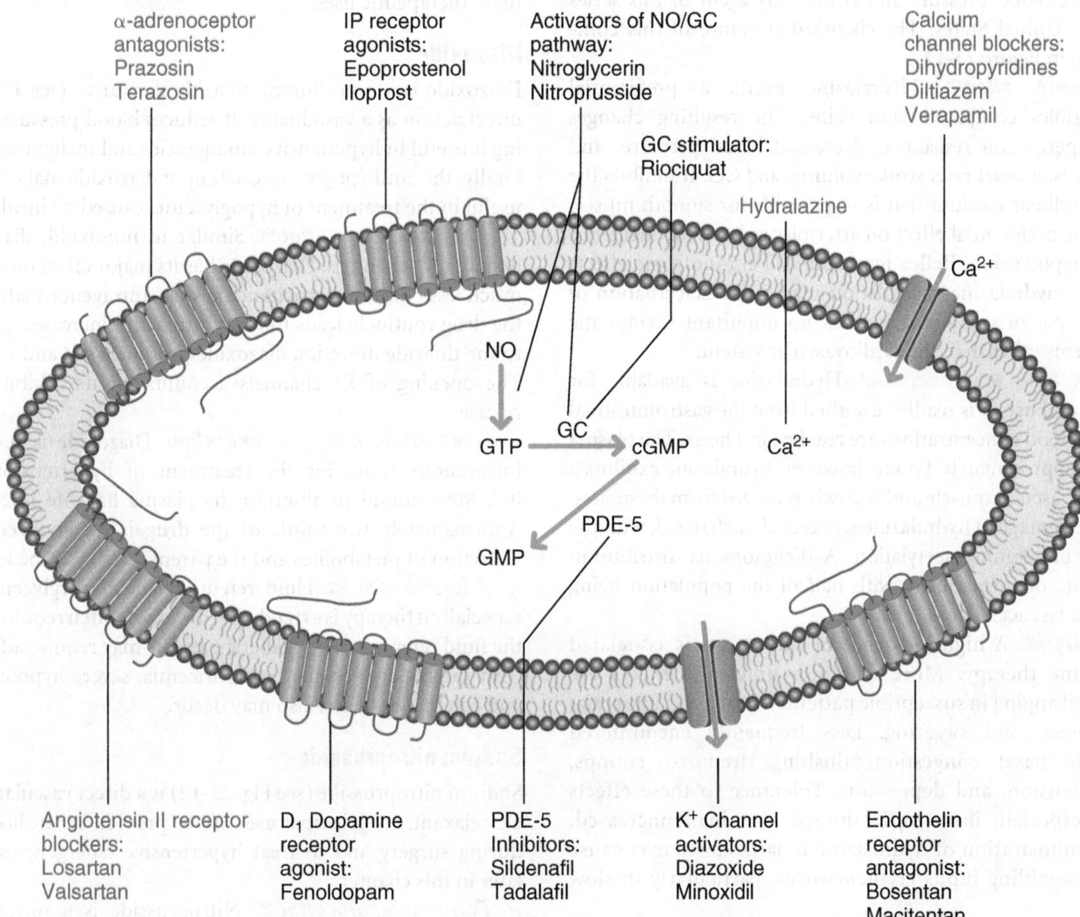

FIG 23-11 Sites of action of drugs that relax vascular smooth muscle. Various drug types that act on the vascular smooth muscle cell are depicted. Individual drug examples are given with each drug class. Drugs shown in red are drugs that are typically used in chronic therapy. The others are used in hypertensive emergencies, refractory cases, or in pulmonary hypertension. Hydralazine inhibits the release of intracellular calcium. *cGMP*, cyclic guanosine monophosphate; *GC*, guanylyl cyclase; *GMP*, guanosine monophosphate; *GTP*, guanosine triphosphate; *IP*, prostacyclin; *NO*, nitric oxide; *PDE-5*, phosphodiesterase-5.

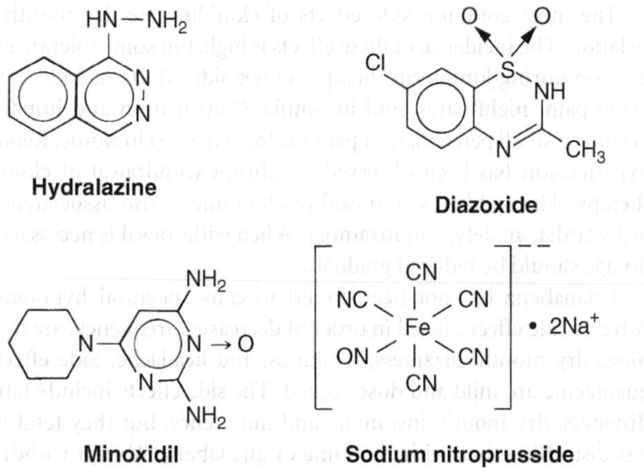

Hydralazine Diazoxide Minoxidil Sodium nitroprusside

FIG 23-12 Structural formulas of some directly acting vasodilators.

relax vascular smooth muscle by inhibiting or stimulating enzymes or membrane-bound receptors that influence contractile responses in a vascular smooth muscle cell.

Hydralazine

Hydralazine is one of a series of phthalazine derivatives that have been shown to reduce blood pressure and is the only agent of this series available in the United States. The chemical structure of this compound is shown in Figure 23-12.

Pharmacologic effects. Hydralazine exerts a preferential effect on arterioles compared with veins. The resulting changes are decreased peripheral resistance; decreased blood pressure; and reflexively increased heart rate, stroke volume, and CO. It inhibits the release of intracellular calcium that is responsible for smooth muscle contraction. The preferential effect on arterioles reduces the incidence of orthostatic hypotension. Reflex inotropic and chronotropic effects that accompany hydralazine vasodilation may cause exacerbation of existing angina pectoris. Hydralazine has no important therapeutic actions on systems other than the cardiovascular system.

Absorption, fate, and excretion. Hydralazine is available for parenteral and oral use. It is readily absorbed from the gastrointestinal tract, and peak blood concentrations are reached in 1 hour. The plasma half-life is also approximately 1 hour; however, hydralazine exhibits a high affinity for vascular muscle and is slowly removed from these sites. Only a small percentage of hydralazine is excreted unchanged, with the major portion undergoing acetylation. A dichotomous distribution exists in the rate of metabolism, with half of the population being characterized as fast acetylators.

Adverse effects. A high incidence of side effects is associated with hydralazine therapy. More common untoward effects are palpitation (and angina in susceptible patients), headache, anorexia, nausea, dizziness, and sweating. Less frequently encountered effects include nasal congestion, flushing, tremors, cramps, postural hypotension, and depression. Tolerance to these effects may develop, especially if the initial dosage is gradually increased. Long-term administration of hydralazine in large doses may cause a syndrome resembling lupus erythematosus, particularly in slow acetylators.

Minoxidil

Minoxidil is another antihypertensive drug that acts chiefly through arteriolar vasodilation. The chemical structure of this piperidinopyrimidine is shown in Figure 23-12. Minoxidil is reserved for use in patients who are refractory to other therapy.

Pharmacologic effects. Minoxidil, similar to other peripheral vasodilators, reduces blood pressure by decreasing TPR. Minoxidil activates K^+ channels, resulting in hyperpolarization, stabilization of the smooth muscle plasma membrane, and reduced contraction. The drug is a prodrug requiring conversion to minoxidil sulfate (a quantitatively minor metabolite) for its vasodilator effect.

The decrease in blood pressure from minoxidil is accompanied by reflex increases in cardiac function, renin secretion, and fluid retention. These potentially adverse responses may be corrected by coadministration of β-adrenergic receptor–blocking agents and diuretics. Minoxidil has no central depressant effects.

Absorption, fate, and excretion. The onset of action of minoxidil after oral administration is rapid, and its hypotensive action is of long duration. This compound is primarily excreted in the urine as the glucuronide conjugate, along with small amounts of the parent compound and hydroxylated derivatives.

Adverse effects. The marked fluid retention caused by minoxidil can lead to congestive heart failure. There are reports of pericardial effusion and cardiac tamponade, sometimes with fatal outcomes. As with other vasodilators, the reflex tachycardia may initiate or intensify angina. Dermatologic reactions and breast tenderness may also occur. Finally, abnormal hair growth, or hypertrichosis, is very common and limits the use of this drug. Topical minoxidil is approved for the treatment of alopecia and baldness, and these indications represent its main therapeutic uses.

Diazoxide

Diazoxide is a non-diuretic thiazide derivative (see Fig. 23-12) with direct action as a vasodilator. It reduces blood pressure rapidly, making it useful in hypertensive emergencies and malignant hypertension. Orally, the antihypoglycemic action of diazoxide makes it occasionally useful in the treatment of hypoglycemia caused by insulin.

Pharmacologic effects. Similar to minoxidil, diazoxide acts by opening K^+ channels. Diazoxide has its major effect on arterioles, with much less effect on capacitance vessels. Intravenous administration of the drug routinely leads to tachycardia and increased CO. In contrast to the thiazide diuretics, diazoxide promotes salt and water retention. The opening of K^+ channels accounts for its inhibition of insulin release.

Absorption, fate, and excretion. Diazoxide is restricted to the intravenous route for the treatment of hypertension. In plasma, it is 90% bound to albumin. Its plasma half-life is 20 to 60 hours. Approximately two-thirds of the drug is metabolized in the liver. Excretion of metabolites and the parent drug is by the kidney.

Adverse effects. Fluid retention and hyperglycemia can occur, especially if therapy is extended. A diuretic is often required to overcome the fluid retention, and diabetic patients may require added therapy to treat the hyperglycemia. Hyperuricemia, severe hypotension, angina, and cerebral ischemia also may occur.

Sodium nitroprusside

Sodium nitroprusside (see Fig. 23-12) is a direct vascular smooth muscle relaxant. Its principal uses are to provide controlled hypotension during surgery and to treat hypertensive emergencies, as described later in this chapter.

Pharmacologic effects. Nitroprusside is a nitrovasodilator. It generates nitric oxide, which activates guanylyl cyclase in vascular smooth muscle. The resulting relaxation of smooth muscle accounts for its antihypertensive response. The drug affects veins and arterioles and reduces preload and afterload. Because capacitance and resistance vessels are dilated, cardiac ischemia and angina are not as frequently associated with nitroprusside as with arteriolar vasodilators.

FIG 23-13 Structural formula of fenoldopam.

Absorption, fate, and excretion. Nitroprusside works rapidly after intravenous administration. It is not used orally. In addition to producing nitric oxide, it is converted non-enzymatically to cyanide by red blood cells and metabolized further to thiocyanate in the liver and kidney. The half-life of nitroprusside is measured in minutes; thiocyanate may persist with a half-life of approximately 3 days. Thiocyanate is excreted by the kidney.

Adverse effects. Adverse reactions can be classified as acute or chronic. Acute effects include a precipitous decline in blood pressure, with resultant sweating, vomiting, headache, nervousness, and palpitation. Metabolic acidosis, methemoglobinemia, and cardiac arrhythmias have occurred. Cyanide accumulation may occur in some individuals, leading to toxicity. Thiocyanate may accumulate in patients with renal insufficiency. Thiocyanate may cause psychosis, muscle weakness, and hypothyroid symptoms.

Nitroglycerin

Nitroglycerin is described in detail in Chapter 21. When given intravenously, nitroglycerin is an effective treatment for perioperative hypertension and to induce controlled hypotension during surgery. Similar in mechanism of action to nitroprusside, nitroglycerin exerts a relatively greater effect on capacitance vessels. Continuous infusion with careful monitoring of blood pressure is required for proper control of blood pressure.

Fenoldopam

Fenoldopam is a vasodilator that is used in emergency situations.

Pharmacologic effects. Fenoldopam (Fig. 23-13) is an agonist at dopamine D_1 receptors. It stimulates D_1 receptors in blood vessels and results in vasodilation, especially in renal vessels. As such, it increases renal blood flow and decreases blood pressure.

Absorption, fate, and excretion. Fenoldopam is given by continuous intravenous administration and has an elimination half-life of approximately 5 minutes. Hepatic metabolism by conjugation accounts for the termination of its pharmacologic effects because the metabolites are inactive. Most of the metabolites are excreted by the kidney.

MISCELLANEOUS DRUGS

Metyrosine (α-methyltyrosine) is an inhibitor of tyrosine hydroxylase, the rate-limiting enzyme in the formation of norepinephrine and epinephrine. Although not recommended for essential hypertension, metyrosine is useful, often in combination with phentolamine, in the pharmacologic amelioration of pheochromocytoma.

Numerous drugs had previously been used to treat hypertension. Drugs such as reserpine, monoamine oxidase inhibitors, *Veratrum* alkaloids, and ganglionic blockers are now rarely if ever used to treat hypertension.

TABLE 23-5 Concomitant Disorders That Favor the Use of Alternative Antihypertensive Drugs

Hypertension Accompanied By	Alternative Drug
Heart failure	β-Blocker
History of myocardial infarction	β-Blocker
Coronary artery disease	β-Blocker
Angina pectoris	β-Blocker or CCB*
Migraine	β-Blocker
Prostate hypertrophy	α_1-Blocker

*Verapamil or diltiazem.

TREATMENT OF HYPERTENSION

Treatment of hypertension often includes pharmacologic and nonpharmacologic approaches for optimal control. Although the latter subject is beyond the scope of this discussion, dietary modification to reduce body weight and decrease Na^+ intake cause demonstrable reductions in blood pressure. Na^+ restriction, even within the well-controlled DASH diet, has been shown to reduce blood pressure. The reduction in blood pressure is proportional to the reduction in Na^+ intake. Restriction of fat intake and alcohol ingestion and cessation of smoking are also important considerations in lessening the dangers of cardiovascular diseases associated with hypertension. Optimal pharmacotherapeutic treatment is based on appropriate diagnosis, proper drug and dose selection, and good patient compliance. Inasmuch as essential hypertension in its early states is asymptomatic, compliance depends strongly on the avoidance of side effects and the simplicity of the therapeutic regimen.

Four drug classes are currently the most common initial drugs used in the treatment of hypertension: **diuretics**, **ACE inhibitors**, **angiotensin II receptor blockers**, and **CCBs**. **β-Adrenergic receptor blockers** are less often used but still are important for the treatment of hypertension, especially in cases of certain concomitant disorders (see Table 23-5). **α_1-Adrenergic receptor blockers** and **aliskiren** are less often used than the β-blockers but are available as substitutes for other antihypertensive drugs or used in combined therapy. Diuretics or ACE inhibitors are considered the most appropriate first choices for many hypertensive patients (Table 23-4).

Therapy needs to be tailored to the patient. When used alone, ACE inhibitors are usually less effective in African American patients than in Caucasians, whereas diuretics may be nearly equally useful in both groups (see Table 23-4). This selectivity of effect correlates with the typically lower contribution of the renin-angiotensin system to hypertension in African Americans and their greater Na^+ sensitivity. Age may also contribute to the response. Certain disease states can also affect the choice of drug. As shown in Table 23-5, a second disorder concomitant with hypertension may dictate a different drug priority.

For initial therapy of hypertension, a low dose of a thiazide-type or thiazide-like diuretic is recommended. An ACE inhibitor is also considered a logical first choice for many patients. When a single drug is ineffective, combination therapy may be required. Drugs such as ACE inhibitors or angiotensin II receptor blockers are commonly used with diuretics, sometimes in combination with additional agents, like the β-adrenergic receptor blockers. Centrally acting antihypertensives can be combined with CCBs with or without a diuretic. Hydralazine, when used, is combined with a β-adrenergic receptor blocker. The addition of the β blocker prevents tachycardia resulting from hydralazine and enhances the antihypertensive response. In addition to their hypotensive effect, the diuretics reduce fluid retention caused by some antihypertensive drugs.

TABLE 23-6 Drugs Used in Acute Hypertension

Drug	Comment
Hypertensive Emergencies (Parenteral)	
Sodium nitroprusside	Often used; requires continuous monitoring
Nitroglycerin	Indicated in patients with ischemic heart disease
Labetalol	Useful in thyrotoxicosis and pheochromocytoma and as a substitute for Na^+ nitroprusside when continuous monitoring is unavailable; contraindicated in patients with systolic heart failure, airway disease, or heart block
Diazoxide	Occasionally used when continuous monitoring is unavailable
Fenoldopam	Has rapid onset and short half-life
Hydralazine	Used in hypertensive states associated with pregnancy
Nifedipine	Short-acting, also used for hypertensive emergencies during pregnancy
Hypertensive Urgencies (Oral Preferred)	
Clonidine	Requires good patient compliance
Captopril	Responses unpredictable
Labetalol	See labetalol above

Severe hypertension almost always requires use of more than one drug. Certain drugs are used only in refractory hypertension. These drugs include guanethidine and minoxidil, each used in combination with a diuretic and other drugs.

Hypertensive Emergencies

In contrast to the gradual increase in blood pressure seen in essential hypertension, a sudden elevation of blood pressure to severely hypertensive levels may sometimes occur. Hypertensive emergencies may arise in the course of any hypertensive disease, including renal hypertension, toxemia of pregnancy, or pheochromocytoma. These situations, regardless of cause, are life-threatening and require immediate reduction of blood pressure. **Parenteral drug administration** is often necessary; however if time permits, oral therapy can be used. Table 23-6 lists drugs used to treat hypertensive emergencies.

Treatment of Pulmonary Hypertension

Pulmonary (arterial) hypertension is a serious and life-threating disease. Although progress has been made in its treatment, life expectancy is still poor. Therapy is aimed at **preventing pulmonary arterial vasoconstriction and dysfunction.** Table 23-7 lists drugs used in treatment and their mechanisms and routes of administration.

Antihypertensive Drug Withdrawal Syndrome

Withdrawal of antihypertensive drug therapy has been associated with several signs and symptoms, depending on the abruptness of the withdrawal, the degree of hypertension, and the drugs involved. The classes of drugs involved in withdrawal reactions include centrally acting agents, β-adrenergic receptor–blocking drugs, neuronal blocking agents, and some vasodilators (e.g., minoxidil, sodium nitroprusside, and nifedipine). Reported responses include rebound hypertension, tachycardia, angina, heart attack, and sudden death.

Recommendations for managing hypertensive patients on drug therapy include encouraging patient compliance and avoiding excessive dosage. To avoid complications, antihypertensive drugs should be withdrawn slowly, and patients should be carefully monitored, especially patients with coronary artery or cerebrovascular disease.

TABLE 23-7 Drugs Used to Treat Pulmonary Hypertension

Drug	Mechanism of Vasodilator Action	Route of Administration
CCBs, e.g., nifedipine, diltiazem	Block calcium channels	Oral
Sildenafil	Inhibits PDE-5	IV
Tadalafil	Inhibits PDE-5	Oral
Epoprostenol (prostacyclin)	Stimulates IP receptor	IV
Iloprost	Stimulates IP receptor	Inhalation
Treprostinil	Stimulates IP receptor	SC, IV, inhalation
Bosentan	Endothelin receptor antagonist	Oral
Ambrisentan	Endothelin receptor antagonist	Oral
Macitentan	Endothelin receptor antagonist	Oral
Riociquat	Stimulates soluble guanylyl cyclase	Oral

CCBs, Calcium channel blockers; *PDE*, phosphodiesterase; *IP*, prostacyclin; *IV*, intravenous; *SC*, subcutaneous.

IMPLICATIONS FOR DENTISTRY

Drug Interactions

Because there are several categories of antihypertensive drugs (each class having a different mechanism of action), there are numerous possibilities for drug interactions. Aspirin and other nonsteroidal antiinflammatory drugs **(NSAIDs) antagonize many antihypertensive drugs.** The antihypertensive effects of ACE inhibitors, ARBs, and aliskiren are reduced by aspirin. In addition, the effect of diuretics is inhibited by NSAIDs. This interaction apparently results from the inhibitory effect of chronic (>5 days) NSAID therapy on prostaglandin synthesis. Prostaglandins are important in maintaining renal blood flow and urine output. NSAIDs also reduce the antihypertensive effect of β blockers. Patients should be advised of this drug interaction; in the event that blood pressure control is lost, substitution with acetaminophen with or without opioid supplementation is advised for pain.

In general, the use of vasoconstrictors in local anesthesia is not contraindicated in hypertensive patients, especially in patients whose blood pressure is well controlled. A possible exception to this statement is a patient receiving an adrenergic neuron–blocking or adrenergic neuron–depleting drug, such as **guanethidine,** or a **nonselective β-adrenergic receptor–blocking drug** such as propranolol. Long-term use of guanethidine-related drugs produces supersensitivity to the actions of exogenously administered catecholamines. **Injudicious use of sympathomimetic amine vasoconstrictors** in local anesthetic solutions could possibly lead to serious disturbances of blood pressure and cardiac rhythm. Nonselective β-adrenergic receptor blockers prevent the decrease in peripheral vascular resistance normally caused by doses of epinephrine used in local anesthesia. Unopposed α-agonistic action may lead to an acute hypertensive episode. To avoid potential complications, the blood pressure of a patient on any of these medications should be taken before and 5 minutes after the injection of a small amount of local anesthetic (e.g., 1 mL of 2% lidocaine with 1:100,000 epinephrine). If no significant reaction is observed, dangerous hypertensive responses to additional local anesthetic are unlikely.

The use of **epinephrine-impregnated retraction cord** is contraindicated in patients with compromised cardiovascular function, including hypertensive patients. Significant amounts of epinephrine can be absorbed, especially if the gingiva is abraded or multiple teeth are involved.

Although not widely used, **centrally acting sympatholytics**, which have a **sedative** side effect, are important to the dentist. In dealing with patients taking these drugs, the dentist must proceed cautiously when using antianxiety agents or other drugs that depress the CNS. In combination with antihypertensives with sedative side effects, these agents may lead to excessive CNS depression. Use of a smaller dose is advised in the premedication of a patient taking methyldopa, clonidine, guanabenz, or guanfacine for hypertension.

Adverse Effects

One adverse effect of significance to the dentist that is associated with antihypertensive medication is orthostatic, or **postural, hypotension**. After being in a supine position, many patients receiving antihypertensive therapy may be unable to compensate adequately for a sudden change in position. Such patients should be observed carefully at the end of dental appointments. Drugs affecting peripheral adrenergic transmission are most likely to cause orthostatic hypotension, although other drugs may also have this action.

Another adverse effect that has implications in dentistry is inhibition of salivary secretion leading to dry mouth. **Xerostomia** is especially common in patients medicated with centrally acting antihypertensive agents (methyldopa, clonidine, guanabenz, and guanfacine).

Hypertension Detection

The American Heart Association has stressed the need for more effective **hypertension detection**, and dentists are encouraged to include blood pressure determinations as a part of routine office visits. Studies indicate that many patients identified by dentists as being hypertensive were unaware of their condition. Most of those identified sought medical attention to treat the hypertension.

Screening for hypertension in the dental office is a simple procedure that can be carried out effectively by auxiliary personnel. Because hypertension is a dangerous but asymptomatic disease in its early stages, the dentist's efforts to identify and aid these patients by its detection are worthwhile. The dentist can advise against abrupt withdrawal from antihypertensive medication and inform the patient of the possible hazards of such action.

ANTIHYPERTENSIVE DRUGS

Nonproprietary (Generic) Name	Proprietary (Trade) Name
Diuretics	
See Chapter 22	
Agents Affecting Adrenergic Function	
Transmitter Synthesis Inhibiting	
Metyrosine	Demser
Neuronal Blocking or Depleting	
Guanadrel	Hylorel
Guanethidine	Ismelin
α-Adrenergic Receptor Blocking	
Doxazosin	Cardura
Phenoxybenzamine	Dibenzyline
Phentolamine	Regitine
Prazosin	Minipress
Terazosin	Hytrin
β-Adrenergic Receptor Blocking	
Acebutolol	Sectral
Atenolol	Tenormin
Betaxolol	Kerlone
Bisoprolol	Zebeta
Carteolol	Cartrol
Esmolol	Brevibloc
Metoprolol	Lopressor, Toprol XL
Nadolol	Corgard
Nebivolol*	Bystolic
Penbutolol	Levatol
Pindolol	Visken
Propranolol	Inderal
Timolol	Blocadren
α-Adrenergic and β-Adrenergic Receptor Blocking	
Carvedilol	Coreg
Labetalol	Trandate
Centrally Acting	
Clonidine	Catapres
Guanabenz	Wytensin
Guanfacine	Tenex
Methyldopa	Aldomet, Amodopa
Direct Vasodilators	
Diazoxide	Hyperstat IV
Hydralazine	Apresoline
Minoxidil	Loniten
Nitroglycerin	Nitro-Bid IV, Tridil
Nitroprusside	Nitropress
Prostacyclin Receptor Agonists	
Epoprostenol	Flolan
Iloprost	Ventavis
Treprostinil	Remodulin, Tyvaso
Selexipag	Uptravi
Dopamine D_1 Receptor Agonist	
Fenoldopam	Corlopam
Endothelin Receptor Antagonists	
Bosentan	Tracleer
Ambrisentan	Letairis
Macitentan	Opsumit
Ca^{2+} Channel Blockers	
Amlodipine	Norvasc
Diltiazem	Cardizem, Dilacor XR
Felodipine	Plendil
Isradipine	DynaCirc
Nicardipine	Cardene
Nifedipine	Adalat, Procardia
Nimodipine	Nimotop
Nisoldipine	Sular
Verapamil	Calan, Isoptin
Angiotensin-Converting Enzyme Inhibitors	
Benazepril	Lotensin
Captopril	Capoten
Enalapril	Vasotec
Enalaprilat	Vasotec I.V.
Fosinopril	Monopril
Lisinopril	Prinivil, Zestril

Continued

ANTIHYPERTENSIVE DRUGS—cont'd

Nonproprietary (Generic) Name	Proprietary (Trade) Name
Angiotensin-Converting Enzyme Inhibitors cont'd	
Moexipril	Univasc
Perindopril erbumine	Aceon
Quinapril	Accupril
Ramipril	Altace
Trandolapril	Mavik
Angiotensin II Receptor Blockers	
Azilsartan	Edarbi
Candesartan cilexetil	Atacand
Eprosartan	Teveten
Irbesartan	Avapro
Losartan	Cozaar
Olmesartan	Benicar
Telmisartan	Micardis
Valsartan	Diovan
Renin Inhibitor	
Aliskiren	Tekturna
Phosphodiesterase-5 Inhibitor	
Sildenafil	Revatio
Tadalafil	Adcirca
Soluble Guanylyl Cyclase Stimulator	
Riociquat	Adempas
Combination Products (Examples)	
Atenolol, chlorthalidone	Tenoretic
Amlodipine, benazepril	Lotrel
Azilsartan, chlorthalidone	Edarbyclor
Bendroflumethiazide, nadolol	Corzide
Betaxolol, chlorthalidone	Kerledex
Captopril, hydrochlorothiazide	Capozide
Hydralazine, hydrochlorothiazide	Apresazide
Methyldopa, hydrochlorothiazide	Aldoril
Propranolol, hydrochlorothiazide	Inderide
Trandolapril, verapamil	Tarka

*Also relaxes vascular smooth muscle by releasing nitric oxide.

CASE DISCUSSION

The doses for both antihypertensive drugs are typical doses. The oral exam indicates that it is unlikely that the cause of the swelling in the pharynx is due to an infection from the teeth or soft tissue of the mouth. The timing of the swelling after the initiation of therapy with the ACE inhibitor, lisinopril, is suggestive of a reaction to that drug. The swelling could be angioedema which, although somewhat rare, typically occurs shortly after therapy is started and is often first noticed 10 to 14 days after the ACE inhibitor therapy is started. Angioedema can be a medical emergency, and the airway can be compromised. The patient should contact his physician immediately. The patient will be taken off the ACE inhibitor in favor of a drug from a different class.

GENERAL REFERENCES

1. Bader M: Tissue renin-angiotensin-aldosterone systems: targets for pharmacological therapy, *Annu Rev Pharmacol Toxicolol* 50:439–465, 2010.
2. Calhoun DA: Hyperaldosteronism as a common cause of resistant hypertension, *Annu Rev Med* 64:233–247, 2013.
3. Drugs for hypertension, *Med Letter*(141)31–39, 2014.
4. Feldman RD, Hussain Y, Kuyper LM, et al.: Intraclass differences among antihypertensive drugs, *Annu Rev Pharmacol Toxicol* 55:333–352, 2015.
5. Frumkin LR: The pharmacological treatment of pulmonary hypertension, *Pharmacol Rev* 64:583–620, 2012.
6. Ghamami N: Time course for blood pressure lowering of dihydropyridine calcium channel blockers, *Cochrane Database Syst Rev* 8, Aug. 31, 2014.
7. James PA, Oparil S, Carter BL, et al.: Evidenced-based guidelines for the management of high blood pressure in adults, Report from the panel members appointed to the Eighth Joint National Committee (JNC 8), *J Am Med Assoc* 311:507–520, 2014.
8. Levine DA, Lewis CE, Williams OD, et al.: Geographic and demographic variability in 20-year hypertension incidence, the CARDIA study, *Hypertension* 57:39–47, 2011.
9. Morisco C, Trimarco B: Angiotensin converting enzyme inhibitors and AT1 antagonists for treatment of hypertension. In *ACEi and ARBS in Hypertension and Heart Failure, Current Cardiovascular Therapy*, 5. New York, 2015, Springer, pp 1–39.
10. Rik HG, Engberink O, Frenkel WJ, et al.: Effects of thiazide-type and thiazide-like diuretics on cardiovascular events and mortality: systematic review and meta-analysis, *Hypertension* 65:1033–1040, 2015.

24

Lipid-Lowering Drugs

George A. Cook

KEY INFORMATION

- Cholesterol is critical for human survival as a membrane component, as precursor to bile acids and steroid hormones, and in lipoproteins for transport of lipid fuels.
- Hyperlipidemia is the major risk factor for the development of atherosclerosis and coronary heart disease.
- Decreasing plasma cholesterol and low-density lipoprotein with lipid-lowering drugs can decrease the incidence of atherosclerosis and coronary heart disease.
- Drugs that inhibit the uptake or synthesis of cholesterol have been the most effective lipid-lowering drugs for most patients.
- Drugs that inhibit the intracellular assembly of lipoproteins are effective as lipid-lowering drugs.
- Familial hypercholesterolemia is the most resistant disease to current lipid-lowering drugs.

CASE STUDY

Your dental patient is a 67-year-old male who has come in for his regular 6-month dental screening. He tells you he is having some muscle pain that feels like flu symptoms, but he is sure he does not have the flu. He asks you for advice. Only two items are remarkable in his medical history. He has a family history of acute myocardial infarction, and he has indicated he is taking only two drugs: simvastatin, 40 mg once a day, and amlodipine, 5 mg once a day. What is your advice to this patient?

INTRODUCTION

The transport of lipids in the blood requires their association with proteins. Fatty acids are transported in association with albumin, and triglycerides derived from dietary fat are transported in large macromolecular, cholesterol-containing particles known as *lipoproteins.* Cholesterol plays an essential role in human life as an important component of cell membranes and a precursor of steroid hormones and bile acids in addition to its role in triglyceride transport. Blood cholesterol levels previously thought to be normal are the cause of premature death, however, from coronary artery disease. Atherosclerosis remains the primary cause of premature death in the United States and in other industrialized countries. The major clinical sequelae of elevated lipoprotein levels, known as *hyperlipidemias* or *hyperlipoproteinemias,* are coronary artery disease, cerebrovascular disease, and peripheral vascular disease. The term *hyperlipemia* (which causes acute pancreatitis) is restricted to elevated plasma triglycerides without elevated cholesterol.

Because the deposition of cholesterol in arteries is a defining feature of atherosclerosis, strategies for its prevention and treatment include methods to reduce plasma cholesterol. Dentists need to understand lipid-lowering drugs as the overall dental patient population of the United States matures, and increasing numbers of patients take these drugs for prevention and therapy of atherosclerosis. Some of these patients may complain of drug side effects and expect their dentist to help. Dentists also need to follow the development of the cholesterol synthesis inhibitors because of their implication in the stimulation of bone formation through inhibited isoprenoid synthesis leading to decreased osteoclast activity and increased osteoblast differentiation.

Guidelines on patient cholesterol management are issued periodically by the Adult Treatment Panel of the National Cholesterol Education Program (NCEP). More recent guidelines have included recommendations for improved lifestyle changes, such as increasing exercise and decreasing consumption of saturated fat and cholesterol, both of which can improve cholesterol levels in some patients without drug therapy.

CHOLESTEROL AND ATHEROSCLEROSIS

Atherosclerosis is caused by development of fatty streaks and plaques in large and medium-sized arteries, especially the aorta, coronary arteries, carotid arteries, renal arteries, and arteries of the legs. Plaques develop in the intimal wall of the vessels after deposition of cholesteryl esters derived from certain lipoproteins. The particular clinical manifestation of atherosclerosis depends on the degree to which the lesions have progressed in a particular part of the vasculature. The presence of atheromatous lesions can have several effects on the circulation to a prescribed area: (1) blood flow may be obstructed by the plaques themselves or by associated thrombi, (2) vascular reactivity and control of blood flow may be lost, and (3) vessels may become weakened and subject to rupture. Observations of initial lesions in young children have shown that this disease begins at an early age and progresses gradually, with clinical symptoms generally appearing much later in life.

Foam cells are a primary characteristic of atheromatous plaques. These cells arise from macrophages that invade the injured arterial endothelium and accumulate large pools of cholesteryl esters from trapped lipoproteins. As with all other cells, macrophages possess a mechanism for converting free cholesterol to cholesteryl esters as a protective mechanism to avoid destabilization of cell membranes due to excessive accumulation of free cholesterol. As macrophages engulf lipoproteins, metabolize cholesterol to cholesteryl esters, and accumulate large numbers of cholesteryl ester-laden vesicles, they obtain a foamy appearance and eventually die and contribute to plaque formation.

TABLE 24-1 Classification and Characteristics of Major Plasma Lipoproteins

Lipoprotein	Major Lipids	Major Apoproteins	Density (g/mL)	Diameter (nm)
Chylomicrons	Dietary triglycerides	B48, CI, CII, CIII, E	<0.98	80-500
Chylomicron remnants	Dietary cholesteryl esters	B48, E		
VLDLs	Endogenous triglycerides	B100, CII, CIII, E	0.98-1.006	30-80
IDLs	Cholesteryl esters, triglycerides	B100, CII, CIII, E	1.006-1.019	25-35
LDLs	Cholesteryl esters	B100	1.019-1.063	15-25
HDLs	Cholesteryl esters	AI, AII*	1.063-1.210	5-12
Lp(a)	Cholesteryl esters	B100, (a)	1.055-1.085	30

HDLs, High-density lipoproteins; *IDLs,* intermediate-density lipoproteins; *LDLs,* low-density lipoproteins; *Lp(a),* lipoprotein(a); *VLDLs,* very low-density lipoproteins.
*HDL serves as a reservoir for C and E apoproteins, transferring them to newly synthesized chylomicrons (in exchange for A apoproteins) and VLDL particles and removing them as these particles are depleted of triglyceride.

The accumulation of foam cells results in a fatty streak visible to the naked eye. Particularly in vascular areas subject to high mechanical shear stresses and turbulent flow, microscopic tearing and disruption of the local endothelium may expose the underlying tissue, resulting in accelerated lipoprotein accumulation, platelet aggregation, and deposition of fibrin. Eventually, an atherosclerotic plaque forms with a thick fibrous cap covering a necrotic center composed of cellular debris and cholesteryl ester deposits.

Lipoprotein Metabolism

Classification of plasma lipoproteins is based on the density of the complexes, with a lower density indicating higher lipid content (Table 24-1). Chylomicrons are the largest particles and possess the greatest proportion of lipid. The other lipoproteins are very low-density lipoprotein (VLDL), intermediate-density lipoprotein (IDL), low-density lipoprotein (LDL), high-density lipoprotein (HDL), and lipoprotein(a). Two separate lipoprotein-producing systems or metabolic pathways are responsible for the transport of lipids (Fig. 24-1): the **exogenous pathway**, producing chylomicrons in the intestinal mucosa from dietary fatty acids and cholesterol, and the **endogenous pathway**, producing VLDL in the liver from fatty acids and cholesterol synthesized de novo by hepatic metabolism of dietary carbohydrates.

A crucial factor in the understanding of physiologic and pathophysiologic aspects of lipoprotein metabolism is the role played by specific **apoproteins**, the proteins associated with lipoprotein particles. Chylomicrons serve to transport dietary lipids to the sites of utilization and storage. Following synthesis in the intestinal mucosal cells, they are transported to the general blood circulation through the intestinal lymphatic system, avoiding the hepatic portal system and thus avoiding immediate metabolism by the liver. The major protein component of chylomicrons is apoprotein B48, which initially plays an entirely structural role in formation and transport. It forms the amphipathic coating of the particle along with unesterified cholesterol and phospholipid, which surrounds the hydrophobic core containing triglycerides and cholesteryl esters and allows the particle to remain suspended in an aqueous environment. On reaching the capillary endothelium of muscle and adipose tissue, the chylomicron triglycerides are rapidly degraded to fatty acids, glycerol, and monoglycerides by the enzyme lipoprotein lipase, which is attached to the luminal surface of endothelial cells of capillaries located in the adipose tissue, skeletal muscles, and heart.

Apoprotein CII serves as a stimulus for endothelial lipase activity. The remaining *chylomicron remnants,* depleted of triglycerides and CII but relatively enriched in cholesterol and apoproteins B48 and E, are released back into the circulation. The **exogenous pathway** terminates in the liver, where the chylomicron remnants are actively taken up by hepatocytes after binding to LRP (LDL receptor-related protein, a member of the LDL receptor family) on the surface of hepatocytes. Apoproteins B48 and E help trigger this receptor-mediated endocytosis. Within the liver, the remnants are digested, releasing the remaining lipids for further metabolism.

The hepatic synthesis of VLDL particles initiates the **endogenous pathway** of lipid transport (Fig. 24-1). VLDL is assembled in the endoplasmic reticulum from endogenously synthesized cholesterol esters, triglycerides, and apolipoprotein B100 by the microsomal triglyceride transfer protein (MTTP). After secretion by the liver, VLDL is subject to attack in peripheral tissues by lipoprotein lipase which is activated by apolipoprotein CII. The resulting IDL particle (or VLDL remnant particle) is greatly reduced in triglyceride content and has two possible fates: a few particles undergo receptor-mediated endocytosis by the liver and lysosomal degradation, but most IDL particles continue further removal of triglyceride by hepatic lipase to yield LDL. The cholesterol content of LDL accounts for the majority of the total plasma cholesterol. Particles of LDL are subject to apoprotein B100–dependent, LDL receptor–mediated endocytosis by various tissues, most importantly the liver. Excess IDL and LDL, through scavenger receptor uptake by intimal macrophages, account for the cholesterol accumulation in atheromatous lesions. There is no evidence that chylomicrons are involved in this disease process.

The synthesis of cholesterol, regulated by the initial enzyme of the pathway (3-hydroxy-3-methylglutaryl coenzyme A [HMG-CoA] reductase), is an energetically expensive process because every carbon atom of cholesterol is derived from intramitochondrial acetylcoenzyme A that would otherwise be utilized for synthesis of ATP in the Krebs citric acid cycle. Maintenance of total body cholesterol is thus a priority. This is exemplified further by the fact that there is no metabolic pathway in the human body for removal of cholesterol other than conversion to bile acids and limited excretion in the feces. Cholesterol is conserved through **enterohepatic cycling** and **reverse cholesterol transport** (see Fig. 24-1) processes that play important roles in energy conservation and become sites of action for some lipid-lowering drugs.

Enterohepatic cycling includes the following processes: (1) synthesis of cholesterol and conversion to bile acids by the liver, (2) secretion of bile acids into the small intestine, (3) absorption of bile acids from the terminal ileum, and (4) transfer through the hepatic portal system and reuptake by the liver. Reverse cholesterol transport is the process by which HDL synthesized by the liver and intestine takes up cholesterol from peripheral cells and transports it back to the liver. HDL cholesterol is sometimes referred to as the "good" cholesterol because it represents the amount of cholesterol being removed from most of the body and because higher levels of HDL cholesterol are associated with decreased risk of atherosclerosis. HDL also assists in the removal of triglycerides from the bloodstream by delivering to chylomicrons and VLDL the C and E apoproteins necessary for their processing.

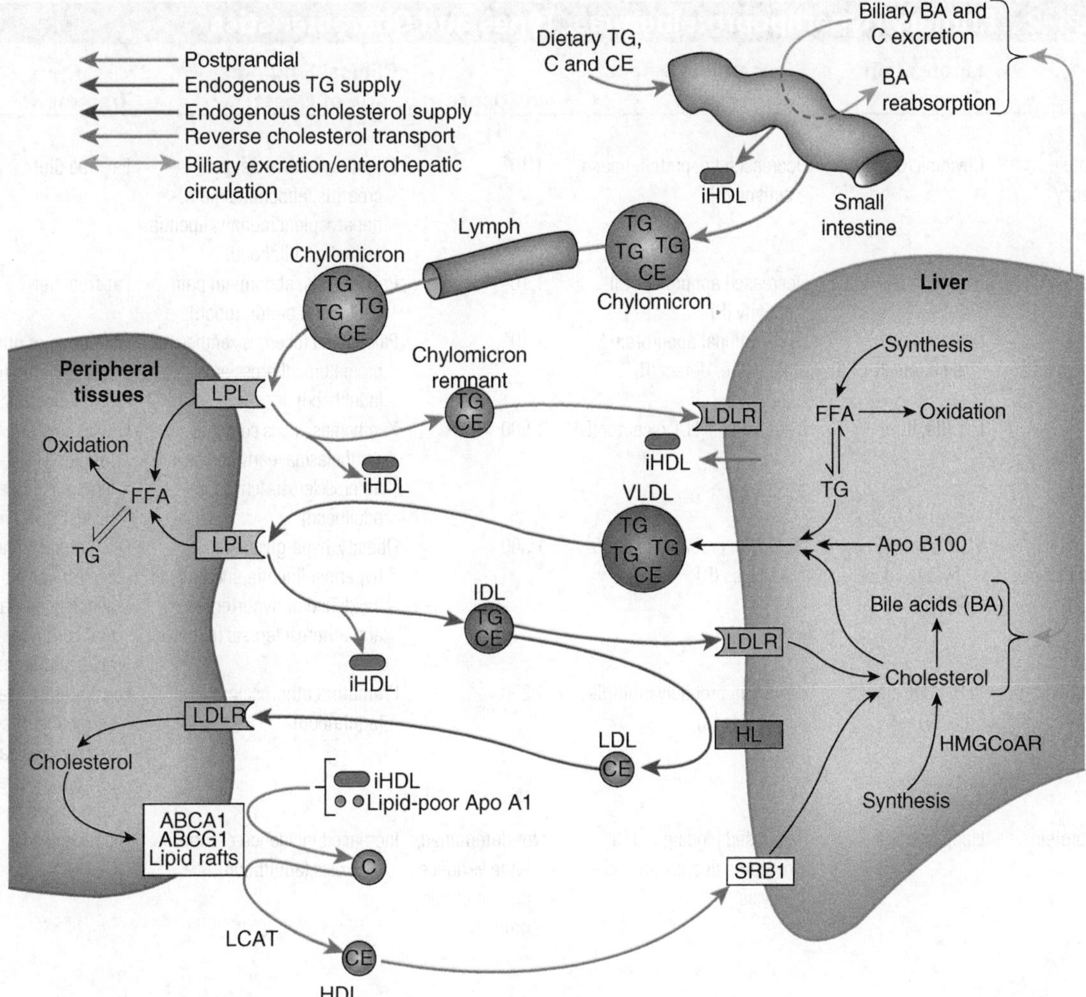

FIG 24-1 Two pathways of lipid transport are shown: The exogenous pathway initiated in intestinal mucosal cells utilizes dietary fat and cholesterol to produce chylomicrons, and the endogenous pathway initiated in the liver utilizes endogenously synthesized TG and cholesterol to produce VLDL. *Apo*, Apolipoprotein; *BA*, bile acids; *C*, cholesterol; *CE*, cholesterol ester; *FFA*, free fatty acids; *HDL*, mature high-density lipoprotein; *iHDL*, immature high-density lipoprotein; *HL*, hepatic lipase; *HMGCoAR*, 3-hydroxyl-3-methylglutaryl coenzyme A reductase; *IDL*, intermediate-density lipoprotein; *LCAT*, lecithin cholesterol acyltransferase; *LDL*, low-density lipoprotein; *LDLR*, low-density lipoprotein receptor family; *LPL*, lipoprotein lipase; *SRB1*, scavenger receptor B1; *TG*, triglyceride; *VLDL*, very low-density lipoprotein. (From Colledge, Nick R, et al: *Davidson's principles and practice of medicine*, 21e, 2010, Churchill Livingstone.)

Role of Lipoproteins in Atherosclerosis

The presence of cholesterol as an integral component of arterial plaques has been known for decades, and many studies have been done to determine whether abnormal concentrations of cholesterol are involved in the origin or progression of plaque formation. These studies have shown that plasma cholesterol concentrations are higher in patients with coronary artery disease than in normal patients, and that the relationship between serum cholesterol concentration and risk of premature death from coronary artery disease is continuous and graded. Furthermore, cholesterol reduction therapy in patients with hyperlipidemia can cause regression of plaque formation in some patients, and it can decrease the mortality rate from atherosclerosis in most patients.

An increase in plasma LDL may be caused either by overproduction of its VLDL precursor or, more commonly, by retarded clearance of LDL from the blood. The plasma half-life of LDL is much longer than the half-life of VLDL. Although LDL receptor–dependent uptake predominates normally, only the alternative phagocytic pathway is available in patients with severe familial hypercholesterolemia, who congenitally lack functional LDL receptors. LDL is the lipoprotein group most directly associated with coronary heart disease. High plasma concentrations of HDL correlate with decreased risk of coronary heart disease.

Hyperlipidemia may be primary (i.e., genetic in origin) or result from dietary factors; disease states such as diabetes mellitus, hypothyroidism, or uremia; drugs such as alcohol, oral contraceptives, or glucocorticoids; or a combination of causes. A summary of various types of primary hyperlipidemias is provided in Table 24-2.

Risk Factors in Atherosclerosis

In addition to high plasma cholesterol, several risk factors have been identified with an increased incidence of atherosclerosis, including hypertension, cigarette smoking, sedentary habits, obesity, diabetes mellitus, hypothyroidism, male gender, and a family history of

TABLE 24-2 Primary Hyperlipoproteinemias: Types and Characteristics

Type	Lipoprotein Elevated*	Biochemical Defect (Inheritance)	Incidence	Clinical Findings (Age of Onset)	Treatment
Monogenic					
Familial lipoprotein lipase deficiency	Chylomicrons (I, V)	Decreased lipoprotein lipase activity (R)	1:10^6	Eruptive xanthomas, pancreatitis, abdominal pain, hepatosplenomegaly, lipemia retinalis (childhood)	Fat-free diet
Familial apoprotein CII deficiency	Chylomicrons, VLDL (I, V)	Decreased apoprotein CII activity (R)	1:10^6	Pancreatitis, abdominal pain (childhood or adulthood)	Fat-free diet
Familial type 3 hyperlipoproteinemia	Chylomicron remnants, IDL (III)	Dysfunctional apoprotein E plus other defect (R)	1:10^4	Palmar and tuberous xanthomas, premature atherosclerosis (adulthood)	Correction of other defect (e.g., hypothyroidism), gemfibrozil nicotinic acid
Familial hypercholesterolemia	LDL (IIa, IIb)	Dysfunctional LDL receptor (D)	1:500	Xanthomas, arcus corneae, xanthelasma, early and severe atherosclerosis (childhood or adulthood)	Low cholesterol and saturated fat diet, HMG-CoA reductase inhibitor, bile acid-binding resin, PCSK9 inhibitors
Familial hypertriglyceridemia	VLDL (rarely chylomicrons) (IV, V)	Unknown; probably multiple subtypes (D)	1:500	Obesity, hyperglycemia, hyperinsulinemia, increased incidence of hypertension and atherosclerosis (puberty)	Low saturated fat diet, correct contributing factors, avoidance of alcohol and oral contraceptives, nicotinic acid, gemfibrozil, fish oils
Multiple lipoprotein-type hyperlipidemia	VLDL, LDL (IIa, IIb, IV)	Unknown; probably multiple subtypes (D)	1:250	Premature atherosclerosis (adulthood)	Low saturated fat diet, correction of contributing factors, avoidance of alcohol and oral contraceptives, lipid-lowering drugs
Lp(a) hyperlipoproteinemia	Lipoprotein(a)	Decreased binding to LDL receptor, decreased fibrinolysis	Not determined; wide variance among ethnic groups	Increased incidence of atherosclerosis (adulthood)	Nicotinic acid
Polygenic					
Polygenic hypercholesterolemia	LDL (IIa, IIb)	Unknown but including normal variation in cholesterol metabolism	1:24	Increased incidence of atherosclerosis (adulthood)	Low cholesterol and saturated fat diet, HMG-CoA reductase inhibitor, bile acid-binding resin, PCSK9 inhibitors

*The electrophoretic pattern, or phenotypic expression, of the lipoproteinemia is indicated in parentheses.
All the monogenic disorders are autosomal.
D, Dominant; *HMG-CoA*, 3-hydroxy-3-methylglutaryl-coenzyme A; *IDL*, intermediate-density lipoprotein; *LDL*, low-density lipoprotein; *Lp(a)*, lipoprotein(a); *R*, recessive; PCSK9, proprotein convertase subtilisin kexin 9; *VLDL*, very low-density lipoprotein.

atherosclerosis or diabetes. As shown in Table 24-2, the clinical manifestations of genetic or familial hyperlipoproteinemias are severe. The lipid-lowering agents discussed in this chapter have proved quite useful in treating many of these disorders and even in reversing the progression of atherosclerosis in patients without specific metabolic defects in lipid metabolism.

Treatment Guidelines from the National Cholesterol Education Program

The primary guidelines from the NCEP for treatment of patients with hyperlipidemia are to increase exercise, decrease saturated fat and cholesterol in the diet, and lower elevated LDL cholesterol levels using drugs. Diabetes also predicts a high risk for coronary heart disease, and these patients benefit from treatment with hypolipidemic drugs. Diabetic patients usually have elevated triglycerides and low HDL cholesterol, requiring different types of drug treatment. Diabetic patients who have confirmed coronary heart disease are at even greater risk and need more specific, aggressive treatment to decrease risk of mortality.

There is also a greater awareness today of numerous individuals in the United States who have a condition known as *metabolic syndrome*, which is characterized by abdominal obesity, elevated fasting glucose, low HDL cholesterol, elevated plasma triglycerides, and high blood pressure. These patients benefit from increased exercise, modified diet, and treatment of lipid abnormalities.

THERAPEUTIC AGENTS

Therapy with drugs that reduce plasma cholesterol is used to delay or reverse the progression of atherosclerosis and decrease the mortality and morbidity rates from the associated clinical manifestations of this disease. Strong evidence supports the idea that correction or lowering of plasma lipid concentrations is beneficial in many instances. These drugs are helpful in treating many familial hyperlipidemias, and they are recommended for use in patients with hyperlipidemias of secondary etiology that cannot be corrected by other means. Lipid-lowering drugs are most frequently administered to patients with a history of

TABLE 24-3 Properties of Lipid-Lowering Drugs

	Lipoprotein Concentrations	Plasma Cholesterol	Plasma Triglyceride	Toxicity	Drug Interactions
Gemfibrozil	↓VLDL, ↓IDL, ↑HDL	↓	↓	Abdominal pain, epigastric pain, diarrhea, nausea, vomiting, flatulence, rash, headache, dizziness, anemia, eosinophilia, leukopenia	Enhanced effect of coumarin anticoagulants; myopathy with HMG-CoA reductase inhibitors
Nicotinic acid	↓Chylomicrons, ↓VLDL, ↓IDL, ↓LDL, ↑HDL	↓	↓	Flushing, pruritus, nausea, diarrhea, glucose intolerance, hyperuricemia, hepatotoxicity	Myopathy, rhabdomyolysis, renal failure with HMG-CoA reductase inhibitors
Cholestyramine, colestipol	↑VLDL (transient), ↓LDL	↓	May increase modestly in some patients	Constipation, nausea, abdominal pain, flatulence, biliary tract calcification, steatorrhea, hyperchloremic acidosis	Decreased absorption of thiazides, tetracycline, phenobarbital, thyroxine, digitalis, coumarin anticoagulants
HMG-CoA reductase inhibitors	↓IDL, ↓LDL, ↑HDL	↓	↓	Headache, flatulence, abdominal pain, diarrhea, rash, increased creatine kinase and other enzyme activities, myopathy	Enhanced effect of coumarin anticoagulants; myopathy, rhabdomyolysis, renal failure with nicotinic acid, gemfibrozil, erythromycin, cyclosporine
Ezetimibe	↓LDL, ↑HDL	↓	↓	Headache, sinusitis, pharyngitis	Cholestyramine binds ezetimibe and lowers its bioavailability; does not alter bioavailability of digitalis or coumarin anticoagulants

↓, Decrease; ↑, increase.

HDLs, High-density lipoproteins; *HMG-CoA*, 3-hydroxy-3-methylglutaryl-coenzyme A; *IDLs*, intermediate-density lipoproteins; *LDLs*, low-density lipoproteins; *VLDLs*, very low-density lipoproteins.

Clofibrate **Gemfibrozil**

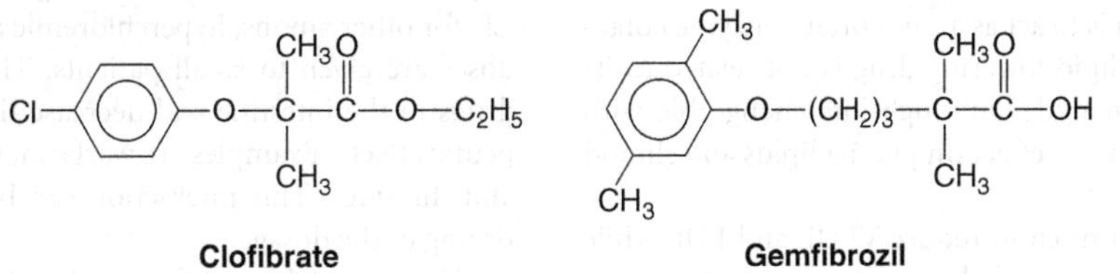

FIG 24-2 Structural formula of the fibric acid derivatives clofibrate (no longer approved for use in the United States) and gemfibrozil.

ischemic heart disease in an attempt to avoid future fatal episodes of myocardial infarction.

The goal of therapy is to reduce lipid levels as much as possible without producing metabolic derangements or adverse drug effects. Altering the diet is generally the initial therapeutic measure, along with correcting any disease state or condition contributing to hyperlipidemia. Increasing HDL by vigorous exercise such as jogging or running is extremely helpful if the patient can manage it. If nonpharmacologic therapy is insufficient, drug administration should be considered depending on determinants such as age, gender, presence of ischemic vascular disease, and coexistence of other risk factors. Even when pharmacologic antihyperlipidemic treatment is instituted, however, nonpharmacologic management, including reduction of dietary cholesterol and saturated fatty acids, weight reduction, exercise, and smoking cessation, remains the cornerstone of therapy.

The following hypolipidemic agents are considered in this chapter: (1) derivatives of fibric acid, including clofibrate and gemfibrozil; (2) nicotinic acid; (3) the bile acid sequestrants cholestyramine and colestipol; (4) inhibitors of HMG-CoA reductase (statins); (5) cholesterol absorption inhibitors; and (6) other agents. The effects of the major drugs on the various classes of lipoprotein are listed in Table 24-3.

The choice of a drug depends on the lipoprotein profile of the patient, the efficacy of the drug in treating the abnormality, and the ability of the patient to tolerate the agent. Drug therapy to reduce plasma LDL concentrations often begins with an HMG-CoA reductase inhibitor, a bile acid sequestrant, or a combination of the two in reduced dosages. Multiple-drug therapy with agents acting through different mechanisms is common if LDL control is not achieved with a single drug.

Fibric Acid Derivatives

One of the first drugs to be approved for the treatment of hyperlipidemia was clofibrate, a derivative of phenoxyisobutyric acid, which is also known as *fibric acid* (Fig. 24-2). Clofibrate is no longer available in the United States because of its association with gastrointestinal cancers. **Gemfibrozil** is safer and more effective than clofibrate, and second-generation fibrates such as fenofibrate are also more effective. These drugs can influence all the lipoproteins, but are most effective in familial type 3 hyperlipoproteinemia and in patients with elevated VLDL concentrations. Fibric acid derivatives act as ligands for the DNA transcription regulator peroxisomal proliferator–activated receptor α (PPARα), modifying rates of synthesis of specific enzymes. They have been shown to increase significantly the activity of extrahepatic lipoprotein lipase, decrease the hepatic synthesis of fatty acids, and increase hepatic fatty acid oxidation in mitochondria and peroxisomes.

Of the more recently developed fibrates, **fenofibrate,** bezafibrate, and ciprofibrate have been developed in Europe; only gemfibrozil and fenofibrate are currently approved for use in the United States. Gemfibrozil is chemically distinct from other fibrates because it has a propylene connector between the phenoxy and isobutyrate ends of the molecule. The drug has been shown to decrease the concentrations of blood triglycerides, cholesterol, VLDL, IDL, and sometimes LDL. It also tends to increase HDL concentrations. In contrast to clofibrate, gemfibrozil has been shown to decrease the incidence of myocardial infarction by 34% over 5 years. Principal side effects of gemfibrozil include abdominal pain, diarrhea, nausea, and vomiting. Less frequent adverse effects are headache, dizziness, anemia, rash, eosinophilia, and leukopenia. Gemfibrozil may also enhance the action of oral anticoagulants and may cause cholelithiasis. When combined with an HMG-CoA reductase inhibitor, muscle damage leading to rhabdomyolysis and myoglobinuria has been reported.

Fenofibrate is the first of the second-generation fibric acid derivatives to be tested in the United States. A potential advantage of the second-generation drugs is their greater ability to reduce LDL concentrations. Side effects include the gastrointestinal disturbances common to all fibrates and the potential for causing cholelithiasis.

Nicotinic Acid

Nicotinic acid (*niacin*) has been recognized since the late 1930s as a member of the vitamin B complex whose deficiency results in the disease pellagra. In 1955, it was reported that doses of nicotinic acid greater than 1 g (i.e., >50 times the recommended daily allowance of niacin as a vitamin) reduce plasma cholesterol concentrations. The function of niacin as a vitamin is to act as an important enzyme cofactor. The action of niacin as a lipid-lowering drug is not related to its function as a vitamin. Nicotinamide, although interchangeable with nicotinic acid as vitamin B_3, has no effect on plasma lipids and should not be used.

Nicotinic acid is used most often to reduce VLDL and LDL while increasing HDL levels. It has been used alone or in combination with other lipid-lowering drugs primarily in patients with extremely high cardiovascular risk. Its mechanism of action seems to involve inhibition of VLDL synthesis through inhibition of adipose tissue lipolysis and inhibition of subsequent delivery of fatty acids to the liver to produce triglycerides for packaging into VLDL particles. Increased clearance of VLDL may also play a role in the mechanism because of elevated lipoprotein lipase activity. Nicotinic acid has the broadest spectrum of activity of the lipid-lowering agents and is potentially useful in most forms of hyperlipidemia.

The major disadvantage of nicotinic acid, which affects 50% or more of the patient population, has been its tendency to produce cutaneous flushing, pruritus, and gastrointestinal distress. An additional side effect in some diabetic patients is increased insulin resistance and hyperglycemia. Extended-release preparations of nicotinic acid marketed in the past few years have made this drug more tolerable to many patients, but they do not eliminate flushing in all patients.

Nicotinic acid is absorbed rapidly, usually reaching a peak plasma concentration in less than 1 hour. The short half-life is primarily due to rapid excretion of unmetabolized nicotinic acid by the kidneys; this necessitates frequent administration of the drug, usually three times a day with meals. Because of the frequent lack of tolerance, doses are started at 100 mg three times per day and are gradually increased at 100-mg intervals until a dose of 1 to 1.5 g is reached. The usual therapeutic dose is 2 to 6 g/day. Extended-release preparations are taken once each day, in the evening, and can be started at a higher dose. These preparations have been shown to have fewer incidences of side effects, even in patients with diabetes.

Bile Acid Sequestrants

Bile acid sequestrants are nonabsorbable anion exchange resins that bind bile acids in the intestinal lumen, prevent their reabsorption, and promote their excretion in the feces. Enterohepatic cycling of cholesterol is markedly reduced by this mechanism, which blocks reabsorption of bile acids from the jejunum and ileum, 90% of which are normally reabsorbed. This increases bile acid excretion rate by 10-fold. Bile acids are synthesized in the liver from cholesterol by 7α-hydroxylase, which is regulated through negative feedback by bile acids. Hepatic cholesterol conversion to bile acids is thereby accelerated, and plasma cholesterol and LDL concentrations are decreased. LDL concentrations are also reduced by these drugs because lower hepatic cholesterol causes upregulation of LDL receptors and hepatic uptake, whereas the VLDL concentration may be unchanged or increased. These resins have no effect in patients with homozygous familial hypercholesterolemia as they have no functioning LDL receptors.

Cholestyramine, colestipol, and **colesevelam** are the three clinically available drugs in this category. They are very large resins that are insoluble in water. The dry resin is mixed with a liquid such as fruit juice and drunk as a slurry. Cl^- is released from the resin as bile acids bind to it, and the released Cl^- is absorbed, but the resin itself is not absorbed. Because it is not absorbed, it has a high safety factor and absence of serious side effects, but the annoying gastrointestinal side effects (nausea, vomiting, abdominal distention, and constipation) limit the use of these drugs. An unpleasant taste adds to the problem of patient compliance with these agents. Because these drugs exchange Cl^- for other anions, hyperchloremic acidosis may develop when large doses are given to small patients. These resins also bind to anionic drugs in the intestine and decrease their absorption and their therapeutic effects. Examples are warfarin, thyroxine, digitalis, propranolol, and thiazides. This interaction can be partially overcome by proper timing of the dosage.

The newest bile acid sequestrant to be approved for use in the United States is colesevelam hydrochloride, which is available in tablet form. Colesevelam has been found to lower LDL cholesterol as effectively as cholestyramine, but it presents less danger of interaction with other drugs such as warfarin through adsorption. There are also somewhat fewer gastrointestinal side effects, and compliance is greater because of the tablet form.

3-Hydroxy-3-Methylglutaryl-Coenzyme A Reductase Inhibitors

The development of drugs that specifically inhibit the biosynthesis of cholesterol has been one of the most important aspects of hypolipidemic drug development. This class of drugs, called the ***statins***, currently includes **lovastatin, pravastatin, simvastatin, fluvastatin, atorva statin, rosuvastatin,** and **pitavastatin**. These agents structurally resemble an intermediate in the **HMG-CoA reductase** reaction (Fig. 24-3) and are potent competitive antagonists of HMG-CoA binding. Numerous clinical studies have now shown these drugs to be the best tolerated and most effective drugs for lowering LDL cholesterol and for reducing stroke, coronary heart disease, and overall mortality. In addition to lowering LDL cholesterol, some studies have shown that statins are useful in reducing triglycerides. Fewer studies have been conducted with patients having low HDL cholesterol, but these have indicated that some statins are effective in elevating HDL cholesterol.

The antihyperlipidemic effect of this class of drugs depends on inhibition of hepatic HMG-CoA reductase, the rate-controlling enzyme in the pathway of cholesterol synthesis (Fig. 24-4). The subsequent depletion of

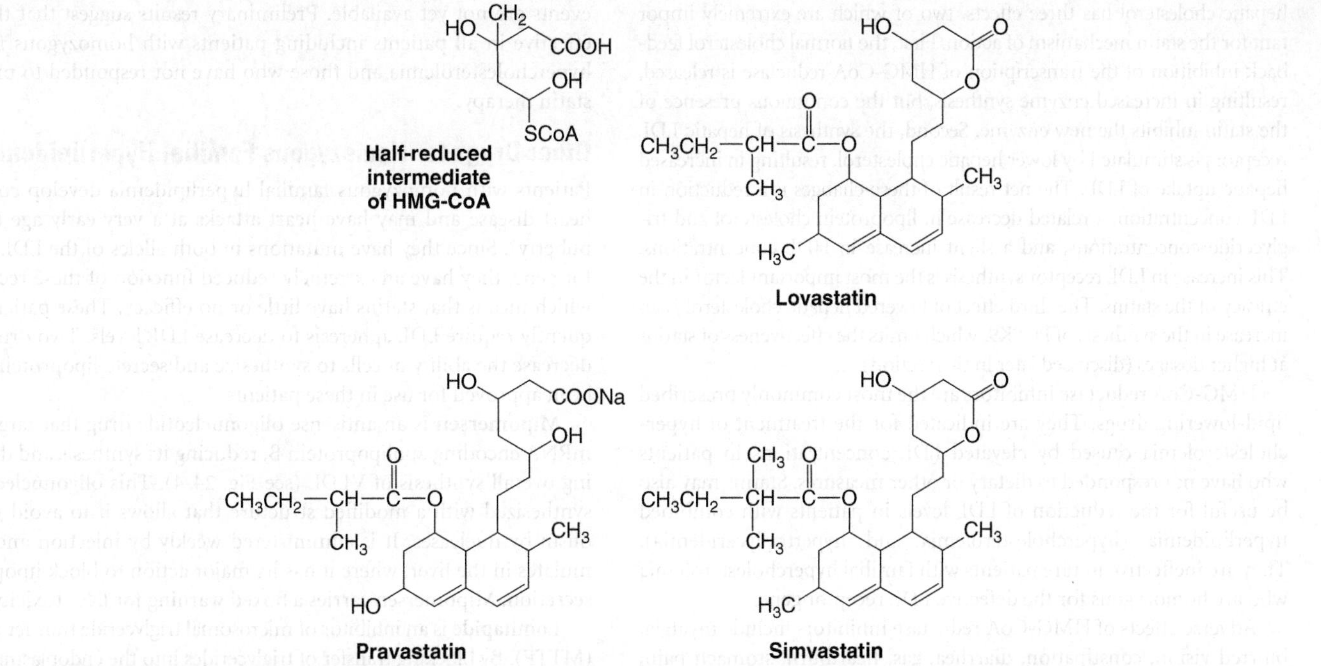

Half-reduced intermediate of HMG-CoA

Lovastatin

Pravastatin

Simvastatin

FIG 24-3 Structural formula of 3-hydroxy-3-methylglutaryl coenzyme A (*HMG-CoA*), half-reduced intermediate, and three HMG-CoA reductase inhibitors.

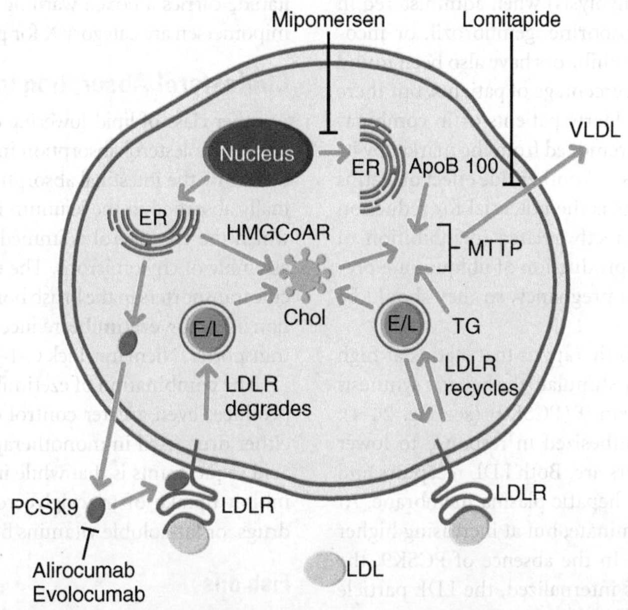

FIG 24-4 Site of action of lipid-lowering drugs acting on the hepatocyte. The synthetic pathway for PCSK9 is shown. **Alirocumab** and **evolocumab** are monoclonal antibodies directed against PCSK9, inhibiting its action on the LDL receptor. PCSK9 causes the LDL receptor to be degraded once it is internalized. (The LDL receptor is recycled to the cell surface in the absence of PCSK9.) **Mipomersen** is an antisense oligonucleotide that blocks the synthesis of ApoB-100 and subsequent lipoprotein. **Lomitapide** inhibits the microsomal triglyceride transfer protein, thus inhibiting ApoB-100-containing lipoprotein production. Both drugs prevent the synthesis of VLDL and eventually LDL. The statins inhibit the synthesis of cholesterol by inhibiting HMGCoAR. *Chol*, Cholesterol; *E/L*, endosome/lysosome; *ER*, endoplasmic reticulum; *HMGCoAR*, 3-hydroxyl-3-methyl glutaryl coenzyme A reductase; *LDL*, low-density lipoprotein; *MTTP*, microsomal triglyceride transfer protein; *TG*, triglyceride; *VLDL*, very low-density lipoprotein. (Modified from Page MM, et al: Recent advances in the understanding and care of familial hypercholesterolemia: significance of the biology and therapeutic regulation of proprotein convertase subtilisin/kexin type 9. *Clin Sci* 129:63-79, 2015.)

hepatic cholesterol has three effects, two of which are extremely impor tant for the statin mechanism of action. First, the normal cholesterol feedback inhibition of the transcription of HMG-CoA reductase is released, resulting in increased enzyme synthesis, but the continuous presence of the statin inhibits the new enzyme. Second, the synthesis of hepatic LDL receptors is stimulated by lower hepatic cholesterol, resulting in increased hepatic uptake of LDL. The net result of these changes is a reduction in LDL concentration, a related decrease in lipoprotein cholesterol and triglyceride concentrations, and a slight increase in HDL concentrations. This increase in LDL receptor synthesis is the most important factor in the efficacy of the statins. The third effect of lowered hepatic cholesterol is an increase in the synthesis of PCSK9, which limits the effectiveness of statins at higher dosages (discussed later in this section).

HMG-CoA reductase inhibitors are the most commonly prescribed lipid-lowering drugs. They are indicated for the treatment of hypercholesterolemia caused by elevated LDL concentrations in patients who have not responded to dietary or other measures. Statins may also be useful for the reduction of LDL levels in patients with combined hyperlipidemia (hypercholesterolemia and hypertriglyceridemia). They are ineffective in rare patients with familial hypercholesterolemia who are homozygous for the defective LDL receptor gene.

Adverse effects of HMG-CoA reductase inhibitors include myalgia, blurred vision, constipation, diarrhea, gas, heartburn, stomach pain, dizziness, headache, nausea, skin rash, impotence, and insomnia. The incidence varies among the different agents, with blurred vision more frequent with lovastatin and pravastatin and impotence and insomnia more frequent with lovastatin. HMG-CoA reductase inhibitors increase the anticoagulant effect of warfarin. Lovastatin has been linked with severe myopathy (rhabdomyolysis) when administered in combination with erythromycin, cyclosporine, gemfibrozil, or nicotinic acid. Other HMG-CoA reductase inhibitors have also been found to produce rhabdomyolysis in a small percentage of patients, but there is increased risk with higher doses in elderly patients or in combination with other drugs. Cerivastatin was removed from the market by its manufacturer because of rhabdomyolysis. Another side effect of statins that may be important in some patients is the potential for reduction in ubiquinone levels. This effect is directly related to inhibition of HMG-CoA reductase which decreases production of ubiquinone precursors. Statins are rated category X in pregnancy, so they should be discontinued prior to conception.

One very important aspect of statin therapy is that statins at high doses become self-limiting because they stimulate the hepatic synthesis of proprotein convertase subtilisin kexin 9 (PCSK9) (see Fig. 24-4). PCSK9 is a serine protease that is synthesized in response to lower hepatic cholesterol just as LDL receptors are. Both LDL receptors and PCSK9 are packaged for export to the hepatic plasma membrane. At low statin levels, LDL receptors predominate, but at increasing higher levels of statin, PCSK9 predominates. In the absence of PCSK9, the LDL receptor/LDL particle complex is internalized, the LDL particle is metabolized, and the LDL receptor is recycled to the plasma membrane to bind more LDL particles. As the synthesis of PCSK9 is stimulated, it is targeted to the plasma membrane where it binds to the LDL receptor. When LDL particles bind to the PCSK9/LDL receptor complex, the ternary complex is internalized, and both the LDL particle and the LDL receptor are metabolized, causing LDL receptor downregulation. This is a normal mechanism that limits the uptake of LDL particles and their associated cholesterol in states of very low hepatic cholesterol. Monoclonal antibodies to PCSK9 can prevent destruction of LDL receptors and might become outstanding drugs in their own right. Two drugs of this type, alirocumab and evolocumab, have been approved by the FDA recently based solely on their ability to lower LDL cholesterol. Data on the ability of these drugs to reduce cardiac events are not yet available. Preliminary results suggest that they are effective in all patients including patients with homozygous familial hypercholesterolemia and those who have not responded to previous statin therapy.

Other Drugs for Homozygous Familial Hyperlipidemia

Patients with homozygous familial hyperlipidemia develop coronary heart disease and may have heart attacks at a very early age (before puberty). Since they have mutations in both alleles of the LDL receptor gene, they have an extremely reduced function of these receptors, which means that statins have little or no efficacy. These patients frequently require LDL apheresis to decrease LDL levels. Two drugs that decrease the ability of cells to synthesize and secrete lipoproteins have been approved for use in these patients.

Mipomersen is an antisense oligonucleotide drug that targets the mRNA encoding apolipoprotein B, reducing its synthesis and decreasing overall synthesis of VLDL (see Fig. 24-4). This oligonucleotide is synthesized with a modified structure that allows it to avoid metabolism by nucleases. It is administered weekly by injection and accumulates in the liver, where it has its major action to block lipoprotein secretion. Mipomersen carries a boxed warning for liver toxicity.

Lomitapide is an inhibitor of microsomal triglyceride transfer protein (MTTP). By blocking transfer of triglycerides into the endoplasmic reticulum, it can diminish assembly of VLDL in the liver and chylomicrons in the intestinal mucosa (see Fig. 24-4). It is administered once daily in capsules taken 2 hours after the evening meal. Patients may have gastrointestinal side effects, but they may also develop more serious liver problems and should be checked regularly for the presence of liver enzymes. Lomitapide carries a boxed warning for hepatotoxicity. Both lomitapide and mipomersen are category X for pregnancy.

Cholesterol Absorption Inhibitors

Another class of lipid-lowering drugs to be developed and approved for use are cholesterol absorption inhibitors. These agents inhibit cholesterol uptake by the intestinal absorptive epithelium. Dietary cholesterol is normally absorbed in the jejunum from bile acid micelles by enterocytes, in which the cholesterol is immediately converted to cholesteryl esters for assembly of chylomicrons. The uptake of cholesterol is mediated by specific transporters in the brush border of these cells. The cholesterol absorption inhibitor, **ezetimibe**, reduces LDL cholesterol. It acts by inhibiting the transporter, Niemann-Pick C-1-like 1 protein (NPC1L1).

The combination of ezetimibe with HMG-CoA reductase inhibitors produces even greater control of hyperlipidemia than is possible with either drug used in monotherapy. An advantage of ezetimibe over bile acid sequestrants is that while inhibiting cholesterol uptake, it does not inhibit uptake of triacylglycerols, bile acids, fatty acids, lipid-soluble drugs, or fat-soluble vitamins by the small intestine.

Fish oils

Evidence exists to support a role for polyunsaturated fish oils in decreasing plasma lipid concentrations. Specifically, the omega-3 polyunsaturated fatty acids (PUFAs), eicosapentaenoic acid (EPA), and docosahexaenoic acid (DHA) can reduce levels of triglycerides through inhibition of the synthesis of VLDL triglycerides and apolipoprotein B, whether consumed as dietary constituents or as purified supplements.

There is some evidence that fish oils can modestly decrease the levels of plasma cholesterol as they substantially decrease triglycerides and VLDL. They can also modestly increase HDL levels. Patients with severe familial hypertriglyceridemia often have significant improvement on a diet high in fish oil. In addition to many over-the-counter preparations of fish oils, there are currently prescription drugs consisting of ethyl esters of EPA and DHA. These are used primarily in combination therapy in patients that have severe hypertriglyceridemia or have triglyceride levels that remain elevated after treatment with other lipid-lowering drugs.

Inhibitors of cholesteryl ester transfer protein

Clinical investigations are currently under way to examine the effects of drugs that inhibit cholesteryl ester transfer protein (CETP). CETP is a protein synthesized in the liver that transfers cholesteryl esters from circulating HDL particles to circulating LDL and VLDL particles. In animals and in humans, the inhibition of CETP causes an increase in HDL cholesterol. Phase III trials are under way for two potential drugs of this type.

COMBINED DRUG THERAPY

Lipid-lowering drugs from the different categories are used in combination for three reasons. First, combined drug therapy may result in a more profound reduction of lipid levels than can be achieved by single-drug therapy. Second, as previously stated, some drugs may elevate certain lipid concentrations; combined therapy with a drug of another category can be used to overcome this unwanted effect. Third, the use of combined drug therapy may allow smaller doses of the drugs to be used than in single-drug therapy, decreasing potential side effects. Examples of multiple-drug therapies having demonstrable value include the combination of a bile acid sequestrant (resin) with either nicotinic acid or an HMG-CoA reductase inhibitor. Other drug combinations that have been shown to be useful include a bile acid sequestrant plus a fibrate, and a resin plus nicotinic acid plus an HMG-CoA reductase inhibitor. Colesevelam plus an HMG-CoA reductase inhibitor may also be a useful combination. The newest combined drug therapy is the use of a cholesterol absorption inhibitor with an HMG-CoA reductase inhibitor. The combination of ezetimibe and atorvastatin has achieved a 50% reduction in LDL cholesterol at low doses (10 mg) of each drug. This result is approximately equal to the effect of 80 mg of atorvastatin alone.

LIPID-LOWERING DRUGS

Nonproprietary (Generic) Name	Proprietary (Trade) Name
Alirocumab	Praluent
Atorvastatin	Lipitor
Cholestyramine	Questran
Colesevelam	WelChol
Colestipol	Colestid
Evolocumab	Repatha
Ezetimibe	Zetia, Vytorin (combination with simvastatin)
Fenofibrate	Tricor, Lofibra
Fish oils (n-3 PUFAs)	Max-EPA, Promega, Sea-omega, Super EPA
Fluvastatin	Lescol
Gemfibrozil	Lopid
Lomitapide	Juxtapid
Lovastatin	Altoprev, Mevacor, Advicor (combination with niacin)
Mipomersen	Kynamro
Nicotinic acid (niacin)	Niacor, Niaspan, Niacin SR, Slo-Niacin
Pitavastatin	Livalo
Pravastatin	Pravachol
Rosuvastatin	Crestor
Simvastatin	Zocor

PUFAs, Polyunsaturated fatty acids.

CASE DISCUSSION

This patient should be advised to make an appointment with his cardiologist very soon to check his medication. Simvastatin is a generic drug used to lower cholesterol that has few side effects but can produce myalgia in some patients, especially at the highest approved dose of 40 mg/day. Continuing myalgia can lead to muscle breakdown and release of myoglobin that can block the renal system (rhabdomyolysis). The myalgia is likely to be exacerbated by the amlodipine he is taking to lower his blood pressure. You should explain to the patient that his cardiologist might want to do some testing and make a change in his medication to avoid this effect, but in the meantime, he must continue to take his medication as prescribed.

GENERAL REFERENCES

1. Aronow WS: Lipid-lowering therapy in older persons, *Arch Med Sci* 11:43–56, 2015.
2. Eckel RH, Cornier MA: Update on the NCEP ATP-III emerging cardiometabolic risk factors, *BMC Med* 12:115–123, 2014.
3. LaRosa JC1, Pedersen TR, Somaratne R, Wasserman SM: Safety and effect of very low levels of low-density lipoprotein cholesterol on cardiovascular events, *Am J Cardiol* 111:1221–1229, 2013.
4. Page MM, Stefanutti C, Sniderman A, Watts GF: Recent advances in the understanding and care of familial hypercholesterolemia: significance of the biology and therapeutic regulation of proprotein convertase subtilisin/kexin type 9, *Clin Sci* 129:63–79, 2015.
5. Ramjee V1, Sperling LS, Jacobson TA: Non-high-density lipoprotein cholesterol versus apolipoprotein B in cardiovascular risk stratification: do the math, *J Am Coll Cardiol* 58:457–463, 2011.
6. Seidah NG, Awan Z, Chretien M, Mbikay M: PCSK9: a key modulator of cardiovascular health, *Circ Res* 114:1022–1036, 2014.
7. Stein EA, Raal FJ: New therapies for reducing low-density lipoprotein cholesterol, *Endocrinol Metab Clin North Am* 43:1007–1033, 2014.
8. Stone NJ, Robinson JG, Lichtenstein AH, et al.: 2013 ACC/AHA guideline on the treatment of blood cholesterol to reduce atherosclerotic cardiovascular risk in adults: a report of the American College of Cardiology/American Heart Association Task Force on Practice Guidelines, *Circulation* 129:S1–S45, 2014.

25

Antianemic and Hematopoietic Stimulating Drugs

Barton S. Johnson

KEY INFORMATION

- Anemia can be a sign of an underlying hematopoietic disorder.
- The three basic parts of hemoglobin are: iron, porphyrin and protein.
- The types of anemia associated with oral manifestations include:
  - Iron deficiency
  - Porphyria
  - Thalassemia, including sickle cell
  - Vitamin B12 and folate deficiency (megaloblastic)
- Hematopoietic stimulating factors include:
  - Erythrocyte stimulating factors
  - Neutrophil stimulating factors
  - Platelet stimulating factors
- Correction of anemic states can occur using a variety of agents including iron supplementation, vitamin supplementation as well as complex methods (e.g., bone marrow transplantation).
- The six classic hematopoietic stimulating agents are:
  - Granulocyte colony-stimulating factor
  - Granulocyte macrophage colony-stimulating factor
  - Stem cell factor
  - Monocyte/macrophage colony-stimulating factor
  - Thrombopoietin
  - Interleukin-3
- Patients with hematopoietic disorders may have signs of:
  - Oral mucositis
  - Intraoral or circumoral viral outbreaks
  - Fungal infections
  - Serious bacterial infections of odontogenic origin

CASE STUDY

Your patient is currently receiving cytotoxic chemotherapy every 2 weeks for stage 4 cancer. He/she tells you that his/her marrow has been hit hard by the regimen, but the oncologist is having him/her use pegfilgrastim each cycle to keep the neutrophil count up. You would like to remove one tooth that is cariously involved and an infective risk. What things should you consider doing differently in this patient?

INTRODUCTION

Hematopoiesis is the intricate system of growth and differentiation of immature pluripotent/multipotent stem cells into all the formed elements of the blood (Fig. 25-1). These stem cells, derived embryologically in the liver and later from bone marrow, divide early in development into either myeloid or lymphoid precursors. The myeloid precursors differentiate into the erythrocytes, megakaryocytes (which give rise to thrombocytes [platelets]), neutrophils, and monocytes. The lymphoid precursors give rise to the T-cell and B-cell lymphocytes, natural killer cells, and all their respective subtypes. The derivation of eosinophils and basophils lies in the myeloid stem line, but it appears to be downstream of the common myeloid precursors. Hematopoietically active bone marrow retains essentially the same mass throughout life, and although cell-producing bone marrow is found in practically all bones through adolescence, it becomes restricted to the vertebrae, sternum, ribs, pelvis, scapulae, parts of the skull, and epiphyseal ends of the long bones after approximately age 20 years.

Hematopoiesis is a dynamic, continuous process because mature cells of the blood have a limited life span in periods of sickness and health. Because of its complexity, ubiquity, and high rate of activity, the hematopoietic system is often the first organ system to show evidence of underlying systemic disease. This chapter discusses the pharmacologic interventions currently available to correct perturbations in marrow function. Conditions such as anemia, thrombocytopenia, neutropenia, and volume depletion and novel approaches to medical care that involve the hematopoietic system are discussed in detail.

ANEMIA

Anemia comprises a multifactorial group of illnesses with a wide range of underlying causes. As a result, ***anemia*** is a generic term indicating only that the concentration of hemoglobin in whole blood is less than normal. Anemia is not a disease, but a sign of underlying disease. When discussing anemia, it is important to diagnose the nature and the cause of the anemia. There are three general categories of diseases that cause anemia: (1) diseases that cause blood loss, (2) diseases that disturb red blood cell production, and (3) diseases that increase endogenous destruction of red blood cells.

Blood loss can occur either acutely, as in hemorrhage from trauma or surgery, or chronically, as with excessive menstrual bleeding or the occult bleeding of esophageal varices or gastric/duodenal ulcers. Disturbed red blood cell production is associated with nutritional deficiencies, disorders that suppress erythrocyte production (such as in aplastic anemia and with some antiretroviral therapies), and myelophthisic (marrow-displacing) diseases. Finally, anemia can be caused by

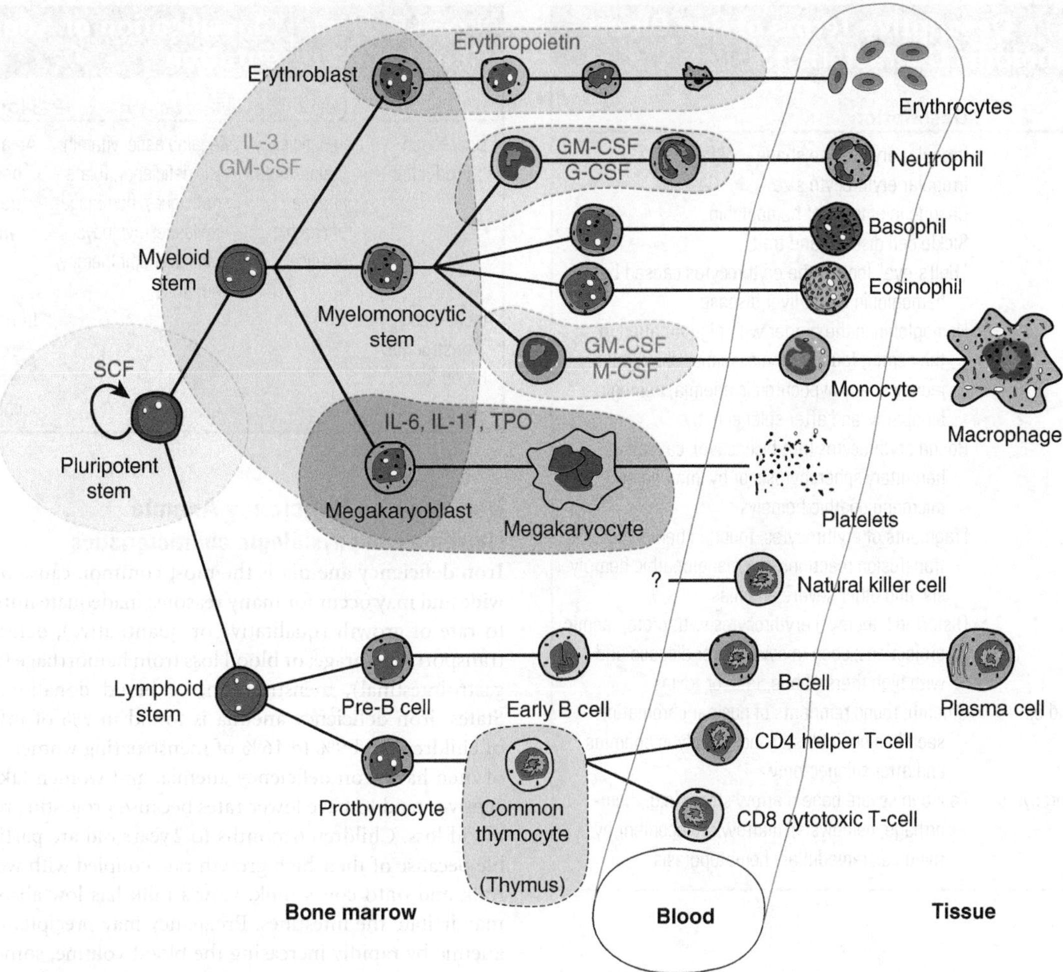

FIG 25-1 Overview of hematopoiesis. *G-CSF*, Granulocyte colony-stimulating factor; *GM-CSF*, granulocyte-macrophage colony-stimulating factor; *IL-3, IL-6, IL-11*, interleukin-3, interleukin-6, interleukin-11; *M-CSF*, monocyte/macrophage colony-stimulating factor; *SCF*, stem cell factor; *TPO*, thrombopoietin.

increased destruction of the red blood cells, such as in sickle cell disease, thalassemia, hemolytic immune reactions, and genetic disorders such as glucose-6-phosphate dehydrogenase deficiency.

When a patient is suspected to have a type of anemia, the first tests to consider are a **simple hematocrit (HCT)** and **erythrocyte count (RBC)**. These two tests tell whether the production-to-loss ratio of red blood cells is normal. The hematocrit is defined as the ratio of red blood cells to the total blood volume. It is expressed as a percentage and is determined by comparing the packed cell volume (which is composed largely of erythrocytes) to the total volume of centrifuged whole blood. Normal values for women are 36% to 45%, and normal values for men are 38% to 50%. In an anemic patient, the hematocrit level is reduced, often into the 20s and in severe cases into the teens or lower. Conversely, the hematocrit increases (referred to as *polycythemia vera* if moderate and *erythroleukemia* if severe) in patients with poor pulmonary function, in patients with some chronic cardiac conditions, in patients with certain marrow tumors, and in patients living at high altitudes. In acute hemorrhage, because plasma and red blood cells are lost together, the hematocrit does not initially reflect the loss until the body or exogenous medical intervention has had the opportunity to replenish the lost plasma volume. In these cases, there may be no indication of a problem until several hours later.

The RBC is a simple determination of the absolute number of red blood cells (in millions) per microliter. Normal values for women are 3.8 to 5.0 million/μL, and normal values for men are 4.4 to 5.6 million/μL.

After anemia has been detected, it can be characterized by evaluating the hemoglobin in the erythrocytes. Normal amounts of hemoglobin per unit volume of blood (assayed on peripheral blood draw) are 15.2 ± 2.2 g/dL for men and 13.7 ± 2.1 g/dL for women. Hemoglobin is the oxygen-carrying component of red blood cells. It comprises three components: iron, porphyrin, and globin. Alterations in any one of these three components can be a cause for a clinical anemia. In normal hemoglobin, iron in the ferrous form (Fe^{++}) is chelated into the middle of the porphyrin chemical ring to yield heme, the nonprotein component of hemoglobin.

The **globin chains** constitute the main protein constituents of hemoglobin. There are four forms of globin chains: α (141 amino acids), β (146 amino acids), δ, and γ (δ and γ are variants of β). Approximately 97% of normal hemoglobin (hemoglobin A) consists of two α and two β chains ($\alpha_2\beta_2$); 1% to 2% consists of the $\alpha_2\delta_2$ combination (hemoglobin A_2). The $\alpha_2\gamma_2$ tetramer forms hemoglobin F, or fetal hemoglobin. Hemoglobin F is the major form during gestation and until approximately 6 months of age. In adults, hemoglobin F makes up less than 1% of normal hemoglobin. One heme ring is accommodated within each of the four structural folds of the tetramer, allowing each molecule of hemoglobin to bind four oxygen molecules.

Hemoglobin accounts for approximately 95% of the dry weight of mature erythrocytes. Any significant changes in hemoglobin are often directly reflected in the way the erythrocytes look or behave grossly.

BOX 25-1 Descriptive Terms of Red Blood Cell Morphologic Characteristics

Term	Description
Poikilocytosis	Irregular erythrocyte shape
Anisocytosis	Irregular erythrocyte size
Polychromasia	Change in amount of hemoglobin
Sickling	Sickle cell disease and trait
Targeting	"Bull's-eye" look to the erythrocytes caused by hemoglobin C and liver disease
Leptocytes	Hemoglobin in the border with pigmentation in the center; found in thalassemia, obstructive jaundice, any hypochromic anemia, hemoglobinopathy, and after splenectomy
Spherocytes	Round erythrocytes (not biconcave), caused by hereditary spherocytosis or by immune or microangiopathic hemolysis
Schistocytes	Fragments of erythrocytes; found in hemolytic transfusion reactions, microangiopathic hemolysis, and other severe anemias
Acanthocytes	Distorted ("thorny") erythrocytes with protoplasmic projections; seen in severe liver disease and with high titers of bile, fats, or toxins
Howell-Jolly bodies	Smooth, round remnants of nuclear chromatin; seen in megaloblastic and hemolytic anemias and after splenectomy
Nucleated erythrocytes	Found in severe bone marrow stress (e.g., hemorrhage, hemolysis), marrow replacement by tumor, extramedullary hematopoiesis

Classically, laboratory analyses for anemia have reviewed erythrocyte size, shape, and color intensity. The size is determined by the mean corpuscular volume (MCV). The *normocytic*, or normal size, range is 80 to 100 fL/cell. Cells that are too small are termed *microcytic*, whereas cells that are too large are termed *macrocytic*. The shape of the red blood cells is also important in diagnosing the cause of anemia. Box 25-1 lists terms that describe various shapes found on a peripheral blood smear. The color intensity of the cell is reflected in the mean corpuscular hemoglobin (normally 26 to 34 pg/cell) and the mean corpuscular hemoglobin concentration (normally 31 to 36 g/dL). These two parameters, along with MCV, collectively referred to as the *red blood cell indices*, are extremely helpful in delineating the causes of a particular anemia.

The various kinds of anemia are classified by their typical effect on the erythrocytes (Table 25-1). When anemia results from a loss of blood (intrinsically from hemolysis or extrinsically from hemorrhage) or because of a decrease in production of normal erythrocytes, the cells are still normal, just fewer in quantity. These anemias are *normocytic* and *normochromic*. When anemia is caused by a decrease in the production of properly formed hemoglobin, the cells tend to be smaller (because hemoglobin comprises such a high percentage of erythrocyte content) and paler in color. These forms of anemia are known as *microcytic* and *hypochromic* and are usually the result of defective or inadequate iron absorption. Forms of anemia that cause the red blood cells to mature incompletely and retain some nuclear DNA content result in larger cells; these are known as *macrocytic* or *megaloblastic* anemia. They generally occur as a result of a deficiency in vitamin B_{12}, folic acid, or both nutrients. In these forms of anemia, the cells may also have a darker or *hyperchromic* color.

TABLE 25-1 Classification of Anemia by Cause and Presentation

	Microcytic	Macrocytic	Normocytic
Decreased production	Iron deficiency thalassemia anemia of chronic disease	Megaloblastic: vitamin B_{12} deficiency, folate deficiency; non-megaloblastic: myelodysplasia, chemotherapy, hepatitis	Aplastic anemia, bone marrow infiltration carcinoma, lymphoma
Increased destruction			Intrinsic hemolysis, extrinsic hemolysis
Blood loss			Acute hemorrhage, chronic hemorrhage

Iron and Iron Deficiency Anemia

Nutrition and physiologic characteristics

Iron deficiency anemia is the most common cause of anemia worldwide and may occur for many reasons: inadequate nutrition in relation to rate of growth (qualitative or quantitative); defective absorption, transport, or storage; or blood loss from hemorrhage (most commonly gastrointestinal), menstruation, or blood donation. In the United States, iron deficiency anemia is found in 7% of infants, 4% to 5% of children, and 9% to 16% of menstruating women. Only 2% to 3% of men have iron deficiency anemia, and women taking oral contraceptives tend to have lower rates because progestins reduce menstrual blood loss. Children 6 months to 2 years old are particularly vulnerable because of their high growth rate coupled with weaning off breast milk and onto cow's milk. Cow's milk has low absorbable iron and may irritate the intestines. Pregnancy may precipitate iron deficiency anemia by rapidly increasing the blood volume, sometimes requiring two to five times the normal intake of iron. According to a World Health Organization technical report, women who have sufficient iron reserves to support the increase in hemoglobin production during pregnancy and who breastfeed their infants are generally capable of meeting their iron needs by diet alone, although supplementation is still recommended. In a nonpregnant, normal, healthy individual, iron reserves and recycling are so effective that even extreme reduction of iron intake may be insufficient to cause severe anemia.

Men average 3.8 g total iron (50 mg/kg) and women average 2.3 g (35 to 42 mg/kg). Approximately 60% to 80% of the iron in the body is incorporated into hemoglobin, while another 10% to 25% is sequestered in reticuloendothelial cells in the storage forms ferritin and hemosiderin. The last 10% to 15% is associated in parenchymal cells with myoglobin. Less than 1% is used in various enzymes, most notably the cytochromes, and trace amounts are linked to the plasma transport protein transferrin. The amount of stored iron varies with intake and demand, averaging 400 mg in women and 1000 mg in men.

The average American ingests 10 to 20 mg of iron per day. Iron is obtained through the diet, most commonly by heme or iron complexed to various organic compounds. Foods considered high in iron (>0.5% by weight) are liver, heart, oysters, egg yolks, and yeast. Other meats and green vegetables have less iron. Absorption of iron from dietary sources is ordinarily 10% efficient or less, but it increases when iron stores are depleted. Therapeutic iron, generally in the form of inorganic salts or complexes, has an even poorer absorption profile than dietary iron because the Fe^{++} must be liberated from the salt before it can be absorbed across the intestinal mucosa.

Iron absorption occurs along the entire length of the intestine, but maximum absorption occurs in the duodenum and proximal jejunum because iron is absorbed primarily as Fe^{++}, and an acid medium favors the breakdown of salts to the ionic form. In the lower portions of the gastrointestinal tract there is a trend toward increasing alkalinity, which favors the formation of less soluble iron salts and complexes. Iron ingested as heme iron is absorbed five to seven times more efficiently than Fe^{++} salts. Iron absorption is hindered by coffee, tea, phosphates, and antacids, particularly calcium carbonate and aluminum or magnesium hydroxide. Absorption of nonheme iron is facilitated by vitamin C. How ethanol interacts with iron is not well elucidated, but approximately 50% of alcoholics exhibit some iron depletion or anemia.

Iron is absorbed by active transport across the intestinal mucosa, where it is converted intracellularly to ferric iron (Fe^{+++}). Depending on the body's acute need for iron, Fe^{+++} is either bound to **transferrin** (destined for the marrow) or converted to **ferritin or hemosiderin** for storage in the intestinal mucosa. Transferrin is a transport that specifically binds two molecules of Fe^{+++} and carries them to the bone marrow and developing erythroblasts. A typical developing erythroblast can process 25,000 to 50,000 transferrin molecules per minute.

A test for transferrin is total iron-binding capacity (TIBC). In a normal adult, approximately 20% to 50% of transferrin is replete with Fe^{+++}. In an iron-deficient individual, transferrin saturation may decrease to 15% or less, and so the *capacity* to bind iron is considerably greater, and the TIBC value increases. Normal values are 250 to 450 µg/dL.

If the body is not in acute need of iron, most of the ingested iron is stored as ferritin. Twenty-four apoferritin monomers bind together to form a hollow spherical shell 130Å in diameter and fenestrated with small pores through which 4000 Fe^{++} atoms can enter. When inside, the Fe^{++} is oxidized to Fe^{+++} and stored in the form of hydrous ferric oxide phosphate. Ferritin, the resulting apoferritin–iron complex, is a very effective storage mechanism, allowing the binding and release of iron to occur rapidly and efficiently. Mature ferritin is found in virtually all cells of the body and in plasma. Although the amount in plasma is small, it reflects the total ferritin stores in the body and is measured to diagnose iron deficiency anemia. Normal values for serum ferritin are 16 to 300 mg/mL in men and 4 to 160 mg/mL in women.

The other minor storage component of iron is hemosiderin. It is found in the monocyte/macrophage system of the marrow and in the Kupffer cells of the liver. Hemosiderin is an insoluble compound that seems to be aggregated ferritin cores partially or completely stripped of the apoferritin protein shell. In pathologic conditions (hemosiderosis), it can be found in large quantities in most tissues of the body.

The concentration of iron in the plasma at any one time represents a balance between the absorption rate, storage capacity, rate of hemoglobin formation, and rate of iron excretion. Iron is remarkably well conserved in the body; less than 0.1% is excreted on a daily basis, or approximately 0.5 to 1 mg/day. The major pathway of iron excretion is through the feces by exfoliation of gastrointestinal cells and their intracellular stores of ferritin when the mucosal cells are replaced by new epithelium. Iron is also lost in considerably smaller amounts by excretion through urine, exfoliation of dermal cells, and perspiration. Menstruation causes the amount of lost iron roughly to double to 2 mg/day. Uncommon sources of iron loss include excessive blood loss or excessive destruction of erythrocytes. Hemorrhage depletes heme iron, whereas excessive turnover of erythrocytes releases it back into the circulation, where it can be recycled. A normal individual can lose a quarter to a third of their erythrocyte mass through hemorrhage without need for iron therapy. Because iron is so well conserved in the body and most people have large reserves, chronically insufficient intake of iron is almost always the cause of iron deficiency anemia.

Pathophysiologic characteristics

Iron deficiency is manifested as signs and symptoms of anemia (pale color, fatigue, tachycardia, tachypnea on exertion). Severe cases, which are rare in first-world nations, may show progressive skin and mucosal changes, such as angular cheilosis and brittle fingernails and toenails. Splenomegaly may be present if hemolysis is occurring. The classic intraoral finding is a red-appearing, sore, smooth tongue caused by atrophy of the dorsal filiform papillae. In very severe cases, Plummer-Vinson syndrome may occur, which is iron deficiency anemia coupled with the formation of esophageal webs and resultant dysphagia. This syndrome is also associated with pharyngeal or esophageal squamous cell carcinoma. Many iron-deficient patients develop pica, an unusual craving for specific foods or unnatural food items (e.g., ice cubes, soil, paint chips) that may or may not contain iron.

The laboratory findings of iron deficiency anemia reflect the severity of the loss. In the first stage, there is a normocytic anemia without changes in erythropoiesis. The ferritin stores are depleting, so the serum ferritin values decrease while the TIBC increases. As anemia progresses and the stores are depleted, the erythrocytes become affected, resulting in a decrease in the MCV, mean corpuscular hemoglobin, erythrocyte count, hemoglobin, and hematocrit.

Iron therapy

The intuitive treatment of any disease state that is accompanied by extreme fatigue, weakness, and loss of color includes increased dietary intake, and the ancient Greeks, Hindus, and other early peoples turned to iron in many forms simply because it represented "strength." Although Sydenham is generally credited with the first rational use of iron (iron filings in wine) for treating anemia in 1681, it was not known that iron was actually present in blood until 30 years later, when Lemery and Geoffry demonstrated its presence. Shortly thereafter, Menghini, an Italian physician, showed that foods with iron actually increase blood iron, but it was not until approximately 1830 that a pill containing iron (ferrous sulfate and potassium carbonate) was introduced into medicine by Blaud, an event that marked the beginning of modern treatment of iron deficiency anemia.

Iron therapy is indicated in iron deficiency anemia; it is contraindicated in anemia of any other cause. Iron is available in the form of Fe^{++} salts (sulfate, gluconate, and fumarate), which are reasonably well absorbed, and an Fe^{+++}-containing compound (iron polysaccharide), which is not as well absorbed. The most commonly used Fe^{++} preparation, and the agent of choice for uncomplicated iron deficiency anemia, is ferrous sulfate. It is normally given in doses (325 mg three times a day) much larger than should theoretically be needed because of its limited absorption (≤15%). The response to oral iron preparations is usually evident in 5 to 10 days and is first manifested by an increase in reticulocytes. Adverse effects associated with orally administered iron are gastrointestinal symptoms (chiefly nausea and vomiting) because of direct irritation of the stomach. The patient will often get black stools as a result of therapy, which may obscure the diagnosis of melena. The drug is unquestionably best absorbed when taken between meals, but gastrointestinal distress is reduced if the medication is taken with meals and if the dose is started at a lower level and slowly increased with time. In general, the hematocrit returns halfway to normal in approximately 3 weeks and is fully corrected in roughly 8 weeks. To replenish iron stores, a course of therapy of 3 to 6 months is generally required.

Although parenteral iron preparations are available, they are not generally used because of the simplicity of oral medication and the much greater risk of serious side effects and higher expense. Iron should be administered parenterally only if the oral preparations are inadequately absorbed or poorly tolerated, such as in patients with enteritis or colitis, or if it is absolutely necessary to replace a serious iron deficit quickly. The classic parenteral form is iron dextran, a sterile colloidal solution of ferric hydroxide and low-molecular-weight dextran, which is administered by intramuscular or intravenous injection. Adverse reactions include pain and straining at the site of injection (intramuscular), urticaria, fever, arthralgia, lymphadenopathy, nausea, and vomiting. Rarely, severe or fatal anaphylactic reactions have occurred after the use of this preparation. Another parenteral form, iron sucrose, is a polynuclear ferric hydroxide sucrose complex. It is believed that the antigenic potential of iron dextran lies in the Fe^{++} and dextran polysaccharides and that this preparation is less allergenic. Iron sucrose is commonly used in patients undergoing renal dialysis who are receiving erythropoietin (EPO) therapy.

Perhaps the most important consideration for the dental professional is the finding that people who are taking oral iron supplements may have altered absorption profiles of other drugs. The **quinolone class of antibiotics, tetracyclines, and thyroid replacement hormones** all form complexes with iron and result in significantly poorer (36% less) absorption profiles. Simply having the patient stagger the iron and the interacting competing medication by ≥2 hours is usually sufficient to avoid this difficulty.

PORPHYRIA

Although iron deficiency anemia is the most commonly encountered form of anemia, it is not the only disorder in which **insufficient functional heme** is produced. The porphyrias, a cluster of disorders that involve decreased or disordered production of the porphyrin ring, can be associated with anemia depending on the variety and severity of the presentation of the diseases. Heme is a major component of hemoglobin, but it is also crucial to several enzyme systems, most notably the large family of cytochrome P450 enzymes involved in steroid synthesis and drug metabolism.

Porphyrin is produced in an eight-step process that occurs in the mitochondria and in the cytosol (Fig. 25-2). The two principal cell types involved are the developing erythroblasts (mature erythrocytes lack mitochondria and are unable to synthesize porphyrin) and the liver hepatocytes. As a result, two general classifications of porphyria exist—erythropoietic and hepatic—that are divided further into nine varieties (Table 25-2), each corresponding to a particular enzyme deficiency in the synthetic pathway of porphyrin. These deficiencies may be genetic in nature or caused by medications.

Acute exacerbations usually occur when there is a significant demand for heme synthesis that cannot be met by the limited enzyme function. Because the heme synthesis pathway is damaged, induction instead leads to the excessive production in the liver of porphyrin precursors, which build up and cause the acute symptoms. This accumulation of protoporphyrins result in neurologic disorders, photocutaneous disturbances, or both.

Probably the most common genetic form of porphyria is **acute intermittent porphyria.** Its mode of transmission is autosomally dominant and results from a partial enzymatic deficiency (<50% of normal) in the third step of porphyrin synthesis. Because synthetic activity is diminished but not lost, most patients remain asymptomatic throughout normal life. Acute exacerbations, which give rise to the name, have highly variable symptoms that last from days to months. The most common presentation is neurologic, including mental changes, seizures, and acute sensory neuropathies such as abdominal pain, chest and back pain, and limb pain. The severity of the pain can be great enough to mimic other

TABLE 25-2 Classification of Porphyrias

Porphyria	Site of Expression	Principal Clinical Feature
Acute intermittent porphyria	Liver	Neurologic
δ-Aminolevulinic acid dehydratase deficiency porphyria	Liver	Neurologic
Hereditary coproporphyria	Liver	Neurologic, photosensitivity
Porphyria cutanea tarda	Liver	Photosensitivity
Variegate porphyria	Liver	Neurologic, photosensitivity
Hepatoerythropoietic porphyria	Liver, bone marrow	Photosensitivity
Congenital erythropoietic porphyria	Bone marrow	Photosensitivity
Erythropoietic protoporphyria	Bone marrow	Photosensitivity
X-linked sideroblastic anemia	Bone marrow	Hemolytic anemia

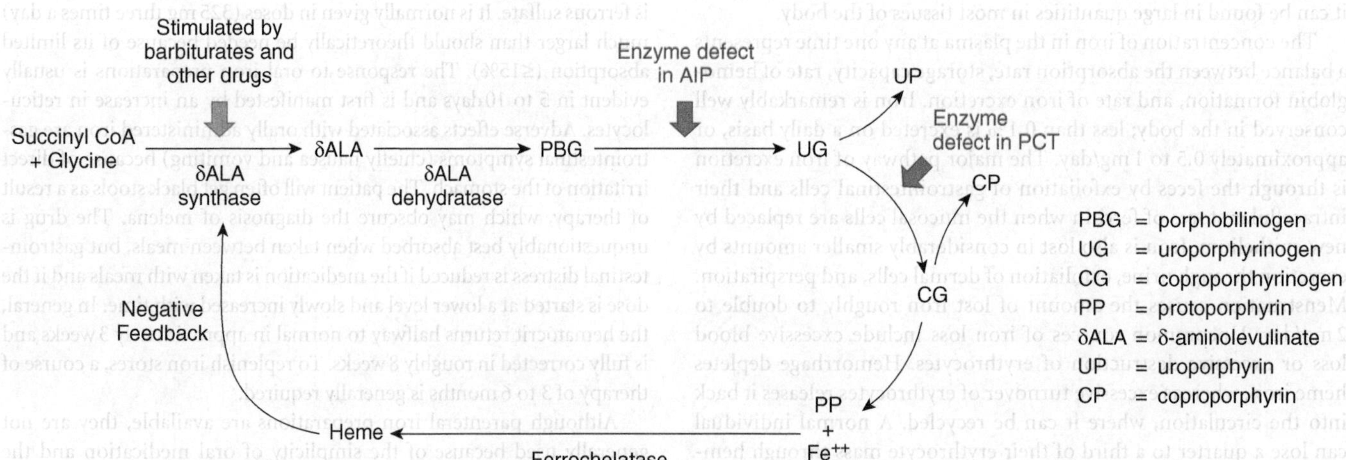

FIG 25-2 Steps in porphyrin synthesis. Products in the synthetic pathway are identified. *Red arrows* identify the enzyme defects for two of the more common porphyrias, acute intermittent porphyria (*AIP*), and porphyria cutanea tarda (*PCT*). ALA synthase is identified as the enzyme activity that is increased with barbiturates and several other drugs.

acute disorders and result in unnecessary surgical intervention such as laparotomy. Motor neuropathies, especially in the cranial nerves, are often seen. Occasionally, motor paralysis of the respiratory diaphragm has resulted in death. Gastrointestinal disturbances—primarily nausea, vomiting, and diarrhea—are common.

Several events can precipitate an attack. Physiologic stressors, such as surgery, excessive alcohol intake, illnesses, and infections, may induce hepatic heme oxygenase, which breaks down heme. Endocrine changes, such as may occur around a woman's menses, or synthetic estrogens and progestins may also induce an attack. More than 1000 medications have been categorized with regard to their porphyrinogenicity, of which a few reactions are well documented and most are still anecdotal. What is accepted is that endocrine properties of the drug, affinity for cytochrome P450, hepatic load, and capacity to modulate nuclear receptors affecting gene transcription all play a role in how porphyrinogenic a drug might be.

Several medications commonly used in dentistry and medicine (Box 25-2) are steroid-based and are metabolized by the cytochrome P450 enzyme system, which leads to increased accumulation of porphyrin precursors. The response of any individual to any of these medications can be highly variable; the proposed unsafe medications should be discussed with the physician on a case-by-case basis. In susceptible porphyric patients, which also includes individuals with hereditary coproporphyria and variegate porphyria, dose reductions or avoidance of specific medications may be necessary.

BOX 25-2 Drugs Considered Safe or Unsafe for Use in Patients with Acute Intermittent Porphyria, Variegate Porphyria, and Hereditary Coproporphyria

Safe	Unsafe or Possibly Unsafe
Acetaminophen	Alcohol
Amitriptyline	Alkylating agents
Aspirin	Azole antifungal drugs
Atropine	Barbiturates (severe)
Chloral hydrate	Carbamazepine
Clorazepate	Chlordiazepoxide
Diazepam	Chlorpropamide
Digoxin	Chloroquine
Diphenhydramine	Clonidine
Glucocorticoids	Dapsone
Guanethidine	Ergots
Hyoscine	Erythromycin
Ibuprofen	Estrogens, synthetic
Imipramine	Food additives
Insulin	Glutethimide
Labetalol	Griseofulvin
Lithium	Hydralazine
Naproxen	Ketamine
Nitrofurantoin	Meprobamate
Opioid analgesics	Methyldopa
Penicillamine	Metoclopramide
Penicillin and derivatives	Nortriptyline
Phenothiazines	Pentazocine
Procaine	Phenytoin
Propranolol	Progestins
Selective serotonin reuptake inhibitors	Pyrazinamide
Streptomycin	Rifampin
Succinylcholine	Spironolactone
Tetracycline	Succinimides
Thiouracil	Sulfonamides (severe)
Vitamins B and C	Theophylline
	Tolazamide
	Tolbutamide
	Valproic acid

Porphyria cutanea tarda is the most common porphyria (part genetic and part acquired) and is representative of the erythropoietic porphyrias. Symptoms commonly include photosensitivity, which results from sequestration of protoporphyrins in the skin and subsequent deposition of iron in the integument. Porphyrin and its precursors undergo photoactivation at 400 nm in the presence of oxygen, causing cellular destruction by release of oxygen free radicals. In skin exposed to light, the porphyrins become photoexcited, and clinically evident cellular damage occurs. Porphyrin-laden erythrocytes also undergo phototoxicity when circulating through light-penetrated tissues. The damage may be sufficient to result in hemolytic anemia.

Management of acute intermittent porphyria has been primarily aimed at avoiding exacerbating conditions. Adequate caloric intake, prompt diagnosis and treatment of infections (including odontogenic and other orofacial infections), and care in not taking medications known to trigger attacks are strategies the patient can use to minimize the risk of developing a crisis. In patients who have photoreactive porphyria, avoidance of sunlight, wearing clothing to cover the skin, and generous use of sunscreen lotion are helpful. Prompt medical intervention including palliative use of opioid analgesics is indicated during porphyric exacerbations.

THALASSEMIA

In addition to problems affecting iron and porphyrin, several disorders of the third component of hemoglobin—the globin chains—can lead to clinical anemia. Grouped together, these disorders are called the *thalassemias.* As discussed previously, normal hemoglobin A is composed of two α-globin and two β-globin chains. When there is a genetic defect in the production of the α chains, the patient has α-thalassemia. Similarly, a defect in the β chains results in β-thalassemia. Sickle cell anemia, although normally addressed as a separate entity, is a variant of β-thalassemia. Thalassemias generally result in a decreased production of their respective protein chains. As a result, hemoglobin synthesis is impaired, and a non-iron-deficient, hypochromic, microcytic anemia ensues.

There are two pairs of genes encoding the α-globin chains, both located on chromosome 16. When all four α-globin genes are defective the condition is incompatible with life. If there is a defective mutation in one of the four genes, the individual is clinically normal but is called a *silent carrier*. If two genes are affected, the patient has *α-thalassemia minor*. The hematocrit is mildly depressed (32% to 40%), and there is a marked decrease in erythrocyte size (MCV 60 to 75 fL). All iron parameters are normal. If three genes are affected, the patient is diagnosed with *α-thalassemia intermedia*, also known as *hemoglobin H disease*. Hemoglobin H is composed of tetramers of β-globin (β_4), resulting from a relative excess of β-globin chains compared with the α chains. Hemoglobin H has a high affinity for oxygen and binds it too tightly for efficient tissue delivery. It is unstable, being prone to denaturation by oxidative medications (e.g., sulfonamides) and infectious conditions. The hematocrit in hemoglobin H disease is markedly depressed (22% to 32%), and the anemia is hypochromic and microcytic in nature (MCV 60 to 70 fL). Clinical signs of the disease include pallor and splenomegaly.

β-Thalassemias exhibit a similar variability in severity based on which mutations in the genome are present. Most β-thalassemias result from point mutations in the gene, which create premature stop codons or cause difficulties with RNA transcription. As a result, the affected β chain may be either reduced (β^+) or absent (β^0). Because the δ or γ forms of hemoglobin can substitute for the β form, β-thalassemias typically have decreased ratios of hemoglobin A ($\alpha_2\beta_2$) and increased ratios of hemoglobin A_2 ($\alpha_2\delta_2$) and hemoglobin F ($\alpha_2\gamma_2$). The total amount of useful hemoglobin is usually severely depressed, however, decreasing oxygen transport capability. Further clinical disease occurs because of a relative excess of α-globin chains, which precipitate and cause damage to the developing erythrocytes and triggers a hyperplastic response by the bone marrow, resulting in increased marrow spaces and subsequent pathologic fractures and osteopenia. Peripherally, the destruction of the red blood cells may lead to a potentially life-threatening hemolytic anemia, splenomegaly, hepatomegaly, and hyperbilirubinemia.

The correct diagnosis of thalassemia is crucial to proper treatment. Mild forms of the disease need no treatment. More severe forms typically require transfusion support and folate supplementation. Iron therapy should be avoided because there is often hemosiderosis/iron overload owing to insufficient complete hemoglobin production. Splenectomy may be required if severe hemolysis is occurring. Finally, allogeneic bone marrow transplantation may be required to correct the defect in severe cases.

Sickle Cell Anemia

Sickle cell anemia is technically a variant of β-thalassemia. A point mutation in the number 6 position of the β-globin chain causes a valine to be substituted for glutamic acid. As an autosomal recessive disorder, *sickle cell anemia* occurs when both alleles are positive for the sickle variant. *Sickle cell trait* occurs in the heterozygous state, where partial penetrance ($\alpha_2\beta^s\beta$) can occur. **The abnormal β chain is designated β^s**, and the resulting tetramer of $\alpha_2\beta_2^S$ is known as *hemoglobin S*. The significance of hemoglobin S is that in the severely deoxygenated state the globin tetramers are capable of coalescing into long, straight, spiral polymers that act as deforming filaments within the red blood cell. The cell loses its typical biconcave disk shape and its inherent pliability that is so important for moving through the microvasculature. These deformed and hardened erythrocytes are much more prone to automembrane damage and hemolysis. Simultaneously, the sickled shape makes them likely to cause microvascular occlusion and endothelial vascular damage.

Sickle cell anemia generally first manifests in the homozygous patient by age 6 months, when hemoglobin F is downregulated and hemoglobin S becomes the dominant form of hemoglobin in the erythrocyte. Many patients with homozygous disease can have normal lives as long as they avoid situations in which moderate–severe hypoxic stress can develop. Acute crises of sickling occur when the globin tetramers are deoxygenated for a sufficient time to allow polymerization into the deforming filamentous form. Small infections, such as odontogenic infections, may or may not cause an acute crisis. Although acidosis can develop, unless the red blood cells are severely hypoxic, they will oxygenate in the lungs before developing significant polymers and distorted cells. If the hypoxic stress is great, such as with more severe infection, acute sickling occurs. The episodes are extremely painful, often lasting several hours to days. Treatment for the acute crisis is aimed at hydration, oxygenation, and resolution of the underlying precipitating factor. Many patients require opioid analgesics to help them through a crisis.

A patient with sickle cell anemia who is prone to repeated acute crises experiences various chronic complications from the disease. The erythrocytes containing hemoglobin S have a shortened life span compared with the erythrocytes containing hemoglobin A, and episodes of sickling accelerate their demise, resulting in a chronic hemolytic-like anemia. The anemia predisposes the patient to diminished oxygen transport capability (furthering the likelihood of a sickling crisis), and the breakdown by-products of the erythrocytes can produce clinical jaundice, hepatomegaly, and splenomegaly. At the same time, chronic and repeated microvascular occlusive episodes can cause renal infarction, stroke, retinopathy, cardiomyopathy, and hepatic damage from occlusive ischemic necrosis. Many patients develop significant microvascular damage in the spleen because of its slow, tortuous microcirculation. In some cases, the spleen ultimately undergoes reactive fibrosis and becomes a small, scarred, essentially nonfunctional organ (autosplenectomy). In severe cases of sickle cell anemia, death can occur from multisystem organ failure.

Two strategies have been used in the long-term management of sickle cell anemia: bone marrow transplantation and pharmacotherapy. Bone marrow transplantation replaces the pluripotent stem cells of the marrow with cells of a person without the genotype, erasing the genetic defect. Although bone marrow transplantation is significantly more predictable than in years past, there is still a significant (>10%) mortality rate associated with the procedure, and the implications of chronic graft-versus-host disease must be weighed. This approach is generally reserved for severe cases that exhibit recurrent sickle crises.

Pharmacologic therapy has shown at least partial success in β-thalassemia and sickle cell anemia. This approach is based on the premise that any measure that increases the quantity of β-like globin molecules in erythrocytes is beneficial. Several antineoplastic agents and erythropoietin (EPO) have been used to stimulate the formation of hemoglobin F. Hemoglobin F transports oxygen as effectively as hemoglobin A, and it circumvents the genetic abnormalities associated with defective β-globin synthesis. In addition, hemoglobin F suppresses the polymerization of hemoglobin S, helping further to reduce the effects of the disease.

VITAMIN B_{12}, FOLATE, AND MEGALOBLASTIC ANEMIA

Deficiency Syndromes

Vitamin B_{12} and folic acid are two nutritional supplements that are crucial to normal DNA synthesis. When one or both of these are deficient, all rapidly dividing cells throughout the body, but especially cells of the bone marrow and gastrointestinal epithelium, begin to have difficulties with proliferation and differentiation caused by inhibition of mitosis and cytokinesis. Primarily, DNA synthesis is impaired; the resulting cells have large RNA-to-DNA ratios, increased cytoplasmic compartments, and unusual immature nuclear forms. In hematopoiesis, the deficiency causes the cells to assume a characteristic macrocytic and often oval or irregular shape that resembles the less mature blast forms—hence the term *megaloblastic anemia*. Protein synthesis is also adversely affected, resulting in substandard cell membranes and shortened life spans, causing the anemia to have a hemolytic component as well.

Although the diagnosis of megaloblastic anemia is most commonly made because of the characteristic changes in erythrocytes, all hematopoietic cell types are affected. Depending on which cell types are adversely affected, there may not only be clinical fatigue caused by erythropoietic depression, but also leukopenia and thrombocytopenia, with an increased potential of infection (particularly in the urinary tract) and hemorrhage.

Although folic acid and vitamin B_{12} have similar effects on the developing erythrocytes, the overall clinical presentations of their respective deficiency states differ greatly. The similarity comes from the sharing of a common biochemical pathway. The major difference is that neurologic manifestations often occur with vitamin B_{12} deficiency but not with folic acid deficiency. Folate deficiency alone is characterized by pallor, anemia, fatigue, and glossitis. Vitamin B_{12} deficiency results in the same signs and symptoms as folate deficiency but also causes inadequate myelin synthesis and epithelial replacement in the gastrointestinal tract. Paresthesias involving the peripheral nerves are the most common presenting symptoms with vitamin B_{12} deficiency. There is also decreased vibration and positional sense. Reflexes may be altered, and motor disturbances, including weakness and loss of sphincter tone, may occur. As the disease progresses, the posterior spinal columns are affected, resulting in difficulty with balance.

In advanced cases, cerebral dysfunction may lead to memory loss, confusion, or dementia and other neuropsychiatric changes. It is crucial to diagnose correctly and treat a vitamin B_{12} deficiency early because most of these neurologic findings can be reversed in the early stages. Patients with more advanced cases have permanent neurologic damage. Severe vitamin B_{12} deficiency is known as *pernicious anemia.* Historically, some anemic patients did not respond to iron supplementation, and their disease was characterized as pernicious, meaning fatal.

Vitamin B_{12}

Nutrition and physiologic characteristics

Vitamin B12 is a generic term for cyanocobalamin and hydroxocobalamin, two stable forms of cobalamin. Cobalamins are unique because they are the only cobalt-containing organic compounds known to occur in nature, and they represent the only known biologic example of a metal–carbon bond. The cobalamins are composed of a nearly planar macrocyclic corrin ring (similar to porphyrin) covalently linked to a trivalent cobalt atom by four coordination bonds in a manner similar to iron binding in heme. As a group, the cobalamins are essential cofactors in several human enzymatic processes that lead to proper DNA formation. A deficiency in them results in a megaloblastic anemia, as the flawed DNA fragments are left in the maturing erythrocyte.

The sole natural and commercial source of cobalamin is synthesis by microorganisms. Many animals can use vitamin B_{12} produced by their own enteric bacteria, but because microbial synthesis in humans is limited to the large intestine (a site too distal for effective absorption) humans must derive their vitamin B_{12} exogenously. Foods rich in vitamin B_{12} include shellfish, such as oysters and clams (>10 µg/100 g tissue), and mammalian organ meats (liver, kidney, and heart). The average daily diet contains 5 to 30 µg of vitamin B_{12}, of which 20% to 30% is absorbed. Daily intake of 1 to 3 µg does little more than compensate for daily loss, but normally more than 1000 times this amount (up to 4 mg) is stored in the liver.

Vitamin B_{12} is quite lipophobic and depends heavily on several transfer proteins to be absorbed from the gastrointestinal tract. When first ingested, the cobalamin liberated from food interacts with ***R proteins*** in the stomach. These "bodyguard" proteins bind tightly to cobalamin and protect it from acidic degradation. As the R protein–cobalamin complex moves into the duodenum and the pH increases, pancreatic proteases degrade the R protein from around the cobalamin. The cobalamin is next adsorbed onto ***intrinsic factor***, an "escort" glycoprotein secreted by the stomach parietal cells that has specific cobalamin-binding properties. The intrinsic factor–cobalamin complex is carried to the ileum, where highly specific receptors on cells of the ileal microvilli transport it across the cell membrane. In the enterocytes, the intrinsic factor is broken down, liberating the cobalamin. Next, a "chauffeur" plasma polypeptide, ***transcobalamin II***, binds the cobalamin to carry the vitamin into the portal bloodstream.

Receptors for this transcobalamin II–cobalamin complex are ubiquitous, but are especially rich in the liver. If the vitamin is needed in the tissues, it is taken up by the respective cells by endocytosis. If there is surplus, the cobalamin is moved to the hepatocytes for storage. Inside the cell, the cobalamin is freed by lysosomal enzymes, and the transcobalamin II is recycled back for reuse.

Normal hepatocyte turnover results in the loss of 3 to 4 µg of cobalamin into the bile each day. The lost vitamin is quickly rebound by intrinsic factor in the small intestine and reabsorbed. Because this enterohepatic circulation is so efficient, very little new vitamin B_{12} is required in the diet each day. As long as the ability of the body to transport cobalamin across the intestinal wall and reabsorb the bile-secreted cobalamin remains intact, a diet completely devoid of vitamin B_{12} may not produce clinical symptoms for many years.

Pathophysiologic characteristics

Vitamin B_{12} deficiency can be difficult to diagnose. Typically, the MCV of the erythrocytes is markedly increased (usually 110 to 140 fL). If there is a concurrent iron deficiency anemia, the combination of microcytic and macrocytic anemias may result in relatively normal-sized cells. Other times, the cells are normocytic for obscure reasons. The peripheral blood smear is abnormal, showing anisocytosis and poikilocytosis, along with the characteristic macro-ovalocytes. Multilobulated neutrophils are typical. Hemolytic changes may also be found. Serum vitamin B_{12} concentrations, normally 150 to 350 pg/mL, are less than 100 pg/mL.

It is rare to see an individual with dietary vitamin B_{12} insufficiency, especially in first-world nations. Only the strictest of vegans who eat no animal and dairy products whatsoever may show dietary insufficiency. Even then, small amounts of vitamin B_{12} may be available in the diet from microorganisms of legumes or exogenous application of cobalamins to grain and cereal products. As previously mentioned, dietary deficiency may take decades to become clinically evident.

A more common difficulty is with malabsorption of dietary cobalamin. In these patients, the transport proteins are defective, so that not only is the primary absorptive capacity decreased or lost, but also the ability of the body to recycle enterohepatic cobalamin is impaired. These patients have a much more rapid onset of symptoms, usually 3 to 6 years. Ileal problems may also lead to vitamin B_{12} deficiency. Luminal stasis may allow significant enteric bacterial overgrowth, leading to blind loop syndrome; the vitamin is "stolen" by the bacteria and is unavailable to the host. Other conditions such as surgical resection, carcinoma, Crohn disease, and other inflammatory bowel disorders may similarly induce a vitamin B_{12} deficiency. Because vitamin B_{12} deficiency results in decreased DNA synthesis of rapidly dividing cells, the enterocytes themselves begin to experience inhibition of mitosis and cytokinesis as the availability of cobalamin declines. As the disease progresses, it becomes increasingly self-perpetuating because the enterocytes become defective and further lose their ability to absorb cobalamin. Pancreatic disease also decreases the absorption of vitamin B_{12} in the small intestine.

Finally, certain drugs can reduce cobalamin absorption. Megadoses of vitamin C may cause vitamin B_{12} to be converted to non-useful analogues, some of which may harbor anti–vitamin B_{12} activity. Long-term exposure to nitrous oxide has been shown in pigs and humans to result in megaloblastic anemia by inhibiting methionine synthase activity. The nitrous oxide irreversibly oxidizes the exposed cobalt atom, and in so doing it permanently inactivates the enzyme.

Therapeutic use

Various preparations are used for vitamin B_{12} therapy, most commonly **cyanocobalamin and hydroxocobalamin**. Both are given by intramuscular or deep subcutaneous injection. Hydroxocobalamin is more highly protein-bound and remains in circulation longer, but the more popular form is cyanocobalamin because hydroxocobalamin has been associated with the development of antibodies to the transcobalamin II–vitamin B_{12} complex.

Initial treatment involves twice-weekly intramuscular injections of vitamin B_{12} for several months. Such treatment brings about a rapid change in the bone marrow from megaloblastic to normoblastic erythropoiesis (usually in 2 to 3 days), with improving relief of glossitis, neuritis, and spinal cord degeneration in several months. As the blood picture improves, the interval between doses can be increased to 2 or 3 weeks. Because the hepatic stores are so great after they are replenished, the patient can eventually be put on maintenance therapy involving an injection every 1 or 2 months, but it must be continued for life. Neurologic damage that is not reversed after 12 to 18 months of therapy must be considered permanent.

Large doses of cobalamin are promptly excreted in the urine and to a lesser extent in the feces. There have been no reports of toxic effects from cyanocobalamin or hydroxocobalamin other than occasional allergic responses to impurities in the preparations.

Folic Acid

Nutrition and physiologic characteristics

In the course of an attempt to isolate vitamin B_{12} to treat another form of megaloblastic anemia peculiar to Hindu women, a different hematopoietic factor, **folic acid (folacin or pteroylglutamic acid)**, was recognized and isolated. Because the hematologic picture produced by vitamin B_{12} deficiency is almost indistinguishable from that of folic acid deficiency, it is not surprising that the paths of discovery of these two essential antianemic factors were so entwined.

Although not usually referred to as such, folic acid fits the definition of a vitamin. It occurs widely in nature as polyglutamate conjugates, but it is an essential human nutrient in microgram quantities. Fresh green vegetables (e.g., asparagus, broccoli, spinach, lettuce) are an excellent source of folic acid. Fruits such as bananas, lemons, and melons have high amounts, and liver, kidney, yeast, and mushrooms are also abundant in folate conjugates. Prolonged cooking destroys folic acid, especially when the conjugates are in dilute aqueous solution.

Absorption occurs primarily in the proximal jejunum, and it depends on specific mucosal membrane conjugates that hydrolyze the dietary polyglutamates to yield folic acid. In the mucosa, folic acid is reduced and methylated to 5-methyltetrahydrofolate before entering the bloodstream. When in tissues, the compound is demethylated to tetrahydrofolate, and conjugated with 1-carbon moieties to yield several active coenzyme forms that are essential for purine and thymidylate synthesis. Tetrahydrofolate is also involved in the conversion reactions of several amino acids. Figure 25-3 illustrates the major metabolic pathways and interactions of folate and vitamin B_{12}.

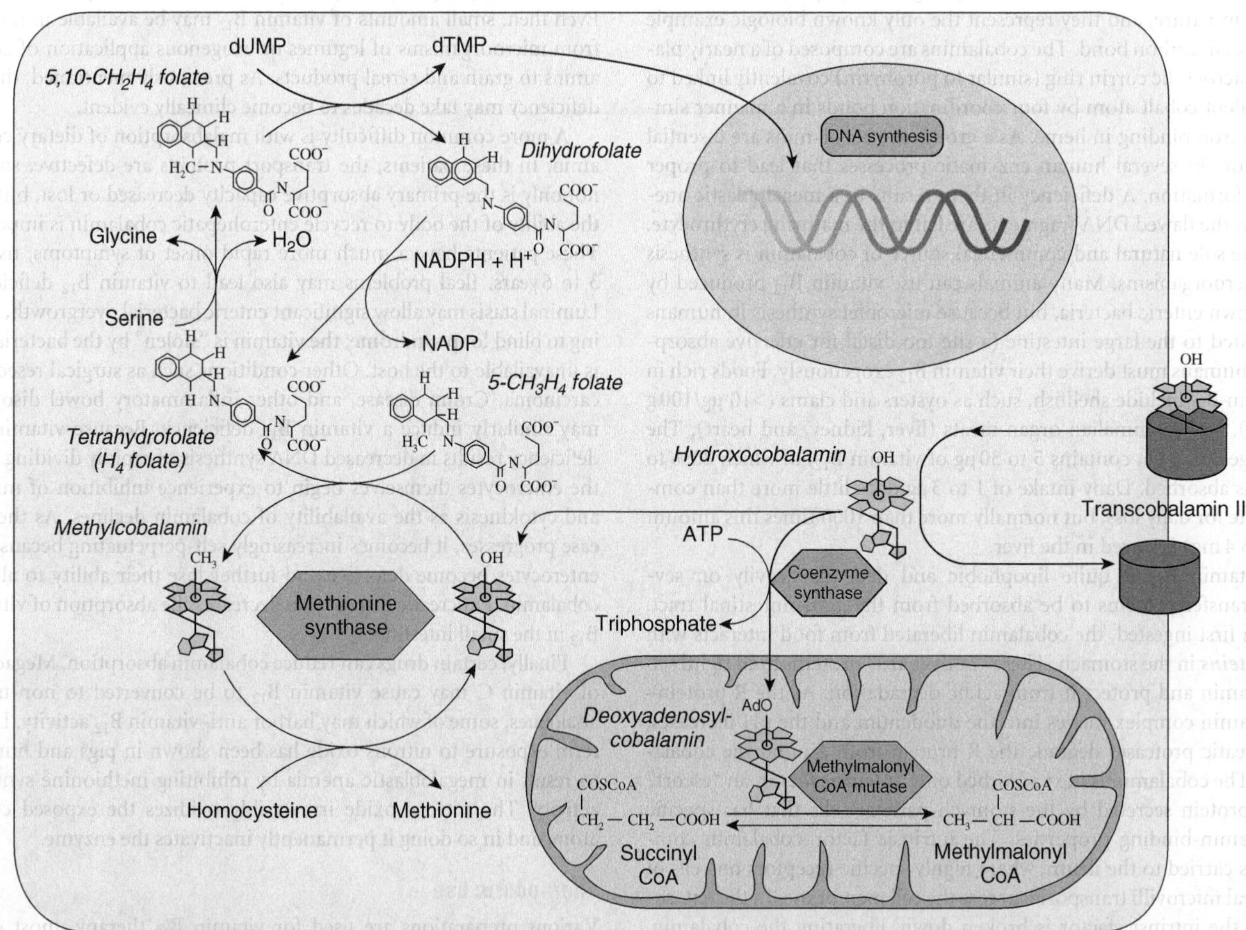

FIG 25-3 Major pathways of folate and vitamin B_{12} metabolism. Dietary folates are converted to 5-methyltetrahydrofolate (*5-CH$_3$H$_4$ folate*). Demethylation by the enzyme methionine synthase yields tetrahydrofolate, an acceptor of single-carbon units in the metabolism of histidine (not shown) and serine. The folate products of these reactions provide carbon units for the synthesis of purines and, as shown for 5,10-methylenetetrahydrofolate (*5,10-CH$_2$H$_4$ folate*), the conversion of deoxyuridylate (*dUMP*) to thymidylate (*dTMP*). Vitamin B_{12}, carried to the cell by transcobalamin II in the form of hydroxocobalamin, is converted to methylcobalamin and deoxyadenosylcobalamin, necessary cofactors for methionine synthase and methylmalonyl CoA mutase. *AdO*, Deoxyadenosyl moiety; *NADP*, nicotinamide adenine dinucleotide phosphate; *NADPH*, reduced nicotinamide adenine dinucleotide phosphate.

The minimum daily folate requirement for humans is approximately 50 µg, but because of incomplete absorption and special requirements for lactating women and certain other individuals, a daily intake of 400 µg of free folate is recommended. Folate is stored and recycled through the enterohepatic pathway similarly to cobalamin. The resorptive process is far less efficient than with vitamin B_{12}, however, and deficient intake may manifest as megaloblastic anemia within a month.

Pathophysiologic characteristics

Folic acid deficiency has the same hematologic profile as cobalamin deficiency. As previously mentioned, folic acid deficiency causes a megaloblastic anemia essentially without neurologic manifestations. In patients who are folate-deficient, serum folate concentrations are less than 3 ng/mL, and erythrocyte folate is less than 150 ng/mL.

Despite the fact that folates are abundant in many foods, deficiency still occurs from many different causes. Various malabsorption syndromes disturb the absorption of folic acid by the intestines. Phenytoin and other antiepileptic drugs, oral contraceptives, and antimalarial drugs may cause folate deficiency by inhibiting folate conjugates in the intestinal wall. The antimetabolites methotrexate and trimethoprim inhibit folate reduction and lead to a megaloblastic anemia with prolonged use.

Elderly individuals and individuals of low socioeconomic status may have an inadequate intake of folate simply from poor nutrition. Overcooking of folate-containing foods, if consistently performed, can lead to folate deficiency. Pregnancy greatly increases the maternal requirement for folate, and a marginal diet can become inadequate to meet the growing demands of the fetus. Maternal folate deficiency, especially before conception, has been implicated in fetal neural tube defects such as spina bifida. Chronic debilitating disease, such as cancer and myeloproliferative disorders, may predispose a patient to folic acid deficiency. Alcoholism and other hepatic diseases are definitely correlated with folate deficiency caused by generally poor nutritional status, malabsorption difficulties across the intestinal wall, and depleted liver stores.

Folate therapy

Folate deficiency can often be treated with simple dietary supplements, such as an additional piece of fresh fruit daily. The vitamin is available in oral tablet form, is included in most multivitamin preparations, and is supplied for injection in the form of sodium folate or the calcium salt of **folinic acid** under the nonproprietary name of **leucovorin**. Leucovorin has been used to counteract the effects of folic acid antagonists (e.g., **the dihydrofolate reductase inhibitors, methotrexate and trimethoprim**) used in cancer or malaria chemotherapy. A study showed that even simple use of folic acid greatly improved the side effects of methotrexate therapy in patients with rheumatoid arthritis, allowing better tolerance of the chemotherapeutic agent. The response to oral folic acid therapy is rapid, and an improvement in the hematologic picture is seen 5 to 10 days after beginning daily administration. Adverse effects directly attributable to folic acid have not been reported.

HEMATOPOIETIC GROWTH FACTORS

Perhaps the most exciting advance in the pharmacologic management of anemia and related disorders has been the introduction of hematopoietic growth factors to the therapeutic armamentarium. Numerous diseases and iatrogenic disorders can cause all or part of a patient's hematopoietic system to produce insufficient cells; the result is usually a pancytopenia with different degrees of individual cell line depression. Examples of causative conditions include the many varieties of leukemia, myeloproliferative disorders, lymphomas, aplastic anemia, and end-stage renal disease. Therapies such as cytotoxic chemotherapy, ionizing radiation, stem cell transplants, and bone marrow transplantation also contribute. Other causes include side effects of medications such as the sulfonamides, phenytoin, zidovudine, and carbamazepine. In the past, the only recourse was to transfuse the patient with whole blood or appropriate replacement components of blood. In severe instances, a bone marrow transplant may have been necessary. Although not a panacea, the introduction of several hematopoietic growth factors has greatly reduced the need for transfusion therapy in many patients with various forms of hematopoietic depression. All these products are derived from their respective human genes that have been subcloned into mammalian, bacterial, or yeast expression systems so that large quantities can be obtained.

Erythropoietin/Darbepoetin

Background and physiologic characteristics

Erythropoietin (**EPO**) was the first growth factor to be identified and successfully cloned into a recombinant vector. The gene is located on chromosome 7q11-22, and the final endogenous protein is a 165-amino acid glycoprotein with a molecular weight of 30,400 Da. Native EPO is formed primarily in the kidneys and, to a smaller degree, in the liver. It is the major humoral regulator of red blood cell production and does not seem to have any effect on other cell lineages.

EPO expression is regulated in the kidney in response to the local oxygen tension by signaling mechanisms that are not well understood but are suspected to involve a membrane-bound, oxygen-sensitive heme protein. The newly formed EPO moves to the bone marrow, where it attaches to EPO receptors on the cell membranes of myeloid stem cells, causing the cells in the presence of other regulatory factors to differentiate into erythroblasts and ultimately into erythrocytes. Once committed to the erythrocytic line, these cells become dependent on continued EPO for their survival. If EPO is removed, the cells die within one or two cell cycles.

Pathophysiologic characteristics

In disease states, EPO synthesis may be disrupted (as in end-stage renal disease), or the protein may be prematurely cleared (as in the anemia associated with rheumatoid arthritis), or the target stem cells may not be responsive to it (as in some myeloproliferative disorders). In all cases of depressed synthesis or accelerated catabolism, the plasma EPO is low. If the problem is decreased tissue responsiveness, plasma EPO levels may be increased 100 times above normal.

Therapeutic use

Two forms of pharmacologic EPO are currently available. The recombinant form of the endogenous glycoprotein known as ***epoetin alfa*** has been available for several years and has been well tolerated. It generally requires intravenous or subcutaneous dosing three times a week. A modified form, **darbepoetin alfa**, requires dosing only once a week. Darbepoetin contains five N-linked oligosaccharide chains instead of only three such chains in epoetin. Its pharmacologic profile is similar to that of epoetin alfa.

Both forms of EPO are currently approved for use in the anemia of chronic renal failure and cancer chemotherapy. A nephrologist once said, "Dialysis saved the chronic renal failure patients' lives, but erythropoietin made them feel better." Prior to erythropoietin therapy, the anemias of chronic renal failure were so great that the patients had little energy to do even simple activities of daily living. Epoetin alfa has also been extensively studied for use in numerous other conditions that result in anemia or pancytopenia for which there is insufficient production of EPO in relation to the metabolic needs of the patient.

One study showed that the use of EPO with supplemental iron significantly improved the health status of patients with congestive heart failure and anemia. Treated patients experienced relative improvements in serum creatinine and left ventricular ejection fraction, resulting in better renal function and a reduced need for diuretics. Correction of anemia has markedly enhanced cardiac function in these patients.

Epoetin alfa has the most consistent effect when plasma EPO is low, but exogenous EPO has also been successful in treating some conditions in which endogenous titers are already high, and the target stem cells seem to be resistant to the effects of the protein. Epoetin alfa is also used in the treatment of chronic anemia associated with acquired immunodeficiency syndrome, but results have been inconsistent. On the positive side, epoetin alfa can often stabilize a patient's hematopoietic profile enough to resume zidovudine therapy. Zidovudine depresses the bone marrow, complicating the anemia to the point at which it may be necessary to discontinue the medication.

Epoetin alfa is sometimes used to prepare patients for autologous blood donation before non-emergent surgery. In these instances, the patient is phlebotomized normally and put on a course of epoetin alfa for a few weeks before surgery. Just before the surgery, patients can be phlebotomized again to maximize the available yield of autologous blood. Epoetin alfa has also been used in patients who require blood products but do not allow transfusions for religious reasons. Epoetin alfa solutions contain human albumin, a blood product. For this reason, these patients may still refuse the therapy unless the diluent can be changed.

Epoetin alfa can be given intravenously and is well absorbed, but the subcutaneous route is preferred because of a greater persistence of each dose in the plasma. (Epoetin alfa has a half-life of 6 to 9 hours after intravenous injection, but 24 to 30 hours after subcutaneous administration.) Less medication needs to be given, resulting in lower cost and fewer adverse effects. Contraindications for its use include uncontrolled hypertension and allergy to albumin or mammalian cell–derived products. Adverse reactions include aggravation of existing hypertension, seizures, headache, and nausea. Failure of epoetin alfa most commonly results from the development of a significant iron deficiency caused by the increased production of hemoglobin. For this reason, close monitoring of the iron stores (TIBC, iron, ferritin) should be performed routinely, with iron supplementation given as necessary. The rate of hematocrit increase should not exceed 4% per week to avoid depleting the iron stores. Clinically significant results are usually seen in 2 to 6 weeks.

Myeloid Growth Factors

Background and physiologic characteristics

Several additional growth factors are currently approved for use by the U.S. Food and Drug Administration. **Granulocyte colony-stimulating factor (G-CSF) and granulocyte-macrophage colony-stimulating factor (GM-CSF)** are crucial to the early and intermediate development of the myeloid line of hematopoiesis. G-CSF is a lineage-specific growth factor for the neutrophil line, whereas GM-CSF is a stimulator for granulocytes and monocytes (with some erythrocyte and megakaryocyte effect as well; see Fig. 25-1). In addition to increasing the numbers of neutrophils, both also activate the neutrophils and monocytes/macrophages in the tissues. Their names are derived from their ability to stimulate colony formation of hematopoietic stem cells when grown in semisolid media.

Recombinant human G-CSF, assigned the nonproprietary name of ***filgrastim***, is synthesized in an *Escherichia coli* bacterial expression system. It is a 175-amino acid polypeptide. A pegylated derivative known as *pegfilgrastim* is produced by covalently linking a large polyethylene glycol moiety to the active polypeptide. The latter version gives extended function. G-CSF binds to cell surface receptors present on the progranulocytes and stimulates them to proliferate and mature. The more differentiated cells are known to have two to three times more G-CSF receptors on their surface, which seems to correlate with increased functional activity in the presence of the drug. Exactly how the G-CSF upregulates transcription in the nucleus is unknown, but part of the therapeutic benefit of this medication is from enhanced neutrophilic activity and increased numbers.

The commercially available form of GM-CSF is a 127-amino acid glycopeptide with a leucine substitution at position 23; ***sargramostim*** is the nonproprietary name. Similar to G-CSF, GM-CSF stimulates terminal proliferation and differentiation of the granulocyte lineage. In contrast to G-CSF, it also stimulates the monocytic lineage. As with G-CSF, the mechanism by which the intracellular changes occur is unknown. It does seem, however, to require interleukin-3 (IL-3) stimulation to obtain a maximal differentiative response.

Several other growth factors have been cloned, purified, and made available for investigational laboratory and clinical use. Among the most important are **stem cell factor (SCF)**, **monocyte/macrophage-colony-stimulating factor (M-CSF)**, **thrombopoietin (TPO)** and its analogues, and **IL-3**. These four, coupled with G-CSF and GM-CSF, round out the six "classic" hematopoietic stimulating agents.

SCF has been assigned the nonproprietary name of ***ancestim***. As the name implies, SCF is crucial for the survival and proliferation of the early pluripotent/multipotent and myeloid/lymphoid stem cells. The immature stem cells produce and "autostimulate" themselves with their own SCF production to maintain a sufficient population of pluripotent/multipotent cells to keep the marrow supplied with adequate precursors for the various differentiation pathways. SCF alone does not push the stem cells toward maturation but maintains their immaturity. When coupled with other growth factors, SCF acts synergistically to "bump" the cells into a committed pathway, where most of these early intermediates begin to lose their need for this particular factor. As the cells continue to move toward maturation, SCF is no longer necessary.

M-CSF, as the name implies, promotes the growth and differentiation of monocyte progenitor cells, but only at high concentrations. More important, however, may be its ability to activate monocyte/macrophage cytotoxicity, as shown by its ability to increase the survival of patients with invasive fungal infections. It remains to be seen how M-CSF may significantly differ in function from GM-CSF.

TPO stimulates the megakaryocytic lineage, which results in increased platelet production by tenfold. The medication so far has been used in cancer chemotherapy patients to hasten platelet recovery after thrombocytopenic nadirs are reached. There are other analogues approved by the FDA, and they function similarly to TPO.

IL-3 is encoded by a gene located near the gene for GM-CSF. Endogenous supply is essentially from activated T cells, mast cells, and natural killer cells. IL-3 is a multilineage, broader-acting hematopoietic growth factor important in initiating early and intermediate stages of hematopoietic differentiation. It seems to be a crucial early trigger for the shift from pluripotent/multipotent stem cells down any of the myeloid differentiation pathways. IL-3 mediates its effects by the retinoic acid (vitamin A) receptors. When "nudged" this way, the cells show irreversible commitment and go on to become one of the myeloid stems that later differentiate into the granulocytic, erythroid, monocytic, or megakaryocytic lineages. IL-3 by itself has little differentiative activity, but it does seem to be involved in the crucial first step to bring stem cells out of the pluripotent/multipotent stage. As the cells mature, they become less dependent on its actions.

Interleukin-11 (IL-11), in the recombinant form of **oprelvekin**, is the first growth factor to gain approval for the management of thrombocytopenia. IL-11 is produced by fibroblasts and stromal cells in bone marrow. It binds to a specific receptor but acts with other growth factors to simulate the growth of myeloid and lymphoid cell lines. The primary therapeutic benefit is a significant decrease in the need for platelet transfusions in patients receiving chemotherapy for nonmyeloid cancers.

Pathophysiologic characteristics

Any of the diseases or therapeutic interventions that adversely affect the hematopoietic system may cause leukopenia, thrombocytopenia, or pancytopenia. Congenital or acquired bone marrow failure states, hematopoietic neoplasms, cancer chemotherapy, and total body ionizing radiation therapy are the most common causes for hematopoietic disruption.

Therapeutic use

Stimulating or accelerating the recovery of the bone marrow (especially the neutrophils) after disease or medical therapy is the primary indication for the myeloid growth factors G-CSF and GM-CSF. Similarly, TPO is being used to hasten the recovery of platelet counts in patients with thrombocytopenia. When so used, the window of immunosuppression and hemorrhagic vulnerability of leukopenic and thrombocytopenic patients has been significantly shortened, greatly improving chances for survival, while decreasing morbidity.

Filgrastim administered intravenously or subcutaneously is generally well tolerated, with the most common side effect being bone pain that clears on discontinuance of the medication. Rare serious reactions include anaphylaxis and splenic rupture. Pegfilgrastim is administered subcutaneously as a single dose after chemotherapy and generally lasts 10 to 14 days.

Sargramostim is administered intravenously. At normal doses, it does not significantly alter the megakaryocyte/thrombocyte or erythrocyte lineages. It does have more severe side effects, however, especially at higher doses. The most common are fever, malaise, arthralgia, myalgia, and increased vascular permeability, which can lead to pleural and pericardial effusions.

SCF generally is given in conjunction with filgrastim and sargramostim. Its use is still limited; side effects associated with its administration include fever, chills, rash, myalgia, injection site irritation, and edema. IL-3 is usually given subcutaneously in daily doses in conjunction with GM-CSF and has been well tolerated.

Oprelvekin is injected daily for 3 weeks after a course of chemotherapy is completed. The therapeutic goal is to reach a platelet count of 50,000/μL. Impaired renal excretion of Na^+ may lead to fluid retention, hypokalemia, pulmonary edema, and atrial arrhythmias.

IMPLICATIONS FOR DENTISTRY

The dentist is often in a unique position as the first health professional to observe manifestations of anemia in a patient. Because the oral signs frequently precede a decrease in hemoglobin below the normal range, the dentist may be able to diagnose the disease before it has caused symptoms warranting medical attention. Because anemia is a sign of an underlying hematopoietic disorder, the blood cells are frequently the earliest biologic indicators of diseases such as cancer, malnutrition, or conditions of drug toxicity. The response may take the form of neutropenia, hemolytic or aplastic anemia, or thrombocytopenia with associated immunosuppression and defective hemostasis leading to spontaneous hemorrhage, internal bleeding, and purpura.

Patients with these difficulties may have **oral mucositis, intraoral or circumoral viral outbreaks, fungal infections, and serious bacterial infections of odontogenic origin**. The dentist should recognize these signs, understand the gravity of the situation, and attempt to ensure that the patient receives proper medical evaluation. Anemic conditions can run the gamut from easily corrected nutritional deficiency states to life-threatening disorders, and the sooner the patient is diagnosed, the better the chances are for correcting the underlying problem.

Patients who are undergoing therapy for these same diseases and taking many of the medications described in this chapter are increasingly encountered in dental practice. The dentist who knows how these medications function and why they are being given is better able to identify the presence or history of a particular disease and to make appropriate decisions about how to manage the patient's overall care.

ANTIANEMIC DRUGS

Nonproprietary (Generic) Name	Proprietary (Trade) Name
Iron Preparations	
Ferrous fumarate	—
Ferrous gluconate	—
Ferrous sulfate	—
Hematopoietic Factors	
Darbepoetin alfa	Aranesp
Epoetin alfa	Epogen, Procrit
Filgrastim (G-CSF)	Neupogen
Oprelvekin	Neumega
Pegfilgrastim	Neulasta
Sargramostim (GM-CSF)	Leukine
Vitamin B_{12} Preparations	
Cyanocobalamin	Nascobal
Hydroxocobalamin	Cyanokit
Folic Acid Preparations	
Folic acid	—
Leucovorin (folinic acid)	—

G-CSF, Granulocyte colony-stimulating factor; *GM-CSF,* granulocyte-macrophage colony-stimulating factor.

CASE DISCUSSION

Pegfilgrastim is a long-acting G-CSF medication. It targets the neutrophilic population of cells and stimulates the bone marrow stem cells to proliferate and keep this critical cell line functional. The fact that the patient needs this medication suggests that not only is the neutrophilic lineage severely affected by the chemotherapy regimen, but perhaps all of the bone marrow is prone to suppression. Before entering any kind of surgical phase on this patient, it behooves you to contact the medical oncologist and inquire about the RBC count, the WBC count, the absolute neutrophil count, the hematocrit and the platelet count. You may find that while the neutrophils are okay (with exogenous stimulation), the patient may have a moderate anemia and thrombocytopenia as well. These may need correction prior to surgery as well. Of course, you will also want to check when is the best time in the chemotherapy cycle for doing the surgery, as the counts will oscillate as the anticancer agents do their job and then are metabolized/eliminated. Perhaps perioperative antibiotics will be indicated. You may also want to consider, if possible, using more conservative approaches to managing the tooth such as endodontic stabilization instead of extraction until the patient is finished with his/her cytotoxic chemotherapy.

GENERAL REFERENCES

1. Handin RI, Lux SE, Stossel TP, editors: *Blood: principles and practice of hematology*, ed 2, Philadelphia, 2002, Lippincott Williams Wilkins.
2. Hillman RS, Ault KA, Leporrier M, Rinder H: *Hematology in clinical practice*, ed 5, New York, 2010, McGraw-Hill.
3. Kaushansky K, Lichtman MA, Beutler E, et al.: *Williams hematology*, ed 8, New York, 2010, McGraw-Hill.
4. Papadakis MA, McPhee SJ, Rabow MW, editors: *Current medical diagnosis and treatment 2015*, Stamford, CT, 2015, Lange Medical Books/ McGraw-Hill.

26

Procoagulant, Anticoagulant, and Thrombolytic Drugs

Barton S. Johnson

KEY INFORMATION

Overview
- The three aspects of the coagulation cascade are:
  - Vascular constriction
  - Platelet adhesion/aggregation/activation
  - Fibrin formation
- Clot remodeling is via plasmin.
- Clot control is designed to prevent extension beyond the site of injury.

Procoagulant drugs
- Medications that can be used to improve hemostasis include:
  - Systemic antihemophilic factors
  - Astringents/styptics
  - Vasoconstrictors
  - Topically applied agents
  - Intrasocket preparations

Fibrin-modulating drugs
- Antifibrinolytic agents such as tranexamic acid and aminocaproic acid slow clot degradation.
- Fibrinolytic agents such as tPA degrade clots rapidly in settings such as stroke and myocardial infarction.

Anticoagulant drugs
- Major antiplatelet agents are:
  - Aspirin
  - Ibuprofen and related drugs
  - Thienopyridines (Clopidogrel and related drugs)
  - GP IIb/IIIa inhibitors
- The indirect thrombin inhibitors are warfarin and warfarin-like drugs.
- The direct thrombin inhibitors are drugs such as dabigatran.
- The factor Xa inhibitors belong to the xaban family.
- Heparin drugs are classified as:
  - Low-molecular-weight heparins
  - Unfractionated heparin

CASE STUDY

Mr. J is a 72-year-old gentleman who presents for care, stating that he wants his remaining teeth removed and replaced with implant-supported removable dentures. Your examination shows that he has 24 remaining teeth, all of which are very carious and effectively non-salvageable. He has a cardiac history that includes a two-vessel coronary artery bypass graft 15 years ago and a balloon angioplasty 2 years ago. He used to take warfarin on a daily basis, but he has recently been switched to dabigatran. He also takes a baby aspirin every day. It is within your skill set to remove the teeth and do the eventual implants, but what considerations should you take with the anticoagulant drugs in preparation for the surgery? Should an intraoperative bleed occur, what options do you have?

INTRODUCTION

The practice of dentistry frequently involves procedures that cause bleeding, and the dentist is often confronted with the need to achieve and maintain hemostasis. The dental practitioner must be familiar with the physiologic processes of hemostasis and the myriad conditions that cause abnormalities of these processes. Complicating matters, modern medicine has developed several therapies for systemic disease that use medications that purposefully alter normal hemostasis. When appropriate, the dentist needs to make alterations in the dosage or scheduling of these compounds before surgery. Only with a clear understanding of the complex process of hemostasis and the various drugs that affect it can the clinician manage patients with inherited or acquired bleeding disabilities safely.

HEMOSTASIS PHYSIOLOGY REVIEW

To understand how the various procoagulant/anticoagulant pharmaceutical drugs interact with the clotting system, it is critical that the dentist have a basic understanding of the physiology of hemostasis. Our surgical approaches constantly cause vascular injury, whether by needle, scalpel, forcep, or bur.

Unlike the trauma setting, in the dental surgical setting, large or intermediate arteries and veins are generally not severed intentionally without prior ligation, but it is common during the extraction of teeth and other oral surgical procedures to sever small arteriolar, venous, and capillary vessels. Extensive blood loss may occur if hemostasis is delayed. The immediate formation of a patent clot requires four distinct yet interdependent steps: (1) vessel constriction; (2) platelet adhesion, activation, and aggregation; (3) cross-linking of fibrin by the coagulation cascade; and (4) limitation of the blood clot to the area of damage only. Later, a fifth step becomes necessary: the controlled breakdown of the clot so that repair and remodeling can occur.

Vascular Constriction

Transection of small arteries and arterioles generally shows a rapid moderate–severe reduction in flow, apparently caused by contraction of vascular smooth muscle initiated directly by the trauma. This initial hemostasis is independent of blood coagulation and platelet agglutination, and it is maintained only for a short period (5 to 20 minutes).

Physiologically, the uninjured vessel wall is lined with endothelial cells that constitutively secrete nitric oxide and prostacyclin, both of which are potent smooth muscle relaxing agents. Nitric oxide and prostacyclin diffuse to the nearby vascular smooth muscle, effect relaxation, and maintain luminal patency. On injury, this secretion is disrupted, and the now unopposed muscle layer reflexively and rapidly constricts, greatly narrowing the lumen. After a few minutes the constriction wanes, and the muscle layers begin to relax again. This brief period of constriction provides a healthy individual sufficient time for the platelets and coagulation cascade to seal the injured site.

Platelet Adhesion, Activation, and Aggregation

Adhesion

The next major event is the adhesion of platelets at the severed edges of the vessel. In normal un-traumatized blood vessels, **platelets** show little tendency to adhere to the endothelium, partly because prostacyclin, again elaborated by the endothelial cells, induces cyclic adenosine 3′,5′-monophosphate (cAMP) synthesis in platelets and inhibits platelet adhesion. Endothelium-derived relaxing factor (**nitric oxide**), also normally secreted by the endothelial cells, is another natural inhibitor of platelet adhesion. Injury to the endothelium, even if the vessel wall remains intact, however, leads to exposure of subendothelial extracellular matrix proteins such as collagen, fibronectin, **von Willebrand factor (vWF)**, thrombospondin, and laminin.

The presence of these proteins, particularly vWF, stimulates a "catch and grab" response in the platelets, causing them to leave the laminar flow of the blood and adhere to the injured area. Platelets have a high density of surface receptors that respond to these proteins, and they undergo an extremely rapid localization to the site of injury, beginning the formation of a thrombus. Two main receptors are involved in adhesion: the glycoprotein **(GP) Ia/IIa** heterodimer, which binds to collagen directly but weakly, and the **GP Ib/IX/V** heterotrimer, which binds with high shear strength to connective tissue vWF associated with the collagen surface (Fig. 26-1). The GP Ib/IX/V–vWF linkage is more of a "tethering" of the platelet to the substrate; later, the adhesion is firmed up by GP IIb/IIIa activation. If vessels without a muscular sheath are severed, the immediate hemostatic action of platelet aggregation is especially important. The true significance of platelets in hemostasis is most evident in the management of patients with thrombocytopenia.

Activation

Activation of platelets is a crucial step in forming a proper thrombus. Activation can occur from various agonists, some of which are strong and others that are weak. Examples include **thrombin, adenosine diphosphate (ADP), thromboxane A_2 (TXA_2)**, 5-hydroxytryptamine (serotonin), epinephrine, vasopressin, fibrinogen, immune complexes, plasmin, and platelet-activating factor. Most plasma-derived agonists exert their effect by numerous G protein–linked membrane receptors. The strongest agonist for platelet activation is binding of vWF to the GP Ib/IX/V heterotrimeric receptors. When one of these receptors is bound by its specific agonist, an intraplatelet protein cascade begins

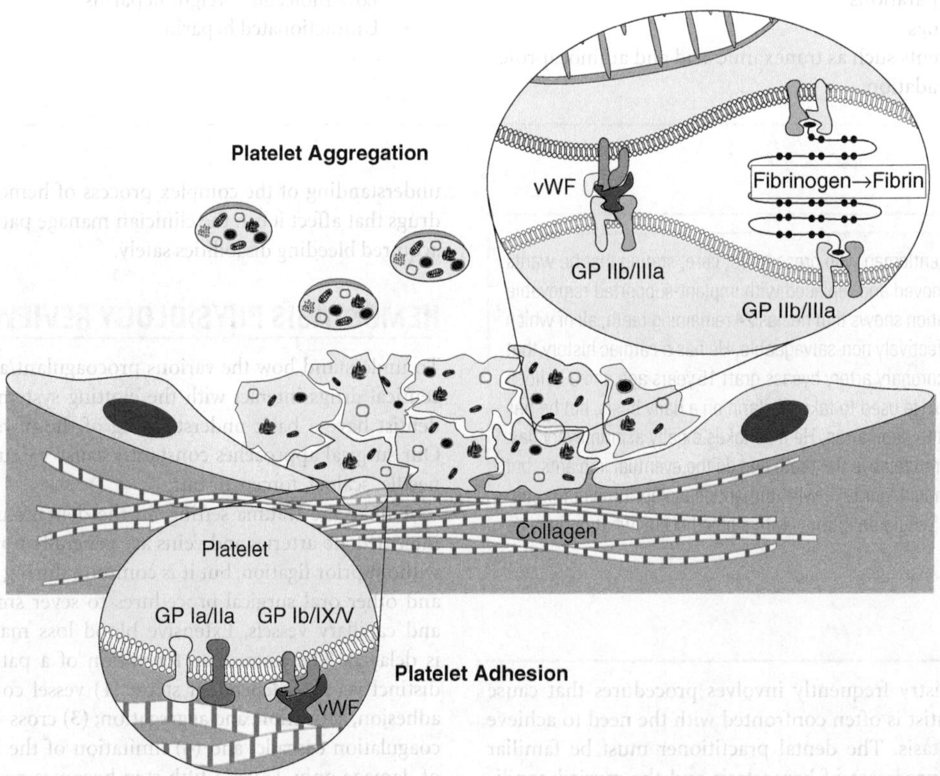

FIG 26-1 Platelet adhesion and aggregation. Exposed collagen at the site of injury stimulates initial weak platelet adhesion by the glycoprotein (*GP*) Ia/IIa receptors. Stronger adhesion follows by the GP Ib/IX/V/vWF complex. Platelet activation is triggered, which leads to initial aggregation by the GP IIb/IIIa receptors binding the GP Ib/IX/V complex. This low-shear bond is later supplanted by a pair of GP IIb/IIIa receptors interacting with fibrinogen to create high-strength mature fibrin "ropes" interconnecting the two, then cross-linking to others. *vWF*, von Willebrand factor.

that ultimately causes activation of Ca^{2+} transporters and movement of Ca^{2+} from stores in the platelet's dense tubular system to the general intracellular matrix. The intracellular increase in Ca^{2+} begins several other changes.

Platelets in the resting state have internal cytoskeletal actin that provides them with a smooth shape; as Ca^{2+} increases, the actin is fragmented into smaller subunits, transforming the normal discoid shape of the platelet to a spherical conformation. These smaller actin subunits are then rapidly reassembled into very-long-chain actin monomers, which cause the platelet to sprout filopods. The filopods are important in ultimate clot retraction. Meanwhile, as the filopods are developing, the increasing intracellular Ca^{2+} concentrations act on cytoplasmic vesicles known as α and dense (or δ) granules (Fig. 26-2), prompting them to rise to the cell surface and degranulate. The dense granules release ADP, adenosine triphosphate (ATP), the vasoconstrictor 5-hydroxytryptamine, Ca^{2+}, and inorganic pyrophosphate. The α granules contain numerous proteins involved in coagulation, adhesion, cellular mitogenicity, protease inhibition, and other functions (Box 26-1). Major proteins released include fibrinogen, coagulation factors, vWF, fibronectin, high-molecular-weight kininogen, plasminogen, plasminogen activator inhibitor-1 (PAI-1), platelet-derived growth factor, additional GP IIb/IIIa, and thrombospondin.

Release of the dense granule **ADP** into the extracellular milieu has an autocatalytic effect on the platelet from which it came while also stimulating nearby platelets. The ADP binds to its own purinergic receptors, most notably **$P2Y_1$ and $P2Y_{12}$**. Activation of both of these receptors is required for maximal aggregation of the platelets to one another. $P2Y_1$ stimulation acts to mobilize Ca^{2+} further (an autocatalytic effect), which leads to further shape change and transient aggregation. $P2Y_{12}$ activation causes inhibition of adenylyl cyclase (blocking conversion of ATP to cAMP), potentiation of secretion by the α and dense granules, and sustained aggregation. ADP also binds the transmembrane protein $P2X_1$, an ion channel receptor linked to influx of extracellular Ca^{2+} into the platelet.

Aggregation

As the activated platelets interact with one another, they begin to aggregate. Aggregation is initiated by the Ca^{2+}-mediated conformational activation **of GP IIb/IIIa**, a heterodimeric transmembrane protein. GP IIb/IIIa is a protein receptor complex unique to platelets and is expressed at extraordinarily high density on the surface of the platelets—some 80,000 to 100,000 per platelet—at an average distance of only 20 nm from one another. Another 20,000 to 40,000 proteins are stored in the α granules and are released onto the surface or within

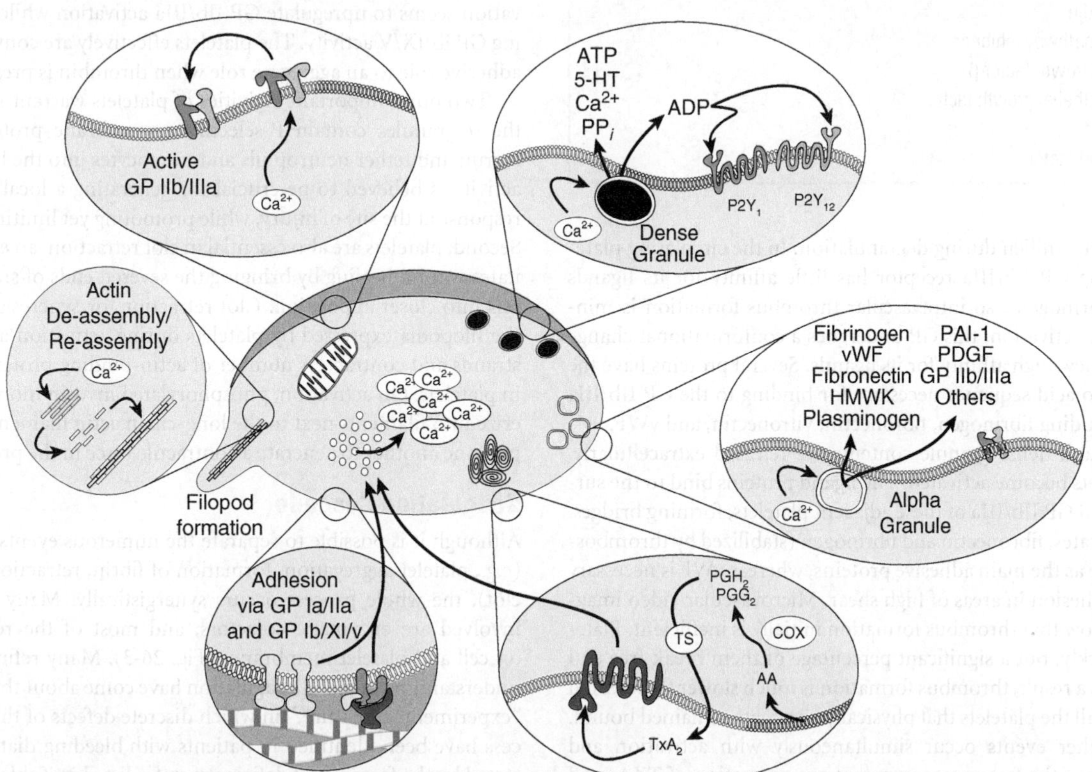

FIG 26-2 Platelet activation. *Lower left, moving clockwise*: contact with the compromised vessel wall by platelet membrane GPs Ia/IIa and Ib/XI/V, stabilized by von Willebrand factor (*vWF*), causes the platelets to become activated and begin moving Ca^{2+} out of their tubular stores. The increased intracellular Ca^{2+} causes actin to break down and reassemble in long chains, resulting in filopod formation. The increase in Ca^{2+} causes conversion of the GP IIb/IIIa from its inactive form to the active form. The dense granules move to the surface and release many activating substances, one of which is adenosine diphosphate (*ADP*). ADP stimulates purinergic receptors $P2Y_1$ and $P2Y_{12}$, both of which accelerate the activation process. The increase in Ca^{2+} also causes a degranulation, resulting in the release of many substances important for further aggregation. Finally, platelet membrane phospholipids yield arachidonic acid (*AA*), which is converted by cyclooxygenase (*COX*) to prostaglandins G_2 (*PGG_2*) and H_2 (*PGH_2*). Thromboxane synthase (*TS*) converts these to thromboxane A_2 (*TXA_2*), which, acting on a G protein–linked receptor, is a potent catalyst of platelet aggregation by accelerating further release of stored platelet Ca^{2+}. *5-HT*, 5-hydroxytryptamine; *HMWK*, high-molecular-weight kininogen; *PAI-1*, plasminogen activator inhibitor-1; *PDGF*, platelet-derived growth factor; *PPi*, pyrophosphate.

BOX 26-1 Contents of Platelet α Granules

α_2-Antiplasmin
α_2-Macroglobulin
Albumin
β-Thromboglobulin
CD63
C1-inhibitor
Endothelial cell growth factor
Epidermal growth factor
Factors V, XI, XIII
Fibrinogen
Fibronectin
GMP 33
High-molecular-weight kininogen
IgA, IgG, IgM
Interleukin-1B
Multimerin
P-selectin
Plasminogen activator inhibitor 1
Platelet factor
Platelet-derived growth factor
Protein S
Thrombospondin
Tissue factor pathway inhibitor
Transforming growth factor-β
Vascular endothelial growth factor
Vitronectin
von Willebrand factor

the local plasma milieu during degranulation. In the circulating platelet, the resting GP IIb/IIIa receptor has little affinity for its ligands (primarily fibrinogen), so intravascular thrombus formation is minimized. Upon activation, this GP undergoes a conformational change that imparts new high affinity for its ligands. Several proteins have the specific amino acid sequence necessary for binding to the GP IIb/IIIa receptor, including fibrinogen, fibronectin, vitronectin, and vWF.

As the α and dense granule contents are released extracellularly, nearby platelets become activated. The ligand proteins bind to the surface-associated GP IIb/IIIa of these adjacent platelets, forming bridges. At low shear rates, fibronectin and fibrinogen (stabilized by thrombospondin) serve as the main adhesive proteins, whereas vWF is necessary for proper adhesion in areas of high shear. Microvascular video imaging studies show that thrombus formation initially is inefficient. Platelets bind quickly, but a significant percentage of them break free and float away. As a result, thrombus formation is much slower than would be the case if all the platelets that physically aggregate remained bound.

Several other events occur simultaneously with activation and aggregation, but the two most important are generation of TXA_2 and platelet-assisted generation of thrombin. Both of these agents accelerate the platelet-activation response. TXA_2 is generated when platelet phospholipases are activated during platelet aggregation, which release arachidonic acid from glycerophospholipids of the platelet membrane. Arachidonic acid is a substrate for cyclooxygenase (COX), yielding the prostaglandin endoperoxides PGH_2 and PGG_2. These prostaglandins are modified by thromboxane synthase to produce TXA_2, which acts at its own protein-linked receptor.

Perhaps the most remarkable effect of platelet activation is the procoagulant activity the platelets impart. In the normally resting platelet, the plasma membrane has negatively charged phospholipids, including phosphatidylserine, sequestered almost exclusively on the inner surface by processes that are not fully understood. When activating ligands bind to the platelet, the resultant increase in intracellular Ca^{2+} causes a membrane enzyme termed *scramblase* to evert the phosphatidylserine to the outer surface, while simultaneously prompting the membrane to form small evaginated microvesicles. Factors Va and VIIIa (discussed subsequently) bind to the phosphatidylserine moieties and recruit factors Xa and IXa. The interaction of these complexes accelerates the conversion of prothrombin to thrombin by a factor of 2.4×10^6. In addition, the binding of activated coagulation factors to the platelets seems to protect the factors from plasma inhibitors, while directing the bulk of the coagulation cascade to the site of injury. The **α granules** contain factors V and IX; factor V is apparently complexed with multimerin, a carrier protein.

As the thrombin is generated, it activates other platelets by stimulating G protein–linked receptors. The thrombin receptors seem to be unique "suicide" receptors, requiring proteolytic cleavage to transmit an activating signal. Thrombin is a serine protease, and it acts on the receptors by cleaving the protein at a serine residue near the amino terminus. The new amino terminus acts as a "tethered ligand" to double back and stimulate the transmembrane protein to activate—hence this receptor has been named a ***protease-activated receptor (PAR)***. There are four such thrombin receptors, PAR-1 through PAR-4; only PAR-1 and PAR-4 are expressed by human platelets. Thrombin-induced activation seems to upregulate GP IIb/IIIa activation while downregulating GP Ib/IX/V activity. The platelets effectively are converted from an adhesive role to an aggregate role when thrombin is present.

Two other important activities of platelets warrant mention. First, the α granules contain P-selectin, a membrane protein that helps recruit and tether neutrophils and monocytes into the local area. This activity is believed to be crucial for generating a local inflammatory response at the site of injury, while promoting yet limiting thrombosis. Second, platelets are also essential in clot retraction, an event that facilitates wound healing by bringing the severed ends of small blood vessels into closer apposition. Clot retraction, or syneresis, occurs when the filopodia expressed by platelets during activation attach to fibrin strands and contract. A number of actin-binding proteins are present in platelets. On activation, phosphorylated myosin monomers polymerize into filaments next to the long-chain actin filaments, which slide past one another to generate a contractile force in the presence of ATP.

Coagulation Cascade

Although it is possible to separate the numerous events of hemostasis (e.g., platelet aggregation, formation of fibrin, retraction of the blood clot), the whole process occurs synergistically. Many of the factors involved are enzymatic cofactors, and most of the reaction occurs on cell and platelet membranes (Fig. 26-3). Many refinements in the understanding of blood coagulation have come about through study of "experiments of nature," in which discrete defects of the clotting process have been identified in patients with bleeding diatheses, as illustrated by the factors and deficiency states listed in Table 26-1.

Initiation of coagulation after injury is a complex process involving an initial pathway of thrombin generation, which autocatalyzes a subsequent burst of additional thrombin generation sufficient to convert fibrinogen to fibrin (see Fig. 26-3). Before the process is described, a brief review of the crucial factors and cofactors and how they function is warranted.

Vitamin K–dependent clotting factors

Synthesized in the liver, the **vitamin K–dependent clotting factors comprise factors II (prothrombin), VII, IX, and X, and protein C.** These five proteins are serine proteases and have similar structural elements. Molecular genetic evidence suggests they all are derived from

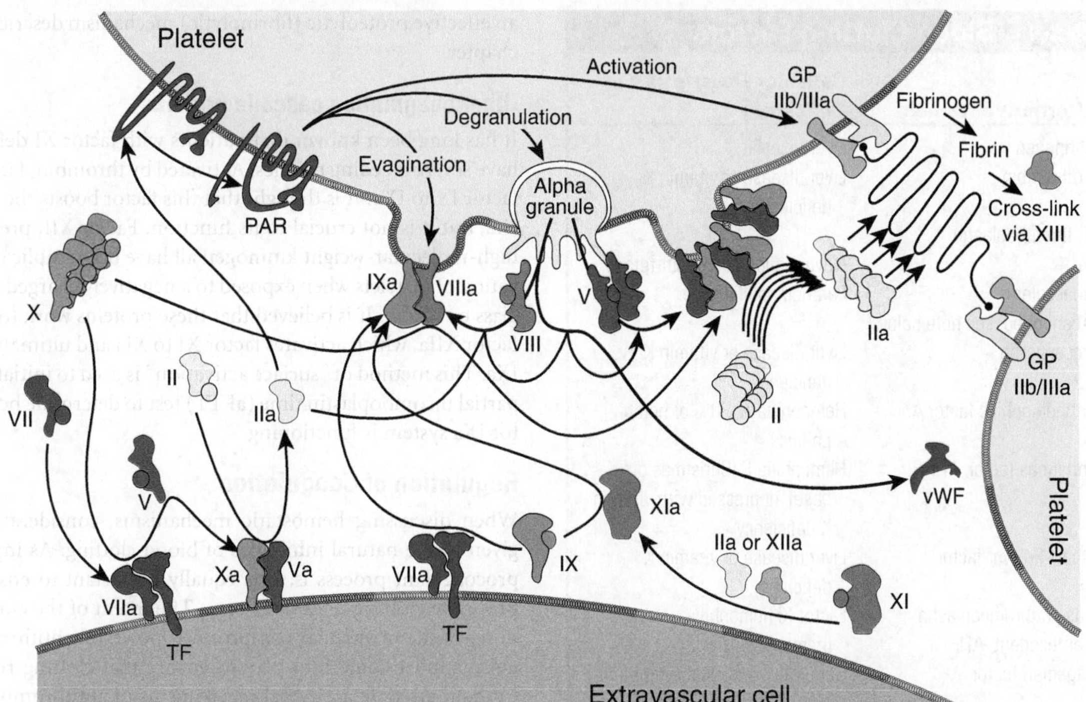

FIG 26-3 Blood coagulation cascade. Tissue factor (*TF*) (factor III) on cell membranes of exposed subendothelial matrix cells combines with circulating factor VIIa (activated by Ca^{2+}) to form an activating complex for factor X and factor IX. Factor Xa, locally bound to the membrane by factor Va, converts prothrombin (factor II) to thrombin (factor IIa). Meanwhile, converted factor IXa diffuses to adjacent platelets, where it is bound to the platelet membrane by factor VIIIa. The complex acts to accelerate factor Xa conversion, leading to additional factor Va binding and ultimately vastly increased thrombin formation. Fibrin, after it is formed from fibrinogen by the proteolytic action of thrombin, is cross-linked and stabilized by factor XIIIa. Thrombin, a serine protease, accelerates the entire cascade by catalyzing cleavage of factor XI to factor XIa, stimulating platelets to activate by the transmembrane protease-activated receptor (*PAR*), and it stimulates conversion of factor XIII to factor XIIIa (not shown). *GP*, Glycoprotein; *vWF*, von Willebrand factor.

a common ancestral precursor gene. They all have a preprotein leader that is cleaved away posttranslationally, leaving an amino-terminal γ-carboxyglutamic acid (Gla) domain with 9 to 12 Gla residues.

The amino terminus Gla domain is crucial for the protein to settle into the lipid membrane and exert its effects locally rather than systemically. To function, the **Gla residues must be carboxylated**, which requires oxygen, carbon dioxide, and vitamin K (see Fig. 26-7). For every glutamate residue carboxylated, one molecule of reduced vitamin K is converted to its epoxide form. A separate enzyme, **vitamin K epoxide reductase**, converts the vitamin K back to the reduced form. This reductase is the target of the warfarin-like anticoagulants and is discussed in greater detail later.

Each of the clotting factors mentioned is a protease that dimerizes with its specific cofactor to allosterically bring out its activity. **Tissue factor (TF)** dimerizes with VIIa (*a* for activated), VIIIa with IXa, and Va with Xa.

Enzymatic cofactors

TF is a protein normally constitutively expressed on the cell surfaces of many **extravascular** cell types. In contrast to the other coagulation cofactors, it is a transmembrane protein homologous to the receptors for interleukin-10 and interferons α, β, and γ. It seems to have procoagulant and signal transduction functions.

When injury occurs and the vasculature gains exposure to cells with TF on their surface, circulating factor VII rapidly binds to TF and undergoes proteolytic cleavage to factor VIIa. **The TF/VIIa complex serves two crucial functions: it cleaves factor X to Xa and factor IX to IXa.**

Newly formed factor Xa rapidly binds to circulating factor V and activates it to Va. The factor Xa/Va dimer settles into the adjacent cellular membrane (via the hydrophobic Gla domain), where it cleaves circulating prothrombin to generate a very small amount of thrombin. This tiny amount of thrombin is insufficient to cleave fibrinogen significantly but, instead, serves four crucial functions that set up the area for a much larger burst of thrombin formation: (1) nearby platelets are activated by their PAR receptors, which causes degranulation; (2) additional factor V is liberated from the platelet α granules and activated; (3) factor VIII is activated and dissociated from vWF; and (4) factor XI is activated. Factor Xa inhibitors are the newest form of anticoagulant medications.

In contrast to the factor Xa/Va complex, activation of factor IXa by TF/VIIa results in an enzyme that is not restricted to the nearby cell surface. As a result, factor IXa diffuses among nearby activated platelets that have placed factors Va and VIIIa on their cell surfaces. The diffusing factor IXa binds tightly to the factor VIIIa cofactor, and this IXa/VIIIa complex efficiently activates additional factor X to Xa. As before, factor Xa then binds to adjacent factor Va, and this time a much larger burst of prothrombin converts to thrombin. This burst is sufficient to begin cleaving fibrinogen and start clot formation.

Fibrinogen and factor XIII

The final phase of blood clotting consists of the **thrombin-mediated proteolytic cleavage of fibrinogen to fibrin.** Fibrinogen consists of a mirror-image dimer in which each monomer is composed of three intertwined and disulfide bond–linked polypeptide chains.

TABLE 26-1 Blood Clotting Factors

Factor*	Alternative Names	Cause or Description of Deficiency
I	Fibrinogen	Liver disease
II	Prothrombin	Liver disease or vitamin K deficiency
III	TF, thromboplastin	
IV	Ca^{2+}	Never deficient without tetany
V	Proaccelerin	Parahemophilia, rare
VI	(Abandoned; see note below)	
VII	Proconvertin	Liver disease or vitamin K deficiency
VIII	Antihemophilic factor A	Hemophilia A, 80% of hemophiliacs
IX	Christmas factor, AHF B	Hemophilia B (Christmas disease), depressed with vitamin K deficiency
X	Stuart-Prower factor	Liver disease or vitamin K deficiency
XI	Plasma thromboplastin antecedent, AHF C	Factor XI hemophilia (hemophilia C)
XII	Hageman factor	Generally no clinical symptoms but may have thromboses, rare
XIII	Fibrin-stabilizing factor, Laki-Lorand factor, fibrinase	Delayed bleeding, defective healing, rare
PF3	Platelet factor 3	Thrombocytopenia
~	Protein C	Liver disease or vitamin K deficiency
~	Protein S	Liver disease or vitamin K deficiency
vWF	von Willebrand factor	vWD types I, IIa, IIb, IIc, III
Pre-K	Prekallikrein, Fletcher factor	
HMWK	High-molecular-weight kininogen	

AHF, Antihemophilic factor; *TF*, tissue factor.
*Roman numerals were assigned in 1958 by the International Committee on Blood Clotting Factors. Factor VI, originally assigned to prothrombin converting principle (prothrombinase) has since been abandoned.

In the dimer, the amino terminus of all six polypeptides meet in the middle of the linear molecule to form the N-terminal disulfide knot, or *E domain*. The carboxy termini of the three polypeptides at each opposite end form a globular protein cluster known as the *D domain*. Between the E and D domains, the polypeptide chains form a helical structure (Fig. 26-4).

Thrombin binds to the central E domain and cleaves off peptides from the knot to expose binding sites in the E domain that match the corresponding D domains of two neighboring fibrinogen molecules. The monomers begin to form a staggered "ladder" protofibril. As the monomers continue to associate, branch points occur that allow the fibrin meshwork to become more like a net and thicken. The initial clot is unstable, being held together primarily by hydrogen bonds. With time, however, the fibrin strands stabilize by becoming covalently bonded by factor XIII. This factor cross-links proteins between the γ-carbon of glutamine in one fibrin strand and the ε-amino group of lysine in the other.

Entrapped in this coagulum "net" are red and white blood cells and intact platelets; the latter promote clot retraction as previously described. These events are followed by the inflammatory processes of organization and wound healing, which require, among other things, an effective proteolytic (fibrinolytic) mechanism described later in this chapter.

Other coagulation cascade proteins

It has long been known that patients with factor XI deficiency do not have severe bleeding profiles. Activated by thrombin, factor XIa cleaves factor IX to IXa. It is thought that this factor boosts the levels of factor IXa, but it is not crucial to its function. Factor XII, prekallikrein, and high-molecular-weight kininogen all have been implicated in the activation of platelets when exposed to a negatively charged surface such as glass or kaolin. It is believed that these proteins work together to yield factor XIIa, which activates factor XI to XIa and ultimately factor IX to IXa. This method of "surface activation" is used to initiate the activated partial thromboplastin time (aPTT) test to determine how well the factor IXa system is functioning.

Regulation of Coagulation

When discussing hemostatic mechanisms, consideration should be given to the natural inhibitors of blood clotting. As important as the procoagulant process is, it is equally important to ensure that inappropriate clotting does not occur. The intent of the clotting system is to seal a site of vascular compromise; powerful antithrombotic mechanisms must come into play to ensure that clotting remains limited to the injured area. Several mechanisms of antithrombosis have been elucidated; they are discussed in detail subsequently and summarized in Figure 26-5.

Strict control of the extremely efficient coagulation cascade is mediated by several proteins that act as natural anticoagulants, all of which rely on the first traces of thrombin from the nearby wound site to activate them. In general, the theory is simple: bind or degrade any activated procoagulant proteins if they escape the site of injury. At the same time, the site of injury must be protected from invasion or inclusion of these same inhibitory proteins.

Because thrombin is the major procoagulant protein, it makes sense that inactivation of it is a high priority. An elegant mechanism exists that, instead of destroying thrombin, uses thrombin to catalyze an important set of anticoagulant proteins, the **protein C/protein S system**. In the microcirculation, where there is a high cell surface-to-volume ratio, the protein C/protein S system predominates. Vascular endothelial cells normally express thrombomodulin on their membranes. **Thrombomodulin** is a transmembrane cofactor protein with no known enzymatic activity. It binds the thrombin that escapes from the surface of nearby platelets but is not carried off in the vascular flow.

Thrombomodulin, as the name implies, alters the conformation of the thrombin and effectively removes its ability to cleave fibrinogen, activate platelets, and activate factors V and VIII. Instead, the new conformation of thrombin imparts a two-thousandfold greater affinity for activation of the vitamin K–dependent protein C. Activated protein C (aPC) has considerable homologous characteristics with the other vitamin K–dependent factors, complete with a Gla domain, hydrophobic domain, and active serine protease domain. The cofactor for aPC is protein S, a membrane-bound protein that has no inherent activity. When aPC is bound, the complex efficiently cleaves and destroys any factors Va and VIIIa that might have been liberated from the platelet surfaces.

Another protein, **antithrombin III (ATIII)**, is a serine protease inhibitor ("serpin") found in the plasma. It inhibits clotting by covalently binding to the active sites of thrombin and certain other serine proteases (factors IXa, Xa, and XIIa). This reaction is normally slow but is accelerated one-thousandfold in the presence of **heparan** sulfate, a proteoglycan synthesized on the surfaces by endothelial cells. (A similar effect is achieved therapeutically by administration of the closely related pharmaceutical agent heparin sulfate.) Although ATIII binds

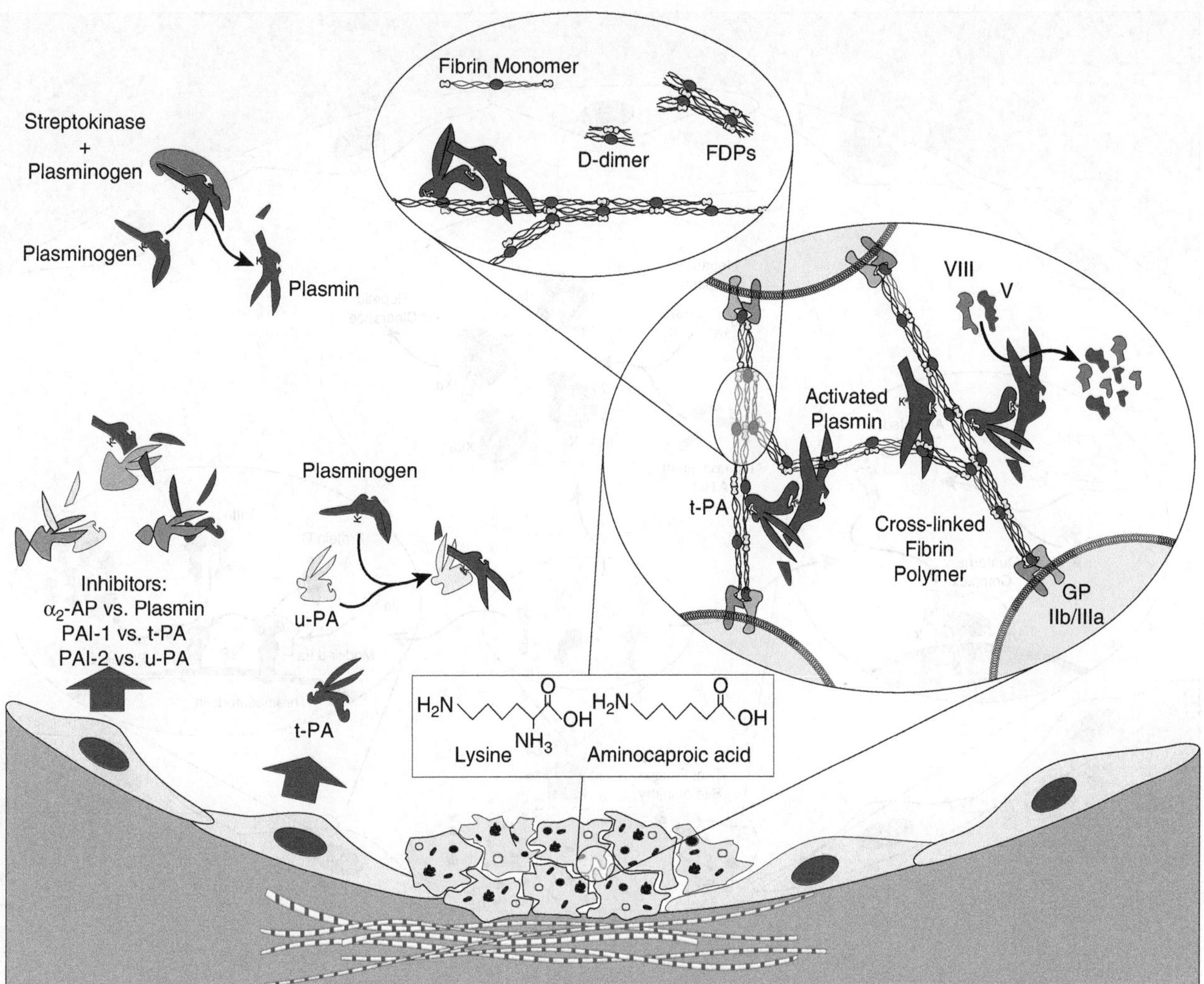

FIG 26-4 Fibrinolysis. Thrombin formation causes adjacent endothelial cells to release tissue plasminogen activator (*t-PA*) and urokinase plasminogen activator (*u-PA*). t-PA adheres to lysine residues on the fibrin molecules and adsorbs plasminogen onto it, also by lysine binding. The proteolytic action of t-PA converts the plasminogen to plasmin at the wound site, whereas u-PA converts it in the free circulation. Plasmin acts to degrade factors V and VIII and proteolytically cleave the fibrin. Various fibrin degradation products (*FDPs*) are liberated, including the D-dimer formed from two fibrin molecule "ends" linked to one fibrin molecule "middle." Aminocaproic acid interferes with plasminogen conversion by occupying lysine-binding sites on t-PA and plasminogen, resulting in antifibrinolysis. The endothelial cells also release several inhibitors: plasminogen activator inhibitor-1 (*PAI-1*), which destroys any free circulating t-PA, and plasminogen activator inhibitor-2 (*PAI-2*), which inhibits u-PA. Both serve to limit the plasminogen activation primarily to the clot site. Another protein, circulating α_2-antiplasmin (α_2-*AP*), neutralizes any free plasmin in the bloodstream, also restricting activity of plasmin to the wound site. Exogenous t-PA functions similarly to endogenous t-PA. Streptokinase combines with plasminogen to create a complex that cleaves other plasminogen molecules to free circulating plasmin. As a result, systemic fibrinolysis is more common with this medication. Not shown is streptokinase formulated with exogenous acylated plasminogen, which spontaneously deacylates on mixing with the plasma to form the same streptokinase–plasminogen complex. *GP*, Glycoprotein.

to these factors without destroying them, reactivation by unbinding probably does not occur physiologically. The ATIII-protease complexes are cleared in the liver. It is believed that ATIII is responsible for complexing with proteases that escape into the circulation.

Finally, **tissue factor pathway inhibitor (TFPI)** (see Fig. 26-5) is a protease inhibitor found in low concentrations in the plasma, mostly bound to circulating lipoproteins or to endothelial cell membrane heparans. It is capable of inactivating factor Xa and the TF/VIIa complex; it must first bind factor Xa before it can bind to the TF/VIIa complex. TFPI seems to be the major inhibitor of free-floating factor Xa, and it may be responsible for shifting the activation of factor IX from the TF/VIIa complex to thrombin-activated factor XI. The inhibitor is found in high concentrations in patients with hemophilia A and B, presumably because fewer substrates are available for TFPI binding. This finding offers one explanation for why hemophiliacs bleed despite normal concentrations of TF, factor VIIa, and factor Xa at the site of injury. TFPI is synthesized in liver and endothelial cells.

PROCOAGULANT AGENTS

In medical and dental practice, it is essential to take appropriate precautions to avoid serious hemorrhage. This admonition is particularly

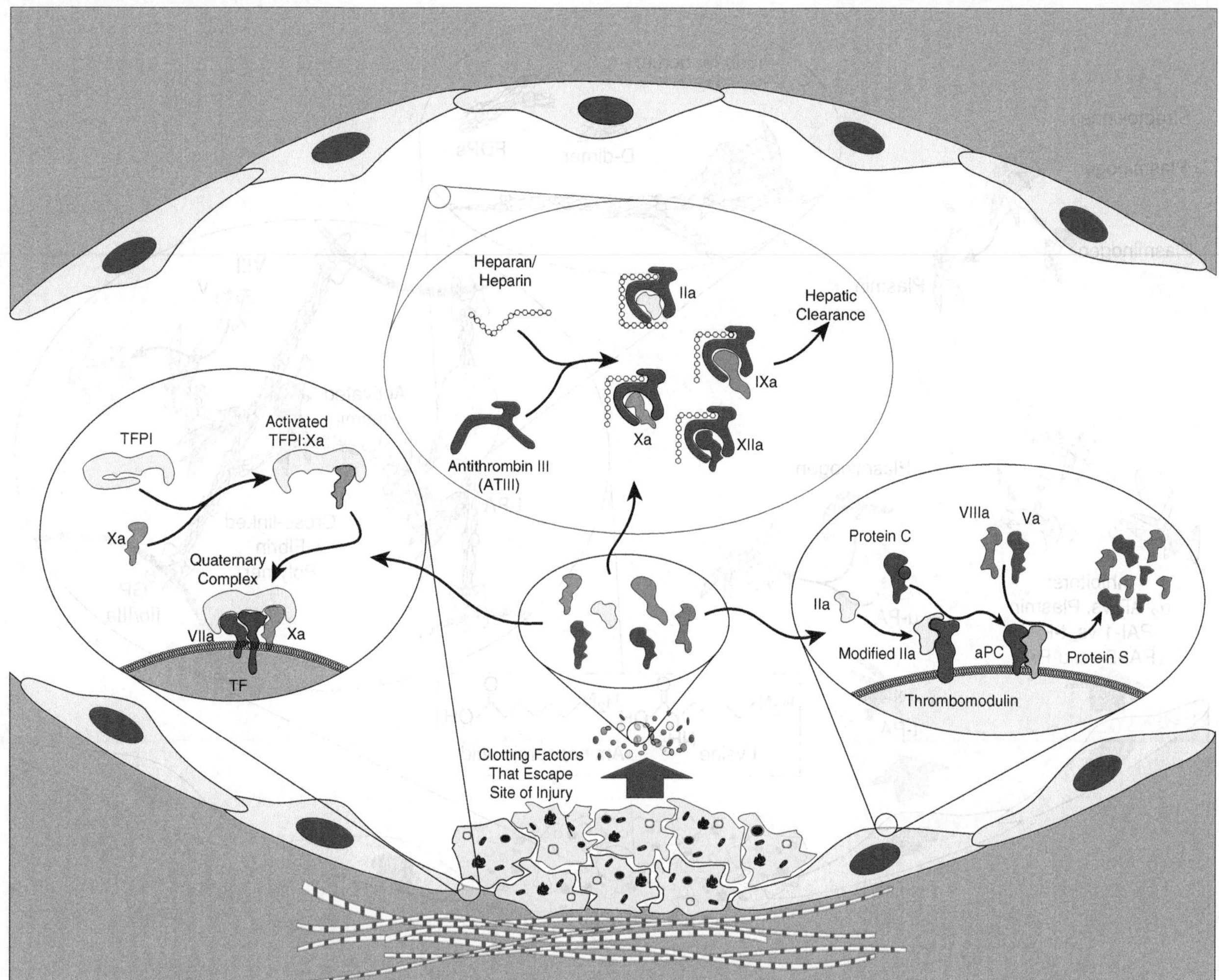

FIG 26-5 The clotting inhibition system: examples of proteins that help limit fibrin formation to the site of the vascular injury by inactivating clotting factors. Antithrombin III (*ATIII*) undergoes conformational change in the presence of heparin/heparan, which allows it to bind and sequester factors IIa (thrombin), IXa, Xa, and XIIa. It is later cleared in the liver. When trace amounts of thrombin bind to thrombomodulin on intact endothelial cell membranes, the thrombin-thrombomodulin dimer undergoes a conformational change that allows it to activate protein C, which is bound to the membrane by protein S to form a protease complex specific for factors Va and VIIIa. Loss of these two factors disrupts the coagulation cascade sufficiently to prevent disseminated intravascular coagulation. A final inhibitor, tissue factor pathway inhibitor (*TFPI*), is first activated by factor Xa and then binds to the tissue factor (*TF*)/VIIa complex to interrupt conversion of additional factor X. *aPC*, Activated protein C.

true for patients with hemophilia, patients with hematopoietic disease, and patients receiving therapies known to affect hemostasis. Precautions, which may include the administration of clotting factors or hospitalization or both, are prudent in these cases. In contrast, normal patients usually require no more than temporary hemostatic assistance (e.g., pressure packs, hemostatic forceps, ligation, or other locally active measures) to facilitate normal hemostasis and allow clotting to occur.

Local Measures

A perplexing hemostatic problem may arise from continued, slow oozing of blood from small arterioles, veins, and capillaries. These vessels cannot be ligated, and measures such as pressure packs and intrasocket preparations, vasoconstrictor agents, and procoagulants must be used. Styptics or astringents, extensively used in the past, are no longer viewed as rational procedures for routine hemostasis in most applications; however, some astringents are commonly used during gingival retraction to aid in controlling the tissue for impressions.

Bleeding caused by dentoalveolar surgery is most often controlled by applying **direct pressure** with sterile cotton gauze. If this treatment is inadequate, the clinician must localize the source of bleeding as originating either within the soft tissues or within the bony structures. Soft tissue bleeding may be controlled by **hemostats, ligation, electrocautery, or application of microfibrillar collagen or collagen sheets** (on broad bleeding surfaces). Microfibrillar collagen, made from purified bovine skin collagen, is used topically to arrest certain hemorrhagic conditions that do not respond to conventional methods of hemostasis. Collagen accelerates the aggregation of platelets and may have limited effectiveness in patients with platelet disorders or hemophilia.

Intrasocket Preparations

Bleeding from bony structures, especially from extraction sockets, can be controlled by various means. If initial attempts to achieve hemostasis with sterile cotton gauze and pressure do not succeed, a gelatin sponge, denatured cellulose sponge, or collagen plug may be inserted within the bony crypt.

Gelatin sponges are intended to be a matrix in which platelets and red blood cells can be trapped. In so doing, the sponges facilitate platelet disruption and can absorb 40 to 50 times their own weight in blood, both of which aid in coagulation. They typically resorb in 4 to 6 weeks. Because they are made of gelatin, they must be applied dry; when moistened, they become difficult to handle. For this reason, many practitioners prefer to use either denatured cellulose preparations or collagen sponge.

Denatured **cellulose** sponge or gauze serves as a physical plug and a chemical hemostatic. The apparent coagulation-promoting action stems from the release of cellulosic acid, which denatures hemoglobin, and these breakdown products help plug the site of injury. However, cellulosic acid, similar to tannic acid, inactivates thrombin; the use of cellulose sponge in conjunction with this procoagulant is ineffective. Two forms of cellulose sponge, oxidized cellulose and oxidized regenerated cellulose, are available. Both these materials cause delayed healing, particularly oxidized cellulose, which notably interferes with bone regeneration and epithelialization. Although regenerated cellulose is said to have less inhibitory action, neither dressing should be left permanently in the wound if it can be removed.

The collagen plug, similar to microfibrillar collagen, serves to accelerate the aggregation of platelets and form a physical barrier. Because it also is usually made from bovine collagen sources, occasional foreign body responses can occur. Overall, the collagen plug generally activates platelets more completely and is the preferred intrasocket product.

Topically Applied Clotting Factors

The most physiologic hemostatic aids are the blood clotting factors themselves. Assuming an otherwise normal clotting system, topical thrombin is often used clinically. It must remain topically applied; if given intravenously, thrombin causes extensive thrombosis and possibly death. **Topically applied thrombin** (particularly in conjunction with a compatible matrix such as gelatin sponge) operates as a hemostatic, particularly if the patient has a coagulation deficiency or is receiving oral anticoagulants, because all that is required for clotting is a normal supply of platelets, fibrinogen, and factor XIII in the plasma. If blood flows too freely, temporary physical hemostasis must be attained before topical thrombin can be of practical value. Recombinant human thrombin is currently available for this purpose.

Fibrin sealant, also sometimes referred to as **fibrin glue**, takes the concept of the application of topical thrombin one step further. Bovine or human thrombin and calcium chloride are mixed in one of two syringes; purified human fibrinogen with factor XIII, aprotinin, and other plasma proteins (fibronectin and plasminogen) are in the second syringe. The two solutions are mixed in a single delivery barrel, where the thrombin cleaves the fibrinogen to fibrin monomers. Initially, they are gelled by hydrogen bond formation, but in 3 to 5 minutes the factor XIII in the presence of Ca^{2+} initiates cross-linking and increases the tensile strength of the clot. As the clot solidifies, the sealant becomes milky white.

The rate of fibrin clot formation depends on the concentration of the thrombin; 4 IU/mL produces a clot in approximately 1 minute, whereas 500 IU/mL requires only a few seconds. The strength of the clot depends on the concentration of the fibrinogen. If used in an area where the clot is likely to break down too soon, or in patients with compromised hemostasis, a protease inhibitor such as **aprotinin can be added to delay fibrinolysis**. Aprotinin functions by inhibiting plasmin, which is generally carried along with the thrombin. The term *glue* arises from the fact that in many medical applications this material has been literally used to adhere tissues together naturally.

Fibrin sealant is commercially available in the United States. The protein fractions are lyophilized and require careful reconstitution at 37° C under sterile conditions; proper mixing of the materials requires approximately 30 minutes to perform. As a result, the emergent use of this material is difficult; typically, it is used more in planned surgeries in patients with known bleeding disorders. It is also an expensive medication; 1 mL of the material costs several hundred dollars. Fibrin sealant works well in stopping the microbleeding and oozing that often accompany dental procedures.

Astringents and Styptics

The terms ***astringents and styptics*** are interchangeable, referring to different concentrations of the same drugs. Many chemicals have vasoconstrictive or protein-denaturing ability, but relatively few are appropriate for dentistry. The suitable preparations are primarily salts of several metals, particularly zinc, silver, iron, and aluminum. Aluminum and iron salts are quite acidic (pH 1.3 to 3.1) and irritating. Iron causes annoying, although temporary, surface staining of the enamel, whereas silver stains may be permanent.

Currently, astringents are generally used in dentistry only to aid hemostasis while retracting gingival tissue. **Aluminum and iron salts** function by denaturing blood and tissue proteins, which agglutinate and form plugs that occlude the capillary orifices. In a rabbit mandible model, when ferric sulfate salts were left in an osseous wound, there was an intense foreign body reaction and delayed healing in many of the experimental sites compared with the control sites. Therefore, it is imperative that if these compounds are used in dentistry, they are used briefly and with copious irrigation and debridement to remove the breakdown products. They should not be applied to areas of exposed osseous material so as to avoid inflammation or complications of retarded healing such as the distressful dry socket. **Tannic acid** (0.5% to 1%) is an effective astringent; it also precipitates proteins, including thrombin, but is often incompatible with other drugs and metal salts used therapeutically. Finally, the use of an astringent in a patient with even a mild bleeding tendency may provide temporary hemostasis but subsequently lead to a larger area of delayed oozing after the chemically affected tissue sloughs.

Vasoconstrictors

Temporary hemostasis may be obtained with adrenergic vasoconstrictor agents, generally epinephrine. Such vasoconstrictors should be applied topically or just under the mucosa only for restricted local effects and for very short periods to avoid prolonged ischemia and tissue necrosis. Because some of the drug is absorbed systemically, particularly in inflamed and abraded tissue, cardiovascular responses may occur. **Epinephrine** solutions and dry cotton pellets impregnated with racemic epinephrine are available for topical application, but other methods to control bleeding are generally preferred.

Systemic Measures

Patients with acquired or genetic bleeding disorders usually have deficiencies in platelet number, platelet function, or faulty or missing clotting factors. Bleeding may develop several hours after trauma or surgery. Uncontrolled bleeding does not generally appear with superficial abrasions, but hemarthrosis and hemorrhage are common with deeper injuries. Thrombocytopenia is frequently drug-induced or associated with other myelogenous diseases; hemophilia disorders are generally inherited. With proper evaluation and supportive therapy (Table 26-2), extensive surgery can usually be accomplished without serious incident.

TABLE 26-2 Procoagulant Preparations Used in the Management of Bleeding Disorders

Nonproprietary (Generic) Name	Proprietary (Trade) Names	Content	Therapeutic Use
Factor VIII Products			
Antihemophilic factor, plasma derived	Humate-P	250, 500, and 1000 IU/vial; contains albumin vWF and small amounts of other proteins	Hemophilia A, vWD
Antihemophilic factor, plasma derived, purified	Alphanate, Hemofil M, Koate DVI, Monarc-M, Monoclate-P	250, 500, 1000, and 1500 IU/vial; contains albumin	Hemophilia A
Antihemophilic factor, recombinant	Bioclate, Helixate, FS, Recombinate	250, 500, and 1000 IU/vial; contains albumin and trace amounts of animal protein	Hemophilia A; patients without HIV or viral hepatitis
Antihemophilic factor, recombinant, albumin-free	Advate, Kogenate FS, ReFacto, Xyntha		
Factor IX Products			
Factor IX complex	Bebulin VH, Profilnine SD, Proplex T	500, 1000, and 1500 IU/vial; also contains significant amounts of factors II, VII, and X	Hemophilia B
Factor IX human complex, purified	AlphaNine SD, Mononine	500, 1000, and 1500 IU/vial; contains small amounts of factors II, VII, and X	Hemophilia B
Factor IX, recombinant	BeneFIX Rixubis Alprolix (Fc Fusion) Ixinity	Varies per manufacturer	Hemophilia B; patients without HIV or viral hepatitis Formulations vary to prolong activity
Factor VIIa Product			
Factor VIIa, recombinant	NovoSeven RT	1, 2, and 5 mg/vial	Hemophilia A or B; patients with inhibitors for factors VIII or IX
Mixed Factor Products			
Anti-inhibitor coagulant complex (factor VIII inhibitor bypassing activity)	Autoplex T, FEIBA VH	≥80 IU/bag; contains other clotting factors; prepared from single donors	Hemophilia A, vWD, hypofibrinogenemia, DIC, Kasabach-Merritt syndrome
Antihemophilic factor, cryoprecipitated	–	≥80 IU/bag; contains other clotting factors; prepared from single donors	Hemophilia A, vWD, hypofibrinogenemia, DIC, Kasabach-Merritt syndrome

Unless otherwise noted, all products are derived from human plasma or, in the case of recombinant products, based on human genes.
DIC, Disseminated intravascular coagulopathy; *HIV*, human immunodeficiency virus; *IU*, international units; *vWD*, von Willebrand disease; *vWF*, von Willebrand factor.

Platelet disorders

Patients with a platelet count of less than 50,000/mm^3 are at risk for surgical or other trauma, but they generally do not exhibit spontaneous hemorrhage until the count becomes less than 20,000/mm^3. Platelet transfusion should be reserved for acute situations because alloimmunization to injected platelets can occur. One unit of platelet concentrate (equal to the platelets derived from 1 U of whole blood) increases the platelet count in adults from 4000/mm^3 to 10,000/mm^3. Platelet recovery is low in patients with hypersplenism and may be undetectable in patients with immune thrombocytopenia. Idiopathic forms may benefit from corticosteroid administration, splenectomy, use of immunosuppressive agents, or (acutely) high doses of intravenous immunoglobulin. Drug-induced disease generally is alleviated by withdrawal of the offending drug. In the case of aspirin or a thienopyridine such as clopidogrel prescribed deliberately to alter platelet function, the relative risks of hemorrhage versus thromboembolism must be considered in relation to the planned procedure.

Hemophilia

All forms of hemophilia are genetically based disorders of coagulation. They may range in severity from mild to moderate to severe; this designation greatly affects what dental interventions can occur. The most common forms of hemophilia result from deficiencies in **factors VIII and IX (hemophilia A and B)**. Although the transmission of both hemophilia A or B is hereditary and X-linked, nearly half of all cases arise spontaneously as new mutations. Any child or adult with newly discovered hemophilia should have counseling with the family as provided by hemophilia treatment centers. Bleeding disorders (especially of the mild variety) are often first discovered after dental procedures, such as extractions or periodontal surgery.

Hemophilia A occurs when there is a deficiency in circulating factor VIII activity. Factor VIII accelerates blood coagulation by serving as a cofactor in the platelet membrane in the enzymatic activation of factor X by the factor IXa/VIIIa complex (see Fig. 26-3). The normal amount of factor VIII antigen averages 100 U/dL. Mild hemophilia occurs when the patient's blood has 5% to 30% of normal factor VIII activity. Moderate disease is defined as showing 1% to 4% factor VIII, and severe hemophilia shows less than 1% factor VIII. Individuals with more than 40% normal factor VIII antigen clot normally.

The gene for factor VIII resides on the long arm of the X chromosome (Xq28), resulting in an X-linked pattern of inheritance. In severe factor VIII hemophilia, gene inversions account for 45% of mutations, whereas other patients have point mutations that often cause a premature stop codon to be inserted, resulting in incomplete mRNA transcription. In general, only males with a faulty factor VIII gene on their only X chromosome show phenotypic expression of severe disease, at a rate of 1 in 10,000. Females who carry an affected X chromosome typically do not show phenotypic disease because the unaffected factor VIII gene on the other X chromosome provides sufficient protein to allow normal clotting. Expression of the normal gene may become depressed during development, however, if key progenitor cells favor the chromosome with the defective gene. The result is that some carrier females are phenotypically mild (or, rarely, moderate) hemophiliacs, with factor VIII concentrations 15% to 25% of normal. Referred to as *symptomatic carriers*, their bleeding tendency is often not discovered until they encounter a significant insult, such as extraction of teeth, orthognathic surgery, or extensive periodontal surgery. For this reason, female relatives of hemophiliacs should have interviews, and possibly blood tests, to determine their carrier status and their factor VIII activity.

Hemophilia B was discovered when it was noted that combining plasma from different hemophiliacs sometimes allowed normal clotting; it was deduced that the second sample corrected the defect in the first. It was later determined that deficiencies in factor IX were responsible for approximately one-fifth of the forms of hemophilia. Older literature refers to factor IX deficiency as *Christmas disease*, named after the surname of the first family studied with this variant of hemophilia.

Similar to hemophilia A, the gene for factor IX is on the X chromosome (Xq27.3) and shows the same familial pattern of expression: affected males and carrier females. Similar to factor VIII deficiency, partial or whole gene deletions or insertions lead to severe hemophilia B, as do nonsense point and some missense mutations. Also similar to hemophilia A, there are mild, moderate, and severe forms of the disease, and female symptomatic carriers occur. Hemophilia A and B are clinically indistinguishable.

Von Willebrand disease

Originally described by von Willebrand in 1926, **von Willebrand disease (vWD)** is an autosomal dominant hemorrhagic disorder resulting from a quantitative or qualitative deficiency of the vWF GP. Males and females are affected equally; the defect is in an autosomal dominant gene located on chromosome 12. vWD may be the most common inherited bleeding disorder, with many cases remaining undiagnosed.

The vWF GP is produced in vascular endothelial cells and megakaryocytes and is stored intracellularly in the α granules of platelets and circulated in the plasma as multimeric polymers. The high-molecular-weight multimers are necessary for normal biologic activity, presumably because of their greater number of ligand-binding domains. vWF has three important functions. The first is to form a tight but noncovalent complex with factor VIII protein, stabilizing and slowing its clearance from the circulation. Second, vWF promotes normal, high-shear platelet adhesion to the subendothelium on injury and exposure of subendothelial matrix proteins. Third, vWF is one of the proteins that binds to the multiple platelet membrane GP IIb/IIIa receptors, along with fibrinogen, to help stabilize the aggregating platelets.

As an aside, ristocetin, one of the first antistaphylococcal antibiotics, was found to cause thrombocytopenia by binding to the platelet membrane and catalyzing the binding of vWF. This resulted in platelet aggregation, thrombus formation, and depletion thrombocytopenia. The antibiotic was removed from clinical use as a result, but is now used as an assay for vWD. By mixing ristocetin, washed platelets, and plasma from the affected patient, an inverse correlation occurs between the amount of functional vWF present in the plasma (originally called *ristocetin cofactor*) and the amount of ristocetin necessary to induce platelet aggregation.

The hematologic disorder in vWD can manifest as either structural or quantitative changes in vWF. Three basic types of disease exist. Type 1 vWD is associated with a mild quantitative defect in the amount of vWF produced. Titers of vWF antigen (total vWF protein) and ristocetin cofactor activity (functional vWF protein) are comparable. This is the most common type (80%) and is most often manifested by mucocutaneous bleeding. Type 2 vWD is a defect in the amount of high-molecular-weight multimers present in the plasma, causing a marked decrease in platelet adhesion but little change in total vWF antigen. There is a high ratio of antigen to ristocetin cofactor activity. Type 3 vWD is characterized by severe bleeding disorders from an essential lack of any vWF, with concomitantly low concentrations of factor VIII and decreased platelet adhesion. This third type is rare, mostly occurring in homozygous or compound heterozygous offspring of parents with mild or asymptomatic variants of vWD.

Treatment

Treatment of either variety of hemophilia or vWD requires the restoration of the appropriate factor so that factor complex **IXa/VIIIa** activity is sufficient. For the treatment of hemophilia A, various factor VIII replacement products are available (see Table 26-2). Because the half-life of factor VIII is 8 to 12 hours, the patient must be reinfused with at least half the original dose at approximately 12-hour intervals to prevent late bleeding from surgical wounds.

Until more recently, the only way to obtain factor VIII was by pooled human blood products. Initially, the most common method was to use cryoprecipitate. Cryoprecipitate is the cold-insoluble (precipitated) protein fraction derived when fresh frozen plasma is thawed at 4°C. It is primarily composed of factor VIII, fibrinogen, and vWF. Classically, it was one of the mainstays of factor VIII hemophilia treatment, but it has virtually disappeared from this use with the development of methods to manufacture recombinant factor VIII. Similar to plasma, cryoprecipitate is not virally inactivated. The most common current use of cryoprecipitate is as a source of fibrinogen for the treatment of disseminated intravascular coagulopathy. Cryoprecipitate is still occasionally used for the treatment of vWD, particularly if it is obtained from a single donor after desmopressin stimulation, but this use is waning.

Modern plasma-derived factor VIII products have greatly reduced the risk of viral transmission by donor screening and viral inactivation protocols. Two methods are currently being used to inactivate viruses: heat and solvent detergent. All viruses that have lipid envelopes are readily destroyed, including HIV, hepatitis B, and hepatitis C. Viruses that do not have lipid envelopes, such as the B19 parvovirus and hepatitis A, can still be transmitted in the solvent detergent or heat-inactivated products. A vaccination for hepatitis A is now available, and patients with hemophilia or vWD are encouraged to receive it early in life.

Some manufacturers additionally purify their factor VIII protein products from the pooled factor VIII proteins on affinity columns, increasing the specific activity of the preparation and decreasing further the risk of viral transmission. Those products are more expensive. One of the factor VIII products, Humate-P, is purified with a process that retains a considerable amount of vWF. Although still occasionally used for factor VIII hemophiliacs, this product has become the favored way to treat bleeds or potential bleeds in patients with moderate–severe vWD and is used mostly for this reason. It has the advantage that it can be manufactured on a large scale, lyophilized for stability and storage, and reconstituted when necessary. It is considered very safe from viral contamination.

Most factor VIII hemophiliacs are now receiving recombinant factor VIII products, particularly if they are HIV and hepatitis virus negative. These proteins are derived from stable transfection of the human factor VIII cDNA into Chinese hamster ovary (CHO) or baby hamster kidney cells, with resultant transcription and protein production. The first-generation products required human albumin to be added to provide stabilization through the purification process; the second-generation and third-generation products are now being made albumin-free. The distinction is important because the albumin adds a small risk for viral contamination. The new products are considered virus-free, have high specific activities, and have been successful in transiently correcting the bleeding disorder. The main difficulty is that in a patient with severe hemophilia with essentially no endogenous protein, the use of this "foreign antigen" product may cause the development of anti-factor VIII antibodies, known in hematology as **inhibitors** and discussed in greater detail subsequently. In most patients who develop them, the inhibitors are low titer and controllable with low-dose daily infusions of factor VIII protein to build immune tolerance over time.

Another approach to the treatment of mild hemophilia A and type 1 vWD was introduced when it was discovered that **desmopressin**, the synthetic 1-desamino-8-D-arginine analogue of vasopressin (antidiuretic hormone), could prevent bleeding in many of these patients. This medication causes endogenous factor VIII, vWF, and plasminogen activator to be released from storage sites on the vascular endothelium. In many patients with mild hemophilia or type 1 vWD, the protein structures are normal, but concentrations are low. With desmopressin, transient increases of two to three times the patient's baseline concentrations can be achieved, which may be sufficient to allow adequate hemostasis during minor surgery. For hemophiliacs who use single donors (usually a parent or sibling) as their sole source of factor product, desmopressin can be given to the donor before donation to double or triple the amount of factor VIII recovered.

The advantage of desmopressin over vasopressin is that it retains the factor VIII–releasing activity but has diminished vasoconstrictor action. Most importantly, desmopressin is devoid of the risk of viral transmission inherent in the blood-derived products. Desmopressin is subject to peptic hydrolysis and is injected or insufflated intranasally. Mild facial flushing is normal during the infusion, with headache, nausea, and lightheadedness as common side effects. Because of its antidiuretic properties, water intake must be restricted for 12 hours to avoid volume overload. (The drug is also used in lower doses as an aid for children with bed-wetting difficulties.)

Historically, factor IX concentrates have been difficult to purify. The most common factor IX preparations are known as **factor IX complex** because, although they have high amounts of factor IX protein, they also contain factors II and X and some factor VII (see Table 26-2). Because of the presence of the excessive extra clotting factors (some partially activated), disseminated intravascular coagulopathy is occasionally a problem. Similar to factor VIII concentrates, they are subjected to various forms of viral inactivation to reduce the transmission of HIV, hepatitis B, and hepatitis C.

Several recombinant factor IX preparations are currently available. Similar to all recombinant products, they are essentially virus-free because they are produced in CHO cells. They vary in how the factor is stabilized, whether by human albumin, the Fc portion of IgG immunoglobulin, or other proprietary methods. The major difficulties in developing these products are the extensive posttranslational modifications the natural protein undergoes. As a result, the manufactured factor IX protein is not as efficacious as the natural factor, so patients often require more protein than the highly purified plasma-derived protein to get sufficient increases in plasma factor IX.

One aspect of blood product replacement therapy that is often overlooked is cost. On average, a patient with severe hemophilia A uses $10,000 to $100,000 worth of factor per year depending on the type of product used and the dose required. Younger hemophiliacs, to avoid potential viral exposure, generally use the recombinant products.

As a hope for the future, correction of hemophilia by gene transfer is being pursued. Gene therapy is in its infancy, but hemophilia is considered one of the more ideal targets for early trials because the active proteins are found in the bloodstream and can be made in just about any tissue as long as they can be released to the blood. It will be interesting to see which hemophilia gene transfer succeeds first. The factor VIII gene is larger and more difficult to transfer, but the resultant protein undergoes much less posttranslational modification than occurs with factor IX.

Inhibitors and ways to circumvent them

A **confounding problem** in treating hemophiliacs is the development of **antibody inhibitors** against the deficient factor. Approximately 5% of patients with severe hemophilia A express a high titer of inhibitor, usually within the first few years of being treated with factor VIII concentrates. Multiple approaches must be used to protect these patients against bleeding crises. The most crucial task is to determine whether the patient carries low-titer or high-titer antibodies. Patients with low-titer antibodies can often be given excessive amounts of factor replacement, depleting the inhibitor antibody sufficiently to allow the remaining factor to promote hemostasis. Although low-titer inhibitors may persist for years, they do not show the typical alloantibody boost response after exposure to human factor VIII concentrates.

In patients with high-titer inhibitors, preventing or reducing hemorrhage risk is crucial. Daily infusion of high-dose, medium-dose, or low-dose factor replacement to induce immune tolerance can be successful. Concomitant administration of immunosuppressant medications may depress antibody formation further. This approach is much more effective with autoantibody inhibitors than with alloimmune responses. A short course of daily intravenous infusion of IgG has sometimes reduced titers as well. After immune tolerance is achieved, most patients require continued low-dose prophylactic factor infusions at least weekly.

When hemophiliacs with high-titer inhibitors require coagulation support, but factor VIII replacement therapy cannot be used, two products may be effective. Factor **VIIa** is a recombinant protein that functions similar to its endogenous counterpart: it combines with TF at the site of injury to stimulate conversion of factors IX and X to their respective activated analogues. Because TF is found only at the site of injury, disseminated coagulation has not been a problem. Also, factor VIIa is not rapidly inactivated by ATIII, giving it a sufficient half-life to allow hemostasis. Because it has a much shorter half-life than either factor VIII or factor IX, **it requires high doses every 2 hours in the dental setting**. The drug has the limitation that its mechanism is to achieve sufficient thrombin formation via the part of the coagulation cascade that is intended for only small amounts of thrombin generation. It seems to work well for initial hemostasis, but there have been difficulties with breakthrough bleeding 48 hours or so after surgery. Concomitant use of local control measures (suturing/collagen) is wise. The current cost of this medication is several thousand dollars per dose.

The other medication that can be used is a procoagulant complex known as FEIBA VH (factor eight inhibitor bypassing activity). The VH form is a vapor-heated concentrate of plasma-derived factors II, VII, IX, and X (the vitamin K–dependent clotting factors) in their inactive and active forms. How this medication corrects the bleeding disorder is unknown, but it is believed the extra factors II and X complex with endogenous factor V and reconstruct the common pathway, eliminating the need for factor VIII. The main difficulty with this medication is that the extra clotting factors can overshoot and cause thrombosis elsewhere in the body. Which product, FEIBA versus factor VIIa, works best in any given patient is unpredictable. Some patients clearly do better with one over the other, but the reason for this is elusive.

AGENTS THAT PROMOTE OR INHIBIT FIBRINOLYSIS

Physiology of Clot Remodeling

Achieving hemostasis is a crucial aspect of the coagulation system, and limiting its spread is another. Remodeling or breaking down clots when they are no longer necessary is a third crucial facet of vascular repair. As healing occurs, it is necessary to remove part or all of

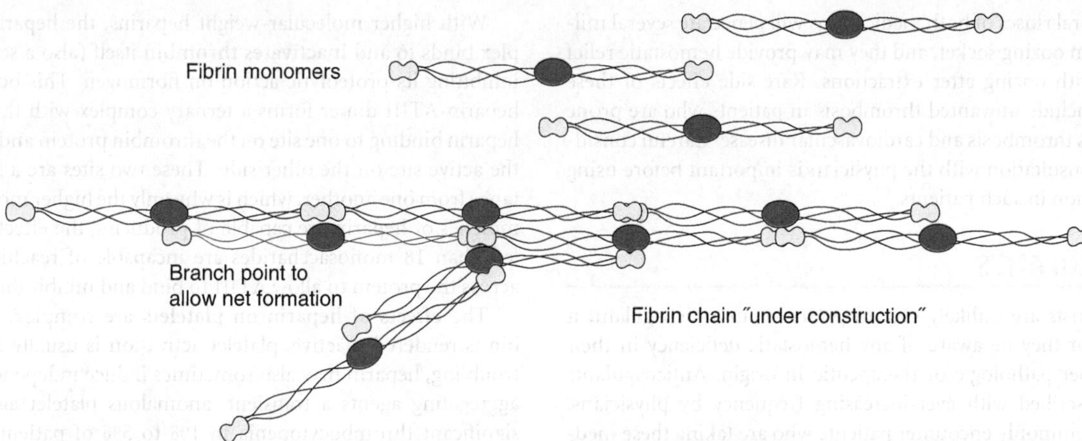

FIG 26-6 Fibrin formation. After conversion of fibrinogen to fibrin, the monomers begin to link together as shown to create staggered "ropes" with branch points. The branch points go on to form the "net," which will be used to capture red blood cells and bring about eventual hemostasis.

the fibrin that has been deposited so that normal blood flow can be restored to the affected tissue. This process is mediated by the **protease, plasmin.** When fibrin is initially deposited (Fig. 26-6), thrombin stimulates adjacent endothelial cells to release **tissue plasminogen activator (t-PA) and urokinase plasminogen activator (u-PA)**.

t-PA is a serine protease that must adhere to the fibrin molecules to function. This binding occurs on lysine residues of the fibrin. When adhered, t-PA binds plasminogen (also at a lysine residue) and cleaves it to liberate plasmin, another serine protease. Plasmin has the ability to bind directly to fibrin. u-PA acts independently of fibrin and instead activates plasminogen to plasmin in the circulation. Plasmin associated with t-PA lyses the fibrin, releasing fibrin degradation products, and degrades factors V and VIII, inhibiting further clotting.

As expected, strict control mechanisms for plasmin activity exist. Without such control, circulating plasmin would cause systemic fibrinolysis and oozing of previously clotted sites. Three proteins are intimately involved. The first, **α_2-antiplasmin (α_2-AP)**, is synthesized in the liver and is efficient at neutralizing any free plasmin circulating in the blood. Binding plasmin to fibrin protects it from attack by α_2-AP, which restricts the activity of plasmin to the wound site. The second control protein, **plasminogen activator inhibitor-1 (PAI-1)**, is synthesized by the endothelial cells in response to thrombin stimulation, with specificity for t-PA. PAI-1 effectively inhibits conversion of plasminogen to plasmin by t-PA, unless the t-PA can "hide" from it by binding to fibrin. The third control protein is PAI-2, which functions similarly to PAI-1, only with specificity for u-PA. The liver also functions to clear the bloodstream of any free active plasmin, further helping to prevent systemic fibrinolysis.

Fibrinolytics

Therapeutic measures designed to induce or facilitate fibrinolysis are available for use in relieving certain types of thromboses, most notably in the event of acute myocardial infarction. These agents may also be valuable in patients with a life-threatening pulmonary embolus, infarctive stroke, or deep venous thrombosis. All these agents function by activating the conversion of plasminogen to plasmin with subsequent natural fibrinolysis. **t-PA (alteplase)** is produced by recombinant DNA techniques. Because t-PA is naturally more fibrin specific than other preparations, it is the first thrombolytic agent recommended by the American Heart Association in the management of myocardial thrombosis. At pharmacologic doses, it imparts some circulating plasminogen conversion, however. A deletion mutation variant of t-PA is available by the nonproprietary name of **reteplase**. It is similar in activity and side effects to t-PA.

Streptokinase, an exotoxin from certain β-hemolytic streptococci, also serves as an activator of plasminogen. It is different from t-PA and u-PA because it is not an enzyme and does not proteolytically cleave plasminogen to plasmin. Instead, it binds noncovalently to plasminogen and confers plasmin-like proteolytic activity on the plasminogen–streptokinase complex. The complex cleaves other molecules of plasminogen, liberating active plasmin. Because streptokinase is an exogenous protein originating in bacteria, there is a higher incidence of adverse and allergic reactions with this medication. A similar medication, **anistreplase** (anisoylated streptokinase plasminogen activator complex), is a combination of streptokinase with an acylated plasminogen, forming an inactive complex that spontaneously deacylates in plasma. The deacylated form is the same as the streptokinase–plasminogen complex previously discussed.

The many available plasminogen activators have made effective treatment possible in reducing ischemic myocardial necrosis if given within 30 to 60 minutes after the onset of chest pain. There is a 47% success rate in thrombolysis if the products are given 1 hour from onset of symptoms. Results are poor if given after a 3- to 6-hour delay.

Antifibrinolytics

In some circumstances, it is advantageous to limit fibrinolytic activity (e.g., after surgery in a hemophilic who may be prone to breakthrough bleeding as the wound heals). Two drugs used for this purpose are aminocaproic acid (sometimes referred to as **ε-aminocaproic acid) and tranexamic acid.** Both competitively inhibit plasminogen and plasminogen activators from binding to fibrin. The usual dose of aminocaproic acid is 50 mg/kg every 6 hours for 10 days. In its tablet forms (500 mg or 1000 mg), this dosage requires the average adult patient to take several tablets every 6 hours. As a result, compliance can be difficult. A concentrated syrup form exists for pediatric use (250 mg/mL), and experience indicates that adult patients generally are more compliant with taking the liquid form of the medication, especially after oral surgical procedures.

Tranexamic acid is roughly eight times more efficient at antifibrinolysis as aminocaproic acid. It is available as an injectable form (Cyklokapron) or as oral tablets (Lysteda). Because the usual dosing is two tablets (650 mg × 2 = 1300 mg) TID, compliance is much better. As a result, it has overtaken aminocaproic acid as the drug of choice in dentistry.

Note that oral rinses of both medications will penetrate several millimeters into an oozing socket, and they may provide hemostatic relief for patients with oozing after extractions. Rare side effects of these medications include unwanted thrombosis in patients who are prone to deep venous thrombosis and cardiovascular disease. Careful consideration and consultation with the physician is important before using either medication in such patients.

ANTICOAGULANTS

Although dentists are unlikely ever to prescribe an anticoagulant, it is essential that they be aware of any hemostatic deficiency in their patient, whether pathologic or therapeutic in origin. Anticoagulants are being prescribed with ever-increasing frequency by physicians, and dentists commonly encounter patients who are taking these medications. There are now three classes of anticoagulants in clinical use: **directly acting agents; indirectly acting agents,** which interfere with the synthesis of coagulation proteins; and **platelet inhibitors,** of which three subclasses exist: **COX inhibitors, GP IIb/IIIa antagonists, and ADP receptor antagonists.** Dentists should be familiar with the pharmacologic features of each class and understand if, how, and when their effects should be modified.

Directly Acting Anticoagulants: Heparins

First extracted by McLean in 1916, **heparin** is a powerful, systemically effective direct-acting anticoagulant. Heparin is a linear mucopolysaccharide primarily composed of repeating units of D-glucosamine in 1,4 glucosidic linkage with d-glucuronic and l-iduronic acids. These disaccharide residues, which are partially esterified (≤40%) with sulfuric acid, make heparin the strongest organic acid normally occurring in the body. About 10 to 15 of these chains, each with 200 to 300 monosaccharide units, are attached to a core protein to give the final proteoglycan as the storage form of heparin in mast cells. Because the polysaccharide chains differ in length, and the sulfation reactions vary, endogenous heparin is a heterogeneous mixture of molecules, with molecular weights ranging from 4000 to 40,000, none of which has been completely characterized. Commercial preparations are made primarily from recombinant DNA techniques.

Heparin is produced endogenously in mast cells, where it is stored in a large macromolecular form complexed with histamine. Heparin and histamine are released together, providing a physiologic example of a fixed-drug combination, the significance of which is not yet fully understood. It has been proposed that adsorbed heparin-like mucopolysaccharides (termed *heparans*) are major contributors to the normally strong electronegative charge maintained by the vascular epithelium. This property is made use of in the manufacture of prosthetic devices such as heart valves, in which ionizable heparin is incorporated into the surface material to inhibit thrombus generation.

Mechanism of action

Heparin interferes with blood coagulation in several ways. Heparin functions by binding tightly to the plasma protease inhibitor **ATIII,** causing a conformational change in the inhibitor that exposes its active site and accelerates its activity a thousandfold. ATIII is a "suicide" protein that covalently binds to several proteases (**factors IXa, Xa, and XIIa**), resulting in the permanent inactivation of the protease and the ATIII protein. As a true catalyst, heparin is not destroyed in this process. The **heparin–ATIII complex** dissociates on binding of a protease to ATIII, releasing intact heparin for renewed binding to another ATIII molecule.

With higher molecular-weight heparins, the heparin–ATIII complex binds to and **inactivates thrombin** itself (also a serine protease), inhibiting its proteolytic action on fibrinogen. This occurs when the heparin-ATIII dimer forms a ternary complex with thrombin by the heparin binding to one site on the thrombin protein and ATIII binding the active site on the other side. These two sites are a significant distance from one another, which is why only the higher molecular-weight moieties of heparin are capable of producing the effect. Molecules of less than 18 monosaccharides are incapable of reaching far enough across the protein to allow ATIII to bind and inhibit thrombin.

The **effects of heparin on platelets** are complex. When thrombin is rendered inactive, platelet activation is usually reduced. More troubling, heparin may also sometimes induce independently of other aggregating agents a transient, anomalous platelet aggregation and significant thrombocytopenia in 1% to 5% of patients. Two varieties of heparin-induced thrombocytopenia (HIT) exist: a relatively benign nonimmune process and an immune-mediated process. The latter, known as type II, can be fatal in 30% of cases. It is believed that complexing of the heparin to platelet factor 4 results in antibody formation and subsequent activation of platelets. In this syndrome, the difficulty is not with bleeding, but with runaway thrombosis. As the platelets activate, they form thrombi, which account for much of the clinical presentation. As the platelets are used up, thrombocytopenia and bleeding occur. Patients with a history of type II HIT are far more likely to have a repeat problem, as would be expected with immunologic phenomena.

Low-molecular-weight heparins

Much research activity has focused on the use of **low-molecular-weight heparin (LMWH)** fractions for the prevention of thrombosis. Unfractionated heparin consists of heterogeneous combinations of various-sized sulfated mucopolysaccharides. Because only high-molecular-weight heparins (heparins with ≥18 specific saccharide sequences) can bind thrombin and inactivate it, attention has turned to LMWHs. They are poor inhibitors of thrombin, but they retain the ability to **catalyze ATIII** to inhibit other serine proteases, most notably **factor Xa.** As a result, they have at least some advantage in that they exert antithrombotic activity without completely destroying the coagulant activity thrombin imparts on factors V, VIII, XII, and XIII. A problem with LMWHs is that they all are prepared by fractionating heparin, and different methods impart different ratios of anticoagulant and antithrombotic activity. **Enoxaparin and dalteparin** currently are the most commonly used medications in this class; the one selected by the physician depends on the degree of anticoagulation desired for the patient.

A synthetic pentasaccharide, **fondaparinux,** similar to LMWHs, has been marketed. This medication is a selective factor Xa inhibitor, and studies have shown that it is more effective than enoxaparin in preventing deep venous thrombosis after hip and knee surgery.

Absorption, fate, and excretion

All available forms of heparin must be administered parenterally because they are highly charged and rapidly hydrolyzed in the gastrointestinal tract. Unfractionated heparin is infused intravenously but may be given by deep subcutaneous or fat depot injection. It should not be injected intramuscularly because of the risk of deep muscle hematoma. Heparin has a dose-dependent biologic half-life of 1 to 5 hours when given intravenously, and it is removed primarily by the liver. When injected subcutaneously, it is absorbed into the systemic circulation so slowly that it rarely is a problem for any kind of dental treatment. **LMWHs** are generally administered **subcutaneously** with once-daily or twice-daily dosing.

Heparin activity is best monitored by the **partial thromboplastin time or the aPTT**, both of which measure drug effects on the intrinsic pathway and are sensitive to low doses of heparin. The partial thromboplastin time is much less sensitive (and often completely normal) to LMWHs. Standardized doses of LMWHs achieve a more consistent anticoagulant effect, reducing the need for monitoring. The prothrombin time (PT), routinely used to monitor oral (indirect-acting) anticoagulants, is also of little value because it does not respond to inhibition of the thrombin-catalyzed part of the coagulation cascade, and heparin is diluted out in the procedure.

Other Directly Acting Anticoagulants

Direct thrombin inhibitors

It has long been known that leeches secrete a potent anticoagulant in their saliva. In many centers, medicinal leeches (*Hirudo medicinalis*) are still used to help patients combat venous thromboembolic events. The active component has been isolated and identified as hirudin, a 65-amino acid polypeptide chain that is a specific direct thrombin inhibitor. It works by stoichiometrically binding to thrombin at two sites: the fibrinogen-binding site and the active protease site. It is the most powerful naturally occurring anticoagulant known.

Hirudin has many advantages over heparin. As a direct thrombin inhibitor, it is able to inhibit clot-bound thrombin that the heparin-ATIII complex cannot reach. As would be expected with a direct inhibitor, it also has caused severe bleeds. A recombinant analogue, **lepirudin**, has been approved for the treatment of thrombosis associated with HIT. Because 50% of patients develop IgG antibodies against the hirudins, aPTT must be monitored closely.

Perhaps the most widely used direct thrombin inhibitor is **bivalirudin**, a semisynthetic analogue of hirudin consisting of 20 amino acids. It competes for the fibrinogen-binding site and the proteolytic site, effectively stopping all cleavage of fibrinogen to fibrin. Bivalirudin differs from hirudin in that it produces only transient inactivation of the thrombin protease site because the thrombin itself slowly acts on the bivalirudin to cleave it, and when cleaved, it "falls off" the thrombin molecule, allowing fibrinogen to bind. This net effect means that it has a relatively short clinical half-life of 1 to 2 hours, but that is advantageous because it can be infused to prevent thrombosis before cardiac surgery and turned off shortly before the case to allow full clotting to occur in a predictable fashion. Bivalirudin was shown more recently to prevent blood clots better than heparin in patients undergoing angioplasty. The drug is primarily cleared via intravascular proteolysis and renal elimination in the urine; it has a significantly longer clinical half-life in patients with moderate–severe renal failure.

Dabigatran (Pradaxa) is a direct thrombin inhibitor available in an oral tablet formulation. It is being used instead of warfarin in many patients due to more consistent anticoagulation, but it has yet to have data on exactly how to manage it in the dental setting. The bleeding risk would, in part, depend on the extent of the dental procedure. A reversal drug for dabigatran, idarucizumab (Praxbind), is now available. Monitoring is generally done with the aPTT.

Factor Xa inhibitors

The newest group of anticoagulants are the **factor Xa (FXa) inhibitors. Rivaroxaban (Xarelto), Apixaban (Eliquis), edoxaban (Savaysa), and Betrixaban** stop the coagulation cascade by binding to FXa and inhibiting the resultant cleavage of prothrombin to thrombin. They have the advantage of rapid onset and relatively short half-lives, which reduces need for "bridging" near surgery. They are generally unmonitored on a routine basis, but the PT and the aPTT will show some effect. Evidence-based guidelines are not available on whether or not discontinuing care prior to dental surgery is necessary, particularly with regard to the extent of the planned surgery and the availability of local control measures (collagen, suturing, etc.), This topic will be discussed in greater detail under dental considerations later in the chapter.

Indirectly Acting Anticoagulants: Warfarin

Discovery of the prothrombin-depressant action of spoiled sweet clover by Roderick in 1929 led to the isolation and synthesis of dicumarol (bishydroxycoumarin) by Campbell and Link in the 1940s. These advances introduced a new era of relatively inexpensive, self-administered oral anticoagulant therapy. Since then, several other **coumarin** compounds (and the similar indanediones) have been introduced, but **warfarin** is the only significant medication in current use.

Mechanism of action

Warfarin acts by competitively **inhibiting vitamin K epoxide reductase,** an enzyme essential for the synthesis of many coagulation factors by the liver. Vitamin K serves as a cofactor in the γ-carboxylation of glutamic acid residues of several proteins, including the **clotting factors II, VII, IX, and X and proteins C and S.** The carboxyglutamic acid moieties formed are able to chelate Ca^{2+}, which promotes conformational change and eversion of hydrophobic domains, allowing the factors to settle into the platelet or endothelial cell membrane and bind cofactors. Vitamin K is oxidized in the carboxylation process and must be reduced enzymatically to regain cofactor activity. Warfarin inhibits this reduction (Fig. 26-7).

The **most sensitive** indicator of vitamin K deficiency or warfarin anticoagulation is the depression of **factor VII.** The PT test best shows factor VII activity and is therefore the monitoring test of choice. Of the four vitamin K–dependent clotting factors, factor VII shows depression first because its half-life is only 4 to 8 hours. Prothrombin, with a half-life of 2 to 3 days, is the last to be diminished.

Adverse effects

Indirect anticoagulants notably produce adverse reactions in the presence of certain drugs and medical conditions. These effects most often arise from interference with vitamin K absorption or metabolism, competition for the drug-binding sites of proteins, or competition for or activation of the hepatic microsomal enzymes responsible for biotransformation. The most important toxic effect of warfarin is unexpected hemorrhage.

Any change in the absorption or availability of vitamin K from the intestine affects the balance between the anticoagulant and **vitamin K** in the liver and is reflected in the PT. In patients with marginal amounts of vitamin K in the diet, depressed bacterial synthesis (such as after antibiotic therapy) of vitamin K in the intestine may affect anticoagulation. Some oral contraceptive agents greatly increase vitamin K_1 absorption in experimental animals.

Warfarin is **highly plasma protein bound** (approximately 99%). This association creates a tremendous reserve of drug in the bloodstream, a very small displacement of which could easily double the concentration of active free drug. Many unrelated compounds that are also highly plasma protein bound theoretically can displace this protein binding and potentiate warfarin's action. Clinically, this effect is thankfully generally mild.

Warfarin is a racemic mixture of an R-enantiomer and S-enantiomer. The R-enantiomer, a weak anticoagulant, is metabolized primarily by hepatic biotransformation using CYP1A2, with CYP2C19 and CYP3A4 providing minor pathways. The S-enantiomer, a potent anticoagulant, is metabolized by CYP2C9. **Medications that either inhibit or induce these various hepatic microsomal enzymes may affect the patient's response to warfarin.** Only trace amounts (approximately 1%) of warfarin are excreted unchanged.

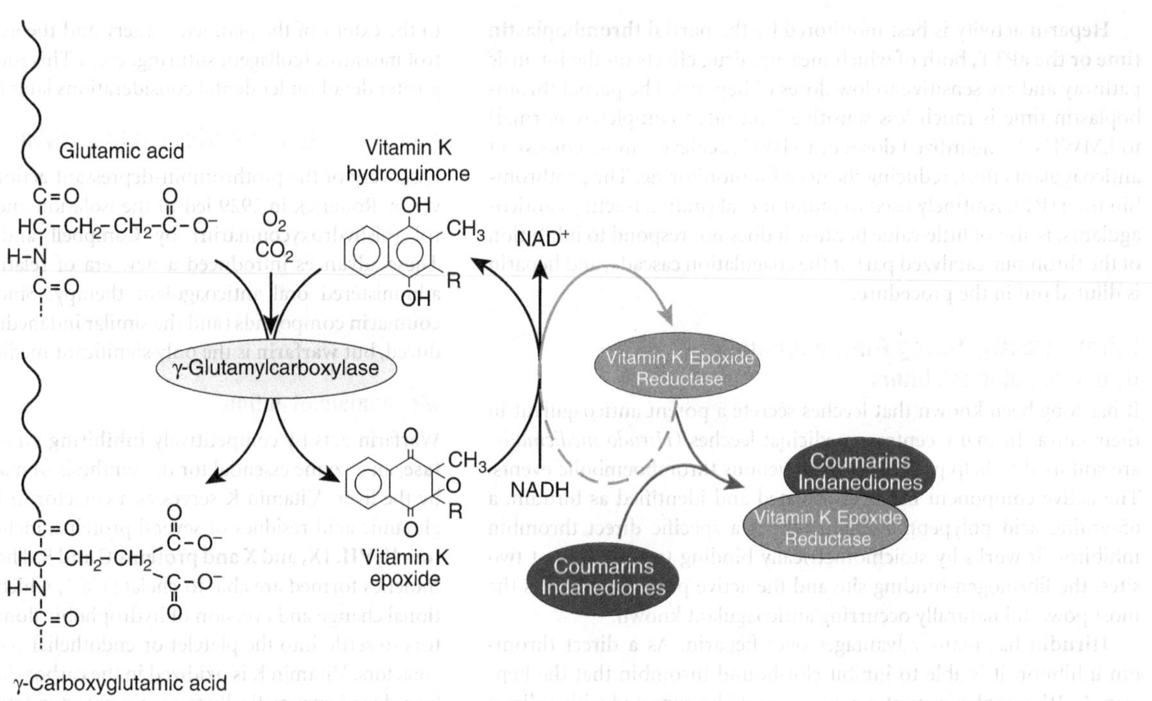

FIG 26-7 Inhibition of synthesis of vitamin K–dependent clotting factors by coumarin and indanedione anticoagulants. In the final posttranslational modification of prothrombin (factor II), factor VII, factor IX, factor X, protein C, and protein S, vitamin K is oxidized to the epoxide in the process of carboxylating glutamic acid residues on the amino end of each protein. The resultant γ-carboxyglutamic acid groups serve to chelate Ca^{2+} ions and conformationally change to expose a hydrophobic domain that settles into phospholipid membranes, anchoring the factors for normal hemostasis. The indirect-acting anticoagulants prevent the restoration of vitamin K by competitively inhibiting vitamin K epoxide reductase, the enzyme responsible for reducing vitamin K epoxide by nicotinamide adenine dinucleotide (*NADH*). *R*, Hydrocarbon side chain of vitamin K.

Many other drug interactions regarding oral anticoagulant agents do not involve vitamin K absorption, carrier protein displacement, or biotransformation. **Aspirin, ibuprofen, and clopidogrel** are representative drugs that inhibit platelet function. When administered concurrently with warfarin, their combined influences on the coagulation cascade may result in uncontrolled bleeding.

Antidotes

Except in situations in which an emergency demands the replacement of whole blood or plasma, the usual antidote for warfarin toxicity is **vitamin K** administered parenterally in high concentrations. Because warfarin inhibits recycling of vitamin K, simple administration of more "fresh" vitamin K obviates the need for recycling the epoxide form immediately. Subcutaneous or intramuscular administration provides obvious improvement in coagulation in 1 to 3 hours, but normal hemostasis may not be achieved for 24 hours.

Similarly, minor correction in an anticoagulated PT is seen if patients ingest significant amounts of **vitamin K** via **their diet**. Liver, broccoli, brussels sprouts, spinach, Swiss chard, collards, and other green leafy vegetables that are high in vitamin K can add enough vitamin K to shift the patient's anticoagulation profile in a few hours after ingestion. This technique is often used by anticoagulation clinics to "fine-tune" a patient before dental surgery if he or she is close to, but not quite under, his or her target PT **international normalized ratio (INR)**.

Kcentra (prothrombin complex concentrate, human) has been recently introduced to more quickly control major bleeding due to vitamin K antagonist therapy. Kcentra contains factors II, VII, IX, and X. The product contains a black box warning about thromboembolic complications. Because of its risks, need for close monitoring, and intravenous use, it is unlikely to be of general use in dentistry.

Anticoagulants: General Pharmacological Characteristics and Therapeutic Uses

The principal pharmacologic actions of directly acting and indirectly acting anticoagulants interfere with some steps in the blood coagulation process. Beyond this, neither directly acting nor indirectly acting anticoagulants have outstanding effects on the cardiovascular, respiratory, or other systems except in the case of warfarin through competition with other drugs for protein binding sites and drug-metabolizing enzymes.

There are many indications in medicine for the use of anticoagulants, including prevention of myocardial infarction, cerebrovascular thrombosis, pulmonary embolism, and venous thrombosis. Clotting protection is necessary for mechanical cardiac valves and during renal dialysis. Cardiovascular compromise, such as that seen in atrial fibrillation or congestive heart failure, causes decreased flow of blood and presents a greater risk for thrombosis in areas of stasis. Atherosclerotic plaques, especially in hypertensive patients, are risks for intimal tears, with resultant thrombus formation. Heparin and oral anticoagulants are useful in the prevention and treatment of these disorders. Oral anticoagulants, classically **warfarin** but now also with the **direct thrombin and FXa inhibitors**, provide sustained forms of therapy. It has become commonplace to see patients treated with anticoagulants for long periods for these various reasons, and anticoagulation clinics are a staple in most medical centers. The dentist must be able to manage such patients appropriately without causing undue harm either from excessive bleeding or from increased thrombosis risk.

Platelet Inhibitors

As is discussed in Chapter 17, drugs that interfere with platelet function are increasingly being recommended for prophylaxis of arterial and venous thrombosis. In recent years, many different agents have been developed and marketed successfully. These agents can be divided into three essential groups: **COX inhibitors, ADP receptor inhibitors, and GP IIb/IIIa inhibitors.** Each has unique characteristics in managing thrombosis via platelet inhibition, and the dentist is likely to find patients with one or more of these medications in their drug profiles.

Cyclooxygenase inhibitors

Aspirin (acetylsalicylic acid) is the prototypic and most commonly recognized COX inhibitor. Inexpensive and readily available, it is prescribed in doses of 81 to 325 mg/day to reduce the risk of myocardial infarction, ischemic stroke, or both. The antihemostatic effect of aspirin is ascribed to irreversible acetylation of COX-1 isozyme. COX-1 is required to synthesize platelet TXA_2 from arachidonic acid. Disruption of this pathway results in decreased platelet aggregation and decreased ADP release. Because platelets are incapable of synthesizing new COX, the inhibition by aspirin lasts for the life of the platelet. When aspirin therapy is used in combination with thrombolytic therapy after acute myocardial infarction, there are significant reductions in mortality and the incidence of major complications.

Adenosine diphosphate receptor inhibitors

As described earlier, ADP binds to its own receptor proteins $P2Y_1$ and $P2Y_{12}$, which results in maximal platelet aggregation. The thienopyridine compounds **clopidogrel and prasugrel irreversibly inhibit the $P2Y_{12}$ receptor** by what is believed to be a covalent bond to the receptor. Both are inactive until metabolized in the liver to their active forms. Because they bind only to the $P2Y_{12}$ receptor, the $P2Y_1$-mediated ADP effects still occur. This results in the platelets still undergoing shape change and transient aggregation, but sustained aggregation and potentiation of granule secretion are impaired. Clinically, patients generally do not have significant hemorrhage from oral surgery if the extent of the surgery is limited and local control measures are used. In more extensive surgeries, stopping the use of these drugs for 24 to 72 hours prior may be advisable. Note that a newer drug, **cangrelor**, is a non-thienopyridine drug that also inhibits the $P2Y_{12}$ receptor in a similar manner to the thienopyridines but has a much shorter half-life.

Glycoprotein IIb/IIIa receptor inhibitors

Activation of GP IIb/IIIa receptors is a crucial near-final step in platelet aggregation, and platelets genetically deficient in these receptors (i.e., Glanzmann thrombasthenia) display a much more profound inhibition of aggregation than platelets altered by the limited effects of aspirin or thienopyridines. As a result, attention has been focused on developing agents that can **antagonize the GP IIb/IIIa receptors.** The first agent, **abciximab**, is a mouse-human chimeric monoclonal antibody protein. The highly variable region of the antibody is from the mouse and is directed against the human GP IIb/IIIa protein complex. The Fc region is human, however, so as to not engender an immunogenic response. No allergic or anaphylactic reactions have been reported, but the medication can result in severe thrombocytopenia.

Molecular analysis of the GP IIb/IIIa receptors indicates that they recognize a specific arginine-glycine-aspartic acid (RGD) sequence found in many of the adhesive molecules to which they bind (e.g., vWF). As a result, peptide analogues have been developed to bind at this RGD sequence and compete for the active sites. (Similarly, the venom of several species of viper contains peptides with similar RGD homologic features; these peptides bind to the GP IIb/IIIa receptors in an antagonistic fashion.) **Eptifibatide** is a currently available example from this group. Rather than an RGD sequence, it has a lysine-glycine-aspartic acid (KGD) sequence that imparts improved specificity for the GP IIb/IIIa receptor.

Other nonpeptide agents that can compete for binding with the GP IIb/IIIa receptor have been developed. Similar to eptifibatide, they have structure and charge characteristics that mimic the RGD sequence and compete for the receptor's docking. **Tirofiban** (a tyrosine derivative) is an example of this kind of medication.

Herbal and Dietary Supplements

There is great academic interest in the surging herbal and dietary supplement use in current society and whether these agents may have pharmacologic action. Many of these agents have been implicated in directly modifying the coagulation status of patients or indirectly interacting with Western medications to increase or decrease their pharmacokinetic profiles. Appendix 2 lists many of these compounds. As more data become available, it will be necessary for the dentist to be knowledgeable about what these medications might do in a patient who requires dentoalveolar or other oral surgery.

IMPLICATIONS FOR DENTISTRY

Surgical Pharmacologic Adjuncts

"Local control measures" is a term often used in the literature to describe non-pharmacologic methods of obtaining or hastening hemostasis. Examples include direct pressure, suturing with or without primary closure, intrasocket sponges of one variety or another, injection of local anesthetic with epinephrine for capillary vasoconstriction, and clotting agents such as fibrin sealants.

In the non-complicated surgical scenario, the best approach by far is to allow a normal, natural blood clot to form without additional intervention. **Direct, firm, sustained gauze pressure**, maintained without "peeking" for 15 to 20 minutes, is generally all that is necessary to successfully stop bleeding in the intraoral environment. If gingival tissues are loose and can be better approximated by suturing, this serves to decrease the socket size and will likely improve the speed of hemostasis.

When a patient has excessive bleeding, the practicing dentist has several options from which to select. While all intrasocket preparations (oxidated cellulose, gelatin, collagen) can help, **collagen** is generally best. Platelets activate with collagen exposure, and the material is considered to be much more natural and therefore kinder to the inflammatory and reparative processes than cellulose or gelatin. As a result, the healing is usually smoother and faster as the body can break down the collagen easily over time. Another option to consider is **topical thrombin or fibrin sealants.** The latter has the disadvantage that it takes 30 to 60 minutes to prepare and so is generally used in the practice of medical surgery for planned events rather than unplanned, urgent bleeding problems. Topical thrombin, on the other hand, can be quickly reconstituted with a sterile solution (usually local anesthetic) and soaked into a collagen plug and placed tightly into the socket in a matter of minutes. This generally stops the bleeding.

If the use of suturing, collagen, and thrombin fail to adequately control the bleeding, the dentist must consider two other possibilities. The first is that the platelets are sluggish and failing to activate appropriately; **transfusion** of a "six pack" (six units) of **platelets** may be necessary. The other option is that the plasmin in the local area is outrunning the clot formation, effectively breaking up the clot as quickly as it is trying to form. In this instance, application of an oral rinse of **tranexamic acid or aminocaproic** acid may be helpful. This scenario is particularly common if the patient presents several hours after the surgery with complaints of excessive oozing from the surgical site.

Of course, if all of these methods fail to control the bleeding, emergent care in a hospital setting may become necessary for both transfusion support and possibly additional surgical intervention to ligate feeder vessels. It must be remembered that many cases of mild hemophilia remain undiagnosed during childhood and only present at the time of the patient's first significant surgical experience, such as removal of teeth for orthodontic reasons or removal of wisdom teeth. Thankfully, in modern dental/medical practice, it is extremely rare to have to deal with true uncontrolled bleeding, and permanent morbidity or mortality is almost unheard of.

Patients Using Anticoagulants

There are no accepted indications for the use of anticoagulants in the practice of dentistry. Many patients requiring dental treatment receive some form of medical anticoagulation therapy, however, for the reasons previously cited. These patients present three kinds of problems to the dentist: (1) without possible modification, their therapeutic regimen may result in excessive bleeding after oral or periodontal surgery; (2) modification of their therapeutic regimen in preparation for surgery may predispose them to thromboembolic events; and (3) they may present a real danger of drug interaction between their anticoagulants and agents commonly used in dental practice, such as some analgesics, antibiotics, and sedatives. It is essential for the dentist to have a complete and thorough knowledge of the patient's drug history and what options are available when treating patients in whom anticoagulant therapy is involved.

Any intended oral surgical therapy in anticoagulated patients requires preliminary planning and consultation with the patient's physician or anticoagulation clinic. **Warfarin is monitored by the INR.** The INR test is performed by adding a source of TF and Ca^{2+} to a patient's citrated blood sample and measuring the time necessary to coagulate the sample. Because various laboratories use TF from different sources (human, rabbit, recombinant), there have been wide variations in the reported values and the resulting amount of anticoagulation. In an effort to normalize the activity of the various forms of TF, a formula has been developed that accounts for the inherent sensitivities of TF and individual laboratory methods. The resultant ratio, the INR, can be compared with any other INR value with high accuracy.

Because the INR is derived from an exponential formula, small changes in anticoagulation result in large changes in the INR value as the anticoagulation progresses. It is generally agreed that for warfarin **a INR value of 2.5 to 3.0** is considered **ideal for most medical conditions.** Prosthetic heart valves and other instances in which more anticoagulation is required generally have a **target value of 2.5 to 3.5.** Although there are no official recommendations from the American Dental Association on the topic of INR and dental treatment, one report recommends that a **INR of 4.0 be used as the upper limit** for simple oral surgical procedures and that a maximum of **3.0 be targeted for procedures likely to result in significant blood loss,** such as multiple extractions with alveoloplasty. Others have agreed that it is unusual to have significant clinical bleeding when the INR is less than 3.0.

If a patient is anticoagulated to a high INR value, the dentist should consult with the physician about the possibility of reducing the anticoagulation to an acceptable INR, as shown in Figure 26-8. A unilateral decision by a dentist to have his or her patient discontinue or decrease coumarin without consulting the physician is at best poor medical practice because medicolegally, even if the warfarin is ultimately decreased, the physician is the appropriate individual to alter and follow the dosages perioperatively. This adjustment may take several days to accomplish. Current medical practice often places the responsibility of the anticoagulation management with an anticoagulation clinic that tracks the INR on a consistent basis, and such a clinic is a reliable resource to help guide the dentist and patient in making therapeutic decisions. Some patients have erratic responses to warfarin, with unpredictable highs and lows in the INR despite the best efforts of the medical team to stabilize it. In these patients, the prudent dentist will obtain a INR on the day of surgery and is prepared to reschedule the appointment if the value is too high to be safe. In the emergent patient, reversal with vitamin K and use of local hemostatic measures (collagen plugs, suturing, topical thrombin, fibrin sealant) may be indicated; in severe cases, the administration of fresh frozen plasma may be necessary.

If the anticoagulant is intravenous **heparin**, the drug may be **withheld by the physician for 1 to 6 hours**. This time interval is dose dependent. If the heparin is to be **restarted after surgery**, typically **waiting at least 1 hour** is advisable to allow time for the clot to form fully. The use of local hemostatic agents may be considered for further hemorrhage control. Note that subcutaneous "maintenance" heparin absorbs into the bloodstream at such a slow rate that it can be effectively ignored in terms of dental bleeding issues.

Patients who are taking an **LMWH** such as enoxaparin present a **dilemma.** Because LMWHs stimulate ATIII to be active against factor Xa but are not very effective against thrombin (factor IIa), the INR and aPTT in these patients are usually normal. A special factor Xa assay (costly and not always available) can be used to monitor these medications. The question arises as to what a dentist should do when patients are using these agents on a daily basis. Data are limited; however, it has been suggested that the LMWH should be **discontinued for 12 hours** before the surgical event. It can be argued, however, that for simple surgical procedures (e.g., dentoalveolar surgery, periodontal surgery), if there is sufficient thrombin generation to maintain the **aPTT at a normal value**, perhaps no adjustment to the regimen needs to be made. Anecdotal evidence supports this latter concept.

Several studies have shown that postoperative bleeding after minor oral surgery, including tooth extraction, is not significantly affected by long-term aspirin therapy. Although such studies are not currently available with respect to thienopyridines such as clopidogrel—either taken alone or with aspirin—an advisory report regarding patients with coronary artery stents states **"there is little or no indication to interrupt antiplatelet drugs for dental procedures."** (See Grines et al., 2007.) This conclusion is based on a paucity of reported bleeding problems after dental procedures, easy access to the affected tissues, and the high effectiveness of local measures in controlling oral bleeding. Should **unusual circumstances** dictate the need to restore platelet function to normal before treatment, withholding antiplatelet drugs for **3 to 7 days** may be necessary because of the irreversible nature of the antiplatelet actions of aspirin and clopidogrel. The patient's physician should be involved in any plan to limit antiplatelet therapy. Local measures coupled with platelet transfusion as required may be necessary if the clinical situation is emergent or too risky to have the patient off these medications for several days.

The **direct thrombin and factor Xa inhibitors** currently have **no data** to suggest how to guide the dentist/oral surgeon in managing patients prior to surgery. Generally if the **aPTT is normal,** it can be argued that it is safer to leave the patients on these medications rather than discontinue them for a period of time, particularly if the extent of planned surgery is minor. If more extensive bleeding is expected, or **if the aPTT is elevated,** consultation with the physician becomes necessary. Generally they will remove the patient from these medications for 2 to 3 days prior to surgery and restart the following day after surgery.

Hemophiliacs

Managing a patient with hemophilia and other coagulopathies has become significantly easier in recent years, but many issues require

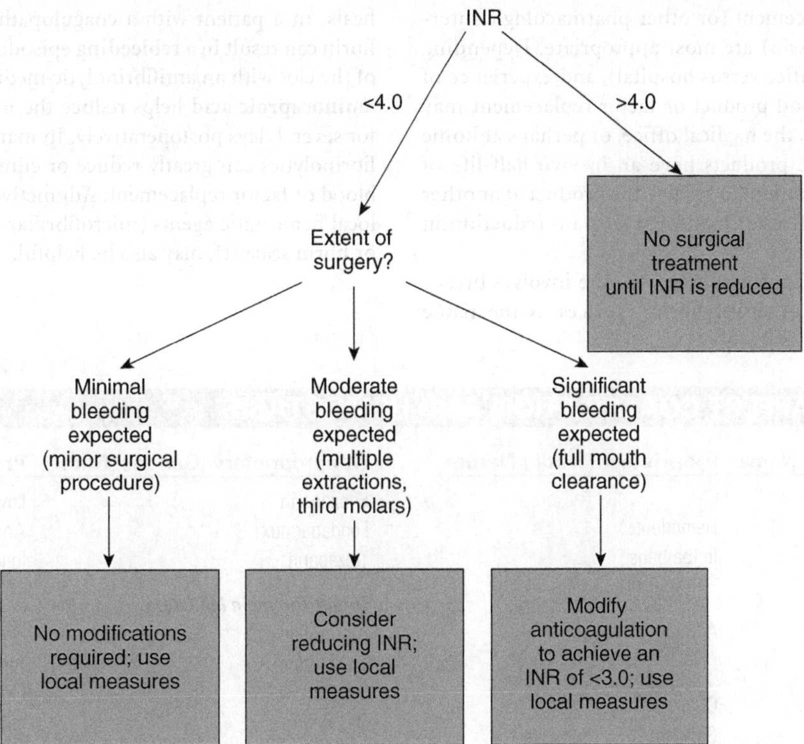

FIG 26-8 Flow chart for determining the appropriateness of dental therapy based on the prothrombin time. *INR*, International normalized ratio. (From Beirne OR, Koehler JR: Surgical management of patients on warfarin sodium. *J Oral Maxillofac Surg* 54:1115–1118, 1996.)

careful consideration before proceeding. The most difficult problem a hemophilic faces outside of dentistry is not the threat of exsanguination from a small laceration but rather the problems encountered from a massive muscle bleed or chronic joint disease resulting from hemarthroses. In dentistry, surgical procedures must be planned so that replacement factor can be given preoperatively and postoperatively. Most patients can now be treated routinely in either the hospital or dental office.

An important issue involves prediction of where an uncontrolled hematoma might develop in the head and neck region. Any potential space that might support the movement of blood through fascial planes toward crucial structures (e.g., the airway or major blood vessels) needs to be considered for "vented" wound management. In these areas, suturing to a tight, primary closure may be contraindicated so as to allow any accumulation of blood to drain preferentially into the oral cavity rather than fill crucial spaces. Conversely, whenever the wound site is sufficiently removed from worrisome dissection paths (e.g., an anterior frenectomy), closure should be sutured tightly to help control localized bleeding. For similar reasons, the dentist must take care that inferior alveolar or posterior superior alveolar nerve block injections of local anesthetic are adequately covered by **factor replacement** to reduce the risk of hemorrhage into muscle or one of the parapharyngeal areas or both. The use of a commercial **intraosseous anesthetic delivery system** (Stabident, X-Tip) is indicated for patients in whom block anesthesia is contraindicated. Profound anesthesia usually can be easily obtained with minimal hemorrhage risk when these systems are used in hemophiliacs.

Associated disorders that commonly occur with hemophiliacs also may affect the delivery of dental care. Hemophiliacs often have joint disorders resulting from **hemarthrosis**. Any spontaneous or trauma-induced bleeding into the synovial space of a joint may cause permanent damage if inflammatory by-products, produced as the blood breaks down, damage the surrounding cartilaginous and bony structures. Knees, ankles, and elbows are most commonly affected, and many hemophiliacs have permanent limitation of motion in their joints by the time they reach adulthood. Joint replacement surgery is common in patients with severe hemophilia. As a result, mobility in and out of the operatory and positioning in the chair itself may be compromised.

Because of the historic necessity of transfusing hemophiliacs with pooled human blood products before recombinant factor replacements were available or the products were treated with heat or solvent detergent to inactivate viruses, many hemophilic patients were infected with HIV, hepatitis B virus, and hepatitis C virus. Seroconversion to HIV began around 1979 and accelerated rapidly until the mid-1980s. Many of these patients have since died. Screening donors began in the 1970s for hepatitis B, in 1985 for HIV, and in 1990 for hepatitis C. This screening has significantly reduced, but not eliminated, the viral risk. Noninfected hemophiliacs (primarily children and teens) are now being given recombinant factor replacements, whereas infected hemophiliacs more often select pooled human-derived, virally inactivated products. In uninfected patients for whom no recombinant factor replacement is available, and especially in families with vWD that is not responsive to desmopressin, the use of single-donor cryoprecipitate (usually a family member) for all necessary transfusions has proved effective in reducing the risk for viral transmission.

When surgical procedures are required in hemophiliacs, it is imperative that the dentist **work closely with a hematologist** well versed in the care of these patients. The dentist should describe the nature of the proposed surgery, the expected amount of bleeding, and the normal postoperative course after the procedure. In this way, the hemophilia treatment center can best plan how much and which kinds of factor replacement (or other pharmacologic intervention, such as desmopressin) are most appropriate. Depending on the training, location (office versus hospital), and experience of the treating dentist, the blood product or factor replacement may be given in the dental office, the medical office, or perhaps at home by the patient. Most of the products have an in vivo half-life of several hours, allowing the patient to receive the product at another site and go to the dental office for treatment with no reduction in hemostatic ability.

The normal healing mechanism of a wound site involves breakdown and reestablishment of newer fibrin matrices as the tissue heals. In a patient with a coagulopathy, the normal breakdown of fibrin can result in a **rebleeding** episode a few days later. Stabilization of the clot with an antifibrinolytic medication such as **tranexamic or aminocaproic acid** helps reduce the incidence of bleeding episodes for several days postoperatively. In many cases, the use of these antifibrinolytics can greatly reduce or eliminate the need for additional blood or factor replacement. Adjunctive measures, such as the use of local hemostatic agents (microfibrillar collagen, suturing, thrombin, or fibrin sealant), may also be helpful.

AGENTS THAT AFFECT COAGULATION AND HEMOSTASIS

Nonproprietary (Generic) Name	Proprietary (Trade) Name
Astringents-Styptics	
Aluminum chloride	Hemodent
Tannic acid	In tea bags
Vasoconstrictor	
Epinephrine	Adrenalin
Topical Procoagulants	
Absorbable gelatin film	Gelfilm
Absorbable gelatin powder	Gelfoam
Absorbable gelatin sponge	Gelfoam, Surgifoam
Absorbable gelatin sponge with thrombin (human)	Gelfoam Plus
Fibrin sealant (human)	Artiss, Tisseel
Gelatin matrix with thrombin (human)	FloSeal
Microfibrillar collagen	Avitene
Oxidized cellulose	Oxycel
Oxidized regenerated cellulose	Surgicel
Thrombin (bovine)	Thrombin-JMI
Thrombin (recombinant)	RECOTHROM
Systemic Procoagulants	See Table 26-2
Fibrinolytics	
Alteplase (t-PA)	Activase
Anistreplase	Eminase
Reteplase	Retavase
Streptokinase	Streptase
Tenecteplase	TNKase
Urokinase (u-PA)	Abbokinase
Fibrinolysis Inhibitors	
Aminocaproic acid	Amicar
Tranexamic acid	Cyklokapron (IV) Lysteda (tablets)
Directly Acting Anticoagulants	
Unfractionated Heparin	
Heparin[†]	—
Low-Molecular-Weight Heparins	
Ardeparin*	Normiflo
Dalteparin	Fragmin
Enoxaparin	Lovenox
Fondaparinux	Arixtra
Tinzaparin	Innohep
Direct Thrombin Inhibitors	
Argatroban	Novastan
Bivalirudin	Angiomax
Dabigatran	Pradaxa
Desirudin	Iprivask
Hirudin	*Hirudo medicinalis*[‡]
Lepirudin	Refludan
Factor Xa Inhibitors	
Apixaban	Eliquis
Betrixaban	
Edoxaban	Savaysa
Rivaroxaban	Xarelto
Indirectly Acting Anticoagulants	
Warfarin	Coumadin
Antidotes for Anticoagulants	
Idarucizumab	Praxbind
Menadiol* (vitamin K_4)	Synkayvite
Menadione (vitamin K_3)	—
Phytonadione (vitamin K_1)	Mephyton
Prothrombin complex concentrate (human)	Kcentra
Protamine sulfate	—
Platelet Inhibitors	
Abciximab	ReoPro
Aspirin	
Cangrelor	Kengreal
Clopidogrel	Plavix
Dipyridamole	Persantine
Prasugrel	Effient
Eptifibatide	Integrilin
Ticlopidine	Ticlid
Tirofiban	Aggrastat
Coagulation Factors	*Listed in chapter*

*Not currently available in the United States.
[†]Available in calcium and sodium salts.
[‡]Organism of origin.

CASE DISCUSSION

Given Mr. J's history of ongoing cardiac issues, it is recommended that you consult with his medical doctor to confirm that his overall health can handle the stress of multiple extractions in the outpatient office setting. If not, then referral to an oral surgeon or hospital dentist who performs the procedure in an operating room with a cardiac anesthesiologist is best. Assuming that he can be managed conservatively, then ordering INR and aPTT tests is indicated. If both of these tests come back within therapeutic limits (INR<3.0 and aPTT normal), then no alteration to his anticoagulation may be necessary. If the managing MD is comfortable stopping the dabigatran for 2 to 3 days prior to the procedure, this will gain you an extra margin of safety. However, if not, then it may be best to keep the patient on the anticoagulant and plan to treat in a controlled hospital setting. It may also be wise to consider phased extractions (a few teeth at a time) rather than attempting to remove all of the teeth in one visit.

Should intraoperative hemorrhage become greater than expected, use of suturing (ideally primary closure) and collagen plugs (+/– reconstituted thrombin) is recommended. Of course, direct firm sustained gauze pressure is always required. This will be effective the vast majority of the time. If this fails to adequately control the bleeding, stop the procedure, and prepare the patient for transport to your local hospital for additional expert management.

GENERAL REFERENCES

1. *AHFS drug information 2015*, Bethesda, MD, 2015, American Society of Health-System Pharmacists.
2. Grines CL, Bonow RO, Casey Jr DE: Prevention of premature discontinuation of dual antiplatelet therapy in patients with coronary artery stents: a science advisory from the American Heart Association, American College of Cardiology, Society for Cardiovascular Angiography and Interventions, American College of Surgeons, and American Dental Association, with representation from the American College of Physicians, *J Am Dent Assoc* 138:652–655, 2007.
3. Hillman RS, Ault KA, Leporrier M, Rinder H: *Hematology in clinical practice*, ed 5, New York, 2010, McGraw-Hill.
4. Kaushansky K, Lichtman MA, Beutler E, et al.: *Williams hematology*, ed 8, New York, 2010, McGraw-Hill.
5. Papadakis MA, McPhee SJ, Rabow MW, editors: *Current medical diagnosis and treatment 2015*, Stamford, CT, 2015, Lange Medical Books/McGraw-Hill.
6. Weitz J: Blood coagulation and anticoagulant, fibrinolytic, and antiplatelet drugs. In Brunton LL, Chabner B, Knollman B, editors: *Goodman & Gillman's the pharmacological basis of therapeutics*, ed 12, New York, 2010, McGraw-Hill.

27

Drugs Acting on the Respiratory System

Karen S. Gregson and Jeffrey D. Bennett

KEY INFORMATION

- Asthma is defined as a chronic inflammatory disorder of the airways associated with airway hyperresponsiveness.
- Symptoms of asthma include episodes of wheezing, breathlessness, chest tightness, and coughing with a widespread, variable, and often reversible airflow limitation.
- Severity of asthma is measured with spirometry.
- The percentage decrease of forced expiratory volume in 1 second (FEV_1) after a methacholine or histamine challenge defines asthma as mild, moderate, or severe.
- Drugs used to treat asthma include short- and long-acting beta adrenergic receptor agonists, corticosteroids, leukotriene modulators, cromolyn, and omalizumab.
- Chronic obstructive pulmonary disease (COPD) is defined as a progressive airflow-limiting disease that is not reversible, which has a component of abnormal inflammatory responsiveness to noxious stimuli.
- Classification of severity of COPD is measured with spirometry.
- The degree by which forced expiratory volume in 1 second (FEV_1) differs from predicted, indicates mild, moderate, or severe disease.
- Treatment guidelines are based on measurements of severity of disease.
- Drugs used to treat COPD include short- and long-acting beta agonists, corticosteroids, phosphodiesterase-4 inhibitors, anticholinergics, and theophylline.

CASE STUDY

Miss G is a 19-year-old patient. She has a history of asthma, which has been classified as mild persistent. She had been taking montelukast 10 mg at bedtime. She rarely uses her albuterol inhaler. However, 2 months ago with the changing weather, she presented to her physician with difficulty breathing. He prescribed prednisone 10 mg daily for 2 weeks. Since that time, her medications have been montelukast 10 mg at bedtime, beclomethasone inhaler 40 mcg q 12 hours, and albuterol inhaler prn. She uses the albuterol about once daily. She denies any illicit drug history; however, she has not previously taken NSAIDs. The patient presents with pain and mild swelling associated with tooth #17. A diagnosis of pericoronitis is made. The site is irrigated with Peridex. This is the third time you have managed an exacerbation of this patient's pericoronitis. You have previously referred the patient to have her partial impacted mandibular third molars extracted. The patient is anxious and has missed more than one prior appointment to have her partial impacted teeth extracted because of her anxiety. How would you manage this patient at this time?

PATHOPHYSIOLOGY OF ASTHMA

Asthma is a chronic inflammatory disease of the airways associated with acute symptoms, exacerbations, and airway remodeling. The acute symptoms, bronchospasm and wheezing, can be reversed by bronchodilators (Fig. 27-1). Exacerbations and airway remodeling are caused by chronic inflammation. Exacerbations can be controlled with antiinflammatory drugs. There is no defined treatment for airway remodeling. Early and late-phase asthma reactions are outlined in Table 27-1. The result of the early phase reaction is bronchoconstriction. The inflammatory mediators released in the late phase play a role in the enhancement of nonspecific bronchial hyperresponsiveness and airway remodeling.

The chronic inflammation seen in the airways in patients with asthma is a complex process in which the whole mucosal immune system appears to be involved. Cell survival in airway tissues plays a role in chronic inflammation. The tissue load in inflammatory sites is controlled by apoptosis of epithelial cells. In asthma the persistence of inflammation is thought to be an alteration of the regulation of apoptosis of epithelial cells. Characteristics of chronic inflammation include epithelial cell shedding and activation, the presence of mixed inflammatory infiltrates and lymphocytes, as well as many other cell types. There is also an increase of inflammatory mediators including endothelins and nitric oxide. The end result of chronic inflammation is remodeling of the airways. Activation of epithelial cells may be important in the regulation of airway remodeling and fibrosis as these cells release fibrogenic growth factors. The airway structural changes include increased thickness of the airway wall and increased muscle mass and mucous glands. Some of the clinical consequences of airway remodeling are increased resistance to airflow, bronchial contraction and bronchial hyperresponsiveness, increased mucus secretion and exudate, and increased surface tension favoring airway closure. While drug therapy does not reverse the effects of airway remodeling, it does decrease the chronic inflammation that plays an important role in this serious complication of asthma.

PATHOPHYSIOLOGY OF COPD

COPD is a progressive condition characterized by irreversible airflow limitation. The major etiologic factor is cigarette smoking (Fig. 27-2). Cigarette smoke is a complex mixture of 4700 compounds including high concentrations of free radicals and other oxidants. Inflammation of the lungs as a reaction to cigarette smoke is characteristic of the disease and is thought to produce lung injury. Symptoms of COPD include chronic cough with sputum

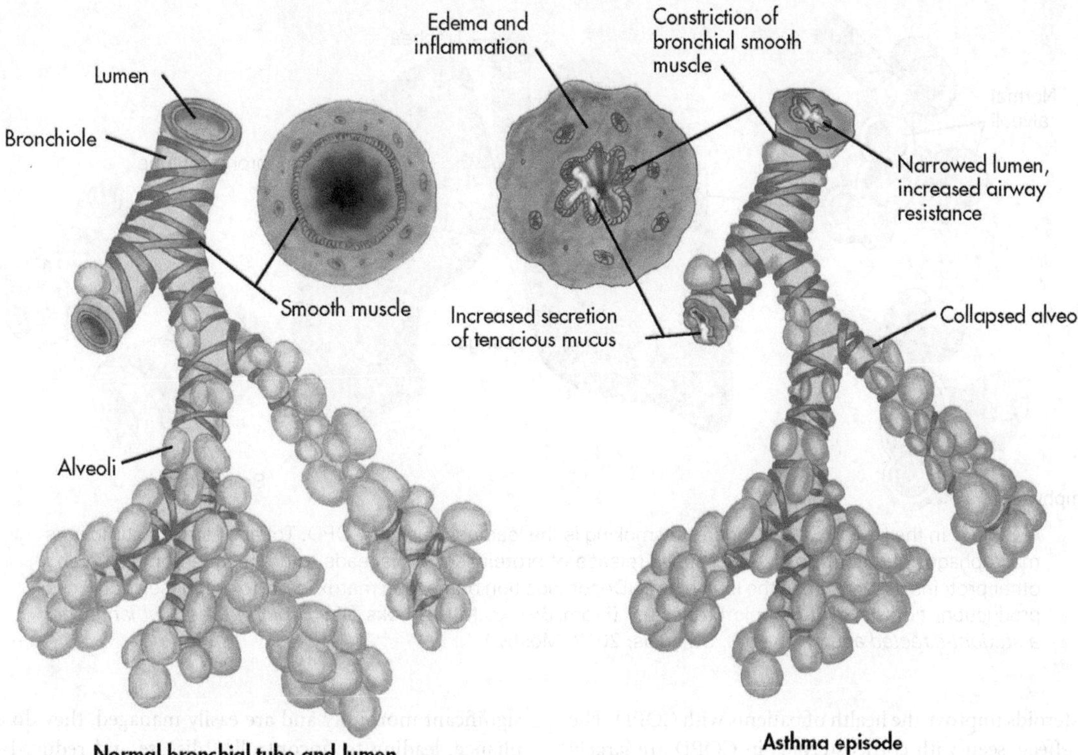

FIG 27-1 Asthma is a reversible, chronic inflammatory disorder of the airways. There is an airway hyperresponsiveness with symptoms of wheezing, breathlessness, chest tightness, and coughing. (From Christensen BL, Kockrow EO: *Foundations of nursing,* ed 6, St. Louis, 2011, Mosby.)

TABLE 27-1 Asthma Pathophysiology: Bronchial Constriction and Airway Inflammation*

Early Phase (10-20 minutes)	Late Phase (6-9 hours)
IgE binds to receptors on mast cells	Activated T_H2 lymphocytes release cytokines that recruit more proinflammatory cells
↓	↓
Mast cells degranulate and release histamine, proteolytic enzymes, cytokines, leukotrienes, and prostaglandins	Eosinophils Mast cells IgE-producing B cells
↓	↓
Bronchoconstriction, vasodilation, and airway inflammation	Airway hyperresponsiveness, edema, mucus production, fibrosis, and airway remodeling

*Sequence of events in the early phase and late phase of asthma. Asthma is caused by airway inflammation and bronchial constriction. Airway remodeling, which results from chronic inflammation and subsequent replacement of normal airway tissue with scar tissue, can weaken lung function and lung growth. While drugs are available to reverse inflammation and promote bronchodilation, drugs that reverse the effects of remodeling are not available.

production and breathlessness upon exertion. There is also a systemic component to the disease involving various organs including skeletal muscle, the central nervous system, and the cardiovascular system. Systemic inflammation intensifies with progression of COPD and has been linked to cardiovascular events, muscle wasting, and colon cancer.

Chronic bronchitis, emphysema, and small airway disease are present in variable degrees in patients with COPD. Chronic bronchitis is an innate immune response to the inhaled toxic particles in cigarette smoke. Emphysema is defined as enlargement of the distal airspaces beyond the terminal bronchioles caused by destruction of the airway walls (see Fig. 27-2). Airway obstruction in the smaller conducting airways is caused by inflammatory mucous exudates.

The presence of CD8+ lymphocytes and CD4+ cells suggests chronic immune stimulation in the airway epithelial cells. Neutrophils and macrophages are found in the sputum, lung parenchyma, and bronchoalveolar lavage fluid from patients with COPD. Each cell type is activated by cigarette smoke. Activation causes the release of reactive oxidant species and proteases by neutrophils. Macrophage activation induces the synthesis and secretion of inflammatory mediators such as tumor necrosis factor α (TNF-α), interleukin 8 (IL-8), monocyte chemotactic peptide-1, and leukotriene B4. Inflammation in the lungs may be further intensified by an imbalance between histone acetylation and deacetylation. Oxidants are believed to interact with histone deacetylase. Nitrosylation of tyrosine residues in histone deacetylase decreases enzymatic activity and leads to an enhancement of inflammatory gene expression through chromatin remodeling.

CORTICOSTEROIDS

Pharmacologic Effects

The pharmacologic effects of steroids on inflammatory lung diseases indicate that they are very effective at controlling symptoms of the disease, but they do not cure the disease. When the steroid dose is reduced or the steroid is discontinued, the symptoms eventually return. In asthma, **corticosteroids reduce airway inflammation and hyperresponsiveness, improve lung function, decrease severity, and reduce the occurrence of acute asthma exacerbations.** Clinical data show

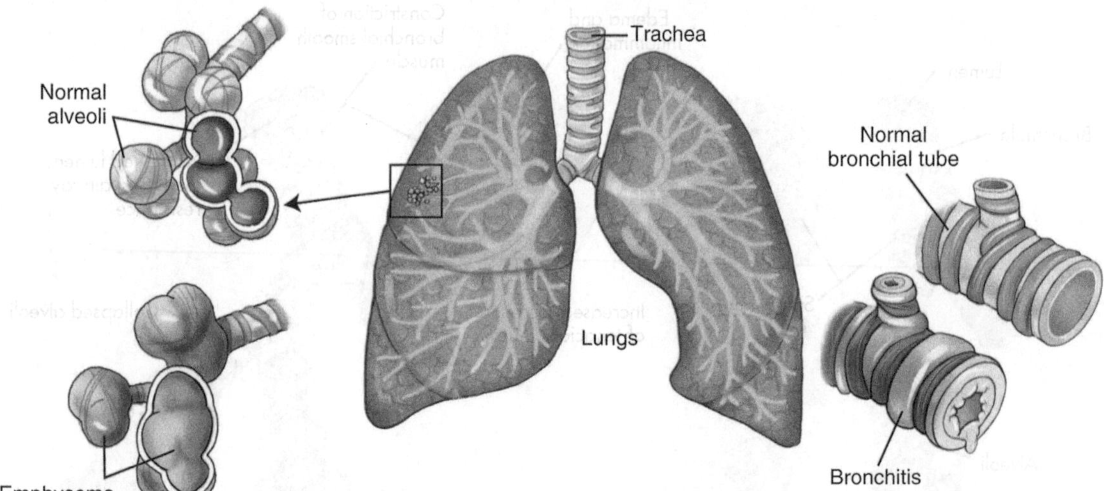

FIG 27-2 In the United States, cigarette smoking is the leading cause of COPD. Tobacco smoke stimulates macrophages and neutrophils and causes release of proteinases. This leads to degradation of elastin and other proteins that compose the lung matrix. Decomposition of the lung matrix leads to emphysema, mucus production, fibrosis, and chronic bronchitis. (From Brooks ML, Brooks DL: *Exploring medical language: a student-directed approach*, ed 8, St. Louis, 2012, Mosby.)

inhaled corticosteroids improve the health of patients with COPD. The pharmacologic effects seen with corticosteroids in COPD are largely the same as seen with asthma, but they also reduce systemic inflammation and reduce the rate of decline of health in patients with COPD.

Efficacy and Safety

The optimal route of administration of corticosteroids for inflammatory lung disease is inhalation. Inhalation delivers the drug directly to the lungs. The corticosteroid acts locally, which minimizes the systemic adverse effects encountered with oral or parenteral administration. Receptor binding affinity is the only pharmacodynamic parameter that varies among the corticosteroids that are available for inhalation. High binding affinity can be considered a desirable trait providing for better efficacy in the lung. High binding affinity can also be detrimental as it can lead to increased systemic adverse effects.

The differences between the inhaled products are dependent upon such factors as formulation, pulmonary and systemic bioavailability, and excretion. Characteristics that enhance the efficacy of inhaled corticosteroids include small particle size and long pulmonary residence time. Solution aerosols formulated with hydrofluoroalkane, and a glucocorticoid such as ciclesonide and beclomethasone dipropionate, have a small mass median aerodynamic diameter (MMAD) of < 2 μm. A small MMAD can have effects on efficacy as the smallest airways have an internal perimeter of 2 μm. MMAD can also have an impact on local adverse effects, as larger particles are more likely to be deposited in the oropharyngeal cavity. Pulmonary residence time is dependent upon two factors: lipophilicity and lipid conjugation. Lipophilic side chains on the D-ring of the steroid portion of the drug slow the dissolution in aqueous bronchial fluid. Lipophilic groups also aid the passage of the drug through the phospholipid bilayer of cell membranes to the receptors in the cell. Lipid conjugation to fatty acids in the pulmonary cells occurs via a reversible ester bond. Esterification provides a slow-release reservoir of the corticosteroid prolonging residence time. This confers a once-a-day dosing schedule to **budesonide** and **desisobutyryl ciclesonide**.

Adverse Effects

The most common adverse effects of inhaled corticosteroids are topical, **oropharyngeal candidiasis,** and dysphonia. While they cause no significant morbidity and are easily managed, they do diminish compliance, leading to uncontrolled disease and reduced quality of life. Less common adverse effects of inhaled corticosteroids are systemic, including adrenal suppression, bone loss, skin thinning, metabolic changes, behavioral abnormalities, weight gain, and decreased linear growth in children. The concentration of the corticosteroid in the blood is a combination of the portion that is swallowed and the portion that is delivered to and absorbed from the lungs.

The safety of inhaled corticosteroids is dependent upon factors such as activation in the lungs, low oral bioavailability, and high protein binding and rapid systemic clearance. While most corticosteroids are inhaled in their pharmacologically active form, **beclomethasone dipropionate** does undergo metabolism in the human lung. Beclomethasone dipropionate is metabolized to beclomethasone-17 monopropionate, which has a relative receptor affinity about 30 times greater than the parent compound. Metabolism in human plasma is quite different from that of human lung. Human lung metabolism involves a simple hydrolysis reaction to the active form. Metabolism in human plasma results in **beclomethasone-21 monopropionate,** which has no binding affinity for the glucocorticoid receptor. This differential metabolism in lung and plasma leads to fewer systemic effects of beclomethasone. **Ciclesonide** is metabolized to dec-ciclesonide by esterases located in human lung. Dec-ciclesonide has a relative receptor binding affinity 120 times that of ciclesonide. Metabolism of ciclesonide in the oropharynx region is very low, resulting in low amounts of active drug entering the systemic circulation by swallowing. Thus, selective activation in the lung can improve the safety profile of an inhaled corticosteroid. The degree of protein binding can also affect the safety of an inhaled corticosteroid. Protein binding to albumin in the blood controls the systemic unbound concentrations and limits adverse effects.

BRONCHODILATORS

Beta-2 Agonists (Long-Acting Versus Short-Acting)

Beta-2 adrenergic agonists are structurally modified catecholamines. Structural modifications confer increased β_2 receptor selectivity, enhanced oral activity, and an extended duration of action after inhalation. Susceptibility to degradation by catechol-O-methyl transferase and reuptake mechanisms in neurons are decreased by structural modifications. There are two types of β_2 adrenergic agonist: short-acting β_2 agonists (SABAs) and the long-acting β_2 agonists (LABAs). The short-acting type has bronchodilatory effects for 4 to 6 hours, exemplified by **albuterol**. The long-acting type has bronchodilatory effects for 12 hours and bronchoprotective effects for 6 to 12 hours. An example is **salmeterol**. Both short-acting and long-acting types were designed along the same structure activity principals. Both albuterol and salmeterol have an identical active moiety, a saligenin head group. However, salmeterol has an extended aliphatic side chain that was designed to anchor the drug in or near the receptor.

There are two theories proposed to explain the increased duration of action of the LABAs. Using site-directed mutagenesis of the β_2 receptor, Green and coworkers (See references) proposed that the aliphatic side chain of salmeterol binds in a second locus of the receptor, termed the exosite, which is separate from the active site. In the second theory, termed the **diffusion microkinetic theory,** the high membrane partition affinity of the two drugs creates a microdepot of the drug near the receptor. The exact nature of the sustained duration of action is likely to relate to aspects of the clinical pharmacology and tolerability of LABAs.

Mechanism of Action

The β_2 adrenergic receptor is a member of the 7-transmembrane receptor superfamily of G protein–coupled receptors. The β_2 adrenergic receptor is linked to an increase in cyclic AMP and activation of protein kinase A (PKA) (see Chapter 1). PKA phosphorylates protein substrates that control calcium effects in smooth muscle cells (see Chapter 21). With decreased calcium availability and decreased sensitivity of airway smooth muscle to calcium, the tissue relaxes passively.

Pharmacologic Effects

Bronchodilation is not the sole pharmacologic effect of β_2 receptor activation. Other effects include reduction of inflammatory cytokine production, suppression of plasma exudation due to receptor presence on postcapillary venules, regulation of fluid balance in alveolar epithelial cells, and reduction of cholinergic neurotransmission. In asthma and COPD, β_2 adrenergic agonists not only cause bronchodilation, but they also offer bronchoprotection, or reduced responsiveness, to noxious stimuli.

Adverse Effects

The most serious adverse effect of β_2 adrenergic receptor agonist use is an increase in sensitivity of the smooth muscle in the lungs to noxious stimuli. Paradoxically, an increased incidence of asthma exacerbations and morbidity and mortality is seen after long-term use of β_2 agonists. This is attributable to the loss of the effects of bronchoprotection and bronchodilation effects of the drugs. This effect is called receptor desensitization, a state of refractoriness that occurs following prolonged exposure to an agonist. The mechanistic basis for receptor desensitization is discussed in Chapter 1. Receptor downregulation is also a related factor that is discussed in Chapter 1. It is not the intermittent, short-acting β_2 agonists, like albuterol, that lead to loss of effect but rather the regular use of the long-acting β_2 agonists. The FDA has required manufacturers of the long-acting β_2 agonists to place a "black box" warning on the physician information for LABAs.

All β_2 agonists are racemic mixtures of R- and S-enantiomers. While the R-enantiomer of albuterol, **levalbuterol**, has 100 times more affinity for the receptor, the S-enantiomer of albuterol is metabolized much more slowly and therefore retained in the lung. Preclinical data indicate that S-albuterol is associated with proinflammatory activity that can lead to bronchial hyperresponsiveness. These activities include an increase in intracellular calcium, an increase in inflammatory stimuli, an increase in eosinophil activation, and recruitment and an increase in mucin production. These proinflammatory activities have led to speculation that the S-enantiomer of **salmeterol** is responsible for the loss of effect seen with long-term use of this drug.

Albuterol

Albuterol, the most commonly prescribed β_2-adrenergic bronchodilator is available in tablet form, as a sustained-release tablet, and as a metered-dose pressurized aerosol. Pulmonary β_2 specificity is greater with aerosol delivery than it is with an oral dose. Adverse reactions to **albuterol** are similar to those of other β_2-adrenergic receptor agonists.

Salmeterol

Salmeterol is a long-acting highly selective β_2-adrenergic agent structurally related to albuterol. Compared with albuterol, salmeterol has greater β_2 receptor selectivity but decreased intrinsic activity. The receptor selectivity and the intrinsic activity differences of the drug minimize cardiac side effects. Salmeterol provides bronchodilation that usually lasts at least 12 hours. Salmeterol is relatively slow in onset (approximately 10 minutes), and maximal bronchodilation takes hours. It is not indicated for the symptomatic relief of acute asthma. Side effects, such as tachycardia, tremor, hypokalemia, and hyperglycemia, are minimal at standard doses.

Incorporating a long-acting β_2 agonist into the therapeutic regimen has several advantages. Clinical trials have shown salmeterol to be more efficacious than albuterol in (1) reducing variation in diurnal peak expiratory flow rates; (2) decreasing nocturnal symptoms, asthma exacerbations, and the need for rescue medications; and (3) increasing overall lung function. The combination of salmeterol with an inhaled corticosteroid has been shown to be beneficial. Several studies have demonstrated that the administration of salmeterol with a lower dose of corticosteroid results in improved pulmonary function compared with a larger dose of corticosteroid administered alone. In addition to the improved physiologic response, the administration of salmeterol decreases the potential of systemic effects of corticosteroids.

OTHER ADRENERGIC AGONISTS

Epinephrine

Epinephrine may be administered by oral inhalations from a nebulizer or metered-dose inhaler. The inhaler is generally favored because it is effective, less expensive, and more portable. The therapeutic effect is weak and transient compared to the longer-acting β_2 agonists resistant to metabolism by catechol-o-methyl transferase (COMT). Signs of overdose include nervousness, restlessness, sleeplessness, bronchial irritation, and tachycardia. Inhalation of recommended dosages may minimize reactions other than bronchodilation. However, patients will frequently have palpitation and tremors that increase with increased use. The occurrence of these signs and symptoms usually limits the use of this drug because patients tend not to tolerate these effects.

Parenteral epinephrine is reserved for acute episodes of asthma requiring immediate relief when inhaled β_2-selective agonists have proved ineffective or could not be effectively administered. In such cases, 0.2 to 0.5 mg may be injected subcutaneously or intramuscularly to produce bronchodilation. Because epinephrine produces α- as well as β-adrenergic receptor stimulation, it can also improve respiration by relieving congestion of the bronchial mucosa.

Interaction Between Corticosteroids and β_2 Agonists

Corticosteroids and β_2 agonists have different mechanisms of action and are used to treat patients with asthma and COPD. Coadministration of the two classes of drugs results in a synergistic effect as each drug enhances the activity of the other. Corticosteroids can protect against receptor desensitization, thereby increasing adenylyl cyclase activity and cAMP accumulation with β_2 agonists. The β_2 receptor gene contains several glucocorticoid response element (GRE) sites in the promoter region, enabling corticosteroids to increase the rate of transcription of β_2 receptors. This effect can offset one of the mechanisms for desensitization, namely receptor downregulation seen in long-term use of β_2 agonists. The efficiency of coupling is increased between the β_2 receptor and G_s after administration of corticosteroids with the resulting increase in the concentration of cAMP in the cell.

Long-acting β_2 agonists can promote the translocation of the corticosteroid receptor to the nucleus even with no corticosteroid present. When a corticosteroid is added, the translocation of the receptor is accelerated, and the rate of GRE-dependent expression of corticosteroid inducible genes is enhanced. An increase in smooth muscle bulk is a pathologic feature of asthma that leads to bronchial hyperplasia and bronchial hyperactivity. Coadministration of β_2 agonists and corticosteroids induces p21, a kinase inhibitor that plays a role in inhibition of proliferation and apoptosis, thus decreasing smooth muscle bulk.

PHOSPHODIESTERASE-4 INHIBITORS

Upregulation of phosphodiesterase-4, the enzyme responsible for degradation of cAMP, is thought to play a role in the loss of effect of β_2 agonists. **Roflumilast** is a phosphodiesterase-4 inhibitor that inhibits the degradation of cAMP, which decreases the number of COPD exacerbations. Adverse effects include changes in mood or behavior problems, including thoughts of suicide or dying, attempt to commit suicide, trouble sleeping (insomnia), new or worse anxiety, new or worse depression, acting on dangerous impulses or other unusual changes in behavior or mood, and weight loss.

ANTICHOLINERGICS

Muscarinic acetylcholine receptors are physiologically important, but medications directed to these receptors are not commonly used because of the difficulty in targeting a specific organ or tissue. The advantage of targeting the respiratory system is in the route of administration, inhalation. The mechanism of action of the anticholinergic drugs in respiratory disease is competitive antagonism of acetylcholine at M_3 muscarinic receptors in the smooth muscle cells of the lungs (see Chapter 6). The result is bronchodilation. Anticholinergic bronchodilators are synthetic quaternary ammonium congeners of atropine; hence, they are poorly absorbed into the bloodstream when given by inhalation. The anticholinergic bronchodilators are classified according to half-life. **Ipratropium** is a short-acting anticholinergic with a half-life of 0.3 hour at M_3 muscarinic receptors. The half-life of **tiotropium**, a long-acting anticholinergic, at M_3 muscarinic receptors is 35 hours. Ipratropium is also used in a combination inhaler with albuterol, which is indicated for use in patients with COPD. It is used four times a day. Tiotropium is also used in patients with COPD, but because of its long half-life, it can be administered once a day. Adverse effects for both drugs are mild, dry mouth, altered taste, and coughing after administration.

THEOPHYLLINE

Mechanism of Action

Theophylline is a naturally occurring plant alkaloid related to caffeine and theobromine. Theophylline causes an increase in the concentration of cAMP in the cell through inhibition of phosphodiesterase-3 and 4. As with the β_2 agonists, an increase in cAMP concentration leads ultimately to a decrease in available calcium in the cell and smooth muscle relaxation. In addition to bronchodilation, theophylline also has antiinflammatory effects, which are exerted through stimulation of histone deacetylases (HDAC). The exact mechanism of action of theophylline on HDAC is not completely understood. This action differs from that of the corticosteroids in that the steroids recruit HDAC to the active transcription site with no direct effect on HDAC activation. There is evidence to suggest that the action of theophylline on HDAC is more direct.

Pharmacologic Effects

Theophylline has been used for over 60 years in asthma and COPD for bronchodilatory effects. Antiinflammatory effects of theophylline include inhibition of the late response to allergen, reduced infiltration of eosinophils and CD4+ lymphocytes into the airways, and a decrease in the concentration of interleukin-8 and neutrophil chemotactic responses. In vitro, theophylline inhibits mediator release from mast cells, reactive oxygen species release from macrophages and eosinophils, and cytokine release from monocytes and T lymphocytes.

Adverse Effects

Theophylline has a narrow therapeutic window with therapeutic plasma concentrations between 10 and 20 mg/L. Above 20 mg/L, serious effects such as ventricular arrhythmias, seizures, and even death can occur. These serious adverse effects may be preceded by headache, abdominal discomfort, increased acid secretion, gastroesophageal reflex, diuresis, repetitive vomiting, and restlessness. Proper dosing of theophylline is dependent upon many patient factors including smoking history, cardiac disease, and hepatic disease. Serum concentration monitoring is often necessary due to the narrow therapeutic window.

LEUKOTRIENE MODIFIERS

Cysteinyl leukotrienes (cysLTs) are a class of lipid molecules that produce smooth muscle contraction and mucus secretion, induce allergic inflammatory cells, modulate cytokine production, influence neural transmission, and alter structure in the airway. Administration of cysLTs to experimental animals and humans produces symptoms that resemble allergic reactions and asthma.

Cysteinyl leukotrienes are produced in mast cells, eosinophils, and macrophages from arachidonic acid. Arachidonic acid is cleaved from membrane phospholipids and metabolized through the 5-lipoxygenase (5-LOX) pathway. Arachidonic acid is oxidized to leukotriene A_4 (LTA_4), which upon conjugation to glutathione is converted to LTC_4. LTC_4 is transported to the extracellular space and cleaved to LTD_4 and LTE_4. LTC_4, LTD_4, and LTE_4 all contain a cysteine residue and are collectively called cysLTs. Previously known as the slow-reacting substance of anaphylaxis, they stimulate airway smooth muscle by interacting with cysLT receptor type 1. It has been shown that they play a role in the inflammatory responses seen in asthma. LTA_4 can also be converted to LTB_4 by epoxide hydrolase in neutrophils and other inflammatory cells. LTB_4 is a neutrophil and eosinophil chemoattractant.

Bronchoalveolar lavage fluid shows an increase in cysLTs in asthmatic subjects after administration of allergen. The increases in cysLTs are not reduced by treatment with inhaled corticosteroids. Increases in cysLTs in the bronchi not only result from noxious stimuli. The drying of the airway and exercise can also stimulate cysLT production. Cysteinyl leukotrienes also interact with inflammatory pathways. Release of cysLTs from mast cells is seen in response to IgE ligation to the cell. Plasma hyperosmolarity and an increase in interstitial fluid volume in exercise-induced asthma and COX-1 inhibition in nonsteroidal antiinflammatory drug-intolerant asthma also cause release of cysLTs. Cysteinyl leukotrienes also promote the generation of chemokines and cytokines from airway smooth muscle, increase the expression of histamine receptors, amplify the effects of tachykinins in the airway, and have a role in the structural changes in the airway seen in asthma. There are two classes of drugs that are used to decrease the effects of the LT pathway in asthma: the leukotriene formation inhibitors and the leukotriene receptor antagonists.

Zileuton, an N-hydroxyurea derivative, **chelates the iron in the active site of 5-lipoxygenase blocking the redox potential of the enzyme** (Fig. 27-3). Zileuton is therefore able to not only block the formation of the but also that of LTB_4. The use of zileuton is not as extensive as that of the leukotriene receptor antagonists probably because of its short half-life and potential liver toxicity. Zileuton is orally bioavailable, with a half-life of 2 hours, and it must be administered 3 to 4 times a day. This can cause problems with patient adherence. Zileuton is contraindicated in liver disease, and liver enzymes must be monitored during therapy.

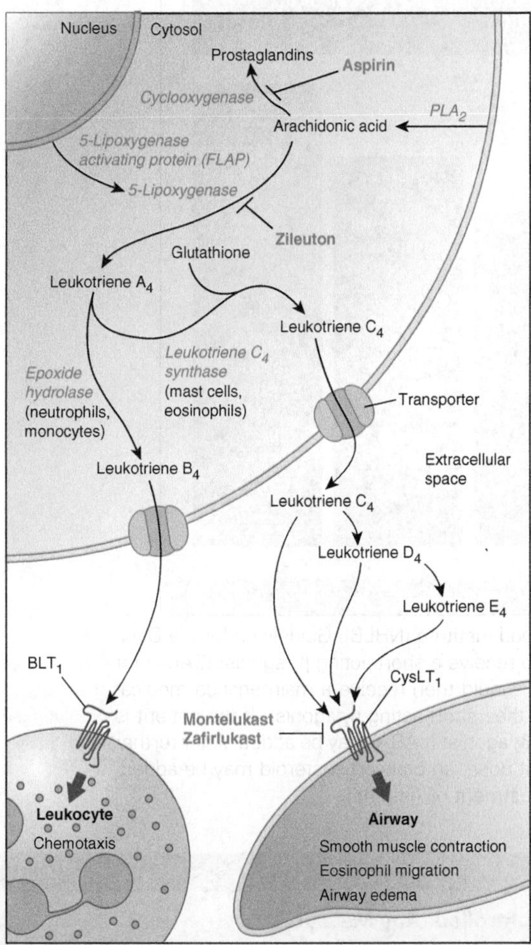

FIG 27-3 Sites of Action of Leukotriene Modifiers. Cysteinyl leukotrienes bind to CysLT1 receptors expressed on airway smooth muscle cells, leading to bronchoconstriction and airway edema. Leukotriene A_4 is converted to leukotriene B_4 by epoxide hydrolase in neutrophils and monocytes. Leukotriene B_4 is transported out of the cell and binds to BLT1 receptors expressed on leukocytes, leading to leukocyte chemotaxis and recruitment. The leukotriene pathway can be inhibited by the 5-lipoxygenase inhibitor zileuton or by the CysLT1 receptor antagonists montelukast and zafirlukast. *PLA_2*, Phospholipase A_2. (From Golan D, Armstrong EJ, Armstrong AW: Principles of Pharmacology: The Pathophysiologic Basis of Drug Therapy, ed. 4, Philadelphia, 2016, Wolters Kluwer.)

Montelukast and **zafirlukast** are **selective antagonists for the cell surface cysteinyl leukotrienes 1 receptor** (Fig. 27-3). They reduce airway hyperresponsiveness, eosinophils, and exhaled nitric oxide. They are orally active and are administered once daily and are generally well tolerated. Elevated levels of cysteinyl leukotrienes are found in chronic asthma with concomitant allergic rhinitis, exercise-induced asthma, and aspirin-sensitive asthma. It has been suggested that the leukotriene antagonists may have a specific role in these conditions.

OTHER DRUGS FOR ASTHMA

Cromolyn

Cromolyn is a non-bronchodilating, nonsteroidal drug used for prophylactic treatment of asthma. It is a synthetic derivative of khellin, the agent in extracts of the *Ammi visnaga* plant that produces smooth muscle relaxation. It is administered by inhalation. Although the mechanism of action is not fully understood, it is known that cromolyn inhibits the release of mediators from mast cells, as well as other inflammatory cells, probably by inhibiting the inflow of Ca^{2+} into the mast cells. The drug inhibits both early and late asthmatic responses and is effective in the long-term treatment of chronic asthma. Other biologic effects, including inhibition of afferent pulmonary nerve fiber receptors that contribute to reflex bronchoconstriction, may also be relevant to its therapeutic action.

Clinically, cromolyn is ineffective in the treatment of acute attacks of asthma, including status asthmaticus. It functions exclusively as a prophylactic agent in the management of chronic symptoms. Maximum benefit is obtained only after 4 weeks of treatment. Cromolyn has also been shown to be useful as a premedication before a challenging exercise, where the drug, similarly to steroids and leukotriene inhibitors, reduces airway hyperactivity. Both long-term and short-term studies have documented clinical improvement in patients taking cromolyn, with a low incidence of adverse effects. Indeed, cromolyn is one of the least toxic medications used for asthma. Most adverse reactions have been mild and have consisted mainly of wheezing, coughing, and dryness of the throat. There have been rare reports, however, of eosinophilia with pulmonary infiltration, pulmonary granulomatosis, and the development of subacute and acute allergic reactions. Generally, any patient who demonstrates a reaction other than a transitory irritative response is removed from cromolyn therapy.

During cromolyn treatment, patients are maintained on regular medication, such as oral bronchodilators. In cromolyn-treated patients receiving corticosteroids, there have been reports of a decreased corticosteroid requirement, which permits many patients to convert from a daily steroid schedule to an alternate-day program or to discontinue steroids completely. A decreased requirement for sympathomimetic and xanthine bronchodilators has also been noted. This mediation-sparing effect is one of the major advantages of cromolyn therapy. Cromolyn is generally available in a metered-dose aerosol unit and in a nebulizer solution. The availability of liquid cromolyn has been a major benefit to many asthmatics, especially young children.

Nedocromil is a drug whose action is very similar the that of cromolyn.

OMALIZUMAB

Immunoglobulin E (IgE) is produced by B cells after sensitization to an allergen. IgE plays a central role in the pathophysiology of allergic responses in patients with asthma. Epidemiologic studies suggest that between 60% and 80% of patients with asthma have rhinitis and 20% to 40% of patients with rhinitis have asthma. Even though the serum concentration of IgE is low, it is highly active due to the large number of high affinity receptors on mast cells and basophils. The binding of IgE to these cells initiates the inflammatory cascade and results in the release of many mediators, including histamine, leukotrienes, and platelet activating factor. The release of these mediators results in airway obstruction by smooth muscle contraction, vascular leakage, and secretion of mucus.

Omalizumab is a murine antihuman monoclonal anti-IgE antibody directed against an epitope on the fragment of IgE that binds to the high- and low-affinity receptor regions. This prevents free IgE from interacting with receptors on cellular targets. The antibody only binds to free IgE, not receptor-bound IgE. Thus the antibody does not cause receptor cross-linking and cell degranulation, which leads to anaphylaxis. The antibody causes a 99% reduction of free IgE. Since there are such a large number of receptors, the binding of omalizumab to IgE alone would not be sufficient to block IgE inflammatory reactions. Omalizumab also downregulates receptor expression on basophils. The reduction in both free IgE and IgE receptors results in inhibition of IgE-mediated inflammation.

The most frequent adverse reaction of omalizumab includes nasopharyngitis, upper respiratory tract infection, headache, and sinusitis. About 0.1% of patients experience urticaria, bronchospasm, hypotension, syncope, angioedema of the throat or tongue, and other symptoms of anaphylaxis. The onset of anaphylaxis can occur 2 to 24 hours after the administration of omalizumab and can occur after any dose. In February of 2007 the FDA required the manufacturer of omalizumab to place a boxed warning on the packaging to alert physicians of the possibility of anaphylactic reaction in patients after administration of omalizumab.

PHARMACOTHERAPY FOR ASTHMA

Patients must avoid tobacco and environmental irritants and allergens. Asthma treatment is progressive in steps and is based on the severity of the disease (Table 27-2 and Fig. 27-4). According to the current National Heart, Lung and Blood Institute (NHLBI) Guidelines

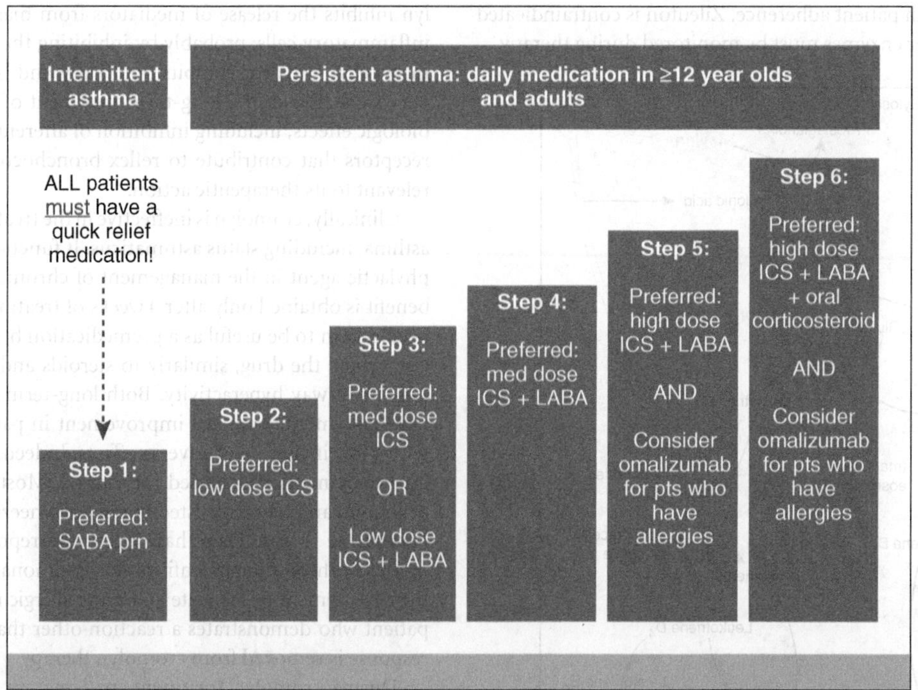

FIG 27-4 According to the current National Heart, Lung and Blood Institute (NHLBI) Guidelines for the Diagnosis and Treatment of Asthma, all patients with asthma should receive a short-acting β_2 agonist (SABA) for quick relief of bronchospasm. Patients with persistent asthma should then receive a maintenance medication, starting with an inhaled corticosteroid (ICS), in addition to their short-acting β_2 agonist. If the patient is not controlled, the ICS dose may be increased and a long-acting β_2 agonist (LABA) may be added. After further increasing the ICS dose and elevating the long-acting β_2 agonist dose, an oral corticosteroid may be added. (Adapted from 2007 NHLBI Guidelines for the Diagnosis and Treatment of Asthma.)

TABLE 27-2 Levels of Asthma Control*

Characteristic	Controlled (All of the Following)	Partly Controlled (Any Measure Present in 1 Week)	Uncontrolled
Daytime symptoms	None (twice or less/week)	More than twice/week	Three or more features of partly controlled asthma present in any week
Limitations of activities	None	Any	
Nocturnal symptoms/awakenings	None	Any	
Need for reliever/rescue treatment	None	More than twice/week	
Lung function (PEF or FEV_1)	Normal	< 80% predicted or personal best (if known)	
Exacerbations	None	One or more/year	One in any week

Adapted from GINA At-A-Glance Asthma Management Pocket Reference, 2006.
*The peak expiratory flow (PEF) is a person's maximum speed of expiration. *FEV1*, Forced expiratory volume in the first second, the volume of air that can be forced out in 1 s after taking a deep breath.

for the Diagnosis and Treatment of Asthma, all patients with asthma should receive a short-acting β_2 agonist (SABA) for quick relief of bronchospasm. Patients with persistent asthma should then receive a maintenance medication, starting with an inhaled corticosteroid (ICS), in addition to their short-acting β_2 agonist. If the patient is not controlled, the ICS dose may be increased and a long-acting β_2 agonist (LABA) may be added. After further increasing the ICS dose and elevating the long-acting β_2 agonist dose, an oral corticosteroid may be added. The use of **omalizumab** is a last resort medication due to the risk of anaphylaxis. It must be administered in a clinic with medical supervision.

Regardless of the severity of asthma, other therapeutic measures may also be used. The prompt administration of antibiotics is indicated for respiratory infections of nonviral origin. Sedatives may be used to minimize emotional stress; expectorants may aid in the removal of secretions.

ASPIRIN-INDUCED ASTHMA

The incidence of aspirin-induced asthma among adult patients with asthma is estimated to be 21%, determined by oral provocation testing. There is an underreporting of aspirin hypersensitivity probably due to either lack of routine aspirin challenge or a lack of recognition by patients of a mild NSAID-induced reaction. Aspirin-induced asthma is more frequent in women than men. It usually begins in adulthood, with the average age of 30 years. Rhinorrhea and nasal congestion are the first symptoms, with complications of nasal polyposis. Approximately 80% of aspirin-induced asthma patients have sinusitis. This syndrome is characterized by asthma, nasal polyps, aspirin reactions, and chronic hyperplastic eosinophilic sinusitis.

The prostaglandin PGE_2 plays a role in aspirin-induced asthma. PGE_2 is proinflammatory in many diseases, but in the lung, it protects against bronchoconstriction during an aspirin challenge. This prostaglandin exerts its activity through the binding of the prostanoid receptor, EP_3. This receptor is expressed on bronchial epithelia and mast cells. Through the EP_3 receptor, PGE_2 inhibits the synthesis of cysteinyl leukotrienes, inhibits the release of mediators from mast cells, and diminishes inflammatory cell influx. PGE_2 is synthesized by cyclooxygenase 1 (COX-1) and 2 (COX-2) in the lung. In the lungs of individuals with aspirin-induced asthma, the expression of COX-2 is diminished. Hence, when COX-1 is inhibited by aspirin or NSAIDs, the concentration of the protective prostaglandin PGE_2 is decreased (Fig. 27-5). COX-2 biosynthesis of PGE_2, also inhibited by aspirin, is insufficient to compensate. Another biochemical difference between patients with asthma who are aspirin intolerant and those who are not is the expression of 5-lipoxygenase. In aspirin-intolerant patients, 5-lipogenase is upregulated; therefore the synthesis of cysteinyl leuko trienes is increased. Aspirin-intolerant patients also express more cysLT receptors on nasal inflammatory cells. While treatment of asthma in aspirin-intolerant patients is essentially the same as aspirin-tolerant patients, leukotriene modifiers, either inhibitors or antagonists, have been reported to be effective in chronic therapy in individuals with aspirin hypersensitivity.

PHARMACOTHERAPY FOR COPD

Recognizing that there is no cure for COPD, the goals of therapy are to prevent disease progression, relieve symptoms, improve health status, prevent exacerbations, reduce morbidity, and minimize adverse effects from treatment. Figure 27-6 illustrates how the severity of COPD is staged and classified into severity groups. The severity groups guide pharmacologic treatment (Table 27-3). Anticholinergics and β_2 agonists cause bronchodilation through different mechanisms. (See earlier.) There is a long history of therapy with a combination of these two drug classes. Combination therapy also allows for lower doses to be administered and therefore minimizes adverse effects from treatment. If the patient has repeated exacerbations, an ICS should be added as regular therapy. Drug therapy is also combined with smoking cessation and pulmonary rehabilitation exercises. As the disease progresses, the patient will require supplemental oxygen therapy.

IMPLICATIONS FOR DENTISTRY

To provide the most effective and safest dental care for the patient with respiratory disease, the dentist must be aware of the patient's history, medication usage, and how the medical problem is being managed. Factors that are important in the patient interview include past history of sudden, severe exacerbations, previous intubation, previous admission to an intensive care unit, two or more hospitalizations or three or more emergency care visits in the past year, comorbidity from cardiovascular disease, frequency of use of a rapidly acting β_2-adrenergic receptor agonist inhaler, and current use of steroids or recent withdrawal from corticosteroids. The use of two canisters per month of a rapid-acting β_2 agonist inhaler is an indication that the respiratory disease is not well controlled. The dentist must also be aware that patient factors can impact the perception of airflow obstruction such as dementia, psychiatric disease, or psychosocial problems. Low socioeconomic status, urban residence, and illicit drug use also put the patient at risk for exacerbation of asthma or COPD. The patient should be asked to bring all medication for the respiratory condition to the dental appointment.

Another consideration is how the patient reacts to dental appointments. Many persons become apprehensive and anxious about impending visits to the dental office. It is known that emotional factors play an active role in precipitating or exacerbating respiratory symptoms. Dental materials that contain powder or the powder in latex gloves can increase the patient's airway obstruction if the particles are inhaled. Some patients may not be able to tolerate a horizontal position in the dental chair for a long period of time.

Analgesic therapy for the patient with asthma must be chosen with care. **Aspirin and aspirin-containing compounds should be avoided if there is a question of patient intolerance or nasal polyps** because asthmatic episodes can be precipitated in some patients in minutes to hours after ingestion of these drugs. Patients with asthma who are unable to tolerate aspirin may also react adversely to other nonsteroidal antiinflammatory drugs (NSAIDs). The analgesics of choice for patients with asthma and aspirin allergy are acetaminophen or opioids, such as hydrocodone. Large doses of morphine can produce bronchial constriction, however, by causing histamine release from mast cells. Opioids also decrease the respiratory drive, which is a dangerous liability to the patient whose airway resistance may be greater than normal.

The hypoxic state seen in patients with COPD can cause oral complications such as difficulty in healing after surgery and difficulty in fighting infection. Difficulty in breathing often forces patients to breathe through the mouth, which can cause xerostomia and the oral problems associated with decreased saliva. Also, many of the medications commonly used in COPD can contribute to dry mouth, such as anticholinergics and beta-agonist inhalers. Patients with advanced emphysema might use portable oxygen with a nasal cannula.

ICS use, especially if improper, can lead to **oral candidiasis.** This is due to reduced oral defenses against infection from residual steroid in the mouth. Patients should rinse their mouths after use to clear any drug remaining there.

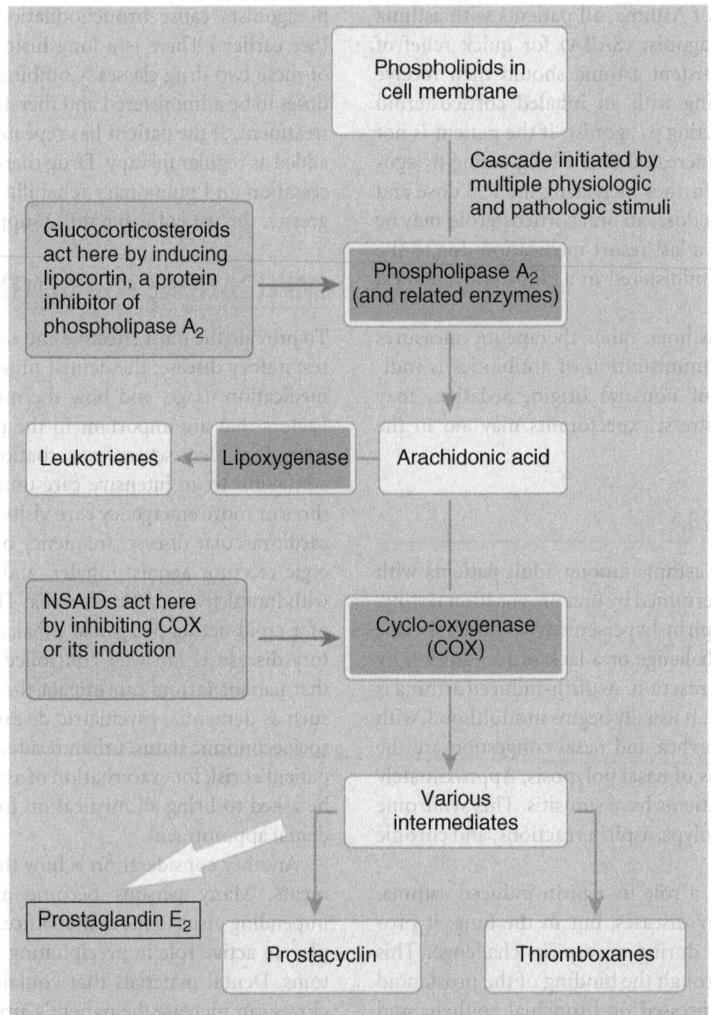

FIG 27-5 Mechanism of aspirin-induced asthma. Arachidonic acid can be catalyzed by lipoxygenase enzymes. These enzymes catalyze the formation of leukotrienes—a class of lipid, inflammatory mediators. Specific to asthma, the cysteinyl leukotrienes, which are produced in mast cells, eosinophils, and macrophages, bind to cysteinyl leukotriene receptors located on airway smooth muscle cells. (See Fig. 27-3.) Upon binding, these molecules stimulate airway edema, smooth muscle contraction, and induction of allergic inflammatory cells. If the patient is taking an NSAID, which blocks the conversion of arachidonic acid to prostaglandins, PGE_2 is not produced, and its protective effect is lost. Moreover, more arachidonic acid is available to be converted to leukotrienes. By blocking cysteinyl leukotriene binding, many of the symptoms related to asthma can be successfully treated. (From Page et al.: *Integrated pharmacology*, ed 2, St. Louis, 2003; Mosby.)

The long-term exposure to cigarettes places the patient with COPD at a greater risk for oral cancer. The dentist should encourage the patient to stop smoking. The ADA has provided guidelines on their Website to assist dentists in approaching the patient to explain the benefits of stopping smoking and to assist the patient in that effort.

MANAGEMENT OF ACUTE BRONCHOSPASM

It is important for the dentist and dental practice employees to be prepared for emergency exacerbations that may occur during a dental appointment. The National Asthma Education and Prevention Program of the National Heart, Lung, and Blood Institute has written guidelines for such situations. The dentist should encourage the patients with respiratory disease to bring their inhalers to all dental appointments. Initial recommended treatment for acute exacerbations is the use of a short-acting β_2 agonist with two to four puffs by a metered-dose inhaler at 20-minute intervals. After initial treatment, the response should be assessed as good, incomplete, or poor. If the response is incomplete or poor, additional therapy with an oral corticosteroid and inhaled anticholinergic will be required with continued treatment with the inhaled short-acting β_2 agonist. For severe episodes, administration of subcutaneous epinephrine 0.2 to 0.5 mg may be required. Patients with an initial poor response might require further treatment in the emergency department.

DRUGS FOR MILD RESPIRATORY ILLNESSES

Numerous drugs are used to provide symptomatic relief of some uncomfortable symptoms of respiratory infection or mild allergies with respiratory symptoms. These include bronchodilators (discussed in previous sections), antitussives, and expectorants. The properties of the antitussives and expectorants are illustrated in Tables 27-4 and 27-5.

COPD severity staging			
Airflow limitation			
Stage	Severity	FEV_1/FVC	FEV_1 (% predicted)
1	Mild	<70%	>80
2	Moderate	<70%	>50 and <80
3	Severe	<70%	>30 and <80
4	Very severe	<70%	<30

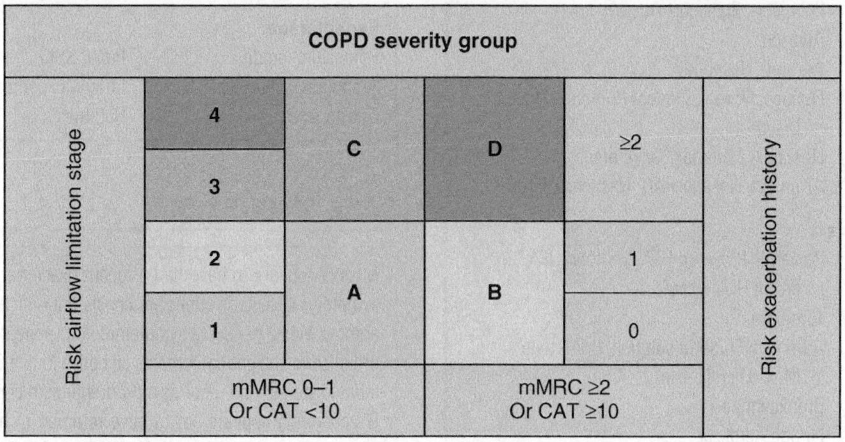

COPD severity group

Risk airflow limitation stage

4
3
C
D
≥2
2
1
A
B
1
0

mMRC 0–1
Or CAT <10

mMRC ≥2
Or CAT ≥10

Risk exacerbation history

FIG 27-6 COPD Severity Staging: Airflow limitation staging is determined by a patient's FEV1. All patients with COPD will have an FEV1-to-FVC ratio of less than 70%. After determining a patient's airflow limitation staging, the next step is to classify a patient's COPD severity group as A, B, C, or D using the bottom table. This bottom table, which is used in clinical practice to guide COPD treatment, takes into account a patient's airflow limitation staging, exacerbation history, and symptom assessment scoring. Group A patients have the lowest risk classification with the fewest symptoms, while group D patients have the highest risk classification with the most symptoms. *CAT*, COPD assessment test (based on a patient questionnaire); *FEV1*, forced expiratory volume in one second; *FVC*, forced vital capacity; *mMRC*, Medical Research Council (mMRC) dyspnea scale (based on the number of dyspnea events).

TABLE 27-3 Drug Choice for COPD Severity Groups*

Group	First Choice Pharmacologic Treatment for COPD
A	PRN short-acting anticholinergic or PRN SAB_2A
B	Long-acting anticholinergic or LAB_2A
C	ICS + (long-acting anticholinergic or LAB_2A)
D	ICS + (long-acting anticholinergic or LAB_2A)

*Group A patients should receive either an as-needed short-acting anticholinergic or an as-needed short-acting β_2 agonist (SAB_2A). In addition to their as-needed (PRN) medication, group B patients should have either a long-acting anticholinergic or a long-acting β_2 agonist (LAB_2A). Group C and D patients should have, in addition to their PRN medication, an inhaled corticosteroid (ICS) plus either a long-acting anticholinergic or a long-acting β_2 agonist. Remember, for patients with asthma, the inhaled corticosteroid serves as the gold standard for preventing exacerbations. In COPD, however, the long-acting anticholinergics and the long-acting β_2 agonists provide better maintenance control. Inhaled corticosteroids are still used in COPD, but since inflammation is only one component of COPD, they are added later in therapy.

TABLE 27-4 Properties of Antitussives

Drug	Class	Mechanism of Action	Adverse Effects/Comments
Codeine	Opioid	Suppression of medullary cough center	Constipation, nausea, some addiction potential
Benzonatate	Structurally related to tetracaine	Inhibits the stretch receptors of the respiratory mucosa	Nausea, constipation, headache, drowsiness, vertigo
Dextromethorphan	Opioid	Suppression of medullary cough center	Few adverse reactions, little addiction potential
Noscapine	Isoquinolone	Suppression of medullary cough center	Nausea, headache drowsiness

TABLE 27-5 Properties of Expectorants

Drug	Actions	Adverse Effects/Comments
Potassium iodide	Little proof of efficacy	Thyroid enlargement and decreased function
Ammonium chloride	Little proof of efficacy	Metabolic acidosis
Guaifenesin	Increased sputum volume, facilitated sputum removal	Nausea, GI upset

DRUGS ACTING ON THE RESPIRATORY SYSTEM

Nonproprietary (Generic) Name	Proprietary (Trade) Name
Corticosteroids (Inhalation or Intranasal)	
Beclomethasone	Beclovent, Beconase AQ, QVAR, Vancenase AQ
Budesonide	Pulmicort, Rhinocort Aqua
Ciclesonide	Alvesco
Flunisolide	Aerobid, Nasalide,
Fluticasone	Flonase, Flovent, Flovent Rotadisk, Flovent Diskus
Mometasone	Nasonex, Asmanex Twisthaler
Triamcinolone	Azmacort, Nasacort AQ, Nasacort HFA
Adrenergic Bronchodilators	
Albuterol	Proventil, Proventil HFA, Ventolin HFA, ProAir HFA, AccuNeb
Bitolterol	Tornalate
Epinephrine	Adrenalin Chloride solution, Primatene Mist, MicroNefrin
Ethylnorepinephrine	Bronkephrine
Formoterol fumarate	Foradil Aerolizer
Isoetharine HCl	—
Isoproterenol HCl	Isuprel
Levalbuterol HCl	Xopenex
Metaproterenol sulfate	Alupent
Pirbuterol acetate	Maxair Autohaler
Salmeterol xinafoate	Serevent Diskus
Terbutaline sulfate	Brethine
Olodaterol	Striverdi Respimat
Vilanterol	
Indacaterol	Arcapta
Anticholinergic Bronchodilators	
Atropine	Day-dose Atropine Sulfate
Ipratropium	Atrovent, Atrovent HFA
Umeclidinium	Incruse Ellipta
Tiotropium	Spiriva
Aclidinium	Tudorza Pressair
Leukotriene Modifiers	
Zafirlukast	Accolate
Montelukast	Singulair
Zileuton	Zyflo
Monoclonal Antibodies	
Omalizumab	Xolair
Combination Inhalers	
Ipratropium and albuterol	Combivent, DuoNeb
Fluticasone, salmeterol	Advair Discus
Umeclidinium, vilanterol	Anoro Ellipta
Fluticasone, vilanterol	Breo Ellipta
Formoterol, mometasone	Dulera
Phosphodiesterase Inhibitors	
Roflumilast	Daliresp
Other Drugs	
Theophylline	Theo-Dur
Cromolyn	
Nedocromil	Alocril, Tilade
Antitussives	
Codeine	—
Benzonatate	Tessalon Perles
Dextromethorphan	Pertussin
Noscapine	—
Expectorants	
Potassium iodide	Pima, SSKI
Ammonium chloride	Efricon Expectorant Liquid
Guaifenesin	Robitussin

CASE DISCUSSION

Miss G appears to have had a recent exacerbation of her asthma. The patient symptoms and medications are consistent with a history of moderate persistent asthma. While her acute symptomatology appears to have resolved with the oral prednisone, the patient remains on both a leukotriene receptor antagonist and an inhaled steroid and requires a β-adrenergic receptor agonist at least daily. Miss G's condition appears not to have returned to her baseline status prior to the exacerbation of her disease. Usually a patient will be maintained on the modified asthmatic medication regimen for 3 to 6 months. At that time the patient's condition will be reassessed, and either the inhaled steroid or leukotriene receptor antagonist will most likely be tapered and ultimately discontinued.

Initial intervention of the pericoronitis is to locally irrigate and debride the area. The site can be curetted and irrigated with chlorhexidine gluconate (Peridex). Antibiotics frequently are not indicated. If tooth #16 is impinging on the inflamed tissue, it too could be extracted to eliminate an aggravating factor. NSAID analgesics are not absolutely contraindicated, but a hydrocodone/acetaminophen combination is an appropriate analgesic that avoids NSAIDS in this patient, who has had a recent exacerbation of her asthma requiring steroids.

The patient had an exacerbation of her asthma 2 months ago. While the patient's condition appears to have improved, her condition has not returned to baseline, and thus she should not be considered to be in optimal and stable condition. For this patient, it may be ideal to manage the pericoronitis medically and delay treatment for an additional month to observe if the patient continues to improve. However, the patient may persist with symptoms consistent with moderate persistent asthma, and this does not preclude her from receiving treatment.

Ideally, the patient should have a good night's sleep prior to the scheduled day of surgery to minimize the aggravating effect of stress on exacerbating a bronchospastic episode. The patient will require some type of sedation management, as her anxiety has interfered with her receiving the necessary care previously. Varying sedative regimens (both enteral and parenteral) may be considered depending on the depth of sedation required. Benzodiazepines are an excellent choice. Oral triazolam, which is an oral benzodiazepine agent, is an acceptable agent that can be administered by the dentist trained in its use. The patient's pulmonary function should have been recently evaluated. Prophylactic administration of the patient's short-acting β_2-adrenergic receptor agonist inhaler (albuterol) prior to beginning the surgery should be considered to minimize an intraoperative bronchospastic episode, regardless of no respiratory findings on auscultation. There is no contraindication to the use of local anesthetic with epinephrine. The patient's albuterol inhaler should be available throughout the procedure and can be used to manage bronchospastic activity despite the prior prophylactic administration. The dentist should have epinephrine 1:1000 for SQ or IM administration available in the emergency cart in the event that the patient has an acute episode that is refractory to the inhaled beta agonist.

GENERAL REFERENCES

1. Barnes PJ: Theophylline: new perspectives for an old drug, *Am. J. Respir. Crit. Care Med* 167:813–818, 2003.
2. Caramori G, et al.: Molecular pathogenesis of cigarette smoking–induced stable COPD, *Annals of the New York Academy of Sciences*, 2015.
3. Deakins KM: Year in review 2014: asthma, *Respiratory Care* 60:744–748, 2015.
4. Green SA, Spasoff AP, Coleman RA, et al.: Sustained activation of a G protein-coupled receptor via "anchored" agonist binding molecular localization of the salmeterol exosite within the β2-adrenergic receptor, J Biol Chem 271:24029–24035, 1996.
5. Frith PA, et al.: Glycopyrronium once-daily significantly improves lung function and health status when combined with salmeterol/fluticasone in patients with COPD: the GLISTEN study—a randomised controlled trial, *Thorax*, 2015.
6. Latorre M, et al.: Differences in the efficacy and safety among inhaled corticosteroids (ICS)/long-acting beta2-agonists (LABA) combinations in the treatment of chronic obstructive pulmonary disease (COPD): role of ICS, *Pulmonary Pharmacology & Therapeutics* 30:44–50, 2015.
7. Navarrete BA, et al.: "Correct use of inhaled corticosteroids in chronic obstructive pulmonary disease": a consensus document, *Archivos de Bronconeumología (English Edition)* 51:193–198, 2015.
8. Naycı, S.A., et al: "Updates in Chronic Obstructive Pulmonary Disease for the Year 2014." 2015.
9. O'Quinn JW, et al.: Omalizumab treatment of moderate to severe asthma in the adolescent and pediatric population, *Journal of Allergy and Clinical Immunology* 135.2, 2015. Abs. 3.
10. Patel M, Shaw D: A review of standard pharmacological therapy for adult asthma–steps 1 to 5, *Chronic Respiratory Disease* 12:165–176, 2015.
11. Stelmach I, et al.: Do children with stable asthma benefit from addition of montelukast to inhaled corticosteroids: randomized, placebo controlled trial, *Pulmonary Pharmacology & Therapeutics* 31:42–48, 2015.

28

Drugs Acting on the Gastrointestinal Tract

David H. Shaw

KEY INFORMATION

- Proton pump inhibitors (PPIs) are administered as inactive prodrugs and irreversibly inhibit H^+, K^+-ATPase (the proton pump).
- PPIs are metabolized by hepatic CYP450 isoenzymes, especially CYP2C19 and CYP3A4, and they may interfere with the metabolism of other medications metabolized by these same enzymes.
- H_2 blockers reduce gastric acid secretion but not as effectively at PPIs.
- Antacids are weak bases that neutralize gastric HCl.
- Anticholinergics may be used in dentistry to modify salivary gland activity.
- Antiemetics act by modifying the action of one or more neurotransmitters (e.g., dopamine, acetylcholine, serotonin, histamine).
- Laxatives used in the treatment of idiopathic constipation act primarily on the intestinal mucosa and contents following one of the following mechanisms of action: wetting agent, stimulant, increase in fluid volume (osmotic), or increase in stool mass (bulk-forming).
- The most efficacious antidiarrheal agents are the opioid derivatives, diphenoxylate and loperamide, which are antagonists to peripheral μ-opioid receptors.
- Chloride channel activators are a relatively new class of drugs that are approved for treating irritable bowel syndrome with predominant constipation (IBS-C) and chronic constipation.

CASE STUDY

A 53-year-old male dental patient is provided extensive restorative dental care that results in significant soft tissue trauma. His medical record shows a history of rheumatoid arthritis and nonsteroidal antiinflammatory drugs (NSAID)-associated peptic ulcer disease. He reports that ibuprofen is helpful in managing his arthritis and that his physician has prescribed dexlansoprazole, taken daily, to reduce his susceptibility to the NSAID-associated stomach irritation. He also reports occasionally taking an over-the-counter (OTC) antacid when experiencing symptoms of hyperacidity. You recognize that the patient will likely experience moderate to significant postprocedural pain requiring pharmaceutical intervention and understand his enhanced gastrointestinal response to NSAID analgesics. How would you manage the expected pain resulting from the restorative care?

Medications that exert an effect on the gastrointestinal tract are among the most frequently used drugs worldwide. Gastrointestinal agents are one of the most commonly cited class of drugs recorded on the medication histories of dental patients along with antihypertensive agents and mood modifiers. Many of these drugs have been discussed in other parts of this book as they have a wider spectrum of activity. The drugs discussed in this chapter are used almost exclusively for their application to gastrointestinal disorders. Included in this group of drugs are PPIs, H_2 antihistamines, antacids, antiemetics, laxatives, antidiarrheal drugs, gastrointestinal stimulants, and chloride channel activators. Some of these drugs are available OTC and may be used at the discretion of the patient.

Dentists may prescribe one of these drugs to modify salivary gland function or reduce medication-induced nausea and vomiting. Knowledge that the patient is taking one or more of these drugs helps the dental provider to better understand the patient's current medical condition, guides treatment decisions such as chair position, and may influence the choice of a dental therapeutic agent. A gastrointestinal disturbance arising during the course of dental treatment may be attributable to, or managed by, one of these agents.

Drugs that act on the gastrointestinal tract and are commonly used in dentistry to modify salivary gland activity or to reduce medication-induced nausea and vomiting are listed in Table 28-1.

GASTRIC HYPERACIDITY, GASTROESOPHAGEAL REFLUX DISEASE, AND PEPTIC ULCER DISEASE

Acid-peptic conditions such as heartburn (pyrosis), dyspepsia (indigestion), gastroesophageal reflux, and **peptic ulcer disease (PUD)** (gastric and duodenal) are often treated with drugs that either reduce intragastric acidity or promote gastrointestinal mucosal defense. In all these conditions, patient discomfort primarily results from the caustic effects of the gastric acid on the esophagus or from overcoming the gastrointestinal mucosal defense system or both. Heartburn is a common term to describe a burning sensation that usually arises from the lower chest area (substernal) and moves upward toward the neck. It most commonly occurs within 2 hours after eating or when lying down or bending over. The symptoms are caused by the abnormal reflux of gastric contents or vapors retrograde into the esophagus. Heartburn that is frequent and persistent is the most common symptom of **gastroesophageal reflux disease (GERD).** GERD is one of the most prevalent digestive diseases among adults. Symptoms arising from GERD, such as heartburn, are among the most common reasons for visits to primary care providers.

PUD is a common, often painful, condition that can seriously affect the quality of life; it is rarely fatal. Peptic ulcers are characterized by spontaneous healing and recurrence. The primary complication is hemorrhage, which may be life-threatening if undetected or ignored.

TABLE 28-1 Drugs Useful in Dentistry That Affect the Gastrointestinal Tract

Therapeutic Use	Drug	Dose (mg)*
Sialagogue	Pilocarpine hydrochloride (Salagen)	5†
	Cevimeline hydrochloride (Evoxac)	30†
Antisialagogue	Atropine sulfate (Sal-Tropine)	0.4-0.6
	Glycopyrrolate (Robinul)	1-2
	Propantheline bromide	7.5-30
Antiemetic	Dimenhydrinate (Dramamine)	50-100
	Meclizine hydrochloride (Antivert)	25-50
	Promethazine hydrochloride (Phenergan)	25
	Metoclopramide (Reglan)	10-15
	Dronabinol (Marinol)	2.5-5.0

*Adult, oral route.
†Discussed in Chapter 6.

Perforation of the gastrointestinal wall, which occurs much less frequently, is a contributing factor in deaths from this disease.

Throughout most of the 20th century, therapy for PUD was directed at suppression of acid secretion or neutralization of secreted acid. This approach was based on the erroneous assumption that ulcers develop only because of increased gastric acid secretion. The primary symptoms of PUD are related to mucosal exposure to gastric acid and pepsin usually caused by *Helicobacter pylori* infection or the breakdown of normal mucosal defenses from the use of NSAIDs. *H. pylori* infects more than half of the world's population and accounts for the majority of stomach and duodenal ulcers. Because only a relatively small percentage of *H. pylori*–infected patients develop PUD in their lifetime, other factors must play a role in the development of this disease. Although *H. pylori* is found in dental plaque and saliva, the relationship between its presence in the mouth and infection in the stomach is not yet clear. The oral cavity may be a permanent reservoir for *H. pylori,* and a person-to-person route is the most probable mode of transmission.

DRUGS USED TO REDUCE GASTRIC ACID AND TREAT PEPTIC ULCER DISEASE

Proton Pump Inhibitors

PPIs are drugs that **irreversibly inhibit H^+/K^+-activated adenosine triphosphatase (H^+, K^+-ATPase,** commonly called the **proton pump**) in the gastric parietal cell (Fig. 28-1), the final common pathway for acid secretion. PPIs have become the drug class of choice for treating acid-related gastrointestinal diseases such as PUD and GERD. PPIs are among the most widely sold drugs because of their outstanding efficacy and safety. Currently, six members of the PPI class are available by prescription in the United States: **dexlansoprazole, esomeprazole, lansoprazole, omeprazole, pantoprazole,** and **rabeprazole** (Table 28-2). Esomeprazole, lansoprazole, and omeprazole are available OTC at a lower dosage. When taken orally, all six agents effectively reduce basal and stimulated acid secretion considerably. They are longer lasting and substantially more potent than histamine H_2-receptor antagonists in the short-term treatment of PUD, GERD, and heartburn. Dexlansoprazole is marketed in a longer lasting dual delayed-release formulation, with two types of granules, each with a coating that dissolves at a different pH. This provides two peak plasma times, but the clinical relevance of this form of release has not been firmly established.

PPIs are administered as inactive prodrugs that accumulate selectively in the acid environment of the secretory canaliculus of the gastric parietal cell. The PPI is rapidly protonated and converted to the active form of

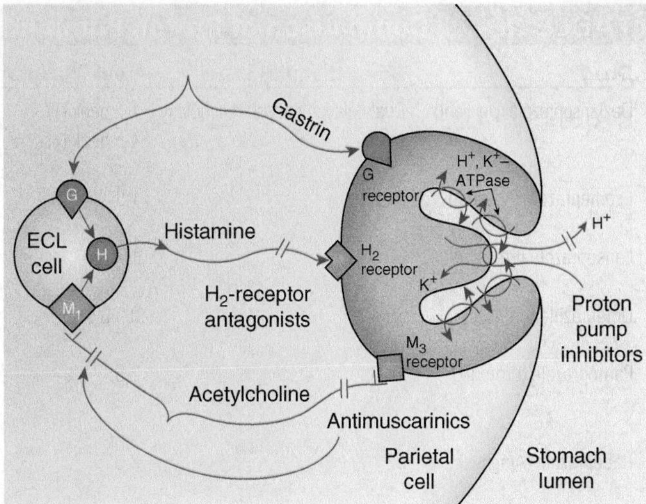

FIG 28-1 The physiologic control of H^+ secretion by the gastric parietal cell, with the site of action of the major antisecretory drugs. Included is an endocrine cell that secretes histamine (enterochromaffin-like [ECL] cell) and an acid-secreting parietal cell.

the drug. Because PPIs bind covalently to active proton pumps, synthesis of new pumps or activation of resting pumps is required to restore activity. This irreversible inhibition of the pump explains why the duration of action of this class extends beyond the elimination half-life of 0.5 to 2 hours (see Table 28-2). Most PPIs are best taken on an empty stomach (food can decrease bioavailability up to 50%) once daily 30 minutes to 1 hour before the first meal of the day so that the peak serum concentration coincides with the maximum activation of the proton pumps. Dexlansoprazole, unlike the other PPIs, lacks the pharmacokinetic and pharmacodynamic drug–food interactions and can be taken with a meal.

The most common adverse effects reported with PPIs are headache, diarrhea, and nausea, but the frequency is only slightly greater than placebo. Long-term use of PPIs may cause a slight increase in serum gastrin. This information led to concerns regarding gastrin-induced neoplasms that have been reported in animal models. PPIs have been used worldwide for close to 40 years and, to date, none have been associated with an increased risk of gastric cancers in patients receiving long-term therapy. Of more recent concern are reports that PPIs, particularly with prolonged therapy, are associated with a decrease in Ca^{2+} and Mg^{++} absorption through induction of hypochlorhydria and with an increased risk to develop community-acquired *Clostridium difficile*–associated disease (CDAD). Acid is also important in releasing vitamin B_{12} from food, and subnormal B_{12} levels have been reported with prolonged PPI therapy.

All PPIs increase gastric pH and may alter the absorption of drugs that are weak bases or acids or formulated as pH-dependent, controlled-release products. Absorption of aspirin, digoxin, and midazolam may be increased, and ketoconazole absorption may be decreased when administered with a PPI. The clinical significance of the alterations is unclear. PPIs can also alter the hepatic metabolism of other medications. All PPIs are metabolized to varying degrees by hepatic P450 cytochromes (CYP450), including isoenzymes CYP2C19 and CYP3A4, and may interfere with the medications metabolized by these same enzymes. Omeprazole has been shown to progressively inhibit CYP2C19 activity with repeated administration and may inhibit the metabolism of diazepam, warfarin (coumadin), and phenytoin. In spite of these concerns, few clinically significant drug interactions have been reported given the enormous popularity of PPIs.

One adverse drug interaction that initiated an FDA warning is the potential interaction between clopidogrel and PPIs. **Clopidogrel** is a

TABLE 28-2 Comparison of Proton Pump Inhibitors

Drug*	Bioavailability (%)	Peak Plasma Time (hr)	Elimination Half-Life (hr)	Primary Route of Excretion
Dexlansoprazole (Dexilant)	Dual delayed-release technology	1-2 peak (1) 4-5 peak (2)	1-2	Hepatic CYP2C19 CYP3A4
Esomeprazole (Nexium)	64-90	1.5	1-1.5	Hepatic CYP2C19
Lansoprazole (Prevacid)	80-85	1.7	1.6	Hepatic CYP2C19
Omeprazole (Prilosec)	30-40	0.5-3.5	0.5-1	Hepatic CYP2C19
Pantoprazole (Protonix)	>77	2-3	1-1.9	Hepatic CYP2C19 CYP3A4
Rabeprazole (Aciphex)	52	2-5	1-2	Hepatic CYP2C19

*Once-daily oral dosing.

TABLE 28-3 Comparison of H_2 Antihistamines

Drug	Bioavailability (%)	Peak Plasma Time (hr)	Elimination Half-Life (hr)	Oral Dose Interval (hr)*
Cimetidine (Tagamet)	60-70	1-3	2	6-24
Famotidine (Pepcid)	40-45	1-3	2.5-3.5	12-24
Nizatidine (Axid)	>90	0.5-3	1-2	12-24
Ranitidine (Zantac)	50-60	2-3	2.5-3	12-24

*For treatment of gastrointestinal disorders (e.g., duodenal or gastric ulcer, heartburn, GERD).

prodrug that is activated by hepatic **CYP2C19**, the same isoenzyme involved, to varying extent, in the metabolism of the PPIs. The concern is that coadministration of clopidogrel and a PPI would reduce the activation of clopidogrel (and its antiplatelet action) in susceptible patients. The clinical relevance of this potential interaction remains a point of debate, but it is recommended that patients taking clopidogrel be prescribed a PPI that has minimal effect on the activity of CYP2C19 (e.g., pantoprazole). The effect of long-term PPI use on cardiovascular health is another area of clinical debate. PPIs may have a negative effect on vascular function leading to an increased risk for myocardial infarction.

PPIs, especially used long-term, may increase the risk of: rebound hypersecretion, bone fracture, and infections, namely, *Clostridium difficle*-induced diarrhea as well as pneumonia.

H_2 Receptor Antihistamines

Histamine is one of the primary mediators of gastric acid secretion, along with acetylcholine and gastrin. The final common pathway is through the proton pump (see Fig. 28-1). As discussed in Chapter 18, H_2 receptors are located on the membranes of acid-secreting parietal cells of the stomach. **H_2 receptor antihistamines** (commonly called **H_2 blockers**) are reversible, competitive antagonists of histamine at the H_2 receptors. The duration and the degree of acid suppression are dose-dependent. These are highly selective agents in that they do not affect the H_1, H_3, or H_4 receptors and are not anticholinergic. **Cimetidine**, the first of these drugs to be used widely, revolutionized the treatment of duodenal ulcers. With the recognition of the role of *Helicobacter pylori* in PUD and the introduction of PPIs, the use of prescription strength H_2 antagonists has markedly declined.

A usual single dose of any of the H_2 antagonists currently available for prescription or nonprescription use in the United States, including **cimetidine**, **famotidine**, **nizatidine**, and **ranitidine** (Table 28-3), inhibits 60% to 70% of total 24-hour acid secretion in a linear dose-dependent manner. These agents are particularly effective in inhibiting nocturnal acid secretion, which is stimulated more by histamine. Food-induced gastric acid secretion is stimulated more by gastrin and acetylcholine and is less inhibited by the H_2 blockers.

H_2 blockers are commonly administered orally as they are rapidly absorbed from the intestines. The antisecretory activity usually begins within 1 hour of administration and persists for 6 to 12 hours. They have an oral bioavailability of 40% to greater than 90% (depending on the degree of first-pass hepatic metabolism), achieve peak plasma concentrations in 0.5 to 3 hours, and are eliminated with a terminal half-life of 1 to 3.5 hours (see Table 28-3). The drugs undergo partial metabolism in the liver; the remainder of the parent drug is eliminated unchanged by the kidney. The duration of effectiveness varies with the drug, dose, and medical condition being treated, ranging from 4 hours for a low dose of cimetidine for hypersecretory disorders to 24 hours for all these agents when used to treat duodenal and gastric ulcers.

Comparative studies of H_2 blockers show that the four drugs in this class are essentially equal in clinical effectiveness regarding ulcer treatment even though they express varying potencies in their ability to block gastrin-stimulated gastric acid secretion in the research laboratory. Cimetidine seems unique among H_2 blockers in exerting biologic effects that are unrelated to gastric H_2 occupancy. **Cimetidine** therapy, particularly when prolonged and at high doses, can cause **antiandrogenic effects**. These reversible effects result from the ability of cimetidine to compete with dihydrotestosterone at androgen-binding sites and to inhibit the CYP metabolism of estradiol. Men treated with high doses of cimetidine for long periods may experience impotence and development of gynecomastia, whereas women may develop galactorrhea. Substitution of ranitidine for cimetidine reverses these effects; no

TABLE 28-4 **Summary of the Major Constituents of Antacids**

Constituent	Neutralizing Capacity	Salt Formed in Stomach	Solubility of Salt	Adverse Effects (Selected)
$NaHCO_3$	High	NaCl	High	Systemic alkalosis, fluid retention
$CaCO_3$	Moderate	$CaCl_2$	Moderate	Hypercalcemia
$Al(OH)_3$	High	$AlCl_3$	Low	Constipation
$Mg(OH)_2$	High	$MgCl_2$	Low	Diarrhea

antiandrogenic effects have been reported after therapeutic doses of famotidine or nizatidine.

Of importance to the dentist is the ability of cimetidine to decrease the hepatic oxidative biotransformation of many other drugs, including lidocaine and diazepam. Cimetidine and ranitidine are ligands for multiple hepatic CYP450 isoenzymes (CYP1A2, CYP2C9, CYP2D6, CYP3A4), with cimetidine exhibiting a much higher affinity and **inhibiting hepatic microsomal enzyme activity** to a much greater extent. The clinical use of ranitidine, famotidine, and nizatidine does not seem to have a significant effect on the metabolism and elimination of other drugs.

The widespread use of cimetidine has revealed various central nervous system (CNS) manifestations (e.g., headache, lethargy, confusion, forgetfulness), especially in elderly patients. Impaired renal function in an older patient may contribute to these reactions. Similar effects have been reported for ranitidine and famotidine but seem to be less common.

Antibiotics

The evidence that PUD (and gastritis and possibly gastric adenocarcinoma) is directly linked to infection by the gram-negative organism *Helicobacter pylori* is now well established. Cultures taken from biopsy material are positive for *H. pylori* in approximately 95% of duodenal ulcer specimens and 75% of biopsy specimens taken from gastric ulcers compared with a roughly 25% incidence in asymptomatic control subjects.

These findings have led to the routine use of antibiotic therapy for the eradication of *H. pylori*–associated ulcers. Significant reductions in clinical symptoms and histologic evidence of ulcers have been achieved. The current cornerstone of therapy for *H. pylori*–associated peptic ulcers involves a triple regimen of a PPI (e.g., **lansoprazole**) with two antibiotics (e.g., **clarithromycin** and either **amoxicillin** or **metronidazole**). This therapeutic regimen has been shown to be highly effective. PPIs not only raise the intragastric pH, but they may also enhance healing through direct anti–*H. pylori* properties. For patients with NSAID-induced PUD, rapid healing is often initiated with the use of a PPI or H_2 antagonist as long as the NSAID is discontinued. Asymptomatic peptic ulceration may develop in people frequently taking an NSAID, and daily administration of a PPI will reduce the incidence of ulcers in these patients.

Gastric Antacids

Gastric antacids are weak bases that buffer or neutralize gastric hydrochloric acid (HCl) to form a salt and water and reduce intragastric acidity. They are commonly used as an OTC remedy for intermittent heartburn and dyspepsia caused by overeating or eating certain foods. Through acid neutralization, antacids also secondarily reduce the proteolytic activity of pepsin, which is completely inactivated at a pH greater than 4. Overuse of antacids is discouraged because excessive neutralization may stimulate acid rebound; this response may be of little clinical significance because the added acid load likely is compensated by the buffers in the antacid. All antacids may affect the absorption of other medications by directly binding to the drug or increasing the intragastric pH, altering the drug's dissolution/solubility. In particular, antacids should not be given within 2 hours of a dose of a tetracycline or fluoroquinolone antibiotic.

Antacids have a rapid onset of action that depends on how fast the product dissolves in gastric acid. In general, antacid suspensions dissolve more easily than tablets or powders for a faster response. The duration of action of an antacid in the stomach is influenced by the gastric emptying time, which is slowed by food in the stomach and patient variability in gastric secretory capacity. In general, antacids taken on an empty stomach have a duration of action of approximately 30 minutes, whereas antacids taken after a full meal may neutralize acid for 3 hours. Four primary compounds are currently used, alone or in combination, in antacid products: sodium bicarbonate, magnesium hydroxide, aluminum hydroxide, and calcium carbonate (Table 28-4). Following is a discussion of these commonly employed compounds used in antacid preparations:

Sodium bicarbonate

Sodium bicarbonate is widely available in the form of baking soda and combination products. It reacts almost instantaneously to neutralize HCl to produce CO_2 and NaCl. The formation of CO_2 results in belching and gastric distention. Sodium bicarbonate is often referred to as a "systemic" antacid because the unreacted fraction is readily absorbed into the general circulation and may alter systemic pH. The potential for Na^+ overload and systemic alkalosis limits its use to short-term relief of indigestion. Na^+ overload resulting from repeated use of large doses may contribute to fluid retention, edema, hypertension, congestive heart failure, and renal failure. Sodium bicarbonate is contraindicated in patients on a low-salt diet.

Magnesium hydroxide

Magnesium hydroxide (Milk of Magnesia) has a rapid onset of action and high neutralizing capacity. It reacts slowly with HCl to form $MgCl_2$ and water without the generation of CO_2. The risk of Mg^{++} overload is low and significant only in patients with impaired renal function. A disadvantage is its laxative effect, and few patients can tolerate it as the sole antacid for any length of time.

Aluminum hydroxide

Aluminum may be administered in several forms (aminoacetate, carbonate, hydroxide, phosphate), but **aluminum hydroxide** gel is the most potent buffer and most frequently used. Aluminum hydroxide dissolves slowly, is poorly absorbed, and reacts with HCl to form $AlCl_3$ and water. As with magnesium hydroxide, no CO_2 is generated. Liquid formulations provide a more rapid response than solid forms. Other than occasional nausea and vomiting, toxicity is rare. The formation of insoluble aluminum salts limits its absorption. Patients with impaired renal function who take aluminum antacids long-term may not clear the Al^{+++} resulting in hyperalbuminemia and accumulation of Al^{+++} in other tissues. The most common side effect is constipation, which may lead to intestinal obstruction. The constipating effect of aluminum-containing antacids is dose-related and can be managed with stool softeners or laxatives or minimized when the drug is taken with magnesium hydroxide. Because Al^{+++} can combine with phosphate in the gut to form insoluble aluminum phosphate, which is then excreted in the feces, prolonged use of large doses of aluminum hydroxide may result in phosphate depletion, particularly when phosphate intake is low. Anorexia, malaise, and muscle weakness are characteristic of phosphate depletion.

Calcium carbonate

Calcium carbonate produces a potent and prolonged neutralization of HCl forming CO_2 and $CaCl_2$. Approximately 90% of the ingested Ca^{2+} forms insoluble salts in the gut and is excreted in the feces. The remaining Ca^{2+} is absorbed into the systemic circulation. Extensive use of Ca^{2+}-containing antacids may cause or exacerbate hypercalcemia, which is characterized by neurologic symptoms and reduced renal function. This effect is rare in healthy patients with normal renal function. Calcium carbonate has a chalky taste and may produce constipation, which reduces its desirability as an antacid. Because some Ca^{2+} is absorbed, Ca^{2+}-containing antacids may be marketed as a source of dietary Ca^{2+}.

Alginic Acid

Alginic acid is not an antacid, but because of its unique mechanism of action, it is added to some antacid preparations to increase their effectiveness in the treatment and relief of the symptoms of GERD. In the presence of saliva, alginic acid reacts with sodium bicarbonate to form sodium alginate. Gastric acid causes this alginate to precipitate, forming a foaming, viscous gel that floats on the surface of the gastric contents. This provides a relatively pH-neutral barrier during episodes of acid reflux and enhances the efficacy of drugs used to treat GERD. Alginic acid products are not indicated for the treatment of PUD.

Simethicone

Simethicone is a defoaming agent used to relieve gas discomfort in the stomach and intestine. It does not have antacid properties, but it may be included in antacid products. Its action is to reduce the surface tension of gas bubbles in the gastrointestinal tract, which allows the gas bubbles to break up and coalesce, facilitating the elimination of the gas by belching or passing through the rectum. The FDA considers simethicone to be safe and effective as an antiflatulent agent.

Sucralfate

Sucralfate, a complex of aluminum hydroxide and sulfated sucrose, is a cytoprotective agent that provides a physical barrier over the surface of a gastric ulcer and enhances the gastric mucosal protective system. Currently, its use in clinical practice is limited because of advances in the treatment of gastrointestinal ulcers and lesions. It has, however, previously been employed to treat several gastrointestinal diseases, including PUD, GERD, and dyspepsia. After oral administration the drug disperses in the stomach and, in the presence of acid, forms a viscous suspension that binds with high affinity at the ulcer site. The negatively charged sucrose sulfate is thought to bind to the positively charged proteins of the ulcer. A physical cytoprotective barrier is produced that covers the ulcer and protects it from further attack by damaging agents such as acid, pepsin, and bile salts.

Although sucralfate possesses no meaningful antacid properties and a precise mechanism of action is unclear, a key element in the acute gastroprotective actions of sucralfate is its ability to maintain mucosal vascular integrity and blood flow. It enhances bicarbonate and mucus secretion, increases mucosal hydrophobicity, and induces an increase in mucosal concentration of prostaglandin—all factors considered important in tissue healing.

Because it is minimally absorbed from the gastrointestinal tract, sucralfate is considered a remarkably safe agent. The most common side effect is constipation (2%) due to the aluminum salt.

Sucralfate may bind to many other drugs and inhibit their absorption, including the fluoroquinolone and tetracycline antibiotics. The use of a topical sucralfate suspension has been advocated in the prevention or treatment of stomatitis caused by chemotherapy or radiation, in spite of equivocal evidence supporting this use.

Prostaglandins

The gastrointestinal mucosa synthesizes a number of prostaglandins, including prostaglandin E. **Misoprostol**, a synthetic prostaglandin E_1 analogue, which is used in the treatment and/or prevention of gastrointestinal ulcers. Although the prostaglandins are crucial in creating the alkaline mucus layer that provides cytoprotective effects on the gastroduodenal mucosa, the ulcer-healing effect of misoprostol and other prostaglandin analogues seems to be caused mainly by the inhibition of acid secretion. These agents interact with a basolateral receptor of the parietal cell that causes the inhibition of adenylyl cyclase. This inhibition results in reduced production of cyclic adenosine 3′,5′-monophosphate, the major second messenger for histamine-induced acid secretion. Misoprostol is approved for prevention of NSAID-induced ulcers in high-risk patients, although PPIs may be as effective and better tolerated. The most common side effects are abdominal pain and diarrhea (>10%); both are dose-related. Misoprostol stimulates contraction of the uterus, which contraindicates its use during pregnancy or in women of childbearing potential. This property makes it effective, however, in women undergoing elective termination of pregnancy by facilitating expulsion of the uterine contents.

Figure 28-2 summarizes various drugs that act on the stomach.

Therapeutic Importance in Dentistry

The diagnosis of GERD may be an important finding when considering if a patient should be reclined in the dental chair. Although it is safe to place most GERD patients supine, some with severe GERD need to be kept at a 45-degree angle for their visit. Asking patients how they sleep (e.g., head higher than feet) can help elucidate what should be done.

A patient history of a gastric or duodenal ulcer provides important information for the dentist because this can influence the choice of a therapeutic agent or time of drug administration. The use of aspirin as an analgesic is contraindicated because of its irritating effect on gastric mucosa; this is particularly true for elderly patients. All NSAIDs share the ulcerogenic property of the salicylates, with the risk of developing NSAID-induced PUD. The risk is increased with increased drug dosage and duration of use. Acetaminophen may be used as an alternative analgesic because it produces minimal damage to gastric mucosa compared with aspirin and other NSAIDs. For acute dental pain in high-risk patients, the cyclooxygenase-2–selective inhibitor celecoxib may also be used. It is efficacious and significantly less ulcerogenic than either aspirin or ibuprofen (see Chapter 17).

As previously mentioned, PPIs may cause sufficient inhibition of gastric acid secretion to reduce the absorption of drugs in which gastric pH influences bioavailability (e.g., ketoconazole, ampicillin). The clinical significance of this interaction has yet to be determined. Likewise, the theoretic risk of increasing the response to diazepam when coadministered with PPIs, especially omeprazole, has shown little clinical significance to date.

Systemic corticosteroids, as used after oral surgical procedures, are potentially ulcerogenic. Even topical steroids used in the management of oral lesions should be avoided in patients with an ulcer

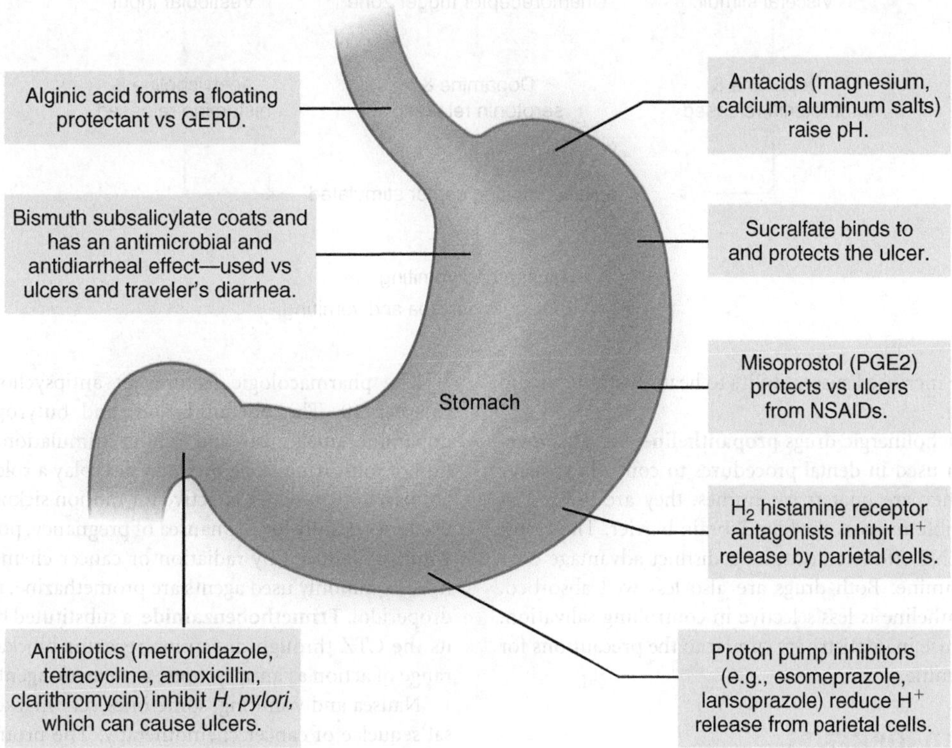
Alginic acid forms a floating protectant vs GERD.
Bismuth subsalicylate coats and has an antimicrobial and antidiarrheal effect—used vs ulcers and traveler's diarrhea.
Stomach
Antibiotics (metronidazole, tetracycline, amoxicillin, clarithromycin) inhibit *H. pylori*, which can cause ulcers.
Antacids (magnesium, calcium, aluminum salts) raise pH.
Sucralfate binds to and protects the ulcer.
Misoprostol (PGE2) protects vs ulcers from NSAIDs.
H_2 histamine receptor antagonists inhibit H^+ release by parietal cells.
Proton pump inhibitors (e.g., esomeprazole, lansoprazole) reduce H^+ release from parietal cells.

FIG 28-2 The mechanism of various drugs that act on the stomach.

because of the possibility that absorption through the mucosa would occur. The choice of a preoperative or postoperative sedative is particularly important for ulcer patients. Diazepam is appropriate for selected patients because, in addition to producing sedation, it can suppress the nocturnal secretion of gastric acid. Absorption of orally administered diazepam, however, may be altered with the concomitant administration of an antacid. For a patient being treated with cimetidine or omeprazole, a prudent choice for sedation might be lorazepam or oxazepam; these are benzodiazepine antianxiety drugs not dependent on hepatic oxidative biotransformation. They are eliminated in the urine as glucuronide conjugates (see Chapter 11), the formation of which is not impaired by either cimetidine or omeprazole.

Treatment with cimetidine for a day or more may cause much higher plasma concentrations of diazepam taken on a regular basis, a more pronounced sedative effect, and slowed elimination of diazepam due to the inhibition of hepatic CYP3A4 by cimetidine. The significance of such cimetidine-induced drug interactions is likely to depend on the patient, however. The manifestations of the diazepam–cimetidine interaction may be clinically insignificant in young adults, but the interaction could be important in elderly patients or in patients on multiple medications. If a course of diazepam therapy is prescribed for a dental patient on cimetidine, dosage reduction should be considered.

As previously mentioned, cimetidine inhibits the hepatic metabolism of lidocaine and presumably other amide local anesthetics. This interaction is of little practical concern in view of the low dosages of lidocaine typically required for intraoral anesthesia and its rapid distribution from the plasma to peripheral tissues.

Aluminum hydroxide gels, Ca^{2+} and Mg^{++} antacids, and sodium bicarbonate impair the absorption of tetracyclines and fluoroquinolones. This action is shared by milk and milk products and seems to result from chelation and an increased gastric pH. Sucralfate can also reduce the absorption of several drugs, including tetracycline, when administered concomitantly. A reasonable general approach for prescribing these vulnerable drugs to a dental patient receiving antacid or sucralfate therapy, or both, would be to separate the administration of each drug by several hours. This approach results in a negligible effect on absorption of the antibiotic.

ANTISIALAGOGUES

The short-term control of salivary flow is often helpful in dental procedures (e.g., occlusal adjustment and impression taking). A dramatic reduction of the secretory function of the salivary glands can be achieved by blockade of acetylcholine at muscarinic receptor sites. The pharmacologic characteristics of the antimuscarinic drugs are presented in detail in Chapter 6, but in summary, these drugs block the action of acetylcholine on the muscarinic receptor sites of effector cells innervated by postganglionic parasympathetic cholinergic nerves. They are used in dentistry to control excessive salivation and during general anesthesia to reduce the incidence of laryngospasm by diminishing respiratory secretions. The recommended oral doses for blocking excessive salivation are small and free of major side effects (see Table 28-1).

The prototypic drugs for this class are the belladonna alkaloids **atropine** and **scopolamine**. Some patients experience side effects such as difficulty in swallowing because of excessive dryness in the mouth and throat and a reduction in sweating. Scopolamine in particular may impair psychomotor activity and is not the drug of choice to reduce salivary secretion in the typical dental setting. The decision to use an antisialagogue depends partly on the patient's medical history. Atropine is contraindicated in patients with prostatic hypertrophy or narrow-angle glaucoma, and the topical use of atropine is absolutely contraindicated in all forms of glaucoma. Atropine should be administered with caution in patients with cardiovascular disease because it can increase the pulse rate and cardiac workload. It may also antagonize the vagal effects of digitalis. Toxic effects are common, particularly

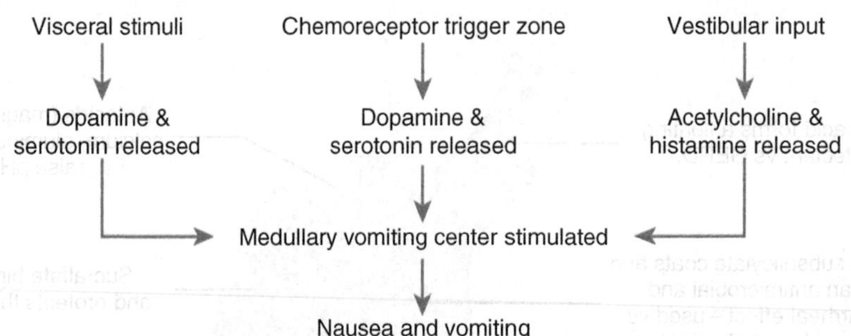

FIG 28-3 Etiology of nausea and vomiting.

in children, who have increased susceptibility to heat prostration from inhibition of sweating.

The synthetic anticholinergic drugs **propantheline** and **glycopyrrolate** have also been used in dental procedures to control excessive salivation. Because they are quaternary amines, they are ionized at body pH and are unable to cross the blood–brain barrier. The resultant freedom from CNS effects constitutes a distinct advantage over atropine and scopolamine. Both drugs are also less well absorbed, however, and propantheline is less selective in controlling salivation. Precautions for their use in dentistry are similar to the precautions for atropine and scopolamine.

EMETICS AND ADSORBENTS

Emetics such as syrup of ipecac have been used in emergent cases of poisoning because they induce forceful emptying of the stomach. The efficacy of emesis in the management of acute poisoning episodes declines when treatment is initiated more than 1 hour after ingestion of a toxic substance. The amount of substance removed from the stomach is inversely related to the duration of time from ingestion to emesis. Ipecac has not been found to be effective in purging the body of poisonous substances. For that reason, the American Academy of Pediatrics does not support the use of ipecac to treat accidental poisonings and manufacturers have stopped production of the ipecac syrup. Instead, the administration of activated charcoal as an adsorbent is preferred because it has been shown to reduce the bioavailability of ingested substances effectively. In all cases in which poisoning is suspected, consultation with the local poison control center should be the first action taken for information needed to determine the appropriate treatment approach.

ANTIEMETICS

Numerous drugs are available that have shown antiemetic action (see Table 28-1). Nausea and vomiting are complex processes that are not yet fully elucidated. The brainstem vomiting center, located in the lateral medullary reticular formation, apparently coordinates the associated motor activities after input from the chemoreceptor trigger zone (CTZ), cerebral cortex, gastrointestinal tract, and vestibular apparatus. The identification of the neurotransmitters and their receptors within these sites has provided a likely target for the disruption of the emetic process (see Fig. 28-3). Cancer chemotherapeutic agents and other chemical stimuli activate the CTZ, an area rich in dopamine D_2 receptors, serotonin 5-HT_3 receptors, and neurokinin 1 and opioid receptors. Motion sickness results from muscarinic and histamine H_1 receptor–mediated response from vestibulocochlear disturbances via cranial nerve VIII. Drugs or drug classes useful as antiemetics include antipsychotics (phenothiazines and butyrophenones), metoclopramide, H_1 antihistamines, anticholinergics, serotonin 5-HT_3 antagonists, neurokinin antagonists, cannabinoids, and corticosteroids.

The pharmacologic features of antipsychotics are discussed in Chapter 10. The phenothiazines and butyrophenones are central dopamine antagonists and inhibit stimulation of the CTZ. Inhibition of muscarinic receptors may also play a role in this activity. Most antipsychotics are not effective for motion sickness, but they are often used successfully for the nausea of pregnancy, postoperative emesis, or vomiting induced by radiation or cancer chemotherapy. Among the most commonly used agents are promethazine, prochlorperazine, and droperidol. **Trimethobenzamide**, a substituted benzamide, also inhibits the CTZ through dopamine receptor blockade and has the same range of action as antipsychotic antiemetic agents.

Nausea and vomiting, sometimes very marked, are almost universal sequelae of cancer chemotherapy. The protracted bouts of severe drug-induced vomiting, which may be only slightly relieved by standard antiemetic therapy, have led to the inability of some patients to complete courses of potentially curative treatment. Chemotherapy-induced nausea and vomiting often responds to high doses of the peripherally and centrally acting dopaminergic D_2 receptor antagonist **metoclopramide**. Peripherally, it also stimulates the release of acetylcholine and sensitizes smooth muscle to acetylcholine. Centrally, it blocks D_2 receptors in the CTZ. In addition, metoclopramide inhibits 5-HT_3 receptors, which may be more responsible for its antiemetic effect. High-dose metoclopramide, similar to other dopamine antagonists, may cause extrapyramidal symptoms and sedation, particularly in young and elderly patients. Prolonged use has been associated with tardive dyskinesia. **Droperidol**, a D_2 dopamine receptor blocker neuroleptic, is an antiemetic used in anesthesia for the prophylactic management of postoperative nausea and vomiting.

As pointed out in Chapter 18, certain H_1 histamine antagonists are effective antiemetics. All possess significant anticholinergic actions that contribute to their antiemetic efficacy. **Diphenhydramine**, **dimenhydrinate**, **meclizine**, and **cyclizine** are especially useful in treating the nausea and vomiting associated with motion sickness, pregnancy, and the postoperative state. These drugs should not be used during pregnancy, however, unless absolutely necessary. The antihistamines are not of significant value in relieving nausea associated with the administration of cytotoxic drugs. **Promethazine**, a phenothiazine antihistamine without significant dopamine-blocking activity, is effective in vertigo and motion sickness. Its sedative action is advantageous in the treatment of postoperative nausea and vomiting. Nonsedating H_1 antihistamines such as loratadine are ineffective against motion sickness because they penetrate poorly into the CNS.

The anticholinergic **scopolamine** is effective in the prevention and treatment of motion sickness, but its oral use is limited by its sedative and antimuscarinic actions. A transdermal sustained-release preparation of scopolamine, when applied to the postauricular area for several hours before need, effectively prevents motion sickness for 72 hours with minimal side effects.

The recognition that 5-HT_3 receptor blockade by high-dose metoclopramide provided antiemetic activity led to the development of several **selective 5-HT_3 receptor antagonists**, including **ondansetron, dolasetron, granisetron,** and **palonosetron.** They are potent, highly selective competitive 5-HT_3 antagonists. 5-HT_3 receptors are found in the gastrointestinal tract and the CNS. These agents are generally well tolerated, although constipation, abdominal discomfort, headache, sedation, dry mouth, blurred vision, and anxiety have been reported by some patients. Extrapyramidal effects, however, have not been reported. At this time, the relative efficacy and safety of the selective 5-HT_3 receptor antagonists have made them drugs of choice for the management of chemotherapy-induced nausea. They are also effective in the prevention and treatment of postoperative and postradiation nausea and vomiting.

Cannabinoids are indicated when conventional antiemetics fail to relieve the nausea and vomiting associated with cancer chemotherapy. **Dronabinol**, or Δ-9-tetrahydrocannabinol, is the main psychoactive constituent in marijuana (see Chapter 39). Evaluation of its use as an antiemetic was undertaken after anecdotal reports that marijuana smokers had less nausea and vomiting in association with cytotoxic agents than other patients. Dronabinol given orally has been shown to be significantly better than placebo and comparable to metoclopramide in reducing chemotherapy-induced vomiting. The use of dronabinol is limited by its tendency to produce acute, and often intolerable, mental disturbances, particularly in older patients who are unaccustomed to marijuana-like side effects.

Corticosteroids, such as dexamethasone and methylprednisolone, have been reported to be effective for cancer chemotherapy–induced nausea and vomiting. The mechanism of this effect is unknown, but it may be related to a reduced synthesis of prostaglandins; prostaglandin E has been shown to induce nausea and vomiting (see Chapter 17). Sedative-hypnotics such as the benzodiazepines may also help prevent anticipated nausea and vomiting associated with chemotherapy; lorazepam is most commonly used.

Aprepitant is a highly **selective neurokinin 1(NK1)-receptor antagonist** employed in combination with 5-HT_3 receptor antagonists and corticosteroids for the prevention of chemotherapy-induced nausea and vomiting. Adding aprepitant greatly improves antiemetic outcomes. This drug is metabolized by CYP enzymes (CYP3A4), and its use may influence the metabolism of other drugs sharing this pathway.

Just as combinations of antineoplastic drugs with different modes of action are used in cancer chemotherapy (see Chapter 36), combinations of different antiemetic drugs are being used to treat the nausea and vomiting associated with the use of antineoplastics. Combinations of antiemetics are often more effective than single-agent therapy because of multiple sites of emetic action by antineoplastic agents and the potential for additive or even synergistic effects of several antiemetics with different mechanisms of action.

Droperidol, metoclopramide, dexamethasone, and 5-HT_3 blockers are useful as antiemetics when used prophylactically to reduce the incidence of postoperative nausea and vomiting. The choice of antiemetic drug given for prophylaxis had little effect on clinical outcome or patient satisfaction.

Alternative treatments, including acupuncture, hypnosis, ginger, and pyridoxine (vitamin B_6), have shown efficacy in several conditions with nausea and vomiting. Widespread acceptance of these alternative therapies awaits confirmation of efficacy from additional studies.

LAXATIVES

Constipation is a common gastrointestinal complaint, affecting millions of people. A large number of these individuals will self-medicate with a laxative or visit their primary care provider seeking relief. Laxatives are used to relieve acute and chronic constipation, treat anorectal disorders (hemorrhoids), and prepare the bowel for examination (colonoscopy). Constipation occurs in all age groups but is especially common in pregnant women and elderly individuals. Most cases are self-limiting or are self-treated with diet. Laxatives are well-known, highly advertised, and the most overused OTC drugs having a therapeutic effect on the gastrointestinal tract. Traditionally, these drugs have been generally classified as stimulants/irritants, saline and osmotic cathartics, bulk-forming agents, stool softeners, and lubricants (Fig. 28-4). Although that taxonomy is used in this chapter, these categories are arbitrary and not reflective of either the pathophysiologic principles or the multiplicity of effects generated by laxatives.

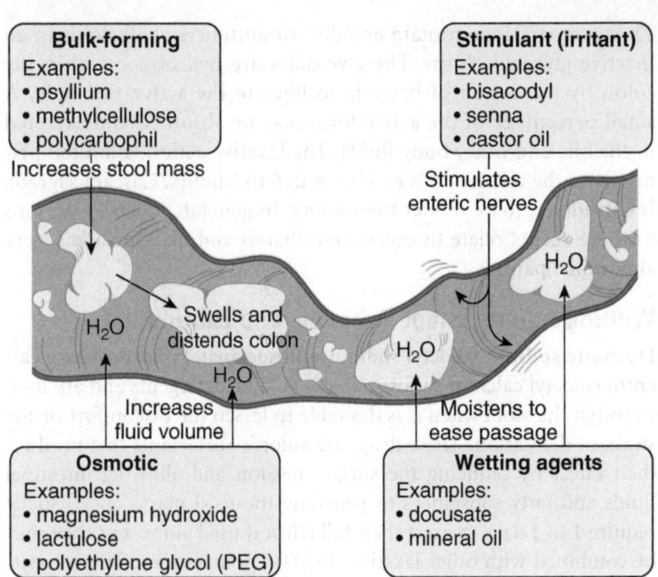

FIG 28-4 The site of action of the major categories of laxatives.

Stimulants

Numerous laxatives belong to the stimulant category. As a group, these drugs are thought to act as a local irritant of the intestinal mucosa that increases propulsive activity. The exact mechanism is not completely understood, but they may increase motility by a selective action on the intramural nerve plexus of intestinal smooth muscle. All the stimulant laxatives increase mucosal permeability, resulting in movement of fluid and electrolytes into the intestinal lumen.

Castor oil is obtained from the seeds of *Ricinus communis* and is hydrolyzed in the small intestine by pancreatic lipase to glycerol and ricinoleic acid, an unsaturated hydroxy fatty acid. Castor oil evokes the secretion of water and electrolytes in the colon and small intestine and increases small bowel peristaltic activity to produce a very prompt cathartic effect in 2 to 6 hours. It is of historic interest but rarely used today.

Phenolphthalein was a widely used stimulant OTC laxative until the FDA banned its use because of reports of its association with carcinogenic tumors in laboratory rats. **Bisacodyl** is structurally related to phenolphthalein and has similar pharmacologic actions. After oral administration, approximately 5% of a therapeutic dose is absorbed from the digestive tract with no apparent systemic effects. The laxative effect is obtained in 6 to 8 hours but can be accelerated by administration in suppository form. The major toxicity is diarrhea with overdosage.

Some of the most extensively used stimulant laxatives are in the anthraquinone group, which includes **senna** and **cascara sagrada.**

These preparations contain emodin (or anthracene) alkaloids in an inactive glycoside form. The glycosides are hydrolyzed within the colon by the action of bacteria to liberate the active principle. A small percentage of the active form may be absorbed and excreted in the bile and other body fluids. The laxative action is limited primarily to the colon and is produced in 6 to 8 hours. Cascara sagrada is considered to be milder than senna. In general, adverse reactions to these agents relate to excessive catharsis and may include severe abdominal pain.

Wetting Agents (Stool Softeners and Lubricants)

Docusate sodium (dioctyl sodium sulfosuccinate) and **docusate calcium** (dioctyl calcium sulfosuccinate) act like detergents and are used to soften the stool when it is desirable to lessen the discomfort or the strain of defecation. These drugs are anionic surfactants that produce their effect by reducing the surface tension and allowing intestinal fluids and fatty substances to penetrate the fecal mass. They usually require 1 to 3 days to exert their full effect if used alone, but they may be combined with other laxatives in OTC preparations. These agents are not believed to interfere with the absorption of nutrients from the intestinal tract, and they are not appreciably absorbed. Docusate is frequently recommended for elderly patients because it is associated with so few side effects. Diarrhea and mild abdominal cramps are the only adverse effects reported.

Mineral oil (liquid petrolatum) may be considered with the surface-active agents because it also softens the stool. Mineral oil acts as a lubricant and coats the intestinal contents, preventing the absorption of fecal water. It produces a cathartic action in 6 to 8 hours after oral administration and 5 to 15 minutes if given rectally. Its use is attended by several potential hazards not associated with the other agents. Prolonged oral use or administration with meals can reduce the absorption of the fat-soluble vitamins (A, D, E, and K). Lipid pneumonia can result from the accidental aspiration of the oil. Mineral oil is absorbed to a limited extent from the intestinal tract; its use with a wetting agent (docusate), which could increase its absorption, is contraindicated. Significant absorption of mineral oil may occur if used repeatedly. The seepage of oil through the anal sphincter may occur and produce pruritus ani or other perianal conditions.

Osmotic Cathartics

Saline osmotic cathartics are salt solutions containing one or more ions that are poorly absorbed from the gastrointestinal tract. Available preparations include Mg^{++} salts (hydroxide, sulfate, or citrate), sodium phosphate (monobasic or dibasic), and sodium biphosphate. The salt solutions osmotically increase the water content of feces and fluid volume in the intestinal lumen; this increases the intraluminal pressure, which exerts a mechanical force to stimulate peristalsis. It has also been postulated that Mg^{++} salts increase colonic motility by causing the release of cholecystokinin. Oral administration of these agents generally results in the production of a fluid to semifluid stool within 30 minutes to 3 hours. If given rectally, laxation occurs in 2 to 5 minutes.

Some absorption of saline cathartics does occur, and consequently systemic effects may be noted. For this reason, Na^+ salts are contraindicated in patients on a low-salt diet and in patients with edema or congestive heart failure. Mg^{++} and K^+ salts are contraindicated in patients with impaired renal function. **Magnesium sulfate** (Epsom salt), which is an effective and frequently used cathartic, may cause serious loss of body water with repeated use. Milk of Magnesia, a suspension of **magnesium hydroxide,** is a widely used OTC preparation. Abdominal cramps and dehydration are reported adverse reactions from saline laxatives.

Several preparations, notably **glycerin**, **lactulose**, and **polyethylene glycol (PEG)**, contain large poorly absorbable or nonabsorbable molecules that produce an osmotic effect resulting in distention and catharsis. Glycerin is used in suppository form to promote defecation. It osmotically dehydrates exposed rectal tissue; the resultant irritation promotes evacuation of the lower bowel within 30 minutes. Lactulose is a semisynthetic disaccharide. In the large intestine, lactulose is metabolized by enteric bacteria to various acids and carbon dioxide. The acidification and increased osmolarity of the bowel contents cause fecal softening and a more normal bowel movement. Two days may be required for a therapeutic effect to occur. Lactulose is also used in patients with liver failure who have developed too much ammonia in their bodies. Lactulose is given orally and rectally to scavenge ammonia ions from the gut lumen and inhibit their absorption. As expected, a side effect is loose stools.

Although PEG acts osmotically to retain water in the gut to produce laxation, it is not metabolized by bowel flora and is not significantly absorbed. In contrast to lactulose, PEG does not produce significant cramps or flatus. These osmotic agents are often the mainstay of therapy for individuals with chronic constipation.

Bulk-Forming Agents

Bulk-forming agents include synthetic fibers (polycarbophil) and natural plant products (**psyllium** and **methylcellulose**). They possess the property of absorbing water and expanding, increasing the bulk of the intestinal contents. The elevated luminal pressure stimulates reflex peristalsis, and the increased water content softens the stool. These agents are not absorbed and do not interfere with the absorption of nutrients from the gastrointestinal tract. Several days of medication may be required to achieve the full therapeutic benefit, although the usual onset of action is 12 to 24 hours. Some patients prefer to add foods such as bran or dried fruit (e.g., prunes and figs) to their diet that exert the same effect rather than use a bulk-forming laxative. These laxatives have the advantage of having few systemic effects and are unlikely to produce laxative abuse. Cellulose agents may physically bind with other drugs if administered concurrently (e.g., salicylates, warfarin, digitalis glycosides) and hinder their absorption. Patients should not take a calcium polycarbophil laxative within 2 hours of taking tetracycline for the same reason.

Laxatives with psyllium come in a powdered mixture containing approximately 50% powdered psyllium seeds and 50% dextrose or sucrose. Sugar-free products are also available. Psyllium seeds are rich in a hemicellulose that forms a gelatinous mass with water. The refined hydrophilic colloid from the seeds is the most widely used form of this agent. Methylcellulose is indigestible and not absorbed systemically. Bloating and flatus have been reported after the use of psyllium products because of bacterial digestion of the plant fibers within the colon.

Opioid Receptor Antagonists

Opioid use for acute and chronic pain often results in constipation by decreasing intestinal motility. This effect is mediated by activation of the μ-opioid receptors in the gastrointestinal tract (see Chapter 16). Two selective μ-opioid receptor antagonists are currently available: **methylnaltrexone** and **alvimopan**. These agents selectively and competitively inhibit the μ-opioid receptors in the gastrointestinal tract without affecting analgesic actions of opioid analgesics in the CNS. This is because these agents do not cross the blood–brain barrier at therapeutic doses. These drugs are only used for the short-term treatment of opioid-induced constipation in patients who have had an inadequate response to other cathartics. Alvimopan is restricted to use in hospitals following a published protocol.

ANTIDIARRHEAL AGENTS

One out of every six illnesses of adults and children involves the digestive system, and diarrhea is one of the most common complaints. Diarrhea occurs when not enough water is removed from the stool during transit, making the stool loose and poorly formed. Commonly used antidiarrheal agents act in one of two ways. They either soak up excess water or decrease intestinal motility, which provides the body more time to absorb the luminal water. Antidiarrheal agents may be used to treat acute diarrhea, although they should be discontinued if the diarrhea worsens despite therapy. They may also be used to control chronic diarrhea associated with conditions such as irritable bowel syndrome (IBS) or inflammatory bowel disease. The following agents have been determined by the FDA to be safe and effective in the treatment of acute nonspecific diarrhea.

Kaolin

Kaolin is a hydrated aluminum silicate with a crystalline structure that allows for a large surface area that adsorbs many times its weight in water. Its use in the treatment of diarrhea is based on its purported ability to absorb fluid, bacteria, toxins, and various noxious materials in the gastrointestinal tract, decreasing stool liquidity and frequency. In the colon, it may act as an adsorbent or protectant, but the adsorption is not selective, and it should not be used in children younger than 12 years without physician approval. If taken together, kaolin may adsorb other medications and reduce their systemic absorption. Few controlled clinical studies showing the efficacy of kaolin have been published, and fewer products containing kaolin as the sole active ingredient are presently available in the United States.

Bismuth Subsalicylate

Bismuth subsalicylate (Pepto-Bismol) is a commonly used OTC agent in the treatment of various gastrointestinal symptoms and diseases, including dyspepsia and acute diarrhea, and in the prevention of traveler's diarrhea. It is the only OTC bismuth compound available in the United States and is estimated to be used by most American households. It is a crystal complex of bismuth and salicylate suspended in a mixture of magnesium aluminum silicate clay. In the stomach, the bismuth subsalicylate reacts with the hydrochloric acid to form bismuth oxychloride and salicylic acid. The salicylate is readily absorbed into the body, whereas the bismuth passes unaltered and unabsorbed into the feces. Caution is advised if patients are taking aspirin or other salicylate-containing drugs concurrently because toxic levels of salicylate may be reached. Bismuth subsalicylate products are not recommended for patients younger than 12 years because of a lack of studies to prove efficacy in young children.

Bismuth is thought to produce its therapeutic actions in part by stimulating prostaglandin, mucus formation, and bicarbonate secretion. It also has direct antimicrobial effects and may bind to enterotoxins, which accounts for its use in the prevention of traveler's diarrhea. In addition, bismuth has been used in the home treatment of gastric ulcers because of its ability to coat the ulcer and other gastric erosions, shielding them from the stomach acid and pepsin. In the treatment of acute diarrhea, the salicylate moiety is thought to inhibit intestinal prostaglandin and Cl^- secretion, leading to a reduction in stool frequency and liquidity. Bismuth subsalicylate has an excellent safety record, and side effects are minor. Bismuth may cause blackening of the stool or harmless black staining of the tongue, which is thought to be caused by the formation of bismuth sulfide from the reaction between the drug and the bacterial sulfides in the gastrointestinal tract. As noted previously, salicylate-induced adverse reactions may occur after the administration of bismuth subsalicylate (see Chapter 17).

Opioid Preparations

Opioids are effective and prompt-acting antidiarrheal agents. As discussed in Chapter 16, opioids enhance tone in the anal sphincter and in segments of the longitudinal muscle of the gastrointestinal tract, while inhibiting propulsive contraction of circular and longitudinal muscle. Opioids cause a marked slowing of fluid movement through the jejunum but produce a minimal effect on the movement of fluid through the ileum or colon. By increasing the contact time of luminal fluid with mucosal cells, therapeutic doses of an opioid increase net intestinal absorption of water and electrolytes, reducing stool volume. Commonly used opioid diarrheals include diphenoxylate and loperamide, which act primarily via peripheral μ-opioid receptors (see Chapter 16).

Diphenoxylate

Diphenoxylate, a Drug Enforcement Administration (DEA) Schedule V (C-V) prescription drug, is a congener of meperidine and was originally synthesized during the search for compounds similar to the opioid analgesics in actions on the gastrointestinal tract but devoid of their CNS effects. The efficacy of diphenoxylate was found to be approximately equal to that of camphorated tincture of opium in patients with diarrhea of various causes. Because diphenoxylate is structurally related to meperidine, there was concern about its abuse potential, but in the several decades of experience with it, diphenoxylate has emerged as having an addiction liability comparable to that of codeine, which is diminished further by the incorporation of atropine (as in Lomotil) and by the low water solubility of diphenoxylate salts, both of which prevent inappropriate parenteral administration.

Various minor side effects have been reported, including abdominal cramps, nausea, weakness, drowsiness, xerostomia, gingival swelling, partial intestinal obstruction, and urinary retention. In patients with inflammatory bowel disease, diphenoxylate has caused toxic megacolon, and it has caused hepatic coma in patients with severe liver disease. Toxic doses have produced respiratory depression and unconsciousness, which can be effectively reversed by the opioid antagonists. Although clinical studies have indicated only minimal, if any, drug interactions during diphenoxylate therapy, the drug may potentially augment the actions of barbiturates, alcohol, opioids, and antianxiety and antipsychotic drugs.

Difenoxin, the principal active metabolite of diphenoxylate, is a DEA Schedule IV (C-IV) prescription antidiarrheal drug that is effective at one-fifth the dosage of diphenoxylate. Atropine is added to the formulation to discourage deliberate misuse of the drug.

Loperamide

Loperamide, a long-acting derivative of haloperidol and diphenoxylate, is the most selective antidiarrheal opioid currently available for clinical use because it has a distribution within the body different from other opioids. Although drugs such as meperidine penetrate the blood–brain barrier and interact with CNS opioid receptors to modify intestinal motor function, only small concentrations of loperamide reach the brain. Its antidiarrheal effect is thought to result mainly from interactions with intestinal μ-opioid receptors. When loperamide is administered orally at therapeutic doses, the effect on the gastrointestinal tract is not accompanied by any significant CNS opioid effect. Large amounts of the drug become concentrated in target tissues along the gastrointestinal tract. One hour after oral administration, 85% of the drug is distributed to the gastrointestinal tract, 5% is distributed to the liver, and less than 0.04% is distributed to the brain.

Loperamide exerts its antidiarrheal effect by altering motor function in the intestine, which results in increased capacitance of the intestine and slowing of intestinal motility; this permits greater absorption of electrolytes and water through the intestine. This action is analogous to that of morphine and codeine. The stimulation of μ-opioid receptors also decreases gastrointestinal secretions, which contributes further to its antidiarrheal effects. Despite differences in distribution and other pharmacologic properties, the action of the traditional opioid antidiarrheal drugs and loperamide seems to be the same: inhibition of propulsion through the intestine.

Adverse effects of loperamide occur infrequently but include abdominal pain and distention, constipation, nausea and vomiting, dry mouth, and drowsiness or dizziness. Allergic reactions, including skin rash, have been reported. In contrast to diphenoxylate and difenoxin, loperamide is available OTC. After years of extensive use, there has been no evidence of drug abuse or physical dependence. It is a safe and effective antidiarrheal agent.

Agents Used for the Prevention and Treatment of Traveler's Diarrhea

Many travelers from the United States acquire a diarrheal illness while visiting developing countries. Worldwide, approximately 20 million episodes of diarrhea occur annually in people traveling from industrial regions to developing countries. The most common infecting organism is enterotoxigenic *Escherichia coli*, which is primarily acquired through fecal contamination of food (e.g., raw vegetables) and water, including ice. The ingested bacteria produce enterotoxins that cause the sudden onset of loose stools, commonly referred to as traveler's diarrhea. This is usually a self-limiting illness lasting only several days. Less common pathogens that may cause this disorder include *Shigella*, *Campylobacter*, *Giardia*, and nontyphoid *Salmonella*.

Several approaches to the prevention of traveler's diarrhea have been evaluated. Because of the potential for drug resistance and adverse reactions, the Centers for Disease Control and Prevention does not recommend prescription of drugs prophylactically; instead, they recommend the traveler begin treatment promptly only when symptoms occur. When prophylaxis is used, once-daily dosing with a fluoroquinolone antibiotic (see Chapter 33) is the recommended treatment of choice. Antibiotics recommended from this group include ciprofloxacin (500 mg), levofloxacin (500 mg), ofloxacin (300 mg), and norfloxacin (400 mg). Rifaximin is a poorly absorbed antibiotic approved for prevention and treatment of traveler's diarrhea caused by noninvasive strains of *E. coli* because the action of this drug is limited to the gut. Azithromycin has been recommended for treatment of traveler's diarrhea in countries where antibiotic resistance is prevalent.

Bismuth subsalicylate has also been shown to be particularly active against mild–moderate traveler's diarrhea, although it is considered less effective than antibiotics. A regimen of 520 mg (1 fluid oz [30 mL] of the liquid suspension or two 260-mg tablets) taken four times a day is effective for the prevention of traveler's diarrhea. If started after the onset of diarrhea, it diminishes the number of loose bowel movements and relieves abdominal cramps. The preparation is well tolerated, and constipation is not a problem. As described previously, the mechanisms of action of bismuth subsalicylate are complex and incompletely understood. Bismuth subsalicylate possesses an antibacterial effect, but this may not be its major action. Salicylate is absorbed, but its exact role is undetermined. Patients on anticoagulants should seek medical advice before using this medication because they may get an additional antiplatelet effect from the salicylate. Travelers taking doxycycline for malaria prophylaxis should not take bismuth subsalicylate because it interferes with the absorption of the doxycycline.

An effective treatment for traveler's diarrhea in most parts of the world consists of loperamide (4 mg loading dose, then 2 mg orally after each loose stool, to a maximum of 16 mg/day) plus a single dose of a fluoroquinolone antibiotic. This regimen usually relieves symptoms within 24 hours. If diarrhea persists after 1 day of therapy, treatment should be continued for 1 or 2 more days.

In countries where traveler's diarrhea is prevalent, what one ingests or avoids ingesting may be as important as chemoprophylaxis in reducing the risk. Common sense is an important preventive measure. Helpful maxims to keep in mind include "boil it, cook it, peel it, or forget it" and the "rule of P's": food is safe if it is peelable, packaged, purified, or piping hot. The U.S. Centers for Disease Control and Prevention has a smartphone app called "Can I Eat This?" to help tourists avoid stomach ailments like diarrhea.

GASTROINTESTINAL STIMULANTS

Drugs that stimulate smooth muscle of the gastrointestinal and urinary tracts are used in the treatment of nonobstructive urinary retention, paralytic ileus, gastrointestinal atony, and postoperative abdominal distention. Cholinomimetic agents such as bethanechol are effective in these situations by promoting gastrointestinal motility (see Chapter 6). Bethanechol is a useful agent because it is resistant to metabolism by cholinesterase enzymes, its relevant actions are essentially stimulatory to the muscarinic M_3 receptors, and its effects on the gastrointestinal tract are much more pronounced than its effects on the cardiovascular system. Previously used for the treatment of GERD and gastroparesis, it is now seldom used because of the introduction of less toxic agents. The side effects of bethanechol are those typical of other cholinergic drugs, but serious adverse reactions are rare with therapeutic doses. This drug is contraindicated in patients with obstructive ileus, obstructive urinary retention, peptic ulcer, bronchial asthma, hyperthyroidism, or serious cardiac disease.

Gastroparesis (gastric stasis) is a clinical syndrome characterized by delayed gastric emptying that leads to debilitation. It is most commonly seen in patients with diabetes mellitus and is characterized by intractable nausea, vomiting, early satiety, abdominal pain, and bloating. Therapeutic success is often elusive. The use of a prokinetic agent is the best option for acute exacerbations and long-term maintenance therapy. **Metoclopramide,** the dopamine D_2 receptor antagonist cited earlier for its antiemetic action, and the macrolide antibiotic erythromycin both have prokinetic actions that are commonly used in the management of gastroparesis. Erythromycin acts as a motilin receptor agonist to stimulate gastrointestinal activity (see Chapter 33). Metoclopramide, possessing cholinomimetic and dopamine antagonist properties, is also useful in this syndrome because the drug stimulates the motility of the upper gastrointestinal tract. Metoclopramide augments esophageal peristalsis, gastric antral contractions, and the rate of intestinal transit. In addition, metoclopramide increases the resting pressure of the lower esophageal sphincter but reduces the resting pressure of the pyloric sphincter. It does not stimulate gastric, biliary, or pancreatic secretions and has little effect on colonic motor activity.

Oral administration of metoclopramide is indicated for relief of symptoms associated with diabetic gastroparesis. The usual duration of therapy is 2 to 8 weeks, depending on the response. An injectable form of metoclopramide is also approved for use in facilitating intubation of the small intestine and the passage of barium into the intestine for radiographic procedures. Of particular concern to the dentist is that the use of opioids or anticholinergic drugs antagonizes the gastrointestinal effects of metoclopramide.

CHLORIDE CHANNEL ACTIVATORS

Two chloride channel activators have been approved for treating **irritable bowel syndrome with predominate constipation (IBS-C)** as well as **chronic constipation: lubiprostone** and **linaclotide.** IBS is the most common disorder diagnosed by gastroenterologists and one of the most common gastrointestinal conditions encountered by family practice physicians. It is characterized by abdominal pain and discomfort in association with altered bowel habits (diarrhea, constipation, or both). Pharmacologic treatment of IBS differs from patient to patient and is directed at relieving abdominal discomfort and improving bowel function. Antidiarrheal agents, especially loperamide, are helpful for patients with predominant diarrhea. Increasing dietary fiber is often helpful for IBS patients presenting with constipation. Increasing dietary fiber (e.g., psyllium) may increase gas production and exacerbate abdominal discomfort, however. For that reason, an osmotic cathartic agent such as Milk of Magnesia is often used to soften stools and increase stool frequency. Low doses of a tricyclic antidepressant (e.g., amitriptyline) that has little effect on mood appear to be helpful for chronic abdominal pain associated with IBS. The mechanism of action is unclear but may be related to the anticholinergic properties of these agents or their action on enteric neurotransmitters such as serotonin.

Lubiprostone stimulates the type 2 chloride channel (ClC-2) in the small intestine. The result is an increase in chloride-rich fluid secretions into the intestine. This stimulates intestinal motility and reduces intestinal transit time. Lubiprostone has very limited systemic absorption with few reported side effects. Nausea is the most common adverse reaction (~30%) and that is reported to be caused by delayed gastric emptying. **Linaclotide** is a 14-amino acid peptide that promotes intestinal chloride secretion; however, it does so indirectly. It binds to and **stimulates guanylate cyclase-C** on the luminal surface of the intestinal epithelium. This action results in an increase in intracellular and extracellular cyclic guanosine monophosphate (cGMP) followed by an increase in activity of the **cystic fibrosis conductance regulator channel**. This leads to increased chloride-rich secretions into the lumen and acceleration of intestinal transit. Linaclotide is poorly absorbed with diarrhea as the most common reported side effect (~20%).

ADVERSE REACTIONS OF THE GASTROINTESTINAL SYSTEM TO DRUGS

The gastrointestinal tract must be considered a target for the adverse side effects of many drug groups, some important to dentistry. Opioid analgesics may produce constipation, nausea, and vomiting. Aspirin-containing analgesic compounds are associated with gastric distress, fecal blood loss, and ulceration. All nonselective cyclooxygenase-inhibiting NSAIDs share the gastric irritation and ulcerogenic action of aspirin. The sedative-hypnotic alcohol chloral hydrate may be prescribed by the dentist for children or elderly patients. A major complaint against its use is the gastric irritation it produces.

Antibiotic agents are often associated with **gastrointestinal distress, especially diarrhea**. Antibiotics, especially agents with a broad spectrum of activity, affect the bacteria that normally exist in the large intestine. As a consequence, antibiotic-associated diarrhea develops. Typically, this diarrhea is caused from an overgrowth of *Clostridium difficile* (*C. difficile*–associated diarrhea). Most antibiotics can cause *C. difficile*–associated diarrhea, but it is most commonly associated with clindamycin, amoxicillin, and the cephalosporins. Many drugs not directly related to dentistry cause a wide spectrum of gastrointestinal effects, including adverse effects on the oral cavity. Taste disturbances, especially in elderly patients, are often drug-induced. **Xerostomia** has been reported to be caused by over 400 medications, including agents from most drug classes. Drugs may also induce various oral lesions (e.g., erythema multiforme) in all age groups. Gingival hyperplasia is a well-known side effect from phenytoin, Ca^{2+} channel blockers, and cyclosporine therapy.

DRUGS ACTING ON THE GASTROINTESTINAL TRACT

Nonproprietary (Generic) Name	Proprietary (Trade) Name (Selected)
Antacids	
Alginic acid, sodium bicarbonate, magnesium carbonate	Gaviscon
Aluminum hydroxide gel	Amphojel
Calcium carbonate	Tums, Alka-Mints
Magnesium hydroxide	Milk of Magnesia
Magnesium hydroxide/aluminum hydroxide	Maalox, Gelusil, Mylanta
Sodium bicarbonate	Bell/ans
Sodium bicarbonate/aspirin	Alka-Seltzer
H_2 Receptor Antagonists	
Cimetidine	Tagamet, Tagamet HB
Famotidine	Pepcid, Pepcid AC
Nizatidine	Axid, Axid AR
Ranitidine	Zantac, Zantac 75
Multidrug Regimen for *H. pylori* Eradication	
Bismuth subsalicylate, metronidazole, tetracycline	Helidac
Lansoprazole, amoxicillin, clarithromycin	Prevpac
Prostaglandin Analogue	
Misoprostol	Cytotec
Proton Pump Inhibitors	
Dexlansoprazole	Dexilant
Esomeprazole	Nexium, Nexium 24HR
Lansoprazole	Prevacid, Prevacid 24HR
Omeprazole	Prilosec, Prilosec OTC
Pantoprazole	Protonix
Rabeprazole	Aciphex
Ulcer-Adherent Complex	
Sucralfate	Carafate
Antisialagogue	
See Table 28-1	
Chloride Channel Activators	
Lubiprostone	Amitiza
Linaclotide	Linzess
Antiflatulent Drug	
Simethicone	Gas-X

Continued

DRUGS ACTING ON THE GASTROINTESTINAL TRACT—cont'd

Nonproprietary (Generic) Name	Proprietary (Trade) Name (Selected)
Antiemetics	
Aprepitant	Emend
Cyclizine	Marezine
Dimenhydrinate	Dramamine
Diphenhydramine	Benadryl
Dolasetron	Anzemet
Dronabinol	Marinol
Droperidol	Inapsine
Granisetron	Kytril
Meclizine	Bonine, Antivert
Metoclopramide	Reglan
Ondansetron	Zofran
Palonosetron	Aloxi
Prochlorperazine	Compazine
Promethazine	Phenergan
Scopolamine, transdermal	Transderm-Scop
Trimethobenzamide	Tigan
Laxatives	
Bisacodyl	Dulcolax
Cascara sagrada	Cascara sagrada
Castor oil	Purge
Docusate calcium	Surfak Liquigels
Docusate sodium	Colace
Glycerin, suppositories	Sani-Supp
Lactulose	Chronulac
Magnesium hydroxide	Milk of Magnesia
Magnesium sulfate	Epsom salt
Methylcellulose	Citrucel
Mineral oil	Milkinol
Polycarbophil	FiberCon
Polyethylene glycol (PEG)	MiraLax
Psyllium	Metamucil, Fiberall
Sennosides	Ex-Lax, Senokot
Antidiarrheal Agents	
Bismuth subsalicylate	Pepto-Bismol
Difenoxin with atropine	Motofen
Diphenoxylate with atropine	Lomotil
Loperamide	Imodium
Opioid μ-Receptor Antagonist	
Methylnaltrexone	Relistor
Alvimopan	Entereg
Naloxegol	Movantik

CASE DISCUSSION

This patient will experience greater postprocedure comfort if prescribed an analgesic. The first consideration should be the recognition of the patient's intolerance to NSAID use demonstrated by his history of severe gastric irritation, including ulcer formation, following NSAID use in managing his rheumatoid arthritis. Therefore, prescribing an NSAID for this patient is contraindicated. The COX-2 selective inhibitor might be prescribed as it is considered stomach friendly, but antacids decrease its absorption, and it has potential interactions with ibuprofen. Acetaminophen with an opioid (e.g., codeine) would both provide the patient adequate analgesia to manage the expected moderate–severe pain without adding to the patient's NSAID drug exposure or interacting with dexlansoprazole or the gastric antacids that are part of his therapeutic regimen.

GENERAL REFERENCES

1. Alexander CF, Moayyedi P, Lacy BE, et al.: American College of Gastroenterology monograph on the management of irritable bowel syndrome and chronic idiopathic constipation, *Am J Gastroenterol* 109:S2–S26, 2014.
2. Anand PS, Kamath KP, Sukumaran A: Role of dental plaque, saliva and periodontal disease in Helicobacter pylori infection, *World J Gastroenterol* 20(19):5639–5653, 2014.
3. Brandt LJ, Prather CM, Quigley EM: Systematic review on the management of chronic constipation in North America, *Am J Gastroenterol* 100:S5–S22, 2005.
4. Candy B, Jones L, Larkin PJ, et al.: Laxatives for the management of constipation in people receiving palliative care, *Cochrane Database of Systemic Reviews*(5), 2015, CD003448, http://dx.doi.org/10.1002/14651858.CD003448.pub4.
5. Furyk JS, Egerton-Warburton D, Meet RA: Drugs for the treatment of nausea and vomiting in adult patients in the emergency department setting (protocol), *Cochrane Database of Systematic Reviews*(9), 2012, CD010106, http://dx.doi.org/10.1002/14651858.CD010106.
6. Gordon M, Naidoo K, Akobeng A, et al.: Osmotic and stimulant laxatives for the management of childhood constipation, *Cochrane Database of Systematic Reviews*(7), 2012, CD009118, http://dx.doi.org/10.1002/14651858.CD009118.pub.2.
7. McQuaid KR: Drugs used in the treatment of gastrointestinal diseases. In Katzung BG, Trevor AJ, editors: *Basic and clinical pharmacology*, ed 13, New York, 2015, McGraw-Hill, pp 1052–1083.
8. Pinto-Sanchez MI, Yuan Y, Bercik P, et al.: Proton pump inhibitors for functional dyspepsia (protocol), *Cochrane Database Systematic Reviews*(7), 2014, CD011194, http://dx.doi.org/10.1002/14651858.CD011194.
9. Shah NH, LePendu P, Bauer-Mehren A, et al.: Proton pump usage and the risk of myocardial infarction in the general population, *PLoS ONE* 10(6):e0124653, 2015, http://dx.doi.org/10.1371/journal.pone.0124653.
10. Wallace JL, Sharkey KA: Drugs affecting gastrointestinal function. In Brunton LL, Chabner BA, Knollmann BC, editors: *Goodman and Gillman's the pharmacologic basic of therapeutics*, ed 12, New York, 2011, McGraw-Hill, pp 1307–1362.

29

Pituitary, Thyroid, and Parathyroid Pharmacology

Gail T. Galasko

KEY INFORMATION

- Vasopressin (antidiuretic hormone), from the posterior pituitary, targets blood vessels and the kidney.
- Oxytocin, also from the posterior pituitary, targets the breast and uterus.
- The principal anterior pituitary hormones discussed in this chapter are prolactin (targets the breast), growth hormone (releases insulin-like growth factor-1 from the liver [IGF-1]), and thyrotropin (targets the thyroid).
- The release of anterior pituitary hormones is controlled by hypothalamic hormones.
- Dopamine and somatostatin are hypothalamic factors that inhibit the release of prolactin and growth hormone, respectively.
- Dopaminergic drugs, somatostatin analogues, growth hormone, and IGF-1 are used therapeutically.
- Thyroid hormones are used to replace a lack of thyroid hormone production.
- Thioamides, such as methimazole, iodides, and ^{131}I, are used to treat hyperthyroidism.
- Control of bone dynamics depends in part on a complex interaction between osteoblasts and osteoclasts.
- Parathyroid hormone (PTH) generally causes calcium release from bone, increases calcitriol (primary active form of vitamin D) synthesis, and decreases calcium excretion while increasing phosphate excretion in the kidney.
- Vitamin D increases calcium and phosphate absorption from the GI tract, and it decreases calcium and phosphate excretion. At physiologic levels, the major effect on bone is indirect, by promoting positive calcium balance.
- Calcitonin and bisphosphonates reduce bone resorption by inhibiting osteoclastic activity.
- IV Bisphosponates are particularly dangerous for dentoalveolar surgery, as they can stop healing indefinitely.
- Other drugs that inhibit bone resorption include denosumab, teriparatide, and estrogens.

CASE STUDY

Mr. K has been your dental patient for 10 years. One year ago, you made complete upper and lower dentures for him. This is his first appointment since final adjustments were made on the dentures. He complains that the dentures no longer fit and seem too big. He wonders if the denture material is not stable and is expanding. Upon oral examination, you observe that his oral hygiene is still excellent but also see that the dentures are loose. The patient seems a little jittery and appears somewhat thinner since last year's appointment. He also seems to be warm most of the time. How should you proceed with the patient's complaint about the ill-fitting denture?

HYPOTHALAMIC AND PITUITARY HORMONES

The pituitary gland consists of an anterior lobe (adenohypophysis) and a posterior lobe (neurohypophysis). It is connected to the hypothalamus, which lies above it, by the stalk that contains neurosecretory fibers and capillaries. The hypophyseal portal system drains the hypothalamus and perfuses the anterior pituitary. Numerous releasing factors or regulating hormones that are produced by the hypothalamus are carried to the anterior pituitary by this portal system. These hypothalamic releasing factors stimulate the anterior pituitary to produce and secrete numerous trophic hormones, which stimulate target glands to produce hormones. The hypothalamic releasing factors, anterior pituitary hormones produced, target glands, and target gland hormones are presented in Table 29-1. Pituitary hormone secretion is regulated by negative feedback. For anterior pituitary hormones, secretion of releasing factors from the hypothalamus is decreased when the concentration of target gland hormones is high and increased when it is low. Vasopressin, oxytocin, growth hormone and related drugs, and prolactin are discussed next. The other pituitary hormones are discussed with their corresponding target organ hormone(s) in this and other chapters. Figure 29-1 shows the pituitary hormones and the hypothalamic factors that control their release.

POSTERIOR PITUITARY HORMONES

The posterior lobe of the pituitary secretes two homologous peptide hormones, vasopressin and oxytocin. These hormones are synthesized in the hypothalamus and transported via the neurosecretory fibers of the stalk to the posterior pituitary, where they are stored and released. Both of these hormones are nonapeptides, and their structures are similar.

Vasopressin

Vasopressin (antidiuretic hormone [ADH]) acts on the **kidney** to increase water reabsorption. It increases total peripheral resistance and has an important role in the long-term control of blood pressure. Vasopressin also has a **vasoconstrictor** action that plays a role in the short-term regulation of arterial pressure. There are two subtypes of vasopressin receptors. V_1 receptors, which are $G_{q/11}$ protein–linked,

TABLE 29-1 Hypothalamic Stimulatory Releasing Factors, Corresponding Anterior Pituitary Trophic Hormones, Target Glands, and Target Gland Hormones

Hypothalamic Hormone	Pituitary Hormone	Target Organ	Hormone Produced
Corticotropin-releasing hormone (CRH)	Adrenocorticotropin	Adrenal cortex	Glucocorticosteroids, mineralocorticosteroids, androgens
GH-releasing hormone (GHRH)	GH (somatropin)	Liver, bone, other tissues	IGFs (e.g., IGF-1)
Gonadotropin-releasing hormone (GnRH)	Follicle-stimulating hormone, luteinizing hormone	Gonads	Estrogen, progesterone, testosterone
Thyrotropin-releasing hormone (TRH)	Thyroid-stimulating hormone	Thyroid	T_4, T_3

GH, Growth hormone; *IGFs*, insulin-like growth factors; T_3, triiodothyronine; T_4, thyroxine.

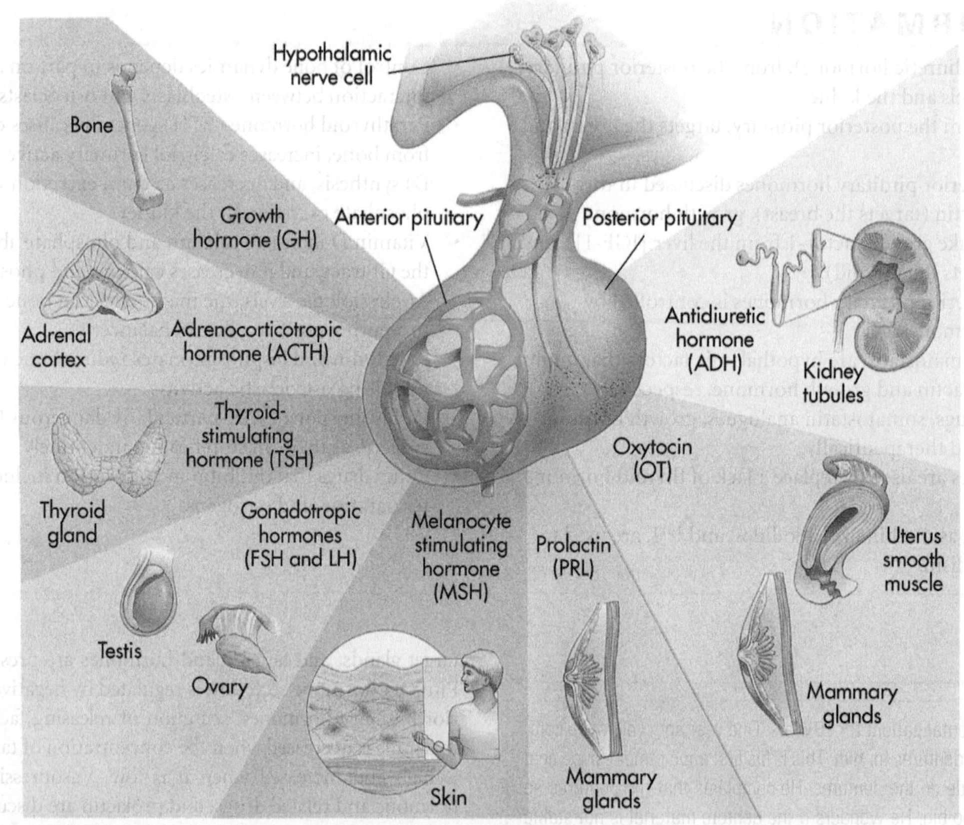

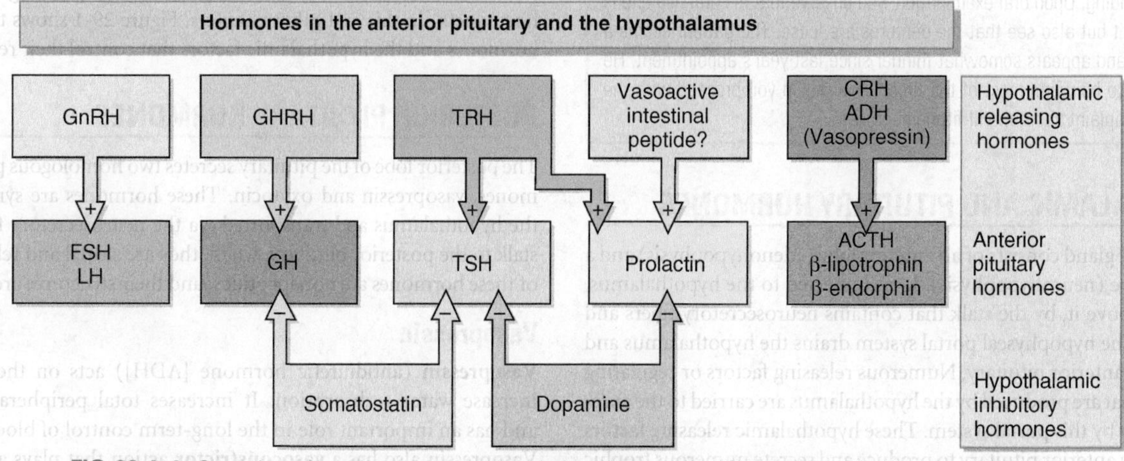

FIG 29-1 **A,** Secretion of anterior and posterior pituitary hormones. (Christensen BL, Kockrow EO: *Adult health nursing*, ed 6, St. Louis, 2011, Mosby.) **B,** Control of secretion of pituitary hormones by hypothalmic hormones. (Bennett PN et al.: *Clinical pharmacology*, ed 11, Edinburgh, 2012, Churchill Livingstone.)

produce their action by stimulation of phospholipase C and formation of inositol triphosphate. This is the pathway responsible for the vasoconstrictor action of vasopressin. V_2 receptors, which are G_s protein–linked, cause **stimulation of adenylyl cyclase** and increase cyclic adenosine 3′,5′-monophosphate (cAMP) formation. Stimulation of V_2 receptors by vasopressin leads to its antidiuretic effect. Lack of ADH leads to diabetes insipidus, resulting in polyuria and polydipsia.

Pharmacokinetics

Vasopressin may be given intravenously, intramuscularly, or intranasally. Because the drug is rapidly metabolized in the liver and kidney, the half-life is approximately 20 min.

Therapeutic uses

Vasopressin (arginine vasopressin) and desmopressin acetate, a long-acting synthetic analogue that acts predominantly at **V_2 receptors**, are used to treat **diabetes insipidus**. The receptors mediating this effect are located on the cells of the collecting duct in the kidney. Vasopressin is also used to control bleeding in certain conditions (e.g., colonic diverticular bleeding). Vasopressin stimulates the release of von Willebrand factor and clotting factor VIII and is used to treat deficiencies of these factors in certain types of hemophilia. **Desmopressin** is also used to **decrease nocturnal enuresis.** Tolvaptan is a vasopressin antagonist that is used in certain cases of heart failure. It is discussed in Chapter 20.

Oxytocin

Oxytocin receptors are $G_{q/11}$ protein–linked receptors that, when stimulated, lead to an **increase in intracellular Ca^{++} and muscle contraction**. Oxytocin causes contraction of uterine smooth muscle and may play a role in the initiation of labor. Oxytocin also stimulates milk ejection in lactating mothers by stimulating myoepithelial cells around the alveoli of the mammary glands. Recent data suggest that oxytocin is a neuropeptide involved in a wide array of social behaviors in diverse species. Maternal bonding, social decision-making, and processing of social stimuli and social memory are enhanced by increased levels of oxytocin.

Pharmacokinetics

Oxytocin has a circulating half-life of 5 min. It is not bound to plasma protein and is metabolized in the liver and kidneys.

Therapeutic uses

Oxytocin is used intravenously for **stimulation of labor** and to **induce postpartum lactation** in cases of breast engorgement.

ANTERIOR PITUITARY HORMONES

Growth Hormone

Growth hormone (GH), also known as somatotropin, is the most abundant of the anterior pituitary hormones. The principal form of GH is a 191-amino acid single-peptide chain with two sulfhydryl bridges. GH for pharmacologic use is produced by recombinant DNA techniques and contains the 191-amino acid sequence of somatotropin, or 192 amino acids consisting of somatotropin plus an extra methionine at the amino terminal end. These preparations are equipotent.

Actions

GH has direct and indirect effects. Its action is through cell surface receptors (JAK/STAT family). The direct actions of GH include **lipolysis in fat cells** and **stimulation of hepatic glucose output**. These effects are opposite to those of insulin. The anabolic and growth-promoting effects of GH are indirect and are **mediated by insulin-like growth factor type I (IGF-I)**. IGF-I stimulates chondrogenesis and skeletal and soft tissue growth. IGF-I increases mitogenesis, increasing cell number rather than cell size. GH-releasing hormone from the hypothalamus stimulates GH release. Somatostatin from the hypothalamus inhibits GH release and release of gastrointestinal secretions.

In contrast to the direct effects of GH, the effects mediated by IGF-I are insulin-like. IGF-I acts through cell membrane receptors that resemble those of insulin. Insulin at high doses may act at IGF-I receptors and vice versa (see Chapter 31). In pharmacologic doses, GH causes an initial insulin-like effect followed by an effect antagonistic to that of insulin.

Pharmacokinetics

Circulating endogenous GH has a half-life of 20 to 25 min, although slow-release forms are available allowing injections once or twice a month. Human GH can be given subcutaneously, with peak plasma levels reached in 2 to 4 h. Metabolism occurs in the liver and the kidney.

Therapeutic uses

GH (somatrem, somatropin) is used in the **treatment of growth failure** in children (pituitary dwarfism), wasting in acquired immunodeficiency syndrome (AIDS), and somatotropin deficiency syndrome. Short-term treatment of GH-deficient adults results in increased lean body mass, decreased fat mass, increased exercise tolerance, and improved psychological well-being. It is sometimes abused by athletes. The GH-releasing hormone analogue sermorelin is used to treat GH deficiency in children who have growth retardation and diagnostically to determine the GH-releasing capacity of the pituitary. **Octreotide, a somatostatin analogue** that inhibits GH release, is approved for use in treating symptoms of **vasoactive intestinal tumors**, metastatic carcinoid tumors, and **acromegaly**. Other uses include AIDS-associated diarrhea and esophageal varices. Lanreotide, another somatostatin analogue, is used to treat acromegaly. Pegvisomant, a competitive antagonist of the GH receptor, is also used to treat acromegaly. Mecasermin is recombinant IGF-1 that is used for IGF-1 deficiency and in certain cases of GH deficiency.

Adverse effects

GH may induce relative insulin resistance. It has been documented to cause diabetes in AIDS patients and decreased insulin sensitivity that is dose-dependent, with a possible increase in type 2 diabetes in children. It may cause scoliosis in children. Arthralgia, especially in the hands and wrist, may occur. Patients may have headaches, especially in the first few months of therapy, and it should be carefully monitored because of the possibility of intracranial hypertension.

Prolactin

Prolactin is an anterior pituitary hormone that is similar in structure to GH. Prolactin increases the growth of the secretory epithelium in the breast and stimulates the production of milk. Although prolactin is not used clinically, the secretion of prolactin can be altered by certain drugs. Because dopamine inhibits prolactin release (Table 29-2), drugs that affect dopamine levels or dopamine receptors in the pituitary affect prolactin release. Bromocriptine and cabergoline are dopamine-receptor agonists that are used to inhibit prolactin release and reduce the size of pituitary prolactin-releasing tumors.

Thyrotropin (Thyroid-Stimulating Hormone)

Thyrotropin (thyroid-stimulating hormone [TSH]) is a glycoprotein hormone consisting of two subunits (α and β). Secretion is pulsatile

TABLE 29-2 Hypothalamic Inhibitory Releasing Factors, Anterior Pituitary Hormones Inhibited, and Target Glands

Hypothalamic Hormone	Pituitary Hormone Inhibited	Target Organ
Dopamine (DA)	Prolactin	Breast
Somatostatin (SS)	Growth hormone	Liver, bone, other tissues

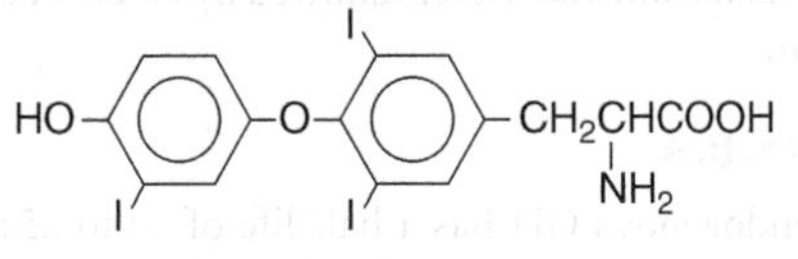

Triiodothyronine (T_3)

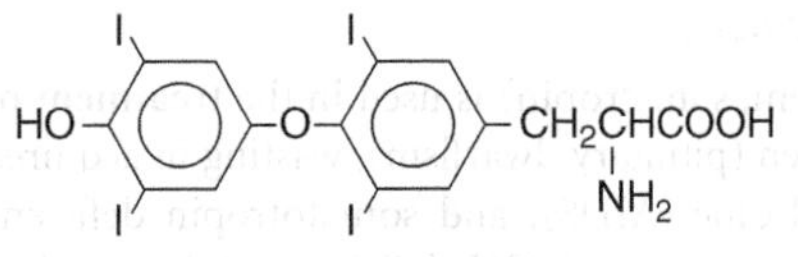

Thyroxine (T_4)

FIG 29-2 Structure of thyroid hormones.

and follows a circadian rhythm, with levels of TSH being highest during sleep at night. TSH secretion is controlled by thyrotropin-releasing hormone (TRH), which is inhibited by thyroid hormone negative feedback. Because TRH is stimulated by cold and decreased by severe stress, TSH is also affected by these conditions. TSH stimulates the thyroid to synthesize thyroglobulin and the thyroid hormones thyroxine (T_4) and triiodothyronine (T_3). An increase in the amount of free thyroid hormone in the circulation results in decreased TSH gene transcription and decreased TSH secretion.

The **TSH receptor** is G protein–coupled. The effects of TSH are mediated by stimulation of adenylyl cyclase and **increased cAMP** (G_s–adenylyl cyclase–cAMP) in the thyroid cell. TSH also causes activation of phospholipase C (G_q-PLC). TSH is used for diagnostic purposes and to stimulate iodine (^{131}I) uptake in some patients with thyroid cancer (see later).

THYROID HORMONES

The active principles of the thyroid gland are iodine-containing amino acid derivatives of thyronine. They are formed from iodinated tyrosine residues. The structures are shown in Figure 29-2.

Synthesis of Thyroid Hormones

The synthesis of thyroid hormones is shown schematically in Figure 29-3. The first step is uptake of iodide by the thyroid gland. This takes place on the basolateral membrane of the cell through the **Na/I symporter,** and it is inhibited by ions of similar size and charge such as perchlorate and thiocyanate. Iodide is transported into the colloid space by means of **pendrin,** an anion transporter located on the apical surface of the thyroid gland cells. (The colloid space is enclosed by the thyroid gland cells.) Iodide is then oxidized by **thyroid peroxidase** at the apical surface resulting in **iodination** of tyrosine residues in thyroglobulin. Thyroid peroxidase also catalyzes the following step, the conjugation or **coupling of iodinated tyrosines** to thyroxine (T_4) or triiodothyronine (T_3).

The ratio of T_4 to T_3 formed is approximately 4:1. Thyroid hormones are released after proteolysis of thyroglobulin. Most of the hormone released is T_4, which is converted to T_3 in peripheral tissues by iodothyronine deiodinases. T_3 is about four times more potent than T_4.

Control of Thyroid Hormone Secretion

The effect of TSH on the thyroid gland is to stimulate the synthesis and secretion of thyroid hormones T_4 and T_3 (see previous discussion). In addition to TSH, the iodine concentration in the blood plays an important role in regulating the uptake of iodide and formation of thyroid hormones in the thyroid gland. Iodination and thyroid hormone release can be inhibited by larger doses of iodides. This is a part of the autoregulatory control of the thyroid.

The **hypothalamic-pituitary-thyroid axis** is stimulated by cold and decreased in severe stress. It is under negative feedback control of the thyroid hormones, which act on the hypothalamus to decrease TRH synthesis and secretion, and on the pituitary to block the action of TRH.

Actions of Thyroid Hormones

Thyroid hormones act by diffusing across the cell membrane and binding to intracellular receptors in target tissues. T_4 is converted to T_3 inside the cell. T_3 has greater affinity than T_4 for the receptors. The action of thyroid hormones leads to an increase in transcription, resulting in synthesis of proteins that produce many of the actions of thyroid hormones. Thyroid hormones are **crucial in normal development and metabolism.** They have a critical effect on growth, partly by direct action and partly by potentiating GH. Thyroid hormones are important for a normal response to parathyroid hormone (PTH) and calcitonin. They are crucial for nervous and skeletal tissues. Thyroid deficiency during development causes cretinism, characterized by mental retardation and dwarfism.

In addition, thyroid hormones are regulators of metabolism in most tissues. **They increase basal metabolic rate and resting respiratory rate.** Thyroid hormones stimulate the heart, resulting in the heart beating more rapidly and with greater force and an increase in cardiac output. Energy use in skeletal muscle, liver, and kidney is also markedly stimulated. T_3 sensitizes the heart to the effects of circulating endogenous catecholamines by a direct effect on Ca^{++} channels, and thyroid hormones cause an increase in myocardial β-adrenergic receptors.

Pharmacokinetics

The thyroid hormones are highly protein-bound; the major plasma-binding protein is thyroxine-binding globulin. They are also bound by thyroxine-binding prealbumin and albumin. The half-life of T_4 is normally 6 to 7 days; this is shortened to 3 to 4 days in hyperthyroidism. T_3 binds more loosely to plasma proteins and has a half-life of approximately 2 days.

THYROID DISORDERS

Worldwide, the most common cause of thyroid disorders is iodine deficiency. In the United States, the leading cause of hypothyroidism is Hashimoto thyroiditis, an autoimmune disease. **Graves disease (diffuse toxic goiter),** also an autoimmune disorder, is the most common cause of hyperthyroidism in the United States.

Hypothyroidism

Thyroid deficiency during development causes **cretinism,** which is characterized by gross retardation of growth and mental deficiency. In an adult, thyroid deficiency results in **hypothyroidism** and, in

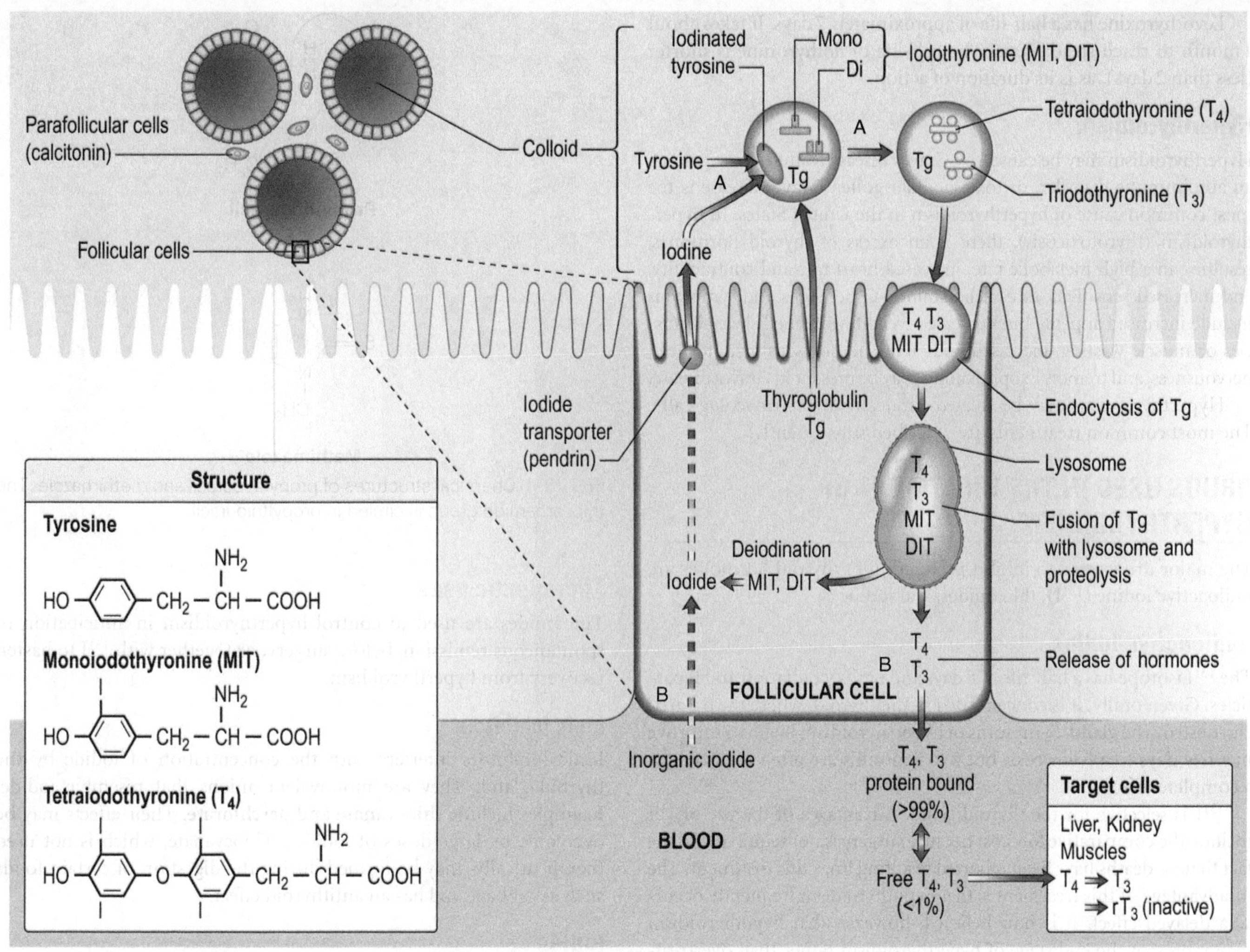

FIG 29-3 Synthesis of thyroid hormones. The sites of action of the thioamides are shown. See text for details. Shown are **A,** sites of inhibition by propylthiouracil and other thioamides and **B,** sites of inhibition by iodide. (Modified from: Kumar P, Clark ML: *Kumar and Clark's clinical medicine*, ed 8, 2012, Saunders.)

more severe cases, myxedema. Hypothyroidism is a common endocrine disorder affecting 1.4% to 2% of women and 0.1% to 0.2% of men. The prevalence of overt and subclinical hypothyroidism is significantly greater in women than in men and increases dramatically in women after age 40 years, affecting 5% to 10% of women older than 50 years. Subclinical hypothyroidism is common, especially among older women. It has been suggested that this condition may be associated with an increased mortality rate, particularly from cardiovascular disease and a subtle decrease in myocardial contractility. Subclinical hypothyroidism is associated with a small increase in low-density lipoprotein cholesterol and a decrease in high-density lipoprotein cholesterol, changes that increase risk of atherosclerosis and coronary artery disease. Cognitive impairment occurs in hypothyroidism, and attention, motor speed, memory, and visual spatial organization all are significantly impaired. In addition, hypothyroidism is an important risk factor for carpal tunnel syndrome.

Signs and Symptoms of Hypothyroidism

Typical **symptoms of hypothyroidism** include lethargy; fatigue; loss of energy and ambition; slowing of intellectual and motor activity; decreased appetite; increased weight; and skin that is dry, cold, and coarse. Hair loss, including loss of the outer third of eyebrows, occurs. Hypothyroid patients have cold intolerance, bradycardia, hypotension, and increased capillary fragility. They also show an exaggerated response to central nervous system depressants such as sedatives and narcotic analgesics.

Replacement Therapy

Animal products include desiccated thyroid, which is composed of animal thyroid glands. Numerous preparations of levothyroxine sodium (T_4) are available. Liothyronine sodium (T_3) and liotrix, a mixture of T_4 and T_3 in a 4:1 ratio, are also available. Synthetic T_4 has a uniform content and a long half-life and is the preferred and most widely used thyroid replacement medication. Because of its greater potential for cardiotoxicity and its shorter half-life, the use of T_3 is controversial and much less frequent. Nevertheless, for some patients, the combination of T_3 and T_4 is better than T_4 alone.

The thyroid hormones are well absorbed after oral administration. Absorption of T_4 may be decreased, however, by food, Ca^{++} preparations, and aluminum-containing antacids. Absorption of T_4 is best if it is taken on an empty stomach in the morning. Absorption of T_3, which is almost completely absorbed, is not affected by food.

Levothyroxine has a half-life of approximately 7 days. It takes about 1 month to reach steady state. The half-life of liothyronine is shorter (less than 2 days), as is its duration of action.

Hyperthyroidism

Hyperthyroidism may be caused by Graves disease (diffuse toxic goiter), an autoimmune disorder, or toxic nodular goiter. Graves disease is the most common cause of hyperthyroidism in the United States. In hyperthyroidism (thyrotoxicosis), there is an excess of thyroid hormones, resulting in a high metabolic rate, increased heart rate and contractility, and increased sensitivity to catecholamines. Other signs and symptoms include increased appetite but decreased weight, weakened skeletal muscles or muscle wasting, increased body temperature, sensitivity to heat, nervousness, and tremor. Exophthalmus may be present in Graves disease.

Hyperthyroidism may be treated surgically or pharmacologically. The most common treatments are described subsequently.

DRUGS USED IN THE TREATMENT OF HYPERTHYROIDISM

The major drugs used to inhibit production of thyroid hormones are radioactive iodine (^{131}I), thioamides, and iodide.

Radioactive Iodine

The ^{131}I isotope has a half-life of 8 days and emits γ radiation and β particles. Given orally, it is concentrated in the thyroid, where the β particles destroy the gland. Symptoms of hyperthyroidism begin to improve in a few days to a few weeks, but 2 to 3 months are often required for a complete effect.

^{131}I is selective for the thyroid gland. Advantages of the use of ^{131}I include the comparative low cost because surgery is not required and the fact that no deaths have been reported resulting from this treatment. The disadvantage of this treatment is that hypothyroidism frequently occurs as a delayed effect. It is now believed, however, that hypothyroidism may represent the end stage of hyperthyroidism rather than overtreatment with ^{131}I. ^{131}I should be avoided in children and pregnant patients. Uptake of low-dose ^{131}I may be used as a test of thyroid function.

Thioamides

Propylthiouracil and methimazole are the most important antithyroid drugs used in the United States within the thioamides (Fig. 29-4). These drugs are related to thiourea and contain a thiocarbamide group that is essential for their antithyroid activity.

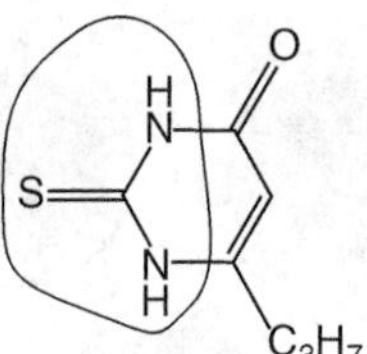

Propylthiouracil

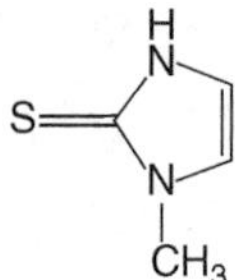

Methimazole

FIG 29-4 Chemical structures of propylthiouracil and methimazole. The thiocarbamide group is circled in propylthiouracil.

Mechanism of action

Thioamides inhibit thyroid peroxidase, decreasing iodide oxidation, iodination of tyrosines, and coupling of iodotyrosyl and iodothyronyl residues (see Fig. 29-3). As a result, less thyroid hormone is synthesized. Propylthiouracil also inhibits the peripheral conversion of T_4 to T_3.

Pharmacokinetics

Thioamides are given orally. Methimazole is distributed throughout body water and has a plasma half-life of 6 to 15 h. An average dose produces more than 90% inhibition of thyroid incorporation of iodide within 12 h, but the clinical response takes weeks to manifest because of the long half-life of T_4 and because there may be stores of hormone in the thyroid that need to be depleted. The actions of propylthiouracil may be seen more quickly because of the inhibition of peripheral conversion of T_4 to T_3.

Adverse effects

Adverse effects include occasional, reversible, yet rapidly developing **agranulocytosis; rashes; pain;** stiffness in joints; paresthesias; and loss or depigmentation of hair.

Therapeutic uses

Thioamides are used to control hyperthyroidism in anticipation of spontaneous remission, before surgery, or together with ^{131}I to hasten recovery from hyperthyroidism.

Ionic inhibitors

Ionic inhibitors interfere with the concentration of iodide by the thyroid gland. They are monovalent anions that resemble iodide. Examples include **thiocyanate and perchlorate.** Their effects may be overcome by large doses of iodides. Thiocyanate, which is not used therapeutically, may be formed during the digestion of certain foods such as cabbage and has an antithyroid effect.

Iodide

Iodide is the oldest remedy for thyroid disorders. Iodine/iodides are required for thyroid hormone synthesis (see Fig. 29-3); however, high concentrations of iodide limit its own transport. In addition, high concentrations of iodide inhibit synthesis of iodotyrosines and iodothyronines (organification) and inhibit thyroid hormone release. These effects, which depend on intracellular concentrations of iodide, are transient. **High plasma iodide concentrations also inhibit release of thyroid hormones.** Iodide has been used preoperatively in preparation for thyroidectomy because it makes the gland less vascular. Iodide is also used together with antithyroid drugs and propranolol to treat thyrotoxic crisis.

Hypersensitivity to iodides is the major adverse effect. Iodism, which is chronic iodine toxicity, has many adverse effects, including unpleasant taste, burning in the mouth and throat, soreness of teeth and gingiva, and increased salivation. Symptoms similar to those of a head cold commonly occur, as do skin eruptions, gastric irritation, and diarrhea. Inflammation of the larynx, tonsils, and lungs and enlargement of the parotid and submandibular glands may occur. Iodide concentrates in salivary glands.

Other Drugs

With excessive thyroid hormone production, such as in thyroid storm, β-adrenergic blockers such as propranolol, or a calcium channel blocker such as diltiazem, can be used to control heart rate. Propranolol also reduces the conversion of T_4 to T_3 in peripheral tissues.

IMPLICATIONS FOR DENTISTRY

Subclinical hypothyroidism and hyperthyroidism are common, well-defined conditions that often progress to overt disease. The clinical presentation of thyroid disorders is often subtle in older adults and may be confused with normal aging.

Hypothyroidism

Hypothyroidism is five to six times more common than hyperthyroidism. **Hypothyroidism affects 7 to 10 times as many women as men,** and the incidence of the disease increases sharply with age in women after age 40 years, affecting 5% to 10% of women older than 50 years. Subclinical states may contribute to hyperlipidemia, cardiac dysfunction, and osteoporosis.

The dentist may be in a position to detect signs and symptoms of subclinical thyroid disease and refer the patient for medical evaluation and treatment; this is very important in hypothyroidism, in which signs and symptoms are subtle and similar to those of depression (Box 29-1). As a result, the disease may not be diagnosed. Subclinical hypothyroidism in younger individuals may manifest as delayed eruption of teeth, malocclusion, and skeletal growth retardation. Other oral manifestations of hypothyroidism include tongue enlargement and scalloping. Hypothyroid patients have increased capillary fragility and show an exaggerated response to central nervous system depressants such as sedatives and opioids.

Clinical hypothyroidism or myxedema may be recognized by a patient's dull expression; puffy eyelids; alopecia of the outer third of the eyebrows; dry, rough skin; dry, brittle, coarse hair; increased size of the tongue; slowing of physical and mental activity; anemia; constipation; and increased sensitivity to cold. In patients with myxedema, stressful situations such as surgery, trauma, or infections may precipitate myxedematous coma. Myxedematous coma is very rare and occurs predominantly in elderly women and has a greater than 50% mortality rate.

Hyperthyroidism

Thyrotoxicosis is characterized by warm, moist skin; a rosy complexion; weight loss; fine, friable hair; and nail softening. Profuse sweating is common in these patients. Achlorhydria may occur, and approximately 3% of individuals affected develop pernicious anemia. Hyperthyroid individuals are **nervous**, emotionally labile, and always moving. They display tremor of the hands and tongue and muscle weakness. In thyrotoxicosis, there is increased bone loss. In these patients, there is also increased stroke volume and heart rate and palpitations. Supraventricular arrhythmias may occur. **Graves ophthalmopathy** may be recognized by eyelid retraction, proptosis, and a bright-eyed stare. Patients who are hyperthyroid are highly sensitive to epinephrine. Propranolol alleviates adrenergic symptoms such as sweating, tremor, and tachycardia.

Oral complications of **thyrotoxicosis include osteoporosis of the alveolar bone.** Dental caries and periodontal disease appear more frequently. In children, teeth and jaws develop more rapidly, and **there is early loss of deciduous teeth and early eruption of permanent teeth. Changes** in the gingiva resulting from hyperthyroidism may lead to ill-fitting dentures.

Barbiturates lower the level of thyroid hormones and should be used cautiously in patients on thyroid replacement therapy.

HORMONES OF CA^{++} HOMEOSTASIS

Parathyroid Hormone (PTH)

The parathyroid glands (there are usually four) are embedded within the posterior surface of the thyroid. The principal cells secrete **PTH,** which is formed by proteolysis of a larger precursor. PTH is a single-chain polypeptide containing 84 amino acids and has a molecular weight of approximately 9500 Da. Loss of the first two amino acids eliminates most biologic activity.

BOX 29-1 Common Signs of Hypothyroidism and Depression

- Depressed mood
- Decreased interests
- Weight gain
- Disturbed sleep
- Muscle weakness/slow speech
- Disturbed concentration and cognition
- Feelings of guilt or inadequacy/inability to cope
- Cold intolerance

Regulation of secretion

The principal factor in **control of PTH secretion** is **plasma Ca^{++} concentration.** High plasma Ca^{++} concentration decreases PTH secretion; low Ca^{++} concentration stimulates it. Ca^{++} regulates PTH secretion by a G protein–coupled, cell surface Ca^{++}-sensing receptor. Phosphate regulates PTH secretion indirectly by forming complexes with Ca^{++}. Increases in phosphate concentration reduce Ca^{++} levels and increase PTH secretion. Calcitriol (1,25-dihydroxyvitamin D_3) directly inhibits PTH secretion by affecting gene transcription.

Pharmacologic effects

PTH regulates Ca^{++} and phosphate, causing an increase in plasma Ca^{++} and a decrease in plasma phosphate concentrations. The primary function of PTH is to maintain a constant extracellular Ca^{++} concentration.

The most important **target tissues for PTH are bone and kidney.** In bone, PTH increases Ca^{++} and phosphate release by increasing bone resorption. It acts on the osteoblast to induce RANK ligand (RANKL), which stimulates osteoclast activity, resulting in **increased bone turnover** (Fig. 29-5). Bone formation and bone resorption are enhanced by PTH. With constant dosing, PTH increases bone resorption. When PTH is given intermittently at low doses, it stimulates cortical and trabecular bone growth. **Teriparatide (recombinant human PTH 1-34)** is used to treat osteoporosis. Agents that reduce osteoclastic activity by acting on osteoblasts often increase the release of osteoprotegerin (OPG) from the osteoblast. Osteoprotegerin binds to RANKL and prevents its action on osteoclasts (see Fig. 29-5). In the kidney, PTH increases reabsorption of Ca^{++} and Mg^{++} and decreases reabsorption of phosphate. **PTH also increases conversion of vitamin D to its active form, 1,25-dihydroxyvitamin D_3 (calcitriol),** which is secreted into the circulation and acts in the gastrointestinal tract to increase the absorption of Ca^{++}.

Pharmacokinetics

PTH has a half-life of minutes, with clearance occurring mostly in the liver and kidney.

Calcitonin

Calcitonin is secreted by the parafollicular cells of the thyroid gland. Calcitonin is synthesized as a prohormone and processed to the hormone. There is considerable species variation in calcitonin. Human calcitonin is a single-chain peptide composed of 32 amino acids and has a molecular weight of 3600 Da. A disulfide bridge between positions 1 and 7 is essential for biologic activity.

Control of Secretion

Elevated extracellular Ca^{++} concentration is the most important stimulator of calcitonin secretion. Calcitonin release is also stimulated by gastrointestinal tract hormones, including cholecystokinin and gastrin.

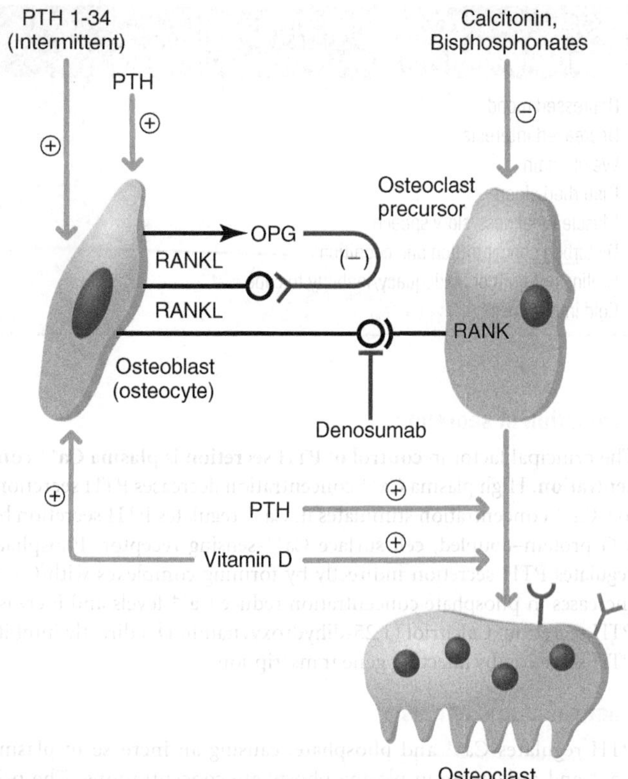

FIG 29-5 Action of several drugs on bone cells. Parathyroid hormone (PTH) stimulates osteoblast and osteocyte action leading indirectly to stimulation of osteoclasts through RANK ligand (RANKL) secretion. (Stimulation of RANK leads to increases in numbers of osteoclasts, resulting in bone breakdown.) The intermittent dosing of PTH 1-34 (teriparatide) stimulates osteoblast formation and activity without the effect on osteoblasts seen with continuous exposure to PTH. The effect of PTH 1-34 is due in part to the synthesis and secretion of osteoprotegerin (OPG). Estrogens (not shown) also have a similar effect on osteoblasts. OPG binds to RANKL, preventing its binding to RANK receptors on osteoclast precursors. At pharmacologic doses, $1,25(OH)_2D$ (most potent vitamin D) has similar actions as PTH. At lower concentrations, vitamin D plays an anabolic effect on bone formation by stimulation of osteoblasts. Denosumab is a monoclonal antibody drug that binds to RANKL and prevents its action at RANK. Many of the effects of intermittent (PTH 1-34) on osteoblasts are similar to estrogens. Calcitonin and bisphosphonates act directly on osteoclasts and osteoclast precursors to inhibit their activity. *$1,25(OH)_2D$*, Calcitriol; *RANK*, receptor activator of nuclear factor kappa-B. (Modified from Dowd F: *Mosby's review for the NBDE*, Part 2, ed 2, St. Louis, 2015, Mosby.)

Actions

Calcitonin acts on G protein–linked cell surface receptors located on target tissues. It reduces plasma Ca^{++} and phosphate concentrations mainly by acting on bone to inhibit **osteoclast** activity and bone resorption (see Fig. 29-5). Calcitonin also acts on the kidney to increase urinary excretion of Ca^{++} and phosphate.

Therapeutic uses

Calcitonin is used in the treatment of **Paget's disease**, in which there is excessive, disorganized bone remodeling, and in some patients with **osteoporosis**. Salmon calcitonin, which is more potent and has a longer half-life than mammalian calcitonin, is typically used in therapy. It is given by injection or nasal spray.

TABLE 29-3 Effects of Parathyroid Hormone and Vitamin D on Bone, Gastrointestinal Tract, and Kidney

Organ	Parathyroid Hormone	Vitamin D
Bone	Low intermittent doses (e.g., PTH 1-34) increase bone formation; higher doses increase bone resorption	Effects depend on dose and various metabolites*
Gastrointestinal tract	Increases Ca^{++} and phosphate absorption (by increased calcitriol production)	Calcitriol increases Ca^{++} and phosphate absorption
Kidney	Decreases Ca^{++}, increases phosphate excretion	Decreases Ca^{++} and phosphate excretion
Overall effect	Increases plasma Ca^{++}, decreases plasma phosphate	Increases plasma Ca^{++} and plasma phosphate

*See text

Adverse effects

Nausea and gastrointestinal tract effects are the most common adverse effects. Rash with itching and swelling may also occur.

Vitamin D

Vitamin D is the name given to two related substances, **cholecalciferol (vitamin D_3)** and ergocalciferol (vitamin D_2). Both substances are active in humans and are able to prevent or cure rickets. Cholecalciferol is formed in the skin from 7-dehydrocholesterol by the action of ultraviolet irradiation; ergocalciferol comes from plants. Vitamin D is also found in dietary products.

The major action of vitamin D is control of Ca^{++} homeostasis. Vitamin D **facilitates absorption of Ca^{++} and phosphate from the small intestine**, interacts with PTH to enhance mobilization of Ca^{++} and phosphate from bone, and **decreases excretion of Ca^{++} and phosphate by the kidney.** In addition, vitamin D has effects **on bone remodeling**. More recent studies suggest that vitamin D may have several other actions, including antiinflammatory properties (downregulation of tumor necrosis factor-α, interleukin-6, interleukin-1, and interleukin-8) and an **antiproliferative effect**. Vitamin D is used to treat rickets, osteomalacia, hypoparathyroidism, to prevent osteoporosis, and topically for the treatment of psoriasis.

The net effect of vitamin D is to increase serum Ca^{++} and serum phosphate. This is different from the net effect of PTH, which is to increase serum Ca^{++} and reduce serum phosphate. The effects of PTH and vitamin D are shown in Table 29-3.

Vitamin D is a prohormone that is a precursor to numerous biologically active metabolites. Cholecalciferol is biotransformed to 25-hydroxycholecalciferol (calcifediol) in the liver and converted further to 1,25-dihydroxyvitamin D_3 (calcitriol), the most potent form (Fig. 29-6). This latter reaction is stimulated by parathyroid hormone and inhibited by a protein synthesized by osteoblast and osteocytes, fibroblast growth factor-23 (FGF-23). Further metabolism to 24,25-dihydroxyvitamin D_3 a less active form, occurs in the kidney. Calcitriol ($1,25(OH)_2D$) (Fig. 29-7) is biologically the most active metabolite of vitamin D.

Receptors for calcitriol are found in various tissues, including bone, gut, and kidney. These are intracellular receptors, as are typical of other steroid hormone receptors. Calcitriol binding to its receptors leads to a selective increase in transcription and production of proteins such

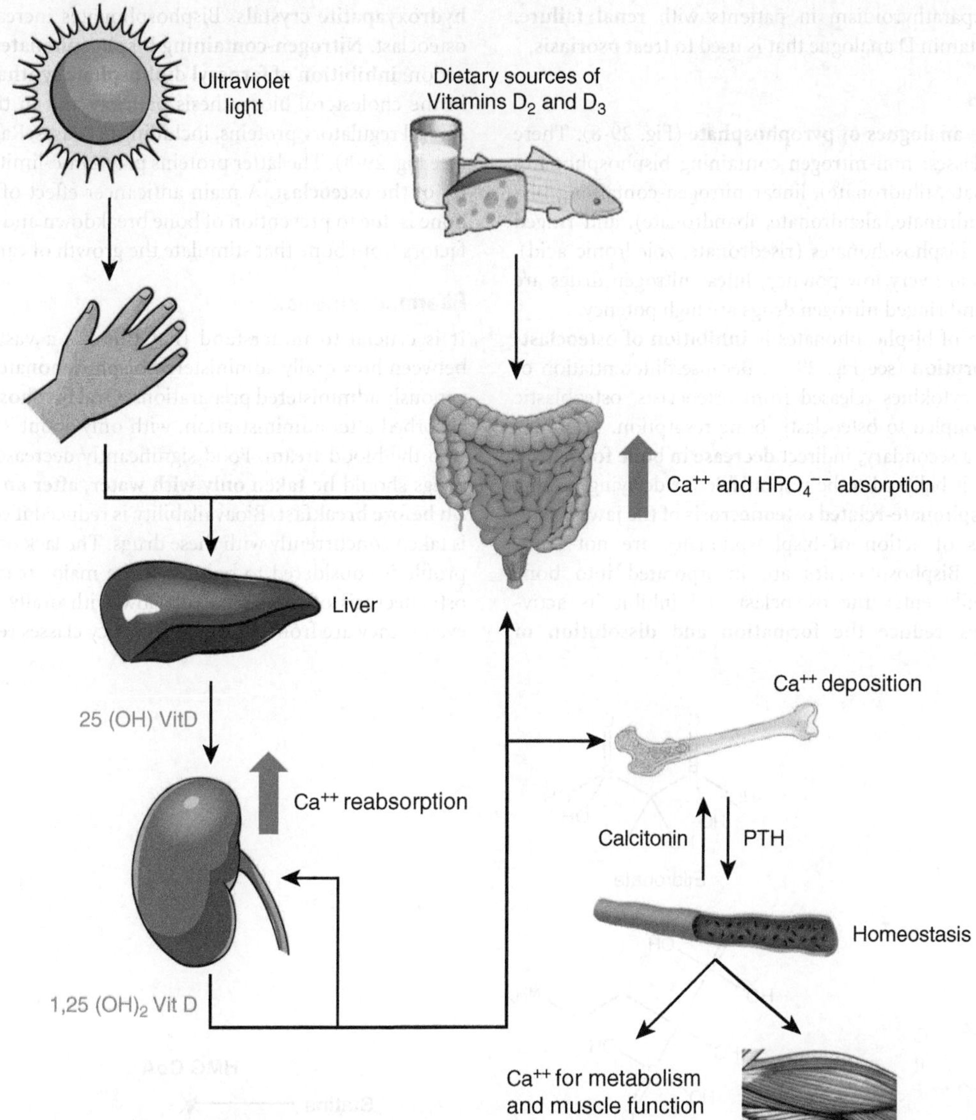

FIG 29-6 Synthesis of 1,25$(OH)_2$ Vitamin D. The effects of parathyroid hormone (PTH) on the synthesis of the most potent vitamin D are shown. (Modified from Kumar V, et al.: *Robbins and Cotran pathologic basis of disease,* ed 8, Philadelphia, 2010; Saunders and Davis JR, Sherer K: *Applied nutrition and diet therapy for nurses,* 2nd ed. Philadelphia: Saunders, 1994.)

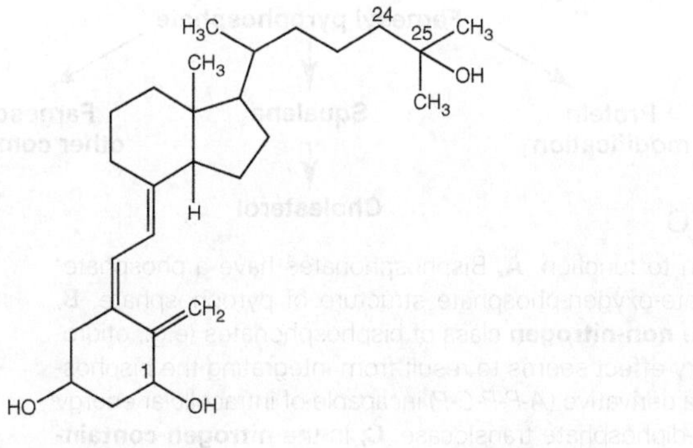

Calcitriol

FIG 29-7 Structure of calcitriol (1,25-dihydroxycholecalciferol).

as Ca^{++}-binding proteins in the gastrointestinal tract. Calcitriol may also act directly on the membrane to alter Ca^{++} flux. In addition to its classic effects (discussed earlier), calcitriol has many other actions, including regulation of PTH secretion, cytokine production, and proliferation and differentiation of numerous cells.

Calcifediol (25-hydroxycholecalciferol) is more potent than calcitriol in stimulating renal reabsorption of Ca^{++} and phosphate. Calcifediol may be the major metabolite involved in the regulation of Ca^{++} flux and contractility in muscle.

High levels of Ca^{++} and phosphate reduce the amount of 1,25-dihydroxyvitamin D_3 produced by the kidney and decrease the amount of 24,25-dihydroxyvitamin D_3. Calcitriol inhibits PTH secretion by a direct action on PTH gene transcription.

Vitamin D is usually given orally. After absorption, vitamin D and its metabolites circulate in plasma bound to vitamin D–binding protein, which is an α globulin. Vitamin D (cholecalciferol) has a plasma half-life of 19 to 25 h but is stored in fat for prolonged periods. The major circulating form is calcifediol, which has a half-life of 19 days. The half-life of calcitriol is 3 to 5 days.

Calcitriol is available for clinical use as vitamin D. Ergocalciferol and cholecalciferol are also available. In addition, doxercalciferol and paricalcitol, analogs of calcitriol, have been approved for treatment of secondary hyperparathyroidism in patients with **renal failure.** **Calcipotriene** is a vitamin D analogue that is used **to treat psoriasis.**

Bisphosphonates

Bisphosphonates are **analogues of pyrophosphate** (Fig. 29-8). There are three distinct classes: non-nitrogen-containing bisphosphonates (etidronate, clodronate, tiludronate), linear nitrogen-containing bisphosphonates (pamidronate, alendronate, ibandronate), and ringed nitrogen-containing bisphosphonates (risedronate, zoledronic acid). Non-nitrogen drugs are very low potency, linear nitrogen drugs are moderate potency, and ringed nitrogen drugs are high potency.

The major action of bisphosphonates is **inhibition of osteoclast-mediated bone resorption** (see Fig. 29-5). Because differentiation of osteoblasts requires cytokines released from osteoclasts, osteoblastic bone formation is coupled to osteoclastic bone resorption. By inhibiting the osteoclasts, a secondary, indirect **decrease in bone formation** occurs. This process is believed to be responsible for delaying healing and creating **bisphosphonate-related osteonecrosis of the jaw.**

The mechanisms of action of bisphosphonates are not completely understood. Bisphosphonates are incorporated into bone matrix and eventually enter the osteoclast and inhibit its activity. Bisphosphonates **reduce the formation and dissolution of hydroxyapatite crystals.** Bisphosphonates increase apoptosis of the osteoclast. **Nitrogen-containing bisphosphonates** have an additional action: **inhibition of farnesyl diphosphate synthase,** a crucial enzyme in the cholesterol biosynthesis pathway and in the isoprenylation of several regulatory proteins, including GTPases, Ras, Rac, Rho, and Cdc (see Fig. 29-8). The latter proteins play a rate-limiting role in the **activity of the osteoclast.** A main anticancer effect of bisphosphonates in bone is due to prevention of bone breakdown and liberation of growth factors from bone that stimulate the growth of cancer cells.

Pharmacokinetics

It is crucial to understand that there is a vast clinical difference between how orally administered bisphosphonates work versus intravenously administered preparations. **Oral bisphosphonates** are poorly absorbed after administration, with only about 2% of the drug taken into the bloodstream. Food significantly decreases absorption. These drugs should be **taken only with water, after an overnight fast, and 2 h before breakfast.** Bioavailability is reduced if coffee or orange juice is taken concurrently with these drugs. The lack of a sizable absorption profile is considered to be one of the major reasons why the risk of osteonecrosis of the jaw is very low with orally administered drugs, even if they are from the higher potency classes (e.g., alendronate and

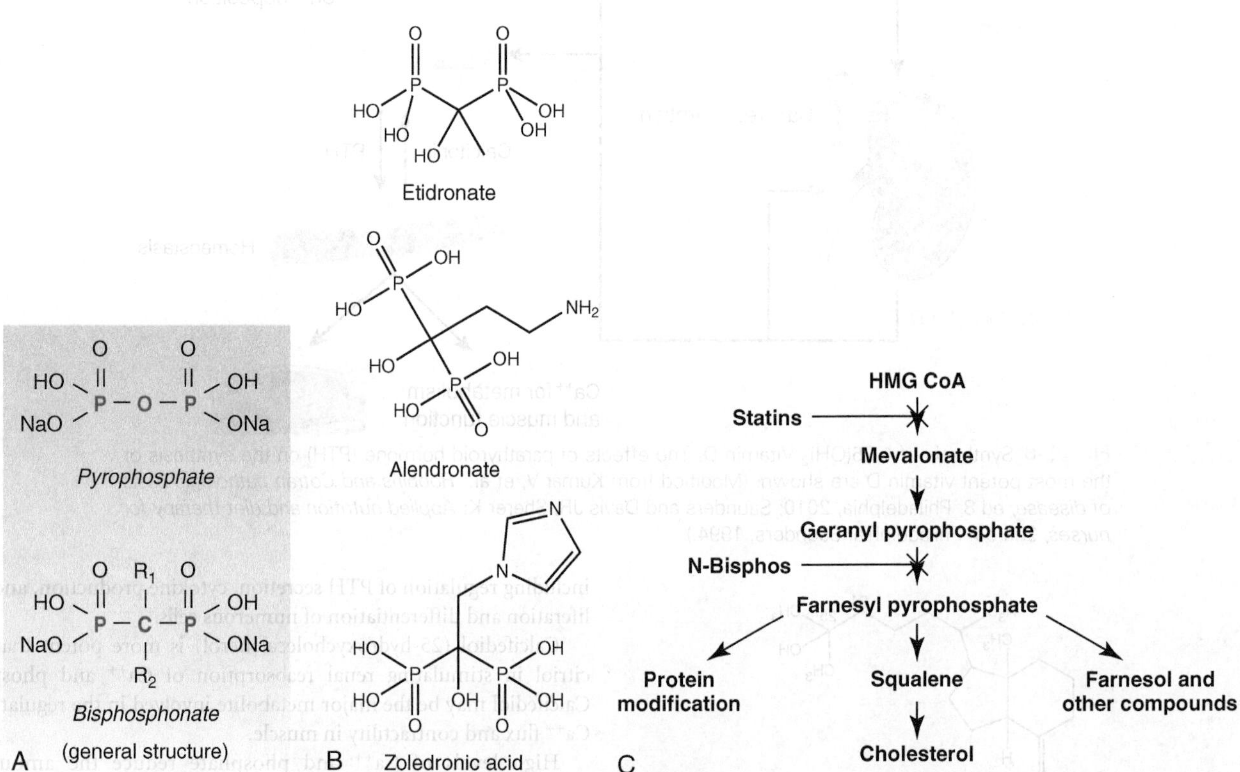

FIG 29-8 Pathways by which bisphosphonates seem to function. **A,** Bisphosphonates have a phosphate-carbon-phosphate structure that mimics the phosphate-oxygen-phosphate structure of pyrophosphate. **B,** Structures of three bisphosphonates are shown. In the **non-nitrogen** class of bisphosphonates (e.g., etidronate, clodronate, tiludronate), the osteoclastic inhibitory effect seems to result from integrating the bisphosphonate into adenosine 5′-triphosphate (*ATP*), yielding a derivative (*A-P-P-C-P*) incapable of intracellular energy transfer by disrupting mitochondrial ATP/adenosine 5′-diphosphate translocase. **C,** In the **nitrogen-containing** bisphosphonates (*N-Bisphos*) (e.g., alendronate, pamidronate, risedronate, zoledronic acid), the mechanism seems to be interruption of a crucial rate-limiting step in the formation of farnesyl pyrophosphate. Ras protein requires farnesylation to be activated. Without Ras activation, cytochrome *c* is released from the mitochondria, which causes caspase-3 activation, an apoptotic signaler. Statin drugs also interrupt this pathway, but not as effectively in bone. The caspase-mediated apoptotic effect seems to be stronger than the ATP analogue effect provided by the non-nitrogen class of bisphosphonates. (**A,** Lehne RA: *Pharmacology for nursing care,* ed 7, St. Louis, 2010, Saunders. **C,** Adapted from Green JR: Bisphosphonates: preclinical review, *Oncologist* 9[Suppl 4]:3–13, 2004.)

risedronate). The **intravenously** administered drugs, pamidronate and zoledronic acid, are estimated to have about 40% of their dose available to the bone after liver conjugation and renal elimination. The **risk for osteonecrosis** becomes much higher with the intravenous forms of these drugs, and in particular with zoledronic acid because of its particularly high potency. Orally administered drugs include alendronate, etidronate, ibandronate, risedronate, and tiludronate.

Bisphosphonates, in contrast to pyrophosphate, are not metabolized and are excreted unchanged in the urine. Plasma levels decrease by more than 95% within 6 h, but the terminal half-life may exceed 10 years because they are slowly released from the skeleton, to which they bind.

Therapeutic uses

Bisphosphonates are used to treat diseases in which there is rapid bone turnover or excessive osteolytic activity. They are used to treat **osteoporosis, Paget's disease, and malignant bone disease**. In the treatment of osteoporosis, alendronate and risedronate have been shown to decrease the incidence of fractures significantly and improve bone mineral density. These two drugs do not have the effect of decreasing bone formation that is seen with etidronate.

In cancer, particularly breast cancer, inhibition of osteolysis has proved to be effective therapy for decreasing metastases to the jaws and malignancy-associated hypercalcemia and for adjunctive therapy in delaying or preventing cancer-related skeletal pain. Therapy reduces the incidence of fractures and may reduce the need for radiation therapy. In Paget's disease, bisphosphonates reduce the rapid bone turnover rate and slow disease progression.

Adverse effects

The most common adverse effects of bisphosphonates are gastrointestinal tract disturbances. **Esophagitis** can occur with oral preparations. To prevent esophagitis, oral preparations are given with liberal amounts of water and with the patient in an upright position. Proton pump inhibitors (see Chapter 28) can also be used. The use of an intravenous form of bisphosphonate such as zoledronic acid is another alternative. Bisphosphonates may cause musculoskeletal pain. Bisphosphonates have been shown to cause **osteonecrosis**, especially in the **mandible** and, to a much lesser extent, the maxilla. There is little evidence that these agents cause significant lesions elsewhere in the body. Although osteonecrosis occurs infrequently, it is most common in patients receiving intravenous bisphosphonate therapy. The risk of developing osteonecrosis in patients taking oral bisphosphonates is estimated to be about one per 100,000 person-years' exposure. For patients who are receiving **intravenous bisphosphonate** therapy for malignant neoplasms, **it is recommended that the dentist avoid extractions unless critically necessary.**

Denosumab

Denosumab is a **monoclonal antibody that blocks RANKL** from binding to its receptor RANK (receptor activator of nuclear factor kappa-β), which is produced by osteoblasts and other cells (see Fig. 29-5). Denosumab is used to **treat osteoporosis and some metastatic cancers in bone** because it prevents the stimulation of osteoclasts. It is given by injection either every 4 weeks or every 6 months, depending on the preparation.

Cinacalcet

Cinacalcet stimulates the calcium-sensing receptor, which results in inhibition of PTH secretion. It is used to treat secondary hyperparathyroidism in adults and to treat parathyroid carcinoma.

IMPLICATIONS FOR DENTISTRY

There is confusion currently in the healthcare community about the effects of bisphosphonates and the risk of **anti-resorptive osteonecrosis of the jaw (ARONJ)**. Here is a summary of what is known:

- The linear non-nitrogen bisphosphonates are rarely used, and are of no clinical concern for ARONJ.
- The oral nitrogen-containing bisphosphonates (linear and ringed) only rarely demonstrate ARONJ. Most of these are used for osteoporosis prevention and the patients using them are considered safe for standard dentoalveolar surgery. However, informed consent must include the rare and remote possibility of ARONJ, which currently has no cure.
- **The IV bisphosphonates** are almost exclusively used to treat Paget's disease and bone-invading cancers such as Multiple Myeloma (plasmacytomas) and metastatic breast cancer. These patients are at a **high risk** for developing ARONJ.
- It is important for physicians to get dental consultations prior to initiating IV bisphosphonate therapy.
- Common accepted ideal dental practice is to do a full dental exam and remove all questionable teeth prior to initiating IV bisphosphonate therapy.
- Most centers agree that after three (3) IV doses of bisphosphonates, no dentoalveolar surgery should be performed **for the rest of the patient's life.** This includes extractions, implant placement, periodontal surgery and apicoectomies. Alternate therapies such as endodontics and conservative periodontal scaling should be employed.
- If a tooth is fractured and absolutely has to come out, ideal therapy is to decoronate it, stabilize the pulp and root canals, and only remove it after it has become completely enveloped in soft tissue. Removing it when still encased in bone brings very high risk of incurable ARONJ.
- "Drug holidays" are contraindicated with the bisphosphonates given their propensity to have half-lives numbered in the years to decades.
- Denosumab is a potent RANKL inhibitor that provides a similar anti-cancer effect. Data indicate that this drug can be removed for 6+ months and then dentoalveolar surgery can be performed with low risk of ARONJ.

CASE DISCUSSION

It is important that the reason for the loose denture be ascertained. The patient should be observed and quizzed as to his overall health. You find that his blood pressure is slightly elevated and his heart rate is 95 bpm. Upon questioning, the patient reports he has recently experienced the following: nervousness, irritable mood, recent weight loss, thinning of his hair, and difficulty in sleeping. Besides these symptoms, you also notice that the patient has a nervous stare.

Before major changes are made in the dentures, it would be best to have Mr. K see his physician for evaluation. Some potential disorders could be considered, for example, cancer or hyperthyroidism. However, the symptoms are more suggestive of hyperthyroidism. (The patient denies any substance abuse.)

At the next dental appointment 2 weeks later, the patient says he has been diagnosed with Graves disease, a common form of hyperthyroidism and has been referred to an endocrinologist who decides to have Mr. K treated with ^{131}I, to be administered in a few days.

Adjustment of the dentures, if needed, should be postponed until the patient has gained euthyroid status. The effect of ^{131}I takes weeks before it achieves its full effect. After about 3 months, the patient's thyroid status can be assessed. He may require a second dose of ^{131}I. More likely the patient will become hypothyroid as a result of ^{131}I, and he will require some supplementation with thyroid hormone. At that time, the patient's denture needs can be reassessed and new dentures made if necessary after the oral tissues have stabilized. In the interim, and if Mr. K's original denture is too unstable, a soft intermediate reline can be placed until the patient's ^{131}I has been excreted or decayed to a safe level. (The ^{131}I radioactive decay half-life is ~8 days.)

HYPOTHALAMIC, PITUITARY, THYROID, AND PARATHYROID DRUGS

Nonproprietary (Generic) Name	Proprietary (Trade) Name
Hypothalamic and Pituitary-Related Drugs*	
Conivaptan	Vaprisol
Desmopressin	DDAVP, Stimate
Lanreotide	Somatuline Depot
Mecasermin (recombinant IGF-I)	Increlex
Octreotide	Sandostatin
Oxytocin	Pitocin, Syntocinon
Pegvisomant	Somavert
Somatrem	Protropin
Somatropin	Genotropin, Humatrope, Nutropin, Nutropin AQ, Norditropin, Saizen, Serostim, Tev-Tropin
Tolvaptan	Samsca
Vasopressin	Pitressin .
Drugs Used to Inhibit Prolactin Release	
Bromocriptine	Parlodel
Cabergoline	Dostinex
Thyroid Hormone and TSH Preparations	
Levothyroxine	Levolet, Levo-T, Levothroid, Levoxyl, Novothyrox, Synthroid, Unithroid
Liothyronine	Cytomel, Triostat
Liotrix	Thyrolar
Thyroid desiccated	Armour Thyroid, Thyrar, S-P-T
Thyrotropin (recombinant human TSH)	Thyrogen
Antithyroid Agents	
Iodide (^{131}I) sodium	Iodotope, Sodium Iodide^{131}I Therapeutic
Methimazole	Tapazole
Potassium iodide	Lugol's solution, Pima, SSKI, iOSAT
Propylthiouracil	PTU
Drugs Affecting Ca^{++} Metabolism	
Bisphosphonates	
Alendronate	Fosamax
Etidronate	Didronel
Pamidronate	Aredia
Risedronate	Actonel
Tiludronate	Skelid
Ibandronate	Boniva
Zoledronic acid	Zometa
Ca^{++} salts	
Calcium acetate	Phos-Ex, PhosLo
Calcium carbonate	Cal-Sup, Os-Cal, Tums
Calcium chloride	–
Calcium citrate	Citracal
Calcium glubionate	Neo-Calglucon
Calcium gluceptate	–
Calcium gluconate	–
Calcium lactate	–
Tricalcium phosphate	Posture
Vitamin D analogues	
Calcipotriene	Dovonex
Calcitriol	Calcijex, Rocaltrol
Cholecalciferol	Delta-D
Dihydrotachysterol	DHT, Hytakerol
Doxercalciferol	Hectorol
Ergocalciferol	Calciferol, Drisdol
Paricalcitol	Zemplar
Other drugs	
Calcitonin (salmon)	Calcimar, Miacalcin, Salmonine
Cinacalcet	Sensipar
Denosumab	Prolia, Xgeva
Parathyroid hormone	Natpara
Teriparatide (PTH 1-34)	Forteo

*Gonadotropins are discussed in Chapter 32.
IGF-I, Insulin-like growth factor type I; *TSH,* thyroid-stimulating hormone.

GENERAL REFERENCES

1. Drugs for post-menopausal osteoporosis, *Med Lett Drugs Ther* 56(1452):91–96, 2014.
2. Heaney RP, Vitamin D: Role in the calcium and phosphorus economies. In 3rd ed., Feldman D, Pike JW, Adams JS, editors: *Vitamin D*, vol 1. New York, 2011, Academic Press. (Chapter 34).
3. Jarnbring F, Kashani A, Bjork A, Hoffman T, et al.: Role of intravenous dosage regimens of bisphosphonates in relation to other etiological factors in the development of osteonecrosis of the jaws in patients with myeloma, *Br J Oral Maxillofacial Surg* 33:1007–1011, 2015.
4. Little JW: Medical management update: thyroid disorders, part I: hyperthyroidism, *Oral Surg, Oral Med, Oral Path, Oral Radiol Endocrinol* 101:276–284, 2006.
5. Pazianas M: Anabolic effects of PTH and the "anabolic window," *Trends Endocrinol Metab* 26:111–113, 2015.
6. Recombinant human parathyroid hormone (Natpara), *Med Lett Drugs Ther* 57(1470):87–88, 2015.
7. Sisson JC, Freitas J, McDougall IR, Dauer LT, et al.: Radiation safety in the treatment of patients with thyroid diseases by radioiodine ^{131}I: practice recommendations of the American Thyroid Association. From the American Thyroid Association Taskforce on Radioiodine Safety, *Thyroid* 21:335–346, 2011.

30

Adrenal Corticosteroids*

Binnaz Leblebicioglu

KEY INFORMATION

- Corticosteroids are released from the adrenal cortex.
- Corticosteroids are induced by various stimulants such as trauma, illness, burns, fever, hypoglycemia, and emotional upset.
- A significant portion of the population uses synthetic glucocorticoids for various reasons. The most common indication is to treat systemic illnesses or conditions that are immunologically based (e.g., asthma and autoimmune diseases). Less common use is for replacement therapy (e.g., treatment of insufficient production of corticosteroids).
- The long-term use of exogenous glucocorticoids may affect circulatory cortisol levels as well as the function of adrenal glands, among other organs.
- Synthetic glucocorticoids such as prednisone and dexamethasone are derived by changing the chemical structure of hydrocortisone or other natural hormones.
- Synthetic glucocorticoids are available in various forms for topical, oral, and parental administration.
- Synthetic compounds are classified based on the differences in duration of action compared to natural hydrocortisone (short-, intermediate-, and long-acting).
- These medications are used in dentistry mainly to treat oral ulcerations, temporomandibular joint disorders, postoperative edema, and allergic reactions.

CASE STUDY

Ms. H is a 50-year-old woman being treated for severe lupus erythematosus. She has long-standing dental phobia and has not been a compliant patient with her dentistry and home-care oral hygiene. As a result, she now has rampant decay on all of her teeth and needs to be converted to dentures. You are recommending full mouth extractions, alveoloplasty, bilateral mandibular tori removal, and four immediate-placement implants (two per arch) to support the future prostheses.

In reviewing her medical history, you note that she is currently taking 30 mg of prednisone per day as part of her therapy for her autoimmune disease. You know that her dental anxiety and postoperative pain experience may increase her stress levels. You know about acute adrenal insufficiency, adrenal crisis, and steroid supplementation. How do you go about managing this patient during the perioperative phase?

HORMONES OF THE ADRENAL GLANDS

The adrenal glands are located in the retroperitoneum superior to the kidneys. Despite their small size, the secretions from these glands play an integral role in kidney function, development, and growth of the body and our overall ability to deal with stress. The adrenal glands are composed of two distinct structures: the outer cortex and the inner medulla.

The hormones produced by the adrenal medulla primarily are **catecholamines** (e.g., **epinephrine** and **norepinephrine**). Catecholamine secretion is increased by adrenocorticotropic hormone (ACTH) and glucocorticoids, but it is also increased by sympathetic nerve stimulation, hypoglycemia, hypoxia, hypercapnic acidosis, hemorrhage, glucagon, histamine, and angiotensin II. Catecholamines have diverse effects throughout the body, but generally their release has been associated with the sympathetic survival "fight or flight" response.

The hormones produced by the adrenal cortex include the **mineralocorticoid** hormones (e.g., aldosterone), **glucocorticoid** hormones (e.g., cortisol), and **gonadal** hormones (e.g., dehydroepiandrosterone). **Aldosterone**, a mineralocorticoid, is primarily involved with regulation of extracellular volume and control of potassium homeostasis, and it has also been implicated in enhanced cardiac muscle contraction, increased vascular resistance, and decreased fibrinolysis. **Dehydroepiandrosterone (DHEA)** and **androstenedione** are weak androgens that can be converted to more potent androgenic or estrogenic hormones by peripheral tissues. **Cortisol**, a glucocorticoid, affects numerous physiologic processes such as metabolism, inflammation, growth, levels of awareness, etc. Optimal functioning of body systems requires that the circulating cortisol levels be maintained within a relatively narrow range. When there are chronic changes in the production of glucocorticoid hormones, pathologic conditions will develop. For example, an excess production of glucocorticoids results in **Cushing disease**, while secretion below the normal range results in **Addison disease.** This chapter will focus on the pharmacologic effects of the glucocorticosteroids.

ADRENAL GLUCOCORTICOSTEROIDS

A Summary of General Physiologic Actions

Using **cholesterol** as a substrate, the adrenal cortex synthesizes and secretes two types of steroid hormones: the 19-carbon androgens and the 21-carbon corticosteroids (Fig. 30-1). The corticosteroids can be classified further on the basis of their major actions. Some of these compounds, such as hydrocortisone (the nonproprietary name for the natural hormone cortisol) (Fig. 30-2), have greater effects on carbohydrate metabolism, as measured by liver glycogen deposition, and they

*The authors wish to recognize Dr. Clarence L. Trummel for this past contributions to this chapter.

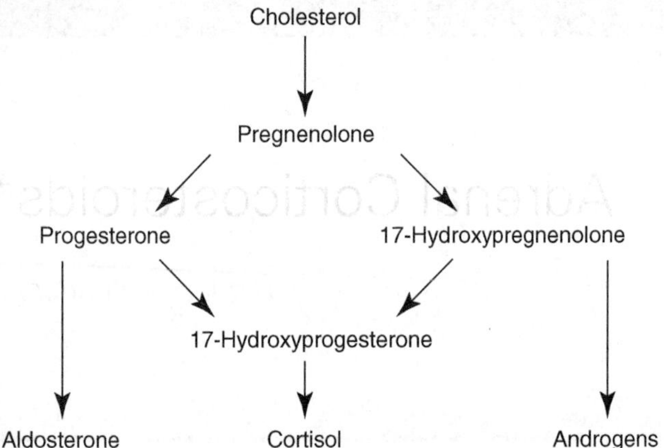

FIG 30-1 Major steps in the synthesis of adrenocortical steroid hormones. All three groups have cholesterol as a common precursor. Cholesterol is derived from several sources, including circulating cholesterol and cholesteryl esters, endogenous stores of cholesteryl esters, and *de novo* synthesis by the gland. Some of the intermediate steps are not shown.

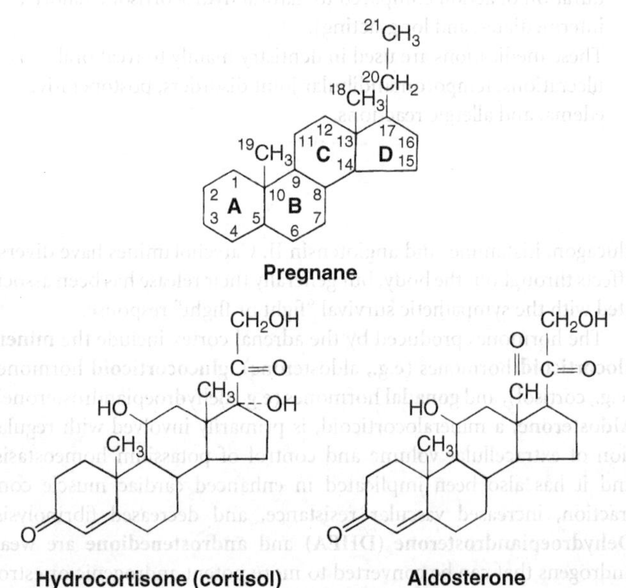

FIG 30-2 Structural formulas of pregnane, the basic corticosteroid nucleus, the prototypic glucocorticoid hydrocortisone, and the mineralocorticoid aldosterone.

are termed **glucocorticoids**. They also possess potent antiinflammatory actions and are used therapeutically for this purpose.

Production of all corticosteroids is highly compartmentalized in the adrenal cortex (Fig. 30-3). The glucocorticoids are produced by the middle layer (zona fasciculata) of the adrenal cortex. The glucocorticoids are not stored to any extent in the adrenal gland but are continuously synthesized and secreted. The total daily production of the major glucocorticoid, **cortisol**, is normally 20 to 25 mg. There is a strong diurnal variation in this process; plasma concentrations of cortisol are several fold higher at 8 am than at 4 pm.

Production of all corticosteroids is directly regulated by the blood concentration of **adrenocorticotropic hormone** (ACTH) secreted by the anterior pituitary gland (Fig. 30-4). Circulating corticosteroids act on the hypothalamus and anterior pituitary to suppress the release of ACTH, completing the control loop linking the pituitary and the adrenal cortex. By this **negative feedback mechanism**, the administration of large doses of exogenous corticosteroids can prevent the tropic

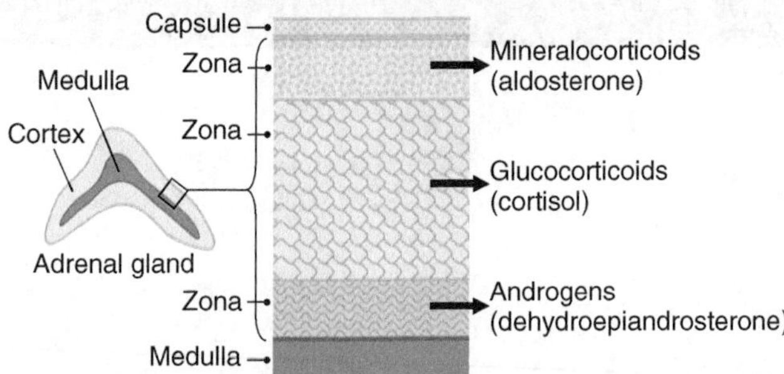

FIG 30-3 Schematic representation of the adrenal cortex and its major hormones. The cortex consists of three histologically and functionally distinct cellular compartments: **zona glomerulosa (outer most), zona fasciculata middle, and zona reticularis (inner most)**. Biosynthesis of the mineralocorticoids (primarily aldosterone), glucocorticoids (primarily cortisol), and some androgens occurs in these compartments.

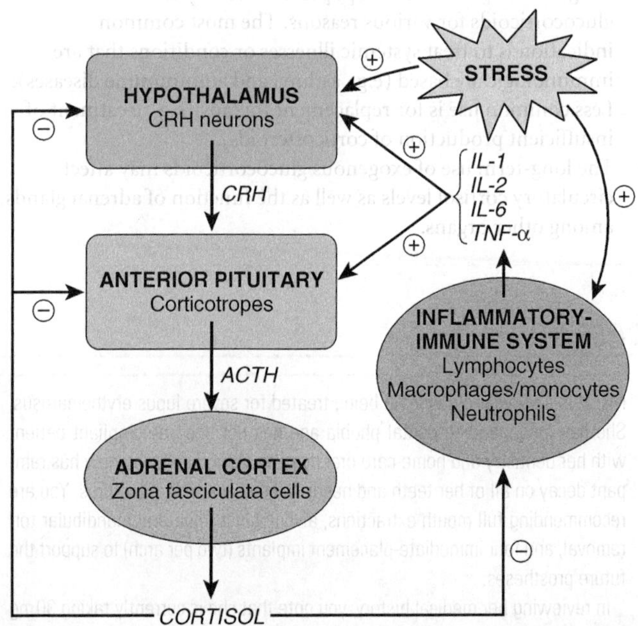

FIG 30-4 Hypothalamic-pituitary-adrenal axis and its relationship to stress and the inflammatory-immune system. Cortisol exerts a negative feedback control on the secretion of corticotropin-releasing hormone (*CRH*) and adrenocorticotropic hormone (*ACTH*). Physiologic or psychological stress increases cortisol secretion directly through neural mechanisms or by activation of the inflammatory-immune system and production of cytokines, including interleukin-1 (*IL-1*), interleukin-2 (*IL-2*), interleukin-6 (*IL-6*), and tumor necrosis factor-α (*TNF-α*). (Modified from Brunton L, Chabner B, Knollman B, editors: *Goodman and Gilman's the pharmacological basis of therapeutics*, ed 12, New York, 2011, McGraw Hill.)

influence of ACTH on the adrenal cortex, completely suppressing the adrenal production of corticosteroids.

Corticosteroids play diverse and complex roles in the body economy of mammalian organisms. They are involved in carbohydrate, protein, lipid, and purine metabolism; electrolyte and water balance; the functions of the cardiovascular, nervous, and immune-inflammatory systems; and the functions of the kidneys, skeletal muscle, bone, and most other organs and tissues. The hormones of the adrenal cortex play a major role in the ability of animals to withstand stressful events. Without the adrenal cortex, life is possible only when food and large amounts of salt and water are regularly ingested, a constant ambient temperature prevails, and infection and other perturbing events are absent.

Most of the diverse actions of corticosteroids seem to be achieved by regulating gene expression. Glucocorticoids enter target cells and bind to cytosolic receptors. These receptors exist in a complex with several proteins, including **heat shock protein** and **immunophilin**. Binding by the hormone or a synthetic analogue alters the conformation of the receptor, freeing it from the associated proteins. The hormone–receptor complex then migrates to the nucleus and binds to the glucocorticoid-responsive elements on DNA of affected genes. The **DNA-binding domain** on the receptor is distinct from the **drug-binding domain**. Gene expression is regulated either negatively or positively to render the characteristic and complex glucocorticoid signature for modification of protein synthesis.

Consistent with the complex mechanism described, the major effects of corticosteroids are not manifested for several hours. Other, less apparent effects are more immediate, however. These likely occur through other receptor mechanisms involving the plasma membrane of target cells.

Absorption, Fate, and Excretion

All the natural and synthetic glucocorticoids except desoxycorticosterone are well absorbed from the gastrointestinal tract. Significant amounts of these drugs may also be absorbed from sites of local application, such as the skin, mucous membranes, and eyes. In normal circumstances, more than 90% of circulating glucocorticoids are bound to plasma proteins, principally an **α-globulin** (corticosteroid-binding globulin, also known as **transcortin**), which has a high affinity but low capacity for these compounds, and **albumin**, which has the opposite characteristics.

Cortisol (hydrocortisone) is rapidly degraded in the liver by reduction, conjugated with glucuronic acid, and excreted in the urine. The plasma half-life of hydrocortisone is approximately 1.5 hours. Synthetic analogues of hydrocortisone generally have longer half-lives; the potent long-acting compound dexamethasone has a plasma half-life of approximately 4 hours and a tissue half-life of approximately 2 days. Because the glucocorticoids act by modifying gene expression, the time course of effect bears little relation to the plasma concentration.

The major metabolic products of corticosteroid metabolism found in the urine, **17-hydroxycorticosteroids** and **17-ketosteroids**, were formerly measured by clinical laboratories to assess adrenal-pituitary function. This method has been largely supplanted by direct measurement of blood cortisol concentrations by radioimmunoassay.

GENERAL THERAPEUTIC USES

Exogenous glucocorticoids and their synthetic analogues are used in medicine for replacement in adrenal insufficiency. They are used more widely for an array of non-adrenal diseases, primarily for their ability to suppress acute or chronic inflammation. In dentistry, glucocorticosteroids are used mainly to reduce the signs and symptoms of excess inflammatory reactions (e.g., treatment of oral ulcers, temporomandibular joint disorders, postoperative symptoms, and anaphylaxis). When corticosteroids are administered in high doses over long periods, severe and even lethal toxicity can result.

Glucocorticoids are used clinically in two ways (Box 30-1). The first and most intuitive is **replacement therapy**. Insufficient production of corticosteroids can result from a defect in the adrenal cortex, anterior pituitary, or hypothalamus; these defects may be congenital or acquired. Depending on the degree of insufficiency, the outcome may be either acute or chronic. The goal in these cases is to reestablish a natural level of circulating steroids for the cells to use daily to maintain homeostasis.

BOX 30-1 Conditions Treated with Corticosteroids

- Adrenal insufficiency (acute or chronic, primary, or caused by anterior pituitary insufficiency)
- Cerebral edema and increased intracranial pressure (brain tumors, meningitis, trauma, cerebrovascular accidents)
- Collagen vascular diseases
  - Lupus
  - Polymyositis
  - Polyarteritis nodosa
  - Chronic granulomatous disorders (sarcoidosis and others)
  - Temporal (giant cell) arteritis
  - Mixed connective tissue disease syndrome*
- Dermatologic conditions
  - Psoriasis
  - Dermatitis (atopic, allergic, irritant)
  - Pemphigus
  - Lichen planus
- Gastrointestinal diseases
  - Ulcerative colitis
  - Crohn's disease
  - Celiac disease
- Hematologic diseases
  - Malignancies (acute and chronic lymphocytic leukemia, lymphoma, multiple myeloma)
  - Hemolytic anemia (autoimmune or drug-induced)
  - Idiopathic thrombocytopenic purpura
- Hepatic diseases
  - Autoimmune hepatitis
- Multiple sclerosis (acute episodes)
- Nephrotic syndrome
- Ocular diseases with inflammatory or allergic components
- Pulmonary disorders
  - Asthma
  - Chronic bronchitis (acute episodes)
  - Aspiration pneumonia
- Rheumatic diseases and joint ailments
  - Rheumatic arthritis
  - Rheumatic carditis
  - Osteoarthritis (intraarticular administration)
  - Bursitis (intracapsular administration)
- Refractory shock (e.g., septic, anaphylactic)
- Solid tumors (e.g., breast)
- Tissue grafts and organ transplants

*Must be differentiated from scleroderma, because of the risks of corticosteroids in scleroderma patients such as renal crisis.

In addition to replacement therapy, glucocorticoids are used on a purely empiric basis in many conditions. These conditions, although varied, are generally characterized by chronic inflammatory and immune phenomena and are associated with tissue destruction and functional impairment. For this reason, it is widely assumed that the salutary effects of glucocorticoid therapy in these diseases are related to **suppression of inflammation and immune reactions**. In none of these conditions do the corticosteroids have specific actions on the basic disease process, despite their ability in some cases to produce dramatic improvement and remission of signs and symptoms. For example, the destructive aspects of the primary disease may continue unchecked; in rheumatoid arthritis, glucocorticoids can effectively relieve the distressing inflammation and pain, but the deterioration of the affected joints progresses. The use of glucocorticoids in other than replacement therapy must be considered palliative.

Because of their lack of specificity and their considerable potential for causing harm, the long-term use of glucocorticoids to treat inflammatory disorders should be viewed with caution. Before glucocorticoids are considered, less toxic and narrower spectrum agents should be used to the maximum extent possible.

When systemic glucocorticoids are used on a long-term basis, they are often administered on alternate days to minimize suppression of the pituitary–adrenal axis. Giving a glucocorticoid every other day between 6 and 9 am mimics the normal diurnal pattern of corticosteroid secretion. Such a regimen seems to lessen suppression of the adrenal cortex and permits increased endogenous corticosteroid production in response to stress. Alternate-day therapy may not adequately control symptoms in some cases, especially in patients with rheumatoid arthritis and ulcerative colitis. Systemic glucocorticoid therapy for less than 1 week usually does not cause significant suppression of pituitary or adrenal function.

THERAPEUTIC USES IN DENTISTRY

Glucocorticoids have limited applications in dentistry. As in medicine, they are used largely to reduce the signs and symptoms of unwanted inflammatory reactions. These potential uses fall into the following general categories: oral ulcerations, temporomandibular joint pain, postoperative sequelae, and allergic reactions.

Oral Ulcerations

A wide variety of ulcerative lesions of the oral mucosa are frequently empirically treated by the topical application of glucocorticoids. Relief of symptoms and abbreviation of the clinical course are usually obtained, regardless of the cause of the ulceration. Applicable conditions are denture-induced and other traumatic ulcers, recurrent ulcerative (aphthous) stomatitis, erosive lichen planus, erythema multiforme, pemphigus vulgaris, benign mucous membrane pemphigoid, and angular cheilitis. Despite their usual salutary effects on signs and symptoms, glucocorticoids do not alter the underlying pathogenesis of chronic ulcerative lesions of the oral mucosa. Although severe disorders with dermatologic and mucosal manifestations, such as pemphigus, are usually treated with systemic glucocorticoids, further improvement of associated oral ulceration may be obtained by topical application of glucocorticoids. Despite the fact that herpetic ulcers may respond favorably, the use of glucocorticoids to treat this condition is contraindicated because suppression of the host response may allow dissemination of the herpes virus. It is important for the clinician to make a careful diagnosis of oral ulcers before instituting glucocorticoid therapy.

The benefit of glucocorticoids applied topically is greatest when the period of contact with the tissue is continuous. Retention at the site of application is difficult in the oral cavity. A partial solution is to apply the drug in a paste that adheres to the mucosa and resists dissolution and displacement. One such vehicle is carboxymethylcellulose in a base of polyethylene resin and mineral oil (Orabase); it is available with or without a glucocorticoid. Symptomatic relief of many oral ulcers, particularly ulcers likely to be of limited duration, may be obtained with the adhesive paste alone.

Temporomandibular Joint Disorders

Pain originating in the temporomandibular joint may have many possible causes, including trauma, bruxism, anatomic anomalies, rheumatoid arthritis, and psychophysiologic disorders. Treatment of such conditions should be conservative and based on careful diagnosis. NSAIDs, antianxiety muscle relaxant drugs, and antidepressants have proved useful for short-term pharmacotherapy. Nondrug approaches include rest, heat, gentle stretching, bite-plane appliances, and occlusal adjustments. In refractory cases of temporomandibular joint pain, or when acute pain is initially so severe that it precludes a course of conservative therapy, intraarticular injection of a glucocorticoid such as prednisolone or dexamethasone may be beneficial. Relief of symptoms may be full or partial, permanent or temporary (especially if the underlying cause of the disorder is not corrected). Although deterioration of the articular surfaces of the joint has been claimed to result from intraarticular injection of corticosteroid, the weight of available evidence does not support such an association. Nevertheless, the best responses to intraarticular injection seem to occur in patients free of radiographic changes in the joint.

Postoperative Sequelae

Glucocorticoids are often used to lessen postoperative complications, mainly reduction of edema and trismus, after dental surgical procedures. A single dose of parenteral dexamethasone (6 to 10 mg) appears to be equally effective to multidose regimens over several days for dental edema and trismus. Although the risk of adverse effects from a short, intensive perioperative course of glucocorticoids is slight, it is uncertain whether the modest benefits typically obtained justify such "prophylactic" use. What is certain, however, is that careful surgical technique is of primary importance in the reduction of uncomfortable postoperative sequelae.

Allergic Reactions

The immunosuppressant and antiinflammatory effects of glucocorticoids may be used to treat the manifestations of various allergic reactions, such as urticaria, contact dermatitis, angioneurotic edema, anaphylaxis, allergic rhinitis and conjunctivitis, insect bites, drug reactions, and serum sickness. H_1 and H_2 antihistamines are major drugs in the treatment of milder reactions involving histamine release (e.g., urticaria). Systemic glucocorticoids become more useful in severe responses. In severe anaphylaxis, although epinephrine is the drug of choice, large doses of glucocorticoids may be beneficial in reducing bronchospasm and laryngeal edema. In this situation, glucocorticoids act to increase the cardiac and vascular effects of catecholamines. In addition, because the maximal effects of glucocorticoids are delayed for several hours after administration, the prolonged duration of action of glucocorticoids can afford added benefit. Thus, the glucocorticoids are not the primary drugs in treating the life-threatening cardiovascular failure of anaphylactic shock; they add a supplemental benefit after the administration of epinephrine.

DIFFERENT FORMS OF GLUCOCORTICOIDS AS MEDICATIONS (TABLES 30-1 AND 30-2)

Preparations

Numerous glucocorticoids are available in various forms for local, oral, and parenteral administration. These include the **natural hormone hydrocortisone and synthetic compounds** prepared by modifying the chemical structures of hydrocortisone and other natural hormones; three of these are shown in Figure 30-5. Relative to hydrocortisone, the synthetic compounds are, in varying degrees, longer acting and more potent. These differences are the basis for classifying glucocorticoids as **short-acting** (<12 hours), **intermediate-acting** (12 to 36 hours), and **long-acting** (>36 hours) (Box 30-2). Representatives of these three categories are **hydrocortisone**, **prednisolone**, and **dexamethasone**. Intermediate-acting and long-acting compounds also have a greater ratio of glucocorticoid to mineralocorticoid activity. Consequently, these agents are preferred for long-term use in the treatment of chronic inflammatory disorders because they cause less disturbance of electrolyte and fluid balance than hydrocortisone.

In the clinical management of inflammatory or allergic disorders, the dosage of glucocorticoids varies widely according to such factors as the nature, severity, and probable duration of the condition being treated and the patient's response. In acute or life-threatening situations, a glucocorticoid should be given in sufficient doses to control the disorder quickly; treatment should be discontinued as soon as possible. In the long-term management of chronic diseases such as rheumatoid arthritis, alternate-day therapy with the minimum dosage that achieves an acceptable reduction of symptoms is the regimen of choice. Table 30-2 lists some of the many different preparations currently available, some of the dosage forms, and a range of doses for a given route of administration. The list at the end of the chapter gives further information on drugs and drug names.

TABLE 30-1 Potencies of Commonly Used Corticosteroids (Relative to Hydrocortisone)

	Liver Glycogen Deposition*	Na^+ Retention
11-Desoxycorticosterone	0	100
Aldosterone	0.1	3000
Cortisone	0.8	0.8
Hydrocortisone	1	1
Prednisolone	4	0.8
Triamcinolone	5	0
Fludrocortisone	10	3000
Dexamethasone	25	0
Betamethasone	25	0

*Generally paralleled by antiinflammatory activity.

ADVERSE EFFECTS (BOXES 30-3 AND 30-4)

Although glucocorticoids are valuable agents in some situations, they have considerable potential to cause greater harm than good. Actualization of this potential depends on, among other factors, the intensity and duration of therapy. A single large dose or a short course of moderate doses of hydrocortisone causes few adverse effects. If more than 20 to 30 mg of hydrocortisone (or its equivalent) is given daily for more than a week, however, some manifestations of **glucocorticoid toxicity** are likely to appear. In general, these manifestations are predictable from our knowledge of the pathologic features of Cushing disease.

Prolonged administration of glucocorticoids (greater than physiologic amounts for >1 week) results in suppression of ACTH from the pituitary and, consequently, suppression of adrenal corticosteroid production; the degree of suppression is dose-related. Abrupt withdrawal or significant reduction of glucocorticoid dosage can precipitate acute adrenal insufficiency. Acute exacerbation of the disease being treated may occur during withdrawal. Cessation or reduction of glucocorticoid therapy must be done slowly and with great caution to permit the recovery of normal pituitary and adrenal function.

Various physiologic stressors, such as acute illness, trauma, pain, anxiety, infection, blood loss, surgery, and general anesthesia, elicit a rapid increase in circulating concentrations of hydrocortisone and other glucocorticoids. This increase is crucial to the success of the body's response to these stresses. In subjects with adrenal suppression resulting from disease or induced by long-term glucocorticoid therapy, any needed surge of glucocorticoid output is impaired. This impairment can very rarely, but quickly, lead to a condition known as **acute adrenal insufficiency,** or **adrenal crisis**. The risk of this condition is a function of the degree of adrenal suppression and the demand for increased glucocorticoid production. Realistically in dentistry, this basically never happens. It is extremely rare in medicine as well, particularly with advanced medical approaches to care.

Should the rare crisis happen, the onset is signaled by any or all of the following: severe nausea, vomiting, and diarrhea, leading to dehydration; chills and fever; sudden penetrating pain in the lower back, abdomen, and legs; profound muscle weakness; extreme lethargy; hypoglycemia;

TABLE 30-2 Commonly Used Corticosteroid Preparations

Nonproprietary (Generic) Name	Proprietary (Trade) Name	Relative Potency	Usual Adult Dose	Route of Administration	Preparations
Hydrocortisone	Hydrocortone	1	20-240 mg/day	Oral	Tablets: 5, 10, and 20 mg
Hydrocortisone acetate	Orabase HCA	1	2-3 times daily	Topical	Paste: 0.5%, containing gelatin, pectin, and sodium carboxymethylcellulose
	Hydrocortone acetate	1	5-50 mg	Intraarticular	Suspension: 25 and 50 mg/mL
Hydrocortisone sodium succinate	Solu-Cortef	1	100-500 mg/day	Intravenous or intramuscular	Powder: 100, 250, 500, and 1000 mg
Prednisone	Deltasone, Orasone	4	5-60 mg/day	Oral	Tablets: 1, 2.5, 5, 10, 20, 25, and 50 mg
Prednisolone	Delta-Cortef	4	5-60 mg/day	Oral	Tablets: 5 mg
Prednisolone acetate	Econopred	4	1-2 drops	Ophthalmic	Suspension: 0.12% and 1%
Triamcinolone acetonide	Kenalog in Orabase	5	2-3 times daily	Topical	Paste: 0.1% with gelatin; pectin, and sodium carboxymethylcellulose in a polyethylene and mineral oil base
Triamcinolone diacetate	Aristocort	5	5-40 mg every 1-8 wk	Intraarticular	Suspension: 25 and 40 mg/mL
Triamcinolone acetate	Kenalog	5	Similar to diacetate	Intraarticular	Suspension: 10 and 40 mg/mL
Dexamethasone	Decadron	25	0.75-9 mg/day	Oral	Tablets: 0.25, 0.5, 0.75, 1, 1.5, 2, 4, and 6 mg
Betamethasone	Celestone	25	0.6-7.2 mg/day	Oral	Tablets: 0.6 mg

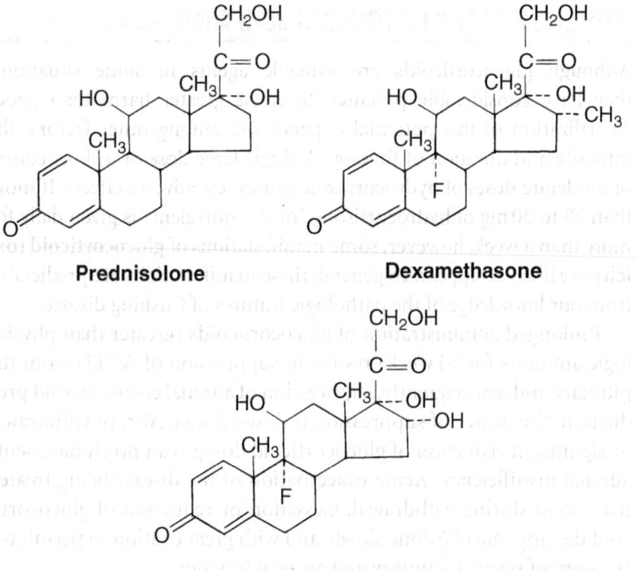

Prednisolone **Dexamethasone**

Triamcinolone

FIG 30-5 Structural formulas of three commonly used synthetic glucocorticoids.

BOX 30-2 Biologic Half-Lives* of Commonly Used Corticosteroids

8-12 hr	Cortisone
	Hydrocortisone
12-36 hr	Methylprednisolone
	Prednisolone
	Prednisone
	Triamcinolone
36-72 hr	Betamethasone
	Dexamethasone
	Paramethasone

*Biologic half-life of a corticosteroid is defined as the period of suppression of the hypothalamus-pituitary-adrenal axis.

hypotension and tachycardia; and tachypnea. These symptoms may be followed by confusion, psychotic manifestations, loss of consciousness, convulsions, cardiovascular and respiratory collapse, and death. True adrenal crisis is a very serious medical emergency, and appropriate and timely intervention is essential. Treatment consists of intravenous glucocorticoids; correction of fluid, electrolyte, and glucose deficits; and vasopressors and other supportive measures as needed.

BOX 30-3 Major Adverse Effects of Glucocorticoid Therapy

Neurologic	Insomnia, agitation, mania, withdrawal syndrome, psychological disturbances, mild (euphoria, nervousness) to pronounced (manic-depressive or schizophrenic psychosis)
Infectious	Increased infection rate due to a depressed host immune response
Vascular	Hypertension, increased atherosclerotic disease risk
Skin and mucosa	Atrophy, acne, thinning of the skin and mucosa, hirsutism, intestinal perforation, pancreatitis, hyperlipidemia, hepatomegaly, poor wound healing
Skeletal	Reduced Ca^{++} absorption, osteoporosis, avascular osteonecrosis, impaired growth in children and adolescents, compression fractures of the vertebrae
Muscular	Myopathy, muscle wasting, changes in body fat distribution (classic cushingoid appearance)
Metabolic	A diabetic-like state including glucose intolerance, obesity, glycosuria
Reproductive	Hypogonadism
Gastrointestinal	Peptic ulcer and related complications such as hemorrhage and perforation
Ocular	Cataracts, increased intraocular pressure

BOX 30-4 The Pharmacologic and Toxic Actions of Glucocorticoids

Carbohydrate and Protein Metabolism	↓Peripheral use and cellular uptake of glucose
	↑Liver glucose synthesis from amino acids (gluconeogenesis)
	↓Protein synthesis in muscle, connective tissues, and skin (anti-anabolic effect)
	↑Blood glucose, liver glycogen, urinary nitrogen excretion
Lipid metabolism	↑Fatty acid release
Electrolyte and water balance	↑Reabsorption of Na^+ from the tubular fluid (leading to edema and hypertension)
	↑Urinary excretion of K^+ and H^+
Antiinflammatory properties	↓Inflammatory response (through the inhibition of specific gene expression)
	↓Production of cytokines
Immune responses	↓T-lymphocyte activation and proliferation
	↓Production of plasma cells
	↓Phagocytosis of antigen by macrophages
	↓Antibody production

IMPLICATIONS FOR DENTISTRY

Patients treated with large doses of glucocorticoids for long periods present potential problems in dentistry. As noted previously, such patients are likely to have a **decreased resistance to infection** and a **poor wound healing response.** Actual or potential sources of infection in the oral cavity, such as carious teeth and inflamed tissues, should be promptly treated. If surgical procedures are necessary, they should be as conservative, atraumatic, and as aseptic as possible. Perioperative antimicrobial prophylaxis may be indicated with some patients.

A second consideration in patients treated with glucocorticoids is **suppression of pituitary adrenal function.** The degree of adrenal suppression depends on the length of treatment, the frequency and manner of administration, and the glucocorticoid preparation used (glucocorticoid potency of individual agents may vary as much as 25-fold; see Table 30-1). As described earlier, an individual with intact adrenal function responds to a stressful situation with an increased release of ACTH and production of cortisol. Patients with suppressed adrenal function are unable to sufficiently increase cortisol production. In assessing the degree of suppression, a good guideline is to assume that any patient who has received 30 mg of hydrocortisone or its equivalent for 4 or more weeks or 80 mg of hydrocortisone for more than 2 weeks has some degree of adrenal suppression. It is a time-honored but completely unproven notion that these patients may develop signs and symptoms of adrenal insufficiency during stressful dental situations (surgery or acute infection). Many scholars suggest that the dose of glucocorticoids be increased during and immediately after treatment in such patients to compensate for the lack of endogenous hormone publication. The recommended dose is typically at least double or triple the patient's maintenance dose, depending on the degree of suppression of adrenal function and the severity of the stressful event. When the period of stress is over, the dose is gradually reduced over several days to the maintenance level. All of this is completely hypothetical and has been shown to not be necessary the vast majority of the time.

A careful review of the literature suggests that patients with glucocorticoid-induced adrenal suppression are at an extremely low risk of acute adrenal insufficiency as a result of routine dental treatment, including most routine (simple and surgical) extractions and periodontal or endodontic surgery. Given this, it is likely quite safe for such patients to forego perioperative glucocorticoid supplementation ("steroid cover"). Patients should be scheduled for an appointment in the morning when circulating cortisol concentrations are the highest and instructed to take their usual dose of corticosteroid within 2 hours of the procedure. More importantly, measures to reduce anxiety such as oral, nitrous oxide, or intravenous sedation are appropriate.

More invasive surgical procedures, such as removal of impacted teeth, bone resection, or quadrant periodontal surgery; lengthy procedures (>1 hour); procedures that may cause considerable blood loss; and any procedure done under general anesthesia constitute more stressful episodes, and they may suggest a medical consultation to determine if corticosteroid augmentation is necessary in a patient with adrenal suppression.

Over the years, there have been regimens providing steroid supplementation for stressful procedures. In modern medical practice, the approaches typically fall into three categories:

1. Add a single dose of additional steroid, either by increasing the oral dose, or providing IM/IV steroids perioperatively. No taper is used. Dexamethasone 6 to 10 mg is the most common agent used in dentistry for this purpose. Medical doctors will commonly use IV hydrocortisone to achieve a similar effect.
2. Increase the preoperative steroid (anywhere from onefold to threefold), either by increasing the oral dose, or providing IM/IV steroids perioperatively. Taper back over several days until the baseline dose is re-achieved. A methylprednisolone dose pack is the most common agent used in dentistry for this approach.

MEDROL DOSE PAK

Day #	Total Tablets per Day	Before Breakfast	After Lunch	After Supper	At Bedtime
1	6	2	1	1	2
2	5	1	1	1	2
3	4	1	1	1	1
4	3	1	1	0	1
5	2	1	0	0	1
6	1	1	0	0	0

3. Do not change the steroid dose at all, and use sedation and quality pain control as the primary approaches to avoid a medical crisis. **This is by far the most common choice when it comes to steroid supplementation (or lack thereof) in the dental arena.**

Because recovery of chronic glucocorticoid-induced adrenal suppression may be slow, patients formerly treated for prolonged periods with glucocorticoids and assumed to have adrenal suppression may need to receive glucocorticoids during stressful situations for 3 to 12 months after cessation of glucocorticoid therapy. Consultation with the patient's physician is essential for the optimal management of a patient who is receiving or has received long-term glucocorticoid therapy.

In contrast to patients who receive replacement therapy, individuals with **hyperadrenalism** present a higher risk for hypertension, osteoporosis, and peptic ulcer. Thus, blood pressure should be monitored and presence of osteoporosis should be investigated. Similarly, analgesics such as aspirin and other NSAIDs should not be the first choice to control postoperative pain for these patients.

CASE DISCUSSION

Dentists should always consider the need for a medical consultation when considering a significant surgery on a patient taking high-dose corticosteroid medications. Most patients, particularly on lower doses of steroids (10 mg prednisone or less), do not need any intervention at all. However, in conjunction with the physician, the team may elect to (1) increase the prednisone for one dose only, (2) increase the prednisone and then taper back to the baseline amount using, perhaps, methylprednisolone dose pack, (3) layer a different steroid for one dose (dexamethasone, for example) at the time of surgery, or (4) more commonly, leave the steroid dose exactly the same.

The stress of the procedure is best managed with moderate benzodiazepine sedation or deep sedation/general anesthesia, and the postoperative pain control is best managed with long-acting local anesthetics and sufficient pain medication (e.g., hydrocodone or oxycodone plus acetaminophen) to make the patient comfortable. Note that aspirin and other NSAIDs such as ibuprofen and ketorolac, while not contraindicated, may increase the risk for peptic ulcer and should be discussed with the physician.

The risk of developing an adrenal crisis is so low that effectively, in this dental setting, it is of little concern.

In this case, one can also consider phased extractions (posterior sextants first, spread over several weeks) and perhaps delaying the placement of the implants until her ability to heal is well assessed.

COMMONLY USED CORTICOSTEROID PREPARATIONS AND PROPRIETARY NAMES

(Respiratory steroids are discussed in Chapter 27.)

Nonproprietary (Generic) Name	Proprietary (Trade) Name
Beclomethasone	Beclovent, Vanceril
Cortisone	Cortone
Dexamethasone	Decadron, Dexone, Hexadrol
Fludrocortisone	Florinef
Flunisolide	AeroBid
Hydrocortisone (cortisol)	Cortef, Hydrocortone, Solu-Cortef
Methylprednisolone	Depo-Medrol, Medrol, Solu-Medrol
Prednisolone	Delta-Cortef, Predalone, Pediapred
Prednisone	Deltasone, Orasone
Triamcinolone	Aristocort, Kenacort, Kenalog

GENERAL REFERENCES

1. Chegini S, Dhariwal DK: Review of evidence for the use of steroids in orthognathic surgery, *Br J Oral Maxillofac Surg* 50(2):97–101, 2012.
2. Dan AE, Thygesen TH, Pinholt EM: Corticosteroid administration in oral and orthognathic surgery: a systematic review of the literature and meta-analysis, *J Oral Maxillofac Surg* 68(9):2207–2220, 2010.
3. Hardy RS, Raza K, Cooper MS: Glucocorticoid metabolism in rheumatoid arthritis, *Ann NY Acad Sci* 1318:18–26, 2014.
4. Leblebicioglu B, Connors J, Mariotti A: Principles of endocrinology, *Periodontology 2000* 61(1):54–68, January 2013.
5. Lee RS, Sawa A: Environmental stressors and epigenetic control of the hypothalamic-pituitary-adrenal axis, *Neuroendocrinology* 100(4):278–287, 2014.
6. Miller CS, Little JW, Falace DA: Supplemental corticosteroids for dental patients with adrenal insufficiency: reconsideration of the problem, *J Am Dent Assoc* 132:1570–1579, 2001.
7. Nicolaides NC, Kyratzi E, Lamprokostopoulou A, Chrousos GP, Charmondari E: Stress, the stress system and the role of glucocorticoids, *Neuroimmunomodulation* 22(1-2):6–9, 2015.
8. Nieman LK: Update in the medical therapy of Cushing's disease, *Cur Opin Endocrinol Diabetes Obes* 20(4):330–334, 2013.
9. Sciubba JJ: Oral mucosal diseases in the office setting, part I: aphthous stomatitis and herpes simplex infections, *Gen Dent* 55:347–354, 2007.
10. Sciubba JJ: Oral mucosal diseases in the office setting, part II: lichen planus, pemphigus vulgaris and mucosal pemphigoid, *Gen Dent* 55:464–476, 2007.
11. Wang AS, Armstrong EJ, Armstrong AW: Corticosteroids and wound healing: clinical considerations in the peri-operative period, *Am J Surg* 206(3):410–417, 2013.
12. Webster JC, Cidlowski JA: Mechanism of glucocorticoid-receptor mediated repression of gene expression, *Trends Endocrinol Metab* 10:396–402, 1999.
13. Yang SL, Marik P, Esposito M, Coulthard P: Supplemental perioperative steroids for surgical patients with adrenal insufficiency, *Cochrane Database Syst Rev* 7(4):CD005367, 2009.

31

Insulin, Oral Hypoglycemics, and Glucagon

Gail T. Galasko

KEY INFORMATION

- Insulin increases glucose uptake into cells, increases glucose use, and decreases glucose production.
- Insulin acts on cell surface receptors that have tyrosine kinase activity, a signaling pathway affecting gene transcription.
- Insulin is used to treat both type 1 and type 2 diabetes.
- Ultrashort-acting insulins are insulin aspart, insulin glulisine, and insulin lispro.
- Regular insulin is short-acting.
- Neutral Protamine Hagedorn (NPH) insulin is intermediate-acting.
- Insulin detemir, insulin glargine and insulin degludec are long-acting.
- Sulfonylureas block ATP-dependent K^+ channels and stimulate the release of insulin from the pancreas.
- Meglitinides (repaglinide and nateglinide) act like the sulfonylureas.
- Metformin stimulates AMP-activated ATPase (AMPK) and reduces blood glucose by several mechanisms.
- Thiazolidinediones (pioglitazone and rosiglitazone) are agonists at the nuclear peroxisome proliferator-activated receptor γ (PPARγ) decreasing gluconeogenesis and increasing glucose uptake into cells.
- Exenatide and sitagliptin are incretin-related drugs and stimulate insulin secretion.
- Canagliflozin is an example of a sodium-glucose co-transporter 2 (SGLT2) inhibitor, which reduces glucose reabsorption in the kidney.
- Pramlintide is an amylin analogue that lowers blood glucose by several mechanisms.
- Acarbose and miglitol inhibit α-glucosidase and delay absorption of carbohydrates.
- The major sign of toxicity from insulin or oral hypoglycemic is hypoglycemia.

CASE STUDY

Ms. DP has been your patient for several years. She is a 67-year-old type 2 diabetic who is being treated with a sulfonylurea. She has arrived for a 3:00 pm appointment, and your receptionist tells you Ms. DP is acting as if she is under the influence and causing disruption in the waiting room. She is slurring her words and acting belligerently. She is taken into one of the operatories and seated. She has a rapid pulse, complains she is dizzy, and appears confused. What could be causing this behavior? What should be done for the patient? How would you advise the patient?

INSULIN AND THE ENDOCRINE PANCREAS

The pancreas has exocrine and endocrine functions. The exocrine system comprises the acinar cells, which secrete digestive enzymes. The endocrine system comprises the islets of Langerhans, which contain four types of cells. Each of these cell types synthesizes and secretes different polypeptide hormones (Table 31-1). Insulin is produced by the β cells, which constitute most (60% to 80%) of the islet and form its central core. The β cell is the primary glucose sensor for the islet.

Insulin is a polypeptide containing 51 amino acids. It is composed of two chains (called the **A and B chains**) that are joined by two disulfide bridges. Insulin is formed by proteolysis of a large, single-chain precursor, proinsulin. In proinsulin, shown in Figure 31-1, the A and B chains are joined by a connecting (C) peptide. Proinsulin is converted to insulin when the C peptide is removed; this occurs within the secretory granules of the pancreatic β cell. Approximately equimolar amounts of insulin and C peptide are stored in the granules and released by exocytosis when the β cell is stimulated. C peptide has no known biologic function, but it can serve as an index of insulin secretion.

Insulin is a member of a family of related peptides known as **insulin-like growth factors** ***(IGFs)***. The receptors for insulin and IGF-I are closely related. Insulin can bind to the receptor for IGF-I with low affinity and vice versa. The growth-promoting actions of insulin seem to be mediated, at least in part, through the IGF-I receptor.

Regulation of Insulin Secretion

Insulin secretion is a tightly regulated process designed to provide stable concentrations of glucose in the blood during fasting and feeding. Regulation of plasma glucose is achieved by the coordinated interplay of various nutrients, gastrointestinal hormones, pancreatic hormones, and autonomic neurotransmitters. A basal secretion of insulin is present during fasting periods. There is a subsequent rapid increase in insulin secretion after ingestion of a meal. Glucose is the principal stimulus to insulin secretion in humans. It is more effective in provoking insulin secretion when taken orally than when administered intravenously.

Actions of Insulin

The classic action of insulin is to decrease the blood glucose concentration. Insulin does this by **increasing glucose uptake into cells, increasing glucose use, and decreasing glucose production**. Liver, muscle, and fat are the important target tissues for regulation of glucose homeostasis by insulin, but insulin exerts potent regulatory effects on other cell types as well. Insulin stimulates glucose transport into muscle and fat by promoting translocation of the intracellular transporter, glucose transporter

TABLE 31-1 Pancreatic Islet Secretions

Cell Type	Hormone Secreted
α (A) cell	Glucagon
β (B) cell	Insulin, amylin (islet amyloid polypeptide)
δ (D) cell	Somatostatin
F (PP) cell	Pancreatic polypeptide
G cell	Gastrin

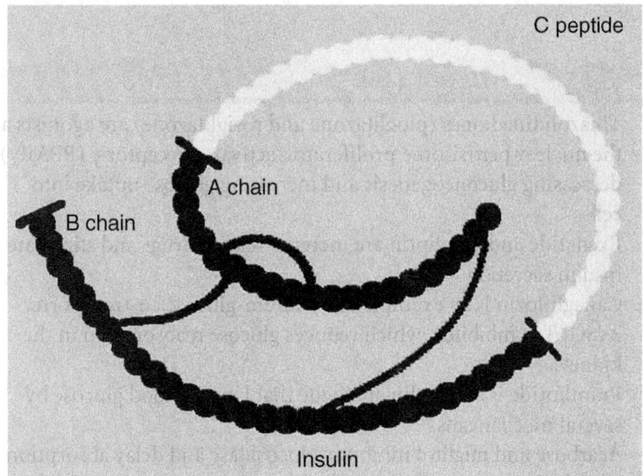

FIG 31-1 Structure of proinsulin. When the connecting (C) peptide is removed, insulin is formed. The A and B chains of insulin are shown in *black*; C peptide is *white*.

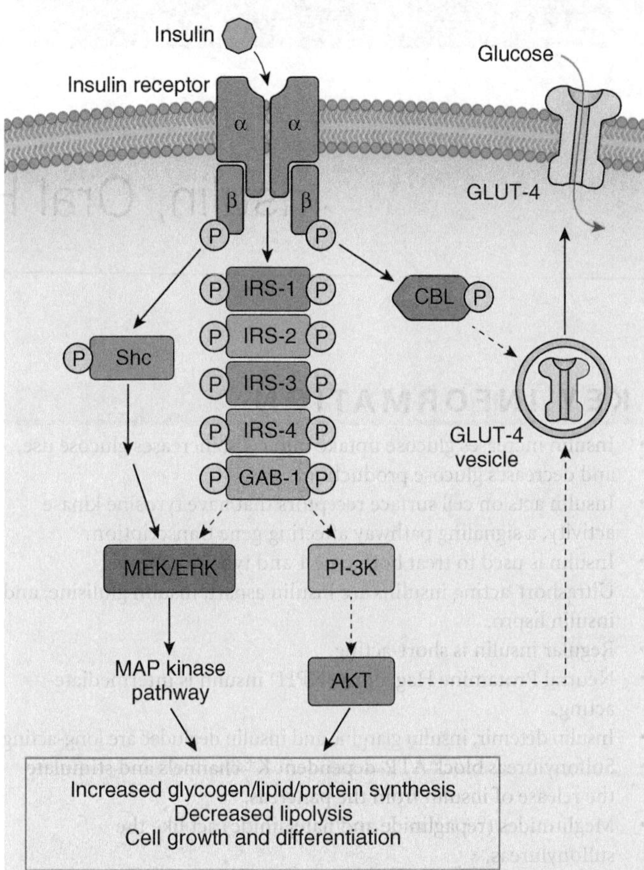

FIG 31-2 Insulin signaling pathways. The action of insulin on its receptor leads to phosphorylation (P) of the receptor and key proteins in the signaling pathways. Effects of insulin occur through numerous mechanisms including enhancing gene transcription and protein synthesis. The translocation of the glucose transporter (*Glut 4*) to the plasma membrane, which is stimulated by insulin, is integral to glucose uptake and subsequent glucose use in cells of key target tissues. *AKT,* Protein kinase B; *CBL,* calcineurin B-like protein; *ERK,* extracellular signal-regulated kinases; GAB-1, Growth factor receptor-bound protein 2-associated binding protein; *IRS,* insulin receptor substrates; *MAP,* mitogen-activated protein; *MEK,* mitogen-activated protein kinase kinase; *PI-3K,* phosphatidylinositol 3′-kinase; *Shc,* Src homology 2 domain-containing. (Modified from Robbins SL et al: The endocrine system, in *Robbins and Cotran Pathologic Basis of Disease,* St. Louis, Saunders, 2010.)

4 (Glut 4), to the cell surface (Fig. 31-2). Insulin does not stimulate glucose uptake into the liver, but it inhibits hepatic glucose production. Insulin inhibits catabolic processes, such as breakdown of glycogen, fat, and protein. It inhibits both glycogenolysis and gluconeogenesis.

Insulin receptors are found on virtually all cells. Activation of the insulin receptor leads to a cascade of phosphorylation and/or dephosphorylation reactions. As a result, **insulin affects the activities of various enzymes involved in intracellular use and storage of glucose, amino acids, and fatty acids.** Glycolysis (use) and glycogen synthesis (storage) are promoted. The effects of insulin are summarized in Table 31-2.

In addition to the short-term metabolic effects, insulin has other, longer term actions. Insulin regulates gene transcription, affecting protein synthesis; it is believed to have important growth-regulating effects in vivo; it increases cell proliferation and differentiation; and it decreases apoptosis.

Pharmacokinetics

Insulin may be given subcutaneously, intravenously (IV), or intramuscularly. Subcutaneous injection of insulin is commonly used in the long-term treatment of diabetes. The kinetics (both absorption and biotransformation) of insulin given exogenously are not the same as those of endogenous insulin secretion. Endogenous insulin is secreted into the portal circulation; injected insulin is delivered into the peripheral circulation. Insulin is biotransformed in various tissues, including the liver, kidney, and skeletal muscle, resulting in the formation of inactive peptides.

Insulin Receptor Interactions

The insulin receptor in mammalian cells is a large transmembrane glycoprotein. It is composed of two α subunits and two β subunits linked by disulfide bonds to form a β-α-α-β heterotetramer. Binding of hormone to the α subunits of the insulin receptor leads to the rapid intramolecular autophosphorylation of tyrosine residues in the β subunits. A series of events is initiated that culminates in a cascade of phosphorylation or dephosphorylation reactions. This activity is shown schematically in Figure 31-2.

Insulin Signaling

There is evidence that insulin acts by synthesis of second messengers that enter the cell to mediate some of the hormone's actions on intracellular enzymes (e.g., phosphorylation, dephosphorylation). These mediators are of the inositolphosphoglycan (IPG) class. IPGs represent a family of second messengers or mediators that are increasingly being implicated as having an important role in signal transduction, not only for insulin, but also for other hormones and growth factors. They are discussed later in this chapter.

TABLE 31-2 **Metabolic Actions of Insulin**

Type of Metabolism	Action of Insulin	Major Target Tissue*
Carbohydrate	Increases glucose transport	Muscle, fat
	Increases glycogen synthesis	Liver, muscle
	Decreases gluconeogenesis	Liver
	Increases glycolysis	Liver, muscle
	Increases glucose oxidation	Fat
Fat	Increases lipogenesis	Liver, fat
	Decreases lipolysis	Liver, fat
	Increases synthesis of triglycerides	Fat
Protein	Decreases protein breakdown	Liver
	Increases protein synthesis	Muscle, various
	Increases amino acid uptake	Muscle, various

*Insulin exerts potent regulatory effects on various cell types in addition to liver, muscle, and fat, the classically important target tissues for glucose regulation.

TABLE 31-3 **Hemoglobin A^{1c} to Estimated Average Glucose Conversion***

HbA^{1c} or A^{1c} (%)	eAG (mg/dL)
6	126
6.5	140
7	154
7.5	169
8	183
8.5	197
9	212
9.5	226
10	240

The formula for conversion is $28.7 \times A^{1C} - 46.7 = eAG$.
eAG, Estimated average glucose.
*Taken from American Diabetes Association Chart. (Accessed July 2016, from: http://professional.diabetes.org/diapro/glucose_calc.)

DIABETES MELLITUS

Diabetes mellitus (DM) is a group of syndromes characterized by hyperglycemia. Virtually all forms of DM are due to either a decrease in the circulating concentration of insulin (insulin deficiency) or a decrease in the response of peripheral tissues to insulin (insulin resistance). The disease has two major forms. Currently, the preferred nomenclature is **type 1** and **type 2 diabetes mellitus.** Older names include **juvenile-onset** or **insulin-dependent DM** for type 1 and **maturity-onset** or **non-insulin-dependent DM** for type 2.

A third form of diabetes, gestational diabetes, occurs during pregnancy and resolves after parturition. Gestational diabetes is important because it is a predictor of type 2 DM (~50% of gestational diabetics develop type 2 DM later in life).

Evidence indicates that the incidence of type 1 and type 2 DM is increasing worldwide. DM is an emerging problem in children and adolescents, particularly minorities.

Type 1 Diabetes Mellitus

There is considerable evidence that type 1 diabetes is an autoimmune disease of the pancreatic β cell, resulting in degeneration. In type 1 diabetes, there is an absolute lack of insulin. Genetic predisposition and environmental components are involved, with the incidence in homozygous twins being approximately 50%. Approximately 5% to 10% of diabetics have type 1 diabetes.

Type 2 Diabetes Mellitus

Approximately 90% to 95% of diabetics have type 2 DM. In type 2 diabetes, target cells are relatively insensitive to insulin. This is known as **peripheral resistance to insulin.** Impaired glucose metabolism in muscle and liver are key features of type 2 diabetes. Genetic predisposition is important in type 2 diabetes; there is greater than 95% concordance in identical twins. While most Caucasian type 2 diabetics are overweight or obese, this occurs in less than half of type 2 diabetics in Asian populations. Type 2 diabetics have impaired glucose taste detection, which may reflect a generalized defect in glucose sensitivity, including the glucose-sensing pancreatic β cells.

Glycosylation of Hemoglobin

Nonenzymatic glycosylation of proteins can occur as a result of elevated blood glucose concentrations. Hemoglobin is glycosylated on its amino terminal valine residue to form the glycosyl valine adduct, termed **hemoglobin A_{1c} (HbA_{1c})** (Table 31-3). Because the half-life of HbA_{1c} is the same as that of red blood cells, the concentration of HbA_{1c} in the circulation can be used to assess the severity of the glycemic state over an extended period (8 to 12 weeks) before sampling.

Insulin Therapy

Insulin is the mainstay for treatment of virtually all type 1 and many type 2 diabetic patients. (**Key Concept: Type 1 DM must be treated with insulin. Type 2 DM may be treated with diet and exercise, oral antihyperglycemic agents, parenteral antihyperglycemic agents, or insulin, alone or in combination.**)

Long-term, insulin is generally given by subcutaneous (SQ) injection. When necessary, insulin may be administered intravenously or intramuscularly. SQ administration of insulin differs from physiologic secretion of insulin in two major ways. First, absorption after SQ administration is relatively slow and does not mimic the normal rapid increase and decrease of insulin secretion in response to ingestion of nutrients. Second, injected insulin diffuses into the peripheral circulation instead of being released into the portal circulation. This may alter both intensity and timing of insulin effects in the liver. Any preferential effect of secreted insulin on hepatic metabolic processes is lost when insulin is given exogenously.

Insulin preparations

Available preparations include human insulins and insulin analogues. Human insulins, so-called because they have the same structure as normal human insulin, are made by genetic engineering (recombinant DNA). In ultrashort-acting insulin analogues (insulin aspart, glulisine, and lispro), amino acids are substituted, or reversed. Long-acting insulin analogues (insulin detemir' glargine and degludec) have groups added. Insulin analogues have been developed to alter the kinetics.

Insulin preparations are classified according to their duration of action into rapid-acting (ultrashort-acting and short-acting), intermediate-acting, and long-acting preparations. Insulin products available in the United States are listed in Table 31-4.

Rapid-acting (ultrashort-acting and short-acting) insulin preparations. Ultrashort-acting insulin preparations—**insulin aspart** (NovoLog), **insulin glulisine** (Apidra), and **insulin lispro** (Humalog)—all

TABLE 31-4 Insulin Preparations

Preparation	Onset	Peak	Duration
Rapid-Ultrashort-Acting			
Insulin aspart (NovoLog)	5-15 min	1-2.5 hr	≤5 hr
Insulin glulisine (Apidra)	5-15 min	0.5-1.5 hr	2-5 hr
Insulin lispro (Humalog)	5-15 min	0.5-1.5 hr	2-5 hr
Rapid-Short-Acting			
Humulin R	30-60 min	2-4 hr	3-7 hr
Novolin R	30 min	2.5-5 hr	3-7 hr
Intermediate-Acting			
Humulin N	1-2 hr	4-12 hr	12-16 hr
Novolin N	1-2 hr	4-12 hr	12-16 hr
Premixed (% NPH/% Regular)			
Humulin 70/30	30-60 min	2-4 hr	≤24 hr
Humulin 50/50	30-60 min	2-4 hr	≤24 hr
Novolin 70/30	30 min	2.5-5 hr	≤24 hr
Premixed			
Humalog mix (75% insulin lispro protamine/25% insulin lispro)	10-30 min	1-2 hr	10-16 hr
NovoLog mix 70/30 (70% insulin aspart protamine/30% insulin aspart)	10-20 min	1-2 hr	10-16 hr
Long-Acting			
Insulin detemir (Levemir)	50-120 min	No peak	18-24 hr
Insulin glargine (Lantus)	1-2 hr	No peak	24 hr
Insulin degludec (Tresiba)	1 hr	No peak	≤24 hr

Kinetics of insulin preparations vary with site of injection.
N, NPH; *R*, regular.

are insulin analogues. They may be used with a pump.* Regular insulins (**Humulin R and Novolin R**) are short-acting preparations. They are soluble, capable of IV use, have a rapid onset, and are dispensed as clear solutions at neutral pH.

Intermediate-acting and long-acting insulin preparations. The intermediate-acting **NPH insulin** preparations contain particles and are cloudy suspensions at neutral pH. **Novolin N** and **Humulin N** are the two preparations available. Both are human insulins of recombinant DNA origin.

Insulin analogues—**insulin glargine** (Lantus), **insulin detemir** (Levemir) and **insulin degludec (Tresiba)**—are soluble, long-acting insulin preparations. Their duration of action is longer, and their time–action profile is flatter (peakless) than NPH insulin preparations. They cause less hypoglycemia at night.

For therapeutic purposes, dosages and concentrations of insulin are expressed in units. Most commercial preparations of insulin are supplied in solution at a concentration of 100 units/mL (approximately 3.47 mg/mL).

Pharmacokinetics

Insulin is generally given by injection, usually subcutaneously. An inhaled form, **insulin human inhalation powder**, is now also available. Absorption of insulin after subcutaneous administration is affected by the site of injection, the subcutaneous blood flow, the volume and concentration of the injected insulin, and the presence of circulating insulin antibodies. Insulin absorption is usually most rapid from the abdominal wall, followed by the arm, buttock, and thigh. Increased subcutaneous blood flow (brought about by massage, hot baths, and exercise) increases the rate of absorption. Soluble insulins may also be given intravenously. The onset of action of insulin after intravenous injection is very fast, but the duration of action is short.

Adverse effects

Hypoglycemia is the most common adverse reaction to insulin. Hypoglycemia may result from an inappropriately large dose, a mismatch between the time of peak delivery of insulin and food intake, increased sensitivity to insulin (e.g., adrenal insufficiency), or increased insulin-independent glucose uptake (exercise). The more vigorous the attempt to achieve euglycemia, the more frequent the episodes of hypoglycemia. The most frequent symptoms of hypoglycemia include sweating, tachycardia, tremor, blurred vision, weakness, hunger, confusion, and altered behavior. Loss of consciousness may follow. Hypoglycemia may be confused with inebriation by onlookers.

With long-standing type 1 diabetes, the mechanisms for counteracting hypoglycemia may be blunted or absent in many patients, putting them at higher risk of developing hypoglycemia. Mild–moderate hypoglycemia may be treated by ingestion of sugar or honey. When hypoglycemia is severe, it should be treated with intravenous glucose or an injection of glucagon.

Adverse effects of inhaled insulin (Afrezza), in addition to hypoglycemia, include risk of acute bronchospasm in patients with chronic lung disease (e.g., asthma, COPD), and it is contraindicated in these patients. Thiazolidinediones may cause fluid retention and heart failure when used together with Afrezza.

ORAL ANTIHYPERGLYCEMIC AGENTS

Sulfonylureas

Sulfonylureas are sulfonamide derivatives (Fig. 31-3). They are traditionally divided into two groups or generations of agents. Second-generation sulfonylureas are considerably more potent than the earlier drugs. Table 31-5 lists sulfonylureas available in the United States.

Mechanism of action

Sulfonylureas are effective only in patients with functioning pancreatic β cells. These drugs stimulate release of insulin by **blocking adenosine 5′-triphosphate (ATP)–dependent K^+ current in pancreatic β cells.** The effects of sulfonylureas are initiated by their binding to and blocking an ATP-sensitive K^+ channel. Glimepiride has been shown to have an additional effect: it increases the sensitivity of peripheral tissues to insulin. This may be true for the other sulfonylureas (especially second-generation drugs) as well. The predominant effect is on insulin secretion.

Pharmacokinetics

Sulfonylureas are well absorbed after oral administration. Glipizide absorption is delayed by food. All sulfonylureas are highly bound to plasma protein (90% to 99%). Plasma protein binding is least for chlorpropamide and greatest for glyburide. Sulfonylureas are metabolized in the liver and excreted in the urine.

The half-lives and extent of metabolism vary considerably among first-generation sulfonylureas. Metabolism of chlorpropamide is incomplete, and approximately 20% of the drug is excreted unchanged, which can be a problem for patients with impaired renal function.

* Insulin lispro, more than the others, may precipitate in pump infusion systems, resulting in unexplained hyperglycemia in patients on continuous subcutaneous insulin infusion therapy.

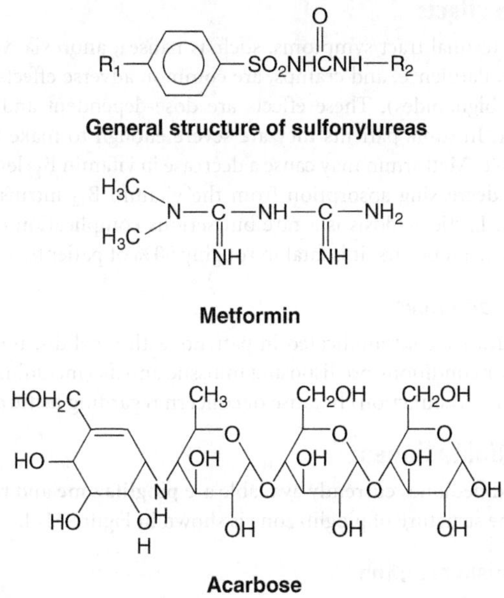

$R_1-C_6H_4-SO_2NHCNH-R_2$ (C=O)

General structure of sulfonylureas

$(H_3C)_2N-C(=NH)-NH-C(=NH)-NH_2$

Metformin

Acarbose

FIG 31-3 Chemical structures of the sulfonylureas, metformin, and acarbose.

TABLE 31-5 Sulfonylureas Available in the United States

Nonproprietary (Generic) Name	Proprietary (Trade) Name	Onset (hr)	Serum Half-Life (hr)	Duration of Action (hr)
First-Generation				
Chlorpropamide	Diabinese	1	36	24-60
Tolazamide	Tolinase	4-6	7	12-24
Second-Generation				
Glimepiride	Amaryl	2-3	9	10-24
Glipizide	Glucotrol, Glucotrol XL	1-3	2-4	10-24
Glyburide	Diaβeta, Micronase, Glynase PresTabs	1-4*	4-10	10-24

*Micronized forms have a faster onset of action.

Therapeutic uses

Sulfonylureas are used to control hyperglycemia in type 2 diabetics who cannot achieve appropriate control with changes in diet and exercise alone.

Adverse effects

Adverse effects are infrequent, occurring in approximately 4% of patients taking first-generation drugs and perhaps slightly less often in patients receiving second-generation agents. The most important adverse effect is hypoglycemia, which, if severe, can lead to coma. Hypoglycemia is a particular problem in elderly patients with impaired hepatic or renal function who are taking longer acting sulfonylureas.

Sulfonylureas have a **sulfonamide structure**, which is the basis for cross-sensitivity with antibacterial sulfonamide drugs. Hypersensitivity reactions occur with some regularity. Other adverse effects of sulfonylureas include nausea and vomiting, occasional hematologic reactions (especially leukopenia and thrombocytopenia, and hemolytic anemia in susceptible patients), cholestatic jaundice, and dermatologic effects. Sulfonylureas are teratogenic in animals (large doses). Patients taking sulfonylureas tend to gain weight, which is a problem in type 2 diabetics, who tend to be obese.

Sulfonylureas have a disulfiram-like effect. In patients who take alcohol concurrently, sulfonylureas may decrease aldehyde dehydrogenase, causing acetaldehyde accumulation (see Chapter 39). As a result, the patient may have flushing, headache, nausea, vomiting, sweating, and hypotension shortly after alcohol ingestion. This reaction is not as likely to occur with a single occasional drink.

TABLE 31-6 Sulfonylurea Drug Interactions

Drugs That Increase the Effect of Sulfonylureas
- Antihistamines (H_2 antagonists)
- Azole antifungals
- Clofibrate
- Mg^{++} salts
- Methyldopa
- Monoamine oxidase inhibitors
- Oral anticoagulants
- Salicylates
- Sulfonamides
- Tricyclic antidepressants
- β-Adrenergic receptor blockers

Drugs That Decrease the Effect of Sulfonylureas
- Ca^{2+} salts
- Corticosteroids
- Diazoxide
- Estrogens
- Phenothiazines
- Sympathomimetics
- Thiazide diuretics
- Thyroid hormones

Drug interactions

As shown in Table 31-6, numerous drugs interact with sulfonylureas by enhancing or decreasing their effect on blood glucose concentration.

Contraindications

Contraindications to the use of sulfonylureas include hypersensitivity to sulfonylureas and drugs that have similar structures (see earlier) and pregnancy. Caution should be exercised in cases of reduced renal or hepatic function. Patients with ketoacidosis should receive insulin, not an oral antihyperglycemic agent.

Meglitinides

Meglitinides that are approved for use in the United States are **repaglinide** and **nateglinide**. The structure of repaglinide is shown in Figure 31-4. These drugs are effective only in patients with functioning pancreatic β cells. Similar to sulfonylureas, they stimulate release of insulin by **blocking ATP-dependent K^+ channels in pancreatic β cells**. They may be used alone or in combination with metformin (see later) and may be given to patients who are allergic to sulfonamides.

Pharmacokinetics

Repaglinide and nateglinide are rapidly absorbed after oral administration. They are metabolized primarily by the liver. Repaglinide peak plasma levels occur within 1 hour, and the plasma half-life is 1 hour. It is recommended that this drug be taken just before each meal. Nateglinide is most effective if taken 1 to 10 minutes before a meal. These drugs offer the advantage of rapid and short-term control over blood glucose.

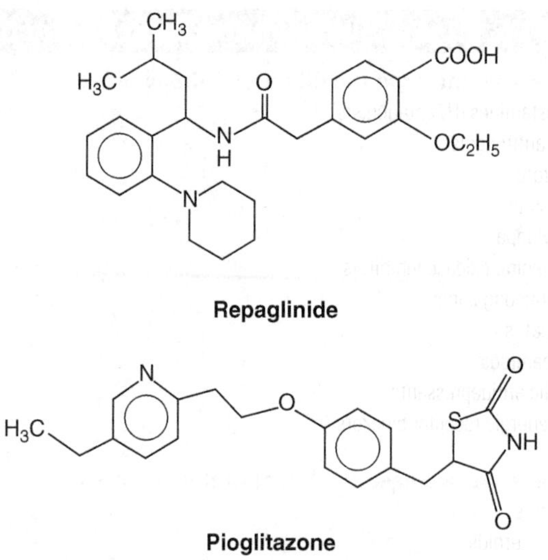

Repaglinide

Pioglitazone

FIG 31-4 Chemical structure of repaglinide and pioglitazone.

Adverse effects

Hypoglycemia is the major adverse effect of repaglinide and is most likely to occur if a meal is delayed or skipped or in patients with hepatic insufficiency.

Drug interactions

Fluconazole, amiodarone, and other cytochrome p450 2D6 enzyme inhibitors may decrease biotransformation and potentiate the effect of nateglinide. CYP 3A4 inhibitors may increase the effects of repaglinide. Nonsteroidal antiinflammatory drugs, salicylates, sulfonamides, and other highly protein-bound drugs may potentiate the hypoglycemic effects of repaglinide.

Biguanides

Metformin is currently the only biguanide approved for use in the United States (see Fig. 31-3). Phenformin and buformin, two other biguanides, are widely used in Europe and elsewhere. Phenformin was withdrawn from the United States in 1977 because of its ability to cause lactic acidosis.

Mechanism of action

The mechanism of action of biguanides differs from that of sulfonylureas or meglitinides. **Biguanides stimulate AMP-activated protein kinase** (AMPK) thereby decreasing blood glucose concentrations by several different actions. They decrease hepatic gluconeogenesis, improve tissue sensitivity to insulin, increase peripheral glucose uptake and use, and decrease intestinal absorption of glucose. Biguanides do not cause hypoglycemia. In addition, patients do not gain weight, in contrast to patients taking sulfonylureas. The action of biguanides does not depend on functioning pancreatic β cells, and they are often used in combination with sulfonylureas and other hypoglycemic agents such as thiazolidinediones.

Pharmacokinetics

Approximately 50% to 60% of an oral dose of metformin is absorbed after oral administration. Food decreases the extent of absorption and delays it slightly. Protein binding is minimal, and metformin is excreted unchanged in the urine by tubular secretion. Approximately 90% is excreted within 24 hours. It has a plasma half-life of approximately 6 hours.

Adverse effects

Gastrointestinal tract symptoms, such as nausea, anorexia, vomiting, diarrhea, flatulence, and cramps, are common adverse effects of metformin (biguanides). These effects are dose-dependent and may be transient. In some patients they are severe enough to make the drug intolerable. Metformin may cause a decrease in vitamin B_{12} levels, possibly by decreasing absorption from the vitamin B_{12} intrinsic factor complex. Lactic acidosis is a rare but serious complication of biguanides. When it occurs, it is fatal in roughly 50% of patients.

Contraindications

Biguanides are contraindicated in patients with renal disease, hepatic disease, or conditions predisposing to tissue anoxia (including cardiopulmonary dysfunction) because of concern regarding **lactic acidosis.**

Thiazolidinediones

Thiazolidinediones currently available are **pioglitazone** and **rosiglitazone**. The structure of pioglitazone is shown in Figure 31-4.

Mechanism of action

Thiazolidinediones act by increasing insulin sensitivity in tissues. They are **agonists at the nuclear peroxisome proliferator-activated receptor-γ (PPARγ)**. PPAR-γ stimulates the transcription for many of the genes responsive to insulin. The thiazolidinediones depend on the presence of insulin for their activity. They decrease hepatic gluconeogenesis and increase insulin-dependent glucose uptake in muscle and fat. They act synergistically with sulfonylureas and metformin.

Pharmacokinetics

Thiazolidinediones are taken orally, once a day, with or without food. The maximal effect is not seen for 6 to 12 weeks. They are metabolized by the cytochrome P450 oxidative enzyme system.

Adverse effects

Thiazolidinediones now carry a **"black box" warning** of congestive heart failure and myocardial ischemia. The risk is greater with rosiglitazone. There is also weight gain and a risk of edema, osteoporosis, and fractures. Hepatotoxicity is also a possible adverse effect.

Drug interactions

Concurrent administration of pioglitazone with oral contraceptives containing ethinyl estradiol and norethindrone can result in decreased plasma concentrations of the contraceptive and can result in loss of contraceptive effect. Cytochromes CYP 2C8 and CYP 3A4 are involved in the metabolism of the thiazolidinediones. Inducers and inhibitors of these cytochrome systems could affect the levels of these drugs.

Incretin-Related Drugs

Incretin-related drugs include **exenatide,** albiglutide, dulaglutide, liraglutide, **sitagliptin,** saxagliptin, and linagliptin (Fig. 31-5). Although the first four drugs are not given orally, these drugs are generally classified with oral antihyperglycemic agents.

It has long been known that oral glucose produces greater release of insulin than intravenous glucose. Two hormones, secreted from the gastrointestinal tract, have been shown to stimulate insulin secretion. They are known as **incretins**. The two compounds are **glucagon-like peptide 1 (GLP-1)**, and glucose-dependent insulinotropic polypeptide. Their secretion is increased by food and elevated glucose levels. GLP-1 has been shown to augment glucose-dependent insulin secretion. It also reduces glucagon secretion, slows gastric emptying, and decreases appetite. GLP-1

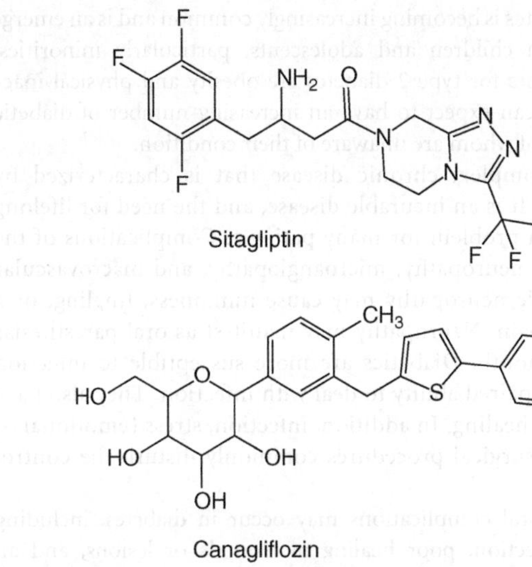

Sitagliptin

Canagliflozin

FIG 31-5 Chemical structures of sitagliptin and canagliflozin.

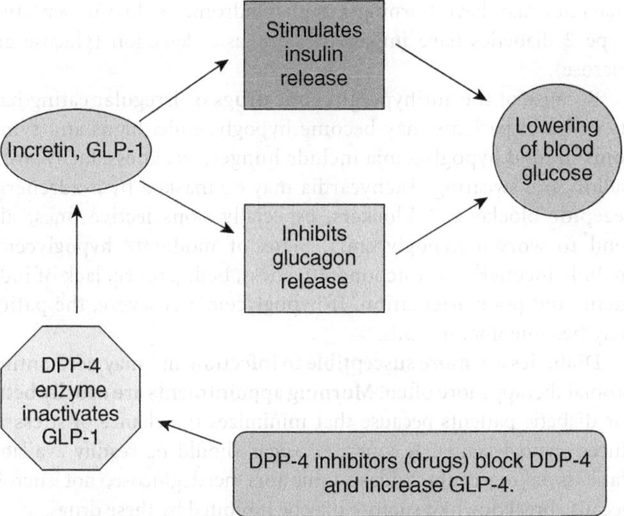

FIG 31-6 Site of action of the incretin-related drugs.

is rapidly inactivated by **dipeptidyl peptidase 4 (DPP-4)**. Exenatide, albiglutide, dulaglutide, and liraglutide are agonists at GLP-1 receptors, but they are resistant to DPP-4. Exenatide is given by subcutaneous injection once a week. Albiglutide and dulaglutide are also injected once a week. Liraglutide is injected once a day.

There are reports of rare cases of hemorrhagic or necrotizing pancreatitis with exenatide. Pancreatitis has also been reported with liraglutide. Sitagliptin, saxagliptin, and linagliptin **inhibit DPP-4**, decreasing the biotransformation of GLP-1. They are given orally. The action of the incretin-related drugs is shown in Figure 31-6.

Sodium-Glucose Co-Transporter 2 (SGLT2) Inhibitors

This class of drugs includes **canagliflozin**, dapagliflozin, and empagliflozin.

Mechanism of action

The SGLT2 inhibitors **block the sodium-glucose co-transporter** 2 that facilitates glucose reabsorption in the kidney. As a result, reabsorption of glucose from the kidney is decreased, renal excretion of glucose is increased, and blood glucose levels are lowered.

Adverse effects

These drugs cause increased incidence of vaginal yeast infections, increased incidence of urinary tract infections, and increased urinary urgency. They may cause hypotension due to intravascular volume depletion. They may increase the incidence of bladder cancer. They may cause hyperkalemia. This class of drugs is not indicated for type 1 diabetics, and they are contraindicated in patients with severe renal impairment or patients with ketoacidosis.

Analogue of Amylin

Pramlintide is an **analogue of amylin** that is approved in the United States. Amylin is a peptide containing 37 amino acids. It is produced by pancreatic β cells and cosecreted with insulin. **Amylin has a role in the maintenance of glucose homeostasis.** It decreases glucagon secretion, slows gastric emptying by a vagally mediated mechanism, and decreases appetite centrally. Pramlintide is an analogue of amylin and has an action similar to amylin. It is used in patients who are being treated with insulin (type 1 and type 2 diabetics). It is given by injection at mealtimes.

MISCELLANEOUS DRUGS IN THE TREATMENT OF DIABETIC PATIENTS

α-Glucosidase Inhibitors

Acarbose and **miglitol** are **α-glucosidase inhibitors** approved for use in the United States. The structure of acarbose is shown in Figure 31-3. α-Glucosidases facilitate digestion of complex starches, oligosaccharides, and disaccharides into monosaccharides, allowing them to be absorbed from the small intestine. α-Glucosidase inhibitors are competitive, reversible inhibitors of intestinal α-glucosidases. Acarbose also inhibits α-amylase. α-Glucosidase inhibitors delay absorption of most carbohydrates. This delayed absorption limits the postprandial increase in glucose. They do not directly affect insulin secretion.

Pharmacokinetics

α-Glucosidase inhibitors are taken at the beginning of meals. Absorption of acarbose is poor. It is metabolized in the gastrointestinal tract, principally by intestinal bacteria. Miglitol is absorbed after oral administration.

Adverse effects

Adverse effects include flatulence, diarrhea, and abdominal pain from the presence of undigested carbohydrates in the lower gastrointestinal tract. These effects tend to decrease with continued use. When given alone, α-glucosidase inhibitors do not cause hypoglycemia. Hypoglycemia may occur, however, with concurrent sulfonylurea therapy. Hypoglycemia should be treated with glucose, not sucrose, because breakdown of sucrose may be inhibited. Miglitol has minor lactase inhibitory activity, but it should not induce lactose intolerance.

Drug interactions

Miglitol decreases plasma concentrations of several drugs, including glyburide and metformin.

Contraindications

Contraindications to α-glucosidase inhibitors include hypersensitivity to these agents, inflammatory bowel disease, and intestinal obstruction.

Inositolphosphoglycans (IPGs)

Evidence suggests that interaction of insulin with its receptor leads to the release of low-molecular-weight IPGs, which enter the cell and act as mediators of insulin action. IPG mediators have been shown to reproduce various short-term effects of insulin. Two families of IPG insulin mediators have been isolated. Myoinositol is a major component of one; chiroinositol is a major component of the other. Studies have shown the presence of hypochiroinositoluria in type 2 diabetics. In addition, there is decreased chiroinositol content and decreased chiroinositol mediator activity in type 2 diabetics. There is evidence that chiroinositol decreases elevated blood glucose concentrations in diabetic monkeys and rats. Studies have also shown that pinitol, which is 3-*O*-methyl chiroinositol, decreases hyperglycemia in a diabetic murine model and in humans with diabetes.

Angiotensin-Converting Enzyme Inhibitors

Angiotensin-converting enzyme inhibitors and angiotensin II receptor blockers have been shown to delay the onset and reduce significantly the progression of diabetic nephropathy. They are given to diabetics to decrease the incidence of these complications of the disease.

GLUCAGON

Glucagon is synthesized in the α cells of the pancreatic islets. It is a 29-amino acid peptide with a molecular weight of approximately 3500 Da. Similar to insulin, it is formed from a larger precursor molecule by proteolytic cleavage. Glucagon binds to specific G_s protein–linked receptors in the liver, causing an increase in adenylyl cyclase activity and production of cyclic adenosine 3′,5′-monophosphate. This ultimately results in an increase in glycogen phosphorylase activity and a decrease in glycogen synthase. Glucagon increases blood glucose concentration by decreasing glycogen synthesis, stimulating breakdown of stored glycogen, and increasing gluconeogenesis in the liver. It does not affect skeletal muscle glycogen, presumably because of a lack of receptors in skeletal muscle. Glucagon has potent inotropic and chronotropic effects on the heart. These are similar to effects resulting from β-adrenergic receptor stimulation.

Pharmacokinetics

Glucagon is rapidly degraded in the plasma, liver, and kidney. Its half-life is 3 to 6 minutes.

Therapeutic Uses

Glucagon may be used in the emergency treatment of severe hypoglycemic reactions (sufficient to cause unconsciousness). It is given parenterally. Glucagon is also used to reverse the cardiac effects of toxic amounts of β-adrenergic receptor blockers.

Adverse Effects

Adverse effects include nausea (usually transient) and vomiting. Glucagon may cause transient tachycardia and hypertension.

IMPLICATIONS FOR DENTISTRY

There are approximately **29.1 million diabetics (approximately 9.3% of the population)** in the United States. About a quarter of diabetics are unaware that they have the disease. In the United States, the annual number of newly diagnosed diabetes cases tripled between 1980 and 2014.

Type 2 diabetes is becoming increasingly common and is an emerging problem in children and adolescents, particularly minorities. Major risk factors for type 2 diabetes are obesity and physical inactivity. Dentists can expect to have an increasing number of diabetic patients, many of whom are unaware of their condition.

DM is a complex, chronic disease that is characterized by hyperglycemia. It is an incurable disease, and the need for lifelong compliance is a problem for many patients. Complications of the disease include neuropathy, microangiopathy, and macrovascular disease. Diabetic neuropathy may cause numbness, tingling, or a deep burning pain. Neuropathy may manifest as oral paresthesias and burning mouth. Diabetics are more susceptible to infection and have an impaired ability to deal with infection. They also have delayed wound healing. In addition, infection, stress (emotional or physical), and surgical procedures commonly disturb the control of diabetes.

Numerous oral complications may occur in diabetes, including xerostomia, infection, poor healing of wounds or lesions, and an increased incidence and severity of caries, candidiasis, gingivitis, periodontal disease, and periapical abscesses. Diabetics often have progressive periodontal disease and may have multiple periodontal abscesses. Diabetics may have burning mouth syndrome or loss of sensation. Type 2 diabetics have impaired sweet taste detection (glucose and sucrose).

Because of the antihyperglycemic drugs or irregular eating habits or both, patients may become hypoglycemic. Signs and symptoms of mild hypoglycemia include hunger, weakness, tachycardia, pallor, and sweating. Tachycardia may be masked by β-adrenergic receptor blockers. β Blockers, especially nonselective ones, also tend to worsen hypoglycemia. Signs of moderate hypoglycemia include incoherence, uncooperativeness, belligerence, lack of judgment, and poor orientation. If hypoglycemia is severe, the patient may become unconscious.

Diabetics are more susceptible to infection and may need antimicrobial therapy more often. **Morning appointments are usually better** for diabetic patients because that minimizes the chance of stress-induced hypoglycemia. A source of sugar should be readily available. Patients taking α-glucosidase inhibitors need glucose, not sucrose, because breakdown of sucrose may be inhibited by these drugs.

TREATING DIABETIC PATIENTS

Blood glucose levels tend to be more stable in the morning, so morning appointments are preferable for diabetic patients. Since **stress** may cause an **increase in blood glucose levels**, short appointments and/or stress reduction techniques may be helpful in preventing an increase in blood glucose levels. Furthermore, it is suggested that the patient's blood glucose should be less than 200 mg/dL before any invasive therapy is started. Diabetics have decreased resistance to infection, so antibiotics, or even prophylactic antibiotic therapy, may be needed. Healing time is frequently prolonged.

Use of epinephrine may cause transient hyperglycemia. This can be minimized by insuring that the patient has taken the usual hypoglycemic medication prior to the appointment and limiting the dose of vasoconstrictor (e.g., 3 cartridges of 1:100,000 epinephrine - adult dose). Glucocorticosteroids also have the potential to raise blood glucose levels.

CASE DISCUSSION

Shakiness, nervousness or anxiety, irritability or impatience, confusion, including delirium, rapid/fast heartbeat, lightheadedness, or dizziness are all signs of hypoglycemia. Contributing to these symptoms is the release of epinephrine when blood glucose falls. Ms. DP's behavior could be due to hypoglycemia.

Ask the patient when she last ate and what did she have to eat as well as her hypoglycemic regimen. Upon questioning the patient, you find out that she had a light breakfast and nothing to eat since then. She has, however, maintained her prescribed regimen for the sulfonylurea. A ready source of glucose (e.g., orange juice, non-diet soda drink, cake icing, or soft candy bar) should be made available to her to bring her blood glucose up (see Chapter 41). A ready source of glucose should be available in the dental office for such an emergency.

You should advise the patient in the future to eat regular meals, including if the patient has a dental appointment that day. Blood glucose levels tend to be more stable in the morning, so morning appointments are preferable for diabetic patients. This should be considered for subsequent appointments for this patient. The patient should also be advised to maintain regular appointments with her physician and to discuss this hypoglycemic incident with him/her.

Since stress may cause an increase in blood glucose levels, short appointments and/or stress reduction techniques may be helpful in preventing an increase in blood glucose levels. Furthermore, it is suggested that the patient's blood glucose should be less than 200 mg/dL before any invasive therapy is started. Diabetics have decreased resistance to infection, so antibiotics, or even prophylactic antibiotic therapy, may be needed. Healing time is frequently prolonged. The use of epinephrine may cause hyperglycemia. Limiting the dose of epinephrine is recommended. (See above.) Glucocorticosteroids also have the potential to raise blood glucose levels.

Of the drugs used in the treatment of diabetes, insulin and sulfonylureas are the most likely to cause hypoglycemia. The tighter the blood sugar control, the more likely hypoglycemia will occur. From 1999 to 2011, there were more hospital admissions related to hypoglycemia than to hyperglycemia among Medicare beneficiaries. Furthermore, 25% of all emergency room hospitalizations for adverse reactions were related to hypoglycemia in older adults. Undesirable health outcomes from hypoglycemia include increased falls and increased incidence of cardiovascular events. As a result of these findings, barring any contraindication, it is now recommended that metformin, long held undesirable in older adults, be used for blood sugar control in type 2 diabetics.

ANTIHYPERGLYCEMIC AND HYPERGLYCEMIC AGENTS

Nonproprietary (Generic) Name	Proprietary (Trade) Name
Antihyperglycemic Agents	
Acarbose	Precose
Acetohexamide	Dymelor
Albiglutide	Tanzeum
Canagliflozin	Invokana
Chlorpropamide	Diabinese
Dapagliflozin	Farxiga
Dulaglutide	Trulicity
Empagliflozin	Jardiance
Exenatide	Byetta
Glimepiride	Amaryl
Glipizide	Glucotrol, Glucotrol XL
Glyburide	Micronase, Diaβeta, Glynase PresTabs

ANTIHYPERGLYCEMIC AND HYPERGLYCEMIC AGENTS—cont'd

Nonproprietary (Generic) Name	Proprietary (Trade) Name
Antihyperglycemic Agents—cont'd	
Insulin	See Table 31-4
Linagliptin	Tradjenta
Liraglutide	Victoza, Saxenda
Metformin	Glucophage, Riomet
Miglitol	Glyset
Nateglinide	Starlix
Pioglitazone	Actos
Pramlintide	Symlin
Repaglinide	Prandin
Rosiglitazone	Avandia
Saxagliptin	Onglyza
Sitagliptin	Januvia
Tolazamide	Tolinase
Tolbutamide	Orinase
Some Combined Preparations	
Empagliflozin + linagliptin	Glyxambi
Glipizide + metformin	Metaglip
Glyburide + metformin	Glucovance
Pioglitazone + glimepiride	Duetact
Rosiglitazone + glimepiride	Avandaryl
Rosiglitazone + metformin	Avandamet
Sitagliptin + metformin	Janumet
Hyperglycemic Agents	
Glucagon	—
Glucose	Insta-Glucose

GENERAL REFERENCES

1. An inhaled insulin (Afrezza), *Med Lett Drugs Therap* 57(1463):34–35, 2015.
2. Davidson JA: The placement of DPP-4 inhibitors in clinical practice recommendations for the treatment of type 2 diabetes, *Endocrine Pract* 19:1050–1061, 2013.
3. De Meyts P, Sajid W, Palsgaard J, et al.: Insulin and IGF-I receptor structure and binding mechanisms. In *Mechanisms of Insulin Action*, New York, 2007, Springer, pp 1–32.
4. Drugs for type 2 diabetes, *Med Lett Drugs Therap* 12(139):17–24, March 2014.
5. Ferrannini E: The target of metformin in type 2 diabetes, *N Engl J Med* 371:1547–1548, 2014.
6. Hardie DG: AMP-activated protein kinase as a drug target, *Ann Rev Pharmacol Toxicol* 47:185–210, 2006.
7. Santos-Paul MA, Neves IL, Neves RS, Ramires JA: Local anesthesia with epinephrine is safe and effective for oral surgery in patients with type 2 diabetes mellitus and coronary disease: a prospective randomized study, *Clinics* 70:185–189, 2015.
8. Scheen A: Pharmacodynamics, efficacy and safety of sodium-glucose co-transporter type 2 (SGLT2) inhibitors for the treatment of type 2 diabetes, *Drugs* 75:33–59, 2015.
9. Tornio A, Niemi M, Neuvonem PJ, Backman JT: Drug interactions with oral antidiabetic agents: pharmacokinetic mechanisms and clinical implications, *Trends Pharmacol Sci* 33:312–322, 2012.
10. Vallon V: The mechanisms and therapeutic potential of SGLT2 inhibitors in diabetes mellitus, *Ann Rev Med* 66:255–270, 2015.

32

Steroid Hormones of Reproduction and Sexual Development

Angelo J. Mariotti

KEY INFORMATION

- Sex steroid hormones are secreted from the ovary, testis, and inner layer of the adrenal medulla cortex.
- The ovary primarily produces estrogens and progestins:
  - estrone, estradiol, estriol,
  - progesterone.
- The testis primarily produces testosterone.
- Estrogens and progestins produce numerous physiologic actions. The most common pharmacologic use of these hormones and their antagonists are for contraception, menopausal therapy, infertility, and hormone-responsive breast cancer.
  - Numerous synthetic estrogens and progestins are used for contraception.
  - Synthesis inhibitors, receptor agonists, and mixed agonists/antagonists (e.g., selective estrogen receptor modulators [SERMs]) are used for estrogen-sensitive carcinomas.
  - Estrogen and progestin agonists and/or SERMs are used in the management of menopause and osteoporosis in women.
- Androgenic compounds have dramatic effects in men and women. The most common pharmacologic use of these hormones and their antagonists are for replacement therapy and management of hormone-sensitive benign and malignant prostate neoplasms.
  - Synthetic androgens are used primarily for testosterone deficiency in boys and men.
  - Antiandrogens are used for prostate cancer, benign prostatic hypertrophy, and hyperandrogenism in women.
- Although the dentist does not prescribe sex steroid hormones or the antagonists, the pervasive presence of these drugs requires the dentist to be aware of the following:
  - biologic responses in the oral cavity,
  - drug interactions (especially concerning antibiotics),
  - some dental materials that may interfere with endocrine function.

CASE STUDY

Mrs. A is a 34-year-old mother of four children whose medical and social history is unremarkable. She is not using any medications except for Necon 10/11 (i.e., biphasic oral contraceptive), which she has taken for the past 9 months for birth control. During the last 6 weeks, she has noticed a growth on her gingiva above the maxillary lateral incisor (Fig. 32-1) that has continued to grow in size with time. In addition, she complains of feeling sick in the morning with anorexia. These signs and symptoms have caused her great concern because it affects the way she eats and looks, and she is worried that the lesion in her mouth may be malignant. What additional information and/or tests would you want to obtain? What is your clinical diagnosis for this condition? How would you treat this condition?

Since the synthesis of sex steroid hormones in the early 20th century, the use of these agents has exploded. Today, steroidal and nonsteroidal compounds with properties of sex steroid hormones are extensively used in the prophylaxis or treatment of disease and for birth control. Although dentists do not typically prescribe these agents, their ubiquitous presence in the population requires a careful understanding of the actions and interactions of sex steroids with other pharmacologic agents and how they affect structures in the oral cavity.

Although sex steroid hormones are essential for reproduction, evidence has accrued that gonadal hormones have a much broader role in human tissues. Androgens, estrogens, and progestins are now believed to be directly or indirectly involved in the regulation of various diverse tissues, such as the brain, heart, kidney, skin, liver, and tissues of the oral cavity (Fig. 32-1). Reports of the effects of sex steroid hormones in the periodontium, a unique structure composed of two fibrous (gingiva and periodontal ligament) and two mineralized (cementum and alveolar bone) tissues, have been noted for more than a century. The actions of sex steroid hormones on periodontal tissues have heightened interest in defining the pharmacologic management of steroid hormone–induced diseases.

STRUCTURE AND FUNCTION

Estrogens

Estrogens, like all sex steroid hormones, are derived from a chemical structure composed of 17 carbon atoms in a four-ring structure (Fig. 32-2). The three naturally occurring and **biologically important estrogens** are **estrone, estradiol,** and **estriol. Estradiol is the most potent estrogen** and is secreted by the ovary, testes, placenta, and peripheral tissues. Estrone is also secreted by the ovary; however, the principal source in women and men is through extragonadal conversion of androstenedione in peripheral tissues. In premenopausal women, the most abundant physiologic estrogen is estradiol; in men and postmenopausal women, the most abundant estrogen in the plasma is estrone. Similar to other lipid-soluble hormones, estrogens are transported in the blood principally bound to carrier proteins,

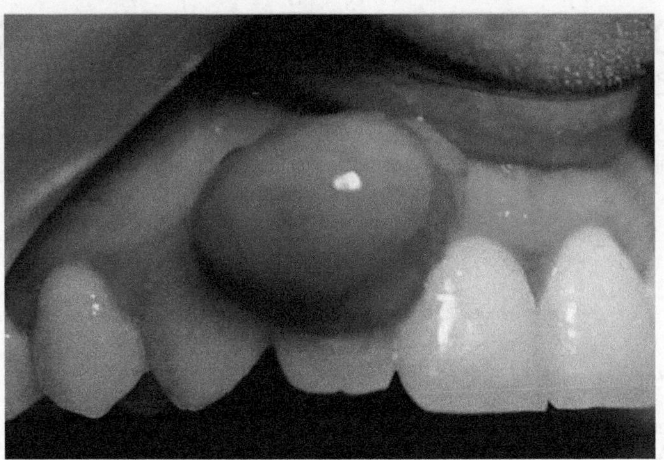

FIG 32-1 The effects of sex steroid hormones can affect the periodontium. (From OSU Division of Periodontology.)

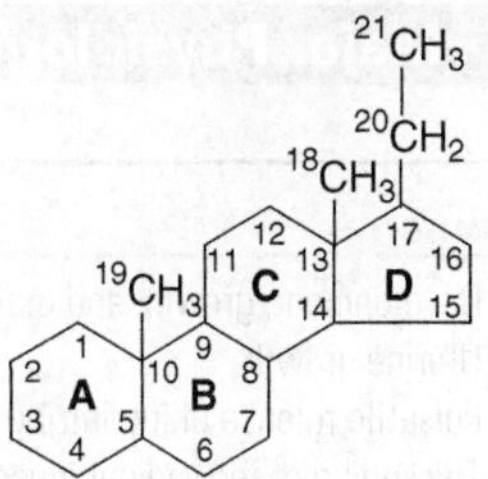

FIG 32-2 Ring structure for pregnane and numbering system for steroids. Progesterone contains 21 carbons. Androgens, estrogens, and some progestins lack carbons 20 and 21. Estradiol and synthetic estrogenic steroids have an aromatic ring A and lack carbon 19.

TABLE 32-1 Indications and Adverse Effects of Common Estrogens, Progestins, and Anabolic-Androgenic Drugs

	Nonproprietary (Generic) Name	Proprietary (Trade) Name	Principal Indications	Adverse Effects
Estrogens	Diethylstilbestrol	Stilphostrol	Prostatic carcinoma	
	Ethinyl estradiol	Estinyl	Prostatic carcinoma; menopausal vasomotor symptoms; estrogen deficiency from surgery, ovarian failure, or hypogonadism; contraception	Serious side effects: thromboembolic disorders, neoplasms (e.g., breast [?], uterine), stroke Other side effects include heavy non-menstrual vaginal bleeding; body aches or pain, chills, cough, difficulty breathing, ear congestion, fever, headache, loss of voice, nasal congestion, runny nose, sneezing, sore throat, unusual tiredness or weakness
	Conjugated estrogens	Premarin	Menopausal symptoms, prevention of postmenopausal bone loss, atrophic vaginitis, hypoestrogenism	
Progestins	Medroxyprogesterone acetate	Provera, Depo-Provera	Dysfunctional uterine bleeding, endometrial carcinoma, contraception	Serious side effects: thromboembolic disorders, heart attacks Other side effects include chest pain, chills, cold/flu-like symptoms, fever, problems with urination, changes in vaginal bleeding, dry mouth, frequent urination, loss of appetite, unusual thirst, changes in nipple redness or swelling of breast, mental depression
	Norethindrone	Aygestin, Micronor, Nor-QD	Dysfunctional uterine bleeding, endometriosis, contraception	
	Norgestrel	Ovrette	Contraception	
Anabolic-androgenic drugs	Danazol	Danocrine	Endometriosis, fibrocystic breast disease, hereditary angioedema	Men: bladder irritation, breast soreness, gynecomastia, priapism, acne, decreased testicle size Women: amenorrhea, oligomenorrhea, virilism (acne, decreased breast size, hirsutism, enlarged genitalia, male-pattern baldness, hoarseness, deepening of the voice) Children: virilism, stunting of linear growth Other side effects: dysphoria, enlarged prostate, irritability, quick to overreact emotionally, trouble concentrating
	Fluoxymesterone	Halotestin	Delayed puberty in boys, hypogonadism, breast cancer	
	Methyltestosterone	Android, Testred, Virilon	Delayed puberty in boys, hypogonadism, breast cancer	
	Oxandrolone	Oxandrin	Catabolic or tissue-depleting processes	
	Testosterone propionate	Testex	Lichen sclerosus, microphallus	

leaving only 2% of the hormone free. Estradiol and estrone are metabolized principally to estriol, which is the major estrogen detected in the urine.

Estrogens may be administered orally, topically, or through intramuscular injections (Table 32-1). Although estradiol is available for enteral administration, it is generally not used in this manner since concentrations in the bloodstream remain low because of extensive hepatic metabolism. The half-life of estrogenic compounds can be increased by synthetic substitutions on the C or D ring of the estrogen molecule. For example, the half-life of estradiol is a few minutes, whereas the half-life of ethinyl estradiol (ethinyl substitution at the C17 position) may be more than 13 hours. Nonsteroidal compounds may also have estrogenic activity; examples of such compounds include diethylstilbestrol, flavones, isoflavones, certain pesticides (e.g.,

TABLE 32-2 **Major Physiologic Effects of Sex Steroid Hormones**

	MAJOR PHYSIOLOGIC EFFECTS	
Hormone	**Women**	**Men**
Estrogens	• Development, growth, and maintenance of secondary sex characteristics • Uterine growth • Pulsatile release of luteinizing hormone from the pituitary • Thickening of the vaginal mucosa • Ductal development in the breast	• The physiologic significance of estrogens is largely unknown, but may be involved in the following: • The regulation of plasma androgen and estrogen levels • Sexual behavior • Bone homeostasis • Spermatogenesis
Progestins	• Glandular endometrial development before nidation • Development of mammary lobules and alveoli • Maintenance of pregnancy (e.g., endometrial gland function, decreased excitability of myometrium, and possible effects on the immune system to decrease rejection of the developing fetus) • Decreases hepatic secretion of very low-density lipoprotein and high-density lipoprotein • Diminishes insulin action • Stimulates the hypothalamic respiratory center • Elevates basal core body temperature at ovulation • Enhances sodium excretion by the kidneys	• Decreases hepatic secretion of very low-density lipoprotein and high-density lipoprotein • Diminishes insulin action • Stimulates the hypothalamic respiratory center • Enhances sodium excretion by the kidneys
Androgens	• The physiologic significance of androgens is largely unknown, but it may be involved in facilitation of human sexual behavior	• Male sexual differentiation of wolffian ducts, external genitalia, and brain in utero • Development of adult male phenotype, including growth and maintenance of male sex accessory organs and anabolic actions on skeletal muscle, bone, and hair • Facilitation of human sexual behavior • Regulation of specific metabolic processes in the liver, kidney, and salivary glands

p,p′-DDT) and plasticizers (e.g., bisphenol A). The biologic activities of estrogens can be found in Table 32-2.

Progestins

Progestins, or steroids that have progestational activity, are derived from a 21-carbon saturated steroid hydrocarbon known as pregnane. **The principal progestational hormone secreted into the bloodstream is progesterone,** which is synthesized and secreted by the corpus luteum, placenta, and adrenal cortex. As with estrogens, most progesterone is transported in the bloodstream by plasma proteins, leaving a small percentage (2%) free. The fate of plasma progesterone depends on hepatic, extrahepatic, and extra-adrenal metabolism. Metabolic inactivation of progesterone to pregnanediol is accomplished by the liver.

Progestins may be administered orally, topically, or through intramuscular injections Progesterone is available for enteral administration; however, it is generally not administered in this manner since concentrations in the bloodstream remain low because of extensive first-pass hepatic metabolism. The bioavailability of progestins can be increased by intramuscular injections in oil, by vaginal suppositories, or by synthetic substitutions of the molecule, which significantly decreases hepatic metabolism. The biologic activities of progestins are principally observed during the luteal phase of the menstrual cycle and pregnancy and can be found in Table 32-2.

Androgens

Androgens are derived from a 19-carbon tetracyclic hydrocarbon nucleus known as androstane. One of the most potent androgenic hormones, **testosterone,** is synthesized by the Leydig cells of the testes, the thecal cells of the ovary, and the adrenal cortex. In men, testosterone is the principal plasma androgen and in target tissues is reduced to **dihydrotestosterone, the mediator of most actions of the hormone.** The irreversible metabolic conversion of testosterone to dihydrotestosterone occurs only in tissues that contain the enzyme **5α-reductase.** Testosterone (but not dihydrotestosterone) can also be aromatized to estradiol by numerous extragonadal tissues (primarily adipose tissue and skeletal muscle), a common route of estrogen production in men. In women, the major plasma androgen is androstenedione, which can be secreted into the bloodstream or converted into either testosterone or estradiol by the ovary.

When secreted into the bloodstream, most androgens are transported to their sites of action by carrier proteins, leaving only 2% free in the blood. Secreted plasma androgens are also metabolized to physiologically weak or inactive molecules consisting of either 17-ketosteroids or polar compounds (diols, triols, and conjugates) for excretion by the kidney or liver.

Androgens may be administered orally, topically, or through intramuscular injections. Testosterone is generally not administered enterally because extensive first-pass hepatic metabolism rapidly reduces plasma concentrations. The bioavailability of androgens is increased by intramuscular injections in an oil vehicle, by transdermal application, or by alkylation at C17, which significantly decreases hepatic metabolism and makes oral administration therapeutically possible. The biologic activities of androgens are manifested in virtually every tissue of the body and can be found in Table 32-2.

MECHANISM OF ACTION

In the bloodstream, sex steroid hormones exist in extremely low concentrations (in the femtomolar to nanomolar range), yet they are

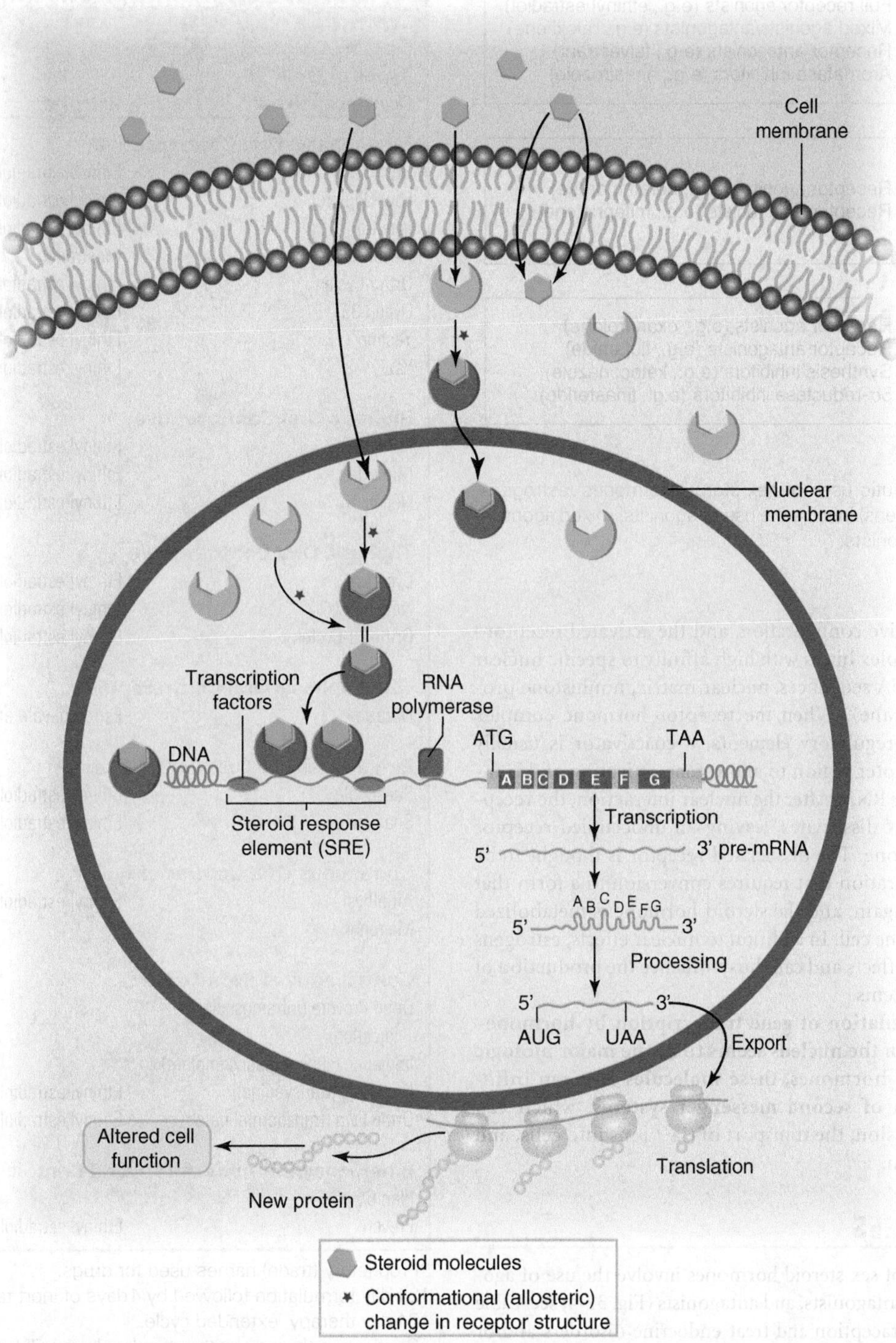

FIG 32-3 The current hypothesis of sex steroid hormone action. DNA domains are shown (ABCDEFG).

capable of regulating differentiation and growth in selected tissues distant from the site of secretion. The actions of sex steroid hormones become even more intriguing when one considers that **the distinct biologic effects of these hormones depend on nominal differences between relatively small (molecular weight approximately 300 Da) molecules.** Testosterone, which is capable of powerful virilizing effects, differs from estradiol by only one carbon atom and four hydrogen atoms. These differences in molecular structure of steroid hormones change biologic activity. **Specificity of hormone response depends on the presence of intracellular proteins or receptors, which specifically recognize and selectively bind the hormone and act in concert with the hormone ligand to regulate gene expression.**

The current hypothesis of sex steroid hormone action (Fig. 32-3) begins with the secretion of the hormones into the bloodstream, where they circulate, principally bound (approximately 98%) to plasma proteins. In the circulation, the unbound or free hormone can enter the cell by diffusion and bind to receptors. These large intracellular protein receptors are located in the nucleus of the cell. When the steroid hormone is bound to the receptor, it transforms

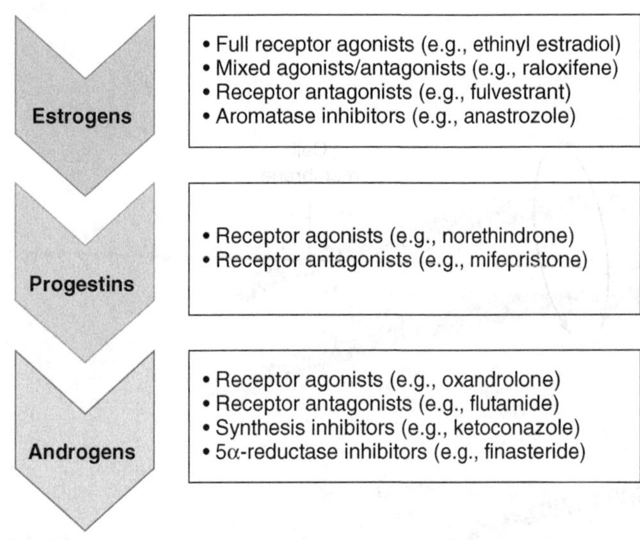

FIG 32-4 The therapeutic uses of sex steroid hormones (estrogens, progestins, and androgens) involve the use of agonists, mixed agonists/antagonists, and antagonists.

the receptor to an active configuration, and the activated receptor–steroid hormone complex binds with high affinity to specific nuclear sites (e.g., discrete DNA sequences, nuclear matrix, nonhistone proteins, nuclear membrane). When the receptor–hormone complex is bound to nuclear regulatory elements, a coactivator is usually recruited to the promoter region to allow gene activation and transcription of messenger RNA. After the nuclear interaction, the receptor–hormone complex dissociates, leaving an unoccupied receptor and the steroid hormone. The dissociated receptor is thought to be in an inactive configuration that requires conversion to a form that can bind the steroid again, and the steroid hormone is metabolized and eliminated from the cell. In addition to nuclear effects, estrogens also have membrane effects and can thus influence the production of second messenger systems.

Although the regulation of gene transcription by hormone–receptor complexes in the nucleus seems to be the major biologic action of sex steroid hormones, these molecules also can influence the production of second messenger systems, which can affect neural transmission, the transport of Ca^{2+} ions into cells, and epithelial cell function.

THERAPEUTIC USES

The therapeutic uses of sex steroid hormones involve the use of agonists, mixed agonists/antagonists, and antagonists (Fig. 32-4; see Table 32-1) to manage contraception and treat endocrine disorders and/or diseases. Some drugs, especially associated with estrogens, have agonist effects that are tissue dependent. This mixed agonist/antagonist effect is the result of the differential tissue distribution of the alpha and beta forms of the estrogen receptor and drug receptor efficacy.

Estrogens

The most common reasons for the prescription of estrogens are for the prevention of conception and to reduce the sequelae associated with declining hormone levels during and after menopause. Oral contraceptives are among the most widely used medications in the world and most often are a combination of an estrogen and a progestin (Table 32-3). **Combination oral contraceptives principally affect conception by suppressing the release of follicle-stimulating hormone and suppressing the surge of luteinizing hormone (LH)** from the anterior pituitary, which consequently prevents ovulation (Fig. 32-5). Other effects of oral contraceptives that reduce conception involve affecting the transport of the egg in the fallopian tubes, as well as reduction in sperm motility and nidation. The estrogen component of combination oral contraceptives usually contains either ethinyl estradiol or mestranol. In these preparations, the estrogen content ranges from 20 to 50 μg pills containing less than 35 μg are usually considered low-dose contraceptives.

TABLE 32-3 Examples of Contraceptive Agents

Types of Oral Contraceptives*	Estrogen	Progestin
Monophasic Oral Contraceptive		
Cryselle	Ethinyl estradiol	Norgestrel
Low-Ogestrel	Ethinyl estradiol	Norgestrel
Loestrin 24 Fe†	Ethinyl estradiol	Norethindrone
Necon 1/50	Mestranol	Norethindrone
Ortho-Cyclen	Ethinyl estradiol	Norgestimate
Ovcon-35	Ethinyl estradiol	Norethindrone
Yasmin	Ethinyl estradiol	Drospirenone
Yaz†	Ethinyl estradiol	Drospirenone
Biphasic Oral Contraceptive		
Kariva	Ethinyl estradiol	Desogestrel
Mircette	Ethinyl estradiol	Desogestrel
Necon 10/11	Ethinyl estradiol	Norethindrone
Triphasic Oral Contraceptive		
Cyclessa	Ethinyl estradiol	Desogestrel
Necon 7/7/7	Ethinyl estradiol	Norethindrone
Ortho Tri-Cyclen	Ethinyl estradiol	Norgestimate
Quadraphasic Oral Contraceptive		
Natazia	Estradiol valerate	Dienogest
Extended-Cycle Oral Contraceptive‡		
Seasonale	Ethinyl estradiol	Levonorgestrel
Seasonique	Ethinyl estradiol	Levonorgestrel
Continuous Oral Contraceptive§		
Amethyst	Ethinyl estradiol	Levonorgestrel
Micronor		Norethindrone
Contraceptives (Non-Oral)		
Depo-Provera (intramuscular injection)		Medroxyprogesterone acetate
Implanon (subcutaneous implant)		Etonogestrel
NuvaRing (transvaginal)	Ethinyl estradiol	Etonogestrel
Ortho Evra (transdermal patch)	Ethinyl estradiol	Norelgestromin
Emergency (Morning-After) Oral Contraceptive‖		
Plan B		Levonorgestrel
Preven	Ethinyl estradiol	Levonorgestrel

*Proprietary (trade) names used for drugs.
†24-day formulation followed by 4 days of inert tablets.
‡84-day therapy, extended cycle.
§Continuous therapy, without a placebo or pill-free period.
‖Postcoital preparation.

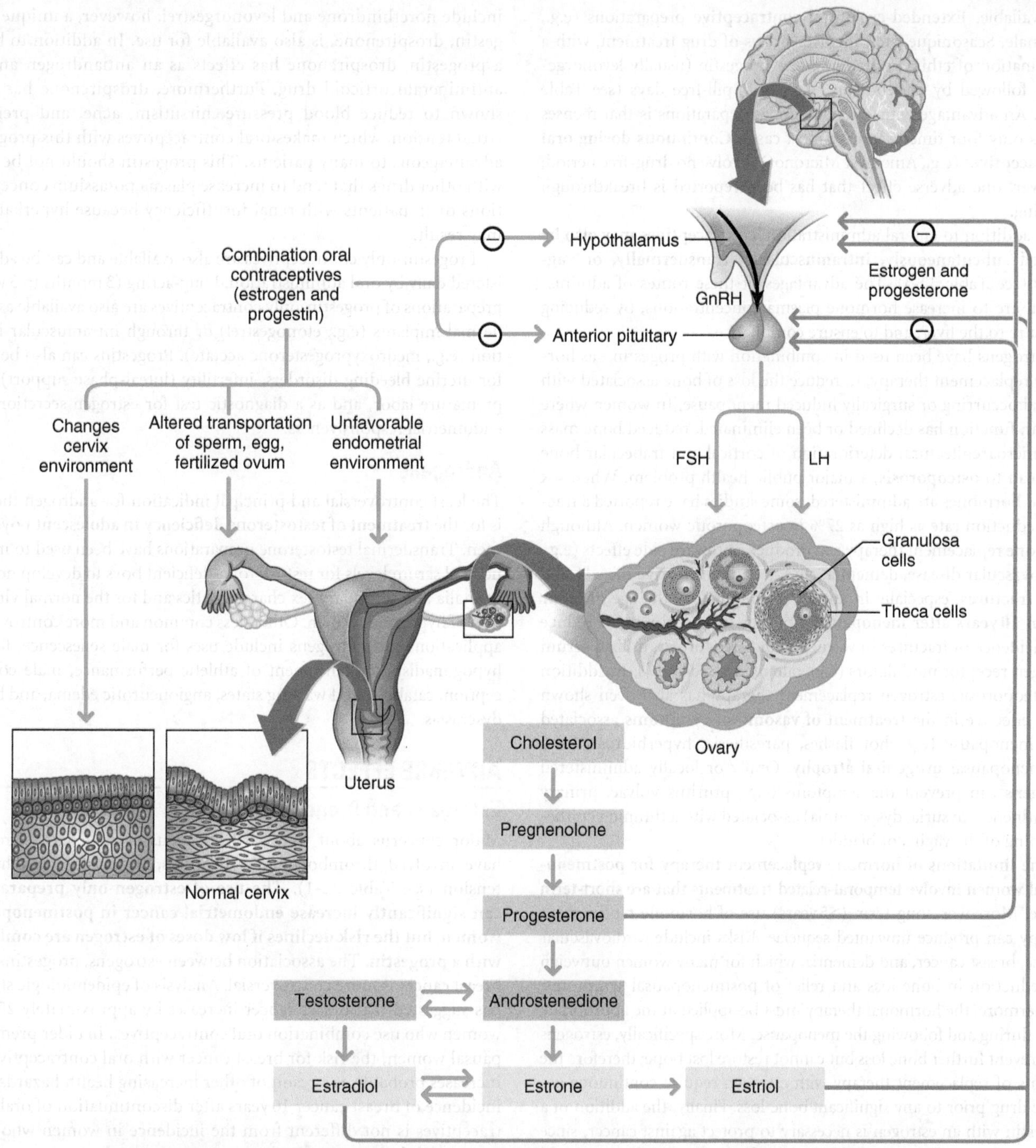

FIG 32-5 Combination oral contraceptives principally affect conception by inhibiting the release of follicle-stimulating hormone (FSH) and suppressing the surge of luteinizing hormone (LH) from the anterior pituitary, which consequently suppresses ovulation.

Combination oral contraceptives include monophasic, biphasic, triphasic, or quadraphasic preparations (see Table 32-3). **Monophasic preparations** (e.g., Cryselle, Loestrin 24 Fe, Ortho-Cyclen, Yaz, etc.) maintain a fixed dose of estrogen and progesterone over a 21-day period; **biphasic contraceptives** (e.g., Kariva, Mircette, Necon 10/11, etc.) maintain a fixed dose of estrogen but increase the progestin dose over a 21-day period; **triphasic preparations** (e.g., Cyclessa, Ortho Tri-Cyclen, Necon 7/7/7, etc.) vary the amounts of estrogen and progestin every 7 days for 21 days, and **quadraphasic preparations** (e.g., Natazia) change estrogen and progestin levels four times in the cycle of use. With exceptions noted in Table 32-3 and discussed later, a 21-day treatment regimen is followed by 7 days of placebo or no drug. Biphasic and triphasic oral contraceptives were designed to approximate more closely the ratios of estrogen and progesterone during the menstrual cycle. The quadraphasic pills can also be used for women with menorrhagia. The progestin in the oral contraceptive protects the endometrium of the uterus against the proliferative action of the estrogen.

In addition to the combination oral contraceptives, extended-cycle oral contraceptives and continuous dosing oral contraceptives are available. **Extended-cycle oral contraceptive** preparations (e.g., Seasonale, Seasonique, etc.) involve 84 days of drug treatment, with a combination of ethinyl estradiol and a progestin (usually levonorgestrel), followed by placebo for 7 days or 7 pill-free days (see Table 32-3). An advantage with extended-cycle preparations is that menses occurs only four times a year in most cases. **Continuous dosing oral contraceptives** (e.g., Amethyst Micronor) involve no drug-free period; however, one adverse effect that has been reported is breakthrough bleeding.

In addition to enteral administration, **contraceptives may also be applied subcutaneously, intramuscularly, transdermally, or vaginally** (see Table 32-3). The advantages of these routes of administration are to increase hormone plasma concentrations, by reducing exposure to the liver, and to ensure compliance.

Estrogens have been used in combination with progestins, as hormone replacement therapy, to reduce the loss of bone associated with natural occurring or surgically induced menopause. In women where ovarian function has declined or been eliminated, reduced bone mass and microarchitectural deterioration of cortical and trabecular bone may lead to **osteoporosis**, a major public health problem. When sex steroid hormones are administered, some studies have reported a fracture reduction rate as high as 27% in osteoporotic women. Although hormone replacement therapy can produce untoward side effects (e.g., cardiovascular disease, dementia, etc.), it can be **effective in reducing bone fractures**, especially in **at-risk women before the age of 60 or within 10 years after menopause.** Another drug regimen, to reduce the incidence of fractures in women with osteoporosis, utilizes serum estrogen receptor modulators (e.g., raloxifene [see later]). In addition to osteoporosis, estrogen replacement therapy has also been shown to be effective in the **treatment of vasomotor symptoms** associated with menopause (e.g., hot flashes, paresthesia, hyperhidrosis) and postmenopausal **urogenital atrophy**. Orally or locally administered estrogens can prevent the symptoms (e.g., pruritus vulvae, urinary incontinence, dysuria, dyspareunia) associated with a thinning epithelial lining of the vagina or bladder.

The limitations of hormone replacement therapy for postmenopausal women involve temporal-related treatments that are short-term in use. Moreover, long-term (>5 years) use of hormone replacement therapy can produce unwanted sequelae. Risks include cardiovascular disease, breast cancer, and dementia, which for many women outweigh the reduction in bone loss and relief of postmenopausal symptoms. Furthermore, the hormonal therapy must be applied at the appropriate times during and following the menopause. More specifically, estrogens can prevent further bone loss but cannot restore lost bone; therefore the benefits of replacement therapy with estrogen require continuous use of the drug prior to any significant bone loss. Finally, the addition of a progestin with an estrogen is necessary to protect against cancer, since estrogen alone will dramatically increase the incidence of endometrial cancer of the uterus in postmenopausal women.

Finally, estrogen can be used to successful treat adolescents when ovaries do not develop and puberty is absent. Treatment with estrogen can promote normal growth of genital structures and breasts and assist in bone growth.

Progestins

Similar to estrogens, **progestins can be used alone or in combination with estrogen for contraception and are used in combination for hormone replacement** in postmenopausal women. The dose of the progestin component for combination oral contraceptives has greater variability because of differences in the potency of the progestin used. In most preparations, the progestin content ranges from 0.1 to 1 mg. Progestins commonly used in oral contraceptives include norethindrone and levonorgestrel; however, a unique progestin, drospirenone, is also available for use. In addition to being a progestin, drospirenone has effects as an antiandrogen and an antimineralocorticoid drug. Furthermore, drospirenone has been shown to reduce blood pressure, hirsutism, acne, and premenstrual tension, which makes oral contraceptives with this progestin advantageous to many patients. This progestin should not be used with other drugs that tend to increase plasma potassium concentrations or in patients with renal insufficiency because hyperkalemia may result.

Progestin-only contraceptives are also available and can be administered daily by oral administration. Long-acting (3 months to 3 years) preparations of progestin-only contraceptives are also available as subdermal implants (e.g., etonogestrel) or through intramuscular injection (e.g., medroxyprogesterone acetate). Progestins can also be used for uterine bleeding disorders, infertility (luteal-phase support), and premature labor, and as a diagnostic test for estrogen secretion and endometrial responsiveness.

Androgens

The least controversial and principal indication for androgen therapy is for the **treatment of testosterone deficiency in adolescent boys and men.** Transdermal testosterone preparations have been used to mimic normal serum levels for testosterone-deficient boys to develop normal genitalia and secondary sex characteristics and for the normal virilization of hypogonadal men. Other, less common and more controversial applications for androgens include uses for male senescence, female hypogonadism, enhancement of athletic performance, male contraception, catabolic and wasting states, angioneurotic edema, and blood dyscrasias.

ADVERSE EFFECTS

Estrogens and Progestins

Major concerns about untoward effects associated with estrogens have involved thromboembolic disorders, neoplasms, and hypertension (see Table 32-1). **The use of estrogen-only preparations can significantly increase endometrial cancer in postmenopausal women, but the risk declines if low doses of estrogen are combined with a progestin.** The association between estrogens, progestins, and breast cancer is more controversial. Analysis of epidemiologic studies has suggested that breast cancer increases by approximately 25% in women who use combination oral contraceptives. In older premenopausal women, the risk for breast cancer with oral contraceptive use increases probably as a result of other increasing health hazards. The incidence of breast cancer 10 years after discontinuation of oral contraceptives is not different from the incidence in women who have never used these agents.

Other untoward consequences associated with estrogen therapy include an increased risk of thromboembolic disorders and stroke. In addition, estrogen therapy has also been implicated in increasing rates of gallbladder disease, nausea, vomiting, breast tenderness, edema, migraine, and endometriosis. Additional evidence indicates a small but significant cardiovascular risk with at least one type of postmenopausal hormone replacement therapy, and this has led to more restricted recommendations regarding such therapy. Untoward effects that are unacceptable to the patient are likely to change treatment strategies and may include other drugs to reduce osteoporosis (e.g., antiresorptive drugs) to either eliminate or create a reduction in the dose of sex hormones used in this age group. **In all instances, development of a rational strategy for prescribing postmenopausal hormone replacement therapy requires careful analysis of benefits**

and risks combined with short-term (less than 5 years) therapy for relieving symptoms of menopause.

In regard to progestins, high blood concentrations can cause blood clots, heart attacks, and strokes, but the more common side effects include changes in vaginal bleeding, dry mouth, frequent urination, loss of appetite, and unusual thirst (see Table 32-1). The less common untoward effects of progestins can cause mental depression, skin rashes, or alterations in the flow of breast milk.

Oral Contraceptives and the Periodontium

Numerous clinical studies from the late 1960s through the early 1980s have described gingival diseases (e.g., gingivitis, gingival enlargement) associated with oral contraceptives in otherwise healthy women. Beginning in the 1970s, it became evident that many of the systemic side effects elicited by oral contraceptives were dose dependent. This realization led to the development of current, low-dose oral contraceptive formulations. Longitudinal clinical studies of women using low-dose oral contraceptives as well as data from a cross-sectional study of the National Health and Nutrition Examination Survey (NHANES) I and NHANES III have not shown an association between current low-dose oral contraceptives and increased levels of gingival disease. **These studies support the premise that current low-dose oral contraceptives have little or no effect on the gingival inflammatory status of women using these drugs.**

Androgens

In men, major untoward effects of pharmacologic doses of androgens include bladder irritation, breast soreness, gynecomastia, and priapism (see Table 32-1). In women, amenorrhea or oligomenorrhea and virilism (e.g., acne, decreased breast size, hirsutism, enlarged genitalia, male-pattern baldness, hoarseness, deepening of voice, etc.) can occur (see Table 32-1). For prepubertal children, virilism is a common untoward reaction of androgens, and stunting of linear growth is possible because of the premature closure of the epiphyses by androgens. Rarely in men and women, hepatic necrosis and hepatocellular tumors may develop in individuals who use 17α-alkylated androgens for a long duration or at high doses.

DRUG INTERACTIONS

Estrogens

Estrogens may increase the effect of corticosteroids. Therefore, the administration of corticosteroids may need to be adjusted in patients taking estrogens because estrogen can increase the therapeutic and toxic effects of corticosteroids. Rifampin, barbiturates, carbamazepine, phenytoin, and topiramate all tend to decrease the effects of estrogens because the former drugs induce liver metabolism of estrogens.

Progestins

Some hepatic enzyme–inducing medications decrease the effect of progestins.

Oral Contraceptives and Antibiotics

Numerous anecdotal observations have suggested that antibiotics (e.g., rifampin, penicillins, tetracyclines, metronidazole, etc.) may reduce oral contraceptive efficacy. For rifampin, its ability to induce liver enzymes increases steroid metabolism, and this can distinctly reduce the efficacy of oral contraceptives. For the other antibiotics, the relationship to and possible effects on oral contraceptive efficacy are not clear-cut. Putative antibiotic-induced mechanisms responsible for reduced efficacy of oral contraceptives include increased urinary and fecal excretion, decreased enterohepatic circulation or intestinal absorption, enhanced fecal excretion, and/or estrogen or progesterone receptors that have been pharmacologically blocked.

Currently, there is no large, prospective clinical trial to determine whether a significant interaction between antibiotics (except for rifampin) and oral contraceptives exists. The American Medical Association Council on Scientific Affairs has reviewed the available literature and suggested that women face a significant risk of oral contraceptive failure when concomitantly using rifampin; whereas, other antibiotics pose a small risk for reducing the efficacy of oral contraceptives. **In all cases, the administration of any antibiotic to a patient using an oral contraceptive should involve informed consent with discussion of the possible interaction between the drugs, counsel about non-hormonal methods of controlling pregnancy, and the design of treatment regimens that are medically appropriate yet take into consideration personal concerns.**

Androgens

The effects of anticoagulants, antidiabetic drugs, insulin, and cyclosporine all are increased with androgens. Hepatotoxic medications pose a greater risk with androgenic agents. The dentist should use caution when prescribing corticosteroids because **concomitant use of androgens and corticosteroids can increase edema and exacerbate existing cardiac or hepatic disease.**

HORMONE ANTAGONISTS AND PARTIAL AGONISTS

Estrogens

Agents that modulate estrogen activity can be categorized into three principal groups: (1) **SERMs**; (2) **full estrogen receptor antagonists**; and (3) **estrogen synthesis inhibitors** (Table 32-4).

SERMs are agents that exhibit agonist, partial agonist, or antagonist activities in different tissues (Fig. 32-6). The pharmacologic goal of SERMs is to provide agonist activity in tissues where estrogen action is desired and to antagonize or elicit no activity in tissues where estrogen activity may be harmful. The selective modulation of estrogenic activity in tissues is possible because of the presence of **two distinct estrogen receptors (α and β forms)** with variable tissue distribution and variable drug affinity to these estrogen receptor forms. Hence, the mixed agonistic activity of these drugs accounts for some degree of selectivity. Raloxifene is an example of SERM that has been approved for the prevention and treatment of osteoporosis. The drug is a partial agonist at estrogen receptors, stimulating estrogen receptors in bone, while inhibiting estrogen receptors in the breast and many other tissues. Similar to raloxifene, tamoxifen, toremifene, and clomiphene are also considered SERMs since they display tissue selectivity of action (see Table 32-4). Tamoxifen has been approved for the adjunctive treatment of breast neoplasms and as a prophylactic agent for women who are at high risk for breast cancer. Toremifene is used for the treatment of metastatic, estrogen receptor–positive breast cancer in postmenopausal women. Clomiphene is a nonsteroidal drug that is distantly related to diethylstilbestrol and continues to be an important drug for the treatment of anovulatory infertility. Clomiphene acts by inhibiting the negative feedback of estrogen on the hypothalamus and pituitary, leading to an increase in the release of gonadotropins resulting in ovulation.

In contrast to the SERMs, fulvestrant is a pure estrogen receptor antagonist. Fulvestrant binds competitively to the estrogen receptor

TABLE 32-4 Examples of Hormone Antagonists

Nonproprietary (Generic) Name	Proprietary (Trade) Name	Classification	Indication
Abiraterone acetate	Zytiga	Inhibitor of testosterone secretion	Adjunctive treatment of prostate cancer
Anastrozole	Arimidex	Aromatase inhibitor	Early and advanced breast carcinoma
Clomiphene	Clomid, Serophene	SERM	Induction of ovulation
Exemestane	Aromasin	Aromatase inhibitor	Early and advanced breast carcinoma
Flutamide	Eulexin	Androgen receptor antagonist	Prostatic carcinoma
Finasteride	Propecia, Proscar	Type II 5α-reductase inhibitor	Benign prostatic hypertrophy, androgenetic alopecia
Mifepristone	Mifeprex	Progesterone receptor antagonist	Early pregnancy termination
Tamoxifen	Nolvadex	SERM	Adjunctive and preventive treatment of breast cancer
Toremifene	Fareston	SERM	Adjunctive treatment of breast cancer
Raloxifene	Evista	SERM	Postmenopausal osteoporosis prevention

SERM, Selective estrogen receptor modulator (also referred to as partial estrogen).

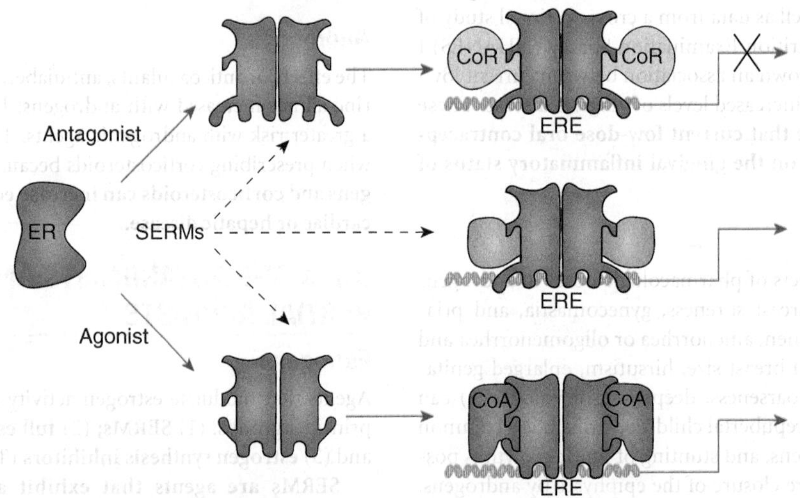

FIG 32-6 Estrogen receptor (ER) pharmacology. Until relatively recently, it was considered that the role of an ER-agonist was that of a "switch," which upon binding converted the receptor into an active state. Antagonists, on the other hand, were believed to function by competitively inhibiting agonist binding, thus freezing the receptor in an inactive state. However, it is now known that the overall conformation of ER is determined by the ligand to which it is bound, which in turn impacts the ability of the receptor to engage functionally different coregulators. Pure agonists enable the interaction of the receptor with coactivators (CoA), while antagonists allow the receptor to interact with only corepressors (CoR). Selective estrogen receptor modulators (SERMs) permit the bound ERs to interact with different subsets of CoAs and CoRs, determined by the overall receptor conformation associated with a given SERM, thereby permitting these drugs to elicit different activities in different tissues. Thus, the cellular response to an ER-agonist complex will be primarily determined by the relative expression level and activity of functionally distinct coregulators in different target tissues. ERE, estrogen response element. (From Wardell SE, Nelson ER, McDonnell DP: From empirical to mechanism-based discovery of clinically useful Selective Estrogen Receptor Modulators (SERMs). *Steroids.* November 2014; 90:30-38, 2014.)

resulting in change in conformation of the receptor and reduced estrogen binding. Fulvestrant is administered as an intramuscular injection to postmenopausal women with hormone receptor–positive metastatic breast cancer who have relapsed or progressed after previous SERM therapy.

Finally, estrogen levels can be affected through the use of therapeutic estrogen synthesis inhibitors. When aromatase, the enzyme responsible for the conversion of testosterone to estradiol, is inhibited, plasma estrogen levels decline. Since aromatase inhibitors do not prevent the ovary from synthesizing estrogens, these drugs are primarily used to treat breast cancer in postmenopausal women, where conversion of androgens to estrogen occur in fat tissue. Aromatase inhibitors (e.g., exemestane, anastrozole, letrozole) have been used for the adjunctive treatment of early stage and metastatic breast cancer patients who have been unresponsive to tamoxifen.

Progestins

Agents that block the effect of progesterone are primarily potent, competitive antagonists of the progesterone receptor (see Table 32-4). Progesterone receptor antagonists, such as mifepristone, can be used as contraceptives and abortifacients and for treatment of endometriosis, leiomyomas, breast cancer, and meningiomas. In the United States, mifepristone is primarily used for the termination of early pregnancy (defined as ≤ 49 days).

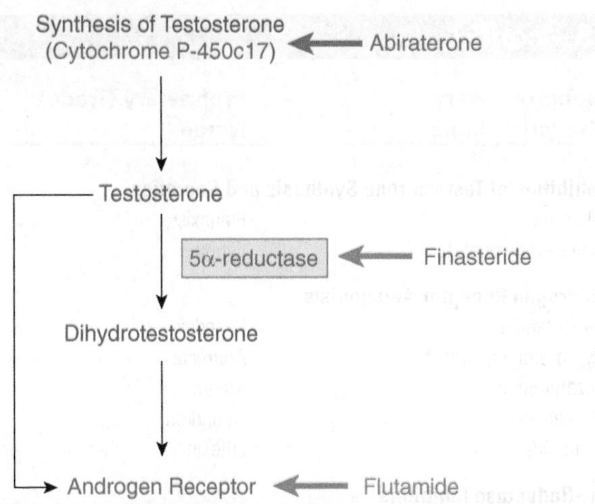

FIG 32-7 Agents that block the effect of androgens can be categorized into three principal groups. Examples of each are shown.

Androgens

Agents that block the effect of androgens can be categorized into three principal groups: (1) **inhibitors of testosterone synthesis and secretion**; (2) **androgen receptor antagonists**; and (3) **5α-reductase inhibitors** (see Table 32-4; Fig. 32-7).

Gonadotropin-releasing hormone (GnRH) antagonists (e.g., cetrorelix acetate, ganirelix acetate, abarelix, etc.) have been effective in reducing the secretion of androgens by inhibiting LH secretion, the hormone responsible for stimulating testosterone synthesis in the testes. Another drug class that inhibits testosterone secretion does so by an entirely different mechanism. More specifically, abiraterone acetate is an inhibitor of cytochrome P-450c17, a critical enzyme in extragonadal and testicular androgen synthesis. Moreover, by inhibiting cytochrome P-450c17, testosterone synthesis is reduced. Abiraterone plus low-dose prednisone improves survival in patients with metastatic castration-resistant prostate cancer.

Potent androgen receptor antagonists, such as flutamide, bicalutamide, enzalutamide, and nilutamide, are used to treat prostate cancer in combination with GnRH antagonists. Spironolactone, an inhibitor of aldosterone, and cyproterone acetate, a progestin, are weak androgen receptor antagonists. Cyproterone is used in some countries to treat advanced prostate cancer. Spironolactone administration may lead to antiandrogenic side effects when it is used for its main purpose as an aldosterone antagonist.

Blocking the conversion of testosterone to dihydrotestosterone is accomplished by inhibiting the enzyme 5α-reductase. Finasteride is an inhibitor of the type 2 isozyme of 5α-reductase, while dutasteride is an inhibitor of type 1 and type 2 isozymes of 5α-reductase. 5α-Reductase inhibitors have been developed for the treatment of benign prostatic hypertrophy. In addition, finasteride is used to treat androgenetic alopecia.

IMPLICATIONS FOR DENTISTRY

The homeostasis of the periodontium is a complex, multifactorial relationship that involves, at least in part, the endocrine system. The assertion that hormone-sensitive periodontal tissues exist relies on several salient observations, including the retention and metabolic conversion of sex steroid hormones in the periodontium and the presence of steroid hormone receptors in periodontal tissues. These biologic findings correlated with clinical observations confirm an increased prevalence of gingival inflammation with fluctuating sex steroid hormone levels that would be consistent with the protective nature of sex steroid hormones in the periodontium. **More specifically, during times of possible vulnerability of the individual, the intensified inflammatory response in the periodontium evoked by sex steroid hormones is necessary to protect both the local and systemic environments by destroying, diluting, or walling off the invading organisms.**

Although the dentist will not intentionally prescribe sex steroid hormones, there are dental compounds that have putative estrogenic activity. Currently, the prescribed use of **Bis-GMA–based resins** for restoration of the dentition has increased the concern of dentists about the safety of what were previously considered inert materials. On the basis of existing research, certain impurities may be present in some Bis-GMA–based resins, and release of impurities from such restorations is potentially estrogenic. Under extreme conditions, these impurities are capable of inducing weak estrogenic effects on target tissues. The amounts of **bisphenol A** that may be present as an impurity or produced as a degradation product from dental restorations, including sealants, are quite small and far below the doses needed to affect the reproductive tract.

Despite not prescribing sex steroid hormones, the dentist will have many patients who present at the office while on these medications. Understanding the pharmacotherapeutics and appropriate therapies to manage patients using oral contraceptives or hormone replacement therapies will influence the health and lifestyles of these individuals.

SEX STEROID HORMONES AND RELATED DRUGS

Nonproprietary (Generic) Name	Proprietary (Trade) Name
Estrogens	
Conjugated estrogens	Premarin
Diethylstilbestrol*	Stilphostrol
Dienestrol	Ortho Dienestrol
Esterified estrogens	Menest
Estradiol	Estrace, Estraderm
Estrogenic substance	Gravigen Aqueous
Estropipate	Ogen
Ethinyl estradiol	Estinyl, in many oral contraceptives
Mestranol	In some oral contraceptives
Quinestrol	Estrovis
Progestins	
Drospirenone	—
Etonogestrel	Nexplanon
Hydroxyprogesterone	Hylutin
Levonorgestrel	Norplant
Medroxyprogesterone acetate	Provera
Megestrol	Megace
Norethindrone	Aygestin
Norgestrel	Ovrette
Progesterone	—
Oral contraceptives	See Table 32-3
Androgens	
Danazol	Danocrine
Ethylestrenol	Maxibolin
Fluoxymesterone	Halotestin
Methandrostenolone	Dianabol

SEX STEROID HORMONES AND RELATED DRUGS—cont'd

Nonproprietary (Generic) Name	Proprietary (Trade) Name
Methyltestosterone	Testred
Nandrolone	Durabolin
Oxandrolone	Oxandrin
Oxymetholone	Anadrol-50
Stanozolol	Winstrol
Testosterone	Striant, Androgel
Testolactone	Teslac
Antagonism of GNRH Receptors, and Inhibition of Release of FSH and LH	
Cetrorelix	Cetrotide
Ganirelix	Ganirelix acetate injection
Selective Estrogen Receptor Modulator (SERM)	
Clomiphene	Clomid
Raloxifene	Evista
Tamoxifen	Nolvadex
Toremifene	Fareston
Pure Estrogen Receptor Antagonist	
Fulvestrant	Faslodex
Antiprogestin	
Mifepristone (RU-486)	Mifeprex
Inhibition of Testosterone Synthesis and Secretion	
Abarelix	Plenaxis
Abiraterone acetate	Zytiga
Androgen Receptor Antagonists	
Bicalutamide	Casodex
Cyproterone acetate*	Androcur
Enzalutamide	Xtandi
Nilutamide	Nilandron
Flutamide	Eulexin
5α-Reductase Inhibitors	
Dutasteride	Avodart, Duagen
Finasteride	Propecia, Proscar
Aromatase Inhibitors	
Anastrozole	Arimidex
Exemestane	Aromasin
Letrozole	Femara

*Not currently available in the United States.

CASE DISCUSSION

To make a definitive diagnosis for Mrs. A, additional medical information concerning her use of oral contraceptives and compliance would be meaningful. Current low-dose formulations of oral contraceptives will not cause gingival enlargements; however, if she is taking multiple pills per day, this may increase her risk for an estrogen-induced pyogenic granuloma. It is more likely that Mrs. A has not been compliant with her oral contraceptive regimen leading to pregnancy (failure rate is 3%), as evidenced by her morning sickness and inability to eat. Even with proper compliance, the failure rate (i.e., unwanted pregnancy) of oral contraceptives is approximately 0.05%. If Mrs. A is pregnant, the gingival lesion would be diagnosed as a pregnancy-associated pyogenic granuloma (i.e., pregnancy tumor). To verify your clinical diagnosis, an excisional biopsy with histologic evaluation would be required to confirm a pyogenic granuloma, as well as a trip by Mrs. A to her OBGYN. Once the pyogenic granuloma is excised, proper oral hygiene and regular visits to the dentist will prevent a recurrence of the lesion.

GENERAL REFERENCES

1. Benagiano G, Bastianelli C, Farris M: Hormonal contraception: present and future, *Drugs Today* 44:905–923, 2008.
2. Edwards J, Li J: Endocrinology of menopause, *Periodontol 2000* 61:177–194, 2013.
3. Helsen C, Van den Broeck T, Voet A, Prekovic S, Van Poppel H, Joniau S, Claessens F: Androgen receptor antagonists for prostate cancer therapy, *Endocr Relat Cancer* 21:T105–T118, 2014.
4. Leblebicioglu B, Connors J: Mariotti: Principles of endocrinology, *Periodontol 2000* 61:54–68, 2013.
5. Mariotti A: The ambit of periodontal reproductive endocrinology, *Periodontol 2000* 61:7–15, 2013.
6. Mariotti A, Mawhinney M: Endocrinology of sex steroid hormones and cell dynamics in the periodontium, *Periodontol 2000* 61:69–88, 2013.
7. Mawhinney M, Mariotti A: Physiology, pathology and pharmacology of the male reproductive system, *Periodontol 2000* 61:232–251, 2013. http://onlinelibrary.wiley.com/doi/10.1111/j.1600-0757.2011.00440.x/abstract.
8. Preshaw PM: Oral contraceptives and the periodontium, *Periodontol 2000* 61:125–159, 2013.
9. Reddy MS, Morgan S: Decreased bone mineral density and periodontal management, *Periodontol 2000* 61:195–218, 2013.
10. Söderholm KJ, Mariotti A: BIS-GMA–based resins in dentistry: are they safe? *J Am Dent Assoc.* 130:201–209, 1999.
11. Wardell SE, Nelson ER, McDonnell DP: From empirical to mechanism-based discovery of clinically useful Selective Estrogen Receptor Modulators (SERMs), *Steroids* 90:30–38, 2014.

33

Pharmacology of Specific Drug Groups: Antibiotic Therapy*

Purnima Kumar

KEY INFORMATION

- The major mechanisms by which antibacterial drugs act are the following:
  - Inhibition of cell wall synthesis
  - Alteration of cell membrane function
  - Inhibition of ribosomal protein synthesis
  - Inhibition of DNA or RNA synthesis or function
  - Inhibition of folic acid synthesis
- Mechanisms by which bacteria become resistant to antimicrobial drugs include these:
  - Enzymatic inactivation of the drug
  - Change in the target of the drug
  - Reducing permeability of the bacterial cell
  - Active drug efflux from the cell
  - Changing growth requirements, bypassing the mechanism of the drug
  - Overproduction of the drug target(s)
- Horizontal gene transfer (one microorganism acquiring DNA from another microorganism) can take place by the following:
  - Transduction
  - Transformation
  - Conjugation
- Adverse antibiotic effects vary from class to class. Some common ones for certain classes include these:
  - Allergies
  - Superinfections, such as pseudomembranous colitis
  - Gastrointestinal adverse effects
  - Renal toxicity
  - Ototoxicity

CASE STUDY

A 20-year-old female college sophomore presents with a complaint of "extremely painful gums" (see Fig. 33-1). The patient also complains of chills for the past two days. You record her temperature at 102 °F. Clinical examination reveals punched-out interdental papillae, gingival bleeding, abundant plaque, and a fetid odor. What is the most likely diagnosis? How would you treat this patient? Would you use systemic medications for treatment? Describe potential and typical adverse effects of your prescription(s).

INTRODUCTION

The modern era of infectious disease began with the first visualization of microbes by Anton van Leeuwenhoek in 1683, the "animicules" of dental plaque scraped from his upper gingiva and killed with salt (the first periodontal chemotherapy). In 1776, Edward Jenner administered the first smallpox vaccination. In 1848, Ignaz Semmelweiss introduced clean surgical operating technique ("gentlemen, wash your hands"). In 1854, John Snow showed the link between cholera and drinking water.

In the 1860s, Louis Pasteur first used the word *germ* for living entities that produced disease, and Joseph Lister used carbolic acid to disinfect wounds. In the 1870s, Robert Koch proved the bacterial causation of anthrax and tuberculosis, and in the 1880s, Pasteur developed anthrax and rabies vaccines. In 1891, Paul Ehrlich showed that antibodies were responsible for immunity. In 1897, Ivanowski and Beiternick discovered viruses. The mosquito vector for yellow fever was described in 1900, *Treponema pallidum* was found to be the cause of syphilis in 1905, human immunodeficiency virus (HIV) was identified in 1983, *Helicobacter pylori* was discovered as a cause of peptic ulcer in 1984, and the West Nile virus was identified in 1999.

In the early 1900s, Paul Ehrlich used the term **magic bullet** for his predicted chemical that would affect only microbial cells and have no effect on mammalian cells. He later used fuchsin and mercury (Salvarsan) to treat syphilis. In 1928, Alexander Fleming serendipitously discovered that a mold, *Penicillium chrysogenum*, lysed staphylococci; this was later developed to its full potential by the isolation of penicillin from *Penicillium notatum* by Florey and colleagues at Oxford in the late 1930s and early 1940s. The first use of penicillin was in 1941 on an English police constable with streptococcal and staphylococcal skin abscesses. In the United States, penicillin was first used in 1942 on Anne Miller, who had streptococcal toxemia of pregnancy. Another ground-breaking event in medical advances was the demonstration in 1935 by Gerhard Domagk that sulfanilamide could be safely used systemically to treat infectious disease. Thus was born the era of antibiotics and anti-microbials, arguably one of the most revolutionary events in the history of mankind.

*The author wishes to recognize Dr. Thomas J. Pallasch for his past contributions to this chapter.

MECHANISMS OF ACTION

By strict definition, antibiotics are chemicals that are derived from microorganisms (commonly yeasts and fungi) and are used to inhibit other microorganisms. Almost all clinically antibacterial drugs are derived from naturally occurring entities, with only few that are entirely synthetically produced (sulfonamides, fluoroquinolones, and oxazolidinones). These drugs are not antibiotics by the narrow definition but are included in the discussion of antibiotics.

Antimicrobials affect the viability of microorganisms by five known processes: (1) **inhibition of cell wall synthesis,** (2) **alteration of cell membrane integrity,** (3) **inhibition of ribosomal protein synthesis,** (4) **suppression of deoxyribonucleic acid (DNA) synthesis, and** (5) **inhibition of folic acid synthesis** (Fig. 33-2). Microbial cell wall synthesis inhibition and membrane effects are extra-cytoplasmic, and inhibition of nucleic acid, protein, and folic acid synthesis are intra-cytoplasmic. Drugs that affect bacterial cell wall or membrane integrity and DNA synthesis are usually, but not always, bactericidal (inducing cell death), and protein and folic acid synthesis inhibitors are usually bacteriostatic (preventing cell growth or replication).

Whether an antimicrobial agent is bactericidal (cidal) or bacteriostatic (static) can also depend on its concentration at the infected site and the particular offending organism because some static drugs become cidal at high concentrations. The previous preference for cidal drugs over static antibiotics (cidal drugs allegedly do not rely on host defenses) has become less distinct because of the appreciation of the long post-antibiotic effects (continued antibiotic activity when the drug blood levels have declined) of bacteriostatic drugs.

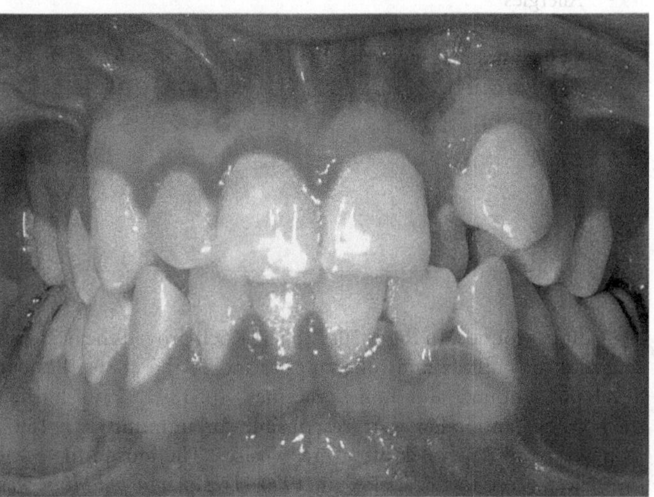

FIG 33-1 Photograph of patient in the case study.

Inhibition of Cell Wall Synthesis

The principal cell wall inhibitors are β-lactam antibiotics and glycopeptides. Bacterial cell walls are rigid and composed of alternating peptidoglycan (murein) units of N-acetyl-D-glucosamine and N-acetylmuramic acid (NAM). These are cross-linked via short peptides by amide linkages to a d-alanyl group on NAM. Various bacterial enzymes (transglycosylases, transpeptidases, carboxypeptidases, endopeptidases) catalyze the formation of the rigid cell wall by incorporating new peptidoglycan into existing peptidoglycan and then cross-linking to form a rigid cell wall. The internal osmotic pressure of the bacterium causes lysis of the bacterial cell because the wall is no longer an effective barrier (see Fig. 33-2).

In addition, in some organisms, an antibiotic may inhibit the inhibitor of an endogenous bacterial autolysin (N-acetyl-muramyl-L-alanine amidase). The autolysin causes the lysis of the bacterial cell wall.

Alteration in Cell Membrane Integrity

A drug may disrupt the integrity of the cell membrane by displacing Ca^{2+} and Mg^{++} from membrane lipid phosphate groups. Cationic antimicrobial peptides are part of humans' natural skin and mucosal defense system and act by disrupting cell wall or membrane integrity by an effect on the gram-negative lipopolysaccharide component that literally puts holes in the wall or membrane (see Fig. 33-2).

Inhibition of Ribosomal Protein Synthesis

Antibiotics may inhibit at either the 30S or 50S ribosomal subunit. This can result in inhibition of initiation of protein synthesis, inhibition of peptidyl transferase, and inhibition of the extrusion of the peptide chain from the ribosome, causing misreading of the mRNA message and other mechanisms (see Fig. 33-2).

Inhibition of Nucleic Acid Synthesis

Mechanisms associated with either RNA or DNA include inhibition of DNA gyrase and topoisomerase IV, inhibition of DNA-dependent RNA polymerase, and damage to DNA (see Fig. 33-2).

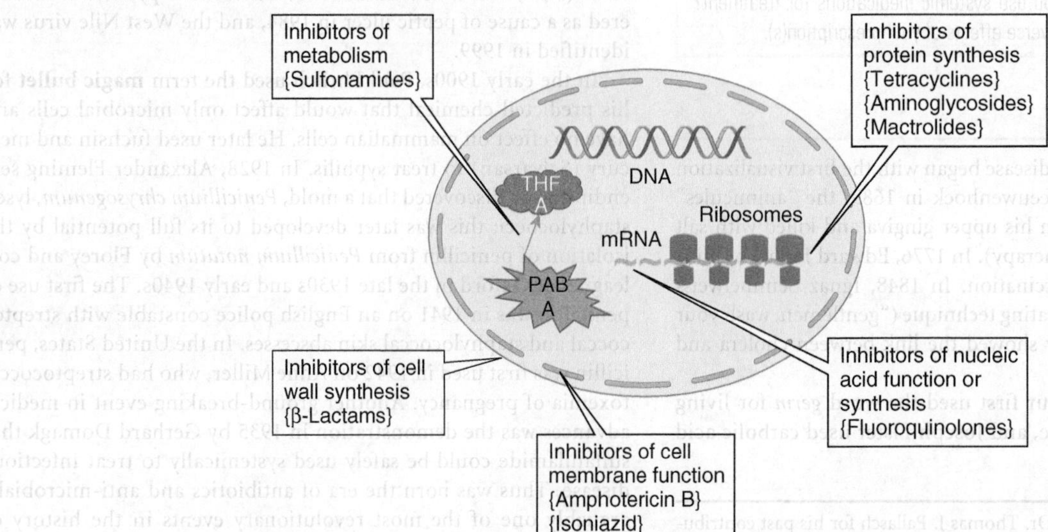

FIG 33-2 Mechanisms of action of antimicrobial drugs and representative drugs.

Inhibition of Folic Acid Synthesis

Sulfonamides and trimethoprim are anti-metabolites that inhibit sequential steps in the bacterial synthesis of folic acid essential for one-carbon transfers in nucleic acid synthesis (see Fig. 33-2).

MICROBIAL RESISTANCE TO ANTIBIOTICS (FIG. 33-3)

Microbial resistance to antibiotics has become a major factor in determining when and which antibiotic is used and dosages and length of administration. It also has spurred renewed interest in antibiotic pharmacokinetics and pharmacodynamics.

Procedures designed to reduce antibiotic-resistant pathogenic microorganisms have been developed, including education of health care providers and the general public, improved handwashing techniques, better hospital infection control, isolation of patients with highly resistant bacteria, control of antibiotic use in hospitals through formularies and pharmacist oversight, and the removal of antibiotics for growth promotion in agricultural animals.

All microbial resistance is local; the patterns and extent of this resistance are determined by the use of antibiotics in a particular community. What is true in Miami may not be true in Los Angeles or in Paris, London, Rome, or New Delhi. If tetracyclines are used widely in the community for acne or Lyme disease, a high resistance level to the drug is likely to be present in that locale. If not, the microbial resistance level is likely to be low. If an antibiotic or its analogue has been used widely in agriculture, this may strongly influence resistance patterns, to the point of rendering a new antibiotic far less useful. In Taiwan, virginiamycin (a streptogramin) has been used for more than 2 decades as a growth promoter in food animals. When quinupristin-dalfopristin, a new streptogramin, was tested on human bacterial isolates before its clinical introduction, more than 50% of some pathogens were already resistant to the drug. Antibiotics are truly societal drugs that cumulatively affect the individual receiving the drug and many others as well.

Microorganisms have developed six known mechanisms to evade the bactericidal or bacteriostatic actions of antimicrobials, as follows: **(1) enzymatic inactivation, (2) modification/protection of the target site, (3) limited access of antibiotic (altered cell membrane permeability), (4) active drug efflux, (5) use of alternative growth requirements, and (6) overproduction of target sites** (see Fig. 33-3).

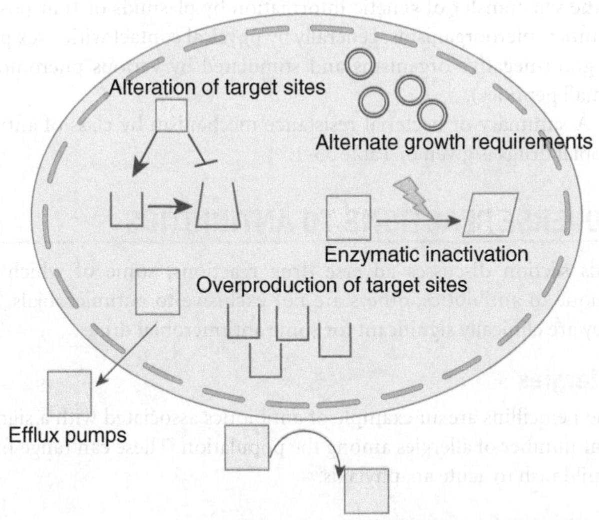

FIG 33-3 Mechanisms by which bacteria can become resistant to antimicrobial drugs.

Enzymatic inactivation is one of the more common methods and is typified by β-lactamase hydrolysis of penicillins and cephalosporins and acetyltransferases that inactivate chloramphenicol, aminoglycosides, and tetracyclines. Altered target sites include ribosomal point mutations for tetracyclines, macrolides, and clindamycin; altered DNA gyrase and topoisomerase for fluoroquinolones; and modified penicillin-binding proteins (PBPs) for viridans group streptococci (VGS) and pneumococci. Most microorganisms have developed ways to alter their cell wall or membrane permeability to limit access of the antibiotic to its receptor by deleting outer membrane proteins or closing membrane pore channels. Altering antibiotic access to the cell interior usually does not confer a high level of resistance on the organism and must be combined with another mechanism for significant resistance potential. Several hundred efflux proteins are available that extrude waste products from the microbial cell but that now have been adapted over time to eliminate antibiotics specifically from the cell interior virtually as fast as they can enter. Enterococci can evade destruction by developing alternative metabolic growth requirements (auxotrophs). Sulfonamide resistance may occur from the overproduction of para-aminobenzoic acid (PABA), and some enteric organisms evade β-lactam antibiotics by overproducing β-lactamase (hyper–β-lactamase producers).

Antibiotic tolerance occurs when the antibiotic no longer kills the microorganism, but it merely inhibits its growth or multiplication. Tolerant microorganisms start to grow after the antibiotic is removed, whereas resistant microorganisms multiply in the presence of the antibiotic. Tolerance is usually caused by the loss of autolysin activity through a failure to create or mobilize the autolytic enzymes. Vancomycin tolerance in *Streptococcus pneumoniae* is unique; a mutation in the sensor-response system controls the bactericidal autolysin activity.

A major factor in the development and maintenance of antibiotic resistance in microbes is that sensitive microorganisms are inhibited, allowing resistant ones to multiply and dominate. Microbial resistance is most likely to occur when subtherapeutic antibiotic doses are used; these are doses that do not kill or inhibit the microorganism, but rather allow it to perceive the chemical as a threat to its survival and to react by mutation to resistance, acquisition, or transfer of resistance genes/virulence factors or induction (expression) of latent resistance genes. The gastrointestinal tract is a massive reservoir for resistance genes readily transferred within and between enteric microbial species, a process greatly enhanced by antibiotics that readily induce the expression or transfer of resistance genes.

SPECIFIC RESISTANCE MECHANISMS

β-Lactamases

The most important acquired mechanism for β-lactam resistance, particularly in gram-negative microorganisms, is the production of various β-lactamases that hydrolyze the β-lactam ring to form a linear metabolite incapable of binding to PBPs.

β-Lactamases have been variously classified by Richmond-Sykes (I to V), Ambler (A to D), and Bush (1 to 4). β-Lactamase enzymes can be chromosomally mediated or easily transferred by transposable elements. The most pressing difficulties with β-lactamases are their widespread dissemination throughout the microbial environment, ability to move between widely disparate organisms, tendency to inhibit new antibiotic agents rapidly, and increasing resistance to β-lactamase inhibitors (clavulanic acid, sulbactam, tazobactam, and avibactam). β-Lactamases have been observed in numerous gram-positive and gram-negative pathogens. The cohabitation of staphylococci and enterococci on human skin in hospitals has likely led to the incorporation of β-lactamases genes into enterococci after the latter organisms had successfully avoided this transfer for billions of years.

Point mutations have appeared more recently in certain β-lactamases, resulting in extended-spectrum β-lactamases in *Klebsiella pneumoniae* that hydrolyze the latest cephalosporins. Certain enteric microorganisms (*Escherichia coli, Citrobacter freundii, K. pneumoniae, Proteus mirabilis*) can produce massive amounts of TEM-1 β-lactamase (hyper–β-lactamase producers) that can overwhelm β-lactamase inhibitors. Metallo-β-lactamases possess the broadest spectrum of inhibitory activity and hydrolyze all β-lactam antibiotics except monobactams (aztreonam) and are not inhibited by any of the β-lactamase inhibitors currently available.

The first plasmid-encoded β-lactamases with the ability to hydrolyze cephalosporins were termed the **extended-spectrum β-lactamases (ESBLs)**. These ESBL microbes were also resistant to aminoglycosides, tetracyclines, and trimethoprim/sulfonamides. ESBLs cause resistance to third-generation cephalosporins (cefotaxime, ceftriaxone, ceftazidime) and monobactams (aztreonam) but are sensitive to cephamycins (cefoxitin, cefotetan) and carbapenems (imipenem, meropenem, ertapenem). These ESBL microbes are horizontally transmitted by mobile genetic elements from food, animals, or family members and induce greater mortality than enteric bacilli without these ESBLs.

Multidrug Antibiotic Efflux Pumps

Certain bacteria can move an antibiotic out of the cell as soon as it enters. Currently, more than 50 such systems have been described, and these cytoplasmic membrane transport proteins (multidrug efflux pumps) have likely evolved to protect the cell from foreign chemical invasion and allow its secretion of cell metabolic products. Efflux pumps operate in *E. coli, Pseudomonas aeruginosa,* staphylococci, *Streptococcus pyogenes, S. pneumoniae, Bacillus subtilis, Pasteurella multocida, Neisseria gonorrhoeae,* mycobacteria, and enterococci. For tetracyclines, these efflux pumps are the major mechanism for resistance and are becoming increasingly so for the fluoroquinolones.

Chromosomal and plasmid-mediated efflux transporter proteins may be quite specific for antibiotics and metabolic product substrates and are regulated by numerous genes and gene products. Repressors are also present and are highly regulated to prevent the accidental overproduction of efflux pumps. Tetracyclines can derepress this system, leading to an overproduction of efflux proteins and increasing resistance to themselves and any other antibiotics carried by these proteins.

Genetic Variations in Bacteria

Microorganisms possess three mechanisms for genetic variation: (1) local nucleotide changes in the genome, (2) rearrangement of genomic sequences, and (3) horizontal acquisition of DNA from other microorganisms (horizontal gene transfer).

Horizontal gene transfer between organisms occurs by **three mechanisms—transformation, transduction, and conjugation**—and use numerous transposable elements that involve mobile genetic elements that are passed from one bacterium to another. These mobile genetic elements include naked DNA, plasmids, bacteriophages, transposons, and integrons.

Plasmids are circular, double-stranded DNA outside the chromosomes. Bacteriophages are viruses that infect bacteria and can mediate genetic transfer. Transposons are DNA segments that cannot self-replicate, but they can self-transfer between plasmids, bacteriophages, and chromosomes. Integrons capture and disseminate genes by site-specific integration of DNA (gene cassettes).

During transformation, bacteria acquire "naked" DNA from their environment to incorporate into their genome. Such genetic transformations are uncommon and require unique circumstances involving genes, binding, uptake, and integration.

Transduction is the movement of DNA from one bacterium to another by a bacteriophage (bacterial virus) intermediary. Conjugation is the self-transfer of genetic information by plasmids or transposons to other microorganisms, generally by physical contact with a sex pilus in gram-negative organisms and stimulated by various pheromones (small peptides).

A summary or bacterial resistance mechanism by class of antimicrobial drugs is given in Table 33-1.

TABLE 33-1 Antibiotic Resistance Patterns

Mechanisms	Antimicrobial Drugs and Examples of Mechanisms
Enzymatic antibiotic inactivation	β-Lactams by β-lactamases Aminoglycosides by aminoglycoside-modifying enzymes Chloramphenicol by acetyltransferases Streptogramins by acetyltransferases Tetracyclines by enzymatic oxidation
Modification/ protection of target site	β-Lactams: altered PBPs Fluoroquinolones: altered DNA gyrase or topoisomerases Rifampin: altered RNA polymerase Sulfonamides: altered dihydropteroate synthase Trimethoprim: altered dihydrofolate reductase Macrolide-lincosamide-streptogramin B aggregate gene (MLS_b): methylation of adenine on 23S rRNA Glycopeptides: change of d-Ala-d-Ala to d-Ala-D-lactate in cell wall Tetracyclines: ribosomal protection
Limiting access of antibiotic	β-Lactams, fluoroquinolones, most antibiotics: altered outer membrane porins Most antibiotics: reduced membrane transport
Active antibiotic efflux	Tetracyclines: TET genes Fluoroquinolones: Nor A genes
Failure to activate antibiotic	Metronidazole: decreased flavodoxin production
Use of alternative growth requirements	Enterococcal auxotrophs
Overproduction of target sites	Sulfonamides: overproduction of PABA Enteric bacilli: overproduction of β-lactamase

PABA, p-Aminobenzoic acid; *PBPs,* penicillin-binding proteins.
From Polk R: Optimal use of modern antibiotics: emerging trends, *Clin Infect Dis* 29:264-274, 1999; Smith H: Host factors that influence the behavior of bacteria pathogens in vivo, *Int J Med Microbiol* 290:207-213, 2000.

ADVERSE REACTIONS TO ANTIBIOTICS

This section discusses adverse drug reactions, some of which are unique to antibiotics; others are not exclusive to antimicrobials, but they are clinically significant for some antimicrobial drugs.

Allergies

The penicillins are an example of antibiotics associated with a significant number of allergies among the population. These can range from a mild rash to acute anaphylaxis.

Antibiotic Resistance

An inevitable effect of the use of antibiotics is the development of resistance on the part of bacteria. On balance, the evidence is substantial that antimicrobial agents at any dose or concentration for virtually any length of time do select for resistance and promote the acquisition and transfer of drug-resistant genes. Many of these species exhibit extraordinary resistance patterns: 50% to 100% of *Salmonella*, staphylococci, and enteric bacilli are resistant to tetracycline, and 32% to 47% are resistant to β-lactams, with 49.7% exhibiting polyantibiotic resistance; 30% of *Staphylococcus aureus* are resistant to ciprofloxacin and 47% to tetracycline; 72% of *Campylobacter* in humans and 99% in chickens and pigs are resistant to ciprofloxacin; and *E. coli* exhibits 70% to 94% resistance to amoxicillin and 62% to 98% resistance to tetracycline. Very low (nanogram/nanomolar) concentrations of antibiotics found in the food chain used in nature to control bacterial ecologic niches induce resistance patterns; subtherapeutic dosages in humans are sufficient to challenge microorganisms and lead to resistance.

The mere presence of a β-lactam antibiotic produces a hundredfold to a thousandfold increase in induction of β-lactamase in microorganisms producing extended-spectrum β-lactamases. *E. coli* carries resistance genes that are not expressed until tetracycline is present. Concentrations of tetracyclines at 0.1 to 1 μg/mL/ per gram in meat cause the dissemination of resistance genes in the human gastrointestinal tract, and 1 μg/mL of tetracycline in drinking water results in a tenfold increase in the transfer of conjugative plasmids from *Enterococcus faecalis* to *Listeria monocytogenes*.

The use of antibiotics can also promote the transfer of resistance genes from one species to another. In oral plaque biofilm, tetracycline resistance genes can be transferred from *Bacillus subtilis* to streptococci, illustrating that non-oral bacteria have the potential to transfer genes to opportunistic oral microorganisms. The self-transfer of *Bacteroides* conjugative transposons can be increased a hundredfold to a thousandfold by the presence of low levels of tetracycline (1 μg/mL).

Oral streptococci can harbor tetracycline resistance genes in dental plaque and disseminate such genes by mobile elements to other microflora: *Enterococcus faecalis*, *Veillonella*, and other streptococci. Salyers and colleagues stated that "the fact that tetracycline acts as an inducer of transfer gene expression illustrates how the use of an antibiotic could accelerate the spread of antibiotic resistance genes not only by selecting for their acquisition but also by stimulating their transfer."

Exposure to antibiotic doses at the low concentrations seen in agriculture and aquaculture, as therapy for inflammatory or other diseases, or for growth effects is a major concern for public health. These antibiotics can make their way into the food and water supply and alter body flora or promote emergence of resistant microbes or the transfer of resistance genes. Perhaps more importantly, the wide use of antibiotics in farm animals leads to organisms that are resistant to one or multiple antibiotics.

Superinfection

A significant and unappreciated adverse effect of antibiotics is the potential to decrease colonization resistance of indigenous anaerobic flora in the digestive tract and other anatomic areas (skin, oral mucosa). The role of colonization resistance is to limit the concentration of potentially pathogenic flora of either an exogenous or endogenous nature in a given body part. Removal of indigenous flora by antibiotics can promote growth of microorganisms not sensitive to the drug (superinfection). Many superinfections result from a reduction in the endogenous microorganisms important for colonization resistance, with the most notable example being antibiotic-induced diarrhea and colitis.

Adverse colonic effects of antibiotics range from simple diarrhea (antibiotic-associated diarrhea) to mucosal inflammatory diarrhea/colitis (antibiotic-associated colitis), with or without associated *Clostridium difficile* (*C. difficile*–associated colitis [CDAC]), to potentially fatal **pseudomembranous colitis (PMC).** Of the 25 million people affected by serious diarrhea annually in the United States, approximately 10% of these cases are the result of antibiotics, particularly broad-spectrum agents. Most of these cases of antibiotic-associated diarrhea are not clinically significant and respond to drug discontinuance and rehydration if necessary.

Any antibiotic is capable of inducing diarrhea, colitis, or PMC, but the most common agent involved is amoxicillin, followed by third-generation cephalosporins and clindamycin. When the colonic flora are disturbed by antibiotics or disease, the colonization resistance of the gastrointestinal tract is reduced by the suppression of natural antagonists of *C. difficile* such as *Bacteroides, Lactobacillus*, pseudomonads, staphylococci, streptococci, peptostreptococci, enterococci, and *E. coli*.

The fear of inducing a potentially fatal case of PMC has led to a reluctance to use clindamycin because early and faulty preliminary data reported a 10% association of PMC with the drug. More recent data indicate that incidence of antibiotic-associated diarrhea and CDAC associated with clindamycin in community use of the drug is very low. The overall risk rate for community-acquired *C. difficile*–associated PMC from retrospective data may be 1 per 10,000 antibiotic prescriptions, and the risk of hospitalization may be 0.5 to 1 per 100,000 patient years. The incidence rate was calculated to be 1.6 per 100,000 persons exposed to ampicillin, 2.9 per 100,000 persons exposed to dicloxacillin, and 2.6 per 100,000 persons exposed to tetracycline, with no antibiotic-associated diarrhea seen in the 1509 patients receiving oral or topical clindamycin.

Statistically, PMC is more likely to occur with amoxicillin than clindamycin. Clinicians should refrain from unnecessary antibiotic therapy in patients within the first 2 months after the elimination of CDAD. Any elective dental procedure requiring antibiotic treatment or prophylaxis would best be postponed for this 2-month period. If antibiotic therapy is required, the use of antibiotics far less commonly associated with CDAD (penicillin V, macrolides) is appropriate.

An example of superinfection in the mouth is the growth of *Candida albicans* as a result of treatment with an antibiotic, especially one with a broad or extended spectrum or metronidazole.

Nephrotoxicity

The kidney is sensitive to the effects of some antibiotics, especially aminoglycoside and peptide antibiotics. Combining two drugs with overlapping toxicity compounds the problem. Mechanisms of renal toxicity involve concentration of the drug in renal tubule cells, leading to the lack of ability to concentrate urine and eventual reduced glomerular filtration rate.

Ototoxicity

Aminoglycosides and peptide antibiotics also are associated with damage and other effects on the eighth cranial nerve leading to vestibular and cochlear dysfunction. Hearing loss, especially high frequency, occurs and can be irreversible due to the concentration of the drugs in the endolymph and perilymph and damage to the cochlea.

Antibiotic-Induced Photosensitivity, Photoallergy, and Phototoxicity

Some antibiotics (along with phenothiazine antipsychotics) are among the most common drugs inducing skin reactions on exposure to sunlight. Photosensitivity may occur in one of two forms: (1) phototoxicity, in which chemicals (drugs) are deposited in the skin, absorb ultraviolet light, and transfer the energy to local tissue, resulting in inflammatory responses, or (2) photoallergy, in which sunlight causes a hapten to become a complete antigen in the skin, eliciting an immediate or a delayed allergic reaction. The signs and symptoms (erythema, urticaria, eczema, lichenoid dermatitis, bullous lesions) may be the same, but the mechanisms are different (photoallergy may need a sensitizing dose unless the drug is continually taken for ≥5 to 10 days). The most common antibiotics that induce photosensitivity are sulfonamides, tetracyclines, and fluoroquinolones. Photosensitivity is managed by discontinuing the drug, avoiding sunlight, and wearing protective clothing.

Long QT Interval Syndrome

Long QT interval syndrome is a cardiac disorder caused by ion channel abnormalities that prolong the time interval between the beginning of the QRS complex and the end of the T wave on the electrocardiogram (see Chapter 19). Antibiotics that have been implicated in the cause of torsades de pointes include fluoroquinolones (gatifloxacin, levofloxacin, moxifloxacin, sparfloxacin), macrolides (erythromycin, clarithromycin), and clindamycin.

The Food and Drug Administration (FDA) Adverse Event Reporting System has found that 77% were caused by macrolides and 23% by fluoroquinolones; 89% to 95% were in older patients; 9% to 13% were fatal; the mean time to the adverse event was 4 to 5 days; and 42% to 62% had cardiac disease, 7% to 11% had renal disease, and 17% had low blood K^+ or Mg^{++} levels. The risk rate has been estimated to be 1 per 1 million exposures to ciprofloxacin, 3 per 1 million exposures to clarithromycin, and 14.5 per 1 million exposures to sparfloxacin (withdrawn from the market in the United States).

Antibiotics and Oral Contraceptives

In response to a few case reports, in the 1980s the FDA issued a warning that antibiotics may interfere with the action of oral contraceptives, potentially resulting in unwanted pregnancies. The proposed mechanisms of reduced contraceptive blood concentrations leading to decreased efficacy include (1) increased urinary/fecal excretion from antibiotic-induced diarrhea, (2) increased microsomal liver metabolism, (3) receptor displacement, (4) reduced gastrointestinal absorption, and (5) reduced enterohepatic circulation. The antibiotic rifampin stimulates the liver metabolism of the oral contraceptives, reducing blood levels. No other experimental data or controlled clinical studies have documented the interference of any other antibiotics with the activity of oral contraceptives.

The reasoning is that some antibiotics, especially broad- or extended-spectrum antibiotics, reduce enteric bacteria that metabolize the conjugated forms of the estrogens and progestins that make up the contraceptive. As a result, less regenerated form of the hormones would be available for reabsorption from the gut, resulting in less effect from the contraceptive. However, several studies document no effect of antibiotics on the blood levels of ethinyl estradiol, norethindrone, and progesterone in patients taking doxycycline (100 mg/day for 7 days), tetracycline (500 mg every 6 hours for 10 days), and ciprofloxacin (500 mg three times/day for 7 days). No effort has been made to determine whether the failure rate of oral contraceptives in women taking antibiotics is greater than the normal failure rate of oral contraceptives in women not taking antibiotics. No official authoritative body has ever examined this alleged drug interaction to investigate the evidence and make a recommendation.

From a purely scientific point of view, no reason exists to believe that any antibiotics other than rifampin interfere with the action of oral contraceptives. From a medicolegal point of view, the dentist may wish to advise a patient taking oral contraceptives and receiving antibiotics to use an additional contraceptive method or practice abstinence during the time the antibiotic is present and for several days after its termination to allow for complete antibiotic excretion (usually five times the half-life of the drug). The oral contraceptive should never be stopped during antibiotic therapy because it is the most effective means of contraception with the exception of abstinence.

The one antibiotic that has been shown to reduce the effect of **oral contraceptives** is **rifampin**. In this case the mechanism is an induction of hepatic metabolism by rifampin. Women taking an oral contraceptive and then prescribed rifampin must use a means of birth control other than an oral contraceptive.

NEW ANTIMICROBIAL APPROACHES

Pharmaceutical companies see new antibiotic development as problematic for economic, regulatory, and scientific reasons. As a result, 10 of the 15 largest drug companies have reduced or eliminated antibiotic research since 1999.

The scientific difficulty with developing new antibiotics is that all the easy targets in bacteria have already been discovered with possibly only a few remaining. Formulating "new" antibiotics that are merely derivatives of existing antibiotics will not solve all the problems of microbial resistance. Entirely new approaches to unique mechanisms of antibiotic action attacking heretofore unknown microbial metabolic processes require a much better basic understanding of microbial life and considerable risk-taking on the part of the pharmaceutical industry.

ANTIBACTERIAL ANTIMICROBIAL DRUGS

Antibacterial drugs are primarily classified according to their chemical class and mechanism of action. They also can be distinguished based on spectrum and adverse effects. In addition to these aspects of antimicrobial drugs, the therapeutic uses, including dental applications, of each class of drugs are discussed.

β-Lactam Antibiotics

Penicillin belongs to the β-lactam family of antibiotics, which remain the most widely used antibiotics in the world. **β-lactams** are composed of five different groups of antibiotics, with the β-lactam nucleus as the common feature: **penicillins, cephalosporins, carbapenems, monobactams, and carbacephems**. Penicillins and cephalosporins are the most important with carbapenems (imipenem, meropenem, ertapenem), monobactams (aztreonam), and carbacephems (loracarbef) reserved for serious infections such as nosocomial (hospital-acquired) infections. β-lactams vary greatly from one another in their spectrum of antimicrobial activity, ranging from an extremely narrow spectrum (e.g., β-lactamase–resistant penicillins) to a very wide spectrum (e.g., imipenem and some cephalosporins).

Penicillins

Penicillin is a generic term for a group of antibiotics that share the β-lactam ring nucleus, similar adverse drug reactions, and similar mechanism of action, but differ in their antibacterial spectrum, pharmacokinetics, and resistance to β-lactamase enzymes.

Classification. Penicillin is a cyclic dipeptide consisting of two amino acids (D-valine, L-lysine), a particular molecular configuration unknown in higher life forms. The synthesis in 1958 of the basic structure of penicillins (6-aminopenicillanic acid) allowed for its manipulation by the addition of various side chains to the β-lactam and thiazolidine rings (Fig. 33-4). Different salts (Na^+, K^+, procaine, benzathine) were also created for pharmacokinetic purposes. On the basis of these modifications, penicillins can be divided into four groups: (1) **penicillin G and penicillin V, (2) antistaphylococcal penicillins that are resistant to β-lactamase produced by staphylococci, (3) aminopenicillins with an extended-spectrum, and (4) extended-spectrum**

penicillins with added activity against gram-negative organisms like *Pseudomonas aeruginosa* (Table 33-2). Some penicillins are combined with a separate β-lactamase inhibitor to protect the penicillin from the enzyme.

Acid-stable penicillins are resistant to break down in stomach acid, indicating their usefulness as oral drugs. Penicillin V, amoxicillin, and dicloxacillin are examples. (Although similar to penicillin V in other ways, penicillin G is acid labile and is not often used orally.) Penicillinase-resistant penicillins are resistant to some β-lactamases. Bacteria, particularly staphylococci, develop resistance to penicillins chiefly through the elaboration of β-lactamase enzymes (penicillinases) that inactivate the penicillins by cleavage of the 6-aminopenicillanic acid nucleus to yield penicilloic acid derivatives (see Fig. 33-4). The production of staphylococcal penicillinase is encoded in a plasmid and may be transferred to other bacteria. Methicillin was the first semisynthetic derivative to be introduced that was stable in the presence of β-lactamase. Subsequently, nafcillin and three isoxazolyl derivatives (oxacillin, cloxacillin, and dicloxacillin) were marketed.

Extended-spectrum penicillins are represented by two groups of penicillin derivatives. One group is the aminopenicillin group: ampicillin, amoxicillin and bacampicillin. The latter is a drug that is rapidly hydrolyzed in vivo to yield ampicillin. The second group contains ticarcillin and piperacillin that exhibit activity against *Pseudomonas* and indole-positive *Proteus* species.

Mechanism of action. Early in the discovery of penicillin, it was noted that the drug acted only on rapidly dividing organisms, and it was later determined that bacterial cell wall precursors (the Park nucleotides) accumulated in sensitive bacteria exposed to the penicillins. Penicillin was determined to be a structural analogue of D-alanine; the final step in the formation of the bacterial rigid cell wall was a **transpeptidation** reaction involving the enzymatic removal of a terminal D-alanine to allow for the formation of the cross-linked **peptidoglycan cell wall** (Fig. 33-5). **β-Lactams are competitive inhibitors** of various enzymes (transpeptidases, carboxypeptidases), collectively termed **penicillin-sensitive enzymes,** or more commonly PBPs. β-lactams promote the formation of cell wall–deficient microorganisms of different shapes (oval, oblong, spherical) depending on the particular PBP affected, which cannot maintain their internal osmotic pressure and eventually burst. The mechanism of action of β-lactams is a classic example of Ehrlich's goal of the "magic bullet," or more specifically a chemical that inhibits a cellular activity present only in bacteria (a rigid cell wall) and not found in mammalian cells.

In some bacterial species, β-lactams have an additional mechanism of action as they activate an enzyme, muramyl synthetase, responsible for the separation of daughter cells after cell division. Activation of this enzyme in the absence of cell division produces lysis of the cell wall (autolysis) and results in bacterial "suicide."

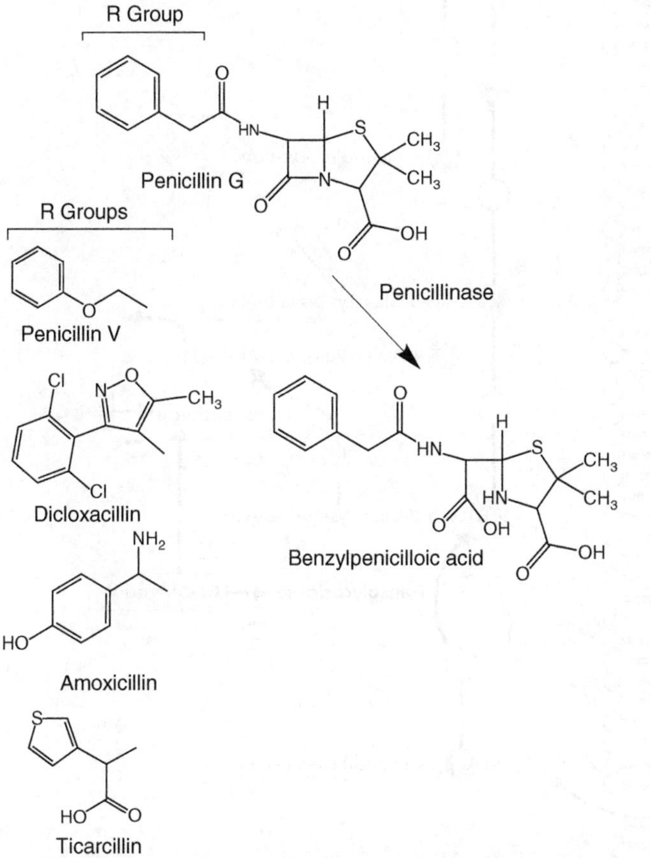

FIG 33-4 Structure of penicillin G and structures of penicillin V, dicloxacillin, amoxicillin, and ticarcillin, as shown by replacement of the R group of penicilloic G. Also shown is the effect of penicillinase in producing the penicilloic acid metabolite, which is inactive as an antimicrobial drug.

TABLE 33-2 Penicillin Groups

Group	Examples	Acid Stable	Spectrum	Penicillinase Resistant
Penicillin G and congener	Penicillin G	No	Narrow	No
	Penicillin V	Yes	Narrow	No
Anti-staphylococcal	Methicillin*	No	Narrow	Yes‡
	Nafcillin	Somewhat‖	Narrow†	Yes‡
	Oxacillin	Yes	Narrow†	Yes‡
	Cloxacillin	Yes	Narrow†	Yes‡
	Dicloxacillin	Yes	Narrow†	Yes‡
Amino-penicillins, extended-spectrum	Ampicillin	Yes	Extended	No
	Amoxicillin	Yes	Extended	No
Extended-spectrum§	Ticarcillin*	No	Extended§	No
	Piperacillin	No	Extended§	No

*No longer used clinically.
†Limited to use against staphylococcal organisms.
‡Resistant to penicillinase from *Staphylococcus aureus.*
§Spectrum includes other gram-negative bacteria (e.g., *Pseudomonas aeruginosa* and indole-positive *Proteus*).
‖Although nafcillin is somewhat acid stable, it is used parenterally.

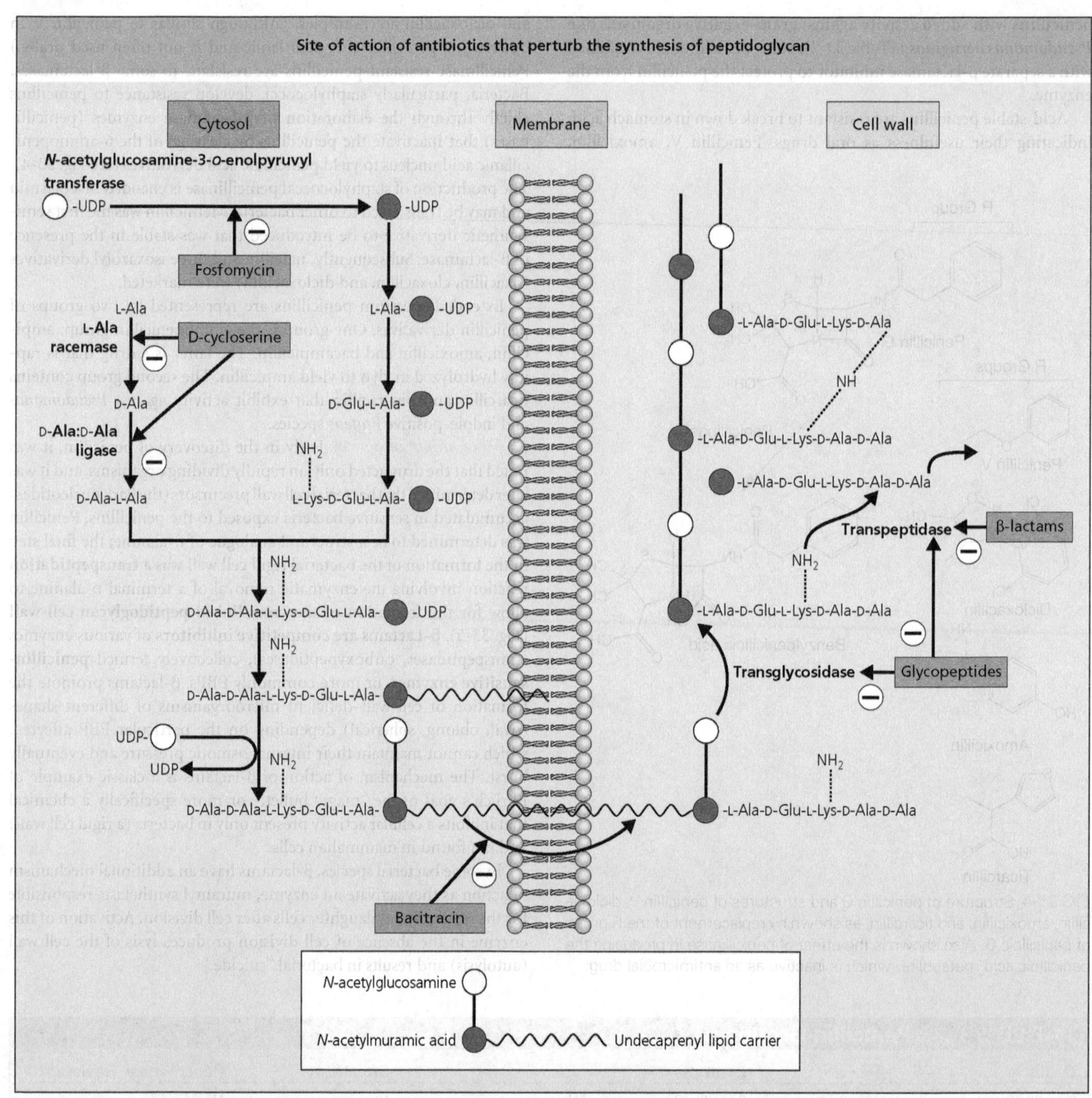

FIG 33-5 Bacterial cell wall synthesis. Details are discussed in the text. The sites of action of various drugs are shown. The lipid carrier that is inhibited by bacitracin is shown as a wavy line. (From Cohen J, et al.: *Infectious diseases*, ed 3, St Louis, 2010, Mosby.)

Considering these mechanisms, it is apparent why consistently high blood levels of β-lactams are required for optimal success (not all bacteria divide at the same time) and why penicillins do not kill rapidly (it takes time for enzyme inhibition and eventual microorganism rupture). This realization that β-lactams kill slowly has raised questions about the mechanism of action in endocarditis prophylaxis: whether they act only (or at all) by microbial killing or rather by cell wall alteration to retard attachment of the bacteria to damaged cardiac valves.

Antibacterial spectrum. Penicillin G and penicillin V are narrow-spectrum antibiotics, showing activity against mostly gram-positive cocci and gram-positive bacilli and gram-negative cocci. Other penicillins have an extended spectrum and greater activity against some gram-negative bacilli.

Penicillin G or penicillin V are drugs of choice against the VGS, *S. pneumoniae, S. Pyogenes, Peptostreptococcus, E. faecalis, Fusobacterium nucleatum, Actinomyces israelii, Clostridium tetani, Clostridium perfringens, Leptotrichia buccalis, N. meningitidis,* and non-β-lactamase–producing *Prevotella* and *Porphyromonas.* Amoxicillin alone or with clavulanate has activity against the same organisms but also *Eikenella corrodens, K. pneumoniae, Enterobacter, Moraxella (Branhamella) catarrhalis, Bacteroides fragilis,* non–methicillin-resistant and (with clavulanate) β-lactamase-producing *Prevotella* and *Porphyromonas E. coli, Haemophilus influenzae, H. pylori,* and *P. mirabilis* (Table 33-3).

TABLE 33-3 Penicillins as Drugs of Choice or Alternative Agents (Penicillin G, Penicillin V, Ampicillin, or Amoxicillin Unless Otherwise Indicated)

*Acinetobacter**
Actinomyces israelii
Bacillus anthracis
*Bacteroides**
*Campylobacter fetus**
Capnocytophaga canimorsus
*Citrobacter freundii**
Clostridium perfringens
Clostridium tetani
Eikenella corrodens
*Enterobacter**
Erysipelothrix rhusiopathiae
Fusobacterium nucleatum
Group A, B, C, and G streptococci
Listeria monocytogenes
Neisseria meningitidis
Pasteurella multocida
Peptostreptococcus micros
*Serratia marcescens**
Proteus mirabilis
Spirillum minus
Streptobacillus moniliformis
Staphylococcus aureus/Staphylococcus epidermidis†
Streptococcus bovis
Treponema pallidum
VGS

VGS, Viridans group streptococci.
*Imipenem/meropenem.
†β-Lactamase-resistant penicillins if methicillin susceptible.
From Handbook of antimicrobial therapy. Choice of antibacterial drugs. *Med Lett Drugs Ther* 20:69-88, 2015; *Facts and comparisons,* St Louis, 2015, Facts and Comparisons.

Amoxicillin and penicillin V are the initial drugs of choice in orofacial infections in nonallergic patients, but they are ineffective against streptococci (VGS) with altered PBPs. The clinical impact of antibiotic failures against these resistant streptococci and gram-negative β-lactamase–producing oral anaerobes is likely to be significant but has yet to be determined by clinical studies. On the basis of the antimicrobial spectrum of penicillin G and V and other clinical characteristics, the drugs are useful in the treatment of numerous diseases (Table 33-4).

Bacterial resistance. Bacteria evade the killing effects of β-lactams by three mechanisms: reduced drug binding to PBPs (altered target sites), hydrolysis by β-lactamase enzymes (enzymatic inactivation), or development of tolerance by the loss of the autolysis mechanism (penicillin becomes bacteriostatic instead of bactericidal). In most species, the principal mechanism is β-lactamase production.

Absorption, fate, and excretion. Penicillin G (benzylpenicillin) is rarely used orally because of its poor gastric absorption rate. Penicillin V and amoxicillin are well absorbed orally, with amoxicillin considerably longer in its half-life (~1 hour vs ~30 minutes). Better oral absorption argues for the use of amoxicillin over penicillin V, but both drugs are effective in microorganism-sensitive orofacial infections and are equally inactive against VGS with altered PBPs.

Procaine penicillin G and benzathine penicillin G are repository forms prepared for intramuscular injection with slow release from the injection site. These preparations extend the plasma level profiles of penicillin (Fig. 33-6). The route of excretion is primarily by the kidneys, with limited liver metabolism. Rapid kidney excretion accounts for the **short half-lives of most penicillins, 90% of which is due to active proximal tubular secretion,** while the remaining 10% is due to glomerular filtration. This is the basis for occasionally extending the half-lives of some penicillins by combining the penicillin with probenecid, which inhibits active tubular transport.

TABLE 33-4 Disease Entities for Which Penicillin G, Penicillin V, and Amoxicillin Are of Major Use

Abscesses, including orodental
Bacteremia (gram-positive)
Endocarditis
Gas gangrene
Mastoiditis
Meningitis
Orodental infections
Osteomyelitis
Pericarditis
Periodontal infections
Pharyngitis
Pneumonia
Rat-bite fever
Scarlet fever
Suppurative arthritis
Syphilis
Vincent's stomatitis
Weil's disease
Wound infections

These diseases are caused by various gram-positive cocci and bacilli and some gram-negative organisms, spirochetes, and anaerobic microorganisms. Susceptibility testing may be essential for some to determine therapeutic mean inhibitory concentrations.

The distribution of the penicillins includes most body fluids but not the humors of the eye or the brain. Penicillin does not pass through the blood–brain barrier unless the meninges are inflamed, such as in meningitis.

β-lactam antibiotics produce time-dependent killing of bacteria, and frequent dosing is required to maintain relatively constant blood levels with as little fluctuation as possible. The killing power of β-lactams is maximum at three to four times the minimum inhibitory concentration (MIC) of susceptible microorganisms. The prime determinant of the efficacy of β-lactams is the length of time the concentration of the drug in the infected area is greater than the MIC of the infecting organism.

To be maximally effective, the serum and tissue concentrations of β-lactams should be greater than the MIC for 50% to 70% of the dosing interval. The current package insert recommends dosing intervals of 6 hours for penicillin V. Penicillin V and penicillin G have an elimination half-life of approximately 30 minutes, and consequently, 6-hour dosing intervals may result in very low serum levels in the last 2 or 3 hours. Continuous intravenous penicillin is receiving greater attention as a way to circumvent this problem.

β-lactamase inhibitors. Currently, four agents are available to bind irreversibly to the catalytic site of susceptible β-lactamases to prevent hydrolysis of β-lactam antibiotics: **clavulanic acid, sulbactam, tazobactam, and avibactam.** Clavulanic acid is derived from *Streptomyces clavuligerus,* sulbactam is a semisynthetic penicillinate sulfone, tazobactam is chemically related to sulbactam, and avibactam is a non-β-lactam inhibitor with broader activity against β-lactamases.

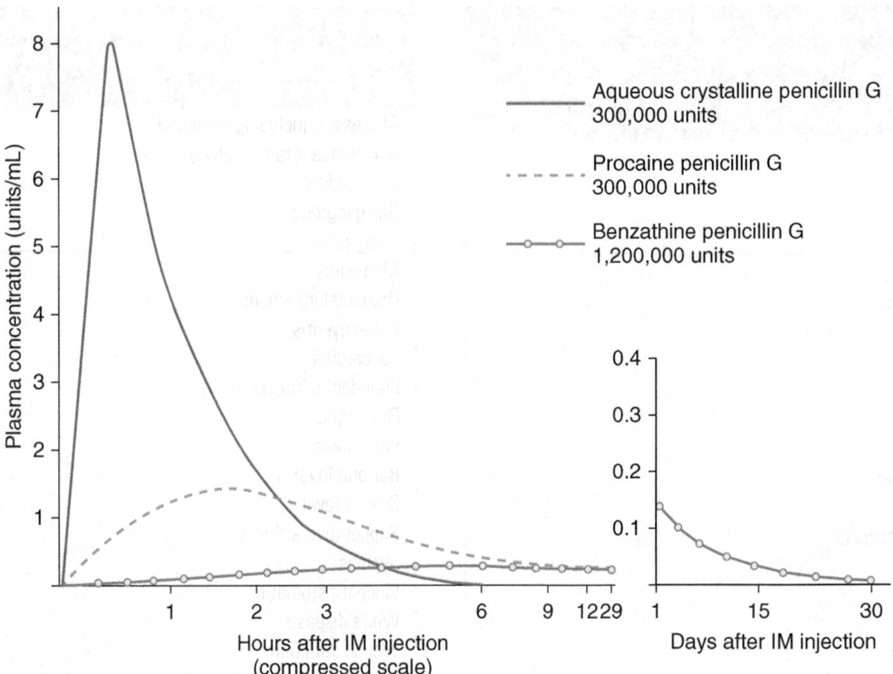

FIG 33-6 Comparative plasma concentrations of penicillin G obtained from soluble versus repository intramuscular (IM) dosage forms.

All β-lactamase inhibitors have the same mechanism of action, which is to bind to the active site of β-lactamases, where they are converted to an inactive product by β-lactamase ("suicide inhibition"). Only clavulanic acid is orally absorbed. Clavulanic acid is combined with amoxicillin, sulbactam with ampicillin, tazobactam with piperacillin, and ceftazidime (see later) with avibactam.

The sole therapeutic use of β-lactamase inhibitors is to prevent the hydrolysis of β-lactam antibiotics in the management of β-lactamase–producing microorganisms responsible for otitis media and sinusitis (*S. pneumoniae, H. influenzae, M. catarrhalis*), nosocomial pneumonia (methicillin-sensitive *S. aureus* (MSSA) or *K. pneumoniae*), intra-abdominal abscesses from β-lactamase–producing anaerobes and other microorganisms, and some upper respiratory tract infections. β-Lactamase inhibitor combinations offer no advantage against non-β-lactamase–producing microorganisms and are ineffective against methicillin-resistant *S. aureus* (MRSA), many coagulase negative staphylococci (CoNS) and enterococci, and the inducible β-lactamases produced by *P. aeruginosa, Serratia marcescens, Enterobacter cloacae, C. freundii*, and *Morganella morganii*. These β-lactamase inhibitor combinations can often be useful as alternative antibiotics against *Bacteroides, M. catarrhalis, E. coli, K. pneumoniae*, indole-positive *Proteus* and others (see Tables 33-3 and 33-5).

Therapeutic uses in dentistry. Because the oral route is the safest, most convenient, and least expensive mode of drug administration, it is favored in the treatment of dental patients. Currently, **penicillin V** and **amoxicillin** are the most frequently prescribed antibiotics for chemotherapy of infections of dental origin.

In some instances, penicillins G and V and amoxicillin are unsuitable for treating oral infections. Some dental infections are caused by β-lactamase (penicillinase)–producing organisms, and in such cases the appropriate antibiotic is a penicillinase-resistant penicillin derivative, erythromycin, or clindamycin. Patients who have been receiving extended prophylactic therapy with penicillin for the prevention of rheumatic fever generally require another antibiotic if they acquire an infection or require endocarditis prophylaxis. Certain periodontal infections are associated with gram-positive and gram-negative aerobic and anaerobic microorganisms, for which an antimicrobial agent with a more extended antibacterial spectrum, such as amoxicillin or more commonly a β-lactam/β-lactamase agent combined with metronidazole, may be the agent of choice.

Adverse effects. The adverse effects of penicillins are allergic and nonallergic in nature.

Allergic reactions to penicillins are common, while allergic fatalities are far less common. Allergy to penicillins ranges from 0.7% to 8% in various studies, with a 0.7% to 4% chance of an allergic reaction (average of 2%) during any given course of penicillin therapy. Most allergic manifestations are maculopapular or urticarial skin reactions.

Penicillin may be the most common cause of anaphylactic death in the United States, accounting for 75% of all cases and 400 to 800 annual deaths. Estimates of severe penicillin anaphylaxis range from 0.004% to 0.015% of individuals exposed and, from the point of view of number of exposures, possibly 1 in 1200 to 1 in 2500 penicillin exposures.

Eventually, 1% to 10% of the general population exposed to therapeutic penicillin has an allergic reaction, with a higher positive history with increased age. The incidence of allergy varies with the route of administration: oral (0.3%), intravenous (2.5%), and intramuscular (5%); the lower incidence by the oral route has been questioned because of limited data.

It is probable that an acute penicillin-allergic reaction is less common in children and elderly patients, but fatal reactions may be more likely in elderly patients because of their compromised cardiopulmonary function. Whether certain individuals are predisposed to penicillin allergy remains unsettled. Risk factors for penicillin allergies include multiple allergies to other drugs, particularly other antibiotics ("multiple allergy syndrome"), or atopic disease (asthma, allergic rhinitis, nasal polyps). Cross-allergenicity exists for all penicillins and, even to a certain extent, other β-lactam antibiotics.

In individuals with a positive history of penicillin allergy, 15% to 40% exhibit allergy on re-exposure to penicillin, and individuals with

TABLE 33-5 Drugs Used to Treat Infections Caused by Specific Microorganisms

Microorganism	Drug of First Choice	Alternative Drugs*
Gram-Positive Cocci		
Staphylococcus species		
Methicillin-sensitive	Penicillinase-resistant penicillin (e.g., dicloxacillin)	A cephalosporin, vancomycin, imipenem, meropenem, clindamycin, a fluoroquinolone, linezolid, tedizolid, daptomycin, telavancin
Methicillin-resistant	Vancomycin ± rifampin	Daptomycin, quinupristin/dalfopristin, linezolid, a fluoroquinolone, doxycycline, trimethoprim-sulfamethoxazole, telavancin, dalbavancin, oritavancin
Streptococcus pyogenes	Penicillin G or V	A cephalosporin, erythromycin, clindamycin, vancomycin, clarithromycin, azithromycin, linezolid, tedizolid, daptomycin, telavancin, dalbavancin, oritavancin
Streptococcus viridans group		
Oral infections	Penicillin G or V	Erythromycin, clindamycin, a cephalosporin
Bacteremia or endocarditis	Penicillin G with or without gentamicin	Ceftriaxone, vancomycin
Streptococci, anaerobic (*Peptostreptococcus*)	Penicillin G or V	A cephalosporin, clindamycin, vancomycin, daptomycin, telavancin
Streptococcus pneumoniae	Penicillin G or V, amoxicillin	A cephalosporin, trimethoprim/sulfamethoxazole, erythromycin, clarithromycin, azithromycin, clindamycin, levofloxacin, gemifloxacin, moxifloxacin, meropenem, imipenem, ertapenem, doripenem, vancomycin, telavancin, a tetracycline
Enterococcus faecalis	Ampicillin, amoxicillin, penicillin G + gentamicin or ceftriaxone	Vancomycin with gentamicin, daptomycin ± gentamicin, linezolid, ampicillin with imipenem (nitrofurantoin or fosfomycin, urinary tract only)
Enterococcus faecium (vancomycin resistant)	Daptomycin (+gentamicin or ampicillin)	Ampicillin + gentamicin, linezolid in combination with other active drug, quinupristin/dalfopristin ± ampicillin (nitrofurantoin or fosfomycin, urinary tract only)
Gram-Negative Cocci		
Neisseria gonorrhoeae	Ceftriaxone	Ceftizoxime, cefoxitin + probenecid, cefixime, cefpodoxime
Neisseria meningitidis	Ceftriaxone, cefotaxime, penicillin G	A fluoroquinolone, meropenem, chloramphenicol
Moraxella (*Branhamella*) *catarrhalis*	A fluoroquinolone, cefuroxime	Trimethoprim-sulfamethoxazole, amoxicillin/clavulanate, erythromycin, clarithromycin, azithromycin, doxycycline, cefotaxime, ceftizoxime, ceftriaxone, cefpodoxime
Gram-Positive Bacilli		
Bacillus anthracis	Ciprofloxacin, doxycycline	Penicillin G, amoxicillin, erythromycin, imipenem, clindamycin, levofloxacin
Clostridium difficile	Metronidazole, vancomycin	Fidaxomicin
Clostridium perfringens	Penicillin G	Clindamycin, imipenem, meropenem, ertapenem, doripenem, metronidazole, chloramphenicol
Clostridium tetani	Metronidazole	Penicillin G, doxycycline
Corynebacterium diphtheriae	Erythromycin	Penicillin G
Corynebacterium jeikeium	Vancomycin	Daptomycin
Gram-Negative Bacilli		
Bacteroides (oropharyngeal strains)	Penicillin G	Cefotetan, cefoxitin, clindamycin, metronidazole, ampicillin-sulbactam, amoxicillin-clavulanate
Capnocytophaga canimorsus	Amoxicillin/clavulanic acid	Cefotaxime, ceftriaxone, ceftizoxime, clindamycin, a fluoroquinolone, imipenem, meropenem, vancomycin, doxycycline
Eikenella corrodens	Ampicillin ± sulbactam, amoxicillin ± clavulanate	Azithromycin, clarithromycin, ceftriaxone, doxycycline,
Escherichia coli	Cefotaxime, ceftriaxone, ceftazidime, cefepime	Ampicillin ± (gentamicin, tobramycin, or amikacin), aztreonam, ampicillin/sulbactam, amoxicillin/clavulanic acid, piperacillin/tazobactam, trimethoprim/sulfamethoxazole, imipenem, meropenem, doripenem, ertapenem, a fluoroquinolone, tigecycline
Fusobacterium species	Penicillin G, penicillin V, metronidazole	Clindamycin, cefoxitin, imipenem, meropenem
Haemophilus influenzae	Cefotaxime, ceftriaxone, trimethoprim-sulfamethoxazole	Cefaclor, cefuroxime, cefotaxime, cefpodoxime, ceftizoxime, ceftriaxone, cefixime, a fluoroquinolone, doxycycline, clarithromycin, azithromycin, ampicillin or amoxicillin ± penicillinase inhibitor
Klebsiella pneumoniae	Cefotaxime, ceftriaxone, cefepime	An aminoglycoside, aztreonam, a fluoroquinolone, imipenem, meropenem, ertapenem, doripenem, amoxicillin/clavulanic acid, ampicillin/sulbactam, piperacillin/tazobactam, ticarcillin/clavulanate, tigecycline, trimethoprim/sulfamethoxazole

Continued

TABLE 33-5 Drugs Used to Treat Infections Caused by Specific Microorganisms—cont'd

Microorganism	Drug of First Choice	Alternative Drugs*
Legionella pneumophila	Azithromycin or ciprofloxacin or other fluoroquinolone	Erythromycin, doxycycline
Leptotrichia buccalis	Penicillin G, penicillin V	Clindamycin, doxycycline, erythromycin
Proteus mirabilis	Ampicillin	An aminoglycoside, a cephalosporin, a fluoroquinolone, ticarcillin/clavulanate, piperacillin/tazobactam, aztreonam, imipenem, meropenem, ertapenem, doripenem, trimethoprim-sulfamethoxazole
Pseudomonas aeruginosa	Ticarcillin/clavulanate or piperacillin/tazobactam ± an aminoglycoside, ciprofloxacin	(Aztreonam, ceftazidime, cefepime, meropenem, doripenem, or imipenem) + an aminoglycoside, levofloxacin
Salmonella typhi	Ceftriaxone, ciprofloxacin, levofloxacin	Amoxicillin, ampicillin, azithromycin, trimethoprim-sulfamethoxazole, chloramphenicol
Shigella species	A fluoroquinolone	Trimethoprim-sulfamethoxazole, azithromycin, ceftriaxone
Other Microorganisms		
Mycobacterium tuberculosis	Isoniazid + rifampin + pyrazinamide ± ethambutol or streptomycin	Amikacin, kanamycin, cycloserine, moxifloxacin, levofloxacin, ciprofloxacin, ofloxacin, capreomycin, kanamycin, ethionamide, para-aminosalicylic acid, bedaquiline (all in combinations)
Actinomyces israelii	Penicillin G, penicillin V	Doxycycline, erythromycin, clindamycin
Nocardia asteroides	Trimethoprim/sulfamethoxazole ± amikacin + imipenem or meropenem	A tetracycline, sulfisoxazole, amikacin, imipenem, meropenem, ceftriaxone, linezolid, cycloserine
Treponema pallidum	Penicillin G	Ceftriaxone, doxycycline
Chlamydia psittaci	A tetracycline	Azithromycin, a fluoroquinolone
Rickettsiae	Doxycycline	Azithromycin, clarithromycin, chloramphenicol
Candida albicans†		
Oral lesions	Clotrimazole, nystatin, miconazole	Itraconazole, fluconazole, posaconazole, caspofungin (all for more serious infections)
Systemic infections	Fluconazole, itraconazole, caspofungin, anidulafungin, micafungin	Posaconazole, amphotericin B
Viruses†		
Herpes simplex		
Orolabial	Acyclovir, famciclovir, valacyclovir	Penciclovir, docosanol
Keratitis	Trifluridine, ganciclovir	
Genital infection	Acyclovir, famciclovir, valacyclovir	
Encephalitis	Acyclovir	
Human immunodeficiency virus (preferred regimens)	**Non-nucleoside reverse transcriptase inhibitor-based regimen** Efavirenz + tenofovir disoproxil fumarate + emtricitabine **Protease inhibitor-based regimen** Atazanavir or darunavir + ritonavir + abacavir + tenofovir disoproxil fumarate + emtricitabine **Integrase strand transfer inhibitor-based regimen** 1. Raltegravir or elvitegravir/cobicistat + tenofovir disoproxil fumarate + emtricitabine 2. Dolutegravir + either abacavir + lamivudine or tenofovir DF + emtricitabine	
Influenza A and B	Oseltamivir, zanamivir	

*Listing does not include all alternative drugs.
†See Chapter 34 for discussion of antifungal and antiviral drugs.
Adapted from the following: Treatment guidelines: Antiviral drugs, *The Medical Letter* 127:19-30, 2013; Abramowicz M, Zuccotti G, editors: Handbook of antimicrobial drugs: drugs for bacterial infections, *The Medical Letter* ed 20, 2015, New Rochelle, NY; Treatment guidelines: drugs for HIV infection, *The Medical Letter* vol. 12, issue 138:7-16, 2014.

a positive history of penicillin allergy have a four to six times greater likelihood of a subsequent reaction than individuals with a negative history. The serum half-life of penicillin IgE antibodies ranges from 10 to more than 1000 days; the risk of recurrent penicillin allergy is higher in individuals with antibodies with long half-lives or repeated penicillin exposures. Few data are available regarding whether the 60% to 85% not exhibiting allergy on re-exposure reacquire the IgE antibodies to penicillin and then have an allergic reaction to the drug on the next (third) exposure by resensitization.

Allergy Testing

Because IgE antibody levels to penicillin are variable, skin testing for penicillin allergy becomes problematic. The incidence of positive skin tests in individuals with a history of penicillin allergy ranges from 4%

to 91% depending on the accuracy of the patient history, the haptens in the test solution, and the time elapsed between the allergic reaction and the skin test.

Penicillin skin testing can be considerably valuable in determining who might have a severe anaphylactic reaction. Approximately 95% of penicillin-allergic individuals form the penicilloyl-protein conjugate (the major antigenic determinant), and approximately 5% form the 6-aminopenicillanic acid and other minor antigenic determinants. Penicillin skin tests with the major and minor antigenic determinants eliciting a negative skin test virtually eliminate the risk for a serious IgE-mediated reaction. A positive skin reaction to the minor determinant mixture indicates a high risk for anaphylaxis.

Penicillins are primarily associated with IgE-mediated (Gell and Coombs type I) allergic reactions, but they may also induce cytotoxic (type II) or immune complex (type III) reactions. Type I signs and symptoms include skin erythema, itching, angioedema, urticaria, wheezing, hypotension, and bronchospasm resulting from mast cell/basophil release of histamine along with other tissue allergic mediators. Type II reactions are caused by circulating IgM or IgG antibodies that attach to blood cells and induce blood dyscrasias, including hemolytic anemia, leukopenia, thrombocytopenia, and aplastic anemia. Type III reactions result from the deposition of soluble immune complexes on blood vessels and basement membranes resulting in serum sickness, vasculitis, and glomerulonephritis. Type IV, delayed-type hypersensitivity reactions are mediated by T lymphocytes. (See figure 3-4.)

Allergic reactions to penicillins can also be classified according to their time of onset. Immediate IgE reactions begin within seconds to 1 hour after drug exposure and are the most life-threatening (it is an allergy truism that the more rapid the onset of the allergic reaction, the more serious the consequences). Accelerated reactions begin 1 to 72 hours after antigen exposure and usually manifest as urticaria or angioedema. Late reactions occur after 72 hours and are characterized by type II and type IV (eczema-like) Gell and Coombs reactions. Of all fatal anaphylactic reactions, 96% occur within the first 60 minutes after penicillin exposure.

Other adverse reactions to penicillins are likely to be autoimmune in origin and have an obscure etiology, including maculopapular rashes, eosinophilia, Stevens-Johnson syndrome, and exfoliative dermatitis. A maculopapular rash is seen in 2% to 3% of patients late in penicillin therapy.

Nonallergic adverse effects. Piperacillin may cause abnormal coagulation times and may produce abnormal liver function test results. Large intravenous doses of penicillins, especially in patients with compromised renal function, may induce hyperexcitability, seizures, and hallucinations. This is due to sufficient drug getting across the blood–brain barrier under these conditions. Amoxicillin is the most common cause of antibiotic-induced diarrhea/colitis because of its spectrum and widespread use. Penicillins are FDA pregnancy category B drugs.

Approximately 5% to 10% of individuals receiving ampicillin or amoxicillin may have a mild pruritic rash, usually beginning on the trunk and extending to the face, extremities, and extensor portions of the knees and elbows. This nonallergic "ampicillin/amoxicillin rash" is not associated with antibody formation and is of unknown cause. It does not seem to increase the risk of true penicillin allergy. The rash may begin 24 hours to 28 days after the drug is begun and may last 90 minutes to 7 days. The incidence of **ampicillin/amoxicillin rash** is 95% to 100% in individuals with cytomegalovirus infection/mononucleosis and 22% in individuals given ampicillin or amoxicillin with allopurinol.

Rare and reversible disorders reportedly associated with penicillins include acute pancreatitis, neutropenia, aseptic meningitis, hepatotoxicity, and increased prothrombin time/international normalized ratio (INR) in patients taking oral anticoagulants either through impaired platelet function or altered gastrointestinal microbial flora. Untoward bleeding may also occur, even in patients not taking coumarin anticoagulants, and is dose-dependent, with a maximum effect 3 to 7 days after penicillin is begun, with a return to a normal bleeding time in 72 to 96 hours; this bleeding has been reported after a dental extraction. The mechanism is likely due to an altered adenosine 5'-diphosphate–mediated platelet aggregation response and is seen most commonly in patients with underlying chronic illnesses associated with hypoalbuminemia and uremia.

Drug interactions. Oral penicillins (penicillin G, penicillin V, amoxicillin) may be antagonized by bacteriostatic antibiotics (tetracycline, erythromycin, clindamycin). NSAIDs and probenecid may increase the serum half-lives of penicillins by decreasing their renal excretion. Individuals taking β-adrenergic blocking drugs, especially nonselective ones, may cause a diminished or nonexistent response to a β-adrenergic receptor agonist given for the treatment of penicillin-induced anaphylactic bronchospasm. Ampicillin or amoxicillin, when taken with allopurinol, can be associated with a non-urticarial rash.

Contraindications. Penicillins are generally contraindicated in individuals allergic to the drugs, but it is well documented that some individuals with a previous allergic history may subsequently tolerate penicillins without allergic manifestations. The best policy is to refrain if possible from penicillin administration to anyone with a positive history. Penicillins may be contraindicated in some individuals taking coumarin anticoagulants because untoward bleeding may occur, but this seems to be highly unpredictable and rare in occurrence. Avoid the concurrent use of amoxicillin or ampicillin with allopurinol.

Cephalosporins

The isolation of the fungus *Cephalosporium acremonium* (now *Acremonium chrysogenum*) in 1948 by Brotzu from the harbor sewage of Sardinia and the subsequent isolation of the active nucleus of cephalosporin C (7-amino-cephalosporinic acid) by Florey and Abraham at Oxford University contributed in large measure to a golden age in antimicrobial chemotherapy. The widespread use of cephalosporins because of their broad antibacterial spectra and low toxicity and allergenicity has resulted in widespread microbial resistance to these agents.

Chemistry and classification (Table 33-6). Cephalosporins are closely related to penicillins, with a six-membered dihydrothiazine ring replacing the five-membered thiazolidine ring of penicillin (Fig. 33-7). Both contain the β-lactam ring, as do the monobactams and carbapenems discussed later. Side chain modification of the 7-APA nucleus has led to differences in antibacterial spectrum, pharmacokinetics, susceptibility to various β-lactamase, affinity for different PBPs, and occasionally adverse reactions.

Cephalosporins are most commonly **classified according to their "generations":** first generation (introduced in the 1960s), second generation (introduced in the 1970s), third generation (introduced in the 1980s), fourth generation (cefepime introduced in 1997), and fifth generation (advanced generation) (ceftaroline, introduced in 2010).

Cephalosporins evolved from early agents primarily active against gram-positive microorganisms (first generation) to agents with a greater gram-negative spectrum (second generation) to agents with greater activity against various nosocomial pathogens, including *P. aeruginosa, B. fragilis,* and organisms producing **extended-spectrum** and ampicillin C (ampC) β-lactamases. The broad spectrum of cephalosporins and their wide use have been major factors in microbial resistance to these agents. Technically, second-generation agents include true cephalosporins and cephamycins (cefoxitin, cefotetan, cefmetazole), which are derived from *Streptomyces* rather than *Cephalosporium.*

TABLE 33-6 Classification and Indications of Cephalosporins by Generations and Other β-Lactam Antibiotics

Cephalosporins	Major Indications
First Generation	
Cefadroxil (Duricef)*	Gram-positive cocci, (but not enterococci or methicillin-resistant *Staphylococcus aureus*) *Klebsiella pneumoniae, Proteus mirabilis, Escherichia coli,* dental prophylaxis (cephalexin, cefazolin)
Cefazolin (Ancef, Kefzol, Zolicef)†	
Cephalexin (Biocef, Keflex, Keftab)*	
Cephalothin (Keflin)†	
Cephapirin (Cefadyl)†	
Cephradine (Velosef)‡	
Second Generation	
Cefaclor (Ceclor)*	Greater effect against some gram-negative organisms than first-generation drugs; cefotetan and cefoxitin have activity against anaerobes
Cefamandole (Mandol)†	
Cefonicid (Monocid)†	
Cefotetan (Cefotan)†	
Cefoxitin (Mefoxin)†	
Cefprozil (Cefzil)*	
Cefuroxime (Ceftin, Kefurox, Zinacef)‡	
Loracarbef (Lorabid)*	
Third Generation	
Cefdinir (Omnicef)*	Penicillin-resistant *S. pneumoniae,* VGS, multidrug-resistant *S. pneumoniae,* enterococci, and some β-lactamase–producing organisms Ceftazidime/avibactam is effective against Enterobacteriaceae, *Pseudomonas aeruginosa,* and organisms producing extended-spectrum β-lactamases
Cefixime (Suprax)*	
Cefoperazone (Cefobid)†	
Cefotaxime (Claforan)†	
Cefpodoxime (Vantin)*	
Ceftazidime (Ceptaz, Fortaz, Tazicef, Tazidime)†	
Ceftazidime/avibactam (Avycaz)†	
Ceftibuten (Cedax)*	
Cefditoren (Spectracef)*	
Ceftizoxime (Cefizox)†	
Ceftriaxone (Rocephin)†	
Fourth Generation	
Cefepime (Maxipime)†	Gram-negative bacteria, cefepime is more resistant to many β-lactamases
Fifth Generation	
Ceftolozane/tazobactam (Zerbaxa)	Similar to third generation drugs, but extended-spectrum β-lactamases; effective vs Enterobacteriaceae, *P. aeruginosa,* other gram-negative bacteria and methicillin-resistant *S. aureus*
Ceftaroline (Teflaro)†	
Other Lactam Antibiotics	
Carbapenems	
Imipenem (with cilastatin in Primaxin)†	Highly resistant gram-negative bacilli, including some anaerobes, *P. aeruginosa, Campylobacter fetus, Citrobacter freundii, Enterobacter, Acinetobacter, Serratia marcescens,* and *Rhodococcus equi,* MSSA, non-penicillin-resistant *S. pneumoniae, Bacillus subtilis, Bacillus cereus, Clostridium perfringens, Bacteroides, E. coli, K. pneumoniae, P. mirabilis,* indole-positive *Proteus, Providencia stuartii, Capnocytophaga canimorsus, Haemophilus influenzae*
Meropenem (Meronem)†	
Ertapenem (Invanz)†	
Doripenem (Doribax)†	
Monobactams	
Aztreonam (Azactam)†	Aerobic gram-negative bacteria, Enterobacteriaceae, *K. pneumoniae, P. mirabilis, C. freundii, Yersinia enterocolitica, Pasteurella multocida, Salmonella, Shigella, Providencia, Neisseria, Haemophilus,* and *P. aeruginosa*

*Oral.
†Parenteral.
‡Oral and parenteral.
Adapted from Asbel LE, Levison M, Cephalosporins, carbapenems, and monobactams, *Infect Dis Clin N Am* 14:435-447, 2000; *Facts and comparisons,* St Louis, 2002, Facts and Comparisons; Karchmer AW, Cephalosporins, In Mandell GL, Bennett JF, Dolin R, editors: *Principles and practice of infectious diseases,* ed 5, New York, 2000, Churchill Livingstone; Marshall WF, Blair JE, The cephalosporins, *Mayo Clin Proc* 74:187-195, 1999; Abramowicz M, Zuccotti G, editors: Handbook of antimicrobial drugs: drugs for bacterial infections, *The Medical Letter* ed 20, 2015, New Rochelle, NY.

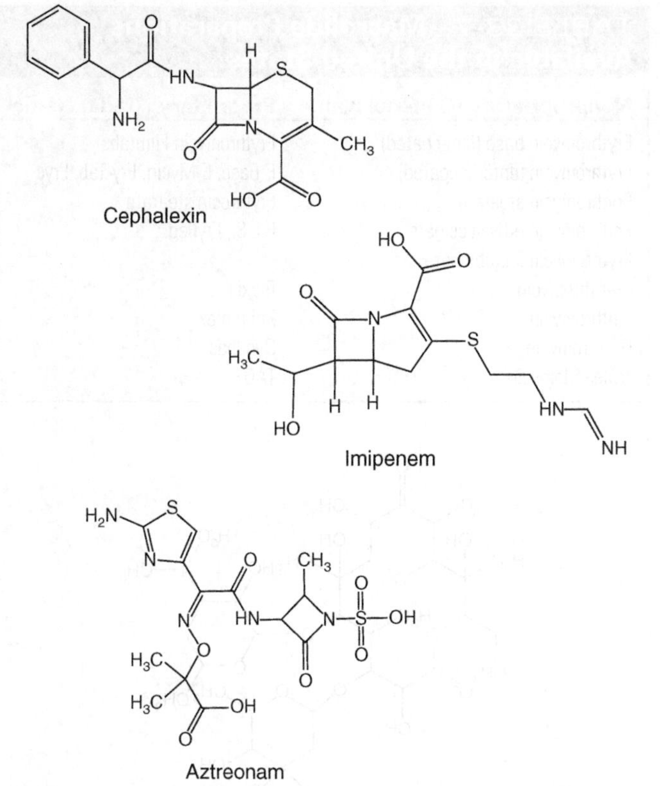

FIG 33-7 Structural formulas for cephalexin, imipenem, and the monobactam aztreonam. Notice the lack of a second ring fused to the β-lactam ring in aztreonam.

Mechanism of action. Cephalosporins possess a mechanism of action **identical to penicillins**: inhibition of bacterial cell wall peptidoglycan synthesis by inhibition of penicillin-sensitive enzymes (transpeptidases, carboxypeptidases) that are responsible for the final three-dimensional structure of the rigid bacterial cell wall. Each bacterial species may have different PBPs, and the affinity of cephalosporins for these PBPs can vary greatly. Most cephalosporins bind to PBP1 and PBP3 of gram-negative organisms, and depending on which PBPs are inhibited, the resulting bacterial cells may take different shapes: oval, round, or filamentous.

Bacterial resistance. The major mechanism of resistance to cephalosporins is the microbial elaboration of various β-lactamases (cephalosporinases). First-generation agents are very sensitive to β-lactamase hydrolysis, with the second to fifth generations more resistant to β-lactamases.

Absorption, fate, and excretion. Oral cephalosporins are generally well absorbed, with all except cefadroxil and cefprozil having their absorption delayed, but not reduced, by food. Cephalosporins are hydrophilic and widely distributed in extracellular fluid, but they do not enter the cells of the immune system (macrophages, polymorphonuclear leukocytes), as do lipophilic macrolides, tetracyclines, and lincosamides. Plasma protein binding is 10% for cephalexin, 25% for cefaclor, 8% to 17% for cephradine, and 80% to 90% for cefazolin and cefoxitin. Excretion of most cephalosporins takes place mainly by glomerular filtration and active tubular secretion in the kidney. The serum half-life is 50 to 80 minutes for cephalexin, 48 to 80 minutes for cephradine, and 35 to 54 minutes for cefaclor. In patients with end-stage renal disease, these half-lives may increase to 19 to 22 hours for cephalexin, 8 to 15 hours for cephradine, and 2 to 3 hours for cefaclor.

General therapeutic uses. Cephalosporins have wide applications in the treatment of infections. The utility of these drugs depends on the generation. Table 33-6 lists indications for the cephalosporins. First-generation drugs are used to treat infections caused by staphylococci and streptococci. They also are useful in surgical and endocarditis prophylaxis. Some gram-negative bacilli, such as *P. mirabilis* and *K. pneumoniae,* may be sensitive. A subset of second generation drugs represented by cefoxitin has good activity against many gram-negative anaerobes.

Third-generation drugs have become prominent in the treatment of **serious gram-negative coccal and bacillary infections**. They are very useful in treating meningitis, pneumonia, gonorrhea, and sepsis from sensitive organisms. Cephalosporins are often given with aminoglycosides for gram-negative bacilli infections. There are significant individual differences between members of the third-generation drugs, and not all indications apply to each member. Cefepime is resistant to many β-lactamases and is effective in treating some gram-negative bacilli that produce β-lactamases. Ceftaroline has activity against methicillin-resistant staphylococci as well as several gram-negative organisms (see Table 33-6).

Therapeutic uses in dentistry. Cephalosporins have good activity against many orofacial pathogens but limited activity against oral anaerobes. These β-lactam antibiotics are also time-dependent agents without significant post-antibiotic effects, and the serum and tissue concentrations of cephalosporins should remain greater than the organism's MIC for at least 60% of the dosing interval to retard organism regrowth as much as possible. Presently, some cephalosporins are choices for **prophylaxis during dental procedures;** however, these drugs are not indicated in acute dental infections unless culture and sensitivity testing indicate otherwise.

Adverse effects. Serious adverse reactions associated with cephalosporins are rare, with the major concern being the potential for cross-allergy with penicillins. Less common adverse reactions include transient increases in liver enzymes, nephrotoxicity, reversible neutropenia, eosinophilia and thrombocytopenia, aseptic meningitis, and disulfiram-like reactions associated with cephalosporins with the methylthiotetrazole side chain (e.g., cefotetan).

The inherent allergic potential of cephalosporins along with their **cross-allergenicity with penicillins** is of major concern. Cutaneous allergic reactions to cephalosporins (rash, pruritus, urticaria) are commonly reported to occur in 1% to 3% of patients. Serum sickness or a morbilliform rash may be seen in children receiving cefaclor. Stevens-Johnson syndrome and toxic dermal necrolysis have been reported.

Anaphylactic reactions to cephalosporins seem to be rare, with an incidence ranging from 0.0001% to 0.1% of individuals exposed. In 9388 patients without a history of penicillin allergy given cephalosporins, two anaphylactic reactions were reported (0.2%). In a retrospective study of 350,000 adverse drug reactions, six fatal cases of cephalosporin-induced anaphylaxis were reported, with three of the six cases in patients with a history of penicillin allergy.

The issue of cross-sensitivity between the cephalosporins and penicillins has never been satisfactorily resolved. Estimates range from 1.1% (the same as the allergy incidence to cephalosporins in the general population) to 18% in the earliest studies. Penicillin-allergic individuals may have a fourfold greater risk of allergy to cephalosporins than individuals not allergic to penicillins; however, penicillin-allergic individuals have a three to four times greater risk of allergy to any drug. No skin test is available to detect cephalosporin allergy, and experience with desensitization is limited and not standardized.

Cephalosporins are generally contraindicated in patients with a positive penicillin skin test to the minor determinant mixture or a history of local or systemic penicillin anaphylaxis (severe urticaria, bronchospasm, hypotension, exfoliative dermatitis), unless cephalosporins are mandated in the management of a life-threatening infection, and anaphylaxis antidotal therapy is readily available.

Drug interactions. Antacids, H_2 histamine receptor antagonists, proton pump inhibitors, as well as iron supplements may reduce the oral absorption of some cephalosporins. Food decreases the oral absorption of cefuroxime and cefpodoxime. Some cephalosporins such as cefotetan may induce a disulfiram reaction with ethanol and may cause hypoprothrombinemia. Nephrotoxicity may be seen with the combination of cephalosporins with aminoglycosides or loop diuretics.

Contraindications. Cephalosporins are contraindicated in patients allergic to these drugs and in individuals with a history of severe penicillin reactions or a positive skin test reaction to the penicillin minor determinant mixture.

Other β-lactam antibiotics

Carbapenems. Carbapenems are derivatives of thienamycin (from *Streptomyces cattleya*) and differ from penicillins by the replacement of the sulfur by a methylene group in the five-membered ring of the β-lactams (see Fig. 33-7). Currently, four carbapenems are available for parenteral use in the United States: **imipenem, meropenem, ertapenem, and doripenem**. Imipenem is combined with cilastatin to reduce the hydrolysis of imipenem by renal dehydropeptidase.

Carbapenems have a **very wide antibacterial spectrum**, have a high specificity for PBP2 of gram-positive and gram-negative microorganisms (resulting in ovoid organisms), and are not hydrolyzed by most β-lactamases. Their indications are listed in Table 33-6.

Microbial resistance to carbapenems is via the loss of an outer membrane protein, resulting in retarding cell wall penetration of the drugs, altered PBPs in *Enterococcus faecium* and MRSA, and hydrolysis by metallo β-lactamases and other β-lactamases.

Carbapenems are classified as FDA pregnancy category B or C drugs, are cross-allergenic with other β-lactams, may increase the level of serum liver transaminases, may induce PMC, and are associated with a 3% to 4% incidence of skin rash. Imipenem, meropenem, and ertapenem are associated with increased central nervous system (CNS) toxicity and seizures. Doripenem has a lower risk of CNS toxicity.

Monobactams. **Aztreonam** is a monocyclic β-lactam (monobactam) lacking the thiazolidine ring of penicillin (see Fig. 33-7). It is available only parenterally. It does not bind to the PBPs of gram-positive or anaerobic microorganisms; its spectrum is limited to aerobic gram-negative species. **Specific organisms are listed in** Table 33-6. Aztreonam is not the initial drug of choice for any infection. It is not indicated in dental infections.

Aztreonam is an FDA pregnancy category B drug and lacks cross-allergenicity with β-lactams. Aztreonam induces β-lactamase production and may be synergistic with the renal toxicity and ototoxicity of aminoglycosides.

Macrolide and Ketolide Antibiotics

Chemistry and classification (Table 33-7; Fig. 33-8)

Macrolide antibiotics are characterized by large 14-membered, 15-membered, or 16-membered lactone rings. Erythromycin, as derived from *Streptomyces erythreus,* was introduced in 1952, and azithromycin and clarithromycin were introduced in 1991 and 1992, respectively. Azithromycin is a 15-membered macrolide with an added nitrogen and N-methylation (making it technically an azalide), whereas clarithromycin is formed by the alkylation of a hydroxyl group of erythromycin (a 14-membered ring). Troleandomycin is a synthetic derivative of oleandomycin, dirithromycin is a prodrug yielding erythromycylamine in the intestine, and telithromycin is a derivative of erythromycin A and a 14-membered macrolide with a 3-keto group substitution.

TABLE 33-7 Macrolide Preparations Available in the United States

Nonproprietary (Generic) Name	Proprietary (Trade) Name
Erythromycin base (film-coated)	Erythromycin Filmtabs
Erythromycin (enteric-coated)	E-Base, E-Mycin, Ery-Tab, Eryc
Erythromycin stearate	Erythrocin stearate
Erythromycin ethylsuccinate	E.E.S., EryPed
Erythromycin lactobionate	—
Clarithromycin	Biaxin
Azithromycin	Zithromax
Dirithromycin	Dynabac
Troleandomycin	TAO

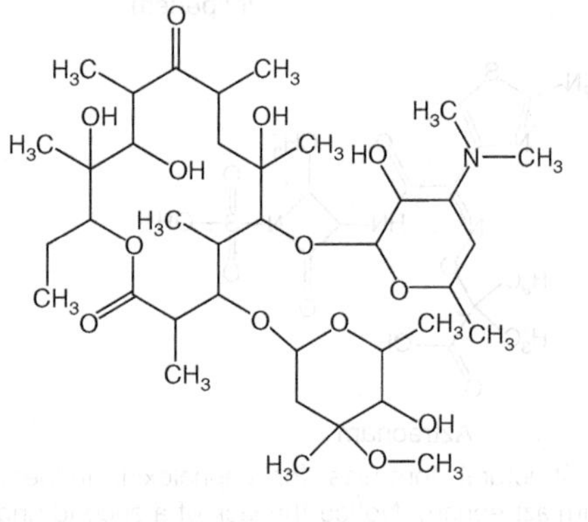

Erythromycin

FIG 33-8 Structure of erythromycin.

Mechanism of action and antibacterial spectrum

The mechanism of action of macrolides is to bind reversibly to the P site of the 50S ribosomal subunit and **inhibit RNA-dependent protein synthesis** by stimulating the dissociation of peptidyl transfer RNA (tRNA) from the ribosome (Fig. 33-9). **Erythromycin** is active against gram-positive aerobic/facultative staphylococci and streptococci, gram-negative anaerobes (*M. catarrhalis, Bordetella pertussis, Legionella pneumophila*), and *Mycoplasma pneumoniae.* It is also **active against organisms listed in** Table 33-8 (**see also** Table 33-5).

Microorganisms generally resistant to macrolides include *H. influenzae, Peptostreptococcus, Aggregatibacter actinomycetemcomitans, Pasteurella, Fusobacterium, Mycobacterium tuberculosis,* MRSA, and Enterobacteriaceae. Marginally affected organisms include *Prevotella* and *Porphyromonas.*

Clarithromycin and azithromycin have special indications because they are more active against some organisms than is erythromycin, or in some cases in which erythromycin is not active. (See Table 33-5.)

Bacterial resistance

The major mechanism for microbial resistance is demethylation of the 2058 residue of the gene coding for the 23S ribosomal RNA peptidyl transferase region, resulting in reduced macrolide binding (ribosomal protection). The *erm* (erythromycin-resistant *methylase*) gene responsible for the ribosomal protection is often associated with tetracycline resistance genes and is frequently combined with the resistance genes for lincosamides (clindamycin) and streptogramins (quinupristin-dalfopristin) to form the macrolide-lincosamide-streptogramin B (MLS_B)

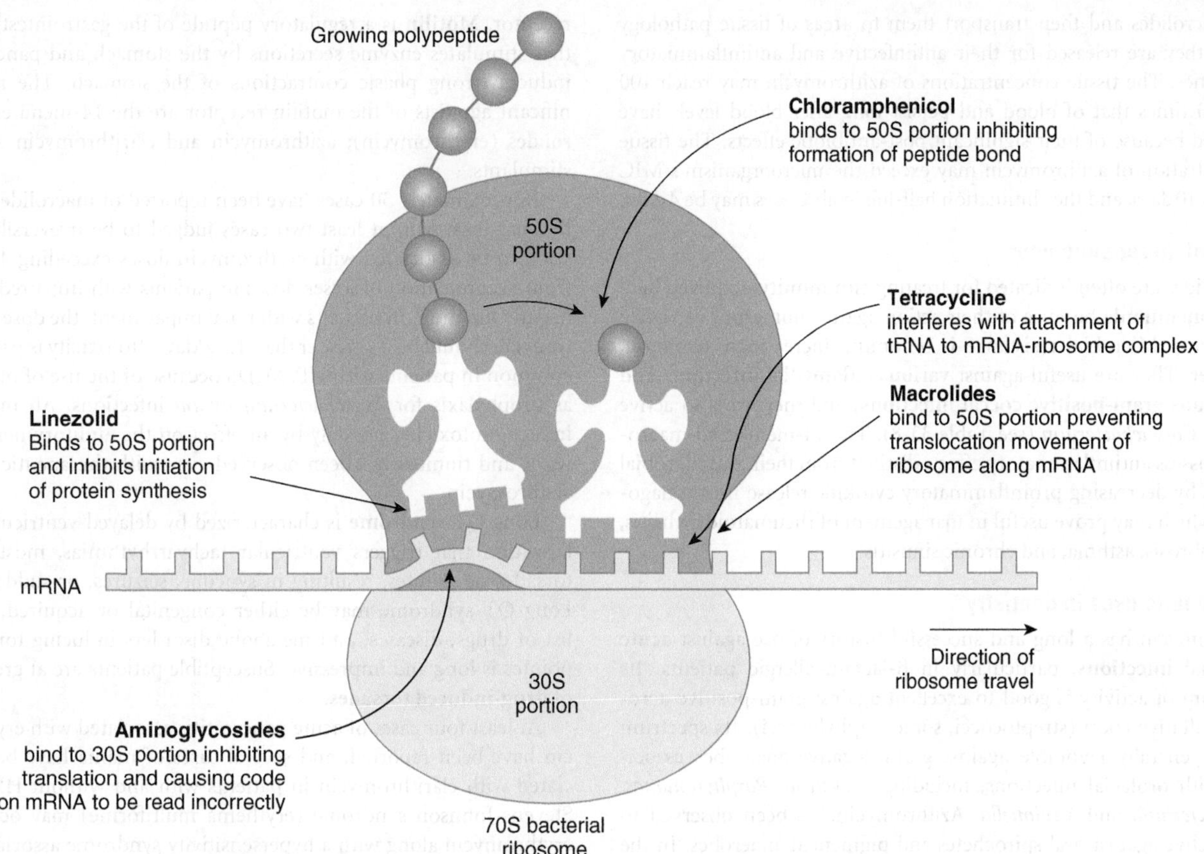

FIG 33-9 Sites of inhibition of bacterial ribosomal protein synthesis by various drugs.

TABLE 33-8 Macrolides as Agents of Choice or Alternative Drugs*

Drugs of Choice	Alternative Agents
Bartonella henselae	*Actinomyces israelii*
Bartonella quintana	*Bacillus anthracis*
Bordetella pertussis	*Borrelia burgdorferi*
Campylobacter jejuni	*Capnocytophaga canimorsus*
Chlamydia trachomatis	*Chlamydia pneumoniae*
Corynebacterium diphtheriae	*Eikenella corrodens*
Corynebacterium jeikeium	*Erysipelothrix rhusiopathiae*
Haemophilus ducreyi	*Leptotrichia buccalis*
Helicobacter pylori	*Mycobacterium leprae*
Legionella pneumophila	*Streptococcus pneumoniae*
Mycobacterium avium	*Streptococcus pyogenes*
Mycobacterium kansasii	
Mycobacterium marinum	
Mycoplasma pneumoniae	
Ureaplasma urealyticum	

*Specific macrolide(s) for most indications are listed in Table 33-5. Drug combinations are used in some cases.

Abramowicz M, Zuccotti G, editors: Handbook of antimicrobial drugs: drugs for bacterial infections, *The Medical Letter* ed 20, 2015, New Rochelle, NY.

aggregate, which confers resistance to all three antibiotic groups simultaneously. Other macrolide resistance mechanisms include active efflux genes encoding for transport efflux proteins and an esterification gene that codes for inactivation of the macrolides by phosphorylation and glycosylation.

Absorption, fate, and excretion

Erythromycin and azithromycin are available for oral and intravenous use, whereas the remaining agents are used only orally. Bioavailability ranges from 10% for dirithromycin to 40% to 50% for azithromycin, clarithromycin, and erythromycin. Food in the stomach may increase or have no effect on the absorption of azithromycin, but the remaining macrolides should be taken 1 hour before or 2 hours after a meal, except for estolate and ethylsuccinate salts of erythromycin, which may be taken without regard to meals. (**Note, however, that the estolate form of the drug has a higher risk of hepatic toxicity.**)

Erythromycin base is poorly resistant to gastric acid and is prepared with enteric coating or as various salts (stearate), esters (ethylsuccinate), or salts of esters (estolate), which protect against gastric acid degradation. Macrolides are best absorbed in the small intestine, and when given orally in standard doses, generally produce adequate tissue MIC concentrations. Erythromycin may have a variable absorption rate. The time to maximum blood concentrations of the macrolides after oral administration is about 2 hours. Impaired renal function may reduce the excretion of the macrolides, with the elimination half-life of erythromycin increasing from 1.6 to 5-6 hours in anuric patients. Clarithromycin and erythromycin are primarily eliminated in the urine, and azithromycin is primarily eliminated in the bile, although erythromycin may also undergo significant biliary excretion. The average serum **half-lives are ~68 hours for azithromycin, 3 to 7 hours for clarithromycin, and ~1.6 hours for erythromycin.**

A remarkable property of macrolides and highly fat-soluble tetracyclines and clindamycin is selective uptake by phagocytic cells and fibroblasts, which function as repository drug depots and as a drug delivery system to areas of inflammation and infection. These cells concentrate the macrolides and then transport them to areas of tissue pathology where they are released for their antiinfective and antiinflammatory properties. The tissue concentrations of azithromycin may reach 100 to 1000 times that of blood and persist long after blood levels have declined because of their significant post-antibiotic effects. The tissue concentration of azithromycin may exceed the microorganism's MIC for 2 to 10 days, and the elimination half-life in abscesses may be 4 days.

General therapeutic uses

Macrolides are often indicated for treating **community-acquired bacterial pneumonia** because of their action against numerous causative organisms. Microbial resistance is becoming increasingly common, however. They are useful against **various chlamydial infections and numerous gram-positive coccal infections,** and they are also active against *Corynebacterium* (see Table 33-8). The 14-membered macrolides possess antiinflammatory effects distinct from their antimicrobial actions by decreasing proinflammatory cytokine release from phagocytes, which may prove useful in management of rheumatoid arthritis, cystic fibrosis, asthma, and chronic sinusitis.

Therapeutic uses in dentistry

Erythromycin has a long and successful history of use against **acute orofacial infections**, particularly in β-lactam–allergic patients. Its spectrum of activity is good to excellent against gram-positive aerobic/facultative cocci (streptococci, some staphylococci). Its spectrum is not generally favorable against gram-negative anaerobes associated with orofacial infections, including *Prevotella, Porphyromonas, Fusobacterium,* and *Veillonella.* Azithromycin has been observed to be effective against oral spirochetes and pigmented anaerobes. In the management of acute periapical abscesses, azithromycin, 500 mg/day for 3 days, has shown comparable efficacy to amoxicillin/clavulanic acid, 625 mg three times daily for 5 to 10 days. Macrolides are also useful for endocarditis prophylaxis. Due to its associated hepatic toxicity, there is no reason for using the estolate form of erythromycin in dental applications.

Clarithromycin is most active against gram-positive anaerobes (*Actinomyces, Propionibacterium, Lactobacillus*), whereas erythromycin is more active than azithromycin for these organisms. Azithromycin has the best activity against gram-negative anaerobes (*Fusobacterium, Prevotella, Porphyromonas, Wolinella, Selenomonas,* and *A. actinomycetemcomitans*). Azithromycin may be more active against streptococci and staphylococci than erythromycin and clarithromycin and has much less propensity for drug interactions. Prolonged use of erythromycin and possibly other macrolides may lead to superinfection with gram-negative enteric bacilli.

Adverse effects

Serious toxicity with macrolides is rare but occasionally significant. The most important adverse effects include epigastric pain, ototoxicity (deafness), ventricular arrhythmias (torsades de pointes), acute pancreatitis, mania, cholestatic hepatitis, hypersensitivity syndrome, and certain drug interactions.

Cholestatic hepatitis is much more common with the **estolate form of erythromycin** than with other forms of erythromycin or other macrolides. This reaction can be misdiagnosed as viral hepatitis. Symptoms usually appear after approximately 10 days of erythromycin use, disappear 2 to 4 weeks after drug discontinuance with no residual effects, and readily reappear with drug readministration. This reaction is less common in children.

The most common serious adverse reaction associated with macrolides, particularly erythromycin, is potentially severe **epigastric pain** resulting from stimulation of the gastric smooth muscle motilin receptor. **Motilin** is a regulatory peptide of the gastrointestinal tract that stimulates enzyme secretions by the stomach and pancreas and induces strong phasic contractions of the stomach. The most significant agonists of the motilin receptor are the 14-membered macrolides (erythromycin); azithromycin and clarithromycin are lesser stimulants.

Approximately 30 cases have been reported of macrolide-induced **hearing loss**, with at least two cases judged to be irreversible. Most seem to be associated with erythromycin doses exceeding 4 g/day or from accumulation of lesser doses in patients with impaired renal or hepatic function. In patients with renal impairment, the dose of erythromycin should be no greater than 1.5 g/day. Ototoxicity is particularly common in patients with HIV/AIDS because of the use of macrolides as prophylaxis for *Mycobacterium avium* infections. All macrolides induce ototoxicity, possibly by an effect on the auditory nerve pathways, and tinnitus has been observed even with therapeutic doses of azithromycin.

Long QT syndrome is characterized by delayed ventricular repolarization that triggers ventricular tachyarrhythmias, most notably torsades de pointes, resulting in syncope, seizures, or sudden death. Long QT syndrome may be either congenital or acquired, and the list of drugs, diseases, and metabolic disorders inducing torsades de pointes is long and impressive. Susceptible patients are at greater risk of **drug-induced torsades.**

At least four cases of acute pancreatitis associated with erythromycin have been reported, and several cases of mania have been associated with clarithromycin in patients with and without HIV/AIDS. Stevens-Johnson syndrome (erythema multiforme) may occur with erythromycin along with a hypersensitivity syndrome associated with azithromycin and clarithromycin consisting of fever, rash, hepatitis, interstitial nephritis, oliguria, and xerostomia. Azithromycin and erythromycin are classified as FDA pregnancy category B drugs, and clarithromycin is classified as an FDA pregnancy category C drug.

Drug interactions

Erythromycin and clarithromycin, primarily through their **inhibition of the liver microsomal enzyme** drug metabolizing and secondarily through their effect on gastrointestinal microbial flora, increase serum levels of fluconazole, ranitidine, alfentanil, benzodiazepines, tacrolimus, theophylline, vinblastine, bromocriptine, buspirone, carbamazepine, cyclosporine, digoxin, disopyramide, ergot alkaloids, felodipine, oral anticoagulants, methylprednisolone, and omeprazole. Azithromycin has much less effect on the liver microsomes. Macrolide blood levels may be increased by fluconazole and decreased by theophylline. Antacids reduce the rate, but not the total amount, of macrolide absorption, and the combination of macrolides and oral contraceptives may result in cholestasis. Bacteriostatic macrolides may interfere with the bactericidal effect of cell wall inhibitors. Concomitant administration with a fluoroquinolone, or pimozide, may lead to torsades de pointes.

After only 3 days of administration, macrolides may seriously reduce digoxin metabolism in the gastrointestinal tract by *Eubacterium lentum,* resulting in digitalis toxicity because the microorganism may metabolize 30% to 40% of the drug. Macrolides may potentiate the anticoagulant effect of oral anticoagulants. Concomitant use of macrolides may increase the myopathy and rhabdomyolysis seen with the "statin" anti-cholesterol agents.

Contraindications

Macrolides are contraindicated in patients with allergy to the drugs in patients with a history of previous allergic cholestatic hepatitis. Macrolides are also contraindicated in combinations with other drugs with which they interact, such as those that induce torsades de pointes.

The maximum daily dose should be 4 g in adults with normal renal function and 1.5 g/day in patients with impaired renal function.

Ketolides

Ketolides (**telithromycin**) are derivatives of erythromycin A specifically designed for activity against bacteria responsible for **community-acquired respiratory tract infections.** Telithromycin is a 14-membered macrolide with a 3-keto group substitution. The oral bioavailability of telithromycin is approximately 55%, with maximum serum concentrations at 1 to 3 hours. The elimination half-life is about 13 hours; the drug has a long post-antibiotic effect and is highly concentrated in white blood cells and pulmonary tissue. It is primarily metabolized in the liver. Telithromycin inhibits bacterial protein synthesis by binding to the 50S ribosomal subunit to inhibit translation at the peptidyl transferase site. The drug also inhibits formation of the bacterial 50 and 30S ribosomal subunits.

Telithromycin is active against a wide spectrum of respiratory pathogens, including *S. pneumoniae, H. influenzae, M. catarrhalis, C. pneumoniae, M. pneumoniae, L. pneumophila*, group A and B streptococci (*S. pyogenes* and *Streptococcus agalactiae*).

The most frequent adverse reactions associated with telithromycin are diarrhea (12% to 20%), nausea (2% to 12%), dizziness (2% to 5%), and headache (2.5% to 5%). A major concern is the drug's association with liver toxicity. Telithromycin is an inhibitor of the liver microsomal enzyme cytochrome P450 system and would be expected to increase blood levels of many drugs. Similar to macrolides, telithromycin may prolong the QT interval. It is classified as an FDA pregnancy category B drug.

Telithromycin has no place in the management of acute or chronic orofacial infections unless dictated by sensitivity testing. Its use is limited in the United States to community-acquired bacterial pneumonia.

Lincosamides

Clindamycin and lincomycin are the only lincosamide antibiotics. Lincomycin was isolated from *Streptomyces lincolnensis* in 1962, and clindamycin (7-chloro-7-deoxy-lincomycin) was introduced in 1966. **Clindamycin** (Fig. 33-10) is used almost exclusively because of its greater efficacy and superior pharmacokinetics.

Mechanism of action and antibacterial spectrum

The receptor site for lincosamides is identical to that of macrolides, chloramphenicol, and streptogramins: the 23S subunit of the 50S bacterial ribosome, resulting in bacteriostatic **inhibition of microbial protein synthesis.** Clindamycin has significant **activity against many gram-positive and gram-negative anaerobic and facultative/aerobic microorganisms.** The major indications are listed in Table 33-9. Clindamycin has indications for some oral infections.

Bacterial resistance

Resistance to clindamycin occurs by three mechanisms: (1) alteration of 23S ribosomal RNA of the 50S ribosomal subunit by adenine methylation (ribosomal protection), (2) an altered single 50S ribosomal protein at the receptor site (receptor alteration), or (3) inactivation in some staphylococcal strains by a nucleotidyl transferase (drug inactivation). Adenine methylation is plasmid mediated and confers MLS_B resistance. The M phenotype macrolide resistance in *S. pneumoniae* does not confer resistance to clindamycin. If erythromycin resistance in staphylococci is inducible and not constitutive, the microorganisms are resistant only to the 14-membered and 15-membered macrolides and remain sensitive to lincosamides, streptogramins, and 16-membered macrolides. Constitutive resistance in staphylococci of the MLS_B type confers resistance to all these antibiotics simultaneously.

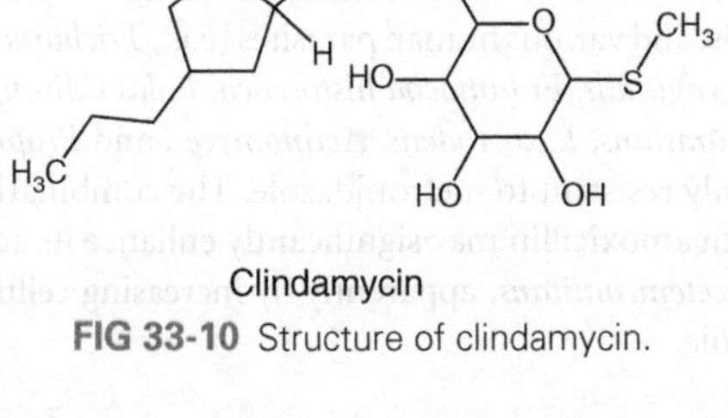

Clindamycin

FIG 33-10 Structure of clindamycin.

Absorption, fate, and excretion

Clindamycin is well absorbed orally with a 90% bioavailability not appreciably reduced by food. The time to oral peak serum levels is 45 to 60 minutes, with an elimination half-life of 2.4 to 3 hours. With renal failure the elimination half-life increases to 6 hours, with a doubling of the serum level. The drug penetrates well into bone but not cerebrospinal fluid; is metabolized primarily in the liver (>90%); and is highly concentrated in the bile, where it may alter colonic flora for 2 weeks after it is discontinued. In a manner similar to macrolides, clindamycin is concentrated preferentially in polymorphonuclear cells, alveolar macrophages, and abscess tissue.

General therapeutic uses

Clindamycin is used in the treatment of certain infections caused by susceptible strains of streptococci, staphylococci, pneumococci, or anaerobes such as *Bacteroides*. Clindamycin may be indicated in the treatment of refractory bone infections. Clindamycin is also useful in treating certain conditions involving anaerobes, such as infections of the female genital tract, pelvic infections, and abdominal penetrating wounds (see Table 33-5). It can also be used in combination for *Pneumocystis carinii* and for toxoplasmosis.

Therapeutic uses in dentistry

Although amoxicillin and penicillin V remain drugs of choice for acute orofacial infections, a resurgence in clindamycin use may be appropriate as the oral microbial resistance to β-lactams continues to increase. It is anticipated that oral microbial resistance to clindamycin will also increase proportionately along with the specter of MLS_B resistance shared with macrolides and streptogramins.

Adverse effects

Minor adverse reactions associated with clindamycin include nausea and vomiting, abdominal pain, esophagitis, glossitis, stomatitis,

TABLE 33-9 Indications for Clindamycin*

Indications
Methicillin-sensitive *Staphylococcus aureus*
Streptococcus pyogenes
Streptococcus pneumoniae
VGS
Peptostreptococcus
Bacillus anthracis
Clostridium perfringens
Actinomyces israelii
Leptotrichia buccalis
Fusobacterium species
Capnocytophaga canimorsus
Bacteroides (oropharyngeal strains)

*Abramowicz M, Zuccotti G, editors: Handbook of antimicrobial drugs: drugs for bacterial infections, *The Medical Letter* ed 20, 2015, New Rochelle, NY.

allergy, reversible increase in serum transaminase levels, reversible myelosuppression, metallic taste, **maculopapular rash** (3% to 10%), and **diarrhea** (2% to 20%, average of 8%). High intravenous doses of clindamycin may result in a neuromuscular blockade similar to that of aminoglycosides.

The major concern with clindamycin has been its purported propensity to cause **antibiotic-induced diarrhea and colitis**, most notably PMC, based on early reports of incidences reaching 10%. It is now apparent that the association of clindamycin with these colonic disorders in outpatient use is less than previously reported, although nonetheless real. Although antibiotic-associated diarrhea is common in the outpatient environment and readily managed by drug discontinuance, serious antibiotic-induced colitis and potentially lethal PMC is more rare.

Care should be taken with patients who have recently recovered from *C. difficile*–associated diarrhea or colitis for 2 months after the cessation of the disease. Any elective dental procedure requiring antibiotic therapy or prophylaxis is best postponed for this 2-month period. If antibiotic therapy is required, antibiotics far less associated with antibiotic-induced diarrhea (e.g., penicillin V, macrolides) are appropriate.

Drug interactions

Clindamycin acts synergistically with nondepolarizing (curare-like) neuromuscular blocking drugs in blocking neurotransmission at skeletal muscle. Oral absorption of clindamycin is slowed by kaolin-pectin antidiarrheal drugs.

Contraindications

Clindamycin is contraindicated in patients allergic to the drug and in combination with curare-like neuromuscular blocking drugs. All antibiotics should be avoided if possible for 2 months after antibiotic-induced colitis.

Metronidazole

Metronidazole (Fig. 33-11) is a synthetic nitroimidazole patterned after a naturally occurring antiparasitic substance that was isolated from a *Streptomyces* species in 1955. The drug was introduced into medicine in 1959 and was quickly found to possess strong trichomonacidal activity. Since then, metronidazole has become the drug of choice for various protozoal infections. A chance observation that the symptoms of acute necrotizing ulcerative gingivitis were relieved in a woman receiving metronidazole for the treatment of vaginal trichomoniasis stimulated research on the drug's antibacterial effects, culminating in its approval in 1981 for the treatment of anaerobic bacterial infections. Its extensive use in treating parasitic diseases worldwide has led to significant resistance to the drug where parasites are a major problem. It was soon discovered that the drug possessed exceptional activity against obligate **anaerobic and microaerophilic microorganisms**, including microorganisms involved in acute orofacial infections, periodontitis, and acute necrotizing ulcerative gingivitis.

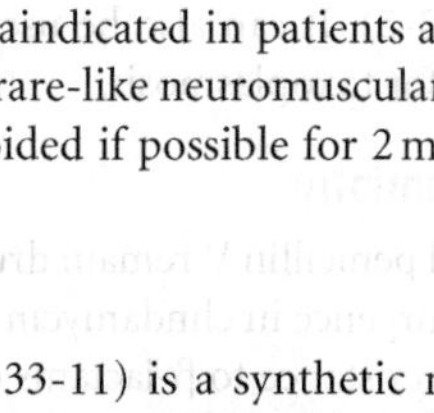

FIG 33-11 Structure of metronidazole.

Mechanism of action and antibacterial spectrum

The antimicrobial activity of metronidazole requires entry into the cell and reduction of its nitro group to produce metabolites that **damage DNA**, eventually inducing cell death. Metronidazole is active only against bacteria that are obligate anaerobes. It is a concentration-dependent rather than time-dependent antibiotic. Because metronidazole metabolites interfere with nucleic acid synthesis, concerns have been raised regarding its potential for mutagenicity, carcinogenicity, and teratogenicity.

Metronidazole penetrates all bacterial cells equally well. In sensitive anaerobes, the nitro moiety of the drug is enzymatically reduced, however, and this metabolite is the active form of the drug. Metronidazole is almost always bactericidal. The drug reacts with bacterial DNA, causing inhibition of DNA replication, fragmentation of existing DNA, and in low doses, mutation of the bacterial genome.

Bacterial resistance

Microbial resistance to metronidazole is limited probably because of its limited clinical use, except in developing countries, where it is widely used to manage parasitic diseases. A notable exception to this generalization is the high level of resistance in *H. pylori* in developed countries. Resistance to metronidazole is chromosomally mediated and plasmid-mediated by a reduction in activity or expression of several genes (*rdx*A, *nim*A, *nim*B) that control nitroreductase activity, which reduces the concentration of active metronidazole metabolites within the microbial cell.

Subinhibitory concentrations of metronidazole may increase resistance rates in various periodontal pathogens, including *Fusobacterium, Prevotella, Porphyromonas,* and *Peptostreptococcus. Bacteroides* strains resistant to metronidazole also acquire enhanced virulence properties.

Absorption, fate, and excretion

Metronidazole is almost completely absorbed from the gastrointestinal tract (oral bioavailability approaches 100%) so that serum levels are essentially the same whether the drug is administered orally or intravenously. Food may delay peak serum levels of metronidazole but not the total amount absorbed. Metronidazole attains a peak blood level orally in 1 to 2 hours, has a wide volume of distribution, has excellent CNS penetration, has **an elimination half-life of 8 hours**, and is biotransformed into five metabolic products, all of which have anti-anaerobic activity. The pharmacokinetics of metronidazole are the same in pregnant and nonpregnant women, its metabolism is reduced in the presence of severe hepatic dysfunction, and its pharmacokinetics are not significantly altered with renal impairment.

General therapeutic uses

The principal medical indications for metronidazole are **anaerobic** abdominal and CNS infections, bacterial vaginosis, protozoan and *H. pylori* infections, and the management of *C. difficile*–associated diarrhea and colitis. Metronidazole is very active against obligate anaerobes (e.g., *Bacteroides, Porphyromonas, Prevotella, Fusobacterium, Peptostreptococcus, Clostridium*), many of which are associated with periodontitis, and various human parasites (e.g., *Trichomonas vaginalis, Gardnerella vaginalis, Entamoeba histolytica, Balantidium coli*). *A. actinomycetemcomitans, E. corrodens, Actinomyces,* and *Propionibacterium* are commonly resistant to metronidazole. The combination of metronidazole with amoxicillin may significantly enhance its activity against *A. actinomycetemcomitans,* apparently by increasing cellular uptake of metronidazole.

Therapeutic uses in dentistry

Metronidazole is highly effective against gram-negative **anaerobic pathogens** responsible for acute orofacial infections and chronic periodontitis. Combination of metronidazole with a β-lactam antibiotic for oral infections may be indicated for serious acute orofacial infections and in the management of **aggressive periodontitis.**

Metronidazole is a concentration-dependent, not time-dependent, antibiotic. The promiscuous use of metronidazole for classic chronic periodontitis is a misuse of the drug and may contribute to the increasing resistance of metronidazole seen with parasites, *H. pylori,* and other microorganisms.

Adverse effects

Minor adverse reactions associated with metronidazole include reversible neutropenia, **metallic taste, dark or red-brown urine,** skin rash, urethral or vaginal burning sensation, gynecomastia, and nausea and vomiting. Rare major adverse reactions include pancreatitis; PMC; **peripheral neuropathy; disulfiram reaction** when combined with ethanol; and CNS toxicity consisting of seizures, encephalopathy, cerebellar dysfunction, paresthesias, mental confusion, and depression. These neurologic reactions generally occur only with high, prolonged, cumulative doses.

Because metronidazole affects DNA synthesis, numerous studies have addressed its potential to cause birth defects. Its use in pregnancy does not seem to be associated with any congenital abnormalities, preterm delivery, or low birth weight in newborns, and the drug has an FDA pregnancy category B classification.

Drug interactions

Barbiturates may reduce the efficacy of metronidazole, **and cimetidine** may reduce its liver metabolism. The concurrent use of **metronidazole and ethanol** may result in acute psychosis and the **disulfiram reaction** (flushing, tachycardia, nausea and vomiting), although for most individuals the risk is minor. Metronidazole may increase lithium blood levels, decrease the body clearance of phenytoin, and significantly increase blood warfarin levels by decreasing its liver metabolism.

Tetracyclines and Glycylcyclines

Tetracyclines (Fig. 33-12) are a group of **broad-spectrum**, bacteriostatic antibiotics that have been extensively used in the treatment of numerous and varied infections. Their widespread use, and often misuse, has resulted in the appearance of many bacterial strains that are resistant to these drugs, which has curtailed their clinical usefulness. Paradoxically, the clinical use of tetracyclines has had a recent resurgence of interest with the growing realization that the drugs may be lifesaving in the treatment of serious nosocomial infections from highly and multiply antibiotic-resistant methicillin-resistant staphylococci. This renewed effectiveness of tetracyclines may be related to the almost complete lack of use of the drugs in hospitals for several decades, possibly leading to the loss of tetracycline resistance genes in this environment. Because of the advent of widespread resistance of *H. pylori* to metronidazole and macrolides, tetracyclines have gained importance in the treatment and prevention of peptic ulcers and gastric cancer and have emerged as a prophylactic agent in the prevention of multidrug-resistant malaria in travelers and the management of community-acquired pneumonia, particularly in penicillin-resistant and macrolide-resistant strains.

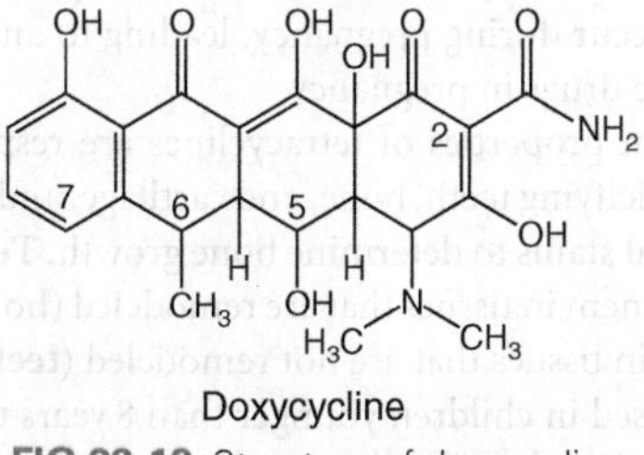

Doxycycline

FIG 33-12 Structure of doxycycline.

Tetracyclines comprise a group of antibiotics with a similar antibacterial spectrum but differing pharmacokinetic properties created by various chemical substitutions on the hydro-naphthacene four-ringed nucleus. Chlortetracycline, oxytetracycline, tetracycline, and demeclocycline constitute the first-generation tetracyclines. Second-generation agents introduced from 1965 to 1972 include minocycline, methacycline, and doxycycline. Glycylcyclines are third-generation agents. The first microorganism clinically detected to be resistant to tetracyclines was a *Shigella dysenteriae* strain in 1953. Today, **doxycycline** is the most commonly used tetracycline (Table 33-10).

Mechanism of action

Tetracyclines inhibit bacterial protein synthesis by **preventing the association of aminoacyl-tRNA with the bacterial ribosome.** The drugs must transverse the gram-negative microbial outer membrane via porin channels or through the gram-positive cell wall in its electronegative hydrophobic form and attach to a single high-affinity binding site on the ribosomal 30S subunit and protein 7 on the 16S rRNA base.

Bacterial resistance

Microbial resistance to tetracyclines is widespread, transposable, inducible, and commonly permanent because their resistance genes are almost always combined in transposable elements with the genes for resistance to other antibiotics (multidrug resistance gene cassettes). Of the three mechanisms for tetracycline resistance (drug efflux, ribosomal protection, and enzymatic inactivation), drug efflux is the most important, with at least 300 different active efflux proteins capable of extruding tetracycline from the bacterial cell.

Tetracyclines are one of the most active chemical inducers of microbial resistance gene expression and downregulate a repressor gene that controls efflux activity for not only tetracyclines but also possibly other antibiotics. Only nanomolar amounts of tetracycline are necessary to de-repress this system and greatly increase antibiotic efflux from bacterial cells. Tetracyclines also promote the mobility of resistance determinants (transfer of resistance genes between bacteria) by stimulating the frequency of bacterial conjugation. Considering these extraordinary properties of tetracyclines to induce and promote microbial resistance not only to themselves but also other antibiotics, it would seem prudent to restrict their use to serious medical infections and restrict their use in most cases of periodontitis, where they may have limited or even undocumented value.

TABLE 33-10 Commercially Available Tetracycline and Glycylcycline Preparations

Nonproprietary (Generic) Name	Proprietary (Trade) Name
Tetracycline hydrochloride	Tetralen, Panmycin, Sumycin, Tetracyn, Tetracap
Oxytetracycline hydrochloride	Terramycin
Demeclocycline hydrochloride	Declomycin
Doxycycline hyclate	Vibramycin, Doxy Caps
Minocycline hydrochloride	Minocin, Vectrin, Dynacin
Glycylcycline	
Tigecycline	Tygacil

Absorption, fate, and excretion

Tetracyclines are adequately but variably absorbed from the gastrointestinal tract with significant differences in bioavailability, as follows: chlortetracycline, 30%; demeclocycline, tetracycline, and oxytetracycline, 60% to 80%; and minocycline or **doxycycline, 95% to 100%.** Dairy products, Ca^{2+}, Mg^{++} and aluminum compounds, and Na^{+} bicarbonate significantly impair tetracycline absorption either by chelation or by altered gastric pH. Their serum protein binding ranges from 20% to 40% for oxytetracycline to 80% to 95% for doxycycline, and the percent excreted unchanged in the urine ranges from 70% for oxytetracycline to 30% to 42% for doxycycline and 12% to 16% for minocycline. With renal impairment, only doxycycline and minocycline do not have increased half-lives and can be administered with reasonable safety. Other tetracyclines may accumulate in conditions of renal impairment, resulting in high blood levels and possible liver necrosis and death.

Tetracyclines are metabolized in the liver to a varying degree depending on the individual drug and are highly concentrated in the bile at levels three to five times higher than serum. More recent tetracyclines are more lipid-soluble with greater tissue distribution than earlier tetracyclines. Enterohepatic circulation and incomplete absorption may lead to high drug concentrations in the feces, particularly with older agents. Doxycycline may be found to some degree in the feces as an inactive form, and it is as yet unknown if this metabolic product is as capable of inducing resistance gene expression or transfer as the parent compound. The serum half-lives of the various agents are 12 to 16 hours for oxytetracycline, tetracycline, and demeclocycline; 14 to 16 hours for methacycline; 11 to 18 hours for minocycline; and **15 to 25 hours for doxycycline.** Peak serum concentrations are reached in 2 hours after the usual therapeutic doses.

General therapeutic uses (Table 33-11 and also see Table 33-5)

Tetracyclines are broad-spectrum antibiotics. Table 33-11 lists some sensitive organisms against which they are used in therapy. Tetracyclines are major drugs in treating **rickettsial diseases,** ***Mycoplasma, Chlamydia*** (treatment of community-acquired pneumonia), *H. pylori,* and *Borrelia.* (*Borrelia burgdorferi* is the causative agent of Lyme disease.)

Many other bacteria nominally within their range of activity should not be treated, at least initially, with a tetracycline because of the numerous resistant strains.

Tetracyclines have been used in the treatment of acne using oral and topical preparations. Tetracyclines are concentrated in the skin and are effective against *Propionibacterium acnes* and may have an antiseborrheic action to reduce skin lipids. Because tetracyclines are deposited in bone, they can be used to measure the rate of bone growth. Other indications include plague, tularemia, cholera, brucellosis, and certain protozoal infections.

TABLE 33-11 Indications for Tetracyclines and Tigecycline

Brucella
*Borrelia burgdorferi**
Borrelia recurrentis
Chlamydia pneumoniae
Chlamydia psittaci
Chlamydia trachomatis
*Ehrlichia chaffeensis**
*Ehrlichia ewingii**
Mycobacterium marinum†
Mycoplasma pneumoniae
*Rickettsiae**
Vibrio cholerae
Vibrio vulnificus
Yersinia pestis
Indications for Tigecycline
Community-acquired pneumonia caused by *Streptoccocus pneumoniae, Hemophilus influenza,* and *Legionella pneumophila*
Intraabdominal and skin infections due to gram-negative rods, streptococcal and staphylococcal bacteria, *Kebsiella, Bacterioides,* and others

*Specifically doxycycline.
†Specifically minocycline.
From Abramowicz M, Zuccotti G, editors: Handbook of antimicrobial drugs: drugs for bacterial infections, *The Medical Letter* ed 20, 2015, New Rochelle, NY.

Therapeutic uses in dentistry

The use of tetracyclines in the management of acute orofacial infections is widely considered inappropriate because of their bacteriostatic activity and extensive microbial resistance. Evidence does not support the use of tetracyclines in the management of chronic periodontitis. Data showing clinical efficacy are lacking, and there is a propensity to induce microbial resistance gene expression and stimulation of drug efflux mechanisms and common association with multiple resistance genes to other antibiotics in transposable elements. Tetracyclines **may** be of use in the management of **localized aggressive periodontitis** and its associated organism, *Aggregatibacter* (formerly *Actinobacillus*) *actinomycetemcomitans.* Tetracyclines also seem to inhibit inflammatory matrix metalloproteinase activity. Tetracyclines may also be used subgingivally. The degree of benefit of the use of tetracyclines in periodontal disease has to be weighed against the risk of developing resistant strains of microorganisms.

Adverse effects

Numerous adverse drug reactions are associated with tetracyclines. Tetracyclines may induce **photosensitivity**; nephrogenic diabetes insipidus (demeclocycline); blood dyscrasias; **liver dysfunction (high doses and especially during pregnancy)**; pseudotumor cerebri and bulging fontanelles (adults and infants); ***C. albicans* overgrowth**; gastrointestinal difficulties (nausea, vomiting, diarrhea, pancreatitis); and various allergic manifestations, including urticaria, serum sickness, angioneurotic edema, and anaphylaxis.

Minocycline in conventional doses is associated with skin, nail, and hair **pigmentation** and a systemic lupus erythematosus–like syndrome, mainly in adolescents taking the drug for acne. This syndrome is usually reversible but may require corticosteroid therapy; however, the absolute risk seems to be low (52.8 per 100,000 uses). Sixteen cases of autoimmune hepatitis have been described.

Minocycline is the only tetracycline that induces **vestibular toxicity** (ataxia, loss of balance), possibly because of its high concentration in the lipid-rich cells of the inner ear. Tetracyclines in general are one of the few groups of drugs that are toxic if ingested beyond their expiration date, inducing a **Fanconi-like syndrome** (azotemia, kidney damage). Tetracycline-induced acute interstitial nephritis may result in acute renal failure. Hepatotoxicity is rare except at high doses and is most likely to occur during pregnancy, leading to an absolute contraindication to the drugs in pregnancy.

The chelation properties of tetracyclines are responsible for their deposition in calcifying teeth, bone, and cartilage, and these drugs have been used as vital stains to determine bone growth. **Tetracycline staining** is not permanent in tissues that are remodeled (bone, cartilage), but it is permanent in tissues that are not remodeled **(teeth)**. Tetracyclines should not be used in children younger than 8 years unless other antibiotics are unlikely to be effective or are contraindicated. Tetracyclines most likely to stain the dentition severely are tetracycline and demeclocycline with oxytetracycline, chlortetracycline, and doxycycline (the least likely), but the magnitude of the staining may depend more on dose and duration than the drug itself. Deposition of tetracyclines in bone and teeth eliminates their antimicrobial activity. Because of the deleterious staining effects on the teeth and the liver, tetracyclines are classified by the FDA as pregnancy category D drugs. Tetracyclines should not be used in pregnancy because of staining of teeth and potential hepatotoxicity.

Minocycline is also able to impart a **grayish discoloration of teeth**, even after tooth formation and eruption. This could at least in part be an extrinsic stain; however, the exact mechanism(s) has/have not been established. This type of staining does not occur with other tetracyclines.

Drug interactions

Tetracyclines and all other antimicrobial ribosomal protein synthesis inhibitors may reduce the efficacy of antibiotic cell wall inhibitors, which rely on cell wall division for their action. **Polyvalent cations** (aluminum, Ca^{2+}, zinc, iron, magnesium, bismuth) may decrease gastric tetracycline absorption by chelation. Na^+ bicarbonate alters the gastric pH and reduces absorption of tetracyclines.

Serum levels of tetracyclines may be reduced from increased hepatic metabolism induced by **barbiturates, carbamazepine, and hydantoins**. The addition of tetracyclines to coumarin anticoagulants (e.g., warfarin) may greatly increase the latter's effect on the INR and lead to serious bleeding episodes. The effect is partially due to the inhibitory effect of tetracyclines on the **intestinal flora that produce vitamin K.**

Contraindications

Tetracyclines are contraindicated in children younger than 8 years, in cases of allergy, **during pregnancy, and during lactation**.

Glycylcyclines

Glycylcyclines are synthetic derivatives of minocycline. **Tigecycline** is the glycylcycline used in the United States. It is effective against some tetracycline-resistant bacteria and other **organisms listed in** Table 33-11. The resistance gene for glycylcyclines is carried on the same transposon as the resistance genes for the macrolides and tetracycline, making the use of glycylcyclines potentially limited.

Fluoroquinolones

Fluoroquinolones were introduced in the 1980s and are C6 fluorine derivatives of nalidixic acid. The terms *fluoroquinolone* and *quinolone* are often used interchangeably; however, this is technically incorrect because nalidixic acid is not a fluoroquinolone, being devoid of the fluorine substitution.

The first fluoroquinolone (norfloxacin) was synthesized in 1978 as a 6-fluorinated derivative of nalidixic acid with a piperazine ring at position 7 (Fig. 33-13). Ciprofloxacin was synthesized in 1981 and marketed in 1986. Newer fluoroquinolones have improved activity against *S. pneumoniae, S. aureus,* gram-positive cocci, anaerobes, *P. aeruginosa,* and various other organisms.

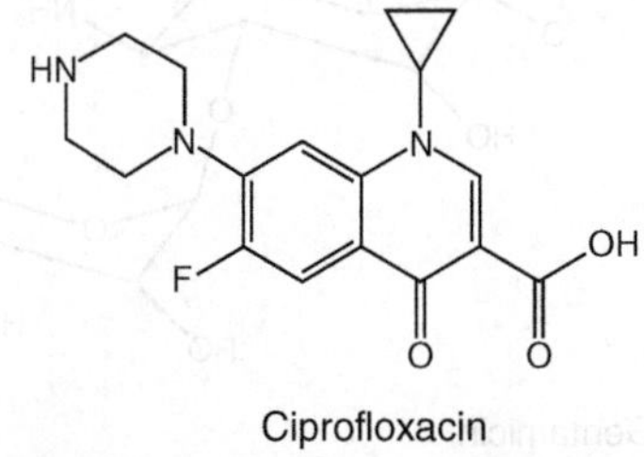

FIG 33-13 Structure of ciprofloxacin.

Mechanism of action and antibacterial spectrum (Table 33-12)

DNA gyrase and topoisomerases are enzymes involved in the crucial processes of DNA replication, transcription, and recombination. **DNA gyrase** has two subunits (A and B) regulated by two genes (*gyr*A and *gyr*B), with topoisomerase IV encoded by *par*C and *par*E genes. Both enzymes are responsible for supercoiling DNA, forming double-stranded DNA, and maintaining DNA in its physiologically stable and biologically active state. **Topoisomerase IV** nicks double-stranded DNA and seals the nicked DNA, whereas DNA gyrase guides the passage of the DNA through the interior of the enzyme complex. Both enzymes are responsible for supercoiling DNA, allowing for its fit into the bacterial cell. Fluoroquinolones stabilize the enzyme complex after strand breakage and before resealing, preventing DNA supercoiling.

Table 33-12 indicates their antibacterial spectra and indications, listing organisms that are sensitive to some or all fluoroquinolones.

Bacterial resistance

Three mechanisms account for microbial resistance to fluoroquinolones: mutations in DNA gyrase and topoisomerase IV, drug efflux pumps, and reduction in microbial outer membrane permeability. The target alterations are accomplished by simple point mutations in DNA gyrase (*gyr*A) and topoisomerase IV (*par*C) and by efflux mechanisms.

TABLE 33-12 Classification of Fluoroquinolones Based on Antibacterial Spectrum

Group	Indications Based on Advantage of Individual Drug
Group I (Urinary Tract Infections)	
Norfloxacin (Noroxin)	Gram negatives, e.g., *K. pneumoniae, E. coli, P. mirabilis, P. vulgaris, Providencia*
Group II (Broad Spectrum)	
Ciprofloxacin (Cipro)	*Pseudomonas aeruginosa, Mycobacterium tuberculosis, Salmonella typhi,* infectious diarrhea, inhalation anthrax
Levofloxacin (Levaquin)	Pneumonia, bronchitis, urinary tract infections, inhalation anthrax, *M. tuberculosis*
Lomefloxacin (Maxaquin)	*Haemophilus influenzae* or *Moraxella catarrhalis* respiratory tract infection, urinary tract infections
Ofloxacin (Floxin)	Pneumonia, urinary tract infections, *M. tuberculosis*
Group III (Greater Gram-Positive Activity)	
Gemifloxacin (Factive)	Streptococci and other organisms causing pneumonia and bronchitis
Sparfloxacin (Zagam)	Streptococci and other organisms causing pneumonia and bronchitis
Group IV (Greater Gram-Positive/Anti-Anaerobic Activity)	
Moxifloxacin (Avelox)	Anaerobes including *Bacteroides,* intraabdominal infections, pneumonia, skin infections, *M. tuberculosis*

Organisms that are sensitive to fluoroquinolones in general include *Mycoplasma pneumoniae, Legionella pneumophila, Chlamydia* species, *Escherichia coli, Haemophilus influenza, Klebsiella pneumoniae, Neisseria gonorrhoeae, Shigella, Proteus mirabilis,* and *Staphylococcus aureus.* Added indications for specific drugs are listed.

Absorption, fate, and excretion

Fluoroquinolones are well absorbed orally with a 70% and 90% bioavailability for **ciprofloxacin and levofloxacin**. Food generally delays the peak concentration of ciprofloxacin and levofloxacin, but it has no effect on **moxifloxacin**. The percent excreted by the kidneys ranges from 27% to 73%, and protein binding ranges from 15% to 35%. Fluoroquinolone half-lives vary, approximately **4 hours** for ciprofloxacin and norfloxacin, **7 to 8 hours** for lomefloxacin and sparfloxacin, and **~14 hours** for moxifloxacin. Pharmacokinetic improvements have included longer half-lives to allow for once-daily dosing and greater volumes of distribution for better tissue penetration. The post-antibiotic effects of fluoroquinolones vary from 1 to 4 hours.

General therapeutic uses

Table 33-12 **identifies differences in indications** based on groups of fluoroquinolones. Fluoroquinolones are used to treat urinary tract infections and bacterial diarrhea (e.g., traveler's diarrhea) because of their activity against many of the causative organisms. Because fluoroquinolones vary in their pharmacokinetics and in their spectra, some, but not all, fluoroquinolones are employed for upper and lower respiratory tract infections, *P. aeruginosa* infections, genital diseases caused by gonococci and *Chlamydia,* legionnaires disease, and tuberculosis.

Therapeutic uses in dentistry

Fluoroquinolones are not indicated for any acute orofacial infections unless dictated by culture and sensitivity tests. Drugs with better antimicrobial spectra are readily available.

Adverse effects

The major adverse effects associated with fluoroquinolones occur in the gastrointestinal tract, CNS, skin, and cartilage. Less common systems involved are the cardiovascular, hepatic, and renal systems. The incidence of each adverse effect may vary among the different drugs because of chemical substitutions on the quinolone nucleus.

Gastrointestinal adverse reactions include nausea and vomiting, dyspepsia and heartburn, and abdominal pain. The heavy use of fluoroquinolones has been associated with **PMC** and diarrhea owing to overgrowth of *C. difficile.* CNS effects include **mild neuropathy** (headache, dizziness, malaise, restlessness, bad dreams) possibly caused by central γ-aminobutyric acid inhibition or activity at the *N*-methyl-D-aspartate receptor. **Dermatologic toxicity** includes rash, pruritus, exfoliative dermatitis, Stevens-Johnson syndrome, and phototoxicity likely caused by dose-related ultraviolet light activation of reactive oxygen from the fluoroquinolones in the skin.

Chondrotoxicity includes arthralgia, joint swelling, tendinitis, and tendon rupture (primarily the Achilles tendon). These disorders are more likely to occur in men, elderly patients, and patients with concomitant corticosteroid therapy, diabetes mellitus, renal failure, other musculoskeletal disorders, or involvement in sports activity. These agents are not approved for children younger than 18 years except for ciprofloxacin.

Other possible adverse effects include induction of a **prolonged QT interval** leading to torsades de pointes, especially with levofloxacin, gemifloxacin, and moxifloxacin. Fluoroquinolones are associated with transient increase in liver enzymes, neutropenia, serum sickness, allergic vasculitis, and renal crystalluria. Because these antibiotics affect DNA, they have been investigated as possible teratogens. At extremely high in vitro doses, fluoroquinolones have induced genotoxicity in the chromosomal aberration test; however, a clinical study of 200 women exposed to ciprofloxacin and norfloxacin during gestation showed no increase in fetal malformations or musculoskeletal defects. Exacerbation of myasthenia gravis has been reported.

Drug interactions

An important drug interaction with fluoroquinolones is the potential increase in CNS toxicity with the concomitant use of **NSAIDs** and methylxanthines. The combination of a fluoroquinolone with tricyclic antidepressants, erythromycin, phenothiazines, and antiarrhythmic agents (quinidine, procainamide, disopyramide) may increase the risk of **torsades de pointes**. Fluoroquinolones may reduce the liver clearance of warfarin and procainamide and increase the toxicity of cyclosporine. Omeprazole may increase fluoroquinolone blood levels, and antacids, sucralfate, and calcium, iron, or zinc supplements may reduce gastric absorption of fluoroquinolones.

Contraindications

Ciprofloxacin should be used with caution during pregnancy and in children. For children younger than 18 years, other fluoroquinolones are contraindicated. Phototoxicity may occur on skin areas exposed to sunlight, and sunscreens are not always effective.

Aminoglycosides

The era of the aminoglycosides began in 1943 with the isolation of streptomycin by Waksman and the subsequent development of kanamycin (1957), **gentamicin** (1963), tobramycin (1968), **amikacin** (1972), and netilmicin (1975).

Chemistry

Streptomycin is produced by *Streptomyces griseus.* Other aminoglycosides are elaborated by various species of *Streptomyces* and *Micromonospora* or, in the case of amikacin and netilmicin, are semisynthetic derivatives of naturally occurring aminoglycosides. As the name implies, these agents consist of a highly polar amino base attached by glycosidic linkage to one or more sugars (Fig. 33-14).

Mechanism of action and antibacterial spectrum

Aminoglycosides bind irreversibly to the 30S ribosome to interfere with the reading of the microbial genetic code and to inhibit protein synthesis. Aminoglycosides are generally bactericidal, and their efficacy in several cases can be greatly enhanced by the concomitant use of cell wall–inhibiting β-lactams and glycopeptides.

The activity of **aminoglycosides** is primarily directed toward **gram-negative bacilli and mycobacteria** (see Table 33-5). The spectrum includes gram-negative enteric bacilli and some other gram-negative bacilli (e.g., *P. aeruginosa* and *Proteus*). There are, however, some differences among aminoglycosides regarding their efficacy toward specific microorganisms. Gentamicin is the most commonly used aminoglycoside, often acting synergistically with ampicillin, penicillin G,

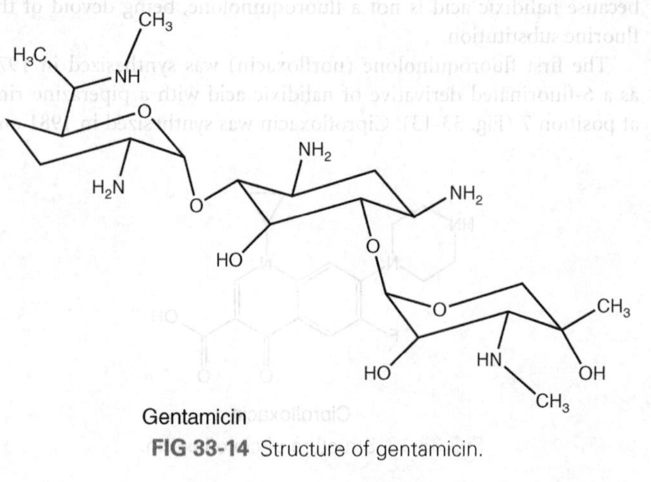

FIG 33-14 Structure of gentamicin.

ceftriaxone, vancomycin, and rifampin. Some original indications for aminoglycosides have been supplanted by safer extended-spectrum β-lactams and fluoroquinolones.

Bacterial resistance

Three resistance mechanisms presently exist for aminoglycosides: ribosomal mutations (less affinity for the 30S ribosome), reduced intracellular transport (primarily in staphylococci and pseudomonads), and, most commonly, plasmid-mediated **aminoglycoside-modifying enzymes** (acetyltransferases, adenyltransferases, and phosphotransferases).

Absorption, fate, and excretion

Aminoglycosides are poorly absorbed orally and do not penetrate well into the CNS, bronchial secretions, or certain microbial cells (e.g., *Rickettsiae, Chlamydiae*), but they are effective intracellularly in the treatment of tuberculosis, plague, brucellosis, and tularemia. Aminoglycosides are classic concentration-dependent antibiotics commonly administered in high parenteral doses repeated after the blood levels have decreased to a low concentration (peak and trough dosing). Single daily dosing is becoming more common, taking advantage of the long post-antibiotic effect of aminoglycosides, a reduction in cost, and lessening of renal toxicity. The normal elimination **half-life of aminoglycosides is 2 to 3 hours**, which can be extended to 24 to 100 hours in end-stage renal disease. Aminoglycosides are excreted primarily by glomerular filtration.

General therapeutic uses

Parenteral aminoglycosides currently available include amikacin, gentamicin, kanamycin, netilmicin, streptomycin, and tobramycin. Kanamycin and neomycin are available for oral use (poorly absorbed) for gastrointestinal infections. Aminoglycosides are primarily indicated for infections caused by **gram-negative aerobic bacteria**, including *P. aeruginosa, Serratia, Klebsiella, Enterobacter,* and *Proteus*. Anaerobic bacteria are insensitive. Aminoglycosides are often combined with a penicillin or cephalosporin for various infections.

Therapeutic uses in dentistry

Aminoglycosides have no uses in orofacial infections unless dictated by culture and sensitivity tests.

Adverse effects

The major adverse effects of aminoglycosides are renal toxicity and **eighth cranial nerve toxicity** (auditory and vestibular ototoxicity). **Nephrotoxicity** is caused by inhibition of an intracellular lysosomal phospholipase in the renal proximal tubules, resulting in aminoglycoside accumulation and subsequent reduced glomerular filtration, reduced water and Na^+ transport, reduced mitochondrial respiration, and reduced renal protein synthesis resulting in renal necrosis. The incidence of some degree of nephrotoxicity can be 10% to 20%.

A primary target for toxicity of aminoglycosides is the hair cells of the inner ear where the initial loss of the outer hair cells eventually damages the inner ear cochlear hair cells (type II). Further damage may occur to the cochlear sensory epithelium and the spiral ganglion cells required for cochlear implants. Vestibular (type I) hair cell damage occurs at the apex of the macula and often earlier than the cochlear hair cell damage. Initial signs and symptoms are hearing loss at the higher frequencies, which increases with dose, duration, and noise exposure. The incidence of cochlear damage may be 15%. Other adverse reactions associated with aminoglycosides include neuromuscular blockade of the curare type, rare blood dyscrasias, headache, dizziness, and urticarial and peripheral neuropathy.

Drug interactions

The nephrotoxicity of aminoglycosides is increased by vancomycin and cephalosporins. Loop diuretics increase auditory toxicity from aminoglycosides. Aminoglycosides **increase the neuromuscular blocking effect of curare-type drugs.**

Vancomycin

Vancomycin is a **glycopeptide** antibiotic, originally isolated from *Streptomyces orientalis* in Borneo in 1956 and introduced into medicine in 1958. Vancomycin is a seven-membered peptide chain with two sugars, vancosamine and glucose. The drug is poorly absorbed from the gastrointestinal tract and causes severe pain when given intramuscularly. It is administered intravenously to treat systemic infections or orally to treat PMC. Its elimination **half-life is ~6 hours,** and it has a post-antibiotic effect of 1.5 to 3 hours.

Mechanism of action and antibacterial spectrum

Vancomycin inhibits gram-positive bacterial **cell wall synthesis** by complexing with the d-alanyl-D-alanine portion of the peptide precursor units to **inhibit the transglycosylase reaction in peptidoglycan synthesis**. This inhibition is at the second stage of bacterial cell wall synthesis before the action of the penicillins at the third stage (see Fig. 33-5). Vancomycin may also affect cytoplasmic membrane permeability and RNA synthesis and, as with the β-lactams, it requires active cell replication. Because of its large molecular size, vancomycin cannot traverse the outer cell membrane of gram-negative bacteria.

The activity of vancomycin is almost exclusively against **aerobic and anaerobic gram-positive** species. Table 33-13 lists several important pathogens that are inhibited by the drug.

Bacterial resistance

Vancomycin resistance is caused by an altered peptidoglycan terminus (d-ala-d-lac instead of the usual d-ala-d-ala), resulting in reduced vancomycin binding and failure to prevent cell wall synthesis. Resistance in vancomycin-intermediate *S. aureus* and glycopeptide-intermediate *S. aureus* may be due to the production of abnormal peptides ("false binding sites") in the cell wall that bind vancomycin and prevent its attachment to its receptor or possibly to an increase of peptidoglycan resulting in thickened cell walls. A form of resistance is seen in *S. pneumoniae* by a unique mutation in the sensor-response system that controls autolysin activity necessary to kill certain bacteria.

TABLE 33-13 Antimicrobial Spectra of Systemic Peptide-Containing Antibiotics

Class	Representative Spectrum
Glycopeptide	
Vancomycin	*Staphylococcus* including MRSA, enterococci, *Streptococcus pneumoniae, Streptococcus pyogenes, Peptostreptococcus,* VGS, *Clostridium difficile, Corynebacterium jeikeium, Bacillus cereus, Bacillus subtilis*
Lipopeptide	
Daptomycin	MRSA, enterococci, *S. Pyogenes, Peptostreptococcus*
Lipoglycopeptides	
Telavancin Dalbavancin Oritavancin	MRSA, enterococci, *S. Pyogenes,* VGS, *Peptostreptococcus, S. pneumoniae*

MRSA, Methicillin-resistant *Staphylococcus aureus*; *VGS,* viridans group streptococci.

General therapeutic uses

Vancomycin is used for serious gram-positive infections caused by such organisms as **methicillin-resistant staphylococci** and *S. pneumoniae.* It is also useful for **non-vancomycin-resistant enterococcal infections**. It is effective in treating enterocolitis caused by *C. difficile*; however, metronidazole should be used for this situation if possible because of the significant risk of promoting vancomycin enterococcal resistance. Vancomycin may also be useful in treating multiple antibiotic-resistant VGS infections (see Table 33-13).

Therapeutic uses in dentistry

Vancomycin has no use in the management of acute or chronic orofacial infections unless dictated by laboratory culture and sensitivity tests.

Adverse effects

Major adverse drug reactions associated with vancomycin include transient or permanent **ototoxicity,** hypotension, reversible neutropenia, **renal toxicity**, skin rash, and **red man syndrome**. The auditory toxicity of vancomycin is dose-dependent and can be exacerbated by the combination with aminoglycosides. Red man syndrome results from the direct histamine release from mast cells manifesting as pruritus; erythematous rash of the head, neck, face, and upper torso; and hypotension mimicking anaphylactic shock. Rapid infusion makes it worse. This glycopeptide-induced anaphylactoid reaction may occur with the first drug exposure, is tachyphylactic in nature, and can be reduced significantly by the slow infusion of vancomycin over a 1-hour period and premedication with antihistamine drugs. To reduce the development of resistant bacteria, vancomycin use is contraindicated or discouraged for routine surgical prophylaxis.

Drug interactions

Vancomycin-induced nephrotoxicity or ototoxicity is increased with the concomitant use of aminoglycosides, and neuromuscular blockade with curare-like agents is enhanced by vancomycin.

Fidaxomicin

Fidaxomicin is a macrolide antibiotic whose spectrum is narrow and limited to gram-positive aerobes and anaerobes. It inhibits RNA polymerase and is bactericidal against ***C. difficile.*** It is given orally to treat colitis due to *C. difficile*. Systemic absorption is minimal when given orally.

Daptomycin

Daptomycin is a cyclic **lipopeptide** bacteriocidal antibiotic. Its causes depolarization of sensitive gram-positive bacteria after binding to their **cell membranes**. Its spectrum includes **MRSA, enterococci, *S. Pyogenes,* and *Peptostreptococcus*** (see Table 33-13). It is administered intravenously and is excreted unchanged by the kidneys. Adverse effects include skeletal muscle damage and peripheral neuropathy.

Lipoglycopeptides

Telavancin, dalbavancin, and oritavancin are intravenous drugs that **inhibit cell wall synthesis in gram-positive cocci,** similar to vancomycin. In addition, telavancin has the additional effect of causing cell depolarization by acting on the cell membrane. The spectrum of these drugs includes **MRSA, enterococci, *S. Pyogenes,*** VGS, *Peptostreptococcus*, and *S.* **pneumoniae** (**see** Table 33-13). The half-lives are telavancin, ~8 hours; dalbavancin, ~6 to 11 days; and oritavancin, ~10 days. Telavancin causes taste disturbances and is linked to QT prolongation and nephrotoxicity. Dalbavancin and oritavancin are associated with GI disturbances and hepatotoxicity. The drugs are used to treat complicated skin and soft tissue infections.

Streptogramins

Quinupristin-dalfopristin, a 30/70 mixture of streptogramins A and B, is approved for intravenous use in the United States.

Mechanism of action and antibacterial spectrum

Quinupristin and dalfopristin bind sequentially to different sites of the 50S subunit of the 70S ribosome to prevent newly synthesized peptide chains from extruding from the ribosome, resulting in cell death. Quinupristin-dalfopristin is used to treat **life-threatening vancomycin-resistant *E. faecium*** (*E. faecalis* is resistant) and **skin** or skin structure infections from ***S. aureus* and *S. pyogenes*.** The drug is additionally approved in the United Kingdom for nosocomial pneumonia. Its spectrum closely resembles that of vancomycin and linezolid.

Bacterial resistance

Microbial resistance occurs by three mechanisms: decreased ribosomal binding by methylation of an adenine residue, drug efflux, and enzymatic inactivation. This resistance belongs to the MLS_B (Macrolide-Lincosamide-Streptogramin B) type, potentially conferring cross-resistance to all these antibiotics.

General therapeutic uses

Quinupristin-dalfopristin should be reserved for life-threatening and multiple antibiotic-resistant infections from *E. faecium,* staphylococci, and some streptococci encountered primarily in the hospital.

Adverse effects

Adverse effects associated with streptogramins include possible severe arthralgias and myalgias, elevation in conjugated serum bilirubin, and significant inhibition of the liver microsomal CYP3A4 drug metabolizing system.

Drug interactions

Streptogramins decrease the liver metabolism of Ca^{2+} channel blockers, immunosuppressant drugs, corticosteroids, several anticancer agents, 3-hydroxy-3-methylglutaryl coenzyme A reductase inhibitors (statins), HIV protease inhibitors, quinidine, nonsedating antihistamines, sildenafil, opioids, and benzodiazepines.

Oxazolidinones

Two oxazolidinones, **linezolid** and **tedizolid**, are totally synthetic antimicrobial drugs.

Mechanism of action and antibacterial spectrum

The oxazolidinones have a unique mechanism of action by binding to the 50S ribosome subunit near the interface with the 30S subunit to prevent the initiation complex required for bacterial translation. This unique mechanism may possibly limit cross-resistance with other antibiotics. Linezolid is approved in the United States for the management of **vancomycin-resistant *E. faecium***; nosocomial and **community-acquired pneumonia** from *S. aureus* and penicillin-sensitive *S. pneumoniae*; and complicated **skin** and skin structure infections from MRSA, MSSA, methicillin-resistant CoNS, *S. pyogenes,* and *S. agalactiae*. Tedizolid has similar indications.

Bacterial resistance

Microbial resistance to linezolid has been detected in isolated cultures of vancomycin-resistant enterococci, *E. coli,* and laboratory strains of *S. aureus*. More recent reports of clinical isolates of *E. faecium* and *S. aureus* resistant to linezolid are disconcerting because the drug has been available only for a short time. The mechanism of resistance seems to be a 62,576T mutation in the gene encoding the central loop domain of 23S rRNA. Tedizolid may be active against certain strains of bacteria resistant to linezolid.

Absorption, fate, and excretion

Linezolid, with a near 100% oral bioavailability, produces peak blood levels at 1 to 2 hours and can be administered parenterally as well. It has an elimination half-life of 4.4 to 5.5 hours and a post-antibiotic effect of 0.6 to 1.4 hours. Tedizolid has a half-life of ~12 hours.

Adverse effects

Approximately 2% to 3% of patients receiving linezolid experience nausea and vomiting, diarrhea, headache, tongue discoloration, taste alteration, fungal superinfections, or very rarely PMC. The most serious adverse reaction is **myelosuppression** (anemia, leukopenia, pancytopenia, thrombocytopenia), which may occur in an average of 2.4% of patients. Linezolid requires weekly blood monitoring tests. The safety of the drug has not been established beyond 28 days of use. It is classified as an FDA pregnancy category C drug. Adverse effects of tedizolid are similar to those of linezolid.

Drug interactions

Linezolid is a weak monoamine oxidase inhibitor and should be used with caution with drugs that release catecholamines and foods containing tyramine. Linezolid may precipitate serotonin syndrome (confusion, agitation, seizures, hypertension, tachycardia, sweating, myoclonus, muscle rigidity, trismus, death), but the clinical significance of this drug effect is as yet unknown. GI disturbances, tachycardia, and hypertension are among the adverse effects associated with tedizolid.

Sulfonamides

The era of effective and safe systemic antimicrobial therapy began in 1932 with the discovery by Domagk that a dye (Prontosil) protected laboratory animals from streptococcal infections. Domagk determined that the active antibacterial portion of Prontosil was sulfanilamide, which was subsequently first used in the United States in 1935. **Trimethoprim** was introduced in 1968 as a synergistic agent **with sulfonamides**, and the combination of **sulfamethoxazole/trimethoprim** is the most commonly used sulfonamide preparation today. The discovery of Prontosil by Domagk ranks with the discovery of the anesthetic properties of nitrous oxide by Wells, the work on penicillin by the Oxford group, and the discovery by Jenner of vaccinations as among the greatest of all medical discoveries.

Chemistry

All the sulfonamides are derivatives of *p*-aminobenzenesulfonamide. Sulfonamides are weak acids with limited water solubility, particularly in solutions of low pH. This property may present problems for the excretion of these drugs in acidic urine.

Mechanism of action and antibacterial spectrum

Sulfonamides and trimethoprim **interfere** with the microbial **synthesis of folic acid** necessary for life in some microorganisms (Fig. 33-15). Mammals acquire folic acid from their diet. Sulfonamides competitively inhibit the incorporation of PABA into dihydropteroic acid, a precursor of dihydrofolate, because the sulfas have a greater affinity for **dihydropteroate synthetase** than PABA. Trimethoprim inhibits bacterial **dihydrofolate reductase** with 50,000 to 100,000 times greater affinity for the bacterial than the human enzyme; this blocks the conversion of dihydrofolic acid to tetrahydrofolic acid, which is important in the synthesis of purines, and DNA. Sulfonamides and trimethoprim inhibit successive steps in the synthesis of folic acid and eventually bacterial nucleotides and DNA.

The trimethoprim/sulfamethoxazole combination is commonly used for respiratory, urinary, and gastrointestinal infections. This combination is used for indications indicated in Table 33-14.

Bacterial resistance

Transferable microbial resistance to sulfonamides and trimethoprim occurs by three principal mechanisms: increased cell permeability barriers and efflux proteins, decreased sensitivity or alterations in target enzymes (dihydropteroate synthase and dihydrofolate reductase), and the acquisition of new target enzymes. Resistance genes for trimethoprim-sulfamethoxazole are carried on transposable elements along with the resistance genes for other antibacterial drugs.

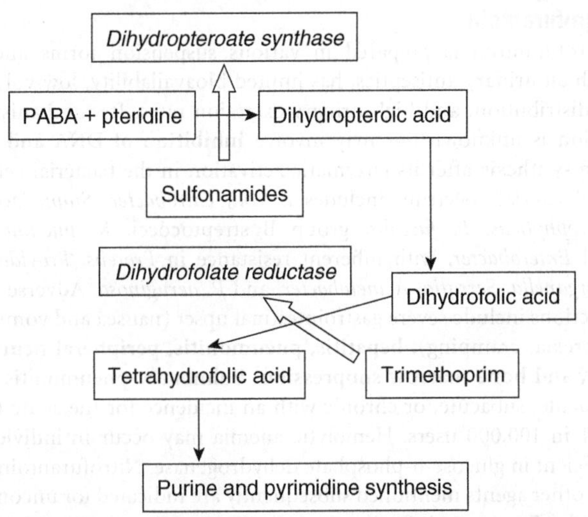

FIG 33-15 Sites of inhibition of folic acid synthesis by sulfonamides and trimethoprim. Note the effect of the two drugs on this common pathway and the effect on purine and pyrimidine synthesis. *PABA*, p-Aminobenzoic acid.

TABLE 33-14 Characteristics of Representative Sulfonamides*

Drug	Half-Life (hrs)	Route	Spectrum
Sulfisoxazole	~6	Oral	*Escherichia coli, Shigella, Yersinia enterocolitica, Burkholderia cepacia, Stenotrophomonas maltophilia, Nocardia, Moraxella catarrhalis,* MRSA, *Streptococcus pneumoniae, Listeria monocytogenes, Bartonella henselae, Brucella, Vibrio cholerae, Mycobacterium marinum, Burkholderia pseudomallei*
Trimethoprim/ sulfamethoxazole	~11/~11	Oral	
Mafenide	—	Topical (burns)	—
Silver sulfadiazine	—	Topical (burns)	—

Nocardia is an indication for sulfisoxazole alone.
*Antimicrobial spectrum corresponds to trimethoprim/sulfamethoxazole, except where noted.

Absorption, fate, and excretion

Sulfonamides are classified **as short-acting, medium-acting, or long-acting.** Short-acting to medium-acting agents include sulfisoxazole, sulfamethoxazole, sulfamethizole, and sulfadiazine. Sulfadoxine is a long-acting agent with an elimination half-life of 100 to 230 hours (it is used in combination with pyrimethamine to treat malaria caused by *Plasmodium falciparum*). Various other sulfonamide preparations include preparations used topically for burns (silver sulfadiazine, mafenide), vaginal preparations, ophthalmic preparations (sulfacetamide), and drugs for the management of ulcerative colitis (salicylazosulfapyridine or sulfasalazine) given orally for local gastrointestinal effects. Oral sulfonamides are 70% to 100% bioavailable (except for sulfasalazine) with a large volume of distribution and **ready penetration into all fluids** and tissues in the body including the CNS. The drugs are metabolized by acetylation and conjugation in the liver and excreted by glomerular filtration.

General therapeutic uses

The primary clinical uses of a sulfonamide alone or trimethoprim/sulfamethoxazole are **genitourinary tract infections, otitis media, acute bronchitis, community-acquired pneumonia, and traveler's diarrhea** from enterotoxigenic bacteria. Two topical sulfonamides, silver sulfadiazine and mafenide, are also used to treat burns. Other sulfonamides are used for ophthalmic and local gastrointestinal indications. There are no indications for sulfonamides and trimethoprim in the management of orofacial infections.

Adverse effects

Approximately 8% of individuals receiving sulfonamides and trimethoprim have some form of adverse reaction, such as nausea and vomiting, **blood dyscrasias**, and **crystalluria** (precipitation in the urine more likely with less soluble preparations such as sulfadiazine). Three to five percent of patients experience allergy in any of its forms from skin rash and pruritus to **major skin eruptions** (Stevens-Johnson syndrome, epidermal necrolysis, exfoliative dermatitis, photosensitivity) to anaphylaxis. Stevens-Johnson syndrome is much more likely to occur with long-acting sulfonamides, which are not available in the United States. Of patients with AIDS, 70% have some form of skin rash and fever from sulfonamides and trimethoprim.

Drug interactions

Trimethoprim and sulfamethoxazole work together synergistically in their antimicrobial effect, increasing the activity and spectrum of the other. Trimethoprim/sulfamethoxazole increases the clinical activity of oral anticoagulants, thiopental, methotrexate, hydantoins, and sulfonylureas, and it decreases the activity of cyclosporine. Sulfonamides are displaced from plasma protein by aspirin, other NSAIDs, and probenecid. PABA (present in some health foods) competes against the effect of sulfonamides.

Contraindications

Contraindications for the use of sulfonamides include **allergy** to sulfonamides and other related drugs, such as **sulfonylureas and thiazide, loop, and carbonic anhydrase inhibitor diuretics**. Health foods and possibly sunscreens containing PABA are contraindicated because PABA competes against the sulfonamide.

Chloramphenicol

Chloramphenicol (Chloromycetin) is a broad-spectrum antibiotic isolated in 1949 from *Streptomyces venezuelae.* It is bacteriostatic and **inhibits** bacterial **protein synthesis** by reversible binding to the peptidyl transferase component of the 50S ribosomal subunit.

Chloramphenicol is a **broad-spectrum antibiotic** whose spectrum includes several gram-positive and gram-negative bacteria, spirochetes, and *Rickettsiae.* Common pathogens sensitive to chloramphenicol include *Salmonella typhi,* other *Salmonella* species, *S. pneumoniae, H. influenzae,* and *N. meningitidis.* The drug is an alternate drug for serious infections such as bacterial meningitis and rickettsial diseases such as Rocky Mountain spotted fever.

The most significant adverse reactions associated with chloramphenicol are **reversible and irreversible bone marrow depression** seen with oral, parenteral, and even topical use. (The drug is absorbed well by any route.) The reversible type is dose-related and possibly caused by inhibition of mitochondrial protein synthesis resulting in anemia, leukopenia, or thrombocytopenia. "Idiosyncratic" bone marrow aplasia is not dose-related; may begin weeks or months after the drug is stopped; and is manifested by an often fatal aplastic anemia, the incidence of which seems to be 1 in 24,500 to 1 in 40,800 patients receiving chloramphenicol by any route of administration. This incidence is 13 times greater than the spontaneous random occurrence of aplastic anemia in the general population. Topical use is associated with a risk of 3 cases in 440,000 uses. The cause of this idiosyncratic **aplastic anemia** is unknown, but it may be due to a genetically determined liver metabolite.

The "**gray baby syndrome**" associated with chloramphenicol is caused by toxicity resulting from the inability of the immature liver of neonates to detoxify the drug by conjugation. The signs and symptoms include abdominal distress, cyanosis, vomiting, circulatory collapse, and possibly death. There are no indications for chloramphenicol in the management of orofacial infections. The drug is rarely used because of its major adverse effects, especially bone marrow aplasia.

Urinary Antiseptics

Nitrofurantoin

Nitrofurantoin is prepared in various suspension forms and, as with all urinary antiseptics, has limited bioavailability, low volumes of distribution, and high urinary excretion rates. Its mechanism of action is unknown but may involve **inhibition of DNA and protein synthesis** after its enzymatic activation in the bacterial cell. Its antibacterial spectrum includes *E. coli, Citrobacter, Staphylococcus saprophyticus, E. faecalis,* group B streptococci, *K. pneumoniae,* and *Enterobacter,* with inherent resistance in *Proteus, Providencia, Morganella, Serratia, Acinetobacter,* and *P. aeruginosa.* Adverse drug reactions include severe gastrointestinal upset (nausea and vomiting, anorexia, cramping), **hepatitis, pneumonitis, peripheral neuropathy, and bone marrow suppression.** Pulmonary pneumonitis may be acute, subacute, or chronic with an incidence for the acute form of 1 in 100,000 users. Hemolytic anemia may occur in individuals deficient in glucose-6-phosphate dehydrogenase. Nitrofurantoin and the other agents mentioned subsequently are indicated for uncomplicated urinary tract infections and cystitis.

Fosfomycin

Fosfomycin is a broad-spectrum bactericidal drug that is converted in the blood to the free acid form of fosfomycin. Its mechanism of action is to **inactivate enolpyruvyl transferase** responsible for the condensation of uridine diphosphate-N-acetylglucosamine with *p*-enolpyruvate, one of the initial steps in microbial **cell wall synthesis** (see Fig. 33-5). The antimicrobial spectrum for fosfomycin includes *E. coli, E. faecalis, Citrobacter, Enterobacter, K. pneumoniae, P. mirabilis,* and *S. marcescens.* Adverse reactions are mild and include diarrhea, vaginitis, rash, and headache. Use of fosfomycin is commonly restricted to only a single dose because of rapid microbial resistance.

Methenamine

The hydrolysis of methenamine, below pH 5.5, results in the liberation of **formaldehyde** as its component. This results in the denaturation of proteins. Methenamine, as the hippurate or mandelate salt to acidify the urine, has a broad spectrum of activity against *E. coli,* staphylococci, and enterococci, with significant resistance in *P. vulgaris* and *P. aeruginosa*. It is used as suppressive or prophylactic therapy in chronic urinary tract infections. Adverse reactions include pruritus, urticaria, nausea and vomiting, cramping, headache, dizziness, proteinuria, hematuria, and precipitation of urate crystals in the urine.

Nalidixic acid

This quinolone antibiotic is used exclusively for the management of urinary tract infections from **gram-negative microorganisms**. (See Table 33-12.) Its mechanism of action is the same as the fluoroquinolones: inhibition of DNA gyrase and topoisomerase IV. The major adverse effects are CNS toxicity (dizziness, weakness, headache, papilledema, and rare seizures and psychosis), blood dyscrasias, photosensitivity, and hemolytic anemia in glucose-6-phosphate dehydrogenase–deficient individuals.

Drugs Used to Treat Tuberculosis

Successful treatment of tuberculosis caused by *M. tuberculosis* became possible only with the advent of chemotherapeutic agents. Multidrug-resistant strains of *M. tuberculosis* have arisen, especially among patients with HIV/AIDS. Because of the rapid development of antimicrobial resistance in strains of *M. tuberculosis,* a combination of agents is always employed for treatment. The primary (first-line) antituberculosis drugs are **isoniazid, rifampin, pyrazinamide, ethambutol, and streptomycin.** (Rifabutin or rifapentine can be used to substitute for rifampin if needed.) (Depending on the reference, streptomycin is classified either as a first-line of second-line drug.) For recurrent infections or cases that exhibit microbial resistance, second-line drugs are available, including ethionamide, cycloserine, amikacin, kanamycin, capreomycin, levofloxacin, moxifloxacin, para-aminosalicylic acid, and bedaquiline. These agents are generally less active and often more toxic than the primary drugs. These drugs are used in combination for active tuberculosis that is drug-resistant.

Until the results of sensitivity tests dictate the regimen, tuberculosis therapy should begin with four drugs: isoniazid, rifampin, pyrazinamide, and ethambutol (or streptomycin) for 2 months, followed by 4 (or 7) months of isoniazid and rifampin. After test results, **typical therapy** consists of isoniazid, rifampin, and pyrazinamide for 2 months followed by isoniazid and rifampin for 4 months, or isoniazid and rifampin for 7 months, the length depending on whether there is a pulmonary cavity on the chest X-ray at presentation and/or a positive sputum culture observed after 2 months of therapy. Other treatment times are recommended for TB meningitis and TB osteomyelitis. Other drug options listed in Table 33-5 are available in multidrug-resistant tuberculosis. The pharmacologic features of isoniazid, rifampin, pyrazinamide, and ethambutol are described here. Streptomycin and other aminoglycoside antibiotics have been previously discussed.

Isoniazid

Isoniazid, the name of which derives from its chemical designation of isonicotinic acid hydrazide, is the most important drug for the treatment and prophylaxis of tuberculosis. Its spectrum of activity is limited, however, to *M. tuberculosis* and one species of atypical mycobacteria, *Mycobacterium kansasii.*

Isoniazid **inhibits the synthesis of mycolic acids**, unique and necessary components of the cell wall of mycobacteria. The drug is bactericidal to actively growing tubercle bacilli but not to dormant organisms. Resistance to isoniazid occurs by spontaneous mutation of the bacterial chromosome at a rate of ~1 in 10^6 divisions. Most established infections can be expected to harbor at least several resistant bacteria. There is no cross-resistance between isoniazid and other antituberculosis drugs except ethionamide.

Isoniazid is well absorbed after either oral or parenteral administration, but the oral route is preferred for reasons of convenience and maximum therapeutic effect. The drug is well distributed into all body fluids, including the caseous material of the tubercle-infected foci. Isoniazid is mainly metabolized in the liver and excreted in the urine as metabolites. Genetic differences in the rate of biotransformation are seen, but these seem to have little effect on therapeutic efficacy. The plasma half-life is prolonged in patients with hepatic dysfunction.

One important adverse reaction with isoniazid is **peripheral neuritis** caused by an isoniazid-induced increase in the excretion of pyridoxine. This adverse effect is more common in **slow acetylators.** This reaction and other symptoms of pyridoxine deficiency can be prevented by prophylactic administration of vitamin B_6 (15 to 50 mg daily). Other adverse effects include allergic reactions (fever, rashes, **hepatitis**), fatal hepatic necrosis (rarely), xerostomia, epigastric distress, hematologic reactions, and convulsions in seizure-prone patients (although administration of isoniazid to patients taking phenytoin has not been problematic except for the potential of pharmacokinetic effects on phenytoin metabolism). A nonallergic hepatitis of some severity has also been reported, and subsequent studies have shown that the incidence of hepatic damage increases with age and in individuals who regularly drink alcohol.

Isoniazid is **also** effective **prophylaxis** against tuberculosis and approved for single-drug therapy for prophylaxis. It is also the most important drug used in tuberculosis therapy for reasons of effectiveness, expense, convenience of administration, and relative safety.

Rifampin

Rifampin is a semisynthetic derivative of one of the rifamycins, a group of macrocyclic antibiotics produced by *Streptomyces mediterranei.* Rifampin is effective against numerous gram-positive and gram-negative bacteria in addition to *M. tuberculosis* and most other species of *Mycobacterium*. Its mechanism of action involves **inhibition of DNA-dependent RNA polymerase.** Mammalian RNA polymerase does not bind the drug, and RNA synthesis in host cells is unaffected. Resistance can develop rapidly to rifampin, frequently in a single step, by alteration of the target enzyme.

Rifampin is generally well absorbed from the gastrointestinal tract after oral administration. The drug is distributed throughout the body and imparts an **orange-red color to the urine**, saliva, sweat, tears, sputum, and feces. It is secreted in the bile and undergoes enterohepatic recirculation, prolonging its half-life. Elimination occurs by hepatic deacetylation and excretion in the urine and feces.

Rifampin may be useful in prophylaxis of tuberculosis in contacts of patients infected with isoniazid-resistant organisms. The drug has proven effective in certain diseases refractory to conventional therapy, such as rifampin in combination as an option in treating resistant *S. pneumoniae* and methicillin-resistant staphylococci.

The incidence of adverse reactions to rifampin is low (4%), and the most common is liver toxicity. Gastrointestinal disturbances, suppression of T-lymphocyte function, neurologic disorders, and various allergic reactions, including soreness of the mouth and tongue, have been reported. Decreased effectiveness of oral anticoagulants, **oral contraceptives,** estrogens, and glucocorticoids have occurred with concomitant administration of rifampin because rifampin induces liver microsomal enzymes. Oral contraceptives are not likely to be effective in a patient taking rifampin.

If rifampin is used sporadically, a flulike syndrome (possibly immune related) may develop, sometimes leading to renal failure, hepatorenal syndrome, hemolysis, and thrombocytopenia. The drug should be taken according to a prescribed regimen. Because rifampin can cause a reddish-orange color in body fluids, staining of soft contact lenses may occur.

Rifabutin

Rifabutin is chemically similar to rifampin and acts by a similar mechanism. Rifabutin is not as potent an inducer of cytochrome P450 enzymes as rifampin and offers the advantage of not interacting with other drugs to the extent that rifampin does. It is useful in treating patients who have HIV/AIDS because it has less interaction with protease inhibitors and non-nucleosidase reverse transcriptase inhibitors. Adverse effects include uveitis and neutropenia but are otherwise similar to those of rifampin.

Rifapentine

Rifapentine is a long-acting rifampin-type drug that has a similar mechanism of action and similar adverse effects. It can be used twice weekly for initial treatment and once weekly during the continuation phase of treatment.

Pyrazinamide

Pyrazinamide is the pyrazine analogue of nicotinamide. It is converted to pyrazinoic acid by bacterial pyrazinamidase. Pyrazinoic acid **inhibits mycolic acid synthesis**, and it disrupts cell wall function. It had widespread use in the 1960s but proved to be hepatotoxic in the doses used and was relegated to secondary status after the development of isoniazid and rifampin. More recently, pyrazinamide in reduced dosage has reemerged as the third most important anti-tuberculosis agent. Resistance to the drug in *M. tuberculosis* infection is associated with the loss of pyrazinamidase activity.

Pyrazinamide is well absorbed after oral administration and is distributed throughout the body. It is metabolized primarily in the liver and excreted largely in the urine.

Pyrazinamide is administered with other anti-tuberculosis drugs to decrease the duration of therapy required to effect a cure of uncomplicated tuberculosis. **Hepatotoxicity** is the most common adverse effect, but this has been less evident with the lower dosages currently used. Other toxic effects associated with current regimens are relatively benign or infrequent. Gastrointestinal disturbances, arthralgias, fever, and rash have been noted. Pyrazinamide may cause **hyperuricemia**, and the drug represents a risk in patients with gout.

Ethambutol

Ethambutol is a synthetic agent that **inhibits arabinosyl transferases**, which are important in cell wall synthesis of sensitive mycobacteria. It is active against *M. tuberculosis* and some other mycobacteria such as *M. kansasii*. Other bacteria are not affected by the drug. Ethambutol is tuberculostatic, and resistance develops, although slowly, if it is used alone.

Ethambutol is given orally because of good absorption from the gastrointestinal tract. Distribution into various body compartments is adequate. The major route of excretion of ethambutol is by renal tubular secretion and glomerular filtration, with the drug appearing in the urine mostly as unchanged drug and as two metabolites. Dosage adjustment is required in the presence of renal impairment.

Adverse reactions to ethambutol are infrequent, the most notable being **optic neuritis**, with symptoms of decreased visual acuity and loss of the ability to perceive the color green. Other adverse effects include gastrointestinal upset; peripheral neuritis; allergic reactions, usually appearing as skin rashes or drug fever; and increased retention of uric acid.

Second-line drugs

A number of **second-line drugs** are used to treat tuberculosis. These are useful in cases of resistance to first-line drugs and include ethionamide, capreomycin, kanamycin, amikacin, para-aminosalicylic acid (whose mechanism is similar to that of the sulfonamides), cycloserine (which inhibits cell wall synthesis), levofloxacin, moxifloxacin, and other fluoroquinolones.

Drugs Used to Treat Leprosy

Although leprosy is rarely seen in the United States, the World Health Organization estimates that 12 million cases exist throughout the world. Leprosy is a bacterial disease caused by the tubercle bacillus *Mycobacterium leprae*. Treatment may be 2 to 4 years or extend throughout the patient's life, depending on the severity and type of disease.

Dapsone is the major drug used in the treatment of leprosy. It belongs to a group of drugs called **sulfones,** which are chemical relatives of sulfonamides. **Dapsone** is bacteriostatic against *M. leprae,* with a mechanism of action similar to that of sulfonamides. Dapsone is used orally. Other drugs, normally used in combination with dapsone, are rifampin and clofazimine. Clarithromycin, minocycline, and ofloxacin may also be effective.

Topical Antibiotics

Bacitracin

Bacitracin is a polypeptide antibiotic derived from *B. subtilis* that functions to **block cell wall formation** by interfering with the dephosphorylation of the lipid compound that carries peptidoglycans to the growing microbial cell wall (see Fig. 33-5). The antibacterial spectrum of bacitracin **is gram positive** and includes staphylococci, streptococci, *Corynebacterium,* and *Clostridium,* with rare resistance seen in staphylococci. Bacitracin is too toxic to be used parenterally but is well tolerated topically. Bacitracin is commonly combined with neomycin and polymyxin B in over-the-counter topical antibiotic preparations, but evidence for efficacy is limited.

Neomycin

Neomycin is an **aminoglycoside** derived from *Streptomyces fradiae* and binds to the 30S ribosomal subunit to inactivate bacterial DNA polymerase and causes misreading of the genetic code to produce lethal proteins. Neomycin has a wide antibacterial spectrum against **gram-positive and gram-negative** bacteria, but it is ineffective against streptococci and *P. aeruginosa.*

Polymyxin B

Polymyxin B was isolated from *Bacillus polymyxa* and functions as a cationic detergent to disrupt the microbial cell membrane, causing a leak in cell constituents. Its spectrum is **gram negative,** and it is particularly useful against *P. aeruginosa.* The drug is not used parenterally because it commonly induces paresthesias, ataxia, and slurred speech.

Mupirocin

Mupirocin has a unique chemical structure composed of a short fatty acid chain linked to monic acid; it **inhibits bacterial RNA and protein synthesis** by binding to isoleucyl-tRNA synthetase to prevent incorporation of isoleucine into bacterial proteins. The antimicrobial spectrum for mupirocin includes staphylococci (MRSA, MSSA), streptococci, anaerobes, and Enterobacteriaceae. The primary use of mupirocin is as a topical application for skin infections, such as **impetigo** due to *S. aureus* or *S. pyogenes.* Mupirocin is also used to reduce or eliminate nasal carriage of staphylococci, particularly MRSA. Its widespread use is associated with an increase in the reinfection rate due to resistance development or reinfection from other body areas.

Retapamulin

Retapamulin belongs to a group of drugs called the **pleuromutilins**. The drug **inhibits protein synthesis** by binding to the 50S ribosomal subunit. Retapamulin inhibits *S. pyogenes* and *S. aureus* (methicillin susceptible). It also has activity against some gram-negative bacteria and many anaerobes. It is used to treat impetigo.

ANTIBACTERIAL ANTIBIOTICS*

Nonproprietary (Generic) Name	Proprietary (Trade) Name
Aminoglycosides	
Amikacin	Amikin
Gentamicin	Garamycin, Jenamicin
Kanamycin	Kantrex
Neomycin	Mycifradin
Netilmicin	Netromycin
Paromomycin	Humatin
Streptomycin	—
Tobramycin	Nebcin
Antituberculosis Drugs (Not Included Elsewhere in This List)	
Aminosalicylate sodium	Tubasal
Bedaquiline	Sirturo
Capreomycin	Capastat Sulfate
Cycloserine	Seromycin
Ethambutol	Myambutol
Ethionamide	Trecator
Isoniazid	Nydrazid
Pyrazinamide	—
Rifabutin	Mycobutin
Rifampin	Rifadin, Rimactane
Rifapentine	Priftin
Topical Antibiotics	
Bacitracin	Baciguent
Mupirocin	Bactroban
Neomycin	Myciguent
Polymyxin B	Aerosporin
Retapamulin	Altabax
Bacitracin with neomycin and polymyxin B	Neosporin
Miscellaneous Agents	
Chloramphenicol	Chloromycetin
Clofazimine	Lamprene
Colistimethate	Coly-Mycin M
Colistin	In Coly-Mycin S
Dalbavancin	Dalvance
Dapsone	
Daptomycin	Cubicin
Fidaxomicin	Dificid
Fosfomycin	Monurol
Lincomycin	Lincocin
Linezolid	Zyvox
Methenamine	Hiprex, Mandelamine, Urex
Metronidazole	Flagyl
Nitrofurantoin	Furadantin, Macrodantin
Oritavancin	Orbactiv
Quinupristin/dalfopristin	Synercid
Tedizolid	Sivextro
Telavancin	Vibativ
Telithromycin	Ketek
Tigecycline	Tygacil
Troleandomycin	TAO
Vancomycin	Vancocin

*Agents not shown here are listed in various tables throughout this chapter.

CASE DISCUSSION

The most likely diagnosis based on the age and circumstances of the patient is acute necrotizing ulcerative gingivitis (ANUG). The patient's chills and temperature indicate that she has signs of a systemic infection, most likely due to the spread of the oral infection. You do two things at the first appointment: (1) debridement and (2) prescribe amoxicillin 500 mg t.i.d. for 7 to 10 days. Although ANUG should be treated by local debridement, you reason that the antibacterial drug is needed to reduce the systemic involvement. Amoxicillin is an extended-spectrum penicillin.

When you begin debridement, the patient may complain of pain. As a result you may use mild ultrasonic scaling to remove some of the supragingival plaque in the first appointment. Before dismissing the patient, you give her instructions on good oral hygiene, proper diet, and, if the patient is a smoker, to enter a smoking cessation program. You instruct the patient to call in three days to check on progress. You find that the patient is much better in three days and then schedule a second appointment to complete the scaling and removal of plaque.

Adverse effects of amoxicillin or other penicillins include allergies that can range from mild to anaphylactic reactions. Amoxicillin is an extended-spectrum antibiotic. This could lead to a superinfection if given for several days. Amoxicillin is usually well tolerated.

GENERAL REFERENCES

1. Abramowicz M, Zuccotti G, editors: Handbook of antimicrobial drugs: drugs for bacterial infections. *The Medical Letter*, ed 20, New Rochelle, NY, 2015.
2. Albert RK, Schuller JL: Macrolide antibiotics and the risk of cardiac arrhythmias, *Am J Respir Crit Care Med* 189:1173–1180, 2014.
3. Bennett PM: Plasmid encoded antibiotic resistance: acquisition and transfer of antibiotic resistance genes in bacteria, *Br J Pharmacol* 153:S347–S357, 2008.
4. Bennett JE, Dolin R, Blaser MJ, editors: *Mandell, Douglas, and Bennett's principles and practice of infectious diseases*, ed 8, New York, Saunders, 2015, Elsevier.
5. Cho H, Uehara T, Bernhardt TG: Beta-lactam antibiotics induce a lethal malfunctioning of the bacterial cell wall, *Cell* 159:1300–1311, 2014.
6. Drugs for bacterial infections, *Med Letter* 11(131):65–74, 2013.
7. Drugs for tuberculosis, *Med Letter* 10(116):29–36, 2012.
8. Leffler DA, Lamont JT: *Clostridium difficile* infection, *N Engl J Med* 372:1539–1548, 2015.
9. Macy E: Penicillin and beta-lactam allergy: epidemiology and diagnosis, *Curr Allergy Asthma Rep* 14:476, 2014 (published online).
10. Salyers AA, Whitt DD: *Bacterial pathogenesis: a molecular approach*, ed 2, Washington, DC, 2002, ASM Press.

34

Antifungal and Antiviral Agents

No-Hee Park, Ki-Hyuk Shin, and Mo K. Kang

KEY INFORMATION

- Antifungal drugs can be used systemically or topically, depending on the drug.
- Antiviral drugs are used to treat influenza infections, ocular herpetic diseases, localized herpes infections, respiratory syncytial bronchitis and pneumonia, hepatitis B and C viral infections, and human immunodeficiency virus (HIV) infection.
- The drug groups available for treatment of HIV infections include nucleoside/nucleotide reverse transcriptase inhibitors, non-nucleoside reverse transcriptase inhibitors, protease inhibitors, integrase strand transfer inhibitors, entry inhibitors, and fusion inhibitors.
- Individuals with HIV infections receive a combination of antiretroviral drugs in an approach called highly active antiretroviral therapy (HAART).
- Herpes simplex virus causes a variety of mucosal lesions that can be treated with enteral acyclovir or topical penciclovir.

CASE STUDY

An 86-year-old patient has come to your office for a reline of her dentures. When you remove the maxillary denture, on the palate you notice white, raised patches that reveal a reddened tender area when they are lightly brushed away. What is your clinical diagnosis and how would you treat this condition?

Major fungal diseases and common causative organisms that are discussed as indications for antifungal drugs are aspergillosis (*Aspergillus fumigatus*), blastomycosis (*Blastomyces dermatitidis*), candidiasis (*Candida albicans*), coccidioidomycosis (*Coccidioides immitis*), cryptococcosis (*Cryptococcus neoformans*), histoplasmosis (*Histoplasma capsulatum*), mucormycosis (many Mucorales such as *Mucor* and *Rhizopus*), sporotrichosis (*Sporothrix schenckii*), and dermatophyte (skin) infections caused by *Epidermophyton, Trichophyton,* and *Microsporum.* Dermatophyte infections are often referred to as tinea infections and identified by the site of the infection (e.g., tinea pedis or athlete's foot).

Antifungal drugs are classified based on chemical category (listed with an example).

- Polyenes (Nystatin)
- Azoles (Itraconazole)
- Echinocandins (Caspofungin)
- Allylamines (Terbinafine)
- Pyrimidine (Flucytosine)
- Oxaborole (Tavaborole)
- Thiocarbamate (Tolnaftate)
- Miscellaneous (Ciclopirox)

ANTIFUNGAL AGENTS

Fungal diseases may take the form of superficial infections involving the skin or mucous membranes, or systemic (deep) infections involving various internal organs. Deep infections are treated with systemically administered drugs. The superficial mycoses, primarily of dermatophytes and *Candida* species, are generally managed with topical drugs. Topical agents considered in this chapter include those with activity against mucocutaneous infections caused by ***Candida albicans,*** the fungus most commonly observed in oral lesions. Often these infections are rather benign, as in denture stomatitis, but they may indicate a serious medical condition such as in immunodeficiency. The systemic fungal infections are subdivided into two groups according to the status of the patient and the type of infecting organism. **Opportunistic mycoses** occur in debilitated and immunocompromised patients, such as those with acquired immunodeficiency syndrome (AIDS), leukemia, or lymphoma, and in patients who are receiving immunosuppressive agents or broad-spectrum antibiotics. The fungi involved include *Candida, Aspergillus,* and *Cryptococcus* species and various Mucorales. They are particularly dangerous and carry a high mortality rate. **Endemic mycoses** are caused by various pathogens distributed unevenly throughout the world and have a relatively low incidence in temperate climates. Examples of endemic mycoses that occur in the United States include blastomycosis, histoplasmosis, coccidioidomycosis, and sporotrichosis.

Common antifungal drugs, their mechanisms of actions, and their indications are listed in Table 34-1. The mechanisms of action of four major drug groups are pictured in Figure 34-1.

POLYENE ANTIFUNGAL DRUGS

The polyene antifungal drugs consist primarily of **amphotericin B and nystatin,** which are a type of the earliest antifungal drugs that became available for clinical uses. These drugs demonstrate a wide spectrum of antifungal activity against common superficial and deep fungal infections, such as candidiasis, aspergillosis, mucormycosis, and cryptococcosis. The primary mode of their antifungal activity results from **binding to ergosterol,** a component of the cell membrane of sensitive fungi (see Fig. 34-1). This binding forms channels in the cell membrane, altering its permeability and causing leakage of Na^+, K^+, and H^+ ions. The polyenes also bind to a lesser extent to cholesterol of

TABLE 34-1 Mechanisms of Action and Clinical Uses of Antifungal Agents

Antifungal Agent	Mechanism of Action	Clinical Uses
Amphotericin B	Binding to ergosterol of fungal membrane	Topical: superficial candidiasis; intravenous: severe, progressive systemic fungal infection*
Nystatin	Binding to ergosterol of fungal membrane	Topical: oral candidiasis
Clotrimazole	Inhibition of ergosterol synthesis	Topical: oral candidiasis, superficial fungal infections†
Fluconazole	Inhibition of ergosterol synthesis	Oral: systemic and localized candidiasis, cryptococcal meningitis, systemic blastomycosis, and coccidioidomycosis
Itraconazole	Inhibition of ergosterol synthesis	Oral: systemic fungal infections,* dermatophyte infections
Miconazole	Inhibition of ergosterol synthesis	Topical: cutaneous candidiasis and vulvovaginitis, superficial fungal infections†
Flucytosine	Inhibition of nucleic acid synthesis	Oral: systemic candidiasis and cryptococcosis
Griseofulvin	Disruption of mitotic spindle	Oral: fungal infections of skin, hair, and nails
Caspofungin	Inhibition of fungal cell wall synthesis	Intravenous: severe, invasive aspergillosis; esophageal candidiasis, candidemia
Micafungin	Inhibition of fungal cell wall synthesis	Intravenous: prophylactic antifungal therapy in neutropenic HSCT patients, esophageal candidiasis, candidemia
Anidulafungin	Inhibition of fungal cell wall synthesis	Intravenous: esophageal candidiasis, candidemia
Tavaborole	Inhibition of amino-acyl-transfer RNA synthetase	Topical: onychomycosis

*Systemic fungal infections include aspergillosis, blastomycosis, candidiasis, chromomycosis, cryptococcosis, coccidioidomycosis, histoplasmosis, paracoccidioidomycosis, mucormycosis, and sporotrichosis. Indications for specific drugs vary.
†Superficial fungal infections caused by pathogenic dermatophytes and yeasts.
HSCT, Hematopoietic stem cell transplant.

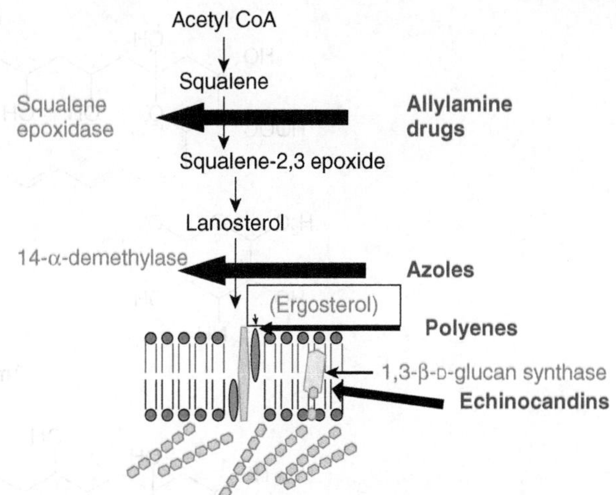

FIG 34-1 Mechanism of action of four classes of antifungal drugs. Allylamines, such as terbinafine, block the synthesis of squalene-2,3 epoxide by inhibiting squalene epoxidase. Azoles, such as itraconazole, block the synthesis of ergosterol by inhibiting 14-α-demethylase. Polyenes, such as amphotericin B, bind to ergosterol and form pores in the membrane. Echinocandins, such as caspofungin, block the synthesis of β(1-3) glucan for insertion into the cell wall by inhibiting 1,3-β-D-glucan synthase. Note that synthesis begins in the membrane to form 1,3-β-D-glucan polymers (bottom) which are crucial components of the cell wall. Other elements of the cell membrane and cell wall are not pictured.

mammalian plasma membrane, which accounts for most of the toxicity associated with their use. Resistance to the polyenes is associated with a replacement of ergosterol with other sterols in the fungal plasma membrane.

Amphotericin B

Amphotericin B is an antifungal agent obtained from *Streptomyces nodosus,* an actinomycetes found in the soil. It is a member of the polyene family of antibiotics, so-called because their structure contains a large lactone (macrolide) ring with numerous conjugated double bonds (Fig. 34-2). The polar hydroxylated portion and the nonpolar hydrocarbon sequence lend an amphophilic character to the molecule. The polyenes are unstable in solution because of the unsaturated chromophore region, which is easily photo-oxidized. Amphotericin B exerts either fungistatic or fungicidal activity depending on the concentration of the drug, the pH, and the fungus involved. Peak activity occurs at a pH between 6.0 and 7.5. Amphotericin B has a **broad spectrum** of antifungal activity and is effective against several fungal organisms including *Candida* species, *Histoplasma capsulatum, Cryptococcus neoformans, Blastomyces dermatitidis,* and *Coccidioides immitis.*

Amphotericin B is not absorbed from the skin or mucous membranes and is poorly and inconsistently absorbed from the gastrointestinal tract. Because of its insolubility in an aqueous media, the drug is reconstituted in a solution of the bile salt deoxycholate immediately before use. For systemic infections, amphotericin B is administered by **slow intravenous infusion** (over a period of 2 to 6 hours each day). The drug is bound in plasma to various lipoproteins and in tissues to cholesterol-containing membranes. Newer preparations (lipid formulations) for systemic use are the following: amphotericin B lipid complex, liposomal amphotericin B, and amphotericin B cholesteryl sulfate complex. The lipid formulations reduce the risk of nephrotoxicity but may provoke more acute toxicity upon IV infusion. The exact metabolic pathway of amphotericin B is not known, but most of the drug is biotransformed and then slowly excreted by the kidney over the next 2 months. Amphotericin B applied **topically** as a 3% cream, ointment, or lotion is useful in the treatment of superficial *Candida* infections. The only adverse effects accompanying the topical application or oral administration of amphotericin B are local irritation and mild gastrointestinal disturbances if swallowed. As an intravenous agent, however, **amphotericin B is the most toxic antifungal in current use. Intravenous amphotericin B causes many side effects** such as hypotension and delirium along with fever, nausea, vomiting, abdominal pain, anorexia, headache, and thrombophlebitis. Hypochromic, normocytic anemia is induced by amphotericin B, and leukopenia and thrombocytopenia occur rarely. Allergic reactions of all types have been reported, including anaphylaxis. All patients receiving intravenous amphotericin B show some degree of **nephrotoxicity**, which may lead to discontinuation of therapy. Permanent damage of the kidneys, however, does not normally occur in patients receiving a cumulative dosage of less than 4 g during a normal therapeutic interval

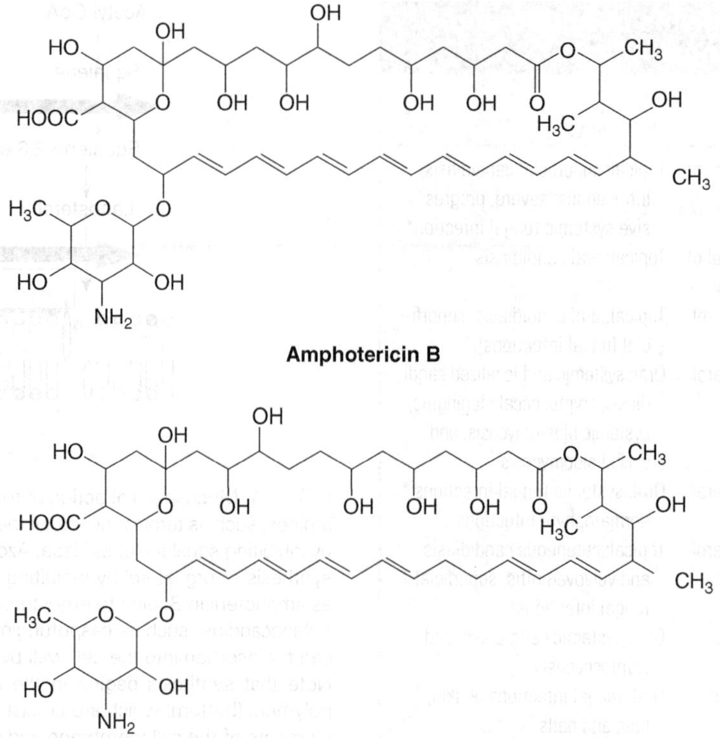

FIG 34-2 Structural formulas of polyene antifungal agents. Nystatin A_1 is one of three compounds found in the commercial nystatin preparation.

of several weeks. Great caution should be exercised when amphotericin B is used with other nephrotoxic drugs. Because amphotericin B can cause **hypokalemia**, it can increase digitalis toxicity. The toxic effects of cyclosporine may also be increased.

Nystatin

The nystatin structure is shown in Figure 34-2. Nystatin is relatively insoluble in water and unstable except as a dry powder.

Nystatin has a spectrum of activity slightly narrower than that of amphotericin B but is nevertheless active against a number of species of ***Candida***, *Histoplasma, Cryptococcus, Blastomyces,* and the dermatophytes *Epidermophyton, Trichophyton,* and *Microsporum.* As with amphotericin B, nystatin is either fungistatic or fungicidal depending on the concentration of the drug present, the pH of the surrounding medium, and the nature of the infecting organism. The mechanism of action of nystatin is also similar to that of amphotericin B. In vitro, some species of *Candida,* such as *C. tropicalis,* can develop resistance to nystatin, but resistance is rarely observed clinically.

Nystatin is not appreciably absorbed from the skin, mucous membranes, or gastrointestinal tract. After swallowing, the bulk of the administered dose appears unchanged in the feces. Because of unacceptable systemic toxicity, nystatin is not used parenterally. Nystatin is used primarily to treat candidal infections of the mucosa, skin, intestinal tract, and vagina. Although the efficacy of oral nystatin for enteric candidiasis has been questioned, topical nystatin remains a drug of choice for the treatment of **candidal infections of the oral cavity** (oral moniliasis, thrush, denture stomatitis) (Table 34-2). It has also been used prophylactically in immunocompromised patients. For the treatment of oral candidiasis, 2 to 3 mL of a suspension containing 100,000 units/mL of nystatin are placed in each side of the mouth, swished, and held for at least 5 minutes before swallowing. This regimen is repeated every 6 hours for at least 10 days or for 48 hours after remission of symptoms. Alternatively, one to two lozenges (200,000 units per each) may be used four to five times per day. For denture stomatitis, nystatin ointment (100,000 units/g) can be applied topically every 6 hours to the tissue surface of the denture. (Other treatments for oral candidiasis are shown in Table 34-2.) Nystatin is well tolerated. Only mild and transient gastrointestinal disturbances such as nausea, vomiting, and diarrhea have occurred after oral ingestion. The major complaint associated with nystatin is its bitter, foul taste.

TABLE 34-2 Treatment Strategies for Oral Candidiasis (Oral Thrush)*

Agent	Formulation	Dosage
Clotrimazole	Oral troches‡	10 mg orally, 5x/day, for 14 d
Nystatin	Oral suspension	4-6 mL (400,000-600,000 U), 4x/day until resolution
Miconazole	Buccal tablets‡	One 50-mg tab per day, placed on the gingiva of the canine fossa above tooth #8 and #9
Itraconazole†	Oral	200 mg daily, for 7-14 d
Fluconazole†	Oral	200 mg on day1, then 100 mg qd, for 14 d
Posaconazole†	Oral suspension	100 mg (2.5 mL) bid on day1, then 100 mg (2.5 mL) qd, for 13 d
Caspofungin†	IV solution	50 mg once/day for 7-14 d, or longer if more severe

*Doses are for adult patients.
†For more serious or extensive infections.
‡Remain in place until dissolved.

AZOLE ANTIFUNGAL DRUGS

The **imidazoles** and **triazoles** comprise the two azole groups of antifungal drugs. The antifungal spectrum of the azole antifungal drugs is broad, including yeasts, dermatophytes, and various species of *Candida, Histoplasma, Blastomyces, Aspergillus,* and *Sporothrix* species. The azoles inhibit the enzyme involved in the synthesis of fungal ergosterol (see Fig. 34-1). More specifically, one of the nitrogen atoms of the azole ring binds to the heme moiety of the fungal cytochrome P450 enzyme **lanosterol14-α-demethylase, thereby inhibiting the conversion of lanosterol to ergosterol**. The triazoles are more selective for the fungal cytochrome P450 enzymes than the imidazoles, accounting for the lower toxicity and fewer drug–drug interactions of the triazoles. The addition of 14-α-methyl sterols such as lanosterol, whose concentrations increase as a result of azole therapy, may disrupt cell membranes of the fungi, even in the presence of ergosterol. Other antifungal actions ascribed to the azole drugs, perhaps related to the changes caused by lanosterol, include inhibition of purine transport, interference with mitochondrial respiration, and alteration of the composition of non-sterol membrane lipids. Acquired resistance to the imidazoles is becoming more common, and it can develop in *C. albicans.* Refractory mucosal candidiasis in immunocompromised patients has been ascribed to the *Candida* species with cross-resistance to clotrimazole and other azole compounds. The structures of representative azoles are shown in Figure 34-3.

Ketoconazole

Ketoconazole is consider the prototype of this group. It **is not often used** for systemic purposes today because it has several adverse effects such as gynecomastia in males and menstrual irregularities in women due to inhibition of synthesis of testosterone and estradiol, respectively. It also inhibits the metabolism of several other drugs with potentially serious drug–drug interactions. Its topical uses are mentioned later.

Itraconazole

Itraconazole is a water-insoluble triazole compound that shows a broad spectrum of antifungal activity, and it is used for several systemic fungal infections. Itraconazole is well absorbed from the gastrointestinal tract when it is given with meals. It is highly bound to plasma proteins (more than 99%), and it has a long half-life (approximately 20 hours after a single dose, up to 60 hours at steady state). Although the concentrations of itraconazole in saliva and cerebrospinal fluid are negligible, tissue concentrations are two to five times higher than that of plasma. The drug is mostly metabolized in the liver and partially eliminated in the bile.

When given in therapeutic doses, itraconazole exerts effective antifungal activity against blastomycosis, histoplasmosis, sporotrichosis, candidiasis, onychomycosis, and other dermatophyte infections. It can be used systemically for **more severe candidiasis**. Itraconazole and related triazoles are more selective for fungal 14-α-demethylase and do

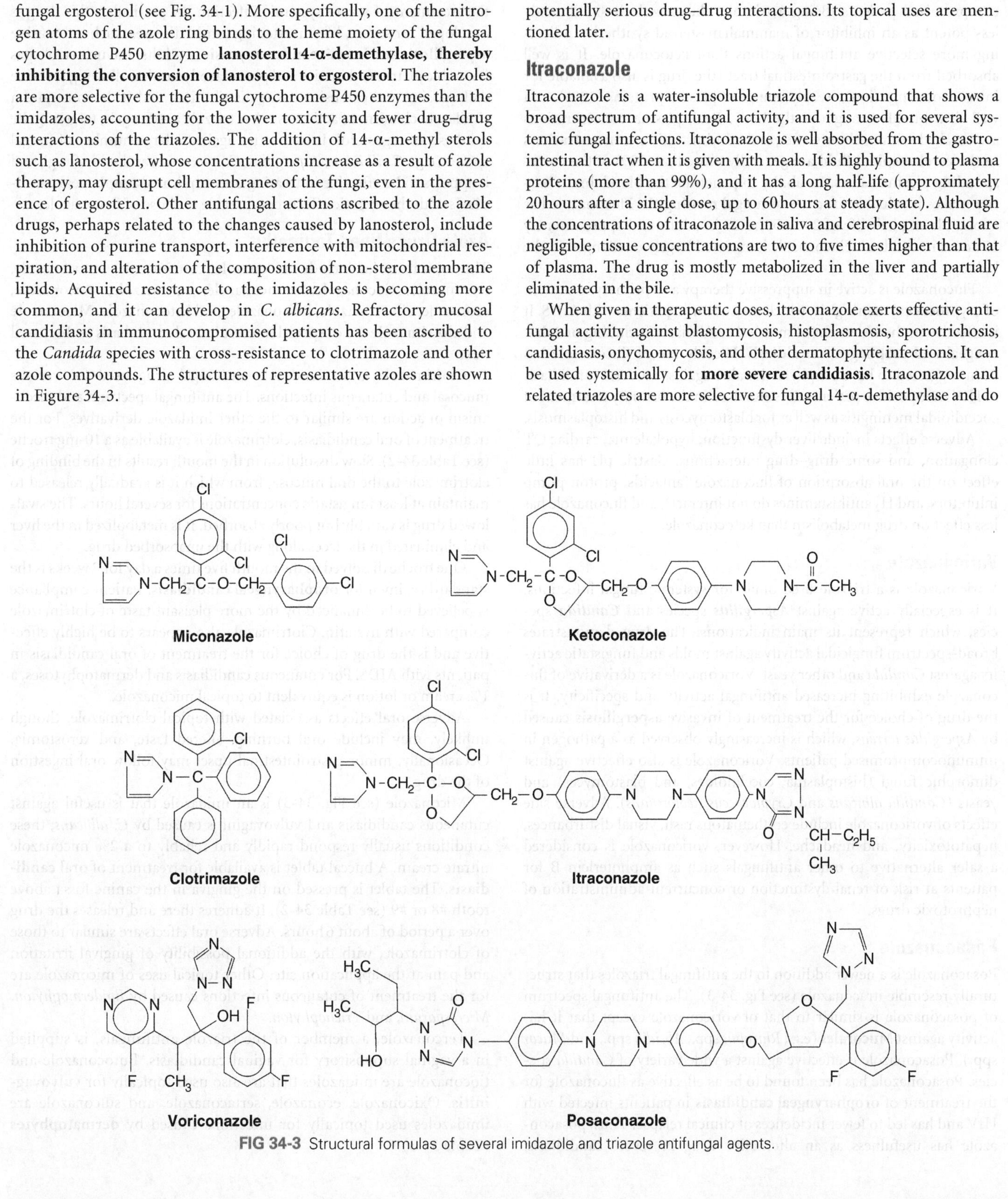

Miconazole

Ketoconazole

Clotrimazole

Itraconazole

Voriconazole

Posaconazole

FIG 34-3 Structural formulas of several imidazole and triazole antifungal agents.

not affect mammalian steroid metabolism as greatly as the imidazoles. Adverse effects include hypokalemia, liver dysfunction, rarely heart failure, and some drug–drug interactions.

Fluconazole

Fluconazole is a water-insoluble fluorine-substituted bistriazole with effective antifungal activity in immunocompetent and immunocompromised patients. Being a triazole, fluconazole is significantly less potent as an inhibitor of mammalian steroid synthesis, indicating more selective antifungal actions than ketoconazole. It is well absorbed from the gastrointestinal tract (the drug is also available for intravenous injection), weakly bound to plasma proteins (12%), and well distributed throughout the body. Peak plasma concentrations are reached within 2 hours after oral administration; **concentrations in the cerebrospinal fluid** are generally more than 50% of the corresponding plasma values. Its ability to penetrate the blood–brain barrier makes it valuable for cases of **fungal meningitis.** Fluconazole has a long plasma half-life of 20 to 50 hours in adults and approximately 17 hours in children. Fluconazole is excreted largely unchanged in the kidney.

Fluconazole is active in suppressive therapy and primary treatment of **cryptococcal meningitis**, which may occur in patients with AIDS. It is effective in the treatment of mucosal candidiasis, including **oropharyngeal and esophageal candidiasis.** Weekly use of fluconazole has been suggested to have prophylactic value against mucosal candidiasis in HIV-seropositive patients. It is also used in the primary treatment of coccidioidal meningitis as well as for blastomycosis and histoplasmosis.

Adverse effects include liver dysfunction, hypokalemia, cardiac QT elongation, and some drug–drug interactions. Gastric pH has little effect on the oral absorption of fluconazole (antacids, proton pump inhibitors, and H_2 antihistamines do not interact), and fluconazole has less effect on drug metabolism than ketoconazole.

Voriconazole

Voriconazole is a triazole used orally for systemic fungal infections. It is especially active against ***Aspergillus*** species and ***Candida*** species, which represent its main indications. The drug demonstrates broad-spectrum fungicidal activity against molds and fungistatic activity against *Candida* and other yeast. Voriconazole is a derivative of fluconazole exhibiting increased antifungal activity and specificity. It is the drug of choice for the treatment of invasive **aspergillosis** caused by *Aspergillus terreus*, which is increasingly observed as a pathogen in immunocompromised patients. Voriconazole is also effective against dimorphic fungi (histoplasma, coccidioides, and blastomyces) and yeasts (*Candida albicans* and *Cryptococcus neoformans*). Adverse side effects of voriconazole include erythematous rash, visual disturbances, hepatotoxicity, and headache. However, voriconazole is considered a safer alternative to other antifungals such as amphotericin B for patients at risk of renal dysfunction or concurrent administration of nephrotoxic drugs.

Posaconazole

Posaconazole is a newer addition to the antifungal triazoles that structurally resemble itraconazole (see Fig. 34-3). The antifungal spectrum of posaconazole is similar to that of voriconazole except that it has activity against **Mucorales** (e.g., *Rhizopus* spp., *Absidia* spp., and *Mucor* spp.). Posaconazole is effective against a wide variety of *Candida* species. Posaconazole has been found to be as effective as fluconazole for the treatment of **oropharyngeal candidiasis** in patients infected with HIV and has led to fewer incidences of clinical relapse. Thus, posaconazole has usefulness as an alternative drug in severe candidiasis. Posaconazole can cause fatigue, nausea, diarrhea, hepatic toxicity, and prolongation of the QT interval.

Isavuconazole

Isavuconazole is the newest addition to the triazole antifungals, approved by the U.S. Food and Drug Administration (FDA) in March 2015, and it represents a broad-spectrum, water-soluble triazole for the treatment of severe systemic infection. In particular, this drug is developed for severe, life-threatening fungal diseases, such as **invasive aspergillosis and invasive mucormycosis** in adults. Isavuconazole has favorable pharmacokinetics and pharmacodynamics, allowing for once daily dosing and extensive tissue distribution, and it demonstrates a similar mechanism of action as other triazole antifungals, targeting the synthesis of ergosterol. It is effective against a large number of fungal species, e.g., ***C. albicans,*** *Aspergillus*, *Cryptococcus*, and other fungi, and it appears to be effective in treating uncomplicated **esophageal candidiasis** with therapeutic effects comparable to those of fluconazole.

Azole Drugs Used Topically

The topical azoles include miconazole, clotrimazole, butoconazole, terconazole, tioconazole, sertaconazole, sulconazole, oxiconazole, econazole, efinaconazole, luliconazole, and ketoconazole. **Miconazole** and **clotrimazole** are of special interest in oral candidiasis as discussed next.

Clotrimazole is an imidazole antifungal drug used for various mucosal and cutaneous infections. The antifungal spectrum and mechanism of action are similar to the other imidazole derivatives. For the treatment of oral candidiasis, clotrimazole is available as a 10-mg troche (see Table 34-2). Slow dissolution in the mouth results in the binding of clotrimazole to the oral mucosa, from which it is gradually released to maintain at least fungistatic concentrations for several hours. The swallowed drug is variably but poorly absorbed. It is metabolized in the liver and eliminated in the feces along with the unabsorbed drug.

One troche dissolved in the mouth five times a day for 2 weeks is the standard regimen for **oropharyngeal candidiasis**. Patient compliance is believed to be enhanced by the more pleasant taste of clotrimazole compared with nystatin. Clotrimazole also appears to be highly effective and is the drug of choice for the treatment of oral candidiasis in patients with AIDS. For cutaneous candidiasis and dermatophytoses, a 1% cream or lotion is equivalent to topical miconazole.

Adverse oral effects associated with topical clotrimazole, though unlikely, may include oral burning, altered taste, and xerostomia. Occasionally, minor gastrointestinal upset may follow oral ingestion of the drug.

Miconazole (see Fig. 34-3) is an imidazole that is useful against cutaneous candidiasis and vulvovaginitis caused by *C. albicans*; these conditions usually respond rapidly and reliably to a 2% miconazole nitrate cream. A buccal tablet is available for treatment of **oral candidiasis.** The tablet is pressed on the gingiva in the canine fossa above tooth #8 or #9 (see Table 34-2). It adheres there and releases the drug over a period of about 6 hours. Adverse oral effects are similar to those of clotrimazole, with the additional possibility of gingival irritation and pain at the application site. Other topical uses of miconazole are for the treatment of cutaneous infections caused by *Epidermophyton, Microsporum,* and *Trichophyton.*

Terconazole, a member of the triazole antifungals, is supplied in a vaginal suppository for vaginal candidiasis. Butoconazole and tioconazole are imidazoles that are also used topically for **vulvovaginitis.** Oxiconazole, econazole, sertaconazole, and sulconazole are imidazoles used topically for infections caused by **dermatophytes** (Table 34-3).

TABLE 34-3 Topical Use of Antifungal Drugs

Class	Drug	Indications	Preparation
Polyene	Nystatin	Candidiasis	Oral rinse, cream, powder, ointment
	Amphotericin B	Cornea, bladder infections	Drops, irrigation
Azole	Miconazole	Candidiasis, tinea infections	Buccal tablet, cream
	Clotrimazole	Candidiasis	Oral troche
	Efinaconazole	Onychomycosis	Solution
	Econazole	Candidiasis, tinea infections	Cream, foam
	Butoconazole	Candidiasis	Cream
	Tioconazole	Candidiasis	Ointment
	Terconazole	Candidiasis	Cream, vaginal suppository
	Oxiconazole	Tinea infections	Cream, lotion
	Sertaconazole	Tinea infections	Cream
	Sulconazole	Tinea infections	Solution
	Luliconazole	Tinea infections	Cream
	Ketoconazole	Tinea infections, candidiasis	Cream, foam
Allylamine	Naftifine	Tinea pedis	Gel, cream
Benzylamine	Butenafine	Tinea infections	Cream
Oxaborole	Tavaborole	Onychomycosis	Solution
Hydroxypyrimidine	Ciclopirox	Tinea infections, candidiasis	Gel, cream, lotion, shampoo
Thiocarbamate	Tolnaftate	Tinea infections	Cream

Tinea infections include tinea pedis, tinea cruris, and tinea corporis. Onychomycosis is infection of the nail bed; toenails most common.

Efinaconazole, a triazole, is used for the treatment of **onychomycosis** and other superficial fungal infections. Efinaconazole is effective against a broad spectrum of fungal species, including *Candida* and *Aspergillus*. There may be extended therapeutic use of this drug beyond onychomycosis in the future.

Luliconazole, an imidazole, is approved for the treatment of tinea infections (see Table 34-3).

Ketoconazole is also used occasionally for tinea infections. It has use in treating certain cases of seborrheic dermatitis.

ECHINOCANDIN ANTIFUNGAL DRUGS

The echinocandins represent a unique class of antifungal drugs (Fig. 34-4) with distinct mechanism of drug action that involves noncompetitive inhibition of synthesis of 1,3-β-D-glucan components of fungal cell walls by **inhibiting 1,3-β-D-glucan synthase** (see Fig. 34-1). The 1,3-β-D-glucan linkages are critical for fungal cell wall synthesis and maintaining the osmotic balance. The echinocandins currently available for clinical uses include caspofungin, micafungin, and anidulafungin. The echinocandins are especially useful for candidal esophagitis and candidemia, *Aspergillus* infections, empirical treatments of febrile neutropenia, and for antifungal **prophylaxis in hematopoietic stem cell transplant** (HSCT) **recipients.**

Caspofungin

Caspofungin is derived from the fermented by-product of *Glarea lozoyenisi*. It is the first of the echinocandins approved by the FDA

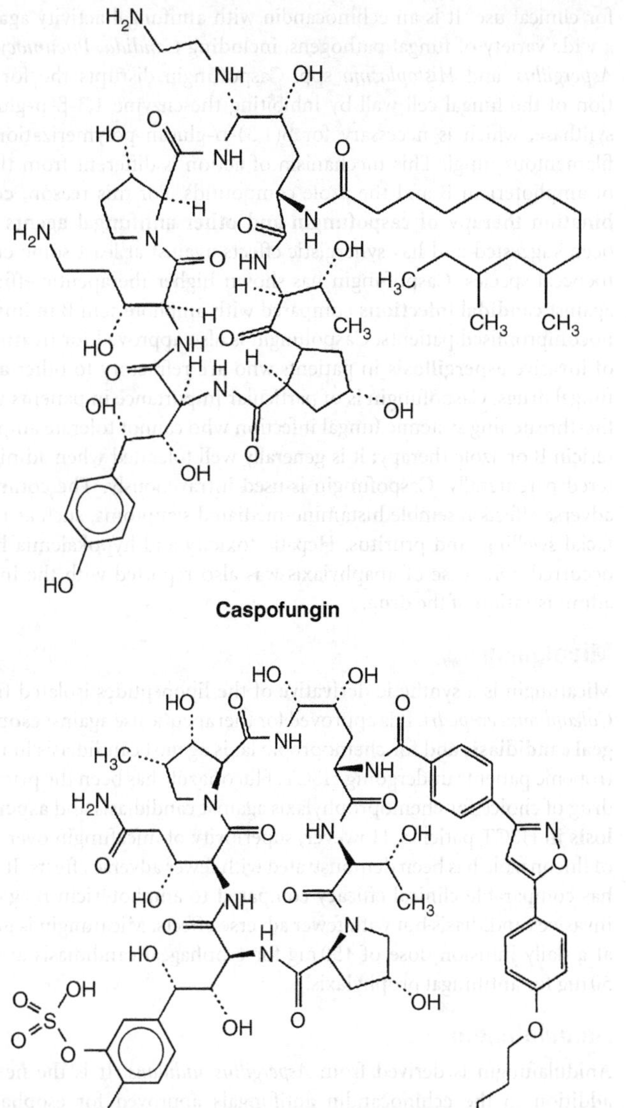

Caspofungin

Micafungin

Anidulafungin

FIG 34-4 Structural formula of echinocandin antifungals.

for clinical use. It is an echinocandin with antifungal activity against a wide variety of fungal pathogens, including *Candida, Pneumocystis, Aspergillus,* and *Histoplasma* spp. Caspofungin disrupts the formation of the fungal cell wall by inhibiting the enzyme 1,3-β-D-glucan synthase, which is necessary for β(1,3)-D-glucan polymerization in filamentous fungi. This mechanism of action is different from those of amphotericin B and the azole compounds. For this reason, **combination therapy of caspofungin and other antifungal agents** has been suggested and has synergistic effects against at least some cryptococcal species. Caspofungin has shown higher therapeutic efficacy against **candidal infections** compared with amphotericin B in immunocompromised patients. Caspofungin is also approved for treatment of invasive **aspergillosis** in patients who are refractory to other antifungal drugs. Caspofungin is of particular importance in patients with life-threatening systemic fungal infection who cannot tolerate amphotericin B or azole therapy; it is generally well tolerated when administered parenterally. Caspofungin is used intravenously. The common adverse effects resemble histamine-mediated symptoms, such as rash, facial swelling, and pruritus. Hepatic toxicity and hypokalemia have occurred. One case of anaphylaxis was also reported with the initial administration of the drug.

Micafungin

Micafungin is a synthetic derivative of the lipopeptides isolated from *Coleophoma empedri*. It is approved for therapeutic use against **esophageal candidiasis** and for chemoprophylaxis against candidiasis in neutropenic patients undergoing HSCT. Fluconazole has been the primary drug of choice for chemoprophylaxis against candidiasis and **aspergillosis** in HSCT patients. However, superiority of micafungin over that of fluconazole has been demonstrated with fewer adverse effects. It also has comparable clinical efficacy compared to amphotericin B against invasive candidiasis but with fewer adverse effects. Micafungin is given at a daily infusion dose of 150 mg for esophageal candidiasis and of 50 mg for antifungal prophylaxis.

Anidulafungin

Anidulafungin is derived from *Aspergillus nidulans*. It is the newest addition to the echinocandin antifungals approved for esophageal candidiasis, candidemia, and invasive candidiasis. Anidulafungin has potent and broad antifungal activity against *Candida* and *Aspergillus* spp., including those resistant to fluconazole. Compared with azole antifungals, anidulafungin is more effective in vitro against ***C. albicans***, *C. tropicalis, C. glabrata,* and *C. krussei*, but not *C. famata* and *C. parapsilosis*. Anidulafungin appears to be more effective than caspofungin against ***Aspergillus***. Large-scale clinical trials confirmed the therapeutic efficacy of anidulafungin against invasive candidiasis and its non-inferiority compared to fluconazole. Anidulafungin is given by intravenous infusion with 100-mg daily maintenance dose for invasive candidiasis and 50-mg daily dose for esophageal candidiasis. A loading dose is also recommended for the first day of treatment.

OTHER ANTIFUNGAL DRUGS

In addition to the aforementioned antifungal drugs, several other antifungal drugs with different and unique mechanisms of action are discussed next. They include flucytosine, thiocarbamate (tolnaftate), allylamines (naftifine and terbinafine), benzylamine (butenafine), oxaborole (tavaborole), and griseofulvin. Flucytosine is used in combination therapy for severe systemic mycosis. The thiocarbamate, allylamines, benzylamine, tavaborole, and griseofulvin are primarily indicated for dermatophytosis.

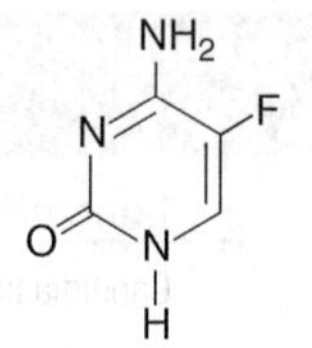

Flucytosine

FIG 34-5 Structural formula of flucytosine.

Flucytosine

Flucytosine, a fluorinated analogus of cytosine (5-fluorocytosine, Fig. 34-5), is a synthetic antimycotic agent orally effective in the treatment of systemic fungal infections, in particular those caused by yeasts. Flucytosine has a limited antifungal spectrum and is mainly effective against *Candida* and *Cryptococcus*. It is also active against some species of *Cladosporium* and *Phialophora*, the latter being etiologic agents for chromoblastomycosis.

Flucytosine is taken up within sensitive fungal cells by cytosine permease, which converts it **to 5-fluorouracil. The 5-fluorouracil is then further metabolized to yield 5-fluorodeoxyuridine monophosphate, a competitive inhibitor of thymidylate synthetase.** The formation of thymidine monophosphate from deoxyuridine monophosphate is thus blocked and the synthesis of DNA impaired. 5-Fluorouridine triphosphate is also formed in fungal cells, leading to the synthesis of defective RNA. Selective toxicity for fungus is achieved with flucytosine because mammalian cells do not readily take up the drug or convert it to 5-fluorouracil.

Flucytosine is indicated for the treatment of **systemic candidiasis and cryptococcosis**; however, resistance to flucytosine frequently develops during therapy of these infections. Mechanisms of resistance include decreased flucytosine uptake by fungal cells (altered permease) and decreased synthesis of the active nucleotide metabolites (decreased deaminase and other enzyme activities). Flucytosine is therefore normally used in **combination with amphotericin B**, which appears to increase fungal uptake of flucytosine and to result in synergistic effects against certain fungal diseases. Perhaps more importantly, coadministration permits reduction in the dose of amphotericin B.

Flucytosine is well absorbed from the gastrointestinal tract, and the peak plasma concentration is attained within 1 to 2 hours after oral administration. The drug is widely distributed throughout the body; it attains a **concentration in cerebrospinal fluid approximately 65% to 90% that of the plasma.** Flucytosine has a half-life of 3 to 6 hours and is excreted unchanged in the urine.

The major toxicity of flucytosine is depression of the bone marrow, resulting in anemia, leukopenia, and thrombocytopenia. This effect is dose related and is reversible. Because flucytosine is excreted mainly through the kidneys, it is advisable to measure the plasma concentration of the drug periodically, especially because it is normally given with the highly nephrotoxic amphotericin B. An elevation of hepatic enzymes in plasma and hepatomegaly occurs in approximately 5% of patients receiving flucytosine. Last, flucytosine may cause nausea, vomiting, diarrhea, and (rarely) severe enterocolitis. These toxic effects may result from the formation and release of 5-fluorouracil by fungi and intestinal microbes.

Allylamine and Benzylamine Antifungal Drugs

The allylamines used as antifungals are **naftifine** and **terbinafine.** Terbinafine is effective against **dermatophytes** (*Microsporum, Trichophyton,* and *Epidermophyton* spp.) and molds (e.g., *Aspergillus* spp.). The allylamines inhibit squalene epoxidase, important in the synthesis of ergosterol (see Fig. 34-1). The accumulation of toxic concentrations of squalene may contribute in large measure to their effectiveness against fungi. The allylamine drugs are used effectively for dermatophytosis of skin and nails. Both drugs are used topically; terbinafine is also given orally for systemic absorption. Terbinafine is highly lipophilic and keratophilic, and thus it accumulates in the stratum corneum of skin and nails. The adverse effects of terbinafine include mild and transient forms of gastrointestinal symptoms, rash, urticaria, and pruritus, but the drug is generally well tolerated.

Butenafine is a benzylamine drug that has the same mechanism of action as the allylamines. It is used topically for the treatment of **dermatophytes.**

Tavaborole

Tavaborole is an oxaborole. The drug **inhibits aminoacyl-transfer ribonucleic acid (tRNA) synthetase**, which is essential in fungal protein synthesis. This mechanism is unique among the antifungal drugs. Tavaborole is used topically to treat onychomycosis, although its spectrum includes fungi other than dermatophytes.

Tolnaftate

Tolnaftate, **a thiocarbamate**, is commonly used as a topical antifungal agent against mild to moderate superficial **dermatophyte** fungal infection in skin and toenails, such as tinea pedis, tinea cruris, tinea corporis, tinea manuum, and tinea versicolor. Tolnaftate is generally not effective against yeasts, such as *C. albicans*. Adverse effects associated with the topical use of tolnaftate are generally mild and may involve allergic contact dermatitis. The mechanism of action may partially involve inhibition of fungal squalene epoxidase. The drug alters hyphae and inhibits mycelial growth in fungi.

Ciclopirox

Ciclopirox is a broad-spectrum hydroxypyrimidine derivative used for dermal infections. It is used topically (see Table 34-3).

Griseofulvin

Griseofulvin is a drug used to treat dermatophytes. It is given orally and absorbed systemically resulting in deposition in keratin precursor cells, where it exerts its antifungal effects. It acts by inhibiting mitosis. It has been largely replaced by other drugs used in the treatment of dermatophyte infections.

TREATMENT OF ORAL CANDIDIASIS

Candidiasis is by far the most common type of oral fungal infection. Regardless of which drug is used, therapy for 2 weeks is required, as summarized in Table 34-2. Even more extended treatment may be necessary. **Clotrimazole**, in the form of oral troches, is highly effective in most cases. On swallowing, however, clotrimazole can cause an increase in plasma concentrations of hepatic enzymes and may rarely lead to hepatitis. **Nystatin** oral pastilles or rinses are also effective. A third choice is a **miconazole** tablet that adheres to the gingiva, releasing the drug (see Table 34-2). For more extensive disease or difficult cases, such as patients with AIDS, systemic antifungal therapy may be indicated. Itraconazole, fluconazole, posaconazole, and caspofungin are systemic choices, as indicated in Table 34-2. In extreme cases, intravenous amphotericin B with or without flucytosine may be considered. The toxicity of amphotericin B must be carefully weighed, and consultation with a specialist in infectious disease is essential. Surgery may be helpful to remove a condensed lesion after medical therapy.

ANTIVIRAL AGENTS

Advances in the pharmacologic control of viral infections have lagged behind achievements in the chemotherapy of other microbial diseases. The reason for this delay, which applies as well to the therapeutic management of neoplastic disorders, has been the difficulty in attaining an antiviral agent with an adequate degree of selective toxicity. Indeed, when the First Conference on Antiviral Agents, sponsored by the New York Academy of Sciences, was held in 1965, there were no more than a half-dozen scientists in the United States who believed that safe and effective antiviral agents could be identified. Because the replication of viruses was known to use metabolic machinery essential for the function of normal cells, it seemed to be nearly impossible to find antiviral agents that would inhibit viral growth without killing the host. Since then, however, many molecular events unique to viral replication have been identified and exploited in the development of selective antiviral agents. Potential points of attack include virus-encoded enzymes and other proteins that appear during viral replication and are different from corresponding cellular enzymes in noninfected cells. Endogenous mediators of antiviral immunity are another potential source of antiviral compounds. Thus, although the issue of selective toxicity of antiviral agents still remains a major challenge, there is now considerable optimism for the future of viral therapeutics, and many safe and effective antiviral agents have been introduced.

More than 32 antiviral agents have been approved for clinical use by the FDA. These drugs include **(1)** oseltamivir, zanamivir, and peramivir for prophylaxis and treatment of influenza A and B infections; **(2)** idoxuridine, vidarabine, and trifluridine for ocular herpetic diseases; **(3)** acyclovir, valacyclovir, penciclovir, famciclovir, docosanol, ganciclovir, foscarnet, cidofovir, and fomivirsen for various systemic and localized herpes infections (e.g., recurrent herpes labialis, oral hairy leukoplakia, cytomegaloviral retinitis, etc.); **(4)** ribavirin, a broad-spectrum agent used to treat respiratory syncytial bronchitis and pneumonia; **(5)** peginterferon, lamivudine, adefovir, entecavir, telbivudine, and tenofovir for chronic hepatitis B viral infection; peginterferon, ribavirin, telaprevir, boceprevir, simeprevir, and sofosbuvir for the treatment of chronic hepatitis C infections; and **(6)** six classes of antiviral agents for the control of HIV infection. Examples of adverse effects of antiviral drugs are in Table 34-4.

Anti-Influenza Viral Agents

Replicative cycles of **influenza virus, a representative RNA virus**, have been extensively studied during the past three decades. After penetrating into the cytoplasm of cells through endocytosis, the viral M2 protein induces an influx of hydrogen ion into the virion from the cytoplasm of the infected cells, resulting in uncoating of virion. This uncoating process induces the release of viral ribonucleoprotein (RNP) complex into the cytoplasm. Then the viral RNAs (vRNAs) enter nuclei of cells and began to replicate, making progeny vRNAs and expressing mRNAs for making structural and nonstructural proteins of the virus. These genomic vRNAs and proteins are assembled to produce virions, which are eventually released from the infected cells. Several antivirals have been developed to disrupt this replicative cycle for the treatment and prophylaxis of influenza caused by influenza virus type A or B. For example, amantadine and rimantadine inhibit the function of M2 protein, and in doing so, they prevent the **uncoating** process of the virus. Oseltamivir, zanamivir, and peramivir are known to inhibit the activity of viral **neuraminidase**, resulting in blocking the release of progeny virus from the infected cells. The primary antiviral spectrum, mechanism of action, and clinical uses of anti-influenza viral agents are listed in Table 34-5.

TABLE 34-4 Some Adverse Effects of Representative Antiviral Drugs

Drug Class	Drug	Side Effect
Anti-influenza drugs	Amantadine	GI effects, insomnia, nervousness
	Oseltamivir	GI effects, headache
Anti-herpes drugs	Acyclovir	GI effects, malaise, fever, headache
	Ganciclovir	GI adverse effects, leukopenia, myelosuppression, peripheral neuropathy
	Foscarnet	Nephrotoxicity, GI adverse effects, fever, anemia
Anti-respiratory syncytial virus drug	Ribavirin	Dysgeusia, insomnia, hemolytic anemia
Antiviral hepatitis (HBV and HCV) drugs	Entecavir (anti-HBV)	Fatigue, nausea, headache, lactic acidosis with fatty liver
	Sofosbuvir (anti-HCV)	Fatigue and headache
	Boceprevir (protease inhibitor for HCV)	Headache, dysgeusia, GI symptoms, anemia, neutropenia, pancytopenia
Anti-HIV drugs	Didanosine (NRTI)	Mitochondrial damage, lactic acidosis with fatty liver, peripheral neuropathy, anemia, myopathy, pancreatitis
	Stavudine (NRTI)	Mitochondrial damage, anemia myopathy, lactic acidosis with fatty liver, peripheral neuropathy, hyperlipidemia
	Efavirenz (NNRTI)	GI symptoms, rash, adverse effects on CNS, liver abnormalities
	Nevirapine (NNRTI)	GI symptoms, rash, headache, hepatitis
	Tipranavir (protease inhibitor)	GI symptoms, rash, hyperlipidemia, liver toxicity, prolongation of PR and QT intervals
	Indinavir (protease inhibitor)	GI symptoms, nephrolithiasis, blurred vision, weakness, prolongation of PR and QT intervals
	Raltegravir (ISTI)	Insomnia, GI symptoms, increase in liver enzymes and creatine kinase
	Maraviroc (entry inhibitor)	GI symptoms, muscle pain, cough, increase in liver enzymes and creatine kinase
	Enfuvirtide (fusion inhibitor)	Pneumonia, hypersensitivity reactions

NRTI, Nucleoside and nucleotide reverse transcriptase inhibitors; *NNRTI*, non-nucleoside and nucleotide reverse transcriptase inhibitors; *ISTI*, integrase strand transfer inhibitor.

TABLE 34-5 Antiviral Spectrum, Mechanisms of Action, and Clinical Uses of Anti-Influenza Viral Agents

Generic Name	Trade Name	Primary Antiviral Spectrum	Mechanism of Action	Clinical Uses
Amantadine	Symmetrel	Influenza A virus	Blockade of uncoating process	Prophylaxis of influenza A infection
Rimantadine	Flumadine	Influenza A virus	Blockade of uncoating process	Prophylaxis of influenza A infection
Oseltamivir	Tamiflu	Influenza A and B virus	Inhibition of viral neuraminidase activity	Prophylaxis and treatment of influenza A and B virus infection
Zanamivir	Relenza	Influenza A and B virus	Inhibition of viral neuraminidase activity	Prophylaxis and treatment of influenza A and B virus infection
Peramivir	Rapivab	Influenza A and B virus	Inhibition of viral neuraminidase activity	Prophylaxis and treatment of influenza A and B virus infection
Vaccine*		Influenza A and B virus	Antibody production	Prophylaxis of influenza A and B virus infection

*There are two types of influenza vaccines in the United States: (1) trivalent inactivated vaccine and (2) a live-attenuated intranasal vaccine. Vaccines are recommended for pregnant women, individuals over 50 years old, persons over 5 years old with chronic medical conditions, caregivers of children under 6 years old, and health care workers. In general, approximately two weeks after immunization, antibodies against influenza virus will reach a protective level and persist for 6 months. A significant proportion of individuals receiving the live-attenuated vaccine will shed vaccine-strain viruses, but the peak titer is below the infectious dose.

Anti-Herpetic Agents

A number of different **herpesviruses** cause diseases in humans. Among them, herpes simplex virus (HSV), varicella zoster virus (VZV), and cytomegalovirus (CMV) are major herpes viruses that cause a variety of infections. They are **DNA viruses.** The viral replication and reproduction in cells are very well known, as depicted in Figure 34-6. HSV causes diseases in the orofacial area, eyes, skin, genital organs, and brain, such as primary herpes stomatitis, recurrent herpes labialis (RHL), herpes keratitis, cutaneous herpetic infections, herpes genitalis, and herpetic encephalitis. Treatment options for RHL are summarized in Table 34-5. The mechanisms of action of anti-HSV drugs, such as vidarabine, are depicted in Figure 34-7.

Primary infection with VZV causes chicken pox in individuals, which may induce zoster after about the age of 60. CMV infection can cause retinitis in 20% to 25% of patients with AIDS and may cause CMV colitis and esophagitis in AIDS patients. With the exception of foscarnet and vaccines, drugs effective against the herpesviruses are purine or pyrimidine analogues that are converted to active nucleotides either by cellular or virus-specific enzymes. Drugs, such as **acyclovir, valacyclovir, and penciclovir**, that are activated by virus-encoded enzymes and inhibit a specific molecular event in viral replication are the most selective agents currently available

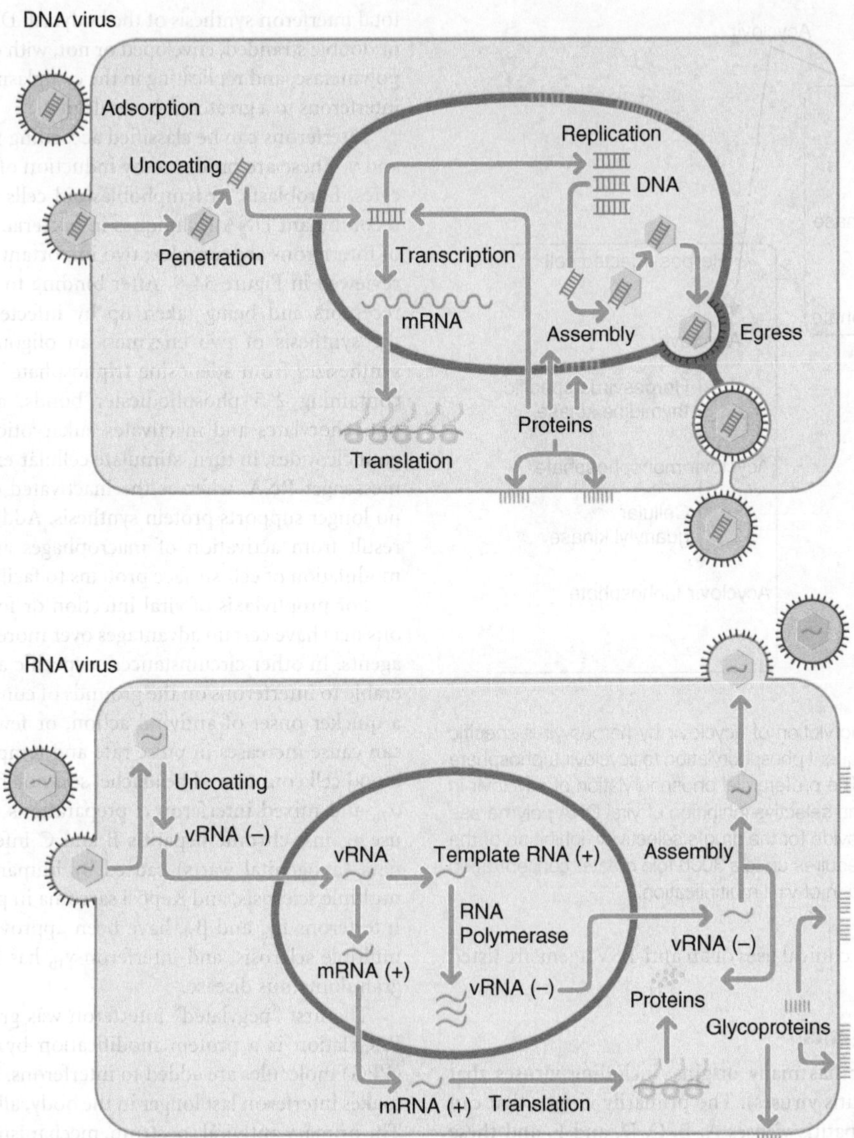

FIG 34-6 Viral replication and reproduction of DNA and RNA viruses.

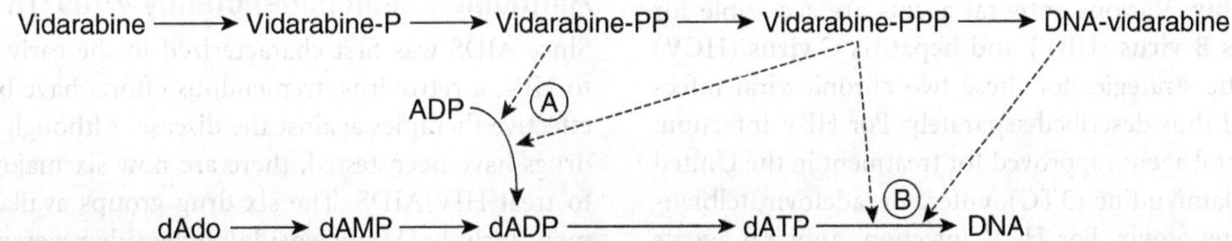

FIG 34-7 Mechanisms of action of vidarabine. *Top,* sequential phosphorylation of vidarabine by cellular enzymes and its incorporation into viral DNA; *bottom,* the conversion of deoxyadenosine (*dAdo*) to deoxyadenosine monophosphate (*dAMP*), diphosphate (*dADP*), and triphosphate (*dATP*) and the synthesis of normal viral DNA. *A,* vidarabine diphosphates (*-PP*) and triphosphates (*-PPP*) inhibit ribonucleotide reductase–dependent production of dADP. *B,* vidarabine triphosphate and vidarabine, incorporated into DNA, block further DNA synthesis by inhibiting the activity of DNA polymerases and terminal deoxynucleotidyl transferase.

(Fig. 34-8). The primary antiviral spectrum, mechanism of action, and clinical uses of anti-herpetic viral agents are listed in Table 34-6.

Anti-Respiratory Syncytial Virus Agents

Winter outbreaks of respiratory tract illness are often the result of respiratory syncytial virus (RSV). In the United States, the season for **respiratory tract illness** generally last 3 to 5 months and peaks in early winter in the South and late winter in the North. People of all ages can contract severe infections of RSV, but it is most common among the very young. It has been estimated that RSV annually accounts for almost 150,000 hospitalizations and 100 to 500 deaths among children in the United States. The primary antiviral spectrum,

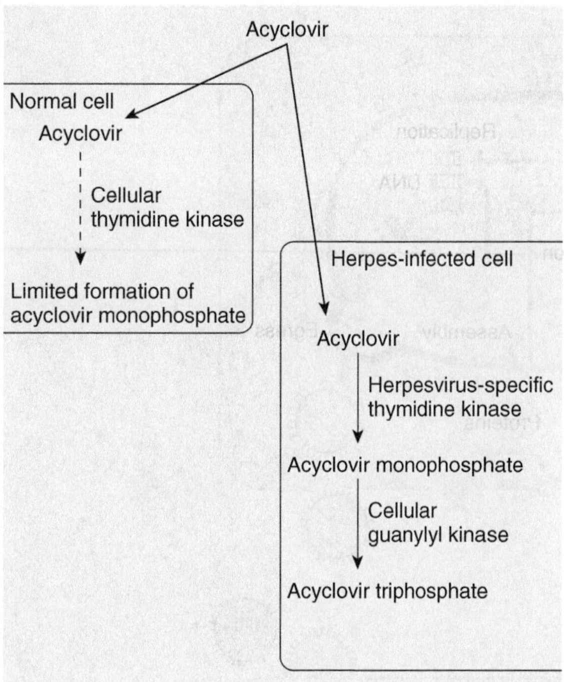

FIG 34-8 Selective phosphorylation of acyclovir by herpes virus-specific thymidine kinase and subsequent phosphorylation to acyclovir triphosphate by cellular guanylyl kinase. The preferential phosphorylation of acyclovir in herpesvirus-infected cells and selective inhibition of viral DNA polymerase by acyclovir triphosphate provide for the drug's selectivity; inhibition of the growth of uninfected cells requires up to a 3000-fold greater concentration of drug than does the inhibition of viral multiplication.

mechanism of action, and clinical uses of an anti-RSV agent are listed in Table 34-7.

Antiviral Hepatitis Agents

Inflammation of the liver has many origins, including viruses that attack the liver (i.e., hepatitis viruses). The primarily viruses that can affect the liver include hepatitis viruses A, B, C, D, and E, and these viruses are responsible for approximately half of all human hepatitis. Viral hepatitis types B (HBV) and C (HCV) cause chronic hepatitis infections throughout the world and are associated with significant morbidity and mortality. Various antiviral agents are accessible for treatment of **hepatitis B virus (HBV) and hepatitis C virus (HCV) infections.** Therapeutic strategies for these two chronic viral infections are different and thus described separately. For HBV infection, there are several antiviral agents approved for treatment in the United States. These include lamivudine (3TC), entecavir, adefovir, telbivudine, clevudine, and tenofovir. For HCV infection, antiviral agents approved for treatment are interferons, ribavirin, sofosbuvir, telaprevir, boceprevir, and simeprevir. There are also two immune system modulators licensed for treatment of HBV in the United States. They are **interferon α_{2a}** and "pegylated" interferon α_{2a} and will be discussed next.

Interferons, used for the treatment of HBV and HCV infections, are glycoproteins secreted by virus-infected cells that promote the establishment of an antiviral state in uninfected cells. In addition to their antiviral activity, interferons regulate cellular functions dealing with cell proliferation and immunologic responses. Although all tissues appear to be capable of synthesizing interferons, cells that are derived from the hematopoietic system (e.g., lymphocytes and macrophages), epithelial cells, and fibroblasts are among the most significant in contributing to the total interferon synthesis of the body. All DNA and RNA viruses, single or double stranded, enveloped or not, with or without virion-associated polymerase, and replicating in the cytoplasm or nucleus, are sensitive to interferons to a greater or lesser degree.

Interferons can be classified according to three major groups: α, β, and γ. These are produced by induction of synthesis in human leukocytes, fibroblasts, or lymphoblastoid cells and, in larger amounts, by recombinant DNA techniques in bacteria. The mechanisms of action of interferons are complex; two important responses to interferon are reviewed in Figure 34-9. After binding to specific plasma-membrane receptors and being taken up by infected cells, interferon induces the synthesis of two enzymes: an oligonucleotide polymerase that synthesizes from adenosine triphosphate a series of oligonucleotides containing 2′,5′-phosphodiester bonds, and a protein kinase that phosphorylates and inactivates eukaryotic initiation factor. The oligonucleotides, in turn, stimulate cellular endonucleases to cleave viral messenger RNA, whereas the inactivated eukaryotic initiation factor no longer supports protein synthesis. Additional antiviral effects may result from activation of macrophages and natural killer cells and modulation of cell-surface proteins to facilitate immune recognition.

For prophylaxis of viral infection or for early treatment, interferons may have certain advantages over more narrow-spectrum antiviral agents. In other circumstances, a specific antiviral agent may be preferable to interferons on the grounds of convenience of administration, a quicker onset of antiviral action, or fewer side effects. Interferons can cause increases in pulse rate and temperature, decreases in white blood cell counts, and headache, somnolence, and malaise. Interferon α_{2b} and mixed interferon α preparations are currently approved for use against chronic hepatitis B and C infections, condyloma acuminata (anogenital warts) caused by human papillomavirus infection, multiple sclerosis, and Kaposi sarcoma in patients with HIV infection. Interferons β_{1a} and β_{1b} have been approved for the management of multiple sclerosis, and interferon γ_{1b} has been approved for chronic granulomatous disease.

The first "pegylated" interferon was granted by the FDA in 2001. PEGylation is a protein modification by which polyethylene glycol (PEG) molecules are added to interferons. In these formulations, PEG makes interferon last longer in the body, allowing less frequent dosing. The primary antiviral spectrum, mechanism of action, and clinical uses of antiviral hepatitis agents are listed in Table 34-8. Adverse effects of representative drugs are listed in Table 34-4.

Antihuman Immunodeficiency Virus (HIV) Agents

Since AIDS was first characterized in the early 1980s and attributed to HIV, a retrovirus, tremendous efforts have been made to develop effective therapies against the disease. Although numerous anti-AIDS drugs have been tested, there are now six major types of drugs used to treat HIV/AIDS. The six drug groups available for clinical treatment include **(1) nucleoside/nucleotide reverse transcriptase inhibitors (NRTIs), (2) non-nucleoside reverse transcriptase inhibitors (NNRTIs), (3) protease inhibitors (PIs), (4) integrase strand transfer inhibitors (INSTIs), (5) entry inhibitors (CCR5 antagonist), and (6) fusion inhibitors.**

One of the first types of drugs used to treat HIV infections was the nucleoside reverse transcriptase inhibitor. NRTIs are analogues of naturally occurring deoxynucleotides. These drugs block the enzymatic function of reverse transcriptase and prevent completion of viral DNA synthesis and multiplication. Unlike NRTIs, nonnucleoside reverse transcriptase inhibitors are not nucleoside analogues and work by noncompetitive inhibition of the reverse transcriptase enzyme, thereby preventing cells from being infected. In spite of the chemical diversity, NNRTIs always bind at the same site of the reverse transcriptase.

TABLE 34-6 Antiviral Spectrum, Mechanisms of Action, and Clinical Uses of Anti-Herpesvirus Agents

Generic Name	Trade Name	Primary Antiviral Spectrum	Mechanism of Action	Clinical Uses
Idoxuridine	Ridinox	HSV	Inhibition of DNA synthesis	Topical use for herpetic keratitis and keratoconjunctivitis
Vidarabine	Vira-A	HSV	Inhibition of DNA polymerase	Topical use for herpetic keratitis and keratoconjunctivitis; treatment of herpes encephalitis
Trifluridine	Viroptic	HSV	Inhibition of thymidylate synthase	Topical use for herpetic keratitis and keratouveitis
Acyclovir	Zovirax	HSV and VZV	Inhibition of DNA polymerase	Treatment of primary and recurrent herpes genitalis, herpetic encephalitis, mucocutaneous herpetic infections in immunocompromised patients, neonatal herpetic infection, and VZV infection, CMV prophylaxis[†]
Valacyclovir	Valtrex	HSV and VZV	Inhibition of DNA polymerase	Treatment of primary and recurrent herpes genitalis, herpetic encephalitis, mucocutaneous herpetic infections in immunocompromised patients, neonatal herpetic infection, and VZV infection, CMV prophylaxis
Famciclovir	Famvir	HSV and VZV	Inhibition of DNA polymerase	Oral use for VZV infection and recurrent herpes infections
Penciclovir	Denavir	HSV	Inhibition of DNA polymerase	Topical use for recurrent herpes labialis
Foscarnet	Foscavir	HSV, VZV, and CMV	Inhibition of DNA polymerase	Treatment of CMV retinitis and acyclovir-resistant HSV and VZV infections
Ganciclovir	Zirgan	CMV	Inhibition of DNA polymerase	Treatment of CMV retinitis and prevention of CMV colitis and esophagitis
Cidofovir	Vistide	CMV and HSV	Inhibition of DNA polymerase	Treatment of CMV keratitis and HSV lesions
Fomivirsen	Vitravene	CMV	Inhibition of DNA synthesis	CMV retinitis
Docosanol	Abreva	HSV	Inhibits fusion of host cell with the herpes viral envelope preventing replication	Recurrent herpes labialis
Vaccine*	Zostavax	VZV	Antibody production	Herpes zoster (shingles)

*The FDA has approved a live-attenuated varicella zoster (VCV) vaccine for prevention of shingles in individuals over 60 years of age. In the United States, more than 90% of adults have had varicella and are at risk of the development of herpes zoster, and more than one million new cases of herpes zoster are reported in the United States each year. It is known that the vaccine enhances VZV-specific cell-mediated immunity that inhibits the reactivation of latent VZV. The vaccine reduces the severity and duration of discomfort and pain caused by herpes zoster by 61%.

[†]Although physicians and dentists have used topical acyclovir for symptomatic relief of recurrent herpes labialis in patients with normal immune systems, there is little evidence of this practice providing real benefits.

CMV, Cytomegalovirus; *HSV*, herpes simplex virus.

TABLE 34-7 Antiviral Spectrum, Mechanisms of Action, and Clinical Uses of Anti-Respiratory Syncytial Virus Agent (Anti-RSV)

Generic Name	Trade Name	Primary Antiviral Spectrum	Mechanism of Action	Clinical Uses
Ribavirin	Virazole	RSV	The triphosphate form of ribavirin, which is the predominant form intracellularly, interferes with viral messenger RNA synthesis; its metabolite, ribavirin 5′-phosphate, inhibits inosine monophosphate dehydrogenase and eventually the formation of guanosine triphosphate	Administered by aerosolization to hospitalized infants and young children with respiratory syncytial virus infections and produces significant reductions in fever and severity of systemic illness*

*It holds promise as an aerosol and oral medication for treatment of influenza, measles, acute and chronic hepatitis, Lassa fever, and a variety of RNA viral infections not commonly seen in the United States. It is an antiviral medicine that is very rarely used to treat people with RSV infections who have a high risk of developing complications.

Another type of drug class used to treat HIV/AIDS patients is the protease inhibitor. HIV protease is a viral enzyme responsible for the cleavage of the Gag and Gag-Pol polyproteins into the enzymes and structural proteins that are required for the final assembly of new infectious virions. In patients with advanced HIV infection, use of a protease inhibitor in combination therapy with other classes of antiretroviral agents significantly improves the survival of patients. After sustained exposure to antiviral agents, viral isolates may develop resistance to one class of drugs and remain susceptible to others. It is therefore preferred to use a protease inhibitor combined with other drugs to avoid drug resistance. Examples of adverse effects of PIs are listed in Table 34-4.

A fourth type of antiretroviral therapy for the treatment of HIV infections interferes with enzymes needed for HIV replication. INSTIs block the action of integrase, a viral enzyme of the HIV type 1, which is involved in integrating DNA, produced from HIV RNA by reverse transcriptase, into the host chromosome, a critical step in the pathogenesis of HIV. Integration of the virally produced DNA into the host DNA is necessary for viral replication. INSTIs are not a cure for HIV or AIDS but are used to prevent HIV from multiplying in the host.

There are two molecular strategies that impede the ability of the HIV to interact with the mammalian cell membrane. The first type is the entry inhibitors that interfere with virus binding to receptors on the outer surface of the cell as it tries to enter. When receptor binding is

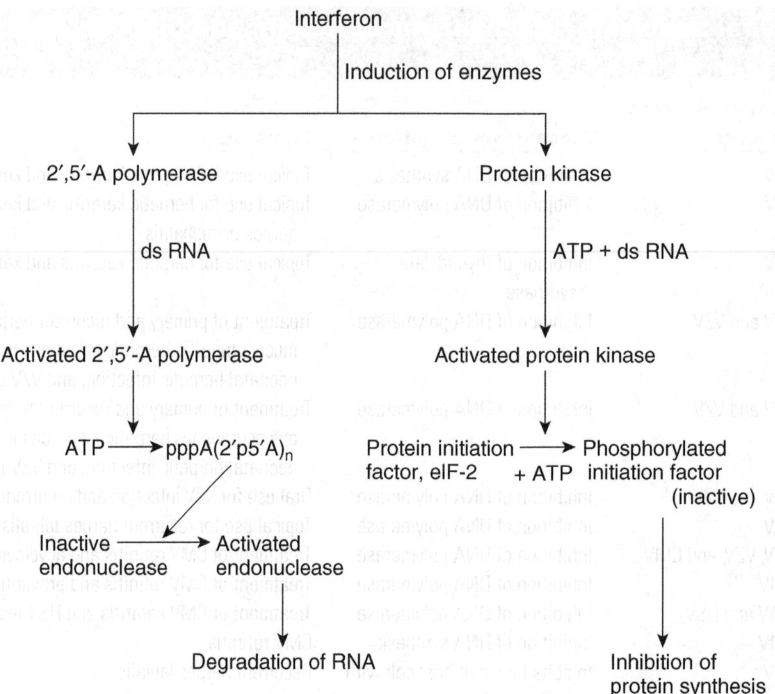

FIG 34-9 Mechanisms of action of interferon. After incorporation into the cell, interferon induces the synthesis of two enzymes, an oligonucleotide polymerase (2′,5′-A polymerase) and a protein kinase, which in the presence of double-stranded RNA (*ds RNA*) leads to a cascade of reactions that inhibit viral replication.

TABLE 34-8 Antiviral Spectrum, Mechanisms of Action, and Clinical Uses of Anti-Hepatitis B Virus and Anti-Hepatitis C Virus Agents

Generic Name	Trade Name	Primary Antiviral Spectrum	Mechanism of Action	Clinical Uses
Lamivudine (3TC)	Epivir	HBV	Inhibits DNA polymerase	HBV infection
Entecavir	Baraclude	HBV	Inhibits DNA polymerase	HBV infection
Adefovir	Hepsera	HBV	Inhibits DNA polymerase	HBV infection
Telbivudine	Tyzeka	HBV	Inhibits DNA polymerase	HBV infection
Clevudine*	Levovir	HBV	Inhibits DNA polymerase	HBV infection
Tenofovir	Viread	HBV	Reverse transcriptase inhibitor	HBV infection
Ribavirin	Copegus	HCV	See Table 34-6	HCV infections
Sofosbuvir	Solvaldi	HCV	Inhibits RNA polymerase	HCV infections
Telaprevir	Incivek	HCV	Protease inhibitor†	HCV infections
Boceprevir	Victrelis	HCV	Protease inhibitor†	HCV infections
Simeprevir	Olysio	HCV	Protease inhibitor†	HCV infections
Interferon α and α2b	Roferon-A and Intron A	HCV and HPV	Stimulation of synthesis of antiviral proteins	Treatment of HBV and HCV and refractory genital warts

*Approved for the treatment of chronic HBV only in some Asian countries, including South Korea and the Philippines.
†Block viral replication by specifically binding to viral proteases and interfering with proteolytic cleavage of protein precursors that are fundamental for the generation of infectious viral particles.

blocked, HIV cannot infect the cell. The drug in this class, maraviroc, is an allosteric inhibitor of the CCR5 receptor. Blocking the CCR5 receptor, which is expressed on the surface of certain human cells, blocks the HIV glycoprotein 120 from associating with the receptor. The CCR5 receptor is an essential co-receptor for most HIV strains and required for the entry process of HIV into the host cell such as human macrophages and T cells. The second type is the fusion inhibitor, enfuvirtide, affecting the virus–membrane relationship. The fusion inhibitor is effective against HIV because the drug binds to a viral envelope glycoprotein, which prevents the fusion between the viral envelope with host plasma membrane, blocking HIV from entering the cell.

Because of the rapidity with which some of these drugs have been developed and approved for marketing, research is ongoing regarding the therapeutic uses and toxic profiles of these agents. An especially promising development from these studies has been the dramatic therapeutic benefits obtained with multiple drug therapy. Examples of adverse effects of the anti-HIV drugs are listed in Table 34-4.

Multiple Class Combination Agents

To prevent strains of HIV from becoming drug resistant, HIV drugs from two or more classes have been combined into a single product. It has been recommended that individuals with HIV infections receive a combination of antiretroviral drugs in an approach called highly active antiretroviral therapy (HAART), which usually combines drugs from at least two different classes. Although there are a variety of drug combinations approved for use in the treatment HIV infections, the National Institutes of Health recommends several different drug combinations to treat people with HIV. These drug combinations include the following:

1. efavirenz (NNRTI), tenofovir (NRTI), and emtricitabine (NRTI)
2. ritonavir-boosted atazanavir (PI), tenofovir (NRTI), and emtricitabine (NRTI)
3. ritonavir-boosted darunavir (PI), tenofovir (NRTI), and emtricitabine (NRTI)
4. raltegravir (ISTI), tenofovir (NRTI), and emtricitabine (NRTI)

The mechanisms of action of anti-HIV agents are listed in Table 34-9.

TABLE 34-9 Mechanisms of Action of Anti-HIV Agents*

Generic Name	Trade Name	Mechanism of Action
Abacavir	Ziagen	Nucleoside analogue reverse transcriptase inhibitor
Didanosine	Videx	Nucleoside analogue reverse transcriptase inhibitor
Emtricitabine	Emtriva	Nucleoside analogue reverse transcriptase inhibitor
Stavudine	Zerit	Nucleoside analogue reverse transcriptase inhibitor
Tenofovir	Viread	Nucleoside analogue reverse transcriptase inhibitor
Zalcitabine	Hivid	Nucleoside analogue reverse transcriptase inhibitor
Zidovudine (AZT)	Retrovir	Nucleoside analogue reverse transcriptase inhibitor
Delavirdine	Rescriptor	Non-nucleotide reverse transcriptase inhibitor
Efavirenz	Sustiva	Non-nucleotide reverse transcriptase inhibitor
Etravirine	Intelence	Non-nucleotide reverse transcriptase inhibitor
Nevirapine	Viramune	Non-nucleotide reverse transcriptase inhibitor
Rilpivirine	Edurant	Non-nucleotide reverse transcriptase inhibitor
Amprenavir	Agenerase	Protease inhibitor
Atazanavir	Reyataz	Protease inhibitor
Darunavir	Prezista	Protease inhibitor
Fosamprenavir	Lexiva	Protease inhibitor
Indinavir	Crixivan	Protease inhibitor
Lopinavir	Kaletra	Protease inhibitor
Nelfinavir	Viracept	Protease inhibitor
Ritonavir	Norvir	Protease inhibitor
Saquinavir	Invirase	Protease inhibitor
Tipranavir	Aptivus	Protease inhibitor
Dolutegravir	Tivicay	Integrase strand transfer inhibitor
Elvitegravir	Stribild	Integrase strand transfer inhibitor
Raltegravir	Isentress	Integrase strand transfer inhibitor
Maraviroc	Selzentry	Entry inhibitor
Enfuvirtide	Fuzeon	Fusion inhibitor

*These drugs were developed primarily to affect the human immunodeficiency virus and to treat people with HIV/AIDS.

ANTIVIRAL THERAPY IN THE ORAL CAVITY

Herpesviruses causes a variety of oral mucosal lesions, including herpetic gingivostomatitis, recurrent intraoral herpes simplex, herpes labialis, herpes zoster (varicella zoster), or the life-threatening eczema herpeticum. Herpetic gingivostomatitis can also manifest in weakened hosts as aphthoid of Pospischill-Feyrter, characterized by rapid expansion of the lesion to the throat and perioral skin. The majority of these HSV-associated viral lesions are routinely treated by oral acyclovir, with intravenous administration in some severe cases. Treatment options for *herpes labialis* are listed in Table 34-10.

Acyclovir is best used as soon as the symptoms begin to appear. The mechanism of action of acyclovir is depicted in Figure 34-8. The intravenous dosage is based on body weight and the type of the lesion. Generally, 5 to 10 mg/kg of body weight is administered intravenously for a 1-hour period and repeated every 8 hours for 5 to 10 days. Long-term suppressive acyclovir therapy is recommended for patients with eczema herpeticum at 200 to 400 mg orally two to three times per day. In addition, supportive therapies for herpetic lesions include antipyretic analgesics, as well as antibiotics and antifungals that help control secondary infections.

Topical 1% **penciclovir** cream is the drug of choice for the control of recurrent *Herpes labialis,* and it may be applied to the lesion every 2 hours during awake hours for 4 days. It reduces the severity of uncomfortableness and significantly shortens the period of lesion by 1 to 2 days.

HSV infection can develop into a more severe and generalized form in AIDS patients. Recurrent herpetic lesions become chronic in these patients, and HSV strains resistant to acyclovir could arise, in which case other anti-herpetic agents, such as **ganciclovir and foscarnet**, may be effective. In AIDS patients, numerous concomitant oral lesions of different viral origins are common. These include the following: **(1)** human papillomavirus infection is almost always noted in these patients, resulting in variants of papillomas, condylomas, and focal epithelial hyperplasia in the oral cavity, **(2)** cytomegalovirus (CMV) is associated with aphthae-like ulcerations in the oral mucosa, and **(3)** oral hairy leukoplakia is an early sign of HIV infection, presumably caused by Epstein-Barr virus in immunocompromised patients. Treatment of oral hairy leukoplakia is rendered only in symptomatic patients and usually involves topical application of a solution of podophyllin resin 25% and acyclovir 800 mg four times daily. Systemic antiretroviral therapy is also provided as described earlier. Oral hairy leukoplakia disappears as a result of drug therapy but normally recurs when the medication is discontinued.

TABLE 34-10 Treatment Options for Recurrent Herpes Labialis (RHL)

Agent	Formulation	Dosage
Penciclovir 1%	Topical	q2hr while awake, 4 d
Acyclovir 5%	Topical	5x/day, 4 d
Docosanol 10%	Topical	5x/day until healing occurs
Valacyclovir	Oral	2 g, q12hr for one day
Acyclovir	Oral	400 mg, 5x/day, 7-14 d
Famciclovir	Oral	1500-mg single dose

ANTIFUNGAL AND ANTIVIRAL AGENTS

Nonproprietary (generic) name	Proprietary (trade) name
Antifungal agents	
Amphotericin B	Abelcet, Amphotec, Fungizone
Anidulafungin	Eraxis
Butenafine	Mentax
Butoconazole	Femstat
Caspofungin	Cancidas
Ciclopirox	Loprox
Clioquinol	Vioform
Clotrimazole	Mycelex
Econazole	Spectazole
Efinaconazole	Jublia
Fluconazole	Diflucan
Flucytosine	Ancobon
Gentian violet	—
Griseofulvin	Fulvicin, Grifulvin V, Grisactin
Haloprogin	Halotex
Itraconazole	Sporanox
Isavuconazole	Cresemba
Ketoconazole	Nizoral
Luliconazole	Luzu
Miconazole	Oravig, Micatin, Monistat-Derm, Monistat i.v.
Micafungin	Mycamine
Naftifine	Naftin
Natamycin	Natacyn
Nystatin	Mycostatin, Nilstat, Nystex
Oxiconazole	Oxistat
Posaconazole	Noxafil
Sertaconzole	Ertaczo
Sulconazole	Exelderm
Tavaborole	Kerydin
Terbinafine	Lamisil
Terconazole	Terazol
Tioconazole	Vagistat-1
Tolnaftate	Aftate, Tinactin
Undecylenic acid	Cruex, Blis-To-Sol
Voriconazole	Vfend
Antiviral agents	
A only-daily combination tablet for HIV	Atripla
Abacavir	Ziagen
Abacavir, zidovudine, and lamivudine (combination)	Trizivir
Acyclovir	Zovirax
Amantadine	Symmetrel
Amprenavir	Agenerase
Boceprevir	Victrelis
Cidofovir	Vistide
Clevudine	Levovir, Revovir
Darunavir	Prezista
Delavirdine	Rescriptor
Didanosine	Videx
Docosanol	Abreva
Dolutegravir	in Triumeq
Efavirenz	Sustiva
Elvitegravir	Vitekta
Entecavir	Baraclude
Famciclovir	Famvir
Fomivirsen	Vitravene
Foscarnet	Foscavir
Ganciclovir	Cytovene
Herpes zoster vaccine	Zostavax
Idoxuridine	Herplex
Imiquimod	Aldara
Indinavir	Crixivan
Interferon α_{2a}	Referon-A
Interferon α_{2b}	Intron A
Interferon α_{n3}	Alferon
Lamivudine	Epivir
Lopinavir	Kaletra
Maraviroc	Selzentry
Nelfinavir	Viracept
Nevirapine	Viramune
Oseltamivir	Tamiflu
Penciclovir	Denavir
Peramivir	Rapivab
Raltegravir	Isentress
Ribavirin	Virazole, Ribasphere, RibaPak, Rebetol, Copegus
Rimantadine	Flumadine
Ritonavir	Norvir
Saquinavir	Invirase
Simeprevir	Olysio
Sofosbuvir	Sovaldi
Stavudine	Zerit
Telaprevir	Incivek
Telbivudine	Tyzeka
Tenofovir disoproxil fumarate	Viread
Trifluridine	Viroptic
Valacyclovir	Valtrex
Valganciclovir	Valcyte
Vidarabine	Vira-A
Zalcitabine	Hivid
Zanamivir	Relenza
Zidovudine	Retrovir

CASE DISCUSSION

Your patient probably has a *Candida* infection of the mouth, and once the diagnosis is histologically confirmed, she must be treated with a prescription of an antifungal medication. The type and duration of treatment depend on the severity of the infection and patient-specific factors such as age and immune status. Generally, oral candidiasis responds to topical application of drugs such as clotrimazole (oral troches) or nystatin (oral suspension).

GENERAL REFERENCES

1. Antifungal drugs: treatment guidelines from the medical letter, *Med Lett issue* 120:61–73, 2012.
2. Collins CD, Cookinham S, Smith J: Management of oropharyngeal candidiasis with localized oral miconazole therapy: efficacy, safety and patient acceptability, *Patience Prefer Adherence* 5:369–374, 2011.
3. Looney D, Ma A, Johns S: HIV therapy—the state of art, *Curr Top Microbiol Immunol* 389:1–29, 2015.
4. Potempa M, Lee SK, Wolfenden R, Swanstrom R: The triple threat of HIV-1 protease inhibitors, *Curr Top Microbiol Immunol* 389:203–241, 2015.
5. Zhu JD, Meng W, Wang XJ, Wang HC: Broad-spectrum antiviral agents, *Front Microbiol* 6:517, 2015.

35

Immunotherapy

Anahid Jewett and Han-Ching Tseng*

KEY INFORMATION

- Inflammation is a mechanism for increasing survival and function of the cells during disease to aid in the restoration of homeostasis.
- T and B cells must undergo several developmental stages to generate receptor diversity.
- T and B cell effector function and generation of memory are important for defense against infection and malignancies.
- Resident and recruited antigen-presenting cells, phagocytes, and natural killer cells have important immunologic roles.
- Increasing costimulation is important to initiate a robust immune response.
- Thymic extracts may induce T cell maturation in patients with an absence of the thymus gland or a defect in its function.
- A possible antigen-delivery strategy to elicit local immune response within the gingiva is the sequestration of candidate antigens into liposomes.
- The effects of a vaccine may be enhanced by incorporation of adjuvants, such as alum.
- Categories of immunotherapy drugs:
  - Agents for active and passive immunization
  - Antitoxins
  - Immunostimulants
  - Immunomodulators
  - Antibodies
  - Immunosuppressants
  - Cytokines
  - Growth factors

CASE STUDY

Mrs. R is your 50-year-old dental patient. It has been one year since her last dental appointment. Five months ago, her physician prescribed prednisone for her rheumatoid arthritis. Upon questioning, Mrs. R indicated that upon referral to a rheumatologist, she was diagnosed with Sjögren's syndrome. The prednisone reduced her joint pain, but she came in to you today complaining about dry mouth. She has to constantly drink water during the day and night to relieve the xerostomia. She also complains of having dry eyes. After examining Mrs. R, you realize that she has several caries and is at risk for periodontal disease. Would you prescribe a drug such as pilocarpine to stimulate the salivary glands and improve Mrs. R's oral condition? What are other therapeutic options for her disease?

Immunopharmacology is the study of the interaction between drugs and the immune system. Immunotherapy is the application of clinical strategies to modulate the activities of certain components of the immune system to improve immune function and to prevent or treat disease. This chapter reviews the immune system with regard to the pathways used toward adaptive, specific immunity that are or can be targeted for immunotherapy and discusses immunotherapeutic strategies that are of clinical importance today or show promise for the future. The pharmacologic manipulation of innate immune mechanisms involved in inflammation is covered in Chapters 17 and 30.

*The authors wish to recognize Dr. Kenneth T. Miyasaki for his past contributions to this chapter. The authors also acknowledge the great help of Ms. Tanya Kavoussi in the preparation of this chapter and the critical review by Dr. Anna Kozlowska. This chapter is dedicated to the memory of Dr. John Yagiela for his insight, passion, and dedication to dental education.

OVERVIEW OF SPECIFIC IMMUNITY

Components of the Immune System

Research in immunology has progressed rapidly over the last three decades. Spanning this period, major technologic feats (e.g., the development of hybridomas for the production of monoclonal antibodies) and major strides in our understanding of the immune system (including elucidation of the role of cytokines and intracellular signaling in immunity) have resulted in significant advances in immunotherapeutics. Today immunopharmacologists use these new insights to pinpoint therapeutic targets among (1) a constellation of cytokines and other growth factors that influence cellular growth, differentiation, and function and (2) myriad receptors responsive to these mediators, specific antigens, or ligands found on other cells.

Cells

The immune system is composed of two major arms: **innate immunity** and **adaptive immunity**. These two components of the immune system differ in the types of effectors, their specificity for antigens, speed of action, and induction of memory. Innate immune cells are the primary initiators of the immune response and support functional activation of adaptive immune effectors. They differ from the adaptive immune effectors by their lack of antigen specificity and their fast-acting capabilities. Unlike the adaptive immune effectors, the innate immune effectors do not generate memory. **The main effectors of the innate immune system are granulocytes, macrophages, and natural**

killer (NK) cells, whereas T and B lymphocytes are the main effectors of adaptive immunity.

All the effectors of the immune system are derived from the bone marrow. Pluripotent hematopoietic stem cells in bone marrow give rise to either myeloid progenitor cells or lymphoid progenitor cells (Fig. 35-1).

Myeloid progenitor cells are the precursors of red blood cells, platelets, granulocytes (polymorphonuclear leukocytes [PMNs]: neutrophils, eosinophils, and basophils), monocyte-macrophages, dendritic cells (DCs), and mast cells and osteoclasts. **Lymphoid progenitor cells** give rise to the T, B, NK/T, and NK cells. Lymphocytes are generated and mature in the bone marrow and thymus, which are considered to be the primary or central lymphoid organs. From there, they travel to reside in secondary or peripheral lymphoid organs, such as lymph nodes, spleen, mucosa-associated lymphoid tissues, gut-associated lymphoid tissues, and bronchus-associated lymphoid tissues.

The various cell types exit the bone marrow at different levels of maturation, circulate through the bloodstream, and may take up residence in specific tissues. Certain cells involved in the body's defense system provide rapid responses, whereas others support slower, adaptive responses. Neutrophils and NK cells exit the bone marrow in a relatively mature state and require very little time to become activated. In contrast, monocytes, DCs, and most lymphoid cells leave the bone marrow in a relatively immature state and complete their maturation at some other tissue site, where they can be activated to respond to local cues.

Lymphocytes circulate between blood and lymphatics continuously. Lymphocytes that have not encountered antigen are called **naïve lymphocytes**; those that have encountered antigen and have become mature are **effector lymphocytes**. Activation of antigen-presenting cells (APCs)—monocytes, B cells, and DCs — is the necessary first step for the induction of adaptive immunity. In adaptive immunity, lymphocytes activated by antigens give rise to clones of antigen-specific cells, which are then selected either positively or negatively. Clonal selection is the central principle of adaptive immunity. The four basic postulates of clonal selection are that **(1)** each lymphocyte bears a single type of receptor with a unique specificity to self and non-self; **(2)** lymphocytes expressing receptors for specificity for self-antigens are deleted at an early stage and therefore are absent from the pool of mature lymphocytes; **(3)** interaction between a foreign antigen and the receptor capable of binding to it leads to lymphocyte activation; and **(4)** the differentiated effector cells derived from an activated lymphocyte will bear receptors of identical specificity to those of the parental cells. In adaptive immunity, unique antigen receptors are generated by gene rearrangement, and signals

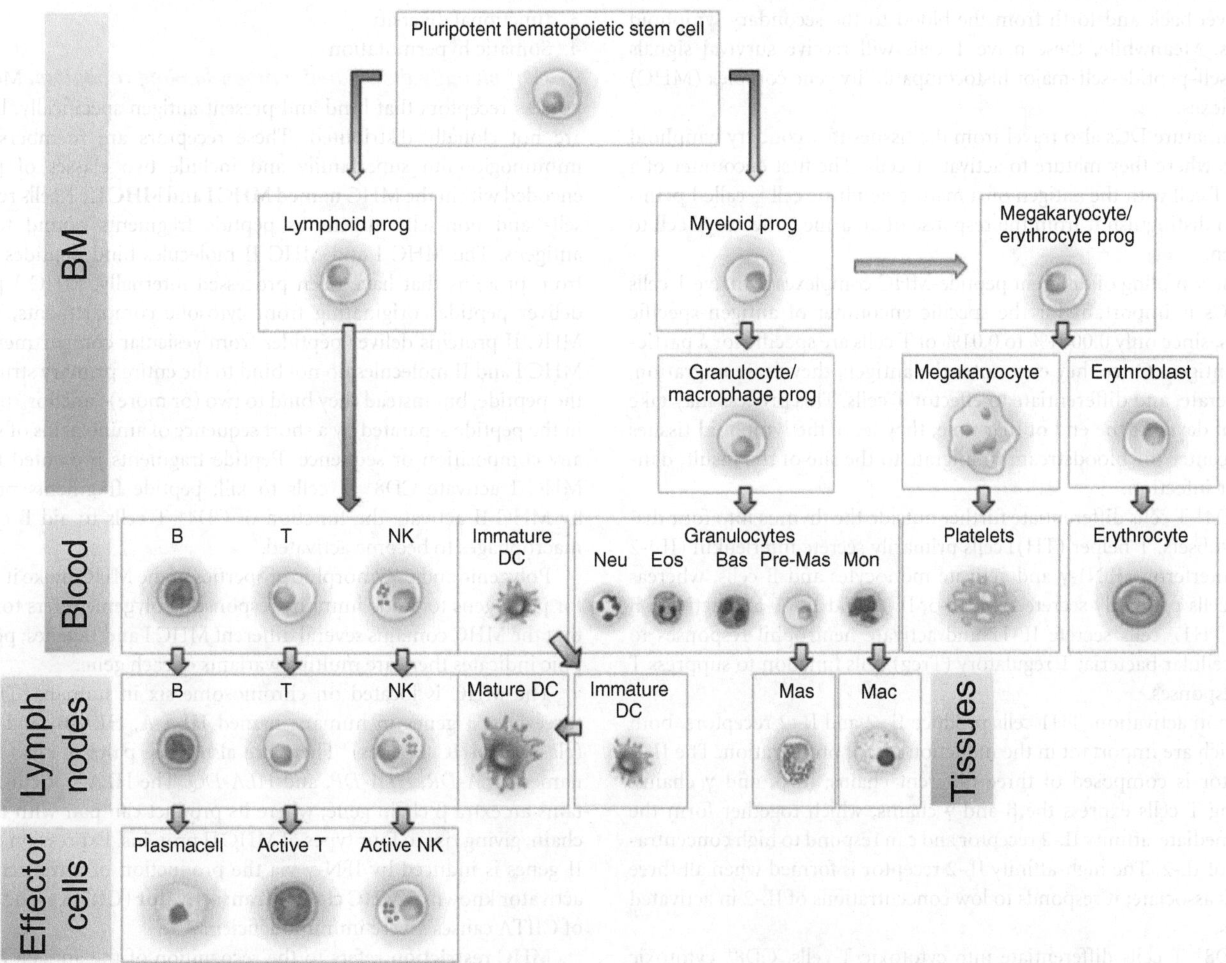

FIG 35-1 Lineage and location of blood cells involved in the immune response. Not shown are the regulatory T cell and the T helper cell TH17. *BM,* Bone marrow; *Prog,* progenitor; *B,* B cell; *DC,* dendritic cell; *T,* T cell; *NK,* NK cell; *Neu,* neutrophil; *Eos,* eosinophil; *Bas,* basophil; *Pre-Mas,* mast cell precursor; *Mon,* monocytes. (Modified from Murphy K: *Janeway's Immunobiology,* ed 8, Garland Science, 2012, Taylor & Francis Group, LLC.)

received through antigen receptors determine the development and survival of lymphocytes. Binding of antigen activates lymphocytes, resulting in the generation of effector cells and the establishment of immunologic memory.

T cells exit the bone marrow as CD3-CD4-CD8–null cells, according to the **cluster of differentiation (CD)** classification of leukocyte antigens, before entering the thymus. In young individuals, the thymus contains large numbers of developing T cell precursors embedded in a network of epithelia known as the thymic stroma, which provides a supportive environment for the developing T cells. T cell precursors proliferate extensively in the thymus, but most eventually are eliminated there. The thymus of a young adult mouse contains 1-2 $\times 10^8$ thymocytes. Although 50 million new cells are generated each day, only two million of these cells survive to leave the thymus. The developmental pathway of T cells in the thymus is the following: early on, CD3-CD4-CD8–null cells develop into $CD3^+pT\alpha CD4^+CD8^+$ (triple-positive) thymocytes. About 95% of triple-positive thymocytes will be eliminated by apoptosis, and the remaining 5% will exit thymus as either $CD3^+CD4^+$ or $CD3^+CD8^+$ double-positive T cells.

Once T cells have completed their developmental stages in the thymus, they enter the bloodstream and then are carried to the secondary lymphoid tissues, such as the lymph nodes or spleen. If they encounter their specific antigen, they will become activated, proliferate, and differentiate to armed effector T cells. Otherwise, they will continue to travel back and forth from the blood to the secondary lymphoid tissues. Meanwhile, these naïve T cells will receive survival signals from self-peptide-self-major histocompatibility gene complex (MHC) complexes.

Immature DCs also travel from the tissues to secondary lymphoid tissues where they mature to activate T cells. The first encounter of a naïve T cell with the antigen on a mature dendritic cell is called **priming**, to distinguish it from the response of an armed effector T cell to antigen.

The sampling of different peptide-MHC complexes by naïve T cells on DCs is important for the specific encounter of antigen-specific T cells, since only 0.0001% to 0.01% of T cells are specific for a particular antigen. Once they encounter the antigen, they cease migration, proliferate, and differentiate to effector T cells. This process may take several days. At the end of that time, they leave the lymphoid tissues and reenter the bloodstream to migrate to the site of the insult, danger, or infection.

$CD4^+$ T cells differentiate further outside the thymus into four distinct subsets. T helper (TH)1 cells primarily secrete interleukin (IL)-2 and interferon (IFN)-γ and activate monocytes and B cells, whereas TH2 cells primarily secrete IL-4, IL-5, IL-6, and IL-10 and activate B cells. TH17 cells secrete IL-17 and activate neutrophil responses to extracellular bacteria; T regulatory (Treg) cells function to suppress T cell responses.

Upon activation, TH1 cells produce IL-2 and IL-2 receptors, both of which are important in the induction of cell proliferation. The IL-2 receptor is composed of three different chains; α, β, and γ chains. Resting T cells express the β and γ chains, which together form the intermediate-affinity IL-2 receptor and can respond to high concentrations of IL-2. The high-affinity IL-2 receptor is formed when all three chains associate; it responds to low concentrations of IL-2 in activated T cells.

$CD8^+$ T cells differentiate into cytotoxic T cells. $CD8^+$ cytotoxic T cells kill virally infected cells or tumor-target cells via two different mechanisms, namely apoptosis and necrosis. Apoptosis is distinguished from necrosis by the intact plasma membrane at the initial stages of programming for cell death, nuclear membrane blebbing, and DNA fragmentation.

Receptors and other cell-surface proteins

Cells involved in specific immunity express various surface glycoproteins to help coordinate their functions and interactions. These glycoproteins include adhesion molecules, cytokine receptors, and receptors that bind and respond to specific antigens and to co-receptors and costimulatory receptors expressed on other cells.

Clonally distributed antigen-specific receptors. As mentioned earlier, T cells and B cells possess receptors that specifically recognize the antigen and are distributed in a clonal manner. These receptors, both members of the immunoglobulin superfamily, are the **T cell receptor (TCR)** mentioned previously and the **B cell antigen receptor (BCR).** Secreted forms of the BCR constitute the immunoglobulins found in plasma, extracellular fluid, and secretions. The BCR and TCR recognize short oligomeric sequences of a molecule and exhibit primary sequence specificity. In addition, the BCR (but not the TCR), which is designed to react with unprocessed antigen, may recognize secondary, tertiary, and quaternary structural features. The diversity of the TCR/BCR repertoire is generated by four main mechanisms:

1. Somatic recombination-variable regions of the receptor chains, which are encoded in several pieces called *gene segments*, are assembled in the developing lymphocytes by somatic DNA recombination (a process known as **gene rearrangement**)
2. Pairing of heavy and light chains of the BCR, or α and β chains of the TCR
3. Junctional diversity
4. Somatic hypermutation

Non-clonally distributed antigen-binding receptors. Most cells possess receptors that bind and present antigen specifically, but they are not clonally distributed. These receptors are members of the immunoglobulin superfamily and include two classes of proteins encoded within the MHC **named MHC I and MHC II.** T cells recognize self- and non-self-antigens as peptide fragments bound to MHC antigens. The MHC I and MHC II molecules bind peptides derived from proteins that have been processed internally. MHC I proteins deliver peptides originating from cytosolic compartments, whereas MHC II proteins deliver peptides from vesicular compartments. The MHC I and II molecules do not bind to the entire primary structure of the peptide, but instead they bind to two (or more) "anchor" positions in the peptide separated by a short sequence of amino acids of virtually any composition or sequence. Peptide fragments presented through MHC I activate $CD8^+$ T cells to kill; peptide fragments presented by MHC II activate the function of $CD4^+$ T cells to aid B cells and macrophages to become activated.

Polygenic and polymorphic properties of the MHC make it difficult for pathogens to evade immune responses. Polygenic refers to the fact that the MHC contains several different MHC I and II genes; polymorphic indicates there are multiple variants of each gene.

The MHC is located on chromosome six in humans. There are three class I genes in humans named **HLA-A, HLA-B,** and **HLA-C** (classical MHC I genes). There are also three pairs of class II genes named *HLA-DR*, *HLA-DP*, and *HLA-DQ*. The HLA-DR cluster contains an extra β chain gene, where its product can pair with the DRα chain, giving rise to four types of MHC II proteins. Expression of MHC II genes is induced by IFN-γ via the production of a transcriptional activator known as **MHC class II transactivator (CIITA)**. The absence of CIITA causes severe immunodeficiency.

MHC restriction refers to the recognition of the antigen by the T cells in the context of self-MHC. Thus a non-self-MHC I presenting the same peptide would not be recognized and would not activate T cells. Non-self-MHC molecules are recognized by 1% to 10% of T cells, an event termed **alloreactivity.** In alloreactivity, recognition of either the peptide antigen (peptide-dominant binding) or the foreign MHC molecule, irrespective of the peptide with which it is complexed (MHC-dominant binding), leads to T cell activation.

Other genes that map to the MHC locus include components of the complement cascade, such as C2, C4, and factor B, and cytokines including tumor necrosis factor (TNF)-α. These genes are referred to as **MHC class III genes.** In addition to highly polymorphic MHC I and II genes, there are many genes encoding MHC I–like molecules that show little polymorphism termed *MHC class Ib*. Some MHC Ib genes (e.g., the MIC gene family) are induced during cellular stress and regulate NK function.

Most individuals are heterozygous at each MHC locus. MHC polymorphism affects T cell recognition of antigen by influencing both the peptide binding and the contact between the TCR and MHC molecule.

Mediators

Numerous water-soluble proteins affect or create specific immune reactions. Two principal groups of interest in immunotherapy are the **cytokines and humoral antibodies.**

Cytokines. Cytokines are produced by a wide variety of cells. They play crucial roles in stimulating the production and function of blood cells of all types and in regulating the differentiation, activation, and suppression of cells involved in specific immunity. Some cytokines are referred to as **interleukins**; cytokines also include **interferons** and **colony-stimulating factors.** Cytokines have local and distant effects and activate cells in an autocrine (causing a self-response) and paracrine (affecting other cells) fashion.

An important feature of cytokine action is that multiple cytokines often work in concert to foster a particular change in cellular activity. The proliferation and differentiation of effector T cells important in cell-mediated immunity (CMI) depend on the interplay of TH1 cytokines such as IL-2, IL-12, and IFN-γ. Activation of B cells for humoral immunity is based on the release of several interleukins (IL-4, IL-5, IL-10, and IL-13) by TH2 cells. TH1 cytokines are important in stimulating B cell differentiation leading to the production of immunoglobulins IgG1, IgG2, and IgG3. TH2 cytokines stimulate IgE and IgG4 production. The actions of selected cytokines are summarized in Table 35-1.

Humoral antibodies. Antibodies synthesized and released by plasma cells directly mediate humoral immunity. As shown in Figure 35-2, the basic immunoglobulin structure consists of two heavy chains and two light chains covalently linked by interchain disulfide bonds. Both chains consist of two or more domains, each defined by a single intra-chain disulfide bond. The heavy chain is composed of three or four constant domains and one variable domain. The light chain incorporates one constant and one variable domain. The relatively flexible hinge regions found in certain immunoglobulins are believed to be remnants of primordial constant domains. Terminal sequences on the amino end of each chain make up the variable regions of the molecule. Within each variable region are hypervariable sequences that are responsible for specific antigen binding. There are two types of light chains: λ and κ. The ratio of λ and κ chains differs in various species, being 1:20 in mice and 1:2 in humans. Sometimes the ratio of λ to κ is used to identify multiple myeloma.

The class of an antibody is determined by its heavy chain. There are five heavy chains or isotypes: IgM, IgG, IgD, IgA, and IgE. IgG is the most abundant subtype and has several subclasses: IgG1, IgG2 (IgG2a and IgG2b), IgG3, and IgG4. The amino terminal region in the variable domain (F domain) of the heavy and light chains (V_H and V_L) binds to antigen, whereas constant domain (C domain) of the heavy and light chains (C_H and C_L) makes up the constant regions.

These domains form the Fc region of the molecule (Fc is the "crystallizable fragment" of a polyclonal immunoglobulin). The Fc region dictates the specific binding of each isotype to different Fc receptors

TABLE 35-1 Selected Cytokines and Their Functional Relationships

Cytokine	Secreted By	Functions
Lymphoid Hematopoiesis		
IL-7	SC	Lymphopoietin-1 Growth of pro-B and pre-B cells Growth of CD4⁻ and CD8⁻T cells
T Cell Stimulating Factors		
IL-1 (α and β)	APC, B, Ep, En	Upregulation of IL-2 receptors on T cells Fever (endogenous pyrogen) Bone resorption (OAF)
IFN-α	B, Ma	Death of virus-infected cells Isotype switching Upregulation of MHC class II Ag
IFN-β	Fb, Ep	Same as for IFN-α
IFN-γ	T	Same as for IFN-α Upregulation of IL-2 receptors
IL-2	T	T Cell proliferation and formation of cytotoxic T lymphocytes
IL-10	T, B	T Cell proliferation Inhibition of cytokine synthesis by TH1 cells Cofactor for mast cell growth Increased B cell expression of MHC class II molecules
B Cell Stimulating Factors		
IL-4	T	Activation of resting B cells Isotype switching (IgG1 and IgE)
IL-5	T	B cell proliferation Isotype switching (IgA, IgM) Eosinophil differentiation factor
IL-6	T, M, Fb	B cell proliferation Death of virus-infected cells
IL-13	CD4⁺ T	Monocytes assume dendritic features Stimulation of B cell differentiation
Tumor Killers and Cell-Mediated Immunity		
TNF-α	Ma	Death of tumor cells Related to IFN-γ and TNF-β Promotion of healing Angiogenesis
TNF-β	T	Death of tumor cells (lymphotoxin)
IL-12	Ma	Stimulation of TH1 cells and CMI Inhibition of TH2 cells and IgE production
Myeloid Factors		
IL-3	L, My	Multiple granulocytic cell type CSF
IL-8	Ma, En	Neutrophil (and lymphocyte) chemotaxis Granulocyte differentiation cofactor
IL-9	T	Erythroid cell precursor growth Mast cell growth
IL-11	SC	Megakaryocyte growth and differentiation
GM-CSF	L, My	Granulocyte/monocyte CSF
M-CSF	L, My	Monocyte CSF
G-CSF	L, My	Granulocyte/erythroid cell CSF
Erythropoietin	RC	Erythroid growth and differentiation

This summary table is not intended to provide a complete listing of all the biologic functions of the cytokines but rather to point out the relationships among them. *Ag,* Antigen; *APC,* antigen-presenting cell; *B,* B cell; *CMI,* cell-mediated immunity; *CSF,* colony-stimulating factor; *En,* endothelial cell; *Ep,* epithelial cell; *Fb,* fibroblast; *G,* granulocyte; *L,* lymphoid cell; *M,* monocyte; *Ma,* macrophage; *My,* myeloid cell; *OAF,* osteoclast-activating factor; *RC,* renal cortex; *SC,* stromal cell; *T,* T cell; *TNF,* tumor necrosis factor.

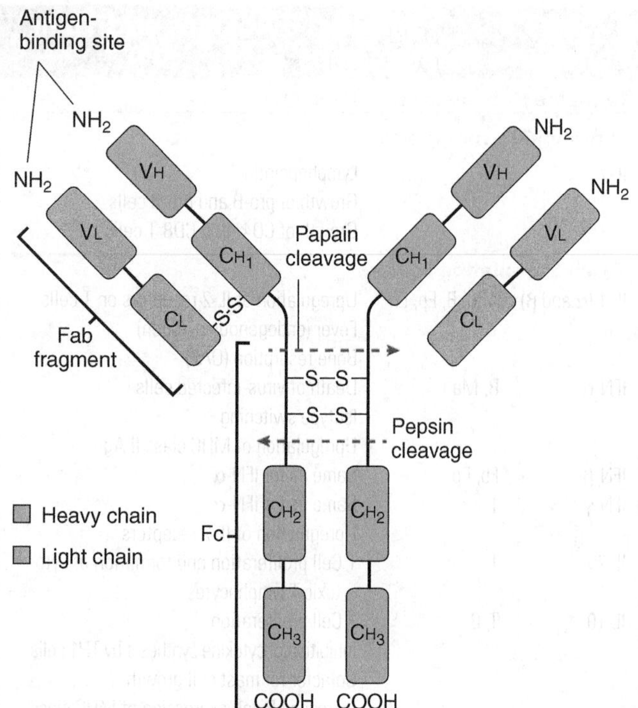

FIG 35-2 Diagram of an IgG antibody, including disulfide linkages. The "crystallization fragment" (*Fc*) of the molecule, formed by portions of the two heavy chains, contains the binding sites for specific cells and for complement; each remaining "antibody fragment" (*Fab*), which consists of one light chain and the remaining portion of one heavy chain, includes the variable regions (*VL* and *VH*) that participate in antibody binding.

on phagocytes, mast cells, and other cells involved in inflammatory reactions. The Fc region also dictates complement activation by IgG and IgM.

There are three discrete regions in the V_H and V_L domains of the antibodies named HV1 (hypervariable 1), HV2, and HV3 (HV3 is the most variable site of each domain). These are separated by structural framework regions (FRs), namely FR1, FR2, FR3, and FR4. The six hypervariable regions in each arm of the antibody that form the antigen-binding site when brought together are complementary to the antigen, thus they are called **complementarity determining regions** or **CDRs**. There are three CDRs: CDR1, CDR2, and CDR3. Antigen molecules contact antibody over a broad area of its surface and bind non-covalently through electrostatic forces, hydrogen bonds, van der Waals forces, and hydrophobic interactions.

Transmembrane and secreted forms of Igs are generated through alternative splicing of heavy chain domains. There are two polyadenylated sites that dictate the generation of transmembrane or secreted forms of Igs. All B cells initially express IgM in its transmembrane form, but upon contact with antigen, they generate the secreted forms and undergo isotype switching to generate other antibodies.

Sequence differences between Ig heavy chains cause the various isotypes to differ in the number and location of their disulfide bonds, the number of attached oligosaccharide moieties, the number of C domains, and the length of the hinge region. The differences between Ig are summarized in Table 35-2.

Each plasma cell produces a unique antibody because of the clonal distribution of the BCR. Initially, the differentiation of B cells to plasma cells results in the production of IgM antibodies. If antigen has also been presented to CD4⁺ T cells by B cells, the T cells can guide B cell differentiation along the memory pathway. In the memory pathway, the isotype may change. Secondary antigen exposure can elicit IgA, IgG, or IgE production. This process of **isotype switching** promotes a more appropriate interplay of antibodies with complement and with myeloid immune cells (e.g., neutrophils, monocytes, mast cells, and eosinophils).

Initiation, Progression, and Termination of Specific Immune Responses

The immune system is normally engaged in the homeostatic regulation of host-derived antigens. Once an antigen receptor is formed, it has to be rigorously tested against self-peptides. Given the incredible number of receptors formed, it is important that those lymphocytes that reach maturity are likely to be useful in recognizing foreign antigens. In general, developing lymphocytes, whose receptors interact weakly with self-antigens or bind antigen in a particular fashion, receive a survival signal. In contrast, lymphocytes with strongly self-reactive receptors must be deleted to prevent autoimmunity through negative selection. The fate of lymphocytes in the absence of any signal is death. In addition, the immune system participates in its more widely appreciated inflammatory function known as the *immune response*.

Immune responses are the measurable alterations in immune system activity after an antigenic perturbation. They are usually initiated by an **immediate inflammatory reaction** resulting from the activation of soluble factors (e.g., complement) found within the extracellular fluid or mediators released by resident leukocytes, especially the mast cells. The immediate inflammatory response signals post-capillary venule endothelial cells to recruit the appropriate acute-phase or chronic-phase leukocytes from the blood. Initially recruited are cells that do not need to progress through proliferation or differentiation to exert an effect, such as neutrophils. Neutrophils are the predominant cells in acute inflammation. Acute inflammation may be followed by slower, chronic inflammation involving less mature cells capable of adaptive cellular differentiation (with or without proliferation). The proliferation and differentiation of clones of cells that recognize the antigen specifically constitute the specific immune response.

The **specific immune responses** involve a series of events (Fig. 35-3), each of which offers a potential site for immunotherapeutic intervention. Included in this series are antigen processing and presentation, T cell activation, lymphocyte differentiation, effector function, and termination. These events occur in response to changes in the intracellular and extracellular concentrations of antigens.

Antigen processing

Antigen processing is the degradation of polymeric antigens into oligomeric units (especially the degradation of a protein into small peptides), which are subsequently bound by MHC I or II molecules. Various hydrophobic peptides and glycolipids can be bound by CD1 antigens, which are related to the MHC I and II molecules.

Intracellular antigens. Processing of intracellular antigens generated within the endoplasmic reticulum or cytosol occurs continuously in all cells. Proteins in the cells become degraded and are replaced by newly synthesized proteins. Degradation of protein occurs in a large, multi-subunit protease-like structure called the **proteasome**. Peptides can further be trimmed in the endoplasmic reticulum (ER) by the help of aminopeptidases. Some proteasomes accept proteins for degradation only if they are tagged by small polypeptides called *ubiquitin*. The peptides generated in the cytosol are transported into the ER where they are bound by nascent MHC I molecules.

Viruses and certain types of bacteria are degraded in the cytosol or in the nuclear compartments before they are presented in the context of **MHC I**. Structurally, MHC I consists of two polypeptide chains: α and β. The α chain is the larger of the two and has three domains: α_1,

TABLE 35-2 **Properties of Immunoglobins**

Name	Properties	Percent of Total Ig	Half-Life (Days)	Distribution	Molecular Weight	Structure
IgA	• Important in specific immunity against supramucosal antigens and in antiinflammatory reactions below the mucosa, as well as caries immunology • 2 subclasses: IgA1 and IgA2 • IgA2 is found in most mucous secretions and constitutes about 40% of total salivary IgA • On a daily basis, ~3 times more IgA is produced than all other immunoglobulins combined • Bound by the polymeric immunoglobulin receptor (pIgR) that enables transportation by transcytosis across the epithelium and into secretions	15	IgA1, 5-9 IgA2, 4-5	Intravascular and secretions	320,000	
IgD	• Role is less clear because it can be co-expressed with IgM on a single B cell • Believed to prevent the induction of B cell tolerance • Protects against parasites	0.2	2-3	Lymphocytes surface	180,000	
IgE	• Important in responses to antigens on secondary exposure • Promotes immediate inflammation; important in initiating acute and chronic inflammation • Enables eosinophils to exert anthelmintic and antiparasitic effects • Has anthelmintic and antiparasitic effects • Production is tightly controlled	0.002	2	Basophils, eosinophils, and mast cells in saliva and nasal secretions	200,000	
IgG	• Principal opsonic antibody important for phagocytosis • Plays a central role in immune responses against submucosal antigens • 4 subclasses: IgG1, IgG2, IgG3 and IgG4 • Fc receptors for IgG are found on neutrophils, monocytes, and DCs	75	21	Intra- and extravascular	150,000	
IgM	• Predominates in neonates and during initial, or primary, immune responses to antigenic challenges, but does not cross placenta • Activates complement • Co-expressed with IgD on the surface of cells • Bound by the polymeric immunoglobulin receptor (pIgR) which enables transportation by transcytosis across the epithelium and into secretions	10	10	Mostly intravascular	900,000	

This summary table is not intended to provide a complete listing of all the functional properties of Igs.
The small round structures represent oligosaccharides.

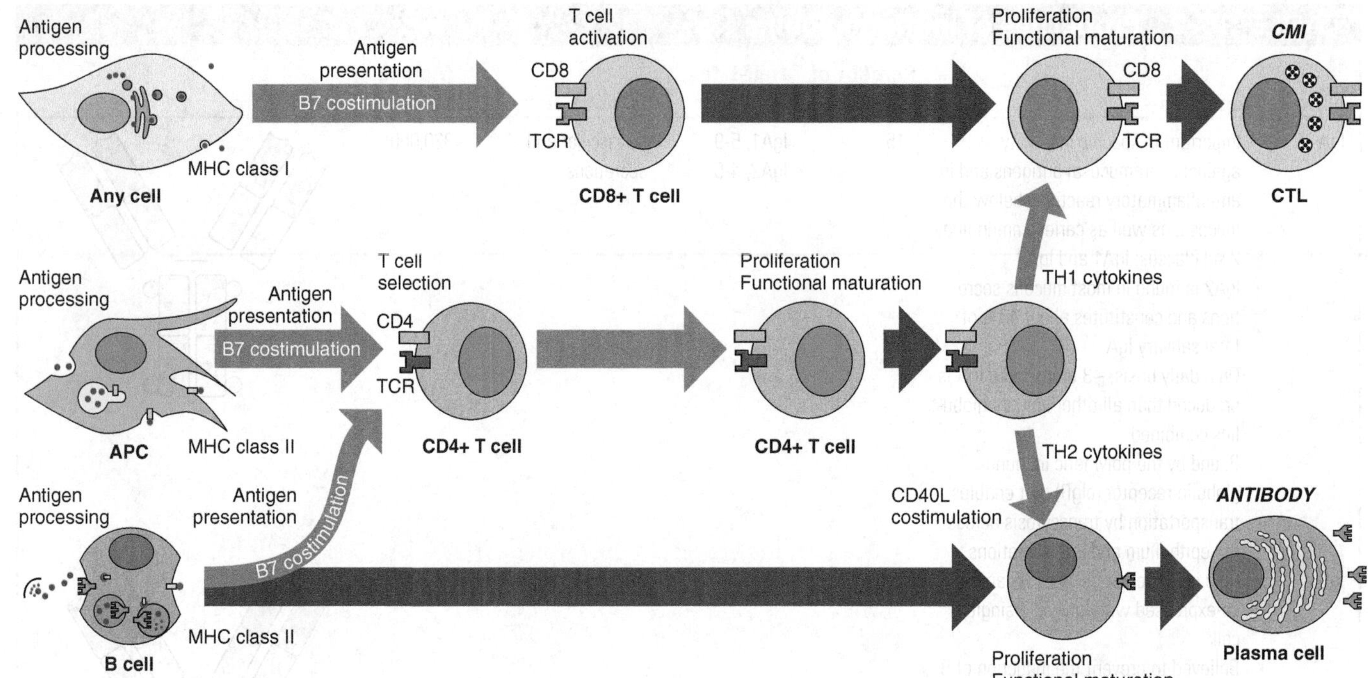

FIG 35-3 Overview of adaptive immune responses. For simplicity, the IL-2 receptor and the TH17 and Treg helper cells are not shown. *APC,* Antigen-presenting cell; *CMI,* cell-mediated immunity; *CTL,* cytotoxic T lymphocyte.

α_2 and α_3. The smaller, non-polymorphic β chain, termed β_2 *microglobulin,* is non-covalently attached to the α_3 domain. Only the α chain spans the membrane. The α_1 and α_2 domains form the cleft that binds to the peptide fragment and are highly polymorphic. Peptides that bind to MHC I molecules are transported from the cytosol to the ER. The peptide-binding site of MHC I is formed in the lumen of the ER and is never exposed to the cytosol. Expression of MHC I on the surface of the cells is unstable unless it is bound to peptide. Mutations at a site where peptides bind to the MHC I protein cause significant decrease in the expression of MHC I on the surface of the cells. Mutations in transporters associated with antigen processing (TAPs) may also not allow for the transport of the peptides from the cytosol to the lumen of the ER.

Newly synthesized MHC I α chains bind to a chaperone protein called *calnexin,* which retains MHC I in a partly folded structure in the ER. When β_2 microglobulin binds the α chain, the complex dissociates from calnexin and then binds to another chaperone, *calreticulin.* A third protein, tapasin, forms a bridge between MHC I molecules and TAP, allowing the transport of the suitable peptide from the cytosol. Most of the chaperone proteins play a role in selecting peptides with higher binding affinity.

Viruses have evolved several means of evading recognition by preventing the appearance of peptide:MHC I complexes at the cell surface. For example, the herpes simplex virus prevents the transport of viral peptides into the ER by producing proteins that bind and inhibit TAP, whereas adenoviruses produce a protein that binds MHC I molecules and retains them in the ER. Cytomegaloviruses accelerate retrograde translocation of MHC I back into the cytosol, where they are degraded.

Extracellular antigens. The majority of pathogenic bacteria and some eukaryotic parasites replicate in the endosomes and lysosomes that form the vesicular system. Pathogens such as *Leishmania* and mycobacteria are picked up by macrophages through endocytosis. The resultant endocytic vesicles gradually become acidified and finally fuse with lysosomes, forming phagolysosomes. These organelles contain acid proteases that become activated at low pH, resulting in degradation of the protein antigen. Among acid proteases are the cysteine proteases **cathepsin** B, D, S, and L. Cathepsin L is the most active of the family. Disulfide bonds also need to be cleaved for peptide processing. Degraded peptides from pathogens are then presented in the context of MHC II molecules to T cells.

Each **MHC II** protein comprises two non-covalently bound chains, α and β, both of which span the membrane. There are two α domains, α_1 and α_2, and two β domains, β_1 and β_2. The α_1 and β_1 domains are very polymorphic and form the peptide-binding locus. The folding of α_1 and β_1 is more open than the α_1 and α_2 domain of MHC I, thus the ends of the peptide fragments are exposed.

Binding of nonspecific peptides to MHC II is prevented by the association of MHC II in the ER with a third polypeptide termed the *invariant chain.* The invariant chain, by forming a trimer with MHC II, covers the antigen-binding groove. Invariant chains also target MHC II to low-pH endosomal compartments where peptide loading can occur. The invariant chain is then cleaved by acid proteases, such as cathepsin S, to generate a truncated form. The subsequent cleavage releases the MHC II molecule leaving a fragment called **CLIP** bound to the MHC II.

Most MHC II molecules are brought to the cell surface in vesicles, which at some point fuse with incoming endosomes where they encounter and bind peptides derived from self- or non-self-proteins. HLA-DM assists in the process by stabilizing MHC II molecules, which would otherwise aggregate. It also catalyzes the removal of CLIP and the loading of the peptide into the groove of the MHC II. HLA-DM, closely related to the MHC II molecule, does not bind to the peptide because its groove is closed. HLA-DM also removes weakly bound peptides, allowing for the binding of high-affinity peptides. Peptides bound to MHC can remain for several days in case the APC does not encounter the target; therefore, increased binding affinity of the peptide to the groove is important.

A second atypical MHC II molecule, called HLA-DO, is produced by thymic epithelial cells and B cells. Unlike HLA-DM, which aids in releasing CLIP and binding peptide, HLA-DO inhibits HLA-DM function and subsequently inhibits antigen loading. The activating capacity of HLA-DM is higher than the inhibiting capacity of HLA-DO because secreted IFN-γ can upregulate HLA-DM but not HLA-DO.

T cell activation

T cell recognition, activation, and effector function depend on **cell–cell contact** mediated by **cell adhesion molecules.** T cells enter the lymph nodes through binding to specialized post-capillary swellings called **high endothelial venules.** The main classes of adhesion molecules involved in lymphocyte interaction are the **selectins, integrins, members of the Ig superfamily, and mucin-like molecules.**

Just as binding of neutrophils to endothelial cells is guided by **chemokines**, migration of naïve T cells into lymphoid tissues is directed by similar molecules, such as secondary lymphoid tissue chemokines. This interaction increases both the affinity and surface expression of integrins on the T cell membranes, which arrests the cells and causes them to move through the endothelial layer to enter the lymphoid parenchyma. The integrin LFA-1, for example, is expressed on all T cells. It binds to Ig superfamily adhesion molecules, such as ICAM-1 and ICAM-2, which are expressed on endothelium and APCs. Binding to LFA-1 allows the leukocytes to migrate through the blood vessel wall in lymph nodes and be able to sample antigen on the surface of APCs. ICAM-3, another adhesion molecule, is expressed only on leukocytes and binds to its partner (DC-sign) on DCs. The binding of CD58 (LFA3) on APCs to CD2 on T cells is yet another example of adhesion molecule interactions.

The initial association of T cells with APCs is mediated by the interplay of multiple adhesion molecules. Binding of LFA-1, ICAM-3, and CD2 on T cells to ICAM-1, ICAM-2, DC-sign, and CD-58 on APCs provides enough redundancy that if one pairing is missing, the T cells can still bind and recognize the specific antigen on the APCs. The transient binding to APCs allows the T cells to sample a large number of MHC:peptide sequences on APCs, and if it recognizes the antigen, signaling through the TCR will significantly increase the affinity of LFA-1 for ICAM-1.

Both signals from **specific antigen and costimulatory molecules** are required for the clonal expansion of T cells. In the absence of costimulatory signals, activation of T cells through antigen receptor will lead to anergy or unresponsiveness. Anergic cells are eventually deleted by cell death. The most highly characterized costimulatory molecules are structurally related glycoproteins belonging to the B7 family. The best-known ones are B7.1 (CD80) and B7.2 (CD86). They bind to the CD28 receptor on the surface of naïve T cells and costimulate in the presence of an antigen receptor. Once a naïve T cell is activated, it upregulates CD40 ligand, which binds to the CD40 receptor on APCs and further activates both the T cells and the APCs. Activated T cells will then upregulate cytotoxic T-lymphocyte–associated antigen-4 (CTLA-4 or CD152), which is similar in structure to CD28 and limits further activation by binding to B7 family costimulatory molecules. This way, activation and proliferation of T cells are regulated.

Resident DCs, such as Langerhans cells, are able to pick up antigen by phagocytosis or macropinocytosis. They can travel and take the antigen to the secondary lymphoid tissues where they lose the capability to phagocytize but gain the ability to present antigen to T and B cells. Both DCs and B cells can bind soluble antigens and present them as peptide:MHC II complexes to T cells. B cells do not express costimulatory molecules constitutively; they need to be activated by bacteria to express B7.1 and B7.2.

The actual recognition of antigen by the TCR is a low-affinity reaction. This characteristic enables many TCRs of a given T cell to interact with the few specific antigens presented by the antigen-presenting cell. Multiple interactions are important because T cell activation depends on the number of TCRs that interact with antigen over time. The factors that influence T cell activation include the number of antigen molecules presented by the antigen-presenting cell, the affinity of the TCR for the antigen, and the number of TCRs. If the interaction with peptide antigen by TCRs is sufficient, the TCRs cluster on the T cell surface and downregulate (the TCRs are probably internalized). With costimulation, activation of TCRs leads to T cell effector function.

In early stages of exposure to antigen, costimulatory signals permit T cells to become receptive to differentiative signals, allowing them to proliferate or mature in function. These signals also block apoptosis. At later stages, the same signals can permit T cells to differentiate terminally, even to the point of death.

Differentiation

After antigen recognition by TCR and BCR, intracellular signaling events allow the T cell to differentiate into **functionally mature cells** (Fig. 35-4). **Much present-day immunotherapy is aimed at this stage of the specific immune response.** Binding of antigen to its receptor leads to the clustering of antigen receptor on lymphocytes, which is the first step in signal transduction. Clustering of antigen receptors leads to activation of intracellular signaling molecules. Protein tyrosine kinases are enzymes that affect the function of other proteins by adding a phosphate group to certain tyrosine residues. Specific growth factors such as c-kit have cytoplasmic domains that contain intrinsic tyrosine kinase activity. T and B cell signaling is different from c-kit signaling since the TCR and BCR do not have intrinsic kinase domains; rather, they rely on the interaction with other tyrosine kinases known as receptor-associated tyrosine kinases.

There are specialized areas within the membrane lipid bilayer that contain high quantities of sphingolipids and cholesterol. These areas are called **lipid rafts.** Signaling molecules associate with lipid rafts. Disruption of the lipid rafts inhibits T and B cell signaling.

Signaling through T and B cells is governed by a complex array of intracellular signaling elements, which can phosphorylate and activate other elements to transduce the signal from the receptor. The receptor-associated protein kinases are localized in the inner surface of the cell membrane and cannot activate their cytosolic targets efficiently unless they themselves are activated. Their activation and subsequent phosphorylation of tyrosines on receptor-associated chains recruits other protein tyrosine kinases, which then transduce the signal. The src-family kinases involved in T and B cell receptor signaling provide an example of this kind of signaling element.

The variant chains of the lymphocyte antigen receptor are associated with invariant accessory chains that mediate the signaling function of the receptor. The BCR is associated with Igα and Igβ invariant chains. The TCR is associated with multiple invariant accessory chains (ε, γ, δ, and ζ). Accessory chains have a structure termed the **immunotyrosine activation motif (ITAM)**, which enables them to signal when the BCR or TCR is bound to the antigen. ITAMs are phosphorylated by src-family receptor–associated tyrosine kinases, which give them the ability to bind to the members of a second family of tyrosine kinases (Syk in B cells and ZAP 70 in T cells). The enzyme activity of each src-family kinase is regulated by the phosphorylation status of its kinase domain and its carboxy terminal region, each having a regulatory tyrosine residue. Phosphorylation of tyrosine in the kinase domain activates the enzyme, whereas phosphorylation at the carboxy terminal tyrosine is inhibitory. Src-family kinases are kept inactive by a tyrosine kinase called *CSK* (c-terminal src kinase), which phosphorylates the inhibitory domain. Since the function of CSK is constitutive in resting cells, src-family proteins remain quiescent until antigen recognition, which then activates a protein tyrosine phosphatase (CD45

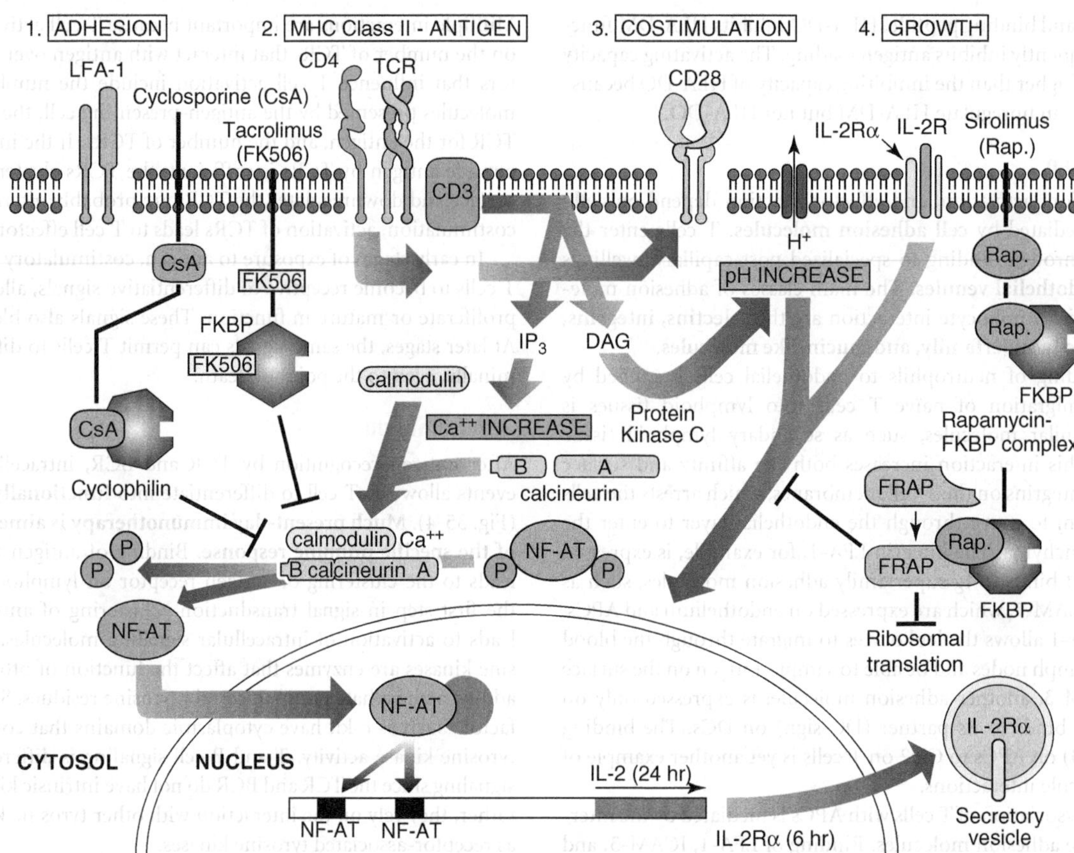

FIG 35-4 Intracellular mediators of T cell differentiation and their inhibition by immunosuppressant drugs. The MAP kinase pathway is not shown. *CsA*, Cyclosporine; *CD*, cluster of differentiation glycoprotein; *DAG*, diacylglycerol; *FKBP*, FK-506-binding protein; *FRAP*, FKBP-rapamycin-associated protein; *IL*, interleukin; *LFA-1*, lymphocyte function-associated antigen-1; *NF-AT*, nuclear factor of activated T cells; *Rap.*, sirolimus; *TCR*, T cell receptor.

that removes the phosphate block from the inhibitory tyrosine and permits activation of the src-family kinases).

Antigen receptor signaling is enhanced by co-receptors that bind to the same ligand. B cell co-receptors are formed by a complex of CD19, CD21, and CD81 proteins. Src-family kinases phosphorylate the ITAMs on Igα and Igβ, and these subsequently recruit Syk to Igβ. *Trans*-phosphorylation of each kinase by the other occurs, and the activated kinases in turn activate phospholipase C-γ (PLC-γ), guanine exchange factors (GEFs), and Tec kinases.

Similar to BCRs, clustering of TCRs and the co-receptors activates CD45, which removes a phosphate from src-family kinases (e.g., Lck) and activates their function, resulting in the phosphorylation of ITAMs. After phosphorylation, ZAP-70 is able to bind and become activated by Lck, which will initiate a signaling cascade leading to the activation of PLC-γ, GEF, and Tec kinases.

PLC-γ is known to cleave membrane phosphatidylinositol bisphosphate (PIP_2), yielding diacylglycerol (DAG) and inositol triphosphate (IP_3). DAG activates protein kinase C (PKC), which in turn stimulates nuclear factor-κB (NF-κB). **NF-κB** usually is complexed with inhibitor proteins collectively called I-κB, which prevent its translocation to the nucleus. NF-κB is an **important transcription factor** for various inflammatory cytokines, and it supports inflammatory aspects of the specific immune response. TNF-α, one of the cytokines whose synthesis is stimulated in part by NF-κB, increases the transcription of NF-κB and its dissociation from I-κB.

IP_3 increases the intracellular Ca^{++} concentration, activating calcineurin, a phosphatase that releases NF-AT (nuclear factor of activated T cells) from a phosphate block. GEFs activate Ras, an important GTPase that activates MAP kinases. The Ras-induced MAP kinases then activate Fos and Jun kinases, which are components of the transcription factor AP-1.

In unstimulated cells, NF-AT is rendered inactive and remains in the cytoplasm by phosphorylation on serine/threonine residues. Ca^{++}-activated calcineurin removes the phosphate block and unmasks the nuclear localization signal, which then directs NF-AT to enter the nucleus of the cell and activate transcription. For NF-AT to remain in the nucleus, the function of glycogen synthase kinase (GSK3) must be inhibited. GSK3 can phosphorylate NF-AT, exporting it back to the cytoplasm. Cyclosporin A and tacrolimus are inhibitors of NF-AT (Fig. 35-4).

Signals from the antigen receptor alter the cytoskeleton to cause changes in cell shape, motility, and secretion. Receptor signaling can be inhibited by interactions with inhibitory receptors expressed on the surface of cells such as NK cells and other lymphocytes.

Natural killer cells

Although we have focused on the function of specific immune effectors T and B cells in this chapter, it is important to emphasize the role of NK cells in immunity since these cells were recently shown to target cancer stem cells; therefore, NK cells are likely to be the key effectors to be used in designing future immunotherapeutic strategies. NK cells arise from the bone marrow and constitute 5% to 15% of total lymphocytes in the peripheral blood. They are known to mediate direct cytotoxicity as well as antibody-dependent cellular cytotoxicity. By producing key cytokines and chemokines, NK cells are known to regulate the

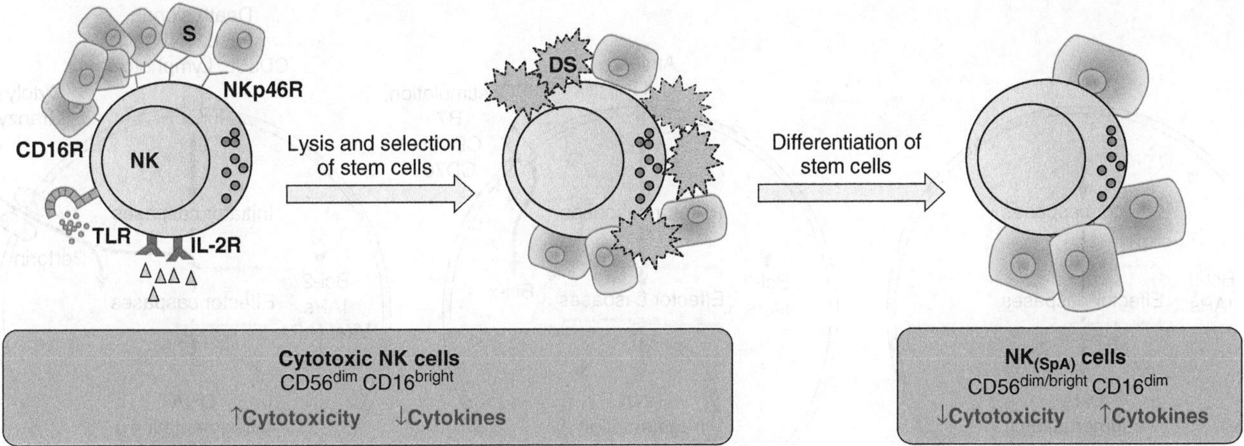

FIG 35-5 Binding and recognition of stem cells by NK cells results in the selection of a subpopulation of stem cells and the promotion of differentiation of selected stem cells. Activation with IL-2, triggering of toll-like receptors, results in the activation of NK cells to mediate cytotoxicity and secretion of cytokines. $CD56^{dim}CD16^{bright}$ NK cell subset is highly cytotoxic and is capable of selecting and lysing cancer stem cells. Whereas, $CD56^{dim/bright}CD16^{dim}$ NK cell subset, which lacks cytotoxicity, is able to secrete high levels of cytokines IFN-γ and TNF-α to support differentiation of selected stem cells. Please note, the receptors shown on NK cells are a partial list of receptors important for the activation of NK cell function. *NK,* NK cells; *NK(SpA) cells,* split anergized NK cells; *TLR,* toll-like receptors; *S,* stem cells; *CD16R,* CD16 receptors; *NKp46R,* NKp46 receptors; *IL-2R,* IL-2 receptors; *DS,* dead stem cells.

functions of other immune cells. Conventional human NK cells are identified by the expression of CD16 and CD56 and by the lack of surface CD3 expression. NK cells mediate their function through a number of important activating and inhibitory cell receptors. It is thought that the balance between activating and inhibitory signals that NK cells receive from their surface receptors determines their functional fate. In addition, the functional fate of these receptors is determined by their intracellular domains for which they either have an immunoreceptor tyrosine-based activation motif (ITAM) or immunoreceptor tyrosine-based inhibition motif responsible for delivering activating or inhibitory signals, respectively.

The association of distinct effector functions with certain NK cell subsets is thought to be developmentally regulated. In this regard, previous studies have identified two distinct subsets of NK cells, namely $CD56^{dim/bright}CD16^{dim}$ and $CD56^{dim}CD16^{bright}$ subpopulations based on their phenotypic and functional analysis. The $CD56^{dim}CD16^{bright}$ NK subset is the major subset in the peripheral blood that mediates cytotoxicity, whereas the $CD56^{dim/bright}CD16^{dim}$ subset constitutes a minor subpopulation of NK cells in the peripheral blood, and its role is in secretion of cytokines. The $CD56^{dim/bright}CD16^{dim}$ subset does not mediate cytotoxicity. The $CD56^{dim/bright}CD16^{dim}$ NK cells are thought to be precursors to the $CD56^{dim}CD16^{bright}$ NK subset. Previous studies have also indicated that NK cells may recognize and become activated by irradiated or stressed cells. The most exciting recent discovery directly relevant to immunotherapy of cancer is the identification of the role of NK cells in recognition, selection, and differentiation of stem cells, in particular cancer stem cells or poorly differentiated tumors (Fig. 35-5). When NK cells interact with tumor cells, they lose cytotoxicity but gain the ability to secrete cytokines, a concept that has been coined split anergy (SpA). The concept of SpA in NK cells and its role in the switch of NK cell function from effector to regulatory cell function and promotion of cellular differentiation have been shown in several recent studies (see Fig. 35-5).

Effector aspects of cell-mediated immunity

In CMI, NK and $CD4^+$ and $CD8^+$ T cells play important roles. $CD4^+$ T cells receive antigen stimulation and costimulation from DCs to secrete key cytokines and growth factors. $CD8^+$ T cells receive antigen stimulation and costimulation from infected or neoplastic cells and become primed to receive proliferative and differentiative signals from $CD4^+$ T cells. $CD8^+$ T cells proliferate and differentiate into cytotoxic T lymphocytes in the presence of TH1 cytokines, such as IL-2, IL-12, and IFN-γ. Unlike T cells, NK cells do not require MHC recognition for their activation, and they can mediate cytotoxicity without prior activation, even though they also respond to TH1 cytokines by increasing cytotoxicity.

Apoptosis. When NK cells or a cytotoxic T lymphocyte recognizes antigen in association with MHC I molecules on virally infected cells or transformed tumor targets, it may induce apoptosis, otherwise known as **programmed cell death.** NK cells or a cytotoxic T lymphocyte does this by presenting the target cell with specific membrane-bound signals delivered by Fas ligand, TNF-α, and APO2 ligand. If the signals are effective, the target cell is induced to die. Target cells express specific TNF-family receptors (TNFRs) for these ligands. Apoptosis, as summarized in Figure 35-6, involves several steps that may be targeted for therapeutic intervention.

Cells possess mechanisms for preventing death by using proteins, such as Bcl-2, and several other inhibitors of apoptosis proteins (IAPs). Bcl-2 is expressed on the membranes of intracellular organelles, including the mitochondria, nucleus, and smooth ER. Bcl-2 and IAPs delay or prevent apoptosis by inhibiting proteolysis mediated by cysteine proteases, termed **caspases,** which are responsive to apoptotic signals. Several viruses (including Epstein-Barr virus, adenovirus, African swine fever virus, and cowpox) produce substances similar to Bcl-2 and IAP, which may help them evade host defenses by preventing apoptosis. Also, B cell lymphomas have been associated with Bcl-2 overexpression. Costimulation of T and B cells induces the expression of apoptosis-inhibiting molecules after antigen stimulation.

Cytolytic activities. A target cell may become resistant to apoptotic signaling mediated by the aforementioned surface ligands, especially if the cell is infected by a virus that produces apoptotic inhibitors. In this case, NK cells and the cytotoxic T lymphocytes must depend on **cytolytic factors** to kill the damaged cell. Within the vesicular

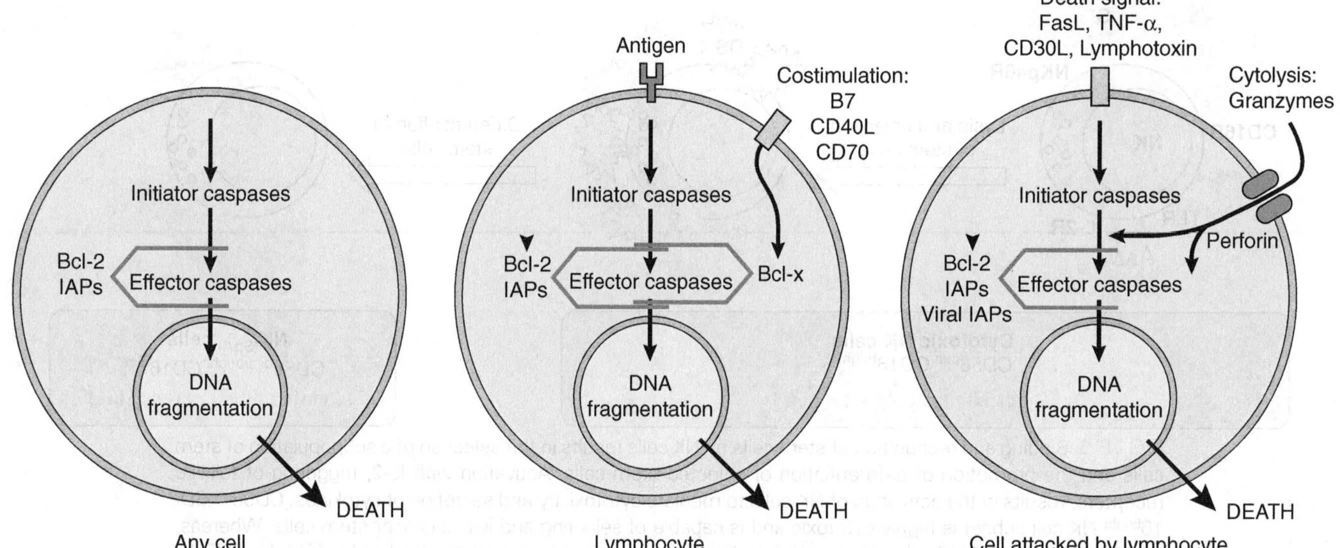

FIG 35-6 Apoptosis and lymphocyte-induced cytolysis. Apoptosis, indicated by the sequence of *arrows*, involves the activation of initiator caspases (e.g., caspase 8), which promotes proteolytic activation of other effector caspases involved in apoptosis. Environmental cues help prevent programmed cellular death by invoking the blocking action (*shaded lines*) of Bcl-2 or specific IAPs or both. Similar molecules (e.g., Bcl-x) inhibit apoptosis in lymphocytes costimulated by members of the TNF family (B7, CD40L, and CD70) and in virally infected cells. Cytotoxic lymphocytes destroy targeted cells either by (1) signaling for apoptosis to occur or (2) releasing perforins and granzymes that activate proteolysis directly. *FasL,* Fas ligand.

components and dense cores of these granules are numerous potentially cytocidal proteins. The vesicles and dense cores are discharged when the cytotoxic granules fuse with the plasma membrane of the NK cell or cytotoxic T lymphocyte.

Granule exocytosis can provide additional death-inducing factors. One factor is **perforin**. Perforin can form polymeric channels in cell membranes. Affected membranes lose their structural integrity, and lysis of the cell soon follows. The second factor is granzyme B. **Granzymes** may gain access to the target cell, either directly by fusion of the granule vesicles or dense core with the membrane of the target cell or because of a sub-lytic quantity of perforin that allows granzymes to gain access to the cytosol of the target cell. When in the cytosol, granzyme B can activate apoptotic proteolysis.

Humoral immunity

Humoral immune responses protect the extracellular spaces of the body from being colonized by pathogenic bacteria and guard against the spread of intracellular pathogens from cell to cell. The **activation of B cells** and their differentiation into antibody-producing plasma cells and memory cells are triggered by the antigen, processes that usually require the assistance of T helper cells.

Antibodies play important roles in active immunity. Antibodies can neutralize the pathogen. Neutralization prevents viruses and intracellular bacteria from binding to specific receptors on the surface of the cells. It also blocks bacterial toxins from gaining access to the cells. Even without neutralization, antibodies can coat the surface of pathogens, thereby enhancing phagocytosis through the process known as **opsonization**. Antibodies support phagocytosis in two ways. First, antibodies bound to the pathogen are recognized by the Fc receptor on phagocytes; second, antibodies activate the complement system, which results in complement binding to the pathogens and recognition by complement receptor on phagocytes.

The BCR binds and delivers antigens to the intracellular compartments where they dissociate. The protein is degraded and returned to the cell surface as peptide bound to MHC II. The MHC II antigen complex stimulates antigen-specific T cells to secrete cytokines and provide costimulatory signals directing mature B cells to become plasma cells and memory B cells.

B cells require two simultaneous signals to become activated. The first signal is the binding of antigen to the BCR. The second signal can occur in either of two ways. In the T helper cell–dependent pathway, the signal is generated by the binding of the T helper cell to the MHC II antigen complex as assisted by CD40/CD40L costimulation. In the T cell–independent pathway, the second signal is caused by the reaction of membrane IgM with a polymeric antigen or by exposure to large concentrations of lipopolysaccharide. In the latter case, the polyclonal activation can activate large numbers of B cells rather indiscriminately.

The B cell co-receptor complex CD19/CD21/CD81 greatly enhances B cell responsiveness to antigen. B cells and T helper cells must recognize epitopes of the same molecular complex in order to interact. This requirement is termed **liked recognition.** Antigenic peptides bound to self-MHC II molecules trigger armed T helper cells to make CD40L and cytokine IL4/IL5/IL6. Isotype switching is decreased in individuals who lack CD40L. Individuals with CD40L deficiency have hyperimmunoglobulinemia M, a disease characterized by an elevation of IgM and a severe deficiency of almost all other isotypes.

In secondary lymphoid tissues, antigen-binding B cells are trapped in the T cell zones and are activated by armed helper T cells. The second phase of the primary B cell immune response occurs when activated B cells migrate to follicles and proliferate to form germinal centers (GCs). GCs are composed mainly of proliferating B cells, with antigen-specific T cells making up 10% of the lymphocytes. Somatic hypermutation, affinity maturation, and isotype switching occur in GC B cells. Negative selection of B cells in GCs keeps the size of the lymphoid tissues manageable.

Antibodies of the **IgA subclass** are particularly important in conferring protection to the **mucosa. IgG and IgM** are important in antibacterial and antifungal host defense, but they can also lead to type II (cytotoxic) and type III (immune complex) immunopathologic reactions (see Chapter 3). Antibodies of the **IgE subclass** not only provide host defense against parasites and worms, but they also can lead to type I immunopathologic reactions (anaphylaxis). Rarely, IgA has been associated with type II immunopathologic conditions. The distinct functional and immunopathogenic attributes of the immunoglobulin isotypes provide another area of potential immunotherapeutic intervention.

Termination of immune responses

Many mechanisms exist to terminate immune responses when they are no longer required. These mechanisms involve the removal of effector cells that are no longer needed and the suppression of activity of remaining cells.

Propriocidal apoptosis. In the later stages of antigen exposure, when the concentrations of proinflammatory cytokines are high, T cells may undergo a form of antigen-induced cell death known as **propriocidal apoptosis.** It may occur as a result of T cell expression of different costimulatory receptors for factors such as B7 proteins. As previously mentioned, the interaction between B7 and CD28 may serve to prepare a cell for early differentiative events in the immune response (resulting in proliferation and functional maturation), but the interaction between B7 and CTLA-4 may prepare a cell for more terminal events (e.g., differentiation leading to functional inhibition and death).

Immune regulation and suppression. Suppression is involved in regulating the balance between humoral and CMI responses and in terminating these responses altogether. Regulating the degree of humoral immune response versus CMI seems related to the activities of $CD4^+$ T cells, whereas terminating responses involve $CD8^+$ T cells. $CD4^+$ T cells of the TH1 phenotype suppress $CD4^+$ T cells of the TH2 phenotype and directly inhibit B cell activity. $CD4^+$ T cells of the TH2 phenotype suppress TH1 activities. $CD4^+$ TH1 T cells also stimulate $CD8^+$ T cells, an event which has been referred to as **suppressor induction.** $CD4^+CD25^+$ Treg cells are key regulators that suppress the function of T cells.

Classically, the $CD8^+$ phenotype has been associated with cytotoxicity and suppressor activity. It is becoming apparent that the suppression mechanism of the $CD8^+$ T cell can resemble its cytotoxic action. $CD8^+$ T cell suppression of specific humoral immunity and the termination of CMI may be accomplished with the CD30 ligand (CD30L). CD30L is a member of the TNF family recognized by CD30 (a member of the TNFR family) found on T cells. In this case, suppression results from the programmed death of the $CD4^+$ T cell.

If there is an imbalance between immune activation and immune suppression, immunopathologic reactions, including immunodeficiency or autoimmunity, may ensue. Suppression pathways thus play a role in two widely differing defective immune states often considered for **immunotherapy: immunodeficiency or autoimmunity**.

Mucosal Immunity

The vast majority of infectious agents invade the human body by one of the mucosal routes. Diarrheal diseases, respiratory infections, parasitic infestations, and diseases such as tuberculosis, measles, hepatitis B, whooping cough, and human immunodeficiency virus (HIV) infection are widespread and continue to cause significant public health problems throughout the world. Another important point regarding the mucosal surfaces is that they are the portal of entry for a great majority of foreign antigens such as food antigens, dusts, pollens, and other materials. In addition, the gastrointestinal tract is colonized by a great number of commensal bacteria, which normally live within their host symbiotically without causing any pathology.

Traditionally, the mucosal immune system has been considered a minor component of the immune system, and to this date, little is known regarding the function of immune cells in mucosa. Because of its size and exposure to a wide variety of foreign antigens, the mucosal immune system perhaps forms the largest and the most important part of the immune system. It contains significant numbers of lymphocytes and produces high amounts of Igs in healthy individuals. It also has many distinctive features. In mucosa, there is an intimate interaction between mucosal epithelia and the lymphoid tissues. Mucosal epithelial cells contain specialized antigen-uptake mechanisms, and most of the lymphocytes have the activated/memory phenotype even in the absence of infection. The mucosa contains large numbers of **regulatory T cells, and they have inhibitory macrophages and tolerance-inducing DCs.** Finally, there is constitutive downmodulation of immune responses to food and other nonpathogenic antigens.

Mucosal-associated lymphoid tissues are located in anatomically defined compartments of the gut. Lymphocytes, macrophages, and DCs are found throughout the mucosa in organized tissues as well as scattered throughout the surface epithelium and an underlying compartment of the connective tissue called the **lamina propria.** Another important feature of the gut mucosa is the existence of specialized epithelial cells called **microfold** (M) cells. These cells are different from the other epithelial cells (e.g., enterocytes in intestines) in that they do not secrete mucus and are the route of entry of foreign antigens. Antigens are engulfed by the M cells and transcytosed via membrane-bound vesicles to the basal cell membrane where they are released into the extracellular compartment. The DCs can then take up the antigen, process it, and present it to naïve, antigen-specific T lymphocytes in Peyer's patches, or they migrate through draining lymphatics to present antigen to naïve antigen-specific T cells in mesenteric lymph nodes. DCs are recruited to the epithelial layer through the action of chemokines.

The mucosal immune system contains large numbers of effector lymphocytes even in the absence of disease. In addition to the organized lymphoid organs in the mucosa, there are other immune effectors that are scattered throughout the mucosa. The majority of those that are in the epithelial layer are mainly $CD8^+$ T cells, whereas in the lamina propria, large numbers of $CD4^+$ as well as $CD8^+$ T cells, plasma cells, DCs, and macrophages can be found. Neutrophils are rare in healthy intestines, but their numbers increase rapidly during an infection. Therefore, healthy intestinal mucosa displays characteristics that are similar to chronic inflammation in response to the intimate interaction between foreign antigens, commensal bacteria, and mucosal immune cells. Because of the function of regulatory immune effectors, a balance is maintained between inflammation and homeostasis during health and disease.

The **trafficking of the lymphocytes** within the mucosa is controlled by the actions of specific sets of **chemokines** and **integrins.** Gut-specific homing is determined by the expression of α_4:β_7 integrin on the lymphocytes, which binds to mucosal vascular addressin MADCAM-1 on the endothelial cells. In addition, the expression of the CCR9 chemokine receptor on lymphocytes is important for attracting lymphocytes to mucosa. Indeed, local production of CCL25 by the gut epithelium, which binds to CCR9, is required for the homing of the lymphocytes to the gut. Only lymphocytes that first encounter antigen in the gut are induced to express gut-specific homing receptors and integrins. This action is mediated by the gut DCs, which impart to lymphocytes the ability to express the α_4:β_7 integrin and CCR9 receptor. These tissue-specific responses explain why vaccination against intestinal infections requires immunization through the mucosal route and not through parenteral routes.

As mentioned previously, IgA is by far the most abundant antibody in mucosal tissues. The ratio of IgA1 to IgA2 in blood is 10:1, whereas in mucosa it is 3:2. Class switching for IgA is under the control of the TGF-β cytokine. IgA2 is resistant to proteolytic cleavage. After secretion of IgA, it will bind to the poly-Ig receptor on epithelial cells and be transported through transcytosis to the apical surface of the epithelial cells. The main function of IgA in mucosa is to prevent the access of pathogen to the mucosal surfaces. Selective IgA deficiency in humans is a common primary immune deficiency in Caucasians, and atopic and autoimmune diseases have been reported in people with IgA deficiency. Most people with IgA deficiency are normal, however, which might result from the fact that IgA can be replaced by IgM.

There are two types of intraepithelial lymphocytes. One has the conventional αβ TCR and co-receptor CD8 (αβ homodimer). These **type a** conventional T cells recognize antigen within the context of MHC I. The second group of lymphocytes has either the αβ or γδ TCR and the CD8αα homodimer. These **type b** T cells do not recognize antigen in the context of MHC I, rather they bind to other ligands, such as MHC Ib. Another non-classical MHC I molecule is the thymus leukemia antigen, which can bind to the CD8αα homodimer with high affinity. The type b T lymphocytes mediate cytotoxicity; they do not undergo positive or negative selection in the thymus.

IMMUNOTHERAPEUTIC AGENTS

Therapies designed to stimulate or replicate endogenous immune reactions have long been used to prevent infectious disease and to treat different types of immunodeficiencies. More recently, attempts have been made to induce immune responses to combat cancer, and specific antibodies have been developed for a wide range of applications.

In certain clinical situations, it is advantageous to temporarily suppress the inflammatory activities of the specific immune system. Organ transplantation is the best example of an instance in which **immunosuppression** is beneficial. Immunosuppression is also helpful in the treatment of autoimmune diseases and other immunopathologic conditions.

Vaccination

The most successful area of immunotherapy has been vaccination, or "**active immunization.**" It was first introduced to Western culture by Jenner in the 18th century, who injected individuals with the cowpox virus to protect them against smallpox. Vaccination is a procedure in which the immune system is exposed to an antigen, such as an inactivated toxin or attenuated pathogen, to elicit antigen-specific clonal expansion (i.e., the proliferation of T cells and B cells that recognize the antigen). Active immunization uses the host's immune system itself to generate antigen-specific immunotherapeutic agents (e.g., antibodies). On subsequent exposure to the actual pathogen, the immune response is of sufficient speed, magnitude, duration, and specificity to prevent the pathogen from causing disease (the secondary response). Clinically, most success has been observed with vaccination designed to elicit humoral immunity rather than CMI.

Caries vaccines

A disease of special interest to dentistry is dental caries. **Vaccines** directed against *Streptococcus mutans* and *Streptococcus sobrinus*—lactic acid bacteria long suspected of being the major cause of dental caries—have been investigated by several laboratories. (See reference Michalek, and Childers) The purpose of these investigations was to induce an immune response that would prevent the adherence or metabolism by these bacteria on the tooth surface. Several types of vaccines have been considered, including (1) oral immunization by whole bacteria or live enteric bacteria that bear antigens of *S. mutans* as a result of recombinant DNA procedures and (2) immunization by various routes using "subunit" vaccines containing isolated antigens (adhesins, glucosyltransferases, dextranases) believed to be involved in cell adherence and plaque formation. Whole cell–based vaccines are anticariogenic in many laboratory animals, including primates.

In humans, **oral immunization** results in the generation of secretory **IgA** antibodies in salivary secretions. Ingested antigens are subjected to partial breakdown within the stomach and small intestine. As described previously, specialized M cell enterocytes in the gut transcytose macromolecular antigens to unencapsulated lymphoid structures known as **Peyer's patches.** Here, in the presence of TH3 T cells, antigen-specific B cells are selected to undergo IgA isotype switching. They eventually migrate to the regional lymph nodes, where they proliferate. IgA-committed progeny enter the blood and are distributed to effector sites, such as the salivary glands, where they produce IgA antibodies for secretion.

Parenteral routes of administration usually lead to **IgG** antibodies that can gain access to the tooth by way of the gingival crevicular fluid. For parenteral administration, subunit vaccines are preferred because antibodies directed against lipoteichoic acid in the cell wall of *S. mutans* may cross-react with human heart muscle. Although purified antigens are effective in preventing caries in gnotobiotic rodents and lower primates, the actual antigenic components; dosage; route of administration; and potential benefits, costs, and adverse effects in humans must be determined before a vaccine can be considered for routine use.

Several modifications to the subunit vaccine approach embellish traditional methods with purified bacterial antigens. Synthetic pieces of a larger antigen, such as glucosyltransferase, have been used as an immunogen. Synthetic peptides derived from a glucan-binding domain of glucosyltransferase or from the amino terminus have also been used. Antisera or monoclonal antibodies raised in laboratory animals against these synthetic domains inhibit glucosyltransferase by 30% to 80%.

Antigen-delivery strategies. Local immune responses can be elicited within the gingiva. The swabbing of gingiva with a 3800 Da component of *S. mutans* in monkeys elicits increases in IgG in the crevicular fluid and secretory IgA in the saliva. From a theoretic point of view, it is difficult to ascribe the IgA response to local (gingival) immunization rather than systemic (enteric) because some antigen must be ingested. From a therapeutic point of view, the method itself may be useful because the swabbing was administered only 10 times over the course of 1 year and resulted in a reduction in *S. mutans* and caries activity.

Liposomes are artificial membrane vesicles that can be prepared to contain hydrophilic solutes internally and hydrophobic molecules within the membrane. One method of increasing antibody responses by gingival immunization has been the sequestration of **candidate antigens (i.e., glucosyltransferase) into liposomes,** permitting the liposomes to desiccate, and administering the dehydrated liposomes to humans. This technique has resulted in salivary IgA2 antibodies against glucosyltransferase, suggesting that dehydrated liposomes may be useful in generating specific salivary immunity against target antigens in the oral cavity.

Genetic engineering provides an especially efficient possibility for delivering a subunit vaccine. A major problem with subunit vaccines has been the inability to maintain sufficiently high amounts of antigen in the gut to stimulate antibody production in a cost-effective manner. Genes for candidate antigens of *S. mutans* have been introduced into "harmless" enteric bacteria. These bacteria can proliferate in the gut, elaborating antigen for a prolonged time compared with a conventional dosage form (e.g., gelatin capsules).

Anti-idiotypic antibodies. During an infection, the body commonly produces antibodies to its own immunoglobulins used to ward off the offending organism. These antibodies, called **anti-idiotypic antibodies**, contain in their hypervariable regions a peptide sequence (idiotope) that is identical with or structurally analogous to an antigenic determinant (epitope) of the infecting microorganism. Injection of these antibodies into a host generates a second set of anti-idiotypic antibodies directed against them. If the injected antibodies are the same allotype as the host, the host forms anti-idiotypic antibodies against only the idiotope. These antibodies also bind to the bacterial epitope. This method can be used to elicit antibodies against virtually any antigenic target. A vaccine containing anti-idiotypic antibodies with idiotopes equivalent to epitopes of streptococcal antigens has reduced caries in the gnotobiotic rat model.

Adjuvants

The effects of a vaccine may be enhanced by incorporation of adjuvants, substances that increase the immune response. The mechanism of action of some adjuvants, such as **alum** (aluminum-containing hydroxides or phosphates), is simply to retard removal of the antigen and to attract lymphoid cells by increasing the inflammatory response (often quite severely) in the immediate area of the vaccine. Many adjuvants, such as complete Freund's adjuvant, that are effective in laboratory tests have not been cleared for routine use in humans because they induce long-lasting necrotic lesions in the area of injection. Alum is the only adjuvant currently approved for use with vaccines (e.g., diphtheria and tetanus toxoids) in humans; however, it is not active with all antigens, and it elicits only humoral responses. In mice, alum adjuvants selectively activate TH2 $CD4^+$ T cells; one of the problems facing immunostimulant therapy has been devising methods to stimulate TH1 and CMI responses.

Bacillus Calmette-Guérin (BCG) is a live attenuated strain of *Mycobacterium bovis* that has been used as a vaccine against tuberculosis since the early part of the 20th century. Similar to complete Freund's adjuvant, it contains mycobacterial derivatives and seems to stimulate CMI. BCG has been shown to stimulate specific tumor immunity in experimental animals, to induce responses in immunodeficient individuals, and to reverse the effects of immunosuppressive drugs. It activates macrophages that produce IL-1. IL-1 stimulates the maturation of $CD4^+$ T cells. BCG has been used experimentally in the treatment of melanoma, hepatoma, leukemia, and bladder cancer; it may also have potential against chronic infections involving immunodeficiency. Severe allergic reactions and shock have occurred infrequently during BCG treatments. Other microbially derived immunostimulants that activate macrophages and should help trigger TH1 responses include extracts of pathogenic bacteria and fungal polysaccharides.

Quil-A is a partially purified saponin extract from plants. It forms immunostimulating complexes with cholesterol and various antigens. The complex may intercalate into the membranes of cells, introducing antigen into the cell cytosol. Humoral immunity and CMI are stimulated by increased MHC presentation.

Enhancement of Costimulation

Because the presentation and recognition of antigen alone are insufficient to initiate an immune response, immunotherapy has also focused on enhancement of costimulation. One method includes the antibody-mediated cross-linking of costimulatory receptors (e.g., CD28 and CTLA-4). It has been shown to enhance T cell activity against tumor targets as measured by increased cytokine output. A second method involves immunization of an individual with tumor cells that have been transfected with a B7 gene plus an MHC II gene, causing the cells to express these protein products constitutively. Such immunization has led to rejection of the tumor at a site distant from the immunization site.

Immunostimulants

Thymic extracts

Primary CMI deficiencies may result from absence of the thymus gland or a defect in its function. Treatment has been directed toward inducing maturation of T cells by using thymic tissue or extracts. In several cases, thymus transplants in humans have corrected CMI deficiencies, with subsequent development of immunocompetence. Immunologically immature fetal thymic tissues are used to prevent graft-versus-host reactions.

Thymic extracts have been used nonspecifically to induce CMI competence. These extracts, including **thymosin**, are usually extracted from calf thymus glands. They consist of a family of non-immunogenic polypeptide hormones. Certain tumors, chronic mucocutaneous candidiasis, and several other diseases caused by primary CMI immunodeficiency have responded favorably to thymosin therapy. Thymic extracts must be administered continually. Although thymosin administration has been found to be of therapeutic benefit, it is still experimental, and its routine use awaits further development.

In Europe, several peptides have been purified or synthesized for experimental use in humans, including thymostimulin, which has proved beneficial in the treatment of hepatocellular carcinoma and chronic obstructive pulmonary disease. These hormones function at different stages of CMI development, inducing the maturation of T cells or differentiation of T cells into functional effectors, such as cytotoxic or suppressor cells.

Levamisole

Levamisole is an anthelmintic drug that possesses nonspecific immunostimulatory properties. In deficient animals and humans, it restores many different immunologic functions, suggesting that it acts on multiple populations of cells, including neutrophils, macrophages, and T cells (but not B cells). Its effects on the immune response and its pharmacologic activity indicate that levamisole is a thymomimetic agent.

Levamisole has been used in the treatment of tumors and other diseases in which there are manifestations of immune dysfunction, including rheumatoid arthritis and Crohn disease. Several investigators have used it successfully in the treatment of recurrent aphthous stomatitis and herpes labialis. It has been suggested that the therapeutic effect of levamisole in aphthous stomatitis, which may have an autoimmune etiology, results from enhancement of suppressor T cells that normally prevent autoimmune responses. It is currently approved for use in the United States as an adjunct to fluorouracil in the treatment of colorectal carcinoma. The combination of levamisole with fluorouracil led to reduced colorectal cancer reoccurrence in comparison with no adjuvant therapy. Treatment with levamisole alone has shown no significant effect on the reduced reoccurrence of the colorectal carcinoma.

Polyclonal Antibody Preparations

Human immunoglobulins

Deficiencies in humoral immunity may result from congenital defects in the production of all or selected immunoglobulin classes, or they may be acquired, as occurs with multiple myeloma. Severe deficiencies in humoral immunity, or hypogammaglobulinemias, require "replacement therapy" consisting of weekly or monthly injections of pooled human immunoglobulins, the dose and frequency depending on the patient's status. These treatments are often accompanied by antibiotics. Selective isotype deficiencies involving individual classes of immunoglobulins are usually less severe because the body may compensate by increased production of other immunoglobulin classes. Selective isotype deficiencies also can be treated with immunoglobulins.

Human immunoglobulin is effective against many common diseases, such as measles and infectious hepatitis, because it is derived from the pooled sera of many individuals, including some who would have contracted these infections in the past and produced protective antibodies against them. Although immunopathologic reactions are possible with allogeneic human immunoglobulins, they are much less a problem than with xenogeneic immunoglobulins, and the risk is greatly minimized by using purified or partially purified IgG. In contrast to most other pooled blood products, human immunoglobulin carries no known risk of HIV or hepatitis B transmission. Intravenous, rather than intramuscular, administration of immunoglobulins is preferable because much larger doses can be infused.

Antisera or purified immunoglobulins may be administered to prevent or treat specific diseases. In some cases, this is referred to as **passive immunization**, a classic term in immunology used to indicate that a donor was immunized with an antigen, and that a recipient host was then injected with the protective antibodies generated by the donor. The injection of antibody obtained from an immune donor into a nonimmune recipient has the advantage of conferring almost instantaneous protection, as opposed to vaccines, which require days or weeks to stimulate a sufficient protective effect. The effects of passive immunization last only **4 to 6 weeks** (equivalent to one to two half-lives of IgG in vivo), however. Human immunoglobulin preparations specifically directed against hepatitis B, cytomegalovirus, rabies, tetanus, infant botulism, respiratory syncytial virus, and varicella-zoster virus are available.

Rh_0(D) immunoglobulin

Rh_0(D) immunoglobulin represents a special case in which passive immunization is used to induce specific immunosuppression for the prevention of **Rh disease.** Rh disease occurs when an Rh-negative woman—one whose red blood cells do not contain the Rh_0(D) antigen—becomes sensitized to the antigen by exposure to the blood of her Rh-positive fetus. On subsequent pregnancies, the mother's anti-Rh antibody passes through the placenta and causes massive destruction of fetal erythrocytes, resulting in hemolytic disease of the newborn.

The injection of anti-Rh antibody into Rh-negative mothers who will give birth to Rh-positive infants is effective in preventing the disorder. The goal of treatment is to prevent mothers from generating anti-Rh_0(D) antibodies. High titers of specific antibody against an antigen specifically inhibit the immune response to that antigen, but the mechanism may be more complex than simple binding of the antigenic stimulus. The injection of anti-Rh_0(D) antibodies may induce the mother to generate a set of antibodies against the variable domains of the injected antibodies. This second set of anti-idiotypic antibodies may impede the interaction of B cells with Rh antigen, cause B cell inactivation or death, or neutralize anti-Rh_0(D)–specific antibodies as they are generated. Such idiotypic–anti-idiotypic inhibitory effects have been shown in laboratory animals. Alternatively, anti-Rh_0(D) antibody may lead to rapid clearance of fetal red blood cells from the mother's circulation by liver macrophages, which would prevent the elicitation of chronic inflammatory reactions necessary for antibody responses.

Antiserum to the Rh antigen is produced in Rh-negative male volunteers. The γ-globulin fraction containing anti-Rh antibody, in the form of Rh_0(D) immunoglobulin (human), must be given within hours of parturition because the fetal erythrocytes carrying the Rh antigen enter the mother's body at this time and induce the immune response that would cause problems in subsequent pregnancies. This specific immunosuppressive treatment has been very successful in preventing Rh disease, and it is now used routinely.

Antitoxins and antivenins

Immunoglobulin preparations that **neutralize toxic compounds**, such as rattlesnake venom and diphtheria toxin, are commonly derived from the sera of horses actively immunized against the noxious substances. The regional availability of these xenogeneic antibody products varies widely depending on the perceived risk of exposure. Being bitten by a poisonous animal outside its normal geographic range can delay the administration of the immunoglobulin antidote and increase the risk of injury or death.

If administered parenterally, xenogeneic (or even allogeneic) sera or immunoglobulins may induce immunity in the recipient against animal (or human) serum antigens. Not only would this response lead to rapid clearance of the antibodies—and circumvent their therapeutic effect—but also it can induce type III immunopathologic reactions such as serum sickness or immune complex disease.

Oral administration of xenogeneic antibodies

The oral administration of xenogeneic antibodies offers one possible strategy for highly precise, cost-effective immunotherapeutics. Cows immunized against cariogenic bacteria exhibit antibodies against those bacteria in their milk. The milk (or whey) can confer protection to individuals consuming that milk in a passive manner. In cows' milk and colostrum, the antibodies are of the IgG1 subclass. *Streptococcus mutans* and caries scores can be reduced in this manner in gnotobiotic animals. Whey from immunized cows also seems to decrease *S. mutans* in human volunteers when it is used as a mouth rinse.

Antithymocyte globulin

Antithymocyte globulin is produced in rabbits and horses by immunization with human thymocytes. It lyses or agglutinates human lymphocytes in vitro and produces lymphocytopenia in vivo. CMI responses are decreased, and allograft survival is prolonged. Antithymocyte globulin is rich in **cytotoxic antibodies** directed against numerous antigens expressed by T cells, including CD2, CD3, CD4, CD8, CD11a, CD18, CD25, CD44, CD45, and HLA (human MHC) class I and II molecules. The immunosuppressive effects are transient, and anti-thymocyte globulin must be given repeatedly. Because the preparation is itself antigenic, however, it can induce an immune response leading to serum sickness. The agent's primary indication is suppression of acute transplant rejection reactions. Studies have shown that the use of a combination immunosuppressive regimen of both anti-thymocyte globulin and cyclosporine as first-line therapy for **severe aplastic anemia** is warranted.

Monoclonal Antibody Preparations

A **monoclonal antibody (MAb)** is an antibody of a **single specificity** produced by cells derived from a single B cell clone. In most cases, the MAb is derived from mice (and is xenogeneic) as illustrated in Figure 35-7. MAbs are increasingly being used diagnostically to assess immunocompetence, to identify infectious diseases, and to monitor the concentrations of hormones and chemotherapeutic agents in the plasma. Some are used as immunosuppressive agents. Their exquisite specificity also makes them ideal guidance systems as carriers for cytotoxic agents (described subsequently). Table 35-3 lists clinically available MAbs and derivatives, their target antigens, and their principal therapeutic indications.

Muromonab-CD3, the first monoclonal antibody to be approved for human use (in 1986), is a mouse MAb that reacts with CD3, a component of the TCR complex (see Fig. 35-4). Antibody binding induces internalization of the TCR. Sensitive T cells die in response to complement activation; other T cells redistribute to non-lymphoid tissues and become significantly less responsive to antigenic challenge.

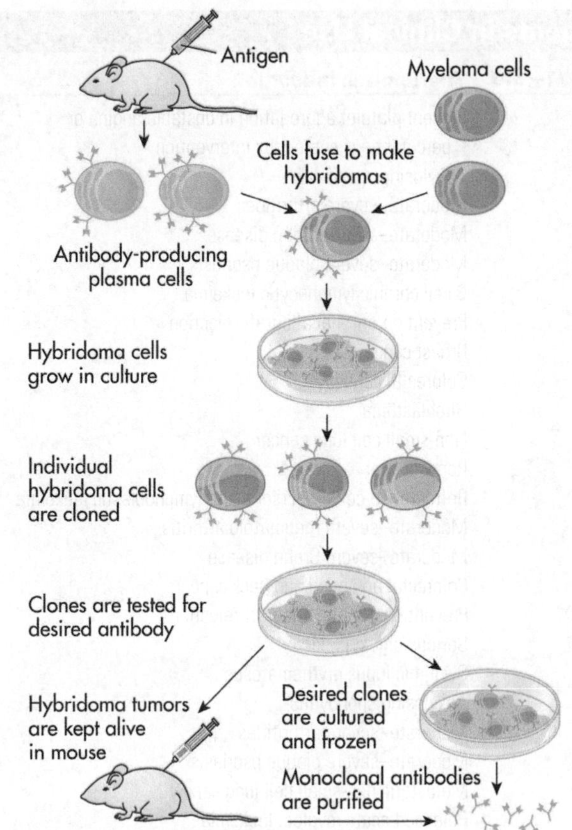

FIG 35-7 Fusion of a normal mouse plasma cell and a myeloma cell results in the formation of a hybridoma with the antibody-forming properties of the plasma cell and the proliferative properties of the myeloma cell. When grown in tissue culture, hybridomas are capable of almost unlimited production of MAb. (From Lewis SM, et al.: *Medical-surgical nursing: assessment and management of clinical problems*, ed 9, St Louis, 2014, Mosby.)

Muromonab-CD3 is highly effective in terminating acute cellular rejection episodes. The major adverse effect of therapy, known as the **cytokine release syndrome,** develops from the stimulation of Fc receptors by CD3-bound MAb. Affected T cells release TNF-α, IL-2, and other cytokines, causing high fever, chills, nausea and vomiting, malaise, weakness, and generalized pain. The syndrome usually begins within 30 minutes of drug injection, lasts for hours, and rarely may produce life-threatening cardiovascular and pulmonary disturbances. Repeated MAb treatment may lead to the development of human anti-mouse antibodies that block the therapeutic effect or sensitize the patient to the drug.

Chimeric antibodies

The most important factor that limits the therapeutic potential of MAbs as a group is their xenogeneic origin, and clinical testing of these reagents has led to some disappointment. One approach to circumvent this problem has been to combine the antigen-specific portions of mouse MAbs with human constant or framework domains (Fig. 35-8). Because the constant region of an immunoglobulin also confers function to an antibody, **chimeric MAb** engineering permits the selection of functional attributes. A chimeric MAb possessing an IgG1 isotype constant region would be most effective in complement activation and antibody-dependent cell-mediated cytotoxicity, whereas a chimeric antibody of the IgA subclass may exhibit antiinflammatory effects.

Basiliximab is a chimeric MAb (60% human, 40% mouse) used to prevent allograft rejection in patients receiving other immunosuppresants. It is directed against the α subunit of the IL-2 receptor on activated T cells (see Fig. 35-4). IL-2 is a major cytokine supporting CMI and organ rejection. In general, the drug is administered only twice; the first dose is infused intravenously within 2 hours before transplantation surgery, and the second is given 4 days later. The only adverse events attributable to basiliximab used in this manner are rare cases of allergic reactions and cytokine release syndrome.

Complementarity-defining region-grafted (humanized) antibodies

Although chimeric MAbs may seem exotic, they have been superseded by a third-generation MAb, the CDR-grafted MAb, more simply known as the **"humanized" MAb.** As described previously, CDR refers to the hypervariable peptide sequences of an antibody that actually bind to an antigen. These hypervariable regions are joined by intervening framework sequences. A CDR-grafted MAb contains rodent hypervariable sequences, human framework sequences, and human constant regions. There is some loss of affinity in humanized MAbs, but it is usually an acceptable tradeoff for the reduced allergenicity. Humanized MAbs are used clinically to prevent rejection of organ transplants. Other diseases in which CDR-grafted MAbs have been used include rheumatoid arthritis, Crohn disease, systemic vasculitis, septic shock, various neoplasms, and viral infections.

Daclizumab is a humanized variant of basiliximab in which the murine (mouse) content of the antibody has been reduced to 10%. As expected, daclizumab is less potent than basiliximab in binding to the α subunit of the IL-2 receptor. A one-time five-dose regimen is used, with the first dose given within 24 hours before transplantation surgery and subsequent doses every 14 days thereafter. Few adverse reactions have been reported for this use of daclizumab; it apparently does not cause cytokine release syndrome.

Conjugated monoclonal antibodies

Immunotoxins are **antibodies coupled with a poison (toxin).** Toxins may be derived from many sources, including plants and microbes (e.g., the lectin ricin, *Pseudomonas* exotoxin, diphtheria toxin). The therapeutic strategy is to have the antibody selectively deliver the toxin to undesirable cells, such as those infected by HIV-1, or participate in immunopathologic reactions. Immunotoxins have also been explored for their potential in cancer immunotherapy (including metastatic melanoma; colorectal, ovarian, and breast carcinomas; non-Hodgkin lymphoma; Hodgkin disease; B cell leukemia; and T cell lymphoma) and immunosuppression in steroid-resistant graft-versus-host disease. Although immunotoxins have been called "magic bullets" capable of pinpoint target destruction, it has become clear that most of these "bullets" are not as accurate as desired and have significant side effects, including vascular leak syndrome, myalgia, aphasia, paresthesia, encephalopathy, neuropathy, thrombocytopenia, liver destruction, renal insufficiency, proteinuria, hypoalbuminemia, dyspnea, hematuria, and tremors. The toxins themselves have proved quite antigenic, eliciting immune reactions in most cases. **Gemtuzumab ozogamicin** is the first immunotoxin to be approved for clinical use. It combines the anti-CD33 antibody gemtuzumab with the anticancer agent ozogamicin. When the agent binds its antigen receptor, it is internalized. The active agent is released to kill the cell. The drug is approved for treatment of acute myeloid leukemia.

Immunotoxins have not been explored extensively as therapeutic agents delivered locally in the oral cavity. Such a strategy might be used to eliminate pathogens selectively or reduce inflammatory activities of

TABLE 35-3 Monoclonal Antibodies and Related Agents in Clinical Use

Non-Proprietary (Generic) Name	Proprietary (Trade) Name	Receptor/Target	Therapeutic Indication
Abciximab	ReoPro	GPIIb/IIIa	Prevent platelet aggregation in unstable angina or percutaneous cutaneous intervention
Adalimumab	Humira	TNF-α	Ankylosing spondylitis Moderate–severe arthritides Moderate–severe Crohn disease Moderate–severe plaque psoriasis
Alemtuzumab	Campath	CD52	B cell chronic lymphocytic leukemia
Basiliximab	Simulect	IL-2	Prevention of renal allograft rejection
Bevacizumab	Avastin	VEGF	Breast cancer Colorectal cancer Glioblastoma Non-small cell lung cancer Renal cancer
Blinatumomab	Blincyto	CD19	Refractory B cell precursor acute lymphoblastic leukemia
Certolizumab	Cimzia	TNF-α	Moderate–severe rheumatoid arthritis Moderate–severe Crohn disease
Cetuximab	Erbitux	EGFR	Colorectal and head and neck cancers
Daclizumab	Zenapax	IL-2	Prevention of renal allograft rejection
Digoxin immune Fab	Digibind	Digoxin	Serious digoxin toxicity
Epratuzumab	LymphoCide	CD22	Systemic lupus erythematosus
Etanercept	Enbrel	TNF	Ankylosing spondylitis Moderate–severe arthritides Moderate–severe plaque psoriasis
Gefitinib	Iressa	EGFR	Metastatic non-small cell lung cancer
Gemtuzumab ozogamicin	Mylotarg	CD33	Relapsed acute myeloid leukemia
Golimumab	Simponi	TNF-α	Ankylosing spondylitis Moderate–severe rheumatoid arthritis Psoriatic arthritis
Ibritumomab tiuxetan	Zevalin	CD20	Non-Hodgkin lymphoma
Infliximab	Remicade	TNF-α	Ankylosing spondylitis Moderate–severe rheumatoid arthritis Moderate–severe Crohn disease Moderate–severe plaque psoriasis Ulcerative colitis
Muromonab-CD3	Orthoclone OKT3	CD3	Acute graft rejection
Natalizumab	Tysabri	α_4-integrin	Relapsing multiple sclerosis
Nimotuzumab*		EGFR	Squamous cell cancer Glioma
Nivolumab	Opdivo	PD-1	Melanoma
Ofatumumab	Arzerra	CD20	Chronic lymphocytic leukemia
Palivizumab	Synagis	RSV F protein	Prevention of RSV disease
Panitumumab	Vectibix	EGFR	Colorectal cancer
Ramucirumab	Cyramza	VEGFR2	Metastatic non-small cell lung cancer Gastric or gastroesophageal junction adenocarcinoma
Rituximab	Rituxan	CD20	Non-Hodgkin lymphoma
Secukinumab	Cosentyx	IL-17	Plaque psoriasis
Tositumomab and iodine I-131 tositumomab	Bexxar	CD20	Non-Hodgkin lymphoma
Trastuzumab	Herceptin	HER2	Metastatic breast cancer
Veltuzumab	hA20	CD20	Non-Hodgkin lymphoma

*Not currently available in the United States. *CD*, Cluster of differentiation (protein); *EGFR*, epidermal growth factor receptor; *HER2*, human epidermal growth factor receptor 2; *IL*, interleukin; *RSV F protein*, respiratory syncytial virus fusion protein; *TNF*, tumor necrosis factor.

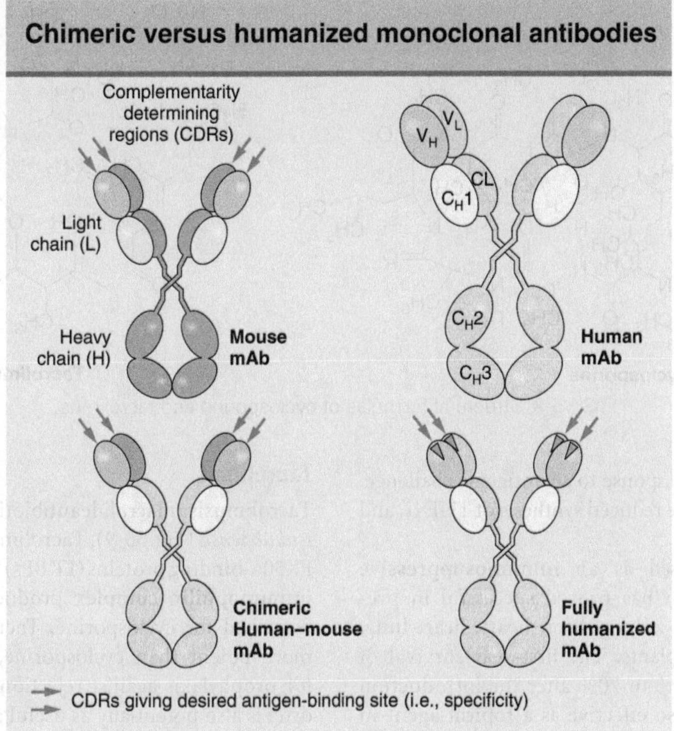

FIG 35-8 Chimeric MAbs are produced by the grafting of the variable regions of rodent immunoglobulin to the constant regions of human immunoglobulin. *Mab,* Monoclonal antibody; *V,* variable regions; *C,* constant regions. (From Floege J, Johnson RJ, Feehally J: *Comprehensive clinical nephrology,* ed 3, Philadelphia, 2007, Mosby.)

the host immune system, and it may not result in the same degree of toxicity observed in systemic administration.

Radioimmunotherapy relies on a similar strategy to deliver radioactive substances in a selective manner for diagnostic or therapeutic purposes. In this case, the potential for tissue damage by the toxin has been replaced by the potential for radiation injury. Inasmuch as several radioimmunotherapeutic agents have been approved for human use, the tradeoff seems favorable.

Ibritumomab tiuxetan, approved in 2002, is a covalently linked conjugate of the MAb ibritumomab and the linker-chelater tiuxetan. Ibritumomab is selective for CD20, a cell-surface antigen expressed by normal B cells and more than 90% of B cell non-Hodgkin lymphomas. Tiuxetan contains a high-affinity binding site that can accommodate either indium-111 (used for diagnostic imaging) or yttrium-90 (used for target cell destruction). A complex administration schedule involving the prior administration of radiation-free MAb is used to limit damage of healthy lymphoid tissue and maximize destruction of lymphoma cells. Common adverse effects include neutropenia and thrombocytopenia. Infection, hemorrhage, allergic reactions, and new malignancies are potentially life-threatening reactions.

Future developments

Contemporary medicine is witnessing an explosive increase in the development of monoclonal antibodies to diagnose and treat disease. Already, monoclonal antibodies constitute the most widely used form of cancer immunotherapy. In the quarter century since the introduction of muromonab-CD3 into clinical practice, slightly more than 20 monoclonal antibodies have been approved for use. Two hundred more are now in clinical trials or awaiting approval. Among these agents are "fully" human monoclonal antibodies (fourth-generation monoclonal antibodies) harvested from mice genetically engineered to produce human antibodies from laboratory bacteria using phage display technology.

Chemolabeled monoclonal antibodies constitute a third strategy for targeting therapeutic agents using monoclonal antibodies. In this case a substance that is not inherently toxic is directed to a specific site where it can produce the desired therapeutic effect. It now seems likely that the early promise to therapeutics represented by the concept of monoclonal antibodies will soon be realized.

Immunophilin Ligands

Cyclosporine (cyclosporin A), **tacrolimus** (FK506), and **sirolimus** (rapamycin) are microbial derivatives now classified as **immunophilin ligands** because they all initially form a complex with cytosolic receptors of the immunophilin family. These drugs seem to have similar but not identical mechanisms of action. Cyclosporine, the first of these agents to gain approval for human use, revolutionized the field of organ transplantation.

Cyclosporine

Cyclosporine was originally isolated from a fungus, *Beauveria nivea.* It is a neutral hydrophobic macrocyclic undecapeptide (Fig. 35-9). Cyclosporine binds immunophilins called **cyclophylins.** The cyclosporine–cyclophylin complex interacts with **calcineurin,** a Ca^{++}-dependent protein phosphatase (see Fig. 35-4). The calcineurin complex is inhibited from dephosphorylating NF-AT, impeding its translocation into the nucleus and impairing transcription important in the earlier phases of immune responses. The immunosuppressive activity of cyclosporine is usually ascribed to its ability to **block IL-2 synthesis**, but the drug also **suppresses macrophage activation and the release of IL-1,** prevents the formation of IL-1 receptors on $CD4^+$ T cells, and blocks the expression of IL-2 receptors on naïve T cells. Increased synthesis of TGF-β inhibits IL-2 activity. The primary outcome is that $CD4^+$ T cells

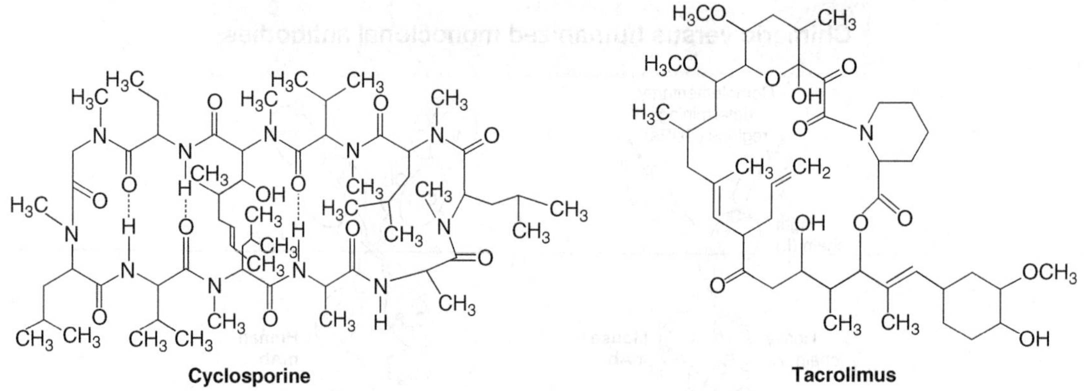

Cyclosporine

Tacrolimus

FIG 35-9 Structural formulas of cyclosporine and tacrolimus.

are not stimulated to proliferate in response to an antigenic challenge. B cell function is also impaired by the reduced synthesis of TNF-α, and mast cell degranulation is blocked.

Cyclosporine is commonly used as an **immunosuppressive agent** to promote graft survival. It has proved successful in preventing rejections of non-matched kidney, liver, heart, heart-lung, bone marrow, and pancreas transplants. The first-year survival of liver transplants increased from 35% to 70% after the introduction of cyclosporine. Cyclosporine is also effective as a topical agent in the treatment of oral lichen planus, and it has been used systemically to treat other autoimmune diseases that may affect oral (bullous pemphigoid, pemphigus) and non-oral (psoriasis, rheumatoid arthritis) tissues. Cyclosporine has proved effective in the treatment of Behçet syndrome (a vasculitis that almost always includes oral aphthous ulcers and uveitis), nephrotic syndrome, inflammatory bowel disease, atopic dermatitis, and endogenous uveitis. Cyclosporine is better tolerated than less selective immunosuppressant drugs. The drug is potentially dangerous, however. The two major adverse side effects associated with long-term use are (1) dose-related renal toxicity, which, including mild forms, may occur in 75% of patients, and (2) hypertension, which is not apparently dose related and occurs in 50% of all renal transplant patients (and is especially common in children). Other side effects include central nervous system toxicity (headache, confusion, depression, seizures), gingival hyperplasia, hirsutism, mild tremor, and hepatotoxicity. The risk of lymphoma and other neoplasias is increased. A topical form of cyclosporine is available to promote tear production in patients with dry eyes due to keratoconjunctivitis sicca.

The precise mechanism of cyclosporine-induced **gingival hyperplasia** is unknown; corrective procedures involve mainly drug titration and surgical intervention. Some studies indicate that cyclosporine therapy results in the selection of fibroblasts with cyclosporine receptors, and it has been proposed that there is an associated immunologic cytokine imbalance.

The absorption of cyclosporine is incomplete and variable among patients. Because interstitial fibrosis of the kidney has been associated with sustained high concentrations of cyclosporine, monitoring of plasma cyclosporine concentrations is necessary. A microemulsion form offers higher and more reliable absorption than the original product. Cyclosporine is **metabolized by CYP3A enzymes**; drugs that induce these enzymes (e.g., carbamazepine, phenobarbital, rifampin) reduce plasma concentrations of cyclosporine, whereas drugs that inhibit them (e.g., erythromycin, ketoconazole, prednisolone) have the opposite effect. Nonsteroidal antiinflammatory drugs, aminoglycosides, and other drugs that cause nephrotoxicity are contraindicated in patients receiving cyclosporine.

Tacrolimus

Tacrolimus is a macrolide antibiotic originally isolated from *Streptomyces tsukubaensis* (Fig. 35-9). Tacrolimus binds to immunophilins known as FK506-binding proteins (FKBPs) (Fig. 35-4). The resulting **tacrolimus-immunophilin complex** produces the same action and effects as described for cyclosporine. Tacrolimus is approximately 100 times more potent than cyclosporine, however. Tacrolimus is approved for prophylaxis against rejection of allogeneic liver transplants. The drug is also potentially as useful as cyclosporine for other conditions. Tacrolimus has been shown to exert profound **antipsoriatic effects,** probably by direct interaction with keratinocytes. Adverse effects of tacrolimus are qualitatively similar to those of cyclosporine except that gingival overgrowth and hirsutism are not observed. Drug interactions are also similar because tacrolimus is metabolized by CYP3A. Tacrolimus ointment is a nonsteroidal topical immunomodulator used specially to treat atopic dermatitis. The prolonged use of this ointment has been found to be safe and effective for the long-term treatment of atopic dermatitis in children.

Sirolimus

Sirolimus, originally known as rapamycin, was originally detected in the fermentation broth of *Streptomyces hygroscopicus.* Sirolimus is a potent immunosuppressant. A structural analogue of tacrolimus, sirolimus binds to the same FKBP receptors (see Fig. 35-4) and is approved for a similar therapeutic indication. Sirolimus has a mechanism of action that is different from cyclosporine or tacrolimus. The sirolimus–immunophilin complex binds not to calcineurin but to a serine–threonine kinase often referred to as **FKBP-rapamycin-associated protein (FRAP).** The FRAP-sirolimus-FKBP complex cannot phosphorylate a set of proteins involved in protein translation important in later stages of the T cell's immune response (i.e., its response to growth factors, IL-2 in particular). It is believed that sirolimus interferes with signals from growth factor receptors, such as the IL-2 receptor (IL-2R), rather than with signals generated by the TCR. In addition to blocking proliferation of T cells, sirolimus affects nonhematopoietic cells and may find applications different from those of cyclosporine or tacrolimus.

Sirolimus is free of nephrotoxicity and neurotoxicity, and it does not promote hypertension. Hyperlipidemia is a common dose-dependent side effect. Anemia, thrombocytopenia, and leukopenia may occur. Combined use of sirolimus with cyclosporine significantly worsens renal function, but a positive drug interaction permits use of reduced cyclosporine doses.

Glucocorticoids

Glucocorticoids such as prednisone and dexamethasone have long been used as immunosuppressive agents, but their mechanism of action has been defined only more recently. As discussed in Chapters 27 and 30, glucocorticoids bind to a soluble intracellular receptor and then enter the nucleus of the cell. Specific glucocorticoid response elements on DNA interact with the glucocorticoid receptor, and **transcription of specific genes is promoted or inhibited**. Several cytokines and other proteins involved in inflammatory reactions are affected. Dexamethasone has also been shown to induce transcription of the I-κB gene. The subsequent increased synthesis of I-κB prevents the translocation of NF-κB from the cytosol to the nucleus. Because NF-κB promotes IL-6 and IL-8 transcription, glucocorticoids are important as antiinflammatory agents and as immunosuppressants. Apoptosis contributes to the rapid decline in peripheral lymphocytes.

Corticosteroids alone or with other immunosuppressive agents that inhibit antibody production and phagocytosis are often used to treat severe type II autoimmune reactions. Corticosteroids are also useful in the treatment of type III immune complex immunopathologic conditions, primarily because of their antiinflammatory properties. In severe cases, another immunosuppressant may be added to block the immune response and allow use of reduced quantities of steroids. The steroids mainly act on CMI. In addition to their lympholytic effects, steroids may interfere with macrophage processing by stabilization of macrophage cell membranes.

Thalidomide and Lenalidomide

Thalidomide, a sedative agent briefly available in Europe more than four decades ago but quickly withdrawn because of its powerful teratogenic effects (see Chapter 3), was approved in 1998 for restricted use by the U.S. Food and Drug Administration (FDA) in the treatment of erythema nodosum leprosum. Although its mechanism of action is unknown, thalidomide decreases excessive production of TNF-α in target patients and downregulates certain surface adhesion molecules involved in leukocyte migration. TH2 cell responses are favored over TH1, yielding increases in IL-4 and IL-5. The drug can be sold only by registered pharmacies, which must obtain informed consent about its use from all patients. Thalidomide should never be used by women who are or may become pregnant; it is also contraindicated in men who are sexually mature and do not agree in writing to the need for using latex condoms when having sexual intercourse with women of childbearing potential. Peripheral neuropathy is an important side effect of the drug.

Lenalidomide is an analogue of thalidomide approved for use in the treatment of certain patients with multiple myeloma or myelodysplastic syndrome. It carries the same prescribing restrictions as thalidomide and is likely to cause neutropenia and thrombocytopenia.

Cytotoxic Drugs

Cytotoxic drugs are of two classes: the first kills lymphocytes, and the second interferes with the proliferative stage of the immune response. The lympholytic drugs are most effective if given before antigen administration. They include the alkylating agents such as cyclophosphamide and phenylalanine mustard. Drugs that impede cellular proliferation include various metabolite analogues that inhibit DNA synthesis. The general pharmacologic characteristics of most of these drugs are discussed in Chapter 36.

Cyclophosphamide

Cyclophosphamide was originally developed for cancer chemotherapy and has been adapted for immunotherapy in the prevention of allograft rejection, control of autoimmune and rheumatoid diseases mediated by antibody, and control of T cell–mediated diseases. Although it is an **alkylating agent**, cyclophosphamide is inactive until it is metabolized within the liver microsomes (the phosphamide ring is hydrolyzed). Cyclophosphamide metabolites are eliminated by the kidney. Liver and kidney function should be considered in the use of this drug. The metabolites of cyclophosphamide exert their effect by alkylating and cross-linking cellular macromolecules, including DNA, ribonucleic acid (RNA), and proteins. Damage to DNA can occur at all stages of the cell cycle, but lethal hits occur mainly in the S phase.

The daily, long-term administration of cyclophosphamide at low therapeutic doses leads to a progressive reduction in circulating lymphocytes, with minimal effect on myeloid cell populations. Within 7 days, B cells, CD4$^+$ T cells, and CD8$^+$ T cells show a 30% to 40% reduction in numbers. Cessation of cyclophosphamide therapy results in a differential rate of recovery of lymphocyte populations. CD8$^+$ T cells recover first, followed by B cells and, finally, CD4$^+$ T cells. Intermittent low-dose administration seems to affect antibody production, but long-term low-dose administration diminishes CMI as assessed by decreased delayed-type allergic reactions. Paradoxic increases in immune activity have also been observed after low-dose cyclophosphamide therapy, attributable to selective depression of T-suppressor cell activity. Cyclophosphamide also depresses myeloid hematopoiesis in the bone marrow, and it has been associated with neutropenia and thrombocytopenia.

Antimetabolites

The purine, pyrimidine, and folate antagonists represent a second group of cytotoxic drugs active against rapidly dividing or metabolizing cells. Included among these are **the purine antagonists azathioprine and 6-mercaptopurine, the pyrimidine antagonist floxuridine, and the folate antagonist methotrexate.** These agents are given with, or within 48 hours of, antigen administration and inhibit cellular proliferation and initial differentiation, usually through inhibition of DNA or RNA synthesis. They all seem to impair CMI and humoral immunity. Originally developed for cancer therapy, these drugs can affect any group of rapidly proliferating cells. Because they are particularly toxic to hematopoietic tissues, they may induce leukopenia (especially neutropenia), thrombocytopenia, and anemia.

Azathioprine. **Azathioprine** warrants special mention because it is used solely as an immunosuppressant. Azathioprine is a prodrug that yields 6-mercaptopurine on intracellular exposure to glutathione and other nucleophilic reactants. Although the pharmacologic features of azathioprine are essentially identical to those of 6-mercaptopurine (see Chapter 36), azathioprine is believed to be a **more selective immunosuppressant.** This advantage may stem from an enhanced uptake or metabolic activation of azathioprine in T cells.

Mycophenolate. **Mycophenolate mofetil** is an ester that is rapidly hydrolyzed to mycophenolic acid, the active form of the drug. The active metabolite is now also available for use. Mycophenolate is an inhibitor of inosine monophosphate dehydrogenase, an important enzyme in purine synthesis. Because lymphocytes depend more on the de novo synthesis of purines than other cells, which can reclaim purines by the salvage pathway, mycophenolate is a more selective immunosuppressant than other cytotoxic agents. CMI and humoral immunity are suppressed, and leukocyte recruitment to inflammatory sites is inhibited.

Slow-Acting, Disease-Modifying Antirheumatic Drugs

One potential immunosuppressive strategy involves the inhibition of selected aspects of antigen processing within the endolysosome or by the proteasome. The antimalarial **disease-modifying anti-rheumatic drugs (DMARDs) chloroquine and hydrochloroquine** seem to have several effects on the immune system, including inhibition of endolysosomal antigen processing. It has been suggested that these weak bases may impair endolysosomal acidification. As a result, individuals treated with chloroquine or hydrochloroquine exhibit diminished antibody formation (including decreased formation of rheumatoid factor, decreased autoantibodies, and decreased total serum IgG and IgA), which is one of the main rationales for their use in Sjögren syndrome and other autoimmune rheumatic diseases.

Gold compounds—gold sodium thiomalate, aurothioglucose, and auranofin—function in part by inhibiting transcription activation. Gold compounds may be active against protein kinase C. As a result, not only are various lymphocyte functions diminished, but also the induction of immune function in nonhematopoietic cells is impaired. In the latter situation, it has been shown that the expression of MHC II molecules by endothelial cells can be inhibited by gold compounds.

Penicillamine and **sulfasalazine** are DMARDs that inhibit proliferation through unknown mechanisms. Penicillamine blocks T cell proliferation in response to IL-1 and blocks IL-1 production by monocytes; sulfasalazine blocks T-mitogen–induced and B-mitogen–induced proliferation of peripheral blood lymphocytes.

Cytokine Therapy

The concept of therapeutics based on the administration of hormones is not new. As more is learned about the activities of immune-induced factors, referred to as *cytokines*, new therapies to increase or decrease immunologic activities will be developed. Currently, over a dozen cytokines have been approved for human use, and others are in clinical trials. In the following discussion, cytokines and soluble cytokine receptors are reviewed in accordance with their principal biologic activities (see Table 35-1).

Hematopoietic growth factors

The hematopoietic growth factors include **colony-stimulating factors**, such as granulocyte colony-stimulating factor, granulocyte/macrophage colony-stimulating factor, monocyte/macrophage colony-stimulating factor, stem cell factor, erythropoietin, and a number of interleukins. Although it is beyond the scope of this chapter to discuss these growth factors, they are used clinically in the treatment of various hematopoietic deficiencies, including neutropenia, anemia, and thrombocytopenia, and they are reviewed in Chapter 25.

Interleukin-1 family

IL-1 occupies the borderland between innate, nonspecific immune responses and adaptive, specific immune responses. Several related molecules, including IL-1α, IL-1β, IL-1 receptor antagonist (IL-1Rα), and their receptors in soluble form, are under consideration for use in immunotherapeutics. IL-1 is produced by many cells, but mainly monocytes/macrophages, in the form of precursor molecules lacking a signal sequence. A large fraction of IL-1α remains inactive in the cytosol of the cell. In contrast, IL-1β is rapidly converted to its active form and released extracellularly in large quantities.

IL-1 can exist in soluble and membrane-associated forms. As a soluble molecule, IL-1 is a factor with wide-ranging systemic effects involving the central nervous system, liver, kidney, hematopoietic system (including neutrophilia and lymphopenia), and vascular system (e.g., promotes leukocyte adherence). The membrane-associated form may be a partially degraded version of IL-1α, which can function as a costimulatory factor for naïve T cells. Some **immunologic effects of IL-1** are listed in Table 35-4. In addition, IL-1β is important as an osteoclast-activating factor and is believed to be involved in **periodontal bone destruction.** IL-1 has cytotoxic activities; it kills melanoma cells, thyrocytes, and β-islet (insulin-producing) cells. IL-1 also induces fever, and as such, it is one of the more important endogenous pyrogens. The pyrogenic effect of IL-1 is blocked by nonsteroidal

TABLE 35-4 Effects of Interleukin-1 on Immune Cells

Target Cells	Effects
Lymphoid Cells	
T cells	Growth factor (primarily owing to its ability to stimulate IL-2)
	Increased IL-2 receptors
	Induction of cytokine synthesis (IL-2, IL-3, others)
	Induction of IFN-γ synthesis
	Chemoattractant
B cells	Growth factor for transformed B cells (B blasts)
	Potentiates B cell growth and differentiation factors (IL-4, IL-6)
	Chemoattractant
NK cells	Facilitates IL-2 and IFN enhancement of tumor cell lysis
	Increases binding of NK cells to targets
	Induces cytokine synthesis (IL-1)
Myeloid Cells	
Neutrophils	Thromboxane synthesis
	Degranulation (secretion)
Monocytes/ macrophages	Induces synthesis of PGE_2, IL-1, and other cytokines
	Induces cytotoxicity
	Colony-stimulating factors
	Stimulates migration

IFN, Interferon; *IL*, interleukin; *NK*, natural killer; *PGE_2*, prostaglandin E_2.

antiinflammatory drugs, suggesting that it depends on the elaboration of cyclooxygenase products.

IL-1Rα, a protein with structural homology to IL-1α and IL-1β, is secreted by monocytes. It is found in the urine of patients with fever or monocytic leukemia. The molecule binds to the IL-1 receptor in competition with IL-1α and IL-1β, but it does not trigger the cellular responses typical of IL-1. IL-1Rα is considered a natural means of blocking excessive IL-1 inflammatory events, which can lead to shock, arthritis, osteoporosis, colitis, leukemia, diabetes, wasting, and atherosclerosis. IL-1Rα has potential therapeutic application in humans, and clinical trials have shown some efficacy in septic shock syndrome and more consistent benefits in rheumatoid arthritis.

Interleukin-1 receptors

The **IL-1 receptor (IL-1R)** is a member of the immunoglobulin superfamily. There are two subtypes of IL-1R. Subtype 1 (IL-1RI) binds IL-1α preferentially and is found on T cells, endothelial cells, keratinocytes, hepatocytes, and fibroblasts. Subtype 2 (IL-1RII) is expressed by neutrophils, monocytes, B cells, and bone marrow cells, and it binds IL-1β preferentially. IL-1RI is more sensitive to inhibition by IL-1Rα than IL-1RII. IL-RII exhibits a very short cytoplasmic domain compared with IL-1RI, suggesting that it may serve as a "decoy" receptor. IL-1R can exist in either a transmembranous form or a soluble form. Soluble receptors exert an antagonistic effect by binding to IL-1. Experiments in mice have shown that recombinant soluble IL-1RI can prolong the survival of cardiac allografts. Much of this survival is attributable to decreased inflammation, rather than to specific immunosuppression. **Anakinra, a recombinant form of IL-1RI,** has been marketed for the **treatment of rheumatoid arthritis** not responding to more traditional DMARDs.

Interleukin-2

Lymphocytotrophic cytokine IL-2 is a glycoprotein produced by TH1 T cells in the presence of APCs. IL-2 is required for IFN-γ production. In specific immune responses, the **main function of IL-2 is to induce T cell proliferation and differentiation**; as such, IL-2 enhances the growth of naïve $CD4^+$ T cells, TH1 $CD4^+$ T cells, and $CD8^+$ T cells. IL-2 can also activate NK cells to form lymphokine-activated killer (LAK) cells. Most immunotherapies involving IL-2 are based on its ability to activate NK cell activity.

The IL-2 receptor is composed of three subunits that form low-, intermediate-, and high-affinity interactions with IL-2.

IL-2 therapy has been explored in various immunodeficiency diseases and cancer, and IL-2 replacement has been effective in treating patients with IL-2 deficiency. The cytokine has been given the nonproprietary name of aldesleukin and has been marketed for the treatment of metastatic renal cell carcinoma (see Chapter 36).

The **NK cell** is believed to be the most important target for IL-2 therapy because depletion of this cell type can negate the protective effects of IL-2 in animal models. The high doses used in cancer chemotherapy are believed to saturate completely the intermediate-affinity IL-2 receptors of NK cells. In animal models, transplanted tumor micrometastases seem to regress when IL-2 is used alone or in combination with LAK cells. In human clinical trials involving advanced melanoma, the coadministration of IL-2 and LAK cells resulted in the complete regression of tumors in approximately 5% of cases and the partial regression (>50% reduction in tumor mass) in 15% of cases. Comparative values for metastatic renal cancer were 4% and 11%. IL-2 therapy has certain inherent problems. IL-2 is a short-range factor designed to influence cells locally. High-dose IL-2 therapy is toxic, and complications lead to a mortality rate of approximately 4%. Adverse effects include capillary leak syndrome (resulting in edema, reduced organ perfusion, and hypotension), cardiac arrhythmias, myocardial infarction, respiratory insufficiency, mental disturbances, and increased infections.

Experimentation with lower dosages has greatly influenced IL-2 immunotherapy. Lower dosages are based on the observation that 10% of NK cells express high-affinity receptors for IL-2; a 500-fold decrease in the IL-2 dose (administered as a continuous intravenous infusion) would still be sufficient to bind to high-affinity receptors. The low-dose regimen was found to produce a gradual, tenfold increase in circulating NK cells without causing significant toxicity. Such low-dose administration of IL-2 has also been used to increase the number of NK cells in patients with HIV infection or advanced cancer.

Subcutaneous administration of IL-2 has been tested as an immunostimulant in individuals with asymptomatic HIV infection. This route leads to an increase in the proportion of T cells expressing IL-2Rs without increasing NK cells or viral proliferation.

Interferons

There are two major classes of interferons: **type 1 interferons** (IFN-α, IFN-β, and IFN-ω) and **type 2 interferon** (IFN-γ). Type 1 interferons are produced by most nucleated cells. IFN-γ is mainly a product of TH1 T cells, $CD8^+$ T cells, and activated NK cells.

Type 1 interferons act by stimulating the phosphorylation of cytosolic proteins termed **signal transducers and activators of transcription (STAT)**. STAT proteins form complexes that enter the nucleus, bind to its designated response element on DNA, and **promote transcription**.

Recombinant forms of IFN-α (interferon alfa-2α, interferon alfa-2β, interferon alfacon-1) and IFN-β (interferon beta-1α, interferon beta-1β) and a purified form from human leukocytes (interferon alfa-N3) have received approval by the FDA for use in the clinical setting, as described in Chapters 34 and 36. IFN-α preparations are indicated in the treatment of **numerous diseases**, including hairy cell leukemia, chronic myelogenous leukemia, condyloma acuminatum, acquired immunodeficiency syndrome–related Kaposi sarcoma, chronic hepatitis B and C, and malignant melanoma. IFN-β preparations are approved for the treatment of remitting and recurring multiple sclerosis. In addition, trials are ongoing for the use of type 1 interferons in numerous other cancers, AIDS, viral infections, papillomas, and angiogenic disorders.

IFN-γ was initially discovered as a result of its antiviral properties, but it also displays antiproliferative effects against tumors. IFN-γ is a glycosylated protein that exists exclusively as a covalently coupled homodimer. It shares very little DNA sequence homology with either IFN-α or IFN-β. The mechanism by which IFN-γ stimulates transcription is similar, however, to that of the type 1 interferons. The resultant effects of its action include (1) stimulation of $CD4^+$ TH1 T cells and macrophages, (2) suppression of antibody production (IFN-γ antagonizes $CD4^+$ TH2 T cells), (3) induction of immunoglobulin class switching, (4) upregulation of MHC II expression by epithelial tumor cells and macrophages (an effect antagonized by prostaglandin E2), and (5) alteration of antigen processing by changing the mix of peptide products produced by the proteasome. IFN-γ, in the form of a single polypeptide chain designated **interferon γ-1b,** is approved for managing serious infections associated with granulomatous disease and delaying the progression of malignant osteopetrosis. It is also useful in the management of rheumatoid arthritis.

TH1 and TH2 Cytokines

In later phases of specific immune responses, one function of cytokines is to regulate the nature of the immune response. **TH1 cytokines** help guide specific immunity against changes in intracellular, **cytosolic antigens**, and **TH2 cytokines** help direct specific immunity against changes in **extracellular antigens**. These TH1 and TH2 responses are mutually inhibitory: the TH1 cytokines IFN-γ and IL-12 inhibit TH2 responses, and the TH2 cytokines IL-4 and IL-10 inhibit TH1 responses. Pharmacologic regulation of the relative proportions of TH1 and TH2 cytokines may provide a way to treat diseases in which an inappropriate TH1 or TH2 response is a component of the disease process.

The types of disorders that may be amenable to cytokine intervention in these later stages include infectious diseases in which there is an inappropriate type of immune response, inflammatory autoimmune diseases, and IgE-mediated allergic diseases. Lepromatous leprosy, nonhealing forms of leishmaniasis, tuberculosis, trypanosomiasis, and certain fungal diseases are infections that may be exacerbated by an inappropriately strong TH2 response. The administration of the TH1 cytokine IFN-γ, as mentioned previously, is approved for this indication.

Experimental allergic encephalomyelitis, a potential animal model for multiple sclerosis, seems to involve an overzealous TH1 response and can be transferred by T cells with the TH1 phenotype. In animals, spontaneous recovery from the disease is associated with an expansion of T cells with the TH2 phenotype; a study in humans with multiple sclerosis suggests that the administration of IFN-γ exacerbates the disease process (to the point where the research had to be terminated). Opposite effects occur with IFN-β, which has FDA approval for the treatment of this form of the disease. The destruction of β-islet cells in insulin-dependent diabetes mellitus has been associated with tissue infiltration by T cells of the TH1 phenotype. For such TH1-mediated disease, it is possible that the administration of TH2 cytokines IL-4 and IL-10 may be beneficial.

IgE-mediated allergic diseases are consistent with the **over-activity of TH2 T cells**. Well-known examples include allergic rhinitis, immediate drug allergies, and life-threatening anaphylaxis resulting from insect stings. The successful long-term treatment of IgE-mediated allergies empirically corresponds with a **shift in antibody isotypes from IgE to IgG**; it is widely believed that various desensitization procedures in which the allergen is injected into the allergic host owe their success to the generation of "blocking antibodies" of the IgG subclass. Bee venom immunotherapy is a good model for such procedures; it is associated with a TH2-to-TH1 shift. The TH1 cytokine profile favors production of IgG rather than IgE. In local tissues, mast cells and basophils are important sources of IL-4. Local therapies currently being explored include anti-IL-4 antibodies and IFN-α.

Short-term desensitization procedures are also available for dealing with IgE-mediated allergies. Occasionally, it may be essential to treat a patient with a certain drug despite a known allergy to that drug (e.g., using penicillin to treat an infection in an individual with a positive skin test indicative of penicillin allergy). Most individuals are not allergic to penicillin itself, but rather to antigens that form by the covalent linkage between the β-lactam ring of penicillin metabolites and certain proteins. In acute desensitization, penicillin is administered in incrementally increasing dosages over 4 to 6 hours. The goal of these therapies is not to cause a permanent reduction in anti-penicillin IgE, but instead to induce rapidly a state of clinical tolerance. The actual mechanism of clinical tolerance is unclear (possible Fc receptor downregulation in mast cells); the end result is a diminished risk of anaphylaxis with only minor urticarial side effects.

Different types of immunotherapy drugs are summarized in Table 35-5. Immunotherapy drugs with specific cancer targets are summarized in Table 35-6.

TABLE 35-5 Drugs Used in Immunotherapy

Non-Proprietary (Generic) Name	Proprietary (Trade) Name
Agents for Active Immunization	
See complete list of vaccines licensed for immunization and distribution in the United States FDA Website: http://www.fda.gov/BiologicsBloodVaccines/Vaccines/ApprovedProducts/UCM093833	
Agents for Passive Immunization	
Botulism immunoglobulin (human)	BabyBIG
Cytomegalovirus immunoglobulin (human)	CytoGam
Hepatitis B immunoglobulin (human)	HepaGam B, HyperHEP B S/D, Nabi-HB
Immunoglobulin (human)	BayGam, Carimune NF, Flebogamma, Gamimune N, Gammagard, Octagan
Palivizumab	Synagis
Rabies immunoglobulin (human)	IMOGAM
Respiratory syncytial virus immunoglobulin (human)	RespiGam
Rh_0(D) immunoglobulin (human)	HyperRho S/D, RhoGAM, WinRho SDF
Tetanus immunoglobulin	HyperTET S/D
Varicella-zoster immunoglobulin	—
Antitoxins	
Antivenin (Crotalidae), polyvalent	—
Antivenin (*Latrodectus mactans*)	—
Antivenin (*Micrurus fulvius*)	—
Crotalidae polyvalent immune fab	CroFab
Rabies immunoglobulin (human)	Hyperab, Imogam
Immunostimulants	
Thymosin*	—
Levamisole*	Ergamisol
Immunomodulators	
Imiquimod	Aldera
Lenalidomide	Revlimid
Mitoxantrone	Novantrone
Thalidomide	Thalomid
Monoclonal Antibodies	
See Table 35-2	
Immunosuppressants	
Abatacept	Orencia
Azathioprine	Azasan, Imuran
Antithymocyte globulin (rabbit)	Thymoglobulin
Basiliximab	Simulect
Belinostat	Beleodaq
Ceritinib	Zykadia
Cyclophosphamide	Cytoxan
Cyclosporine	Gengraf, Neoral, Sandimmune, Restasis
Daclizumab	Zenapax
Dinutuximab	Unituxin
Glatiramer	Copaxone
Ibrutinib	Imbruvica
Idelalisib	Zydelig
Lenvatinib	Lenvima
Lymphocyte immunoglobulin, antithymocyte globulin (equine)	Atgam
Melphalan	Alkeran
Mercaptopurine	Purinethol
Methotrexate	Rheumatrex Dose Pack, Trexall
Muromonab-CD3	Orthoclone OKT3
Mycophenolate mofetil	CellCept
Mycophenolic acid	Myfortic
Olaparib	Lynparza
Palbociclib	Ibrance
Panobinostat	Farydak
Pembrolizumab	Keytruda
Prednisone	Sterapred
Sirolimus	Rapamune
Tacrolimus (FK506)	Prograf
Trametinib	Mekinist
Slow-Acting Disease-Modifying Antirheumatic Drugs	
See Chapter 17	
Cytokines	
Aldesleukin (IL-2)	Proleukin
Anakinra	Kineret
Denileukin diftitox	Ontak
Interferon alpha-2a	Roferon-A
Interferon alpha-2b	Intron A
Interferon alpha-n3	ALFERON N
Interferon alfacon-1	Infergen
Interferon beta-1a	Avonex, Rebif
Interferon beta-1b	Betaseron, Extavia
Interferon gamma-1b	Actimmune
Peginterferon alpha-2a	Pegasys
Peginterferon alpha-2b	PEG-Intron
Siltuximab	Sylvant
Hematopoietic Growth Factors	
See Chapter 25	
Therapy for Allergic Reactions	
See Chapters 18, 27, and 30	

*Not currently available in the United States.

TABLE 35-6 Immunotherapy for Cancer Treatment*

Non-Proprietary (Generic) Name	Proprietary (Trade) Name
Adenocarcinoma of the Stomach or Gastroesophageal Junction	
Trastuzumab	Herceptin
Ramucirumab	Cyramza
Basal Cell Carcinoma	
Vismodegib	Erivedge
Brain Cancer	
Bevacizumab	Avastin
Everolimus	Afinitor
Breast Cancer	
Everolimus	Afinitor
Trastuzumab	Herceptin
Pertuzumab	Perjeta
Ado-trastuzumab emtansine	Kadcyla
Cervical Cancer	
Bevacizumab	Avastin
Colorectal Cancer	
Cetuximab	Erbitux
Panitumumab	Vectibix
Bevacizumab	Avastin
Regorafenib	Stivarga
Ramucirumab	Cyramza
Dermatofibrosarcoma Protuberans	
Imatinib mesylate	Gleevec
Endocrine/Neuroendocrine Tumors	
Lanreotide acetate	Somatuline Depot
Head and Neck Cancer	
Cetuximab	Erbitux
Gastrointestinal Stroma Tumor	
Imatinib mesylate	Gleevec
Sunitinib	Sutent
Regorafenib	Stivarga
Giant Cell Tumor of the Bone	
Denosumab	Xgeva
Kaposi Sarcoma	
Alitretinoin	Panretin
Kidney Cancer	
Bevacizumab	Avastin
Sorafenib	Nexavar
Sunitinib	Sutent
Pazopanib	Votrient
Temsirolimus	Torisel
Everolimus	Afinitor
Axitinib	Inlyta
Leukemia	
Tretinoin	Vesanoid
Imatinib mesylate	Gleevec
Dasatinib	Sprycel
Nilotinib	Tasigna
Bosutinib	Bosulif
Rituximab	Rituxan
Alemtuzumab	Campath
Ofatumumab	Arzerra
Obinutuzumab	Gazyva
Ibrutinib	Imbruvica
Idelalisib	Zydelig
Blinatumomab	Blincyto
Liver Cancer	
Sorafenib	Nexavar
Lung Cancer	
Bevacizumab	Avastin
Crizotinib	Xalkori
Erlotinib	Tarceva
Gefitinib	Iressa
Afatinib dimaleate	Gilotrif
Ceritinib	LDK378/Zykadia
Ramucirumab	Cyramza
Nivolumab	Opdivo
Lymphoma	
Ibritumomab tiuxetan	Zevalin
Denileukin diftitox	Ontak
Brentuximab vedotin	Adcetris
Rituximab	Rituxan
Vorinostat	Zolinza
Romidepsin	Istodax
Bexarotene	Targretin
Bortezomib	Velcade
Pralatrexate	Folotyn
Lenalidomide	Revlimid
Ibrutinib	Imbruvica
Siltuximab	Sylvan
Idelalisib	Zydelig
Belinostat	Beleodaq
Melanoma	
Ipilimumab	Yervoy
Vemurafenib	Zelboraf
Trametinib	Mekinist
Dabrafenib	Tafinlar
Pembrolizumab	Keytruda
Nivolumab	Opdivo
Multiple Myeloma	
Bortezomib	Velcade
Carfilzomib	Kyprolis
Lenalidomide	Revlimid
Pomalidomide	Pomalyst
Myelodysplastic/Myeloproliferative Disorders	
Imatinib mesylate	Gleevec
Ruxolitinib phosphate	Jakafi

Continued

TABLE 35-6 Immunotherapy for Cancer Treatment*—cont'd

Non-Proprietary (Generic) Name	Proprietary (Trade) Name	Non-Proprietary (Generic) Name	Proprietary (Trade) Name
Neuroblastoma		**Soft Tissue Sarcoma**	
Dinutuximab	Unituxin	Pazopanib	Votrient
Ovarian Epithelial/Fallopian Tube/Primary Peritoneal Cancers		**Systemic Mastocytosis**	
Bevacizumab	Avastin	Imatinib mesylate	Gleevec
Olaparib	Lynparza		
		Thyroid Cancer	
Pancreatic Cancer		Cabozantinib	Cometriq
Erlotinib	Tarceva	Vandetanib	Caprelsa
Everolimus	Afinitor	Sorafenib	Nexavar
Sunitinib	Sutent	Lenvatinib mesylate	Lenvima

*Includes some enzyme inhibitors such as tyrosine kinase inhibitors and hedgehog pathway inhibitor.

Engineered TCR, CAR/T, TIL, and NK therapies

Due to recent advances in immunotherapeutic strategies and the demonstrated effectiveness of such therapies in arresting or inhibiting disease progression, immunotherapy is now regarded as one of the main strategies for cancer treatment. T cells engineered to express tumor-specific T cell receptors (TCRs) with high affinity for tumor antigens are currently being used in clinical trials of patients with relapsed tumors. Chimeric antigen receptor T (CAR/T) cells that combine both antibody-like recognition site with T cell activating function is also a novel therapeutic direction with promising results. Tumor infiltrating lymphocytes (TILs) have been isolated and expanded ex-vivo for infusion in cancer patients. NK cells can be expanded and delivered to patients for the elimination of cancer stem cells that seed the cancer, along with their use in promoting differentiation of the remaining tumors for the inhibition of cancer metastasis.

Although impressive results were obtained by strategies previously indicated in certain cancer patients, it is still unclear whether such treatments will deliver long-lasting remissions in patients. In addition, toxicities associated with the treatments have halted the effort for the continuous infusion of these cells for the complete elimination of the tumors. Future studies will be directed toward designing cellular therapies, which will be specific to tumors and will have long-term persistence of engineered cells in the patients with low overall toxicities. Until then, cancer patients will continue receiving monoclonal antibodies to immune checkpoints such as PD-1 and CTLA-4 that have shown efficacy in treating the tumors in a selected group of patients. Future strategies will not only use the engineered and expanded T, CAR/T, TIL, and NK cells, but also they will combine such treatments with a number of immune checkpoint inhibitors.

CASE DISCUSSION

The symptoms of dry mouth, dry eyes, and rheumatoid arthritis are typical of Sjögren syndrome. To alleviate dry mouth, Mrs. R can chew on sugarless candy or dried fruit to stimulate the production of saliva. Mrs. R's physician, or you, can also prescribe pilocarpine or cevimeline to increase saliva production. A saliva substitute is a useful option. All of these strategies assume sufficient functional salivary gland tissue to generate saliva. Moreover, there appears to be no contraindication or drug–drug interaction that would preclude the use of pilocarpine or cevimeline. By repairing carious teeth and increasing saliva secretion, Mrs. R's oral health should improve, and her increased risk for future dental cavities will subside.

Mrs. R should be referred to an ophthalmologist for treatment of dry eyes. Several strategies are available to Mrs. R to relieve dry eyes associated with Sjögren syndrome. Mrs. R can preserve her natural tears by wearing wraparound glasses to reduce evaporation of tears due to contact with air and wind. She can also use over-the-counter artificial tears to temporary relieve her dry eyes; however, if the extent of dry eyes is severe, her physician can prescribe cyclosporine ophthalmic eye drops or recommend a punctal occlusion procedure to slow down the drainage of tears by inserting a small plug into the tear ducts.

Mrs. R should be encouraged to see her rheumatologist regularly. If Mrs. R's joint pain worsens, her physician can adjust the NSAID or glucocorticoid (such as prednisone) dose. A class of medications called DMARDs, which includes hydroxychloroquine (Plaquenil), azathioprine (Imuran), cyclophosphamide (*Cytoxan*), mycophenolate (CellCept), and methotrexate (*Rheumatrex*), can control joint inflammation. Another class of medication called TNF inhibitors, which includes infliximab (Remicade), etanercept (Enbrel), and adalimumab (Humira), are available for rheumatoid arthritis. Currently, no biologic therapies have been approved for Sjögren syndrome as such, but rituximab (Rituxan) and monoclonal antibodies specific for CD20 (HuMax-CD20, veltuzumab, ofatumumab) and CD22 (Epratuzumab) are currently under clinical investigation. A strong understanding of immunotherapy will aid in the development of new immunotherapy drugs for patients suffering from Sjögren syndrome, as is Mrs. R.

GENERAL REFERENCES

1. Ahmadzadeh V, Farajnia S, Feizi MA, Nejad RA: Antibody humanization methods for development of therapeutic applications, *Monoclon Antib Immunodiagn Immunother* 33:67–73, 2014.
2. Choi J, et al.: Structure of the FKBP12-rapamycin complex interacting with the binding domain of human FRAP, *Science* 273:239–242, 1996.
3. Cronstein BN: Second-line antirheumatic drugs. In Snyderman R, Gallin JI, editors: *Inflammation: basic principles and clinical correlates*, Philadelphia, 1999, Lippincott Williams & Wilkins.
4. Dinarello CA: Modalities for reducing interleukin 1 activity in disease, *Trends Pharmacol Sci* 14:155–159, 1993.
5. Dinarello CA: Interleukin-1: a proinflammatory cytokine. In Gallin JI, Snyderman R, editors: *Inflammation: basic principles and clinical correlates*, Philadelphia, 1999, Lippincott Williams & Wilkins.
6. Goldstein AL, Low TL, McAdoo M: Thymosin alpha1: isolation and sequence analysis of an immunologically active thymic polypeptide, *Proc Natl Acad Sci* 74:725–729, 1977.
7. Jewett A, Tseng HC: Potential rescue, survival and differentiation of cancer stem cells and primary non-transformed stem cells by monocyte-induced split energy in natural killer cells, *Cancer Immunol Immunother* 61:265–274, 2012.
8. Jewett A, Tseng HC: Tumor microenvironment may shape the function and phenotype of NK cells through the induction of split anergy and

generation of regulatory NK cells. In Shurin M, Umansky V, Malyguine A, editors: *The tumor immunoenvironment*, Springer, 2013, pp 361–384.
9. Michalek SM, Childers NK: Development and outlook for a caries vaccine, *Crit Rev Oral Biol Med* 1:37–54, 1990.
10. Murphy KM, Weaver C: *Janeway's Immunobiology*. ed 9, New York, 2016, Garland Science.
11. Ohno M, Natsume A, Wakabayashi T: Cytokine therapy, *Adv Exp Med Biol* 746:86–94, 2012.
12. Tseng HC, Jewett A, Cacalano N: Split anergized Natural Killer cells halt inflammation by inducing stem cell differentiation, resistance to NK cell cytotoxicity and prevention of cytokine and chemokine secretion, *OncoTarget* 6:8947–8959, 2015.
13. Von Boehmer H, Melchers F: Checkpoints in lymphocyte development and autoimmune disease, *Nat Immunol* 11:14–20, 2010.

36 Antineoplastic Drugs

Karl K. Kwok, Erica C. Vincent, and James N. Gibson

KEY INFORMATION

- The goal of chemotherapy is to eradicate every viable tumor cell without significantly damaging normal host tissue.
- Classic chemotherapy agents are not tumor cell–specific and kill all cells actively undergoing cell division, resulting in the unintended destruction of normal host cells.
- Alkylating agents prevent cell division by reacting with DNA and RNA.
- Alkylating agents are composed of six major chemical classes that include nitrogen mustards, alkyl sulfonates, ethylenimines, triazines, tetrazines, and nitrosoureas.
- Antimetabolites serve as fraudulent substrates for biochemical reactions, either inhibiting synthetic steps or becoming incorporated into molecules and interfering with cellular function or replication.
- The three classes of antimetabolites include folic acid analogues, purine analogues, and pyrimidine analogues.
- Antitumor antibiotics are antibiotics that have been found to exert antineoplastic activity because of their cytotoxic properties. These substances operate in part by binding with DNA to produce irreversible complexes that inhibit cell division.
- The antineoplastic activity of vinca alkaloids has been attributed to their capacity to arrest cell division in metaphase by binding to the microtubule protein, tubulin, that forms the mitotic spindle.
- Hormone agonists and antagonists are used for cancer therapy by mimicking or blocking hormone action.
- The activity of certain enzymes involves inhibition of protein synthesis in tumor cells.
- Platinum agents are heavy metals that cause DNA strand breaks and inhibit DNA synthesis.
- Podophyllotoxins are plant derivatives that inhibit the action of topoisomerase II and cause DNA strand breaks in tumor cells.
- Camptothecins are plant derivatives that produce cytotoxic effects via inhibition of topoisomerase I, which causes single-strand breaks in DNA.
- Taxanes (from plant derivatives) and epothilones (from myxobacterium metabolites) cause disruption of microtubule function and induce tumor cell cycle arrest.
- Differentiating agents (e.g., retinoids) aim to direct the less differentiated cancer cell to resume a process of normal maturation.
- Biologic response modifiers are used to assist the body's natural ability to kill cancer cells or to minimize adverse effects on normal cells.
- Targeted antineoplastic therapy is a form of molecular medicine that targets the specific molecular pathways in tumor cells to eradicate them without harming normal host cells.
- Antineoplastic agents are rarely used as single entities for the treatment of cancer and many are used concomitantly or in sequence as a combination therapy.
- Oral complications of cancer therapy may result directly from the cytotoxic effects (direct toxic effects) of the drugs on oral tissues (including salivary glands) or result from therapy involving distant tissues (indirect toxic effects).

CASE STUDY

Your new patient, Mrs. P, has been referred to your office from the oncologist for an oral lesion on her mandible. Mrs. P has been receiving Zometa (zoledronic acid) for 18 months for bone metastases emanating from her breast cancer. Upon oral examination, you find an area of exposed bone that is approximately 3 mm by 4.5 mm on the lingual surface of her mandible next to her first molar. She reports that it has been present for the past three months, and although she is not in pain, she wants to know what it might be. She is considering discontinuing her monthly Zometa treatment because of the exposed bone in her jaw. What pharmacologic recommendations can you provide for her?

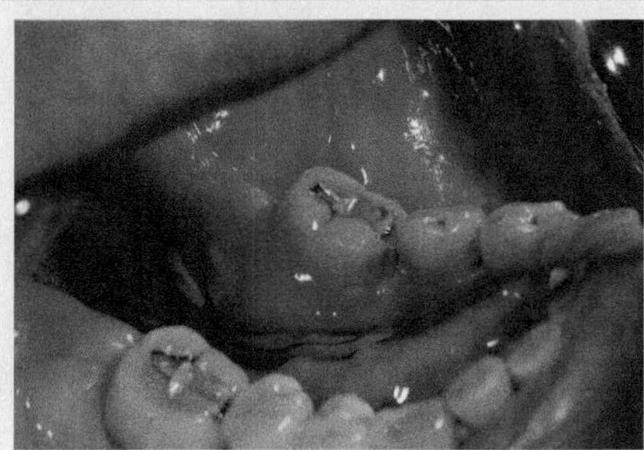

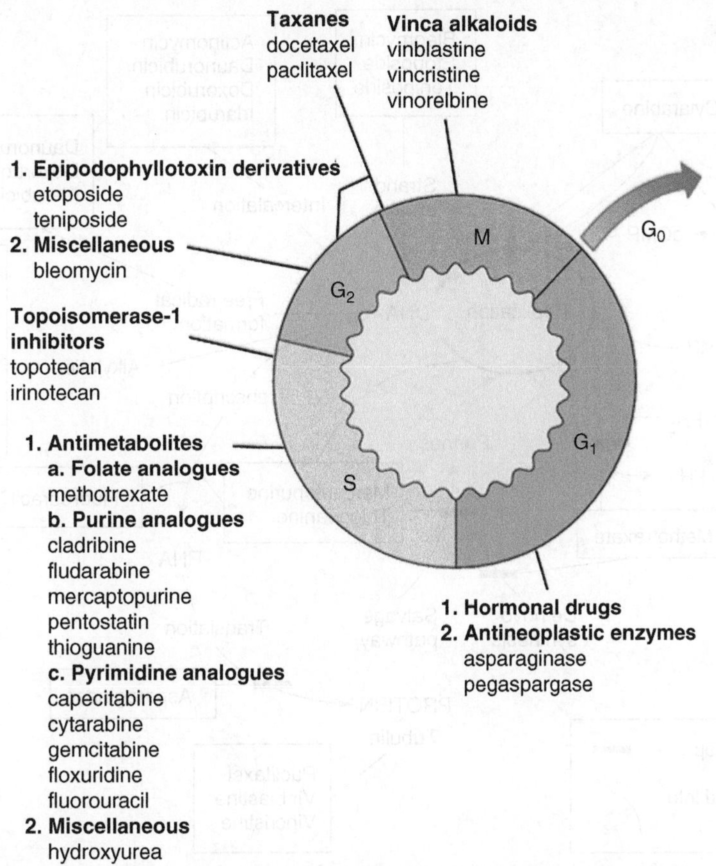

FIG 36-1 Cell cycle sites of antineoplastic activity. G_0, Resting phase; G_1, period before DNA synthesis, during which the enzymes necessary for DNA synthesis are synthesized; G_2, period of specialized protein and RNA synthesis and the manufacture of mitotic spindle apparatus; *M*, mitosis; *S*, DNA synthesis, during which DNA is replicated. (From Lilley LL, Harrington S, Snyder JS: *Pharmacology and the nursing process*, ed 7, St. Louis, 2014, Mosby.)

The role of antineoplastic drugs in cancer treatment has greatly expanded in the past few decades. Antineoplastic drugs are often used as the primary means of treatment to cure some malignancies such as testicular cancer, leukemias, and lymphomas. These agents can also be used in conjunction with surgery and/or radiation to prevent relapse or recurrence of various malignancies and in the palliative setting to reduce symptoms of disease and prolong survival. Research has resulted in the development and approval of new agents, more effective applications of existing agents, and the use of adjunctive drugs to overcome resistance and minimize drug toxicity.

The past decade has also brought about a greater depth of research and understanding of the molecular biology of cancer cell growth. Many mechanisms of cellular growth stimulation and retardation and the actions of growth modulators have been discovered. Gene rearrangements and mutations and their resultant influences on cell growth are being elucidated. These discoveries provide many new targets for the management of abnormal cell growth, and they have resulted in multiple new approaches to cancer therapy and several new classes of drugs. Antineoplastic regimens that contribute to the goal of eliminating and destroying tumor cells now include **traditional chemotherapeutic drugs** (e.g., alkylators, antimetabolites, steroids, plant alkaloids, and other agents), **biologic response modifiers, novel targeted agents, hormonal therapies**, and **agents used specifically to protect the patient from the toxic effects of these drugs.**

PRINCIPLES OF CANCER CHEMOTHERAPY

The goal of chemotherapy is to eradicate every viable tumor cell without significantly damaging normal host tissue. Attaining this goal requires that the tumor be inherently sensitive to the chemotherapy agents prescribed, that the tumor receptor sites be exposed to adequate concentrations of active drug for sufficient periods, and that the host cells be resistant to the effects of the chemotherapy drugs. **Classic chemotherapy agents are not tumor cell–specific and kill all cells actively undergoing cell division, resulting in the unintended destruction of normal host cells in the gastrointestinal tract, bone marrow, hair follicles, and other tissues.**

Chemotherapy drugs kill or impair susceptible tumor cells by blocking a drug-sensitive biochemical or metabolic pathway. Some, such as cell cycle phase–specific antimetabolites, act by inhibiting DNA synthesis and are most effective against rapidly dividing cells. Others, such as alkylating agents, act by interfering with nucleic acid function and protein production throughout the entire cell division cycle and are effective against both proliferating and resting cells (Figs. 36-1 and 36-2). All chemotherapy drugs are extremely cytotoxic with low margins of safety. Incorporating the current understanding of tumor biology, the patient's physiologic status, and the drug's pharmacologic features, the principles that govern the useful application of cancer chemotherapy include the following:

1. The **tumor must be susceptible** to the drugs selected for treatment. Not all tumors are responsive to the same agents.

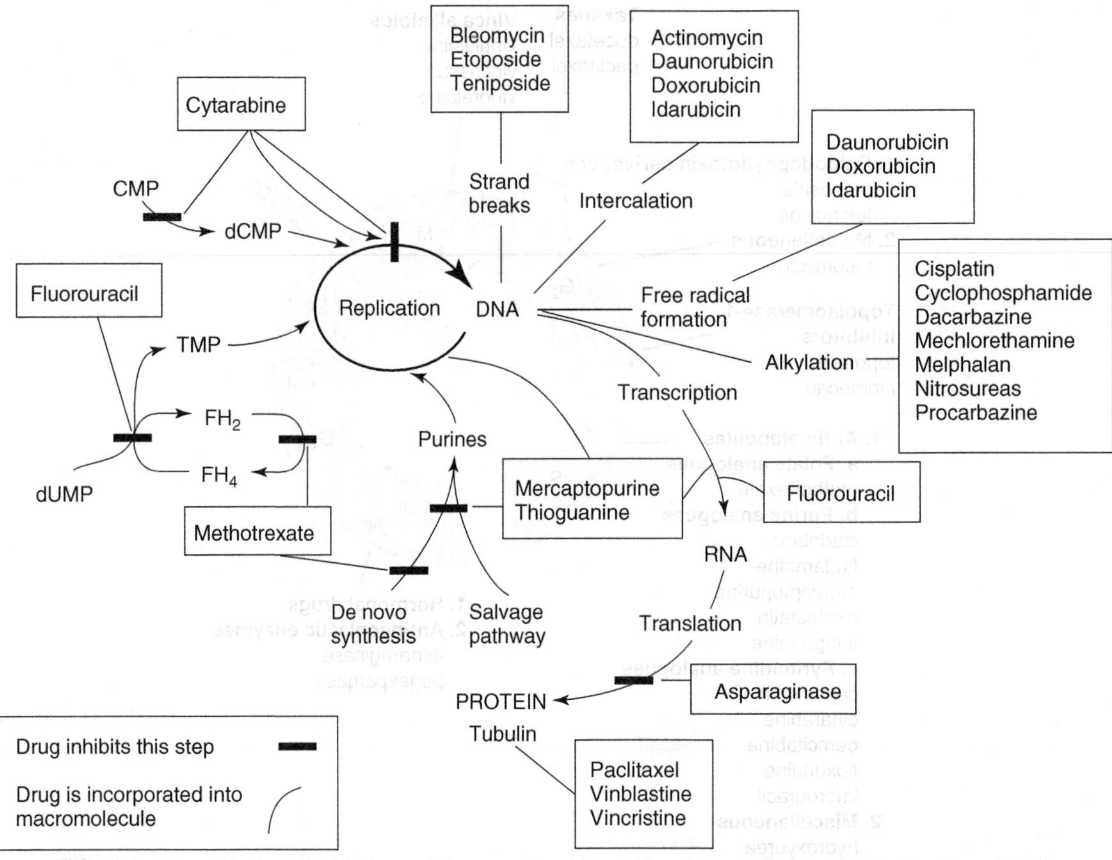

FIG 36-2 Potential sites of inhibition and incorporation of select antineoplastic agents into the biosynthetic pathways of nucleic acids and proteins. *CMP,* Cytosine monophosphate; *dCMP,* deoxycytosine monophosphate; *dUMP,* deoxyuridine monophosphate; *FH_2,* dihydrofolate; *FH_4,* tetrahydrofolate; *TMP,* thymidine monophosphate.

2. The drugs or methods of administration must **not have intolerable local or systemic toxicity** that would prevent the completion of an adequate course of treatment.
3. The dosages and schedules for the drugs must be calculated to maximize the contact with the tumor cells, and the **drugs must be present in sufficient concentration** during the crucial periods of the cell's metabolic cycle.
4. **Cancer chemotherapy is more effective when the tumor mass is small** than when the tumor cell burden is high. A larger fraction of the tumor cell population is undergoing active division in a small tumor mass, and the blood supply is more plentiful, allowing for increased sensitivity and delivery of the drugs. Debulking by surgery or irradiation reduces tumor cell burden and can induce resting cell populations into active cell division, increasing the growth fraction of the tumor and thus the sensitivity to chemotherapy.
5. **Anticancer drugs kill cells according to first-order kinetics.** Even a drug that destroyed 99.99% of the tumor cells would leave a substantial number of tumor cells intact if the initial quantity was large. Because survival of a few or perhaps even a single malignant cell may lead to tumor regrowth, chemotherapy is generally given in cycles to maximize tumor cell reduction. The optimal interval between cycles is determined by the time required to allow for sufficient bone marrow recovery without allowing significant tumor regrowth.
6. The administration of combinations of **antineoplastic drugs takes advantage of the different mechanisms of action.** By using agents that act at different phases of the cell cycle, synergistic effects and an increase in the collective antitumor effect may be obtained without an increase in undesirable side effects. Combination chemotherapy may prevent or slow the development of resistant cancer cells.
7. **Cancer cells may build up resistance** to a previously effective drug, which then becomes ineffective. Such resistance has been ascribed to various causes, including decreased drug penetration resulting from a reduction in tumor blood supply, drug-provoked mutations, enzyme alterations, and acquired resistance through natural selection of tumor cells insensitive to the drug. The therapeutic potential of antineoplastic drugs may be enhanced by active antitumor defense mechanisms in the host. Immunotherapy given with chemotherapy, either concurrently or sequentially, may boost the tumoricidal effect of certain drugs.

CHEMOTHERAPEUTIC DRUGS

Antineoplastic Alkylating Agents

Alkylating agents are composed of six major chemical classes: (1) nitrogen mustards (chlorambucil, cyclophosphamide, estramustine, ifosfamide, mechlorethamine, melphalan, and bendamustine), (2) alkyl sulfonates (busulfan), (3) ethylenimines (thiotepa), (4) triazines (dacarbazine), (5) tetrazines (temozolomide), and (6) nitrosoureas (carmustine, lomustine, and streptozocin). They all share the common chemical characteristic of forming alkyl radicals, which form covalent linkages with nucleophilic moieties such as the phosphate, sulfhydryl, hydroxyl, carboxyl, amino, and imidazole groups. This radical formation **allows them to react with organic compounds such as DNA**

and RNA and proteins essential for cell metabolism and protein synthesis. By binding these groups, they also prevent cell division by cross-linking strands of DNA.

Alkylating agents are not cell cycle specific, although they are **most destructive to rapidly proliferating tissues** and seem to cause cellular death only when the cell attempts to divide. Because they produce irreversible changes in the DNA molecule, alkylating agents are mutagenic, teratogenic, and carcinogenic in addition to being oncolytic. Alkylating agents are also radiomimetic because they produce morphologic damage in cells similar to the damage caused by radiation injury. Infections are a common adverse outcome in patients receiving these agents owing to their myelosuppressive and immunosuppressive properties. They vary greatly in lipid solubility, membrane transport, pharmacokinetic properties, and in clinical application. The adverse effects and clinical applications of alkylating agents are summarized in Table 36-1.

Nitrogen mustards

Mechlorethamine. Mechlorethamine was the first nitrogen mustard introduced in clinical practice and the progenitor of antineoplastic alkylating agents. It is still used systemically in the treatment of Hodgkin's disease; in combination with vincristine, procarbazine, and prednisone; and topically to treat mycosis fungoides. The drug is a vesicant that produces severe local tissue necrosis unless administered through a running intravenous infusion. This irritant effect is used to control intractable pleural effusions caused by intrapleural malignancies. In such instances, the drug is administered by intracavitary injection into the pleural space. Usually given intravenously, this drug is highly reactive and has a short stability and biologic half-life. The acute side effects of nitrogen mustard are nausea and vomiting, and these usually begin within 30 minutes after injection and persist for 8 hours.

Bendamustine hydrochloride. Bendamustine hydrochloride (Treanda) is an intravenously administered bifunctional mechlorethamine derivative with alkylator and purine antimetabolite activity. This bifunctional agent may have an advantage to overcome cross-resistance with other alkylating agents. Bendamustine has been studied in combination with rituximab in the management of patients with indolent or mantle cell lymphoma and has shown significant activity. It has been approved more recently for the treatment of chronic lymphocytic leukemia and continues to be studied in many other tumor types, including breast cancer and sarcomas. The most common adverse effects (occurring 15% to 20% of the time) include neutropenia, thrombocytopenia, anemia, pyrexia, nausea, and vomiting.

Chlorambucil. Chlorambucil is given orally for chronic lymphocytic leukemia, indolent non-Hodgkin's lymphoma, carcinoma of the ovary and breast, and multiple myeloma. The drug is well absorbed and rapidly metabolized, but its route of excretion is uncertain. Chlorambucil is generally well tolerated with minimal gastrointestinal toxicity in the usual doses.

Cyclophosphamide. Cyclophosphamide is a cyclic mustard that resulted from attempts to produce an alkylating agent with greater selectivity for neoplastic tissues than the original nitrogen mustard mechlorethamine. Cyclophosphamide is a broad-spectrum agent and is valuable in induction, maintenance, and remission therapy for non-Hodgkin's lymphoma, leukemias, prostate, lung, breast, and ovarian cancers. It is also used in high doses as part of the conditioning regimen for bone marrow transplants. Cyclophosphamide has excellent immunosuppressive properties and is thus useful in severe rheumatoid arthritis, allograft rejection, and other autoimmune disorders. The drug may be administered orally or intravenously and is metabolized to the active compounds phosphoramide mustard and acrolein by the liver. Acrolein is a metabolic by-product that is toxic to the bladder, producing hemorrhagic cystitis and dysuria that can be minimized by vigorous hydration, frequent bladder emptying, and administration of the chemoprotectant mesna. Cyclophosphamide is very myelosuppressive, manifested primarily as leukopenia.

Ifosfamide. Ifosfamide is a nitrogen mustard differing from cyclophosphamide only in the location of a chloroethyl moiety. This intravenous drug is also a prodrug that must be metabolized by the liver cytochrome P450 (CYP) system to the active alkylating agent ifosfamide mustard and other toxic metabolites (acrolein and chloroacetic acid). Ifosfamide has a broad spectrum of antineoplastic activity. Although ifosfamide has several significant toxic effects, the dose-limiting toxicity is hemorrhagic cystitis. The high incidence of this toxicity requires uroprotection with aggressive hydration, frequent bladder emptying, and the concurrent use of mesna, a uroprotective agent. Mesna contains a free sulfhydryl group that reacts with and inactivates the toxic metabolite acrolein.

Melphalan. Melphalan is a phenylalanine mustard that is available orally for treatment of multiple myeloma and carcinomas of the ovaries and breast. Melphalan is erratically absorbed from the gastrointestinal tract, and to overcome this pitfall, intravenous melphalan is utilized for the high doses prescribed for bone marrow transplant conditioning regimens. When high-dose melphalan is administered, it carries a high risk of mucositis, especially when combined with total body irradiation. To minimize the severity of mucositis, patients are counseled to eat ice chips to restrict blood flow to the oral mucosa and reduce drug delivery to this area (often referred to as cryotherapy).

Alkyl sulfonates

Busulfan. Busulfan historically was used almost exclusively in the control of chronic myelogenous leukemia. Today, it is used mostly in high-dose conditioning regimens for bone marrow transplants. A slow-acting sulfur mustard that is well absorbed after oral administration, busulfan is rapidly cleared from the blood and excreted in the urine as inactive metabolites. It has bone marrow–suppressive effects similar to other antineoplastic alkylating drugs; however, with busulfan, the myelosuppression can be quite prolonged.

Ethylenimines

Thiotepa. Thiotepa (triethylenethiophosphoramide) is an alkylating agent that has produced favorable results in breast and ovarian cancers, lymphoma, and rhabdomyosarcoma. It is clinically used in standard doses for the treatment of superficial bladder cancer, where it is directly instilled into the bladder lumen. This agent has also been used to control malignant effusions, and high doses are used in bone marrow transplants. After intravenous infusion, most of the drug is excreted unchanged in the urine.

Triazines

Dacarbazine. Dacarbazine (DTIC) is an artificially synthesized congener of the naturally occurring purine precursor 5-aminoimidazole-4-carboxamide. Originally developed as an antimetabolite, DTIC is N-demethylated in the liver to yield an effective alkylating derivative (called 5-[3-methyltriazen-1-yl]imidazole-4-carboxamide [MTIC]). After intravenous administration, the drug is extensively metabolized and renally excreted. DTIC has an elimination half-life of approximately 5 hours. The drug is most effective in the management of malignant melanoma, soft tissue sarcomas, and Hodgkin's disease. Nausea and vomiting are the predominant side effects, with an onset in the first few hours that may persist for several days. Fatal hepatic damage has occurred rarely.

TABLE 36-1 Classification of Available Antineoplastic and Associated Drugs

Class or Type of Agent	Nonproprietary (Generic) Name	Proprietary (Trade) Name	Adverse Effects*	Stomatitis†	Clinical Applications
Alkylating Agents					
Nitrogen mustards	Chlorambucil	Leukeran	Myelosuppression, pulmonary fibrosis, dermatotoxicity, hepatotoxicity	0	Chronic lymphocytic leukemia, Hodgkin's disease, lymphosarcoma, ovarian cancer, seminoma
	Cyclophosphamide	Cytoxan	Immunosuppression, myelosuppression, dermatotoxicity, hemorrhagic cystitis, GI enterotoxicity, hepatotoxicity, alopecia, SIADH	+	Hodgkin's disease; lymphoma; leukemia; multiple myeloma; sarcoma; testicular, prostate, lung, breast, and ovarian carcinoma
	Estramustine	Emcyt	Myelosuppression, cardiovascular toxicity, GI enterotoxicity, gynecomastia	+	Prostate cancer
	Ifosfamide	Ifex	Myelosuppression, nausea and vomiting, hemorrhagic cystitis, lethargy, confusion	+	Testicular carcinoma, sarcoma, ovarian carcinoma
	Mechlorethamine	Mustargen	Myelosuppression, nausea and vomiting, tissue necrosis, alopecia, neurotoxicity	0	Hodgkin's disease, lymphoma, mycosis fungoides
	Bendamustine	Treanda	Myelosuppression, nausea and vomiting, hypersensitivity reactions, fever	0	Chronic lymphocytic leukemia
	Melphalan	Alkeran	Myelosuppression, GI enterotoxicity, pulmonary fibrosis, dermatotoxicity, teratogenicity, SIADH	0	Multiple myeloma, ovarian carcinoma
Alkyl sulfonate	Busulfan	Myleran	Myelosuppression, nausea and vomiting, pulmonary fibrosis, dermatotoxicity, cataract formation, gynecomastia	0	Chronic myelocytic leukemia, polycythemia vera
Ethylenimine derivative	Thiotepa	Thioplex	Myelosuppression, infertility, dermatotoxicity, nausea and vomiting	0	Carcinoma of breast, ovary, and bladder; rhabdomyosarcoma
Triazene derivative	Dacarbazine	DTIC	Nausea and vomiting, fever, myelosuppression, alopecia, hepatotoxicity, dermatotoxicity	0	Melanoma, Hodgkin's disease, sarcoma
Tetrazine derivative	Temozolomide	Temodar	Myelosuppression, GI enterotoxicity	+	Brain tumor, melanoma
Nitrosoureas	Carmustine	BiCNU	Myelosuppression, GI enterotoxicity, hepatotoxicity, nephrotoxicity, pulmonary fibrosis	0	Hodgkin's disease, brain tumor, lymphoma, melanoma, multiple myeloma
	Lomustine	CeeNu	Myelosuppression, GI enterotoxicity, hepatotoxicity, nephrotoxicity, pulmonary fibrosis	0	Hodgkin's disease, lung and brain tumors, multiple myeloma, melanoma
	Streptozocin	Zanosar	Nausea and vomiting, nephrotoxicity, hypoglycemia, hepatotoxicity, fever, myelosuppression	0	Islet cell carcinoma of the pancreas
Antimetabolites					
Folic acid analogue	Methotrexate	Trexall	Myelosuppression, mucositis, nausea and vomiting, pulmonary fibrosis, nephrotoxicity, neurotoxicity	++	Choriocarcinoma; carcinomas of head, neck, breast, and lung; lymphocytic leukemia; sarcoma; trophoblastic tumor; testicular and bladder tumors; psoriasis
	Pemetrexed disodium	Alimta	Myelosuppression, rash, nausea and vomiting, neuropathy and myalgias, stomatitis, pharyngitis	++	Malignant pleural mesothelioma, non-small cell lung cancer
Purine analogues	Mercaptopurine	Purinethol	Myelosuppression, nausea and vomiting, hepatotoxicity, immunosuppression	++	Acute leukemia, chronic myelogenous leukemia
	Thioguanine	Tabloid	Myelosuppression, hepatotoxicity, nausea and vomiting	++	Acute leukemia, chronic myelogenous leukemia
	Fludarabine	Fludara	Myelosuppression, nausea and vomiting, alopecia	++	Chronic lymphocytic leukemia
	Clofarabine	Clolar	Myelosuppression, nausea and vomiting, hepatotoxicity, systemic inflammatory response syndrome, cardiotoxicity	0	Acute lymphocytic leukemia
	Nelarabine	Arranon	Myelosuppression, nausea and vomiting, cough, dyspnea, neurologic toxicities, progressive multifocal leukoencephalopathy	0	T-cell acute and lymphoblastic leukemia and lymphoma
	Pentostatin (2′-deoxycoformycin)	Nipent	Nephrotoxicity, CNS depression, nausea and vomiting	0	Hairy cell leukemia
	Cladribine (2-CDA, 2-chloro-deoxyadenosine)	Leustatin	Myelosuppression	0	Hairy cell leukemia

TABLE 36-1 Classification of Available Antineoplastic and Associated Drugs—cont'd

Class or Type of Agent	Nonproprietary (Generic) Name	Proprietary (Trade) Name	Adverse Effects*	Stomatitis†	Clinical Applications
Pyrimidine analogues	Cytarabine	Cytosar-U	Myelosuppression, nausea and vomiting, hepatotoxicity, dermatotoxicity, CNS, conjunctivitis	++	Acute leukemia, lymphoma, chronic myelogenous leukemia
	Capecitabine	Xeloda	GI enterotoxicity, myelosuppression, dermatotoxicity, neurotoxicity, hepatotoxicity	++	Colorectal cancer, metastatic breast cancer
	Fluorouracil	Adrucil	GI enterotoxicity, myelosuppression, dermatotoxicity, neurotoxicity	++	GI adenocarcinoma; carcinoma of lung, breast, ovary, prostate, cervix, bladder, head and neck
	Floxuridine	FUDR	GI enterotoxicity, myelosuppression, dermatotoxicity, hepatotoxicity, neurotoxicity	++	Hepatic metastases from GI adenocarcinomas, carcinomas of head and neck
	Gemcitabine	Gemzar	Myelosuppression, fever and flulike symptoms	0	Adenocarcinoma of the pancreas
Vinca Alkaloids					
	Vincristine	Oncovin	Neurotoxicity, SIADH, dermatotoxicity, GI enterotoxicity, alopecia	+	Hodgkin's disease; lymphocytic leukemia; chronic myelogenous leukemia; Wilms tumor; sarcoma; multiple myeloma; cancer of breast, cervix, lung, and ovary
	Vinblastine	Velban	Myelosuppression, GI enterotoxicity, neurotoxicity, SIADH	+	Hodgkin's disease; lymphoma; cancer of breast, bladder, and testis; Kaposi sarcoma
	Vinorelbine	Navelbine	Myelosuppression, GI enterotoxicity, neurotoxicity	+	Non-small cell lung carcinoma, breast carcinoma
Antibiotics					
	Bleomycin	Blenoxane	Pulmonary toxicity, GI enterotoxicity, skin reactions, anaphylaxis, fever	+	Testicular cancer, Hodgkin's disease, lymphoma, sarcoma, squamous cell carcinoma of head and neck, GI tumors
	Dactinomycin (actinomycin D)	Cosmegen	Myelosuppression, GI enterotoxicity, dermatotoxicity, tissue necrosis	+	Wilms tumor, rhabdomyosarcoma, Ewing sarcoma, neuroblastoma, testicular carcinoma, osteosarcoma, choriocarcinoma
	Daunorubicin, liposomal daunorubicin	Cerubidine, DaunoXome	Myelosuppression, cardiotoxicity, GI enterotoxicity, alopecia, tissue necrosis, radiation recall reaction	+	Acute leukemia
	Doxorubicin, liposomal doxorubicin	Adriamycin, Doxil	Myelosuppression, cardiotoxicity, GI enterotoxicity, alopecia, tissue necrosis, radiation recall reaction	++	Acute leukemia; sarcoma; Hodgkin's disease; neuroblastoma; bladder cancer; carcinoma of lung, GI tract, endometrium, ovary, thyroid, and breast; Wilms tumor; multiple myeloma
	Epirubicin	Ellence	Myelosuppression, cardiotoxicity, GI enterotoxicity, dermatotoxicity	++	Breast cancer
	Idarubicin	Idamycin	Myelosuppression, alopecia, cardiotoxicity, nausea and vomiting	+	Acute leukemia
	Mitomycin	Mutamycin	Myelosuppression, pulmonary toxicity, alopecia, tissue necrosis, GI enterotoxicity	+	Carcinoma of head, neck, lung, GI tract, breast, cervix, and bladder
	Mitoxantrone	Novantrone	Myelosuppression, hepatotoxicity, GI enterotoxicity, cardiotoxicity	+	Acute leukemia, chronic myelogenous leukemia, lymphoma, breast and ovarian cancer
Hormone Agonists and Antagonists					
Adrenal corticosteroids	Prednisone, prednisolone	Deltasone, Delta-Cortef	Peptic ulcer, hypokalemia, hyperglycemia, psychosis, osteoporosis, infections, fluid retention	0	Hodgkin's disease, lymphocytic leukemia, multiple myeloma, breast cancer, hypercalcemia
Androgens	Fluoxymesterone, testolactone	Halotestin, Teslac	Masculinization, edema, alopecia, acne, hypercalcemia	0	Metastatic breast cancer
Estrogens	Chlorotrianisene, diethylstilbestrol, ethinyl estradiol	TACE, Stilphostrol, Estinyl	Gynecomastia, breast tenderness, edema, thrombosis, depression	0	Postmenopausal carcinoma of breast, carcinoma of prostate
Progestins	Hydroxyprogesterone, medroxyprogesterone, megestrol	Delalutin, Depo-Provera, Megace	Edema, alopecia, hirsutism, genitourinary toxicity, neurotoxicity	0	Metastatic endometrial carcinoma, renal and breast carcinoma

Continued

TABLE 36-1 Classification of Available Antineoplastic and Associated Drugs—cont'd

Class or Type of Agent	Nonproprietary (Generic) Name	Proprietary (Trade) Name	Adverse Effects*	Stomatitis[†]	Clinical Applications
Adrenal suppressant	Aminoglutethimide	Cytadren	Hypotension, fever, myelosuppression, neurotoxicity, masculinization	0	Carcinoma of adrenal cortex and breast, Cushing syndrome
Aromatase inhibitors	Anastrozole, exemestane, letrozole	Arimidex, Aromasin, Femara	Nausea, vomiting, hot flashes, GI enterotoxicity, hepatotoxicity, hypertension	0	Advanced carcinoma of breast
Gonadotropin-releasing hormone analogues (agonists)	Goserelin, leuprolide	Zoladex, Lupron	Hot flashes, tumor flares, impotence, amenorrhea, vaginal bleeding, osteoporosis	0	Carcinoma of prostate and breast
Gonadotropin-releasing hormone analogues (antagonists)	Degarelix	Firmagon	Hot flashes, impotence, osteoporosis, hepatic injury, arthralgias	0	Carcinoma of prostate
Antiestrogen	Tamoxifen, toremifene	Nolvadex, Fareston	GI enterotoxicity, hot flashes, tumor flare, vaginal discharge, ocular toxicity	0	Postmenopausal carcinoma of breast, metastatic melanoma
	Raloxifene	Evista	Hot flashes, GI enterotoxicity	0	Breast cancer, osteoporosis
Antiandrogens	Bicalutamide	Casodex	Gynecomastia, nausea, hot flashes	0	Carcinoma of prostate
	Flutamide, nilutamide	Eulexin, Nilandron	Gynecomastia, nausea	0	Carcinoma of prostate
	Enzalutamide	Xtandi	Gynecomastia, hot flashes, seizures	0	Carcinoma of prostate
	Abiraterone	Zytiga	Diarrhea, hot flashes, arthralgias, hyperaldosteronism (fluid retention, hypertension, hypokalemia)	0	Carcinoma of prostate
Miscellaneous Classes					
Enzymes	L-asparaginase, PEG-L-asparaginase	Erwinaze, Oncaspar	Acute hypersensitivity, reaction, fever, hepatotoxicity, coagulation defects, GI enterotoxicity	0	Acute lymphocytic leukemia
Platinum complexes	Cisplatin	Platinol	Nephrotoxicity, ototoxicity, nausea and vomiting, GI enterotoxicity, neurotoxicity, acute allergic reactions	0	Carcinoma of testis, prostate, cervix, ovary, endometrium, lung, bladder, head and neck; sarcoma; neuroblastoma
	Carboplatin	Paraplatin	Myelosuppression, GI enterotoxicity, neurotoxicity	0	Testicular and ovarian carcinoma, head and neck cancers, lung cancer
	Oxaliplatin	Eloxatin	Pharyngolaryngeal dysesthesia, paresthesias, peripheral neuropathy, diarrhea, myelosuppression	0	Colorectal cancer
Other Drugs					
	Altretamine	Hexalen	GI enterotoxicity, neurotoxicity, myelosuppression	0	Ovarian cancer
	Arsenic trioxide	Trisenox	GI enterotoxicity, dermatotoxicity, cardiotoxicity, leukocytosis, retinoic acid syndrome	0	Acute promyelocytic leukemia
	Bexarotene	Targretin	Rash, headaches, hypothyroidism, photosensitivity, hypertriglyceridemia, hypercholesterolemia	0	Cutaneous T-cell lymphoma
	BCG, intravesical	TheraCys	Cystitis, flulike symptoms, infections	0	Superficial bladder cancer
	Hydroxyurea	Hydrea	Myelosuppression, alopecia, GI enterotoxicity, rare neurologic disturbances	+	Chronic myelogenous leukemia, sickle cell anemia, polycythemia vera
	Mitotane	Lysodren	GI enterotoxicity, neurotoxicity, hematuria, cystitis, dermatotoxicity, adrenal insufficiency	0	Carcinoma of adrenal cortex
	Porfimer	Photofrin	Photosensitivity, GI enterotoxicity, cardiotoxicity, anemia, fever	0	Endobronchial cancer, esophageal cancer
	Procarbazine	Matulane	GI enterotoxicity, myelosuppression, CNS depression, dermatotoxicity, disulfiram reactions	+	Hodgkin's disease, lymphoma, multiple myeloma
	Thalidomide	Thalomid	Neurotoxicity, dermatotoxicity, fever, GI enterotoxicity, tooth pain, dry mouth, tongue discoloration, taste changes, venous thromboembolism, teratogenicity	0/+	Melanoma, multiple myeloma, renal cell carcinoma, erythema nodosum leprosum
	Lenalidomide	Revlimid	Neuropathy, somnolence, constipation, myelosuppression, venous thromboembolism, teratogenicity	0	Multiple myeloma, myelodysplastic syndrome, mantle cell lymphoma

TABLE 36-1 **Classification of Available Antineoplastic and Associated Drugs—cont'd**

Class or Type of Agent	Nonproprietary (Generic) Name	Proprietary (Trade) Name	Adverse Effects*	Stomatitis[†]	Clinical Applications
Other Drugs—cont'd					
	Pomalidomide	Pomalyst	Neuropathy, somnolence, constipation, myelosuppression, venous thromboembolism, teratogenicity	0	Multiple myeloma
	Tretinoin	Vesanoid	Headache, xerosis, cheilitis, teratogenicity, arthralgia, myalgia, leukocytosis, retinoic acid syndrome	0	Acute promyelocytic leukemia
Natural Products					
	Paclitaxel	Taxol	Myelosuppression, alopecia, hypersensitivity reaction, neuropathy, bradycardia	0	Metastatic carcinoma of ovary and breast
	Docetaxel	Taxotere	Myelosuppression, hypersensitivity reaction, neurologic toxicity, fluid retention	0	Advanced breast carcinoma
	Ixabepilone	Ixempra	Myelosuppression, peripheral neuropathy, mucositis, and diarrhea	+	Breast cancer
	Etoposide	VePesid	Myelosuppression, nausea and vomiting, hypersensitivity reaction	0	Carcinoma of testis and lung, Hodgkin's disease, lymphoma, lung cancer, sarcoma
	Teniposide	Vumon	Myelosuppression, alopecia, neuropathy, nausea and vomiting	0	Acute lymphocytic leukemia, lymphoma, carcinoma of lung and breast
	Irinotecan	Camptosar	Diarrhea, myelosuppression, nausea and vomiting	0	Metastatic carcinoma of colon or rectum
	Topotecan	Hycamtin	Myelosuppression, nausea and vomiting, flulike symptoms	0	Metastatic carcinoma of ovary
DNA Demethylation Agents					
	Azacitidine	Vidaza	Myelosuppression, nausea and vomiting, diarrhea, and mucositis	+	Myelodysplastic syndrome
	Decitabine	Dacogen	Myelosuppression, nausea and vomiting, rash, headache, edema, hyperglycemia, hypokalemia, hypomagnesemia	0	Myelodysplastic syndrome
Biologic Response Modifiers					
	Interferon alfa-2a, interferon alfa-2b, interferon alfa-n3	Roferon-A, Intron-A, Alferon-N	Fever, myalgia, GI enterotoxicity, neurotoxicity, myelosuppression	0	Hairy cell leukemia, chronic myelogenous leukemia, Kaposi sarcoma, chronic hepatitis
	Aldesleukin (IL-2)	Proleukin	Fever, fluid retention, hypotension, respiratory distress, capillary leak syndrome, nephrotoxicity, rashes	0	Metastatic renal cell carcinoma
	Levamisole	Ergamisol	Flulike symptoms, nausea and vomiting	0	In combination with fluorouracil for colorectal cancer
Protectants					
	Amifostine	Ethyol	Hypotension, nausea and vomiting	0	Administered before cisplatin to reduce incidence of nephrotoxicity, before radiation therapy for head and neck cancer to reduce xerostomia
	Dexrazoxane	Zinecard	Abnormalities in liver and renal function test results, additive myelosuppression	0	In combination with doxorubicin therapy in breast carcinoma to reduce incidence of cardiomyopathy
	Filgrastim, sargramostim	Neupogen, Leukine	Fever, myalgia, bone pain, pericardial effusions	0	Prevent chemotherapy-induced neutropenia, increase neutrophil counts and prevent infections
	Leucovorin	Wellcovorin	Hypocalcemia	0	Methotrexate rescue, used with fluorouracil to increase activity of chemotherapy agent
	Oprelvekin	Neumega	Edema, dizziness, dyspnea, fatigue, arthralgia, myalgia, palpitations	0	Prevention of chemotherapy-induced thrombocytopenia

Continued

TABLE 36-1 Classification of Available Antineoplastic and Associated Drugs—cont'd

Class or Type of Agent	Nonproprietary (Generic) Name	Proprietary (Trade) Name	Adverse Effects*	Stomatitis†	Clinical Applications
Protectants—cont'd					
	Palifermin	Kepivance	Skin rash, tongue thickening	0	Prevent and reduce mucositis after high-dose chemotherapy
	Mesna	Mesnex	Nausea and vomiting	0	In combination with ifosfamide or cyclophosphamide to prevent hemorrhagic cystitis

*Myelosuppression includes a suppression of blood cell–forming elements resulting in leukopenia, thrombocytopenia, and anemia. GI enterotoxicity includes nausea, vomiting, diarrhea, and mucosal damage. Dermatotoxicity includes cutaneous toxicities such as pigmentation, rashes, erythema, and exfoliation. Neurotoxicity includes peripheral neuropathy, pain, paresthesias, altered sensorium, decrease in sensory and motor activity, and paralytic ileus. Hepatotoxicity includes liver dysfunction such as drug-induced hepatitis, transient elevation of transaminases, bile stasis, cholangitis, and veno-occlusive disease. Cardiotoxicity includes myocardial damage, congestive heart failure, and arrhythmias. Nephrotoxicity may manifest as renal insufficiency or acute renal tubular necrosis.
†Stomatitis: 0, rare; +, occasional; ++, frequent or common.
CNS, Central nervous system; *GI*, gastrointestinal; *SIADH*, syndrome of inappropriate antidiuretic hormone secretion.

Tetrazines

Temozolomide. Temozolomide is the first imidazotetrazinone derivative used in clinical practice. Similar to DTIC, temozolomide is metabolized to MTIC, which is ultimately converted to the cytotoxic methyldiazonium ion. Temozolomide has advantages over DTIC: it can be administered orally, and it does not require hepatic conversion to MTIC because temozolomide is spontaneously converted to the active metabolite at physiologic pH. Temozolomide penetrates tissues well and is able to cross the blood–brain barrier, allowing it to be used to treat brain tumors such as astrocytoma and glioblastoma multiforme, an aggressive primary brain tumor. Temozolomide has also been used to treat malignant melanoma. The major toxic effects associated with this alkylating agent include myelosuppression, nausea, vomiting, headache, and fatigue.

Nitrosoureas

Carmustine and lomustine. Two nitrosoureas, carmustine and lomustine, decompose in the body to yield reactive intermediates that act as classic alkylating agents, causing strand breaks and cross-links in DNA. They also produce isocyanates that inhibit DNA repair and RNA synthesis. Carmustine is administered intravenously, whereas lomustine is given orally. Both are rapidly metabolized and slowly excreted in the urine. Nitrosoureas are characterized by their lipophilicity and their ability to cross the blood–brain barrier. This property is useful in the treatment of brain tumors. Each typically produces a delayed bone marrow suppression that becomes apparent in 3 to 6 weeks and lasts for an additional 2 to 3 weeks. Other common side effects include nausea and vomiting in most patients within 2 to 6 hours after administration.

Streptozocin. Streptozocin is a naturally occurring anticancer antibiotic that has a mechanism of action similar to that of nitrosoureas. Unlike carmustine and lomustine, streptozocin does not readily cross the blood–brain barrier, and it is not strongly myelosuppressive. Streptozocin is unique in its special affinity for the islet cells of the pancreas. The drug is diabetogenic in animals and effective against metastatic insulinomas in humans. Streptozocin should be administered intravenously with care because it is a vesicant. It is one of the most emetogenic agents and requires adequate premedication with antiemetics. Potentially fatal renal toxicity and hepatotoxicity have occurred.

Antimetabolite Agents

Antimetabolites bear a marked structural resemblance to folic acid and to the purine and pyrimidine bases involved in the synthesis of DNA, RNA, and certain coenzymes. They differ in molecular arrangement from the corresponding metabolite to a degree sufficient to **serve as fraudulent substrates for biochemical reactions**, either inhibiting synthetic steps or becoming incorporated into molecules and interfering with cellular function or replication. Antimetabolites characteristically **exert their major effects during the S phase** (DNA synthesis phase) of the cell cycle. This activity interferes with the growth of rapidly proliferating cells throughout the body: the bone marrow, germinal cells, hair follicles, and lining of the gastrointestinal tract. **Oral mucosa toxicity is an especially prominent feature of these agents.** Three classes of antimetabolites exist: folic acid analogues, purine analogues, and pyrimidine analogues.

Folic acid analogues

Folic acid is an essential vitamin that is converted into metabolically active tetrahydrofolic acid by the enzyme dihydrofolate reductase. Tetrahydrofolic acid participates in the synthesis of purines, thymidylate, and ultimately nucleic acids by transferring methyl groups to nucleotide precursors.

Methotrexate. Methotrexate is the 4-amino, 10-methyl analogue of folic acid and a potent inhibitor of dihydrofolate reductase. This inhibition results in the decreased conversion of dihydrofolate to tetrahydrofolate and impaired synthesis of thymidylic acid and inosinic acid. Deficiencies of these acids retard DNA and RNA synthesis. Protein synthesis is also inhibited because reduced folates are cofactors in the conversion of glycine to serine and homocysteine to methionine.

Methotrexate is readily absorbed from the gastrointestinal tract and is primarily excreted in the urine. There is some enterohepatic recycling of methotrexate, which extends the elimination half-life of the drug and is responsible for most of the marrow and gastrointestinal toxicity. Methotrexate is very hydrophilic and tends to distribute into "third space" fluid accumulations such as ascitic, pleural, or peritoneal fluids that can potentially act as a drug reservoir. The presence of these clinical features or renal failure or both contributes to increased toxicity.

Depending on the indication, methotrexate may be administered by many different routes with a variable dosing range. Administered orally, the drug is often used to treat rheumatoid arthritis and psoriasis. Intrathecal administration is used to treat central nervous system (CNS) tumors, and intraarterial administration is used for regional therapy of head and neck cancers. Given intravenously and intramuscularly, methotrexate is a valuable therapeutic agent in some forms of leukemia, choriocarcinoma, lymphoma, sarcoma, testicular tumors, and carcinoma of the breast and lung. The drug is also used in very high doses for adjuvant and salvage therapies for osteosarcoma, leukemia, and CNS lymphoma. High-dose therapy with methotrexate requires monitoring of serum blood concentrations and the use of **folinic acid "rescue."** The folinic acid (e.g., citrovorum factor, calcium folinate, leucovorin) bypasses the blockade of dihydrofolate reductase in normal cells and may reduce the incidence and severity of mucositis and myelosuppression. Other non-tumoricidal applications of methotrexate include its use after allogeneic bone marrow transplants to prevent graft-versus-host disease, to treat systemic lupus erythematosus, and in steroid-dependent asthmatic patients to decrease asthmatic symptoms.

Methotrexate is subject to many important drug interactions. Highly plasma protein-bound drugs such as salicylates, sulfonamides, and phenytoin may displace methotrexate from its protein-binding sites and result in greater toxicity. Organic acids such as salicylate and probenecid inhibit the renal tubular secretion of methotrexate, resulting in delayed drug clearance and toxicity. Penicillins can also compete with methotrexate for renal tubular secretion. In patients receiving high-dose methotrexate, the concurrent use of nonsteroidal antiinflammatory drugs (NSAIDs) should be avoided because this drug class can also reduce renal blood flow and increase the risk of nephrotoxicity. While the exact mechanism of the interaction is unknown, proton pump inhibitors (PPIs) have also been shown to delay methotrexate clearance.

Dose-limiting toxic effects of methotrexate include bone marrow depression manifested by leukopenia and thrombocytopenia; a very painful stomatitis with mucosal and epithelial ulceration; pharyngitis and dysphagia; esophagitis; gastroenterocolitis; and proctitis with associated watery and bloody diarrhea. Large doses can be nephrotoxic, and long-term treatment with methotrexate can lead to changes in hepatic function.

Pemetrexed disodium. Pemetrexed disodium is an antifolate that attacks multiple enzyme targets, including dihydrofolate reductase, thymidylate synthase, and glycinamide ribonucleotide formyl transferase. By inhibiting the formation of precursor purine and pyrimidine nucleotides, pemetrexed prevents the formation of DNA and RNA required for the growth and survival of normal cells and cancer cells. Pemetrexed is approved for treatment of malignant pleural mesothelioma and non-squamous histologic subtypes of non-small cell lung cancer (NSCLC). Vitamin supplementation with folic acid (1 mg daily) and vitamin B_{12} (1000 µg intramuscularly every 9 weeks) is required to minimize the hematologic toxicity as well as the risk of stomatitis with this agent. Steroid treatment with dexamethasone (4 mg twice a day on the day before, the day of, and the day after pemetrexed therapy) is used to help limit skin rashes. The most common side effects are hematologic, rash, nausea, and vomiting. Occasionally, chest pain, edema, and hypertension may be seen in patients, and neuropathy and myalgias occur in 29% and 13% of patients, respectively. Stomatitis has been reported in nearly 20% of patients treated with pemetrexed.

Pralatrexate. Pralatrexate is the newest antifolate to be developed and is approved for the treatment of peripheral T-cell lymphoma. It was designed to have increased affinity for reduced folate carrier 1 as well as folylpolyglutamate synthetase, resulting in increased intracellular transport and cytotoxic metabolites, respectively. Pralatrexate also has increased affinity for other enzymes involved in folate metabolism compared to methotrexate. As with pemetrexed, vitamin supplementation with folic acid (1 mg daily) and vitamin B12 (1 mg injection every 8 to 10 weeks) is recommended to limit myelosuppression and mucositis. The most common side effects of pralatrexate are mucositis, myelosuppression, rash, diarrhea, and fatigue.

Purine analogues

Mercaptopurine and thioguanine. The mechanism of action of the thiopurines, mercaptopurine and thioguanine, have not yet been fully established. Presumably, they affect the incorporation of purine derivatives into nucleic acids. The analogues are converted in the body to the ribonucleotide form, which interferes with the conversion of inosinic acid into the nucleotides adenine and guanine and ultimately result in the inhibition of DNA and RNA synthesis. They also inhibit de novo biosynthesis of purines from the small molecule precursors (glycine, formate, and phosphate) leading to fraudulent DNA production.

Orally administered mercaptopurine is readily absorbed but undergoes extensive first-pass metabolism by the liver. After intravenous injection, the plasma half-life is approximately 90 minutes. The drug is metabolized by methylation in the liver and by the hepatic enzyme xanthine oxidase. Concurrent administration with allopurinol, a xanthine oxidase inhibitor originally developed to increase the anticancer effect of mercaptopurine, requires a 50% reduction in the dose of mercaptopurine. Allopurinol is of little clinical value in this setting because it also increases the toxicity of mercaptopurine. Currently, mercaptopurine is used mainly for maintenance of remission in acute lymphocytic leukemia. The chief toxic effect is myelosuppression. Pulmonary fibrosis, hepatitis, and pancreatitis may rarely occur. Thioguanine has activity, toxicity, and clinical applications similar to those of mercaptopurine.

Fludarabine. Fludarabine (2-fluoro-ara-AMP) is an analogue of adenosine. This injectable purine antagonist is quickly dephosphorylated in the plasma, enters the cell, and is converted to the triphosphate form. This false nucleotide inhibits ribonucleotide reductase and DNA polymerase, resulting in the inhibition of DNA synthesis. Fludarabine is indicated for the treatment of B-cell chronic lymphocytic leukemia in patients who have not responded to traditional therapy with an alkylating agent. It has also been used for treatment of non-Hodgkin's lymphoma, hairy cell leukemia, cutaneous T-cell lymphoma, and acute myeloid leukemia. Fludarabine is primarily excreted by the kidneys and has a long plasma half-life of approximately 10 hours. Transient myelosuppression and immunosuppression, with an increased risk of opportunistic infections, seem to be the major toxicity at current doses. With high doses, irreversible neurotoxicity (confusion, seizures, and blindness) may occur weeks to months after treatment.

Pentostatin. Pentostatin is an antimetabolite isolated from *Streptomyces antibioticus*. This purine analogue is an inhibitor of adenosine deaminase, which converts adenosine to inosine. This inhibition apparently leads to inhibition of methylation and other reactions. Cytotoxic treatment with pentostatin results in the accumulation of deoxyadenosine 5′-triphosphate, reducing purine metabolism and inhibiting DNA synthesis. The drug exhibits activity in nonreplicating and dividing cells. Pentostatin is quickly distributed to all body tissues after administration; the plasma half-life is 2.6 to 9.4 hours, with the majority of the drug recovered in the urine unchanged. Pentostatin has been most active in the treatment of hairy cell leukemia; it also has activity in patients with chronic lymphocytic leukemia. Toxicity is dose-dependent, with acute renal failure and CNS side effects being the most severe.

Cladribine. Cladribine is an adenosine deaminase–resistant purine substrate analogue toxic to lymphocytes and monocytes. It is most often used in the treatment of hairy cell leukemia and acute myeloid leukemia. The major dose-limiting toxicity is myelosuppression.

Clofarabine and nelarabine. Clofarabine and nelarabine are purine nucleoside antimetabolites approved for the treatment of acute lymphocytic leukemias. Clofarabine is converted intracellularly by deoxycytidine kinase to the 5′-monophosphate metabolite, then via monophosphokinases and diphosphokinases to the active 5′-triphosphate form. The clofarabine 5′-triphosphate inhibits DNA synthesis through its action on ribonucleotide reductase and DNA polymerases. Clofarabine is approved for the treatment of pediatric patients with relapsed or refractory acute lymphocytic leukemia after at least two prior treatment regimens. It is also being studied for other malignancies, including the treatment of acute myeloid leukemias in adults. The principal toxicities associated with clofarabine are nausea, vomiting, hematologic toxicity, febrile neutropenia, hepatobiliary toxicity, infections, and renal toxicity. Clofarabine can also produce a syndrome manifested by the rapid development of tachypnea, tachycardia, hypotension, shock, and multiorgan failure called systemic inflammatory response syndrome, which is similar to a capillary leak syndrome. Cardiac effects include tachycardia and left ventricular systolic dysfunction.

Nelarabine is a prodrug of the deoxyguanosine analogue 9-beta-D-arabinofuranosylguanine (ara-G). Nelarabine is demethylated to ara-G and activated to the active 5′-triphosphate, ara-GTP. The active ara-G is incorporated into the DNA resulting in inhibition of DNA synthesis and cell death. There is a preferential accumulation in T-cells, and nelarabine is approved for the treatment of patients with T-cell acute lymphoblastic leukemia and lymphoma who have not responded to or have relapsed after treatment with at least two other chemotherapy regimens. A major adverse effect associated with nelarabine resulting in a "black box" warning involves neurologic events that include severe somnolence, convulsions, peripheral neuropathies, and paralysis. Other adverse effects include fatigue, bone marrow suppression, gastrointestinal side effects, and some pulmonary complaints of cough and dyspnea. Rarely, patients have experienced blurred vision while receiving nelarabine. The combination of nelarabine and adenosine deaminase inhibitors, such as pentostatin, should be avoided because this combination may result in a decreased conversion of nelarabine to its active substrate, decreasing its efficacy and potentially changing the adverse effect profile of both drugs.

Pyrimidine analogues

Fluorouracil and floxuridine. The fluorinated pyrimidines fluorouracil and floxuridine are converted intracellularly to 5-fluoro-2′-deoxyuridine monophosphate (FDUMP). FDUMP is a potent antimetabolite that binds to and inhibits thymidylate synthetase, inhibiting formation of thymidylic acid and impairing DNA synthesis. 5-flurodeoxyuridine triphosphate (F-dUTP) may also be incorporated into DNA, producing single-strand breaks and contributing to its cytotoxicity. Fluorouracil metabolism also produces a critical intermediate, 5-fluoroxyuridine monophosphate (5-UMP), which is subsequently tri-phosphorylated and incorporated into RNA, interfering with its cellular functions.

Fluorouracil is used most often for treatment of gastrointestinal adenocarcinomas, breast cancer, and ovarian cancer. Activity has also been reported in bladder and prostate cancer. The drug is usually given intravenously as a bolus injection or as a prolonged continuous infusion for days to weeks. Continuous infusion is advantageous because the plasma half-life of the drug is short (10 to 20 minutes), and the drug (similar to other antimetabolites) works primarily in the S phase of the cell cycle. Continuous infusion provides for prolonged exposure of tumor cells to the drug and the opportunity for cell populations not in the S phase to cycle into that sensitive phase. The toxicity profile of fluorouracil depends on the method of administration. Given as a continuous infusion over a 96-hour period, the dose-limiting toxicity is mucositis, whereas intravenous bolus results in more bone marrow suppression. Notably, many common chemotherapy regimens utilize both bolus and continuous infusion fluorouracil so patients often experience both types of toxicity. Patients that are deficient in the enzyme dihydropyrimidine dehydrogenase experience more severe toxicity, specifically diarrhea and neutropenia. Fluorouracil can be administered topically to treat actinic keratoses and noninvasive skin cancers. In addition, it can be used to improve efficacy of radiation therapy in head and neck cancers by working as a radiosensitizer. Folinic acid (leucovorin) has been combined with fluorouracil to enhance the inhibition of thymidylate synthetase leading to increased efficacy and toxicity.

Floxuridine, the deoxyribonucleoside of fluorouracil, exerts a more direct inhibition of thymidylate synthetase than fluorouracil. The drug must be given by continuous infusion because it is rapidly catabolized in vivo. Floxuridine administered intraarterially is indicated for gastrointestinal adenocarcinomas that have metastasized to the liver and has produced beneficial results in the treatment of head and neck carcinoma, although fluorouracil is now the preferred agent in this setting. The adverse effects of fluorinated pyrimidines may be quite severe. Stomatitis, pharyngitis, dysphagia, enteritis, and diarrhea can be life-threatening. Myocardial ischemia caused by coronary artery vasospasm has been described with fluorouracil.

Capecitabine. Capecitabine (5′-deoxy-5-fluoro-N-[(pentyloxy)carbonyl]-cytidine) is an oral prodrug of 5-fluorouracil used in the treatment of advanced breast and various gastrointestinal cancers. Capecitabine is hydrolyzed in the liver and ultimately converted to the active drug 5-fluorouracil. Its spectrum of activity and pharmacokinetic profile are similar to infusional fluorouracil. Side effects of capecitabine include severe diarrhea, stomatitis, and some mild nausea and vomiting. Severe hand-foot syndrome (palmar/plantar erythrodysesthesia) and other dermatologic changes have been reported.

Cytarabine. Cytarabine (cytosine arabinoside) is an analogue of 2′-deoxycytidine that inhibits DNA polymerase activity after being incorporated into DNA as a fraudulent nucleotide, resulting in impaired DNA synthesis. Cytarabine is primarily a cell cycle S phase–specific agent. When given intravenously, the drug is rapidly cleared from the blood by deamination in the liver, with a plasma half-life of 5 to 20 minutes. With these properties, continuous infusion is often the preferred route of administration. Cytarabine crosses the blood–brain barrier, achieving cerebrospinal fluid concentrations of 40% to 50% of those in the plasma. This feature allows for the treatment of CNS disease with systemic high-dose therapy. Cytarabine may be administered intrathecally and produces high concentrations that decline slowly because of the absence of cytidine deaminase in the CNS. Cytarabine is the most active single drug available for the treatment of acute myelogenous leukemia in adults, producing about a 25% incidence of complete remission if given as monotherapy. It is often used in combination with other agents for synergistic activity. It also exhibits modest activity against lymphomas. The major side effect is myelosuppression. High doses produce nausea and vomiting, mucositis, diarrhea, cerebellar toxicity, and keratoconjunctivitis.

Gemcitabine. Gemcitabine (difluorodeoxycytidine) is a cytosine analogue that is useful in many types of solid tumors, and it is indicated for use in advanced stages of breast, pancreatic, ovarian, and non-small cell lung cancer. Gemcitabine's dose-limiting side effect is myelosuppression, predominately thrombocytopenia. Transient febrile reactions and a flulike syndrome have been commonly reported, along with rare cases of pulmonary toxicity.

Antitumor Antibiotics

Numerous substances originally isolated as **antibiotics have been found to exert antineoplastic activity** because of their cytotoxic properties. These substances, produced naturally by various *Streptomyces* species, operate in part by binding with DNA to produce irreversible complexes that inhibit cell division. Various other possible mechanisms for cytotoxicity have been proposed for these agents. **Antitumor antibiotics can damage cells in different phases of the cell cycle**, behaving as non-phase-specific agents. Semisynthetic derivatives and liposomal encapsulation of some of these compounds have been developed in an effort to reduce toxicity but retain the cytotoxic potency of the parent compound.

Dactinomycin

Dactinomycin (actinomycin D) is a crystalline antibiotic composed of a phenoxazone chromophore and two cyclic peptide chains obtained as a product of fermentation by *Streptomyces parvulus*. The drug intercalates into DNA between adjacent guanine–cytosine base pairs and inhibits DNA-directed RNA synthesis. Dactinomycin is rapidly distributed into tissues and has a prolonged terminal half-life. The drug apparently is not metabolized, but it is primarily excreted in the bile. Dactinomycin is the most commonly used for the treatment of pediatric tumors, such as Wilms tumor, Ewing sarcoma, and embryonal rhabdomyosarcoma, and it is of considerable value in treatment of choriocarcinoma and testicular tumors. This agent is highly emetogenic, and mucositis is the dose-limiting toxicity. Extravasation from the vein causes severe tissue necrosis.

Anthracyclines

Anthracyclines are antitumor antibiotics initially developed from compounds produced by *Streptomyces*. This class includes daunorubicin, doxorubicin, idarubicin, and epirubicin as well as liposomal formulations of daunorubicin and doxorubicin. These agents exert their cytotoxic effects through several proposed mechanisms. First, the planar structure of the molecule allows for intercalation between DNA base pairs, thereby disrupting DNA and RNA synthesis. These agents also act as topoisomerase II inhibitors, resulting in double-strand DNA breaks during DNA replication. Finally, oxygen free radical generation is believed to be responsible for some of the toxicity of anthracyclines.

Anthracyclines are associated with myelosuppression, mucositis, radiation recall, red/orange discoloration of urine, and tissue necrosis if there is extravasation during administration. The cardiotoxicity that can be seen with these agents is believed to be due to free radical generation and presents either as acute arrhythmias or more commonly as a delayed cardiomyopathy. The risk of developing cardiomyopathy increases dramatically after exceeding a given lifetime dose of anthracyclines (i.e., 400 mg/m^2 in the case of doxorubicin).

Daunorubicin. Daunorubicin is a cytotoxic anthracycline antibiotic produced by *Streptomyces peucetius* subsp. *caesius*, which is also the source of doxorubicin and idarubicin. Daunorubicin is most useful in the treatment of acute myelogenous leukemia and acute lymphocytic leukemia. The drug is extensively tissue bound with a long elimination half-life. The major route of elimination is through biliary excretion, with some urinary excretion.

Doxorubicin. Doxorubicin differs from daunorubicin by one hydroxy group. Doxorubicin is commonly used in a broad range of malignancies including but not limited to leukemia, lymphomas, breast cancer, and sarcoma. Doxorubicin is rapidly cleared from the plasma and concentrates in the tissues. Urinary excretion is low, rarely accounting for more than 10% of the administered dose; in contrast, biliary excretion is high. As plasma concentrations of doxorubicin and its metabolites are markedly elevated, and the rate of elimination is greatly prolonged in the presence of severely impaired liver function, dose reduction should be considered in patients with hepatic impairment.

Liposomal encapsulated forms of doxorubicin and daunorubicin are now available. They allow for increased plasma circulation time and the possibility of enhanced antitumor activity and decreased cardiomyopathy. They also differ from conventional formulations in respect to indications and are used in Kaposi sarcoma related to acquired immunodeficiency syndrome (AIDS), advanced breast and ovarian cancer, and multiple myeloma.

Epirubicin. Epirubicin is a semisynthetic derivative of doxorubicin that is approved for use in patients with breast cancer and demonstrates activity in gastric and esophageal malignancies as well as soft tissue sarcomas. Epirubicin has also been evaluated for its intravesical use in superficial bladder cancer. Epirubicin is metabolized in the liver but also undergoes extrahepatic metabolism. Most of epirubicin's metabolites are eliminated through the biliary system, but up to 20% to 30% are eliminated in the urine.

Idarubicin. Idarubicin is an analogue of daunorubicin lacking the methoxy group on the C4 position of the aglycone. This drug is used for the treatment of acute myelogenous leukemia and some types of lymphoma.

Anthracenedione

Mitoxantrone. Mitoxantrone, an anthraquinone antibiotic, is a synthetic drug with antibacterial, antiviral, antiprotozoal, and immunomodulating properties. Its antineoplastic activity results from intercalation to DNA and inhibition of topoisomerase II, producing DNA strand breaks. Unlike anthracyclines, mitoxantrone has a much lower potential for free radical generation, resulting in a lower risk of cardiotoxicity. It is clinically active against prostate cancer that is resistant to hormonal therapies, acute leukemias, lymphomas, as well as relapsing-remitting multiple sclerosis. The drug can impart a blue-green color to the urine for up to 24 hours after administration; bluish discoloration of the sclera may also occur.

Bleomycin

Bleomycin is an antibiotic complex of several glycopeptides derived from *Streptomyces verticillus*. The cytotoxic action of bleomycin has been attributed to DNA scission and fragmentation with inhibition of usual DNA repair mechanisms. RNA and protein synthesis seem to be inhibited as well. Bleomycin is rapidly cleared from the blood and concentrated in the liver, lungs, spleen, kidneys, and epithelial tissue. Approximately 80% is excreted in the urine within 24 hours. Bleomycin is cell phase specific, having its major effects on cells in the G_2 and M phases of the cell cycle.

The main clinical applications of bleomycin are in the treatment of squamous cell carcinoma of the head and neck, testicular tumors, and Hodgkin's lymphoma. Bleomycin is also used to treat malignant pleural effusions by direct instillation into the pleural space. The major attractive features of bleomycin include minimal nausea and vomiting, almost no myelosuppression, and lack of local tissue toxicities. This favorable toxicity profile accounts for the inclusion of bleomycin into many combination chemotherapy protocols. The major dose-limiting toxicity is pulmonary, manifesting as interstitial pneumonitis that might progress to pulmonary fibrosis and fatal pulmonary insufficiency. This toxicity is associated with a cumulative lifetime dose of more than 400 units, age older than 70 years, underlying pulmonary disease, chest irradiation, and high supplemental oxygen exposure. Some reports suggest an increase in oxygen-induced pulmonary complications in patients previously treated with bleomycin. For anesthesia and postoperative periods, it is recommended that elevated inspired oxygen concentrations should be administered only when clearly indicated.

Mitomycin

Mitomycin is derived from *Streptomyces caespitosus*. After intracellular activation, mitomycin inhibits DNA synthesis by reacting with

DNA in the manner of the alkylating agents. When combined with fluorouracil or nitrosoureas, mitomycin has been effective against gastrointestinal, head and neck, breast, cervix, and lung carcinomas. Mitomycin is also commonly used in bladder cancer as an intravesicular instillation. When given intravenously, severe toxicity to the bone marrow (neutropenia and thrombocytopenia), reaching a maximum in about 3 to 4 weeks, and to the gastrointestinal tract (nausea, vomiting, oral ulceration, and diarrhea) are the dose-limiting toxicities. Pulmonary toxicity and hemolytic uremic syndrome are also dose related. Intravesicular use may cause dysuria, bladder spasms, suprapubic pain, mild hematuria, and rarely has been associated with bladder fibrosis or contracture.

Vinca Alkaloids

Vinblastine, vincristine, and vinorelbine

Vinblastine and vincristine, the two older alkaloids in clinical use, are derived from asymmetric dimeric compounds extracted from the shrub *Vinca rosea*. Vinorelbine, a second-generation vinca alkaloid, is a semisynthetic derivative of vinblastine. The antineoplastic activity of vinca alkaloids has been attributed to their capacity to **arrest cell division in metaphase by binding to the microtubule protein, tubulin, that forms the mitotic spindle.**

These drugs are metabolized in the liver and excreted mainly by the biliary and intestinal tracts. Vinblastine and vincristine are of major value in treating ALL, Hodgkin's lymphoma, and other lymphomas. Vinorelbine is used in the treatment of NSCLC, breast, cervical, and ovarian cancers. The toxicity profile of the various vinca alkaloids differs despite their similar structure. The dose-limiting toxicity of vincristine is neurotoxicity manifesting as peripheral sensory and autonomic neuropathy, including constipation, ileus, paresthesias, neuropathic pain, and it may progress to loss of deep tendon reflexes. Vinorelbine and vinblastine primarily cause neutropenia (platelets and red blood cells are relatively spared) with much less neurotoxicity than vincristine. Vinblastine is associated with more mucositis than the other agents. All vinca alkaloids are associated with alopecia and are potent vesicants, and extravasation requires immediate attention. Vinca alkaloids must never be given intrathecally; doing so results in an ascending paralysis that is universally fatal.

In 2012, a liposomal formulation of vincristine was approved for treatment of relapsed ALL in patients who do not have a Philadelphia chromosome mutation. The liposomal encapsulation increases the duration of therapeutic levels of vincristine in the body and may be associated with less severe neurotoxicity compared to traditional vincristine. This allows higher doses to be utilized.

Hormone Agonists and Antagonists

The role of hormonal manipulation for cancer therapy was initially explored in 1896, when ovariectomy was first used in the treatment of breast cancer. Because they share commonality of their steroid ring structure, adrenocorticosteroids, estrogens, antiestrogens, androgens, progesterones, and gonadotropin-releasing factors each have a role in therapy for certain cancers.

Glucocorticoids

Glucocorticoids are widely **used in combination with other antineoplastic drugs** in the treatment of acute and chronic lymphocytic leukemia, lymphomas, and multiple myeloma. They are also useful for various types of **supportive care needs of patients** with cancer, such as reducing hypercalcemia associated with bony metastases, management of spinal cord compression, antiemetic therapy, and pain management. Dexamethasone, prednisone, and methylprednisolone are the most commonly utilized glucocorticoids for these various oncologic indications, varying in their potency, biologic half-life, and mineralocorticoid activity. Short-term use of these agents is commonly associated with insomnia, gastritis or indigestion, and elevated blood glucose. Prolonged use, as is seen with treatment of many of the aforementioned oncologic indications, can be associated with skin thinning, a Cushingoid appearance, hypertension, osteoporosis, immune suppression, and rarely avascular necrosis.

Drugs affecting sex hormone status

Sex hormones, tamoxifen, and toremifene. Estrogens are useful in the treatment of advanced prostatic carcinoma and as adjunctive treatment in select patients with postmenopausal breast carcinoma. Although the mode of action is unknown, the therapeutic response in breast cancer is correlated with the presence of estrogen-binding receptor sites within the tumor. The **selective estrogen receptor modulator**, tamoxifen, is beneficial in patients whose adenocarcinoma of the breast depends on circulating hormones for growth, indicated by positive estrogen or progesterone receptor status. Tamoxifen has also been used in endometrial carcinoma and ovarian cancer. The side effects seen with this oral agent include an initial flare in disease activity, bone pain, or hypercalcemia; this is associated with efficacy of the medication. Additional side effects include hot flashes, sweating, nausea and vomiting, and increased risk for thromboembolism. Tamoxifen is metabolized by the cytochrome P450 enzyme system within the liver, resulting in its conversion to more potent metabolites. Many selective serotonin reuptake inhibitor (SSRI) antidepressants have been shown to inhibit this hepatic metabolism, leading to reduced efficacy of tamoxifen. Toremifene is a chlorinated derivative of tamoxifen shown to possess similar efficacy and tolerability as tamoxifen. Toremifene's main advantage is that its metabolism is not affected by SSRIs and may be safely combined with these agents. Androgens are effective in some cases of metastatic breast cancer. Progesterone agents such as megestrol are effective in metastatic endometrial, breast, and renal cell carcinoma.

Anastrozole, letrozole, and exemestane. Anastrozole and letrozole are **nonsteroidal, reversible inhibitors of the aromatase enzyme and prevent the conversion of androgens to estrogens** (Fig. 36-3). Exemestane differs in that its structure is steroidal in nature, and it irreversibly inhibits the aromatase enzyme. These agents are indicated for first- and second-line hormonal therapy in postmenopausal women with hormone receptor–positive breast cancer. Randomized clinical trials comparing 5 years of each of the aromatase inhibitors with 5 years of tamoxifen have demonstrated superior survival rates in postmenopausal women receiving the aromatase inhibitor. Recent randomized trials have also demonstrated additional survival benefits in women who receive 5 years of therapy with an aromatase inhibitor following an initial 5 years of tamoxifen therapy.

Aromatase inhibitors are generally well tolerated. Common adverse effects include nausea, vomiting, arthralgias/myalgias, and hot flashes. There are high rates of osteopenia/osteoporosis in women receiving aromatase inhibitors (as well as those receiving tamoxifen therapy). As a result, women prescribed these therapies require calcium and vitamin D supplementation, and some may be receiving bisphosphonate therapy for prevention/treatment of osteoporosis.

Leuprolide and goserelin. Leuprolide (a nonapeptide) and goserelin (a decapeptide) are synthetic analogues of naturally occurring gonadotropin-releasing hormone (GnRH). They have **potent GnRH-agonist properties during short-term or pulsatile therapy**, but they paradoxically **inhibit gonadotropin secretion and suppress ovarian and testicular steroidogenesis during long-term administration by inducing a negative feedback loop** with the pituitary gland. Because

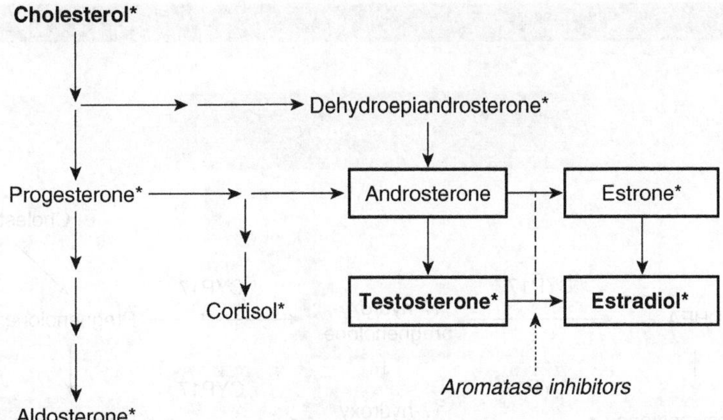

FIG 36-3 Aromatase inhibitor site of activity in the steroidogenic pathway. Aromatase inhibition prevents biologic conversion of androstenedione to estrone and testosterone to estradiol. *Biologically active hormones.

of these inhibitory effects, these agents interfere with the growth of hormone-dependent tumors. GnRH agonists are used clinically for the palliative treatment of advanced carcinoma of the prostate and are valuable in the control of breast cancer. The initial surge of hormone release caused by these agents can induce pain at the site of the tumor or hypercalcemia, which is known as "tumor flare." More common side effects include hot flashes, erectile dysfunction, and gynecomastia. Long-term use can cause osteoporosis and metabolic changes (hypercholesterolemia and hyperglycemia).

Degarelix. Degarelix is a subcutaneous GnRH antagonist approved for treatment of advanced stages of prostate cancer. The main difference between degarelix and the GnRH agonists is that the antagonistic property of degarelix on the pituitary gland does not induce the initial surge of luteinizing hormone and follicle stimulation hormone seen with the GnRH agonists. Side effects of degarelix are similar to those of leuprolide and goserelin only without the risk of "tumor flare."

Abiraterone. Abiraterone is a selective inhibitor of 17 alpha-hydroxylase/C17,20-lyase (CYP17), an enzyme produced by the testes, adrenal glands, as well as prostate cancer cells. Inhibition of CYP17 prevents conversion of cholesterol into testosterone and other androgens within these tissues, shrinking hormone-sensitive prostate cancer cells. Common side effects of abiraterone include fatigue, diarrhea, arthralgias, and hot flashes. As a consequence of abiraterone's effects on the enzymatic conversion of cholesterol (Fig. 36-4), patients may also experience side effects of hyperaldosteronism (hypertension, hypokalemia, and fluid retention). Alternatively, abiraterone reduces levels of circulating cortisol, mandating concomitant administration of prednisone to prevent symptoms of adrenocortical insufficiency.

Flutamide, bicalutamide, nilutamide, and enzalutamide. Flutamide is a nonsteroidal antiandrogen that competes directly for testosterone receptor binding sites in prostate cells. This agent is indicated for prostate cancer when used in combination with a GnRH agonist, and it can help prevent the "tumor flare" phenomenon associated with the GnRH agonists. Adverse reactions include diarrhea, hot flashes, gynecomastia, and decreased libido. Bicalutamide and nilutamide are nonsteroidal antiandrogen agents similar to flutamide and are also used in combination with a GnRH agonist or orchiectomy for advanced prostate cancer. Nilutamide has rarely caused interstitial pneumonitis and affects the eyes' ability to adjust to changes from light to dark conditions, such as driving from daylight into a dark tunnel. Enzalutamide is a second-generation antiandrogen that, unlike the other agents in this class, exhibits no agonistic properties at the androgen receptor. It is similarly used in conjunction with a GnRH agonist to treat castration-resistant prostate cancer. Side effects of enzalutamide are largely the same as with first-generation antiandrogens with the additional risk of seizures.

Enzymes

Asparaginase

Asparaginase is an enzyme that catalyzes the hydrolysis of L-asparagine to L-aspartic acid and ammonia. Asparaginase products are isolated from different types of bacteria, namely *Escherichia coli* and *Erwinia chrysanthemi*. They **inhibit protein synthesis in tumor cells** by depriving them of the amino acid asparagine. This drug is phase specific, with the greatest activity in the G_1 phase of the cell cycle. Clinical use is confined presently to acute lymphocytic leukemia. Asparaginase products may produce acute hypersensitivity reactions with hypotension, sweating, bronchospasm, and urticaria. Other effects in patients taking L-asparaginase include the possibility of hepatitis, pancreatitis, and altered production of coagulation factors resulting in either increased bleeding or increased clotting risk. A second formulation of asparaginase is pegaspargase (PEG-L-asparaginase), which has polyethylene glycol covalently linked to the asparaginase structure to decrease immunogenicity and to prolong its half-life.

Platinum Agents

Cisplatin

Cisplatin (*cis*-diamminedichloroplatinum or CDDP) is a heavy metal complex containing a central atom of platinum surrounded by two chloride ions and two amino groups in the *cis* position. The compound has biochemical properties similar to bifunctional alkylating agents in that it produces **interstrand and intrastrand cross-links in DNA, inhibiting its synthesis and causing DNA strand breaks.** Cisplatin is not a cell cycle phase–specific agent. The drug is most effective in the treatment of carcinoma of the testis and ovary, transitional cell bladder neoplasia, small cell and non-small cell lung cancer, and head and neck cancers. It is also used as a radiosensitizer when given concurrently with radiation therapy.

After intravenous injection, cisplatin is excreted primarily in the urine. Severe emesis is the dose-limiting toxicity; however, newer antiemetic agents usually allow for the completion of therapy. Nephrotoxicity, presenting as renal tubular necrosis, is another major dose-limiting side effect that requires normal saline hydration to minimize its incidence. The agent can be ototoxic, causing initially high-frequency and later complete hearing loss, and long-term use produces peripheral neuropathy. Bone marrow suppression is rare with typical doses, but high doses can cause leukopenia. Concurrent

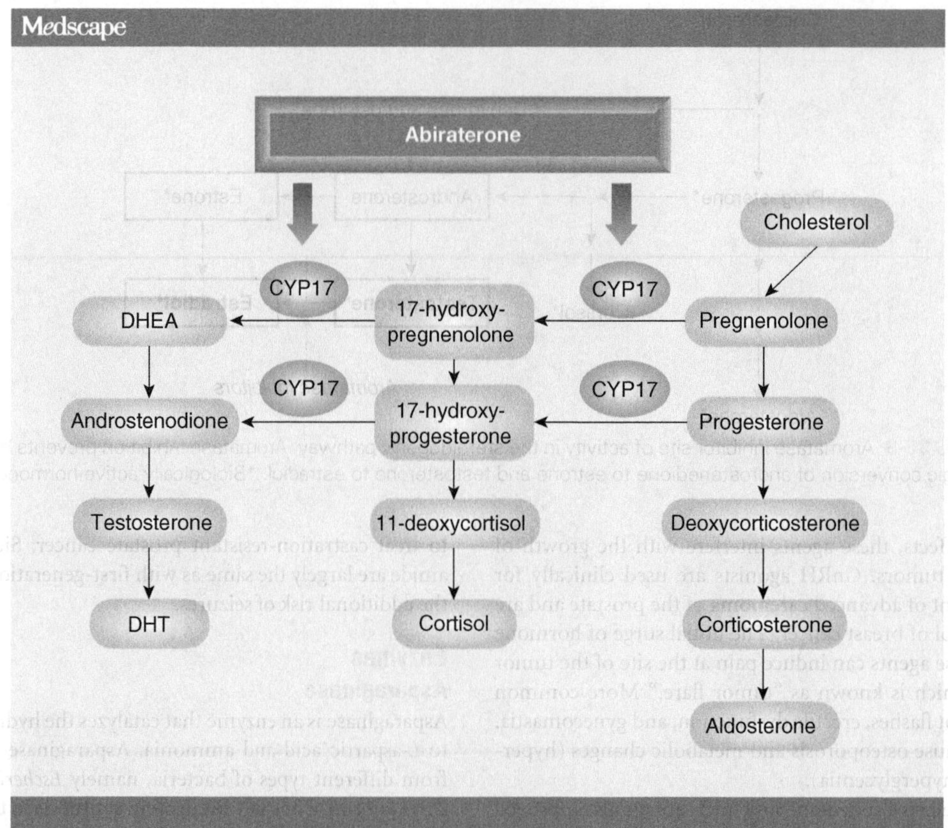

FIG 36-4 Abiraterone's inhibition of CYP17 blocks multiple steps in the enzymatic conversion of cholesterol to androgen derivatives. As a consequence of CYP17 inhibition, the cholesterol bioconversion pathway is shunted toward formation of excess aldosterone and less cortisol and androgens. Adverse effects may result from the resulting hyperaldosteronism and hypocortisolism. (From Agarwal N, Hutson TE, Vogelzang NJ, Sonpavde G: Abiraterone acetate: a promising drug for the treatment of castration-resistant prostate cancer, *Future Oncology* 6(5):665–679, 2010.)

administration of amifostine with cisplatin may reduce the cumulative renal toxicity associated with repeated administration in patients with advanced carcinoma of the ovary and NSCLC.

Carboplatin

Carboplatin is a second-generation platinum complex designed to maintain antitumor efficacy while decreasing nephrotoxicity, ototoxicity, and neurotoxic effects. The emetogenic potential of carboplatin is less than that of cisplatin. The major dose-limiting side effect is myelosuppression, with thrombocytopenia being more significant than leukopenia. Carboplatin is active in small cell and non-small cell lung cancer, ovarian carcinoma, head and neck carcinomas, and a variety of other malignancies.

Oxaliplatin

Oxaliplatin is a third-generation platinum derivative that possesses the additional mechanism of blocking DNA replication and transcription. Oxaliplatin is approved for the treatment of patients with advanced colorectal cancer when administered in combination with fluorouracil and leucovorin. It is also active in gastroesophageal carcinomas, ovarian, pancreatic, and breast cancers, as well as select hematologic malignancies. The toxicity profile of oxaliplatin includes a unique, acute neuropathy as well as the traditional chronic neuropathy that characterizes the other platinum agents. The acute neuropathy is characterized by cold-induced paresthesia of the hands, feet, and perioral area; jaw tightness; and laryngopharyngeal dysesthesia. These symptoms can occur during the infusion or within hours after administration and resolve once the affected area is warmed. Symptoms of chronic peripheral neuropathy may also be aggravated by exposure to cold.

Podophyllotoxins

Etoposide

Etoposide, a semisynthetic derivative of the mandrake plant substance podophyllotoxin, **induces DNA strand breaks by inhibiting the action of topoisomerase II** and producing free radicals. It is indicated for the first-line treatment of small cell lung cancer and for refractory testicular cancer. It is also active against various sarcomas, acute leukemias, NSCLC, and lymphomas. Myelosuppression, nausea, and vomiting are the most common adverse effects. High doses of etoposide can cause significant hypotension and alcohol intoxication, owing to the fact that it is dissolved in ethanol due to poor aqueous solubility. Etoposide phosphate is a prodrug formulation of etoposide. This formulation has greater solubility, allowing for more rapid infusion with less hypersensitivity and hypotensive reactions.

Teniposide

Teniposide has a similar mechanism of action to etoposide, but with higher potency. Current uses include treatment of refractory childhood leukemias and neuroblastoma. Myelosuppression is dose-limiting, and severe allergic reactions have been reported. Teniposide, similar to etoposide, is poorly soluble in water and is thus supplied in an alcohol-based solution.

Camptothecins

Topotecan and irinotecan

Topotecan is a semisynthetic analogue of camptothecin. Camptothecin is isolated from an ornamental tree, *Camptotheca acuminata*, found in China. Camptothecins produce their cytotoxic effects via **inhibition of topoisomerase I, which causes single-strand breaks in DNA.** Topotecan is indicated for the treatment of metastatic ovarian carcinoma, relapsed and refractory cervical cancer, and as second-line therapy for small cell lung cancer. Topotecan in combination with cytarabine is also used to treat advanced myelodysplastic syndromes and acute myelogenous leukemia. The major dose-limiting side effect is myelosuppression.

Irinotecan, another derivative of camptothecin, is indicated for use in colorectal carcinomas. Irinotecan in combination with fluorouracil/leucovorin has become a standard regimen for first- or second-line therapy in advanced stages of colorectal cancer. The major side effects of topotecan include myelosuppression, diarrhea requiring aggressive medical management, and symptoms of cholinergic excess (salivation, lacrimation, diaphoresis, and abdominal cramping).

Taxanes and Epothilones

Paclitaxel

Paclitaxel is another naturally derived product. Originally extracted from the bark of the western yew tree, *Taxus brevifolia*, paclitaxel **promotes polymerization and stabilization of microtubules and inhibits their depolymerization, halting cell replication in M phase.** It is poorly soluble in water and is formulated in a Cremophor El (polyoxyethylated castor oil) and alcohol vehicle. This vehicle is believed to be responsible for the high incidence of infusion reactions seen with paclitaxel administration. These reactions may manifest as dyspnea, hypotension, bronchospasm, urticaria, and erythematous rashes. Due to the high risk of hypersensitivity reactions, prophylactic premedication with steroids and H_1 and H_2 antihistamines is recommended. Prolonging the infusion may also help reduce the likelihood of severe hypersensitivity reactions, but longer infusions of paclitaxel are also associated with more severe myelosuppression. The antineoplastic activity of this drug is broad, and the current approved use of paclitaxel includes treatment of metastatic carcinoma of the ovaries and breast. A novel formulation of paclitaxel is available that consists of paclitaxel bound to albumin, eliminating the need for Cremophor El, resulting in significantly fewer hypersensitivity reactions compared to conventional paclitaxel. Albumin-bound paclitaxel is approved for metastatic breast cancer, NSCLC, and first-line therapy of pancreatic adenocarcinomas when combined with gemcitabine.

Docetaxel

Docetaxel is an antineoplastic agent belonging to the taxane family. It is a semisynthetic preparation derived from the needles of yew plants. Its mechanism of action is similar to that of paclitaxel. Docetaxel is indicated for the treatment of locally advanced breast cancer, non-small cell lung, prostate, gastric, and head and neck cancers. Docetaxel has a toxicity profile similar to that of paclitaxel, with hypersensitivity reactions requiring premedication with 3 days of dexamethasone beginning the day before therapy. Hypersensitivity reactions to docetaxel are often attributed to the solubilizer polysorbate 80; this different vehicle allows for some patients who have reactions to one taxane to receive the other without issue. Fluid retention and cutaneous toxicity occur more frequently than with paclitaxel, but there are fewer cardiac arrhythmias and myalgias.

Ixabepilone

Ixabepilone is the first of the class of epothilones to be approved. Epothilones A and B are more potent than the taxanes in their **binding of microtubules and in causing cell cycle arrest.** Ixabepilone is a semisynthetic analogue of epothilone B and has demonstrated activity in paclitaxel-resistant breast cancer. It is approved for monotherapy or in combination with capecitabine for treatment of patients with metastatic or locally advanced breast cancer resistant to treatment with an anthracycline and a taxane. Major toxicities associated with ixabepilone are peripheral neuropathy, myelosuppression, stomatitis, diarrhea, and arthralgias.

Miscellaneous Agents

Hydroxyurea

Hydroxyurea **inhibits DNA synthesis by blocking the action of ribonucleoside diphosphate reductase.** Hydroxyurea is readily absorbed from the gastrointestinal tract and penetrates various tissues throughout the body, including the CNS. Elimination is mainly by urinary excretion. Hydroxyurea is used principally to treat chronic myelogenous leukemia, myeloproliferative disorders, and to reduce rapidly increasing peripheral blast counts in acute leukemia. Hydroxyurea is also used in sickle cell disease to prevent pain crises and minimize the need for blood transfusions. High doses most often produce myelosuppression and megaloblastic anemia.

Procarbazine

Procarbazine, a derivative of methylhydrazine, was originally synthesized for its use as an antidepressant. **Its cytotoxic activity is likely due to inhibiting transfer of methionine's methyl groups into transfer RNA, preventing protein synthesis as well as DNA and RNA synthesis.** Procarbazine is most active against Hodgkin's disease and is modestly effective in CNS malignancies, other lymphomas, and multiple myeloma when given in combination with alkylating agents and vinca alkaloids. Nausea and vomiting occur with high doses, and hematologic toxicity in the form of leukopenia and thrombocytopenia occurs within 3 to 4 weeks of administration. Because procarbazine is a mild monoamine oxidase inhibitor (MAOI), patients should be warned about concurrent use of tyramine-rich foods, antidepressants, CNS depressants, and other drugs that are known to interact significantly with MAOIs. Procarbazine is reported to have some degree of disulfiram-like activity, so alcoholic beverages should be avoided during treatment with procarbazine.

Thalidomide, lenalidomide, and pomalidomide

Thalidomide was used in Europe and Canada in the 1950s as an anxiolytic, antiemetic, and sedative drug until it was discovered to cause major teratogenic effects. This agent was not approved for use in the United States at that time because of a potential for irreversible neurotoxicity after long-term use. In the late 1990s thalidomide was approved by the FDA for the treatment of Hansen disease (leprosy), and it has since been utilized in many other conditions, such as AIDS-related apthous stomatitis, rheumatoid arthritis, and refractory chronic graft-versus-host disease. Thalidomide has also become a revolutionary treatment for multiple myeloma. The mechanism of thalidomide's activity is complex and still not well understood, but it involves **two major effects: antiangiogenesis and immune system modulation.**

Angiogenesis, as stated previously, is an important mechanism for tumor growth and formation of metastases. On inhibition of angiogenesis, the tumor cells starve without the necessary nutrient supply. In addition, thalidomide can inhibit tumor necrosis factor-alpha production, stimulate T-cell proliferation, and modulate interferon and interleukin-2 release. The role of each of these mechanisms in its antineoplastic effect is unknown. Thalidomide's efficacy in multiple myeloma led to its approval as a first-line treatment option in this disease when combined with dexamethasone, with or without a third agent. The most frequent dose-dependent adverse effects include sedation, rash, neuropathy, and constipation. Thalidomide has also been shown to increase the risk of developing venous thrombosis, and it is recommended that high-risk patients receive anticoagulation therapy while taking thalidomide. Because of the risk of birth defects, patients and physicians must be enrolled in a drug company program to be able to take or prescribe thalidomide.

Lenalidomide and pomalidomide are both structural analogues of thalidomide, and they possess similarly complex mechanisms of action. Lenalidomide is approved for treatment of multiple myeloma in combination with dexamethasone, and more recently, it won approval for treatment of refractory mantle cell lymphoma and select patients with myelodysplastic syndromes. Pomalidomide is indicated for the third-line treatment of multiple myeloma in patients who have previously received lenalidomide and a proteasome inhibitor (e.g., bortezomib). Adverse effects of lenalidomide include myelosuppression, fatigue, constipation, and somnolence. While lenalidomide also carries the risk of peripheral neuropathies and venous thromboembolism, they are less likely than with thalidomide. Pomalidomide possesses a side-effect profile more similar to lenalidomide, with the additional risk of confusion. Similar to thalidomide, patients taking these agents and prescribing physicians must be enrolled in a program aimed at preventing birth defects.

Decitabine and azacitidine

Decitabine and azacitidine are both **inhibitors of DNA methylation.** Hypomethylation of DNA results in the reactivation of genes that have been previously silenced, allowing for return of normal function to oncogenes and tumor suppressor genes. Decitabine is a deoxycycline and cytarabine nucleotide derivative that inhibits the process of DNA methyltransferase after being incorporated into the DNA, whereas azacitidine can be incorporated into DNA and RNA. Azacitidine is also a nucleotide analogue and is incorporated in place of cytidine, where it acts as a direct and irreversible inhibitor of DNA methyltransferase. Both of these agents have been approved for the treatment of myelodysplastic disorders and have shown promise as lower-intensity treatment options for patients with acute myeloid leukemia. The major adverse effects of these drugs are myelosuppression, resulting in thrombocytopenia, neutropenia, and infection. Common gastrointestinal side effects include mild nausea and vomiting and mucositis. Other effects include liver dysfunction and creatine elevations.

Bisphosphonates

The bisphosphonates, zoledronic acid and pamidronate, have been used to manage hypercalcemia of malignancy and for **bone pain associated with metastases arising from breast, prostate, and lung carcinomas and multiple myeloma.** The use of these agents has had a favorable impact on the natural history of these diseases, improving quality of life by decreasing pain and skeletal fractures. Side effects include fevers, flulike syndromes, decreased renal function, and hypocalcemia as well as the development of antiresorptive agent-induced osteonecrosis of the jaw (ARONJ) (See chapter 29).

Differentiation Agents: Retinoids and Arsenic Trioxide

Several classes of compounds have the potential in vitro and in vivo to have a differentiation effect on the malignant clone of cancer, allowing for growth and maturation of the immature, cancerous cells and restoring more normal cellular processes. Among these compounds are the retinoids, including some commercially available and experimental agents such as isotretinoic acid (13-*cis*-retinoic acid), 9-*cis*-retinoic acid, all-*trans*-retinoic acid, bexarotene, etretinate, and the arotinoids. Retinoid effects seem to result from changes in gene expression mediated through specific intracellular receptors. **Retinoids play crucial roles in normal development and physiologic functioning. They are also capable of inhibiting cell growth, inducing differentiation, and inducing apoptosis in various tumor cell lines.**

Tretinoin

Tretinoin is the commercial formulation of all-*trans*-retinoic acid. This agent has been the most successful differentiating agent used in the treatment of acute promyelocytic leukemia. Genotypically, these leukemic clones have a characteristic translocation between the long arms of chromosome 15 and 17, which results in fusion between a gene that encodes RARα (retinoic acid receptor alpha) and a gene known as *pml*. **The *pml*/RARa fusion protein functions as an oncogene and blocks differentiation of myelocytes at the promyelocyte stage.** Orally administered tretinoin induces differentiation and apoptosis of malignant promyelocytes. Tretinoin, similar to most retinoids, is teratogenic and should be avoided during pregnancy. Common side effects include dry skin, exfoliation, xerostomia, and cheilitis. A rare but potentially lethal dose-limiting toxicity is known as **retinoic acid syndrome**, or **differentiation syndrome**, which consists of fever, chest pain, dyspnea, hypoxia, pulmonary infiltrates, and pleural or pericardial effusions.

Bexarotene

Bexarotene is a retinoid that selectively activates RXR (retinoid X receptor). The approved indication for bexarotene is for the treatment of refractory cutaneous T-cell lymphoma. Bexarotene causes lipid abnormalities in the majority of patients, requiring monitoring and possibly treatment. Other side effects include headache, liver damage, hypothyroidism, rash, dry skin, leukopenia, and nausea.

Other retinoids

Of all the retinoids, isotretinoic acid (13-*cis*-retinoic acid) has undergone the most extensive clinical examination. The activity of this agent alone in established cancers is limited. It has been used to reverse oral leukoplakia in heavy tobacco users. The duration of clinical response is brief, and most patients have a relapse if the drug is stopped. Isotretinoic acid has also demonstrated activity in treating the childhood malignancy neuroblastoma when used in combination with intensive chemotherapy, radiation, surgery, and autologous stem cell transplantation. Isotretinoic acid commonly causes xerostomia, dry skin, lipid abnormalities, headaches, and arthralgias. Rare complications include bleeding and inflammation of gingival tissue, hearing difficulty or tinnitus, and inflammatory bowel disease. Isotretinoin is highly teratogenic and patients (both male and female), prescribers, and dispensing pharmacies must enroll in a company-funded program that tracks attestations that patients are not pregnant and using appropriate birth control.

Arsenic trioxide

The development of arsenic trioxide (As_2O_3) has revolutionized the treatment of acute promyelocytic leukemia (APL). Clinical trials have demonstrated that arsenic trioxide, in combination with all-*trans*-retinoic acid, produced higher response rates and improved survival compared to traditional chemotherapy for most patients with APL. The proposed mechanisms of activity of this agent include induction of apoptosis by activation of cysteine proteases (caspases) and initiation of differentiation of leukemic promyelocytes into mature white blood cells. The adverse effects attributed to arsenic trioxide in clinical trials consisted of lightheadedness during infusion, fatigue, musculoskeletal pain, hyperglycemia, and peripheral neuropathy. The frequency of oral complications from this treatment is low and includes sore throat, oral blisters, and dry mouth. A more serious but rare side effect is a presentation similar to "differentiation syndrome," described earlier. Cardiac side effects include QTc interval prolongation on electrocardiogram.

Biologic Response Modifiers

It has long been understood that the immune system has a role to play in the development and suppression of certain malignancies. As a result, there is much interest in developing agents targeting these pathways. Known as the fourth modality of cancer therapy, **biologic response modifiers are used to assist the body's natural ability to kill cancer cells or to minimize adverse effects on normal cells.**

Interferons

Two types of human interferon, interferon alfa-2a and interferon alfa-2b, have been produced by recombinant DNA techniques and marketed for cancer chemotherapy. Each agent is a protein chain of 165 amino acids, differing from each other only at a single amino acid residue. A purified form of interferon-α, prepared from human plasma, is also available under the nonproprietary name of **interferon alfa-n3.**

These agents exert antiviral, immunostimulant, and antiproliferative properties by binding to specific cell membrane receptors; however, the exact mechanism of action remains to be elucidated. They are currently being used to treat hairy cell leukemia, Kaposi sarcoma, chronic hepatitis, chronic myelogenous leukemia, melanoma, and other malignancies in combination with chemotherapy and as biologic response modifiers in other nonmalignant diseases.

Interferons are given by subcutaneous, intravenous, or intramuscular injection and have plasma half-lives of 4 to 8 hours. They are hydrolyzed in the kidney, and metabolites are largely reabsorbed from the glomerular filtrate. Numerous side effects have been associated with their use. Most patients have a flulike syndrome with fever, chills, myalgia, fatigue, and headache. Loss of appetite is also common, and patients may have nausea, vomiting, and diarrhea. Dermatologic and CNS disturbances (e.g., ataxia, confusion, depression) occur in few patients.

Aldesleukin

Aldesleukin (interleukin-2 [IL-2]) is a recombinant product produced by a genetically engineered *E. coli* strain. **IL-2 has numerous immunoregulatory properties, including enhancement of lymphocyte mitogenesis, lymphocyte cytotoxicity, induction of killer cells (natural and lymphokine activated), and induction of interferon-γ production.** IL-2 is administered by intravenous infusion and is metabolized and eliminated by the kidneys. The plasma half-life of IL-2 is short (approximately 90 minutes). Currently, IL-2 is used for the treatment of adults with metastatic renal cell carcinoma and metastatic melanoma. High-dose IL-2 treatment has produced some long-lasting complete responses or partial remissions in these diseases. The major toxicities of IL-2 are associated with capillary leak syndrome, resulting in clinically significant hypotension, weight gain, fluid retention, pulmonary edema, and acute renal dysfunction with oliguria or anuria. Some of the common side effects (e.g., chills and fevers) can be reduced with appropriate premedication. Pruritic rashes are also common.

Sipuleucel-T

Sipuleucel-T is the first commercially available **cancer vaccine.** It is an autologous product prepared from a patient's own antigen-presenting cells that have been cultured with prostate antigen protein (PAP). When reinfused into the patient, these cells induce T-cell mediated immunity to attack tumor cells expressing PAP. Sipuleucel-T is approved for use in asymptomatic advanced prostate cancer. The most common toxicities of sipuleucel-T are infusion reactions, occurring in up to 70% of patients, manifesting as chills, fever, fatigue, hypoxia, and hypertension. Other toxicities include increased risk of deep vein thrombosis, stroke, and myocardial infarction.

Ipilimumab

Ipilimumab is a recombinant human IgG1 immunoglobulin monoclonal antibody targeting the cytotoxic T-lymphocyte–associated antigen 4 (CTLA-4). **Blocking CTLA-4 allows for enhanced T-cell activation and proliferation allowing for the body's own immune system to seek out and kill malignant cells** (Fig. 36-5). Ipilimumab is approved for use in metastatic melanoma and is being studied in a number of other

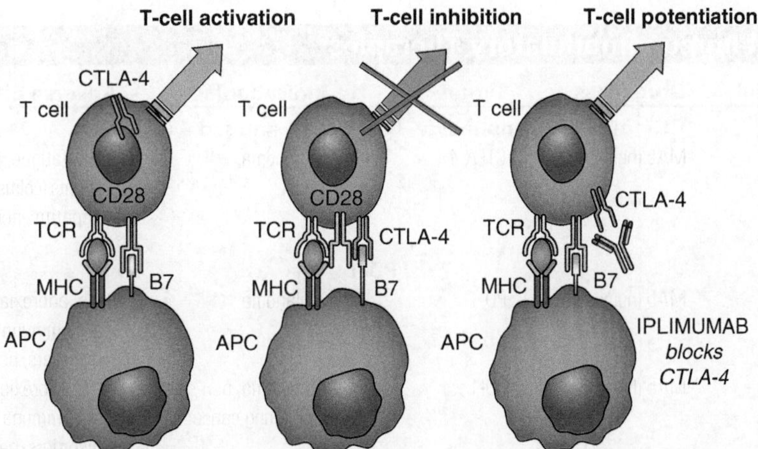

FIG 36-5 Mechanism of action for ipilimumab. Cytotoxic T-lymphocyte antigen-4 (CTLA-4) is a negative regulator of T-cell activity. Image 1: T-cell activation requires two separate stimulatory signals. The first signal occurs when the T-cell receptor (TCR) binds to the major histocompatibility complex (MHC) of an antigen-presenting cell (APC). The second signal, or co-stimulatory signal, occurs when the CD28 receptor of T cells binds the B7 ligand of APCs. Image 2: CTLA-4 is a naturally occurring T-cell receptor that, when bound by B7 on APCs, prevents the co-stimulation required for T-cell activation and suppresses T-cell activity. Image 3: ipilimumab is a monoclonal antibody designed to bind CTLA-4 and prevent its binding of B7, allowing for T-cell activation and potentiation to occur, allowing for enhanced immune-mediated destruction of tumors. (From Saijo N: Present status and problems on molecular targeted therapy of cancer. *Cancer Research and Treatment: Official Journal of Korean Cancer Association* 44(1):1–10, 2012. http://dx.doi.org/10.4143/crt.2012.44.1.1.)

solid tumors. The toxicities associated with ipilimumab can primarily be attributed to its immune stimulating effects. These immune-mediated adverse effects, which can be severe and fatal, include dermatitis, endocrine disorders, enterocolitis, hepatitis, and neuropathies (Table 36-2). For severe symptoms corticosteroids are recommended to attenuate the immune stimulation causing the toxicity.

Nivolumab and pembrolizumab

These monoclonal antibodies represent a novel class of immune-modulating therapies, known as anti-PD-1 inhibitors (programmed cell death-1). **They bind to the PD-1 receptor, preventing the ligands PD-L1 and PD-L2 from binding, resulting in disruption of T-cell regulation and activation.** Without the inhibitory effects of PD-L1 and PD-L2 the antitumor effects of T cells are enhanced (analogous to the immune-checkpoint inhibition of ipilimumab). Nivolumab has been approved for use in metastatic melanoma and NSCLCs, whereas pembrolizumab is approved only for metastatic melanoma; both are being studied in a number of other solid tumors. The most common toxicities associated with these agents are primarily immune-mediated reactions and may manifest as colitis, pneumonitis, hepatitis, nephritis, or hyper/hypothyroidism (see Table 36-2). As with ipilimumab and IL-2 therapy, very durable responses have been seen in a portion of patients responding to anti-PD-1 inhibitors.

Blinatumomab

Blinatumomab is an agent for the treatment of refractory Philadelphia chromosome negative, B-cell ALL that possesses a novel mechanism of action. **It is a bispecific T-cell engager (BiTE), targeting CD19 on malignant B cells and CD3 on normal host T cells, upregulating cytotoxic T-cell activity.** This upregulation of T-cell activity leads to production of cytokines and T-cell proliferation resulting in lysis of CD19-positive B cells. Adverse effects of blinatumomab can mostly be attributed to the cytokine storm resulting from T-cell proliferation, including fever, headache, nausea, hypotension, and increases in transaminases and bilirubin. Neurotoxicity, ranging from confusion and coordination problems to encephalopathy and seizures, has been seen in a significant portion of patients. Corticosteroids or the anti-IL-6 antibody tocilizumab may be of benefit in mitigating these adverse events, but robust clinical experience is currently lacking.

Filgrastim, sargramostim, and oprelvekin

Thrombocytopenia and neutropenia are important dose-limiting toxicities of chemotherapy that can potentially delay treatment or require reduction in the total dose delivered to the patient. Prevention or reduction in the duration and severity of bone marrow toxicity enables patients to receive full-dose chemotherapy as scheduled, with the intent of maximizing efficacy of the prescribed regimen.

Colony-stimulating factors, such as filgrastim (granulocyte colony-stimulating factor; G-CSF) and sargramostim (granulocyte-macrophage colony-stimulating factor; GM-CSF), are approved to ameliorate the neutropenia induced by chemotherapeutic agents. They shorten the overall period of neutropenia, reduce the number of febrile episodes, and decrease the need for broad-spectrum antibiotics. They are also used to mobilize stem cells from the bone marrow into the peripheral blood to allow for apheresis collection for stem cell transplants. Two newer formulations of growth factors have been approved by the FDA for similar indications: tbo-filgrastim and filgrastim-sndz. These represent the first biosimilars approved for use in the United States and are expected to demonstrate similar efficacy and tolerability as filgrastim. Adverse effects of these agents are usually flulike symptoms, fever, chills, and bone pain. Pleuritis, pericarditis, and splenic rupture have rarely been reported.

Oprelvekin is a recombinant interleukin-11 (IL-11) indicated to mitigate and shorten the thrombocytopenia produced by intensive chemotherapy in non-myeloid malignancies. IL-11 is an endogenous cytokine that participates, along with other growth factors, in stimulating megakaryocytes and their precursors in the bone marrow. Oprelvekin prevents severe thrombocytopenia and decreases the need for platelet transfusions in cancer patients receiving highly myelosuppressive chemotherapeutic regimens. The widespread use of oprelvekin is limited, however, by its adverse effect profile and cost. Administration of oprelvekin leads to significant fluid retention, which

TABLE 36-2 Select Immunomodulatory Therapies

Generic Name (Brand Name)	Drug Class	Target	Indication(s)	Adverse Effects
Cytotoxic T-Lymphocyte–Associated Antigen 4 (CTLA-4)				
Ipilimumab (Yervoy)	MAb (human)	CTLA-4	Melanoma	Rash, fatigue, fever, vitiligo, autoimmune-related events (colitis, hypopituitarism, thyroid disorders, hepatitis, neuropathy)
PD-1				
Pembrolizumab (Keytruda)	MAb (humanized)	PD-1	Melanoma	Rash, anorexia, myalgias, diarrhea, autoimmune-related events (colitis, thyroid disorders, hepatitis, pneumonitis)
Nivolumab (Opdivo)	MAb (human)	PD-1	Melanoma, non-small cell lung cancer	Rash, anorexia, myalgias, diarrhea, autoimmune-related events (colitis, thyroid disorders, hepatitis, pneumonitis)
Bispecific T-Cell Engager (BiTE)				
Blinatumomab (Blincyto)	MAb (mouse)	CD19 of B cells & CD3 of T cells	Ph- ALL	Cytokine release syndrome (fever, hypotension, liver injury, weakness, nausea), neurologic toxicity (tremor, dizziness, encephalopathy, confusion, seizures, coordination disorders), myelosuppression, infection

ALL, Acute lymphoblastic leukemia; *CTLA-4*, cytotoxic T-lymphocyte–associated antigen 4; *MAb*, monoclonal antibody; *PD-1*, programmed cell death-1; *Ph-*, Philadelphia chromosome negative.

may cause other complications such as peripheral edema, dilutional anemia, palpitations, dyspnea, headache, and atrial arrhythmias. Headache, myalgia, arthralgia, and fatigue are also reported frequently.

Palifermin

Palifermin is a human keratinocyte growth factor and binds to the keratinocyte growth factor receptor, which results in proliferation, differentiation, and migration of epithelial cells. It is FDA approved to decrease the incidence and duration of severe oral mucositis in patients with hematologic malignancies receiving myelotoxic therapy that requires hematopoietic stem cell support that is expected to result in severe mucositis. This injectable growth factor is given daily for 3 days before and 3 days after chemotherapy. In a clinical trial in autologous transplant patients, it reduced the duration of World Health Organization grade III and IV mucositis from 9 to 6 days and incidence from 98% to 63%. Palifermin has also been studied for use with chemotherapy agents such as fluorouracil, which can increase the risk of mucositis, and for the prevention of high-dose methotrexate–induced oral mucositis, where it may reduce the incidence, severity, and duration of the lesions. Palifermin's current role is to prevent or decrease the duration of mucositis in stem cell transplant patients, but sufficient evidence does not yet exist to recommend use in non-transplant chemotherapy regimens. Owing to its effects on epithelial cells, the main toxicities of palifermin are mucocutaneous in nature: edema, rash, oral/perioral dysesthesia and thickness, taste alterations, and tongue discoloration and thickening.

TARGETED ANTINEOPLASTIC THERAPY

Researchers constantly strive to find the "magic bullet" to cure cancer. In the process of discovering new molecules with anticancer activity, the molecular mechanisms and cellular processes have become better understood. **The idea of targeting a specific molecular pathway in the tumor cell cycle originated from the limitations of traditional antineoplastic drugs such as nonselective toxicity, drug resistance, and suboptimal success rates.** Over the past few years, many new drugs have been developed that fall into the category of targeted therapy and are summarized in Table 36-3. Tyrosine kinase inhibitors, monoclonal antibodies, histone deacetylase inhibitors, and proteasome inhibitors target a specific receptor or pathway in malignant cells. They are used as single agent or combination therapy to eradicate specific types of tumor cells, increase response rates, and slow the progression of cancers.

Tyrosine Kinase Inhibitors

One of the first types of targeted therapy to be developed was the tyrosine kinase inhibitors (TKIs). **These agents bind to and inhibit various cell surface receptors made of glycoproteins that span the cellular membrane and transduce intracellular responses, typically related to cell cycle regulation or other functions critical for malignant cell growth.** While these agents would ideally be developed to target one specific tyrosine kinase, they often have multiple targets. This can lead to off-target toxicities associated with their use. Another challenge in the development of TKIs is acquired resistance to these agents. The challenge of overcoming resistance to TKIs has led to the development of newer agents as well as investigation of different dosing schedules and combination therapy.

Monoclonal Antibodies

Another common class of targeted agents is that of the monoclonal antibodies (MAbs). MAbs are single immunoglobulin antibodies or fragments specific to a targeted surface antigen or ligand. **MAbs that target cell surface antigens may inhibit tumor cell growth by preventing receptor–ligand interaction,** via **cell-mediated cytotoxicity, or through targeted delivery of traditional chemotherapy agents as part of an antibody-drug conjugate.** Monoclonal antibodies are classified as mouse, chimeric, humanized, or fully human based on the proportion of mouse versus human components. Utilizing humanized or fully human MAbs reduces the formation of human anti-mouse antibodies, which are often responsible for serious infusion reactions and possibly reduced efficacy due to immune complex formation and inactivation of the infused MAb. Infusion reactions are common with MAbs, and many require specific premedication prior to infusion and/or specific titration of the infusion rate to be administered safely. Refer to Figure 36-6 for further information on the general mechanisms of TKIs and MAbs.

Philadelphia Chromosome (BCR-ABL) Inhibitors

Chronic myeloid leukemia (CML) develops as a result of a chromosomal translocation between the chromosomes 9 and 22 (also known as t(9; 22) or Philadelphia chromosome) resulting in an abnormal gene product, BCR-ABL. BCR-ABL is a constitutively active tyrosine kinase present in hematopoietic cells but not in other tissues, making it an attractive target for drug therapy. The first TKI developed to **inhibit the abnormal BCR-ABL kinase** was imatinib, and its success led to not only the development of other BCR-ABL TKIs but to the boom of targeted therapies as a whole. BCR-ABL TKIs also illustrate the challenge of overcoming resistance that often develops to targeted therapies. There are now numerous mutations associated with imatinib failures, and second- and third-generation BCR-ABL TKIs have been developed that are effective in treating patients with these resistant clones. Most recently, ponatinib was approved for treatment of CML with the T315I mutation, which had previously been resistant to all available agents.

Epidermal Growth Factor Receptor Inhibitors

The presence of mutated epidermal growth factor receptors (EGFRs) in various cancer types has been associated with increased cellular proliferation. There are multiple subtypes of EGFR, one of which, HER2, will be discussed separately. Currently, **EGFR inhibitors** are approved for the treatment of NSCLC, colorectal cancer, and head and neck cancers and include both TKIs and MAbs. In NSCLC the best response has been seen in patients who have an EGFR mutation, while in colorectal cancer, those with EGFR-positive tumors that are KRAS wild type have a better response than those with KRAS mutations, which seem to impart resistance to EGFR-targeted therapy. One unique side effect of EGFR inhibitors is a distinctive acneiform rash occurring in a large proportion of patients. The rash usually develops over the first 1 to 3 weeks of therapy and may wax and wane or completely resolve over the course of therapy. The rash occurs most often in areas of skin with sebaceous glands such as the scalp and face, particularly the nose and cheeks. There is some evidence that development of an acneiform rash may correlate with better response to therapy, but this has not been definitively established. Examples of anti-EGFR MAbs and TKIs, along with indications and common side effects, can be found in Table 36-3.

Vascular Endothelial Growth Factor Inhibitors

In order to grow in size, solid tumors require increased blood supply to survive and maintain their accelerated replication rate. Vascular endothelial growth factor (VEGF) stimulates endothelial cell proliferation, especially in areas of ischemia. Many solid tumors have upregulated production of VEGF to increase tumor vascularization, allowing for continued growth. **VEGF-targeted therapies, both MAbs and TKIs, have been developed to target the VEGF ligand as well as the**

TABLE 36-3 **Targeted Therapies**

Generic Name (Brand Name)	Drug Class	Target	Indication(s)	Adverse Effects
			BCR-ABL	
Imatinib (Gleevec)	TKI	BCR-ABL, PDGF, SCF, c-kit	Ph+CML, Ph+ALL, GIST, MDS	Nausea/vomiting, bone marrow suppression, edema, fatigue
Dasatinib (Sprycel)	TKI	BCR-ABL, SRC, c-kit, EPHA2, PDGFRβ	Ph+CML, Ph+ALL	Bone marrow suppression, QTc prolongation, edema, cardiomyopathy
Nilotinib (Tasigna)	TKI	BCR-ABL, c-kit, PDGFR	Ph+CML, Ph+ALL	Bone marrow suppression, QTc prolongation, edema, hyperglycemia
Bosutinib (Bosulif)	TKI	BAC-ABL, SRC	Ph+CML	Bone marrow suppression, QTc prolongation, edema, pancreatitis, decreased bone density
Ponatinib (Iclusig)	TKI	BCR-ABL, VEGFR, FGFR, PDGFR, EPH, SRC, KIT, RET, TIE2, FLT3	Ph+CML, Ph+ALL	Bone marrow suppression, arrhythmias, arterial and venous thrombosis, heart failure, hepatotoxicity
			EGFR	
Erlotinib (Tarceva)	TKI	EGFR	Non-small cell lung, pancreatic	Acneiform rash, diarrhea, pneumonitis, cardiac events (CVA/MI)
Afatinib (Gilotrif)	TKI	EGFR, HER2, HER4	Non-small cell lung	Acneiform rash, diarrhea, decreased LVEF, pneumonitis, keratitis
Cetuximab (Erbitux)	MAb (chimeric)	EGFR	Colorectal (KRAS wild type), head and neck	Acneiform rash, nausea, diarrhea, infusion reaction, hypomagnesemia
Panitumumab (Vectibix)	MAb (human)	EGFR	Colorectal (KRAS wild type)	Acneiform rash, nausea, diarrhea, keratitis, hypomagnesemia, hypocalcemia
			VEGF	
Bevacizumab (Avastin)	MAb (humanized)	VEGF	Cervical, colorectal, glioblastoma, ovarian, non-small cell lung, renal cell	Hypertension, VTE, bleeding, impaired wound healing, heart failure, proteinuria, GI perforation
Ziv-aflibercept (Zaltrap)	Fusion protein	VEGF-A, VEGF-B, PIGF	Colorectal	Hypertension, proteinuria, hemorrhage, VTE, diarrhea, impaired wound healing, GI perforation
Ramucirumab (Cyramza)	MAb (human)	VEGFR 2	Colorectal, gastric, non-small cell lung	Hypertension, hypothyroidism, proteinuria, hemorrhage, impaired wound healing, GI perforation
Sunitinib (Sutent)	TKI	PDGFRα, PDGFRβ, VEGFR1, VEGFR 2, VEGFR3, FLT-3, CSF-1R, RET	GIST, PNET, renal cell	Hypertension, skin discoloration, diarrhea, myelosuppression, bleeding, mucositis, GI perforation, hypothyroidism, QTc prolongation, hepatotoxicity, impaired wound healing
Sorafenib (Nexavar)	TKI	VEGFR 1, VEGFR 2, VEGFR 3, CRAF, BRAF, PDGFRβ, c-KIT, FLT3	Hepatocellular carcinoma, renal cell, thyroid	Hypertension, hand-foot syndrome, rash, diarrhea, hepatotoxicity, myelosuppression, bleeding, impaired wound healing, GI perforation, QTc prolongation
Pazopanib (Votrient)	TKI	VEGFR 1, VEGFR 2, VEGFR 3, PDGFRα, PDGFRβ, c-KIT, Lck, C-Fms	Renal cell, soft tissue sarcoma	Hypertension, hair discoloration, hand-foot syndrome, hyperglycemia, diarrhea, myelosuppression, hepatotoxicity, heart failure, hemorrhage, QTc prolongation, VTE, hypothyroidism, impaired wound healing, GI perforation
Regorafenib (Stivarga)	TKI	VEGFR 1, VEGFR 2, VEGFR 3, PDGFRα, PDGFRβ, KIT, RET, FGFR 1, FGFR 2, TIE2, DDR2, TrkA, Eph2D, RAF-1, BRAF, $BRAF^{V600E}$, SAPK2, PTK5, Abl	Colorectal cancer, GIST	Hypertension, hand-foot syndrome, electrolyte abnormalities, myelosuppression, bleeding, hepatotoxicity, GI perforation
Lenvatinib (Lenvima)	TKI	VEGFR 1, VEGFR 2, VEGFR 3, PDGFRα, FGFR1, FGFR 2, FGFR 3, KIT, RET	Thyroid	Hypertension, hand-foot syndrome, hemorrhage, diarrhea, QTc prolongation, hepatotoxicity, GI perforation, VTE
			ALK	
Crizotinib (Xalkori)	TKI	ALK, HGFR, RON	Non-small cell lung (ALK+)	Edema, neuropathy, diarrhea, lymphocytopenia, neutropenia, visual disturbances, QTc prolongation, bradycardia, hepatotoxicity
Ceritinib (Zykadia)	TKI	ALK, IGF-1K, InsR, ROS1	Non-small cell lung (ALK+)	Neuropathy, acneiform rash, diarrhea, hyperglycemia, anemia, hepatotoxicity, increased serum creatinine, QTc prolongation, visual disturbances

Continued

TABLE 36-3 Targeted Therapies—cont'd

Generic Name (Brand Name)	Drug Class	Target	Indication(s)	Adverse Effects
			BTK	
Ibrutinib (Imbruvica)	TKI	BTK	CLL, mantle cell lymphoma, Waldenström macroglobulinemia	Rash, diarrhea, myelosuppression, musculoskeletal pain, fever, atrial fibrillation
			PI3K	
Idelalisib (Zydelig)	TKI	PI3Kδ	CLL, follicular NHL	Rash, diarrhea, myelosuppression, cough, fever, hepatotoxicity
			mTOR	
Everolimus (Afinitor)		mTOR	Breast cancer, PNET, renal cell carcinoma, subependymal giant cell astrocytoma	Stomatitis, asthenia, headaches, anorexia, rash, diarrhea, abdominal pain, dyslipidemias, hyperglycemia, pneumonitis, immunosuppression
			HDAC	
Vorinostat (Zolinza)		HDAC1, HDAC, HDAC3, HDAC6	Cutaneous T-cell lymphoma	Alopecia, hyperglycemia, diarrhea, muscle spasms, proteinuria, increased serum creatinine, myelosuppression, QTc prolongation, VTE
Romidepsin (Istodax)		HDAC	Cutaneous T-cell lymphoma, peripheral T-cell lymphoma	Hypotension, fever, electrolyte abnormalities, myelosuppression, QTc prolongation
Panobinostat (Farydak)		HDAC	Multiple myeloma	EKG changes, arrhythmia, electrolyte abnormalities, diarrhea, myelosuppression, hepatotoxicity
Belinostat (Beleodaq)		HDAC	Peripheral T-cell lymphoma	QTc prolongation, rash, hepatotoxicity, anemia, thrombocytopenia
			HER-2	
Trastuzumab (Herceptin)	MAb (humanized)	HER-2 subdomain IV	HER-2+ breast and gastric cancers	Diarrhea, decreased LVEF, infusion reaction, interstitial pneumonitis
Pertuzumab (Perjeta)	MAb (humanized)	HER-2 subdomain II	HER-2+ breast cancer	Diarrhea, decreased LVEF, infusion reaction
Ado-trastuzumab emtansine (Kadcyla)	ADC	HER-2 subdomain IV, plus microtubule inhibitor	HER-2+ breast cancer	Peripheral neuropathy, xerostomia, stomatitis, thrombocytopenia, hepatotoxicity, decreased LVEF, interstitial pneumonitis
Lapatinib (Tykerb)	TKI	HER-2, EGFR	HER-2+ breast cancer	Acneiform rash, diarrhea, mucositis, hepatotoxicity, decreased LVEF, QTc prolongation, interstitial pneumonitis
			BRAF	
Vemurafenib (Zelboraf)	TKI	BRAF (V600E and V600K mutation)	Melanoma with V600E mutations	Rash, skin photosensitivity, arthralgias/myalgias, fever, nausea, diarrhea, QTc prolongation, hepatotoxicity, pancreatitis, cutaneous squamous cell carcinomas and keratoacanthomas, uveitis and blurred vision
Dabrafenib (Tafinlar)	TKI	BRAF (V600E and V600K mutation)	Melanoma with V600E or V600K mutations	Rash, hand-foot syndrome, fever, hyperglycemia, arthralgias/myalgias, diarrhea, myelosuppression, QTc prolongation, hepatotoxicity, pancreatitis, uveitis and blurred vision, cutaneous squamous cell carcinomas and keratoacanthomas, non-cutaneous malignancies
			MEK	
Trametinib (Mekinist)	TKI	MEK1 & MEK2	Melanoma with V600E or V600K mutations	Rash, acneiform rash, fever, stomatitis, hypertension, hyperglycemia, decreased LVEF, myelosuppression, hemorrhage, venous thromboembolism, retinal pigment epithelial detachment, interstitial pneumonitis, cutaneous squamous cell carcinomas and keratoacanthomas
			JAK	
Ruxolitinib (Jakafi)	TKI	JAK1 & JAK2	Myelofibrosis, polycythemia vera	Myelosuppression, fatigue, hepatic transaminitis, increased cholesterol and triglycerides, non-melanoma skin cancers, withdrawal syndrome

TABLE 36-3 Targeted Therapies—cont'd

Generic Name (Brand Name)	Drug Class	Target	Indication(s)	Adverse Effects
			Proteasome Inhibitors	
Bortezomib (Velcade)		26S proteasome	Multiple myeloma, mantle cell lymphoma	Herpes virus reactivation, peripheral neuropathy, diarrhea, myelosuppression, hepatic injury
Carfilzomib (Kyprolis)		20S proteasome	Multiple myeloma	Infusion reactions, tumor lysis syndrome, herpes virus reactivation, peripheral neuropathy, diarrhea, myelosuppression, hepatic injury
			PARP	
Olaparib (Lynparza)	TKI	PARP1, PARP2, PARP6	Ovarian cancer	Anemia, fatigue, nausea, vomiting, headache, myalgias, and occasionally mucositis
			CDK	
Palbociclib (Ibrance)		CDK4, CDK6	Estrogen receptor+, HER-2(−) breast cancer	Stomatitis, myelosuppression, infections, fatigue, alopecia, nausea, diarrhea, peripheral neuropathy, venous thromboembolism
			Cell Surface Antigen-Targeted Monoclonal Antibodies	
Rituximab (Rituxan)	MAb (chimeric)	CD20	CD20 + NHL and CLL	Infusion reactions, hepatitis reactivation, infections due to immunosuppression, myelosuppression
Ofatumumab (Arzerra)	MAb (human)	CD20	CD20 + CLL	Infusion reactions, hepatitis reactivation, infections due to immunosuppression, myelosuppression
Obinutuzumab (Gazyva)	MAb (humanized)	CD20	CD20 + CLL	Infusion reactions, hepatitis reactivation, infections due to immunosuppression, myelosuppression
Ibritumomab-yttrium-90 (Zevalin)	MAb-radiation conjugate	CD20-targeted radiation (beta particles)	CD20 + NHL	Infusion reaction, prolonged myelosuppression, infection, rash (including Stevens-Johnson syndrome)
Alemtuzumab (Campath)	MAb (humanized)	CD52	B-cell CLL	Infusion reactions, myalgias, rash, severe and prolonged immunosuppression (increased viral, fungal, and bacterial infections), thyroid disorders, secondary malignancies
Gemtuzumab ozogamicin (Mylotarg)	ADC	CD33, plus the alkylating agent calicheamicin	Acute myeloid leukemia (but withdrawn from market)	Infusion reactions, myalgias, acute respiratory distress, mucositis, prolonged myelosuppression, hepatic injury
Brentuximab vedotin (Adcetris)	ADC	CD30, plus the microtubule inhibitor monomethyl auristatin E (MMAE)	Hodgkin's lymphoma, anaplastic large cell lymphoma	Neuropathy, rash, nausea, diarrhea, myelosuppression, myalgias, hepatic injury

ADC, Antibody-drug conjugate; *ALL,* acute lymphoblastic leukemia; *ALK,* anaplastic lymphoma kinase; *BTK,* Bruton's tyrosine kinase; *CDK,* cyclin-dependent kinase; *c-FMS,* transmembrane glycoprotein receptor tyrosine kinase; *CLL,* chronic lymphocytic leukemia; *CML,* chronic myeloid leukemia; *EGFR,* epidermal growth factor receptor; *FGFR,* fibroblast growth factor receptor; *GIST,* gastrointestinal stromal tumor; *HDAC,* histone deacetylase; *HER-2,* human epidermal growth factor receptor 2; *HGFR,* hepatocyte growth factor receptor; *IGF-1K,* insulin-like growth factor 1 receptor; *InsR,* insulin receptor; *JAK,* Janus-associated kinase; *Lck,* leukocyte-specific protein tyrosine kinase; *MAb,* monoclonal antibody; *MDS,* myelodysplastic syndrome; *MEK,* mitogen-activated extracellular kinase; *mTOR,* mammalian target of rapamycin; *NHL,* non-Hodgkin's lymphoma; *LVEF,* left ventricular ejection fraction; *PARP,* poly ADP ribose polymerase; *PDGF,* platelet-derived growth factor; *PI3K,* phosphatidylinositol 3-kinase; *PIGF,* placental growth factor; *Ph+,* Philadelphia chromosome positive; *PNET,* pancreatic neuroendocrine tumors; *RON,* Recepteur d'Origine Nantais; *SCF,* stem cell factor; *TKI,* tyrosine kinase inhibitor; *VEGF,* vascular endothelial growth factor. *VTE,* venous thromboembolism.

associated VEGF receptors. VEGF inhibitors are usually associated with stabilization of disease when used as monotherapy and have been approved for use in a number of malignancies including glioblastoma, colorectal, ovarian, non-small cell lung, renal cell, thyroid, hepatocellular carcinoma, gastrointestinal stromal tumors (GIST), and pancreatic neuroendocrine tumors (PNET). VEGF inhibitors have several class effect toxicities including hypertension, venous thromboembolism, GI perforation, hemorrhage, and impaired wound healing.

Due to the risk for impaired wound healing and hemorrhage, VEGF inhibitors are not recommended prior to elective surgery. While the optimal duration between surgery and most VEGF inhibitor therapies has not been established, the package insert for the MAb bevacizumab recommends withholding bevacizumab therapy for at least 28 days pre-surgery and to not reinstate treatment for at least 28 days postsurgery and until wounds have fully healed. Some sources have recommended discontinuation as long as 6 to 8 weeks prior to surgery. Many small molecule TKIs also have anti-VEGF effects as part of their mechanism of action, like sunitinib, a drug approved for the treatment of kidney cancer and GIST. The guidelines for its use relative to surgery are less defined. Some have suggested cessation of sunitinib therapy 1 week before surgery and restarting after wound healing has commenced, or at least 1 week postsurgery.

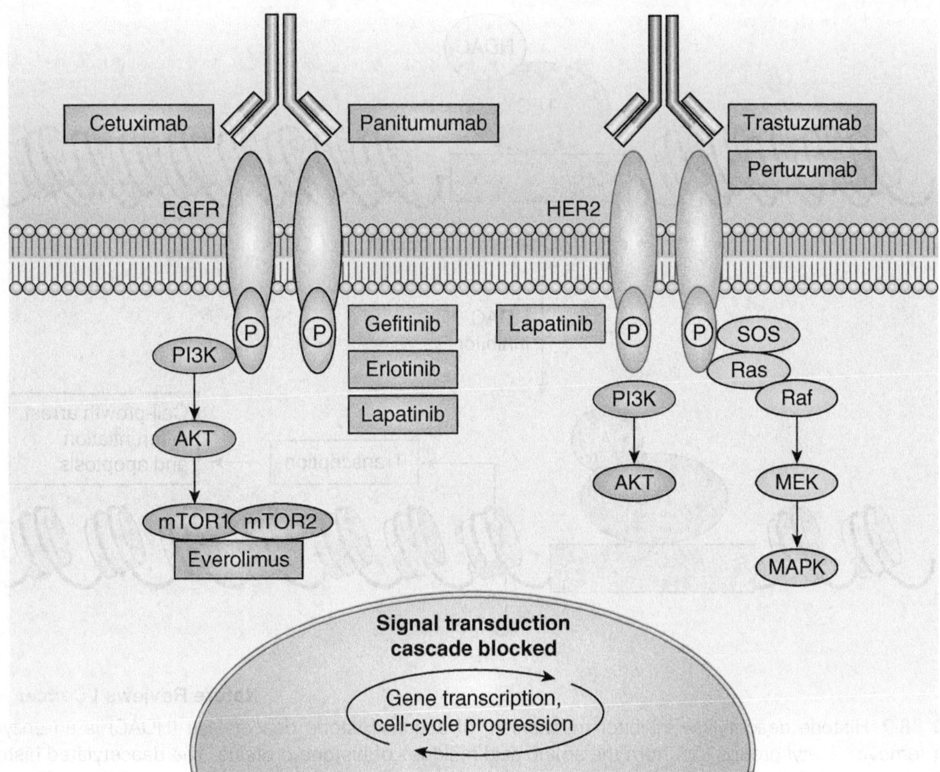

FIG 36-6 Malignant cells possess dysregulated signaling pathways that result in excessive growth and replication, as well as impaired mechanisms for cellular destruction (apoptosis). Advances in molecular biology have elucidated several of these overly active molecular pathways, allowing for potential targets for anticancer therapies. Epidermal growth factor receptor (EGFR) and human epidermal growth factor receptor 2 (HER2) are two transmembrane tyrosine kinases that are often upregulated in certain malignancies. Monoclonal antibodies (e.g., cetuximab, panitumumab, trastuzumab, and pertuzumab) inhibit activation and downstream signaling of these receptors by binding to their extracellular domains or by binding and neutralizing the receptor's endogenous ligand and preventing dimerization and activation of the associated receptor. Tyrosine kinase inhibitors (e.g., gefitinib, erlotinib, and lapatinib) prevent the intracellular phosphorylation of the transmembrane tyrosine kinase, preventing activation of the downstream cascade of intracellular signaling molecules. (From Okines A, Cunningham D, Chau I: Targeting the human EGFR family in esophagogastric cancer, *Nature Reviews Clinical Oncology* 8:492–503, August 2011.)

Anaplastic Lymphoma Kinase Inhibitors

A small percentage of patients (2% to 7%) with NSCLC have an abnormal gene rearrangement involving the anaplastic lymphoma kinase (ALK) oncogene. ALK mutations generally do not overlap with other more common mutations in NSCLC, such as EGFR or KRAS, and they tend to be more common in never-smokers or light smokers with adenocarcinoma histology (up to 30%). Two agents are currently available that **target the ALK fusion protein**, crizotinib and ceritinib, and they are recommended as first-line therapy in patients with metastatic ALK-positive NSCLC. These agents are capable of producing response rates of up to 60% in advanced disease and have improved progression-free survival. Refer to Table 36-3 for adverse effects.

Bruton's Tyrosine Kinase Inhibitors

Bruton's tyrosine kinase (BTK) is a signaling molecule early in the B-cell antigen receptor (BCR) cascade. **Inhibition of BTK disrupts BCR signaling and leads to apoptosis in cells driven by chronic BCR signaling.** The pathogenesis of a number of B-cell malignancies including diffuse large B-cell lymphoma, mantle cell lymphoma, follicular lymphoma, and B-cell chronic lymphocytic leukemia (CLL) has been linked to BCR activity. Ibrutinib is the first BTK inhibitor to become commercially available, and it is approved for CLL, mantle cell lymphoma, and Waldenström macroglobulinemia. Side effects associated with this daily oral TKI include thrombocytopenia, diarrhea, neutropenia, upper respiratory infections, rash, arthralgia, nausea, sinusitis, and stomatitis. Initiation of ibrutinib also causes a marked, benign lymphocytosis in the majority of patients that typically occurs early in therapy and can persist for up to 23 weeks. It is important to note that this lymphocytosis does not indicate a suboptimal response to therapy.

PI3K and mTOR Inhibitors

Phosphatidylinositol 3-kinase delta (PI3Kδ) is another signaling molecule in the BCR cascade, downstream of BTK. **Idelalisib is an inhibitor of PI3Kδ that has been shown to inhibit BCR-mediated cell proliferation** and has been approved for CLL and follicular lymphoma. In CLL, idelalisib in combination with rituximab improved 24-week progression-free survival (93% versus 46%) and 12-month overall survival (92% versus 80%).

The mammalian target of rapamycin (mTOR) kinase is another drug target located downstream in the PI3K pathway. Everolimus is an inhibitor of mTOR and is approved for the treatment of postmenopausal hormone receptor–positive, HER2-negative breast cancer patients, advance PNET, renal cell carcinoma, and subependymal giant cell astrocytomas (SEGA). Common side effects associated with this agent include stomatitis, asthenia, cough, headaches, anorexia, rash, diarrhea, and abdominal pain. Everolimus is also a potent

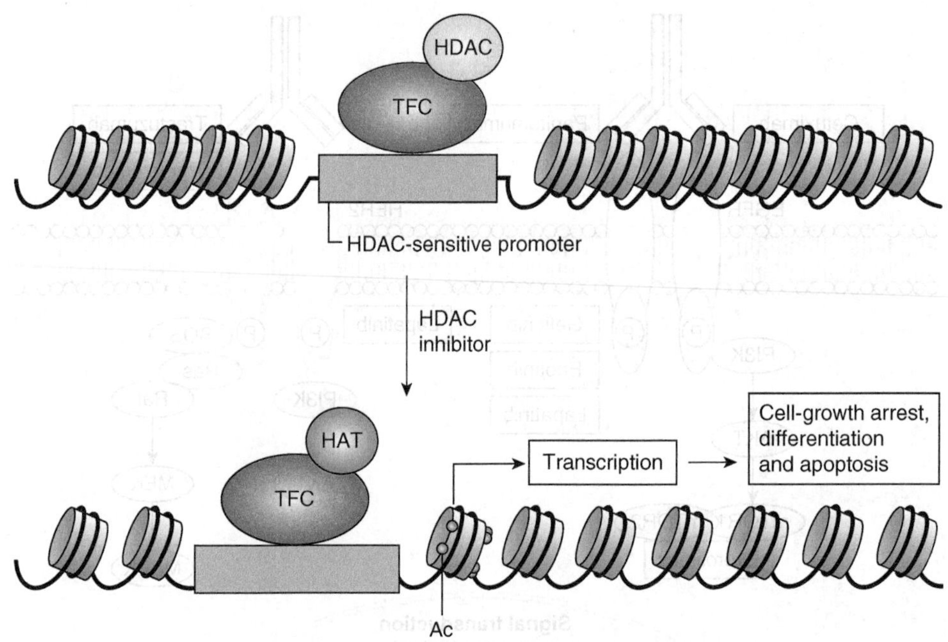

FIG 36-7 Histone deacetylase inhibitor mechanism of action. Histone deacetylase (HDAC) is an enzyme that removes acetyl groups (Ac) from the amino acid residues of histone proteins. The deacetylated histone is then able to tightly wrap DNA around it, preventing gene transcription of the wrapped DNA by the transcription factor complex (TFC) and halting protein production of the silenced gene. HDAC inhibitors allow histone acetylation by the enzyme histone acetyltransferase (HAT) and thus promote gene transcription. The cytotoxic properties of HDAC inhibitors are not fully understood, but it is thought that by regulating gene transcription these agents may silence oncogenes and allow for transcription of tumor suppressor genes, impeding the rapid growth of malignant cells. (From Marks PA, Rifkind RA, Richon VM, Breslow R, Miller T, Kelly WK: Histone deacetylases and cancer: causes and therapies, *Nature Reviews Cancer* 1: 194–202, December 2001; http://dx.doi.org/10.1038/35106079.)

immunosuppressant used to prevent allograft rejection in liver and renal transplantation, and thus it increases the risk of opportunistic infections.

Histone Deacetylase Inhibitors

Histone acetylation and deacetylation are important processes in regulating gene expression, making the genes more available or less available for transcription. **Histone deacetylase (HDAC) enzymes collapse the DNA around histones and reduce gene transcription.** Deregulation of histone acetylation has been shown to play a part in the development of several hematologic and solid tumor malignancies, allowing expression of oncogenes that stop apoptosis or inhibit other cellular pathways (Fig. 36-7). HDAC inhibitors are thought to cease the expression of oncogenes and to reactivate apoptosis, cellular differentiation, and tumor suppressor genes. They halt cell cycle progression at G_1 and G_2-M phases, degrade chromatin, and may also inhibit angiogenesis. Several HDAC inhibitors have been approved, primarily for use in cutaneous T-cell lymphoma, peripheral T-cell lymphoma, and multiple myeloma. These agents are being studied in a number of other malignancies including AML, MDS, and non-Hodgkin's lymphoma.

Human Epidermal Growth Factor Receptor-2 Inhibitors

The human epidermal growth factor receptor-2 (HER2) oncogene is part of the EGFR family of cell surface receptors. Presence of HER2 overexpression occurs in up to one-third of breast cancers and has been shown to result in more aggressive disease and carry a higher risk of relapse compared to tumors that do not overexpress HER2. **Development of HER2 inhibitors, including MAbs and TKIs, have helped offset the worsened prognosis associated with HER2-positive breast cancer** and have greatly improved survival compared to historical counterparts. In 2013, ado-trastuzumab emtansine was approved for use in patients with HER2-positive breast cancer who have experienced disease progression while receiving trastuzumab. This agent is an antibody-drug conjugate in which trastuzumab is linked to an antimicrotubule agent called DM1. This novel mechanism allows for more targeted delivery of the cytotoxic agent to cells that overexpress HER2, helping minimize off-target toxicity. More recently, HER2 overexpression has been shown to contribute to the pathogenesis of certain gastric tumors, and trastuzumab has been approved for treatment of these cancers. See Table 36-3 for adverse effects of HER2-inhibiting agents.

BRAF and MEK Inhibitors

Various malignancies have been shown to possess mutations within the mitogen-activated protein kinase (MAPK) pathway (consisting of RAS-RAF-MEK-ERK kinases). Notably, a substantial proportion of melanomas harbor mutations within the RAF family of kinases, with the V600E and V600K mutations of BRAF representing the most common among them. **Vemurafenib and dabrafenib are two TKIs that have been developed to specifically target cells containing these mutations, inhibiting BRAF kinase activity and downstream signaling, eventually leading to arrest in cellular proliferation and division.** (BRAF is a member of the RAF family.) Both of these agents are approved for malignant melanoma owing to their impressive response rates in treating this disease. Unfortunately, the benefit seen with these drugs has proven to be short-lived, with an average time to disease progression of about 6 months. In vitro data suggests that the transient benefit of BRAF inhibitors is likely due to malignant cells upregulating other kinases in the MAPK pathway, specifically MEK kinases, to overcome the inhibition of upstream BRAF kinases. It is postulated that amplification of MEK kinase activity could also be responsible for the high rates of low-grade, secondary skin cancers seen with BRAF inhibitors.

In an effort to prolong duration of response seen with BRAF inhibitors, sequential blockade of the MAPK pathway has been studied with combination BRAF and MEK inhibitor therapy. Trametinib, an inhibitor of both MEK1 and MEK2 kinases, when combined with dabrafenib has demonstrated improved response rates in malignant melanoma and a longer duration of response (9.4 months compared to 5.8 months) compared to dabrafenib alone. Interestingly, the incidence of secondary skin cancers was also lower in the combination group (7% versus 19% in the dabrafenib only group).

Janus-Associated Kinase Inhibitors

Myelofibrosis is a myeloproliferative neoplasm characterized by splenomegaly with resulting constitutional symptoms, cytopenias due to fibrosis of bone marrow, and heightened risk of acute myeloid leukemia. In the early 2000s, it was discovered that the Janus-associated kinase-signal transduction and transcription (JAK-STAT) intracellular signaling cascade is dysregulated in all patients with myelofibrosis. A particular JAK mutation, JAK^{V617F}, is present in about half of these patients and has become the target of ruxolitinib, a novel TKI therapy. While initially hoped to reverse disease pathogenesis, ruxolitinib monotherapy has been incapable of producing disease remission. Ruxolitinib has, however, offered significant reductions in spleen size of patients with myelofibrosis with resulting improvement of symptoms such as abdominal pain, early satiety, shortness of breath, and fatigue. Newer data also suggest an improvement in overall survival of patients who receive ruxolitinib, likely due to improvements in performance status. Notably, patients without the specific JAK^{V617F} mutation may also benefit from ruxolitinib therapy. See Table 36-3 for adverse effects.

Proteasome Inhibitors

The proteasome is a protein complex located within all eukaryotic cells to help regulate protein synthesis and destruction. Normally the proteasome degrades unnecessary or damaged proteins within the cell into amino acids that can be further incorporated into new proteins. **The proteasome inhibitors, bortezomib and carfilzomib, impair this amino acid recycling that eventually impairs normal cell cycling, gene expression, and stress-response mechanisms leading to cellular apoptosis.** The proteasome inhibitors have revolutionized the therapy of multiple myeloma, and they have been studied in other hematologic malignancies such as mantle cell lymphoma. These agents are associated with cumulative peripheral neuropathy, which can lead to dose reduction and changes in therapy. They also cause high rates of herpes virus reactivation, necessitating prophylaxis with an antiviral medication such as acyclovir or valacyclovir. See Table 36-3 for other side effects.

PARP Inhibitors

PARP inhibitors target the enzyme poly ADP ribose polymerase (PARP) and are being investigated in several types of malignancies. **PARP is a protein involved in repairing single-stand breaks in DNA; inhibitors of this enzyme prevent DNA repair and allow accumulation of single-strand breaks.** During DNA replication, these single-strand breaks result in double-strand breaks when the DNA helix unwinds. Patients with tumors harboring mutations in homologous recombination repair enzymes BRCA1, BRCA2, and PALB2 (e.g., some ovarian and breast cancers) are unable to repair these double-strand breaks, and affected cells enter apoptosis. PARP inhibitors are most promising in the treatment of breast and ovarian cancers, given relatively high rates of BRCA1/2 mutations in these malignancies. Olaparib is the first PARP inhibitor approved for treatment of refractory ovarian cancer possessing a BRCA mutation. The side effect profile of olaparib includes anemia, fatigue, nausea, vomiting, headache, myalgias, and occasionally mucositis.

Cyclin-Dependent Kinases Inhibitors

Cell cycle dysregulation is a hallmark alteration of cancer cells. **Cyclin-dependent kinases (CDK) are a group of kinases involved in controlling a cell's progression through the cell cycle.** Two of these proteins, CDK 4 and 6, regulate the progression from the G_1 to S phase of the cell cycle and are the target of the TKI palbociclib. Palbociclib is approved in combination with letrozole for the first-line endocrine-based treatment of postmenopausal women with estrogen receptor–positive, HER2-negative breast cancer. This agent is also being studied for management of refractory hormone-receptor positive breast cancer in an attempt to overcome mechanisms of endocrine resistance. Toxicities of palbociclib include myelosuppression, risk of infections, fatigue, alopecia, nausea, diarrhea, peripheral neuropathy, and stomatitis. Palbociclib may also impart a greater risk of venous thromboembolism.

Cell Surface Antigen-Targeted Monoclonal Antibodies

Hematologic malignancies (leukemias and lymphomas) can arise from any stage of differentiation in the hematopoiesis cascade. While the particular type of hematologic malignancy can sometimes be surmised through visual examination under the microscope, the morphologic appearance is not always sufficient to subcategorize the particular type of cancer. Advances in immunohistochemistry (IHC) have allowed for more precise diagnosis by exposing tissue samples to various antibodies directed against cell surface molecules/antigens known to be expressed on specific cells. The antigen–antibody reaction is then visualized in one of a variety of manners.

One group of cell surface molecules used in IHC is the cluster of differentiation (CD) family. Each stage of hematopoiesis has its own unique sequence (or thumbprint) of CD molecules that can be used to identify it. Within the past couple of decades, this predictable **expression of CD molecules on various hematologic malignancies has allowed for therapeutic targeting of the malignancy with monoclonal antibodies (MAbs).** One of the most successful examples of this treatment modality is that of rituximab. Rituximab targets CD20, which is expressed on the majority of B cells (with the exception of early pro-B cells or mature plasma cells), and it has shown great activity in treating CD20-positive B-cell leukemias and lymphomas.

The majority of CD-targeted MAbs exert their cytotoxic properties by binding to a particular CD-antigen and then "flagging" the bound cell for destruction by the body's immune system (e.g., natural killer cells, eosinophils, or the complement system). There are also certain MAbs that have been conjugated to a chemotherapeutic agent possessing a more traditional cytotoxic mechanism, such as an alkylating agent, that is then released into the bound malignant cell (termed antibody-drug conjugates, or ADCs). These ADCs allow for more targeted delivery of potent chemotherapeutics to malignant cells, allowing for improved efficacy and reduced toxicity of the conjugated chemotherapeutic (Fig. 36-8). A similar tactic has been employed with ibritumomab-yttrium-90, in which a monoclonal antibody is bound

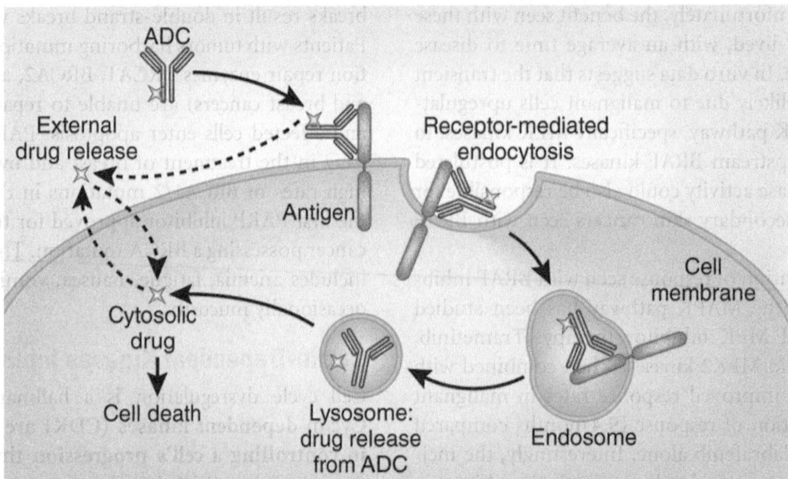

FIG 36-8 Antibody-drug conjugates (ADC) are designed to deliver highly toxic chemotherapeutic agents specifically to malignant cells, sparing normal cells from damage. The ADC consists of a monoclonal antibody (targeted against antigens present on tumor cells) bound to a cytotoxic agent by a peptide linker. Once the antibody binds to its specific antigen, the entire ADC is internalized by the cell via endocytosis. Cellular lysosomes then act to degrade the peptide linker connecting the antibody and cytotoxic agent, releasing the cytotoxic agent within the cell to exert its anticancer effects. ADCs are not a perfect technology, and there is some risk of extracellular release of the cytotoxic agent, which probably accounts for some of the off-target toxicities of these drugs. (From Senter PD, Sievers EL: The discovery and development of brentuximab vedotin for use in relapsed Hodgkin's lymphoma and systemic anaplastic large cell lymphoma, *Nature Biotechnology* 30, 631–637, 2012; http://dx.doi.org/10.1038/nbt.2289.)

to a radiation-emitting molecule (yttrium-90) to deliver "targeted" radiation to malignant cells expressing CD20. Refer to Table 36-3 for specific cell surface antigen-targeted MAbs, their adverse effects, and indications for use.

COMBINATION THERAPY

The previously discussed **drugs are rarely used as single entities for the treatment of cancer.** Choriocarcinoma is one of only a few malignancies that can be cured with a single agent (doxorubicin). **Resistance of tumor cells to chemotherapy may explain poor initial responses and relapses during monotherapy.** A hypothesis for tumor resistance has been proposed. Resistant tumors exhibit either inherent resistance or acquired resistance. The possible mechanisms of acquired resistance include defects in the resistant cells, transport, or activation of the chemotherapeutic prodrug to the active species. Also involved may be an alteration of the DNA repair, gene amplification, altered nucleotide pool, increased salvage pathways, and development of pleiotropic drug resistance or multidrug resistance. Research is ongoing to better understand and overcome tumor resistance.

The current chemotherapeutic approach to prevent resistance is similar to the approach described for combination chemotherapy: (1) **use agents with different cell cycle specificity, mechanisms of action, toxicities, and potential combinations for synergy** and (2) **administer the drugs in intermittent courses and at maximal tolerated doses to maximize cell kill**, allow for host recovery, and avoid prolonged drug-free intervals. The dose intensity of a regimen is a well-recognized variable for response and cure in sensitive tumors. The use of alternating non–cross-resistant regimens may improve outcome further, as seen with the ABVD regimen (doxorubicin [Adriamycin], bleomycin, vinblastine, and dacarbazine), alternating monthly with the traditional MOPP regimen (mechlorethamine, vincristine [Oncovin], procarbazine, prednisone) for the treatment of advanced Hodgkin's disease. This regimen was made more dose-intensive by combining the two regimens into a monthly cycle MOPP/ABV hybrid program. The ultimate dose-intensive regimens include high-dose chemotherapy, with or without irradiation, requiring bone marrow transplantation or peripheral stem cell reinfusion to rescue the host from total marrow aplasia. Antineoplastic agents are often more successful when used in combination with radiation therapy and surgery for the treatment of tumors such as head and neck carcinomas. Combination regimens containing cisplatin and fluorouracil are used simultaneously with radiotherapy to render the tissue radiosensitive and as a postoperative adjunct to destroy micrometastases that may have escaped destruction during local surgery.

Targeted therapy approaches are being incorporated into combinations with more traditional chemotherapy agents, as they add a different mechanism of cytotoxicity. Combinations such as rituximab plus CHOP (cyclophosphamide, hydroxydaunomycin, vincristine [Oncovin], prednisone) for non-Hodgkin's lymphoma have been shown to be more effective than chemotherapy alone and have become the standard of care. Other combinations, such as TKIs and chemotherapy, have also proven to be more successful than chemotherapy alone in treating certain diseases. More studies are needed to establish the place of targeted therapy and chemotherapy combinations in cancer treatment to optimize outcomes.

Potential Drug Interactions and Relative Contraindications

Most antineoplastic drugs have a narrow therapeutic index. Although drug interactions may enhance or diminish the antitumor effects and result in improvement or treatment failure, drug interactions may also increase or decrease the side-effect profile of the antineoplastic drug. Caution must be used when prescribing other therapeutic agents to patients undergoing active anticancer therapy. Interactions may occur between antineoplastic drugs and drugs that have no antineoplastic effects. One example is the relative contraindication for the use of NSAIDs, such as ibuprofen and aspirin, in patients who may be thrombocytopenic from myelosuppressive chemotherapy regimens. NSAIDs may affect platelet function and increase gastrointestinal irritation, increasing the bleeding risk in patients with a low platelet count. Other drug–drug interactions may occur from changes in absorption, clearance, or excretion of the antineoplastic drugs; changes in protein binding; or through the induction or inhibition of isoenzymes of the CYP450 system that metabolize the particular antineoplastic substrate or its metabolites.

Not all the metabolic pathways and interactions for antineoplastic agents have been identified. Many antineoplastic agents are substrates for metabolism by the CYP3A4, CYP2B6, and CYP2D6 isoenzymes. Concurrent use of an antineoplastic agent and the inhibitors of these and other hepatic isoenzymes may potentially delay elimination of the antineoplastic agent and enhance its activity or toxicity. An example of inhibitors of the CYP3A4 isoenzyme is the commonly used antifungal drug, fluconazole, which may possibly increase blood levels of cyclophosphamide, a substrate of a CYP3A4 isoenzyme. This antineoplastic agent is also metabolized by the CYP2B6 isoenzyme, so the metabolism of cyclophosphamide is only partially affected by the inhibitory effects of fluconazole. The antibiotic erythromycin can increase the toxicities of vincristine, likely through inhibition of vincristine's metabolism by CYP3A4. Although many analgesics (e.g., oxycodone and morphine) are substrates for metabolism by CYP isoenzymes, no clinically significant drug interactions from CYP isoenzyme effects on these analgesics and antineoplastic drugs have been reported.

Many antineoplastic drugs are excreted by the kidney. Nephrotoxic drugs may increase the toxicity of these agents by delaying drug elimination. Methotrexate is an antifolate antimetabolite with a wide spectrum of activity. It is a weak acid and is eliminated by tubular secretion in the kidney. Its renal clearance may be decreased by drugs that inhibit or compete for the tubular secretion of methotrexate or by reduced renal blood flow resulting from inhibited prostaglandin synthesis. Drugs that decrease methotrexate elimination include salicylates, NSAIDs, PPIs, probenecid, sulfonamides, and the penicillins. The toxic effects associated with delayed elimination of methotrexate include pancytopenia and mucositis. The risk of this interaction is considerably less with low-dose methotrexate used for rheumatoid arthritis. During methotrexate therapy, acetaminophen, opioids, or celecoxib, a cyclooxygenase-2 inhibitor, should be considered as alternatives to salicylates and NSAIDs for analgesia.

Some interactions result from pharmacodynamic mechanisms. Procarbazine is a weak MAOI. Caution should be taken in the administration of indirect-acting sympathomimetics (e.g., amphetamines and pseudoephedrine) while the patient is taking procarbazine to prevent potentially dangerous hypertensive episodes. Direct-acting sympathomimetics such as epinephrine, isoproterenol, and norepinephrine do not seem to interact to the same degree. While receiving procarbazine, the ingestion of ethanol should be avoided as it may result in a disulfiram-like reaction: flushing, headaches, nausea, and hypotension.

Other drugs with harmful interactions include warfarin and antineoplastic agents such as 5-fluorouracil, capecitabine, and ifosfamide; close monitoring of the international normalized ratio is necessary to prevent life-threatening bleeding. Many interactions have been reported, and consideration should be given to interactions that can result in clinically significant effects. Not all drug–drug interactions require avoidance of such therapeutic agents. In some cases, dosages may be titrated and patients monitored to minimize the risk.

IMPLICATIONS FOR DENTISTRY: ORAL COMPLICATIONS OF CHEMOTHERAPY

These various advances in cancer therapy are lifesaving, but they often have significant morbidity and complications. Considerable attention is now being paid to the medical significance of complications of cancer therapy and the effects these complications have on quality of life. Studies have shown that the oral complications of cancer therapy can significantly interfere with the course of cancer therapy, adversely affect general quality of life, and increase the cost of care. In addition, a number of chronic orofacial complications can significantly affect long-term quality of life and oral function after cancer therapy. Successful prevention and treatment of the oral complications of cancer therapy can reduce pain, suffering, and disability while decreasing the risk of complications that may interfere with ongoing cancer therapy or result in lifelong functional compromise.

TABLE 36-4 Oral Complications of Cancer Chemotherapy

Direct Toxicities	Indirect Toxicities
Oral mucositis	Myelosuppression
Salivary gland dysfunction	Neutropenia, immunosuppression
Neurotoxicity	Anemia
Trigeminal nerve neuropathies	Thrombocytopenia
Taste dysfunction	Infection
Dentinal hypersensitivity	Viral (HSV, VZV, CMV, EBV, other)
Temporomandibular dysfunction	Fungal (candida, aspergillus, other)
Myofascial pain	Bacterial
Temporomandibular joint dysfunction	Gastrointestinal mucositis
Dental and skeletal growth and development (pediatric patients)	Nutritional disturbances
Abnormalities in dentition	Nausea and vomiting
Changes in jaw development	Acidic damage to oral tissues
Osteonecrosis related to bisphosphonate therapy	Heightened gag reflexes

In general, the therapeutic effects and toxicities of cancer chemotherapy arise from damage to rapidly dividing cancer and normal cells. Only a few anticancer agents can specifically target cancer cells. Consequently, most cancer chemotherapeutic agents inadvertently damage normal tissues of the body. Because the growth fraction for cancer is usually much higher than most normal tissue compartments, there is a quantitative difference in damage to the cancer cells compared with normal cells. Although systemic toxic effects of cancer chemotherapy usually result from damage to rapidly dividing cells, some toxicities result from damage that is not specifically related to cell division.

Oral complications of cancer therapy may result directly from the cytotoxic effects (direct toxic effects) of the drugs on oral tissues (including salivary glands) or result from therapy involving distant tissues (indirect toxic effects). The clinical presentation of complications generally represents the results of complex interactions among multiple factors. These oral complications are listed in Table 36-4.

A number of factors affect the clinical expression of oral toxic effects of chemotherapy, the most prominent being which chemotherapeutic agent is administered along with its dose and schedule. The high turnover rate of oral mucosal tissues puts them at risk for the cytotoxic effects of many antineoplastic agents. Direct mucosal damage may be accentuated by many factors, including (1) salivary gland dysfunction, which compromises the barrier and lubricating functions provided by saliva; (2) mucosal trauma or irritation (e.g., from normal oral function, medications, and mouth breathing); and (3) infections caused by indigenous oral flora (especially opportunistic oral pathogens), acquired pathogens, and the reactivation of latent herpesviruses that cause local and systemic complications in patients who become immunosuppressed.

TABLE 36-5 Agents Studied for Oral Mucositis

Class of Agent	Agent	Status MASCC/ISOO* Guideline Regarding Management of Oral Mucositis
Cryotherapy	Ice chips placed in the mouth starting 5 minutes before administration of chemotherapy and replenished as needed for 30-60 minutes, depending on half-life of agent	Recommended during administration of bolus chemotherapy with 5-fluorouracil, ledertrexate, and melphalan
Growth factor	IV keratinocyte growth factor-1 (Kepivance, Amgen)	Recommended in patients with hematologic malignancies receiving high-dose chemotherapy and total body irradiation before autologous stem cell transplantation; FDA approved in this population
	IV fibroblast growth factor-20 (Velafermin, CuraGen)	Development for chemotherapy-induced mucositis recently halted because of negative results from clinical trials
Antiinflammatory agents	Benzydamine hydrochloride mouth rinse	Recommended for patients receiving moderate-dose RT, based on previous evidence, but not FDA approved; phase III trial halted because of negative results of interim analysis
Antioxidants	IV amifostine (Ethyol, MedImmune)	No guideline; insufficient evidence of benefit for radiation-induced oral mucositis
	Topical N-acetyl cysteine (RK-0202, RxKinetix)	Currently in clinical trials for radiation-induced oral mucositis
Promoters of healing	Topical glutamine (Saforis, MGI Pharma)	Currently in clinical trials for chemotherapy-induced oral mucositis
Antimicrobial agents	Antimicrobial lozenges	Not recommended for prevention of radiation-induced oral mucositis
	Systemic acyclovir and analogues	Not recommended for prevention of chemotherapy-induced oral mucositis
	Chlorhexidine mouth rinse	Not recommended for prevention of radiation-induced oral mucositis or for treatment of chemotherapy-induced oral mucositis
Topical coating agents	Topical sucralfate	Not recommended for prevention of radiation-induced oral mucositis
Laser therapy	Laser	Suggested when necessary technology/training is available in patients receiving high-dose chemotherapy or chemoradiotherapy before hematopoietic cell transplant

*Multinational Association for Supportive Care in Cancer and the International Society of Oral Oncology.
FDA, Food and Drug Administration; *RT,* radiation therapy.

Direct Oral Toxic Effects

Oral mucositis

The terms **oral mucositis** and **stomatitis** were often used interchangeably in the past, but they do not reflect identical processes. **Stomatitis** is a more general term and is applied to any inflammatory condition of the oral tissues, regardless of cause, including infections and autoimmune disorders. The term **oral mucositis** is increasingly being applied to inflammation and breakdown of the oral mucosa resulting from damage caused by chemotherapeutic agents or radiation therapy. Oral mucositis is the preferred term to represent the direct mucosal toxicity of cancer therapies on oral mucosal tissues.

Oral mucositis is a significant problem in patients receiving chemotherapy for solid tumors. It has been reported in **20% to 40% of patients receiving conventional chemotherapy** and may affect up to 80% of patients receiving high-dose chemotherapy prior to hematopoietic stem cell transplantation. Oral mucositis can be very **painful** and can significantly **affect nutritional intake, mouth care, and quality of life.** In patients immunosuppressed because of chemotherapy, increased severity of oral mucositis was found to be significantly associated with an increased number of days requiring total parenteral nutrition and parenteral narcotic therapy, increased number of days with fever, incidence of significant infection, increased time in the hospital, and increased total inpatient charges. A reduction in the next dose of chemotherapy was twice as common after cycles with mucositis than after cycles without mucositis. Mucositis is not only a concern for pain and suffering, but it can also cause dose-limiting toxicity of cancer chemotherapy with direct effects on patient survival.

Management of mucositis currently is focused on palliation of pain and efforts to reduce the influence of secondary factors on mucositis. Based on an extensive systematic review of the literature, the Mucositis Study Group of the Multinational Association for Supportive Care in Cancer and the International Society of Oral Oncology (MASCC/ISOO) has developed clinical practice guidelines for the management of mucositis. These guidelines are discussed subsequently and addressed in Table 36-5.

Pain control is provided through various strategies, including topical anesthetics, mucosal coating agents, and systemic pain medications. Focal application of topical anesthetic agents is preferred over widespread oral administration for many reasons. Generalized oral mucosal anesthesia carries the risk of accidental mucosal trauma. Generalized rinsing with anesthetics also may reduce or eliminate the gag reflex, which may increase the risk of aspiration pneumonia. Systemic absorption or swallowing of anesthetics from ulcerated mucosa can result in systemic toxicity, depending on the agent and the dose that is swallowed. However, when mucositis becomes extensive, intentional generalized topical applications of anesthetics are often used to reduce pain.

A common approach to managing oral mucositis is to use a combination solution that includes many different agents, such as topical anesthetics, coating agents, and antifungal drugs. When using these rinses, the clinician faces numerous considerations, as follows:

1. Are all the agents necessary? Topical antifungals have not been shown to be effective for prophylaxis, especially in immunosuppressed patients. Is a topical coating agent necessary, or would a simple topical anesthetic suffice? Are the agents collectively compatible?
2. Are all the agents and their non-active ingredients well tolerated? Diphenhydramine elixir contains alcohol, coloring, and flavoring agents, all of which can irritate damaged mucosa.

3. Have the medications been compounded in the correct proportions, and is the patient using an adequate volume for appropriate dosing? Does compounding reduce the concentration of each agent to a suboptimal level?
4. What is the cost/benefit ratio for the rinse, and are the added pharmacy costs for compounding a combination rinse offset by significantly improved effectiveness and convenience compared with single agents? Because the primary goal of these rinses is to provide pain relief, this can be an important consideration.

When topical pain control strategies become inadequate for controlling pain, systemic analgesics are necessary. Opioids are usually the drugs of choice. Various delivery systems such as time-release oral tablets, dermal patches, and suppositories can also be used to provide adequate pain relief.

The combination of long-term indwelling venous catheters and computerized drug administration pumps to provide patient-controlled analgesia has significantly increased the ability to control severe mucositis pain while reducing the dose and side effects of opioid analgesics.

Multiple studies have shown that good oral hygiene plays an important role in the management of oral mucositis. The MASCC/ISOO guidelines recommend use of a standardized oral care protocol including brushing with a soft toothbrush, flossing, and use of non-medicated rinses (e.g., saline or sodium bicarbonate rinses). Patients and caregivers should be educated regarding the importance of effective oral hygiene.

Various agents have been studied to prevent oral mucositis or to reduce its severity, including cryotherapy, growth factors, antiinflammatory agents, antibacterial agents, promoters of healing, and mucosal coating agents. Table 36-5 lists selected agents studied more recently for oral mucositis.

Salivary gland dysfunction

Saliva has an important role in maintaining oral health. **Although the effects of ionizing radiation on salivary gland tissue have been well documented, the corresponding effects of cancer chemotherapy have not.** Overall, the studies on effects of various chemotherapeutic agents on salivary gland function have produced inconsistent results, with trials showing varied effects on flow rate, sialochemistry, and dry mouth complaints. No histopathologic investigations of major salivary glands have been reported, but a postmortem study showed minor salivary gland damage after the administration of various chemotherapeutic agents, with changes evident in the first 3 weeks after chemotherapy administration followed by gradual healing with minimal or no sequelae several weeks to months after therapy. Clinical observations support the contention that alterations in salivary function associated with cancer chemotherapy are generally reversible, in contrast to the alterations seen after salivary gland exposure to radiation therapy.

Patients with salivary gland dysfunction should be assessed to determine whether they are receiving other drugs that can alter salivary function (e.g., anticholinergics, antiemetic drugs, or tricyclic antidepressants). Oral dryness can also be exacerbated by mouth breathing, oxygen administration, or dehydration.

Attempts to manage salivary gland dysfunction can have beneficial effects on the quality of oral health of cancer patients. Frequent rinsing with normal saline can help keep mucosal surfaces moist, clear debris, and stimulate salivary gland function for short periods. Saliva replacements (mouth-wetting agents) may provide temporary symptomatic relief. Saliva substitutes may be useful. Other strategies to stimulate salivary glands include the use of "taste stimulation" with sugar-free gum or candies and regimens that use cholinergic drugs. Cevimeline and pilocarpine which directly stimulate salivary glands, can be useful for treating xerostomia when functional salivary gland tissue remains. Increasing the ingestion of moist foods (e.g., flavored gelatins), sauces, and gravies can ameliorate the discomfort of eating. Dry or cracked lips should be kept lubricated with agents such as lanolin-based creams and non-perfumed, non-medicated skin moisturizing agents. The use of antibiotic-containing topical agents on the lips may be indicated to prevent secondary infection, especially in immunosuppressed patients.

Neurotoxicity

Direct neurotoxicity from cancer chemotherapy has been noted with certain chemotherapeutic drugs (most commonly the microtubular agents vincristine and vinblastine and taxol). **This neurotoxicity may result in severe, deep-seated, throbbing mandibular or maxillary pain that can mimic dental pathology (i.e., toothache).** Neurotoxicity is generally considered a dose-limiting complication for these drugs, and prompt diagnosis is important. Appropriate dental/periodontal examinations (including tooth vitality testing as necessary) must be performed to rule out pulpal or periodontal sources of pain. Opioid-containing analgesics may be useful in controlling pain, and the use of neurologically active medications may be considered. The neurotoxicity may be transient and generally subsides shortly after dose reduction or cessation of chemotherapy.

Tooth thermal hypersensitivity is occasionally reported by patients after chemotherapy. Symptoms usually resolve spontaneously within a few weeks to months after the discontinuation of chemotherapy. Topical brush-on fluorides, desensitizing toothpastes, and dentin varnishes can be helpful in reducing or eliminating symptoms.

Taste dysfunction is a neurosensory problem that can be associated with cancer chemotherapy. Taste receptors are neuroepithelium-derived cells, with a turnover rate of approximately 10 days. They generally regenerate if not irreversibly damaged. In addition, the damage to olfactory receptor cells must be considered when a patient has taste dysfunction. Aberrations in taste perception can vary from hypergeusia to hypogeusia to dysgeusia. Some patients simultaneously report several different symptoms: hypergeusia with some tastes and dysgeusia with others. Patients receiving cancer chemotherapy occasionally report a bad taste that results from the diffusion of drug into the oral cavity, known as "venous taste phenomenon."

Temporomandibular joint and myofascial pain disorders may manifest as facial pain, headache, temporomandibular joint dysfunction, and occasionally ear or throat pain. The myofascial-based complaints generally result from clenching or bruxing in response to stress, sleep dysfunction, or occasionally CNS toxicity from certain medications. The short-term use of muscle relaxants or anxiolytic agents plus physical therapy (i.e., moist heat applications, massage, and gentle stretching) often resolves these problems. Occlusal splints can be used while sleeping to help patients with more persistent clenching/bruxing tendencies and who present with pain on awakening.

Alterations in dental and skeletal growth and development

As the number of long-term survivors of childhood cancer has increased, the risk for damage to developing dental and skeletal structures from cancer therapies has become apparent. **Chemotherapy-related damage to developing teeth includes hypoplastic dentin and enamel, shortened and conical roots, taurodontic-like teeth, microdontia, incomplete enamel formation, and complete agenesis of teeth.** Eruption patterns may be altered, and changes in alveolar, mandibular, and maxillary bone growth and development can have orthodontic and cosmetic implications. The addition of radiation to treatment protocols (e.g., cranial irradiation for leukemia, etc.) significantly increases the risk for damage to developing teeth.

Osteonecrosis of the jaws related to bisphosphonate therapy

Osteonecrosis of the jaws (ONJ), also called antiresorptive agent-induced osteonecrosis of the jaw (ARONJ) and medication-related osteonecrosis of the jaw, is an oral complication in patients receiving bisphosphonate or RANKL inhibitor therapy. Although this complication has also been reported in patients receiving antiresorptive agents for osteoporosis, cancer patients are at significantly higher risk. The complication must manifest as exposed bone in the mandible or maxilla for at least 8 weeks and may sometimes be accompanied by infection, pain, and swelling. **The risk for ARONJ seems to be related to a combination of (1) the antiresorptive potency of the bisphosphonate administered, (2) the amount and duration of the antiresorptive drug used, and (3) the occurrence of situations requiring bone to heal or remodel.**

Studies have shown that the risk for ARONJ in patients receiving oncologic doses of bisphosphonates or RANKL inhibitors is similar. The occurrence of ARONJ has been reported to be elevated following dental extractions in patients receiving these agents for delaying or preventing skeletal-related events in patients with bone metastases from primary tumors (e.g., breast, prostate, etc.).

All patients treated with antiresorptive drugs should receive a dental examination and be informed about the potential adverse oral effects of these drugs. Patient management should be directed at reducing future needs of dentoalveolar surgery. It is also very **important to establish meticulous preventive dental regimens for patients.** Each preventive dental regimen should be customized to patient needs. In general, these regiments should include patient education, oral hygiene home care routines to reduce dental caries and periodontal disease, elimination of habits that can increase dental disease (e.g., smoking, alcohol, etc.), and a schedule for routine visits to a dentist. Refer to Chapter 29 for further discussion of ARONJ.

Indirect Oral Toxic Effects

Although direct toxic effects are generally the most visible oral complications of cancer chemotherapy, indirect oral effects can potentially be of more concern. The most important indirect toxicities are oral infections associated with myelosuppression and immunosuppression associated with damage to myelogenous stem cells and cellular elements of the immune system. Preexisting oral and dental infections can spread, with the oral cavity serving as the point of entry for organisms into deeper tissues and the systemic circulation. Other indirect toxic effects to the oral cavity are thrombocytopenia, anemia, and GI toxicity (i.e., nausea, vomiting, and alteration in absorption of nutrients).

Oral mucosal infections

The risk for infection increases as the degree and duration of immunosuppression increase. In addition, as immunosuppression worsens, the classic signs and symptoms of oral infection (e.g., redness, swelling, pain) may be reduced because of the same diminished immune responses. Patients who receive cancer therapy can have chronic low-grade oral infections (periodontal disease and endodontic infections) that can become serious infections when the patients become immunocompromised, yet these infections may also go undetected longer because of a lack of cellular response by the immune system. Because of the myelotoxic effects of many cancer therapies, as the neutrophil and platelet numbers decrease, many cancer patients are instructed to stop tooth brushing and flossing when blood counts decrease below certain thresholds. Stopping oral hygiene may unfortunately increase the risk of oral infection.

Fungal infections can occur via superficial colonization by *Candida* species, especially ***Candida albicans,*** and is a common finding in cancer patients receiving chemotherapy. As the degree and duration of immunosuppression increase in patients receiving myelosuppressive/immunosuppressive therapy, there is a distinct increase in the risk for invasive oral fungal infections such as aspergillosis and mucormycosis and numerous other invasive fungal organisms. Yeast and fungal organisms generally have low infectivity, but with changes in the local or systemic immunity, they can pose a significant infectious risk.

Factors affecting oral colonization and infection risk include alterations in competing oral bacterial flora (most commonly associated with the use of systemic antimicrobials), decreased salivary gland flow rates, and immunosuppression. The latter is especially related to neutropenia. Alteration in host oral bacterial flora in cancer patients with myelosuppression supports increased candidal colonization. With the development of new strategies to prevent and treat fungal infections, however, the fungal organisms associated with oral infections are changing. The widespread use of fluconazole prophylaxis has been associated with increasing numbers of *Candida glabrata* (*Torulopsis glabrata*) and *Candida krusei* infections that may have decreased sensitivity to fluconazole and other antifungal agents.

Cochrane systematic reviews have addressed the efficacy of various antifungal drugs in prevention and treatment of oral candidiasis in cancer patients. Nystatin, although commonly used, was found to be ineffective, possibly because it is not absorbed in the GI tract. Drugs partially absorbed from the GI tract, such as topical clotrimazole or miconazole, were found to be effective and can be useful for superficial oral infection. Persistent or locally invasive infection (including atrophic and erythematous candidiasis), especially when a risk exists for systemic spread, should be treated with appropriate systemic agents. Systemic azoles (e.g., fluconazole, itraconazole) that are fully absorbed in the GI tract are very effective against the organisms and generally considered the most effective way to prevent or reduce fungal colonization and subsequent infection. These drugs are secreted in saliva; salivary concentrations of fluconazole are directly proportional to plasma concentrations. It has been suggested that systemic antifungals may be less effective for oral candidiasis in patients with decreased salivary production because of reduced oral delivery of the drug through saliva. In one study, salivary concentrations of fluconazole were not found to correlate to response to therapy, however; this area requires further research.

The treatment of disseminated candidal infections remains difficult and can be complicated by the presence of azole-resistant organisms. Amphotericin B and echinocandins (e.g., caspofungin) are the systemic antifungals of choice for severe deep mycoses, especially in immunocompromised patients. Organisms that can cause serious oral infections in immunocompromised cancer patients include *Aspergillus*, *Mucor*, and *Rhizopus*. These infections often have a nonspecific appearance and can be confused with other oral toxic effects. Diagnosis depends on laboratory tests, and systemic therapy must be instituted immediately because these infections can spread systemically and lead to fatal outcomes.

Viral infections from the herpes group viruses can cause significant oral disease in patients receiving cancer chemotherapy. **Herpes simplex virus (HSV), varicella zoster virus (VZV), cytomegalovirus (CMV), and Epstein-Barr virus (EBV) are recognized causes of oral lesions in cancer patients.** Most infections with HSV, VZV, and EBV represent reactivation of latent virus, whereas CMV infections can result from either reactivation of latent virus or newly acquired virus. Other viruses causing oral lesions in cancer chemotherapy and hematopoietic cell transplant patients are adenovirus, coxsackieviruses, and human herpesvirus. The diagnosis of viral lesions in the mouth can be made through direct immunofluorescent examination of scrapings from lesions, through viral culture, and sometimes through examination of biopsy material with immunohistologic stains specific for each virus.

Finally, **bacterial infections** can have a broad display of untoward effects in the mouth. The different environmental niches of the oral cavity—mucosal surfaces, periodontal sulci, and tooth surfaces—harbor a wide array of organisms. In immunosuppressed patients, the potential for acquisition of non-oral bacteria must also be considered. As with fungal and viral infections, the risk for bacterial infection increases as the severity and duration of immunosuppression increase. Neutropenia is the primary risk factor predisposing to bacterial infection, with risk increasing significantly when the neutrophil count decreases to less than $500/mm^3$. Antibiotic prophylaxis is indicated in these situations. As infectious disease protocols and antibiotics have evolved, the pressures on the oral microflora have been constantly altered. Over the years, oral flora in cancer patients have shown a shift from a risk for overgrowth by primarily gram-negative enteric bacilli (e.g., *Pseudomonas*, *E. coli*, *Serratia*, and *Klebsiella*) to the reemergence of a risk for infection primarily from gram-positive organisms, especially streptococcal and staphylococcal species. Mucositis and mechanical disruption in the oral mucosa can create a point of entry for oral bacteria, and oral colonization or secondary infection of the oral tissues can increase the severity and course of oral mucositis.

Chlorhexidine oral rinses can promote a decreased rate of colonization by bacteria in and around teeth and reduce gingival infections. Although topical chlorhexidine (0.12%) is effective in reducing gram-positive bacterial colonization and associated periodontal infections, studies using chlorhexidine to diminish the severity and duration of mucositis have produced inconsistent results, with some studies showing benefit and others showing no benefit.

Oral hemorrhage

Hemorrhage from oral tissues in patients receiving cancer therapy can result from thrombocytopenia, loss of coagulation factors from disseminated intravascular coagulation or liver disease, mucosal infections (including gingivitis and periodontitis), and trauma. **Spontaneous mucosal petechiae and gingival bleeding may be observed when the platelet count decreases to less than $20,000/mm^3$.** Damage to mucosal tissues, such as damage resulting from oral HSV infections, increases the risk of bleeding. Trauma associated with oral function can also induce minor hemorrhage.

Oral hemorrhage in cancer patients with thrombocytopenia is rarely a debilitating complication, although its occurrence can be alarming to patients, caregivers, and family. Local measures center on forming an adequate clot and protecting the clot until healing has occurred. Direct pressure applied by moist gauze or gauze soaked in topical thrombin can be used. A vasoconstrictor such as epinephrine can help with initial control, but rebound vasodilation can occur as the drug's effect wears off. Clot-forming agents, such as those made from microfibrillar collagen hemostatic products (Avitene Hemostat, INSTAT), fibrin glue, and chitosan (HemCon), can also be used to organize and stabilize clots. Platelet transfusions are usually not required except for patients whose platelet counts are profoundly suppressed, resulting in insufficient clot formation and repeated significant bleeding episodes. Aprotinin or aminocaproic acid can be used adjunctively to promote coagulation, especially when platelet transfusions are marginally effective in controlling bleeding.

Gastrointestinal effects: nutritional disturbances, nausea, and emesis

A frequent and often significant site of toxicity of cancer chemotherapy is the GI tract. As it does with the oral mucosa, chemotherapy can damage the rapidly proliferating mucosal lining of the stomach and intestines. The resulting mucositis can lead to significant discomfort (cramping, pain), diarrhea, ulceration, and disruption in the absorption of nutrients. In addition, gastric injury plus CNS toxicity from chemotherapy can cause patients to have frequent and profound nausea and emesis. This complication can significantly affect the patient's quality of life during and after cancer chemotherapy.

In addition to the effect of emesis on the quality of life is the negative influence on oral nutrition intake and the potential damage to oral tissues after emesis; the pH of oral tissues can decrease to approximately 2.0. In the presence of mucositis, the exposure of compromised mucosa to this acidic fluid can potentially damage the tissues further. Also, the vigorous tongue movements usually associated with chemotherapy-associated emesis can result in increased trauma to the tongue and floor of the mouth as these tissues move against incisal and occlusal surfaces.

Protocols to reduce or prevent nausea and vomiting during chemotherapy have become remarkably effective. Often initiated prophylactically, these therapies can minimize the problem and ensure patient comfort. Strategies often combine approaches that target the GI mucosa and the CNS nausea and vomiting centers. The nausea and vomiting associated with chemotherapy can result in adverse conditioning such that normal smells, tastes, and other associated stimuli can induce nausea and vomiting; even just driving by the clinic or hospital where the therapy was administered can be a trigger. Patients may even develop an aversion to swallowing their own saliva, tooth brushing, or wearing removable dental appliances. These conditions may also trigger a heightened gag reflex. Systematic deconditioning strategies can generally help control or eliminate this problem and allow for the resumption of routine oral care.

SUMMARY OF ORAL COMPLICATIONS OF CHEMOTHERAPY

The oral cavity is highly susceptible to the direct and indirect toxic effects of cancer chemotherapy and therapeutic ionizing radiation. Stabilization of oral health before treatment and supportive oral and dental care are crucial components of the patient's overall management, affecting all phases of therapy. Oral complications occurring during and after therapy can profoundly add to the suffering of the patient, adversely affect the success of therapy, and significantly increase the overall cost of care. Oral care should be preventive and therapeutic to minimize oral and associated systemic complications.

Oral complications of chemotherapy are generally acute (i.e., during therapy) and resolve shortly after the cessation of therapy. Consequently, **the dentist must clearly understand the specifics of the proposed therapy and the potential oral problems based on the patient's current oral health and develop a plan that covers all phases of therapy**.

CASE DISCUSSION

First and foremost, you must discuss with Mrs. P the risks and benefits of using antiresorptive agents. All drugs have a risk of use and a benefit that is derived by the patient. These antiresorptive drugs, such as zoledronic acid, are extremely important in reducing the number of and delaying the onset of skeletal-related events. The benefit is that zoledronic acid can improve the quality of life and reduce the chance of mortality of the patient. The oral risk is that the patient may develop an ARONJ. Although ARONJ can be disconcerting to the patient, it is managed by the dentists and will, in most cases, allow the patient to have normal, pain-free occlusal function. The risk of death from an ARONJ is negligible when compared to the mortality associated with bone metastases.

GENERAL REFERENCES

1. Adorno-Cruz V, Kibria G, Liu X, Doherty M, Junk DJ, Guan D, Hubert C, Venere M, Mulkearns-Hubert E, Sinyuk M, Alvarado A, Caplan AI, Rich J, Gerson SL, Lathia J, Liu H: Cancer stem cells: targeting the roots of cancer, seeds of metastasis, and sources of therapy resistance, *Cancer Res* 75(6):924–929, March 15, 2015, http://dx.doi.org/10.1158/0008-5472.CAN-14-3225.
2. Al-Ansari S, Zecha JA, Barasch A, de Lange J, Rozema FR, Raber-Durlacher JE: Oral mucositis induced by anticancer therapies, *Curr Oral Health Rep* 2:202–211, 2015.
3. Applegate CC, Lane MA: Role of retinoids in the prevention and treatment of colorectal cancer, *World J Gastrointest Oncol* 7(10):184–203, October 15, 2015, http://dx.doi.org/10.4251/wjgo.v7.i10.184.
4. Barillet M, Prevost V, Joly F, Clarisse B: Oral antineoplastic agents: how do we care about adherence?, *Br J Clin Pharmacol* 80(6):1289–1302, December 2015, http://dx.doi.org/10.1111/bcp.12734. Epub 2015 Oct 28.
5. Carreras Puigvert J, Sanjiv K, Helleday T: Targeting DNA repair, DNA metabolism and replication stress as anti-cancer strategies, *FEBS J*, October 28, 2015, http://dx.doi.org/10.1111/febs.13574.
6. Cook AM, Lesterhuis WJ, Nowak AK, Lake RA: Chemotherapy and immunotherapy: mapping the road ahead, *Curr Opin Immunol* 39:23–29, December 24, 2015, http://dx.doi.org/10.1016/j.coi.2015.12.003.
7. Di Lauro L, Barba M, Pizzuti L, Vici P, Sergi D, Di Benedetto A, Mottolese M, Speirs V, Santini D, De Maria R, Maugeri-Saccà M: Androgen receptor and antiandrogen therapy in male breast cancer, *Cancer Lett* 368(1):20–25, November 1, 2015, http://dx.doi.org/10.1016/j.canlet.2015.07.040.
8. Lalla RV, Bowen J, Barasch A, Elting L, Epstein J, Keefe DM, McGuire DB, Migliorati C, Nicolatou-Galitis O, Peterson DE, Raber-Durlacher JE, Sonis ST, Elad S: Mucositis Guidelines Leadership Group of the Multinational Association of Supportive Care, MASCC/ISOO clinical practice guidelines for the management of mucositis secondary to cancer therapy, *Cancer* 120:1453–1461, 2014.
9. Mariotti A: Bisphosphonates and osteonecrosis of the jaws, *J Dent Educ* 72:919–929, 2008.
10. National Cancer Institute: *Oral complications of chemotherapy and head/neck radiation.* Available at: http://www.cancer.gov/cancertopics/pdq/supportivecare/oralcomplications/healthprofessional. Accessed January 19, 2016.
11. Robinson A, Scully C: Pharmacology: new therapies and challenges, *Br Dent J* 217(6):258–259, 2014.

PART III

Special Subjects in Pharmacology and Therapeutics

37

Medications for Management of Chronic, Non-Odontogenic Pain

Robert L. Merrill and Raymond A. Dionne

KEY INFORMATION

- Pharmacologic treatment of orofacial pain disorders involves knowledge of many different classes of medications.
- The neurotransmitters associated with the reticular activating system (serotonin, norepinephrine, dopamine, and acetylcholine) mediate both pain and sleep.
- The mechanisms of chronic pain are similar in the three categories of chronic orofacial pain.
- Pharmacologic agents that can be used to manage orofacial pain conditions in one pain category may be useful for pain in the other categories.
- Tricyclic antidepressants are used for pain relief in certain situations and can induce sleep affecting serotonin and adrenergic receptors by blocking reuptake (Chapter 10). These medications are commonly used in the medical community to treat headache disorders, neuropathic pain disorders, and musculoskeletal pain disorders.
- Other classes of antidepressants do not have the same impact on pain as the tricyclic antidepressants but are often used as adjunctive therapy in chronic pain to treat the depression and anxiety that are a result of the pain.
- Antiseizure medications are used to treat both neuropathic pain disorders and headache disorders.

CASE STUDY

A 64-year-old woman was referred to the orofacial pain clinic by her dentist for a toothache that has persisted for 4 months despite dental interventions including remaking a crown and root canal therapy, all without benefit. She described the pain as a continuous, deep, aching, and burning pain in the left posterior mandibular teeth. She was not aware of any relieving or aggravating factors. Acetaminophen or ibuprofen did not help the pain. She indicated that she could chew on the left side without pain. The pain seemed to worsen in the evening, making it difficult to get to sleep. What is your diagnosis and treatment plan for this patient?

INTRODUCTION TO PHARMACOLOGIC MANAGEMENT OF CHRONIC PAIN

The management of chronic pain differs from the management of acute pain. In general, the emphasis in dentistry is acute pain management with more limited experience in the diagnosis and management of chronic pain. An unfortunate sequela of this is that patients with chronic pain conditions are seen first by clinicians who attempt to treat the chronic pain condition with acute treatment protocols, often resulting in tooth loss and/or unnecessary surgery. The Commission on Dental Accreditation recognizes orofacial pain as a specialty of general dentistry, and there are now 13 orofacial pain programs in dental schools around the United States that focus on chronic pain management. Treatment of chronic pain requires physical medicine, as well as pharmacologic and psychological management protocols to address the pain problems effectively. The basic classification of orofacial pain syndromes primarily involves non-odontogenic pain disorders within the rubrics of neuropathic, neurovascular, musculoskeletal pain disorders, and sleep-related breathing disorders. The pharmacologic management of the disorders within each of these categories may involve using similar medications due to the commonality of pain mechanisms, pathways, neurotransmitters or neuromodulators, and receptors among the various categories of pain.

This chapter will not discuss the use of opioids for chronic pain other than to indicate that in cases of intractable pain resulting from cancer or other conditions such as chronic neuropathy due to failed temporomandibular surgery, long-term use of opioids may be the only option for helping the patient, although this is rare because opioids generally are less effective in treating neuropathic pain than several other drugs.

Classification of Orofacial Pain

The scope of disorders associated with orofacial pain is large and includes musculoskeletal disorders (e.g., TMDs), neuropathic disorders (e.g., trigeminal neuralgia), and neurovascular disorders (e.g., headaches) (Table 37-1).

Since basic pain mechanisms are shared among the three general categories, including both peripheral and central mechanisms, there is a significant overlap with the medications used to treat the various conditions. In addition, when treating chronic orofacial pain disorders, other factors and comorbidities may need to be addressed to optimize treatment, necessitating use of psychiatric and/or sleep medications.

The Trigeminal Nerve and Its Role in Orofacial Pain

The trigeminal nerve conducts pain sensation to the central nervous system (CNS) as shown in Figure 37-1. Nerve fibers in the trigeminal nerve also innervate **blood vessel in the dura and pia mater** where **vasoactive** and **inflammatory** actions occur. There are complex relationships between serotonin (Fig. 37-2) and other mediators, and these are important in many aspects of orofacial pain.

DRUGS FOR THE TREATMENT OF MUSCULOSKELETAL PAIN

The optimum management of musculoskeletal pain employs both physical medicine modalities and pharmacologic management with the emphasis placed on physical medicine. Centrally acting skeletal muscle relaxants are indicated for relief of acute painful musculoskeletal conditions of local origin, but they should be used only as an adjunct to a physical medicine program that includes physical therapy, moist heat and ice, and other nonpharmacologic therapies. There are few studies demonstrating the efficacy of muscle relaxants, and many clinicians are skeptical about their widespread use because of a lack of evidence of benefit apart from the sedative effects of the drugs. There are many causes for muscle spasms, and muscle relaxants are not effective for all causes.

The **sedative effect** generated by most of the muscle relaxants may provide the most benefit. Sleep and pain are closely tied together. Patients who do not sleep well tend to have more hyperalgesia the next day, and patients who sleep better have less pain. **Histamine** is released from the tuberomamillary nucleus in the hypothalamus and is a neurotransmitter that modulates wakefulness. Additionally, histamine may be involved in muscle pain and muscle fatigue, and blocking the histamine activity may relieve muscle stiffness and muscle pain. Furthermore, when the histamine receptors are blocked centrally, sleepiness is enhanced. This may be the main benefit of muscle relaxants with antihistaminic activity contributing to the sedative effect.

TABLE 37-1 Classification of Orofacial Pain

Disorder	Examples
Musculoskeletal	Myalgia, myofascial pain
	TM joint disorders, e.g., disc displacements ± reduction
	Arthritides, e.g., osteoarthritis, rheumatoid arthritis, capsulitis
Neuropathic pain	Trigeminal neuralgia, other chronic pain
Neurovascular disorders	Tension-type headache
	Migraine
	Cluster headache

Muscle Relaxant Drugs

The following drugs are generally considered to have muscle relaxant capabilities, and most have anticholinergic and antihistaminic side effects (Table 37-2).

Nonsteroidal Antiinflammatory Drugs (NSAIDs)

Most of the NSAIDs are similar in action; their use in orofacial pain is usually limited to acute conditions. NSAIDs are often used long-term for **temporomandibular joint arthritides**, but not without adverse effects. Besides altering platelet function, long-term use of NSAIDs may risk a detrimental effect on the endogenous reparative process within the joint as well as other systemic adverse effects. For the most part, NSAIDs are used as temporary measures to stabilize acute flare-ups of pain, and long-term use is not usually recommended. Selective COX-2 inhibitors (e.g., celecoxib) were developed to avoid the adverse effects of dual COX-1/COX-2 inhibitors but were recognized to have the potential for increased incidence of cardiovascular events and stroke, as well as marginal activity in the treatment of TMD, and they should only be considered in patients where a dual COX-1/COX-2 inhibitor is contraindicated. Although any NSAID can provide relief from pain and inflammation, three NSAIDs are discussed next because of unique qualities or delivery systems.

Ketorolac

Injectable ketorolac is effective for managing acute inflammatory pain conditions as well as being a preemptive agent after procedures that are likely to cause postprocedure inflammation, such as

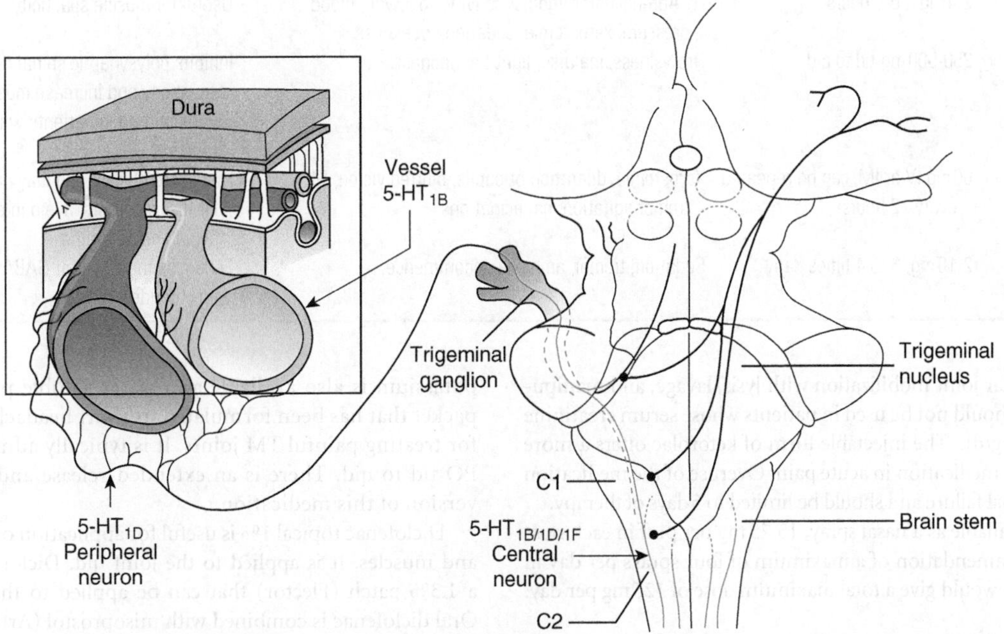

FIG 37-1 Trigeminal nerve and its role in orofacial pain. The innervation of the dura matter by the ophthalmic (1st) branch of the trigeminal nerve. Vessels contain serotonin (5-HT_{1B}) receptors, while the nerves contain 5-HT_{1D} receptors. Afferent fibers synapse in the trigeminocervical complex, which extends from the trigeminal nucleus caudalis to the dorsal horns of C1 and C2 and contains $5\text{-HT}_{1B/D/F}$ receptors. Second-order neurons project to more rostral brain areas, such as periaqueductal grey and thalamus. (See Fig. 37-2.) (From McMahon SB, Kolzenburg M: *Wall and Melzack's textbook of pain*, ed 5, 2006, Churchill Livingstone.)

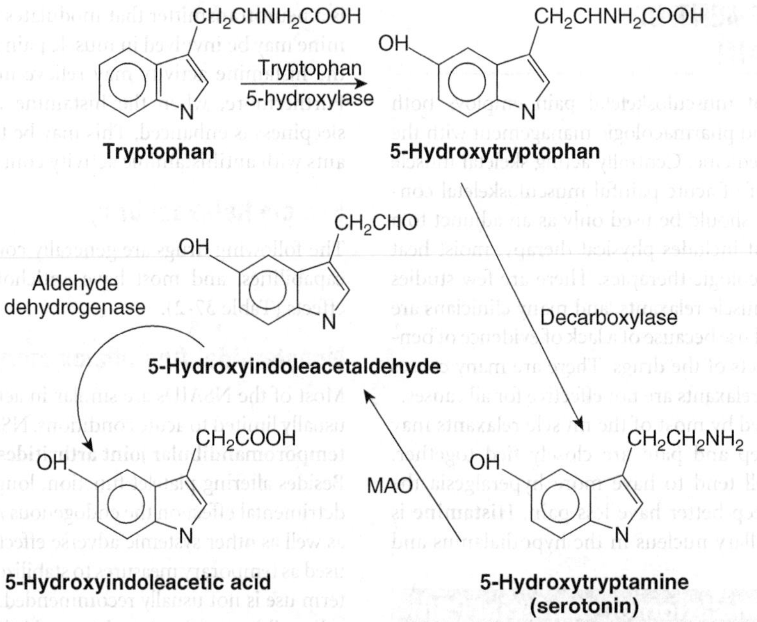

FIG 37-2 Biosynthesis and metabolism of serotonin. MAO, Monoamine oxidase.

TABLE 37-2 Muscle Relaxant Drugs

Generic Drug	Dose	Adverse Effects	Other Comments
Cyclobenzaprine	5-10 mg tid	Weight gain, cardiac arrhythmias; caution in elderly	Normalizes quality and duration of sleep
Carisoprodol	250-350 mg tid and at bedtime	Ranked 54th of 234 abused drugs; metabolized to meprobamate, a major tranquilizer; seizures	
Methocarbamol	500 mg tid	Seizures, drowsiness, nausea blurred vision	Most effective for muscle spasticity
Metaxalone	800 mg/day to 800 mg bid to tid	Leukopenia, hepatotoxicity, rash, dizziness, headache nausea	Use with caution in patients with hepatic impairment
Baclofen	10 mg/day to 20 mg tid	Confusion, blurred vision, abdominal pain, and fatigue	Not metabolized in liver
Tizanidine	2-4 mg q 6-8 hours	α_2-Adrenoceptor agonist activity, so lowers blood pressure; xerostomia, sedation, weakness	Useful for muscle spasticity
Chlorzoxazone	250-500 mg tid to qid	Drowsiness, malaise, light-headedness	Inhibits polysynaptic spinal reflexes to reduce spasticity and increase muscle mobility; use with caution in patients with compromised liver function
Orphenadrine	60 mg IV or IM, can be repeated every 12 hours	Xerostomia, dilatation of pupils, blurred vision, GI, tremor agitation, hallucinations	Histamine blocker and may have activity on NMDA receptors; avoid in patients who have to avoid antihistamines
Diazepam	2-10 mg, 3 to 4 times daily	Sedation, tremor, amnesia, incontinence,	Enhances the effect of GABA at $GABA_A$ receptors on chloride channels

temporomandibular joint mobilization with lysis, lavage, and manipulation. Ketorolac should not be used in patients whose serum creatinine is greater than 5 mg/dL. The injectable form of ketorolac offers a more rapid and effective medication in acute pain. Overuse of the medication can cause acute renal failure and should be limited to 5 days of therapy.

Ketorolac is available as a nasal spray, 15.75 mg per puff in each nostril, with the recommendation of a maximum of four sprays per day in each nostril, which would give a total maximum dose of 126 mg per day.

Diclofenac potassium

Diclofenac is particularly useful as a topical agent for painful TMJ capsulitis and myalgia associated with TMD. It comes in three different delivery systems: oral, a topical gel, and a topical patch. Diclofenac potassium is available as a 50-mg tablet. It can be dosed tid to qid with a maximum daily dose of 200 mg. Diclofenac potassium is also available as a water-soluble powder in a 50-mg packet that has been formulated to abort headache. It is very useful for treating painful TM joints. It is typically administered at 50 mg PO tid to qid. There is an extended-release and a delayed-release version of this medication.

Diclofenac topical 1% is useful for application on painful TM joints and muscles. It is applied to the joint qid. Diclofenac also comes in a 1.3% patch (Flector) that can be applied to the painful area bid. Oral diclofenac is combined with misoprostol (Arthrotec) to limit the amount of GI irritation caused by diclofenac.

Naproxen sodium

Naproxen sodium is one of the preferred NSAIDs for treatment of TMJ. Naproxen sodium is usually dosed at 500 mg bid due to its longer half-life.

Adrenocorticosteroids

Adrenocorticosteroids are useful in the treatment of **acute inflammatory pain**, headache, and some neuropathic pain. Corticosteroids are effective in treatment of cluster headache and for intractable migraine that has not responded to other forms of therapy. Normally, a high initial dose of steroid is given, and then the drug is tapered over a 1- or 2-week period. Steroids are used in topical, oral, and injectable forms.

Steroids are thought to act through a number of mechanisms on chronic pain syndromes; for example, steroid modulation of γ-aminobutyric acid ($GABA_A$) receptors located outside the blood–brain barrier suppresses neurogenic inflammation and (calcitonin gene-related peptide) CGRP- and (substance P) SP-induced plasma extravasation. Injectable and oral steroid therapy is effective in management of **acute and chronic temporomandibular joint inflammation.** Intraarticular corticosteroids reduce pain and swelling associated with **inflammatory disease of both muscles and joints.** Patients who have inflamed temporomandibular joints are typically started on a protocol including soft diet, moist heat, NSAIDs, and possibly steroids to suppress the joint inflammation.

Cortisone and hydrocortisone injected into the joint are beneficial, but they tend to diffuse out of the joint rapidly, thereby not giving a sustained effect. The disodium phosphate ester of betamethasone is used with the insoluble acetate ester form, imparting a rapid effect from the phosphate ester and a sustained effect from the acetate ester. Triamcinolone acetonide and triamcinolone hexacetonide also have very low solubility and a long duration. Up to three injections may be given in a joint, but there should be an interval of 4 weeks between injections.

DRUGS FOR NEUROPATHIC PAIN

The current understanding of neuropathic pain includes a number of disorders that are not discussed in detail here. Trigeminal neuropathy is grossly broken down into disorders involving peripheral and central sensitization mechanisms. The treatment of neuropathy requires an understanding of all these condition and mechanisms. **Trigeminal neuralgia is the most common neuropathy seen in the orofacial region.** The discussion of those disorders will focus on trigeminal neuralgia, with a brief discussion of some other neuropathic pain syndromes.

The antiseizure medications remain the mainstay for treating these conditions along with neural blockade where appropriate. For **trigeminal neuralgia** and **glossopharyngeal neuralgia, antiseizure drugs** are still regarded as the **gold standard for treatment** because of their superior clinical efficacy.

Antiseizure Drugs

The mechanisms responsible for the action of antiseizure medications are variable and depend on the type of medication. The medications most effective for trigeminal neuralgia are use-dependent Na^+-channel blockers; however, these medications are not usually the most effective for the other chronic peripheral and central neuropathies.

Carbamazepine

Carbamazepine is considered the gold standard for the management of trigeminal neuralgia, but it is also used to treat other neuropathic pain conditions. The primary mode of action of carbamazepine is thought to be its action as a use-dependent **Na^+-channel blocker**, inhibiting repetitive neuronal discharge. Structurally, it is similar and related to tricyclic antidepressants.

Before taking carbamazepine, the patient should have baseline laboratory values for liver function and complete blood count, platelet, and differential. An extended-release form of carbamazepine is available. This medication only requires a twice-per-day dosing schedule, which is more convenient for the patient and aids in compliance. Initially, liver function tests should be obtained every 30 days to check liver response to the medication. Carbamazepine induces CYP3A4 and other subfamilies of the cytochrome P450 system, causing increased metabolism of the drug with lowered serum levels. The result of this effect is noted after 1 to 2 weeks of therapy and requires increasing the dose to obtain better pain control. The inductive effect also reduces the effect of several other drugs.

Oxcarbazepine

Oxcarbazepine is structurally similar to carbamazepine, and its mechanism may involve similar use-dependent inhibition of voltage-dependent Na^+ action potentials. Oxcarbazepine does not induce liver microsomal enzymes and therefore does not decrease its own half-life or the half-lives of other drugs. Compared to carbamazepine, oxcarbazepine has an increased tolerability and safety margin. It does not require liver enzymes or complete blood count monitoring, but electrolytes should be checked for Na^+ concentrations, as oxcarbazepine can induce hyponatremia. Oxcarbazepine can be titrated more rapidly than carbamazepine, which is a distinct advantage for patients in an acute phase of trigeminal neuralgia.

Gabapentin

Gabapentin has been used for seizures since the mid-1980s but did not become available in the United States until the 1990s. Gabapentin is a structural analogue of GABA and was developed as a GABA agonist; however, its mode of action is not through action on GABA receptors. Gabapentin decreases hyperalgesia in the formalin test, a model for centralized neuropathy. It has been hypothesized that the **$\alpha_2\delta$ subunit of voltage-dependent Ca^{2+}** channels maintains mechanical hypersensitivity in neuropathic pain, and recent studies have shown that gabapentin selectively interacts with these units to reduce activity; however, this may not correlate with its therapeutic effects.

Gabapentin crosses membrane barriers using the L-amino acid transporter system. A small amount is also known to cross by passive diffusion. It concentrates in the brain cytosol at a ratio of 10:1 compared with the extracellular space. An analgesic effect is attained rapidly but its anticonvulsant effect is delayed, indicating probable different mechanisms for the two effects.

Gabapentin is excreted unchanged in the kidney. It has few interactions with other medications, and the side-effect profile is relatively benign compared with the other antiseizure drugs.

Valproic acid

Valproic acid was the first antiepilepsy medication approved by the Food and Drug Administration for migraine. Valproic acid is structurally different from other anticonvulsants, and its mechanism of antiseizure and analgesic action is related to **inhibition of Na^+ channels, inhibition of T-type Ca^{2+} channels,** and **facilitation of GABAergic neurotransmission** by inhibiting GABA aminotransferase and activating glutamic acid decarboxylase. In seizures, valproic acid may have direct effects on neuronal membranes, inhibiting kindling and reducing excitatory neurotransmission by the amino acids (see Chapter 12). Valproic acid is also used as a mood stabilizer in manic-depressive disorders.

Lamotrigine

Lamotrigine is a novel anticonvulsant drug that is useful for trigeminal neuralgia through its action as a Na^+-channel blocker. The cellular mechanism of **Na^+-channel blockade** is the same mechanism by which carbamazepine and phenytoin exert their action; however, it is unlikely that Na^+-channel blockade is lamotrigine's only cellular mechanism.

Topiramate

The antiseizure drug topiramate is a monosaccharide derivative that modulates voltage-dependent Na^+ conductance, potentiates GABA-evoked currents, and blocks the kainate and α-amino-3-hydroxy-5-methyl-4-isoxazole propionate (AMPA) subtypes of the glutamate receptor. The Na^+-channel effect and blocking of the metabotropic AMPA and kainate receptor may account for this medication's ability to suppress trigeminal neuralgia and other neuropathic pain states. Topiramate has been shown to have antihyperalgesic and antinociceptive activity in animal models of neuropathic pain. Topiramate is FDA approved for partial onset seizures, primary generalized tonic-clonic seizures, and migraine prophylaxis.

Side effects include sedation, dizziness, nervousness, ataxia, nausea, weight loss, metabolic acidosis, kidney stones, secondary narrow angle-closure glaucoma, sedation, and some weight loss. The sprinkle capsule formulation allows topiramate to be taken with a tablespoon of soft food if needed. Important drug interactions of topiramate with carbamazepine, phenytoin, and valproate can decrease topiramate levels due to increased clearance. Topiramate may increase the clearance of phenytoin and valproate and reduce the effectiveness of oral contraceptives. One of the modest side effects of topiramate is weight loss, approximately 6 kg after 12 to 18 months of use. It has been observed that the weight changes are greatest in patients with more weight to lose. Generally, the weight is gained back after 18 months.

Phenytoin

Phenytoin was the first antiseizure medication used to treat neuropathic pain. Its mode of action is similar to carbamazepine. Phenytoin suppresses ectopic discharge of neuromas when applied topically. This effect is probably moderated by a reduction in high-frequency repetitive firing of action potentials by **blocking Na^+ channels**. Phenytoin is available orally and as an intravenous preparation that has been shown to be beneficial in managing acute flare-ups of neuropathic pain.

Pregabalin

Pregabalin is the first antiepileptic drug approved by the FDA since 1999. It has been approved for the treatment for painful diabetic neuropathy and post-herpetic neuralgia and recently was approved for the treatment of fibromyalgia. Pregabalin is an active S-enantiomer of racemic 3-isobutyl gamma-aminobutyric acid. The mechanism of action for pain is still to be determined. **Similar to gabapentin**, it is not metabolized in the liver and has no interaction with cytochrome P450 isoenzyme system and has no known drug–drug interactions. The most common side effects are dizziness and somnolence. Pregabalin has been shown to improve slow-wave delta sleep and may be useful in sleep disorders associated with poor-quality delta sleep. In these cases, taking the majority of the dose at bedtime can be useful. Pregabalin has been designated as a Schedule V controlled substance because of its potential for abuse and dependence. Patients with neuropathy are started at 50 mg three times daily and may be titrated up to 300 mg daily within 1 week based on efficacy and tolerability. It is generally dosed at one-third to one-sixth the dose of gabapentin and is considered more potent than gabapentin. Most patients taking pregabalin only need to be dosed two times per day. Generally, pregabalin can reduce both neuropathic pain and anxiety associated with it within 1 week of initiation.

Tiagabine

Tiagabine is a potent and selective GABA reuptake inhibitor with antiallodynic effects noted in rodent models of neuropathic pain. The antinociceptive effect was related to inhibition of GABA reuptake and resultant **increased extracellular GABA** levels. Because pretreatment of experimental animals with a $GABA_B$ receptor antagonist eliminated the antinociceptive effect of tiagabine, $GABA_B$ receptors may be involved in the tiagabine effect. The antiallodynic effects are dose dependent, with significant increases in threshold response to tactile stimulation. For trigeminal neuralgia, tiagabine is used as an add-on drug in combination with another antiseizure medication when better control of the pain is needed.

Levetiracetam

Levetiracetam could be a useful medication for trigeminal neuralgia. It is not metabolized in the liver. Although the side-effect profile is relatively benign, the drug has some potential psychiatric side effects that may limit its use. It is associated with aggressive behavior, hostility, suicidality, and psychosis.

Zonisamide

Zonisamide is a sulfonamide antiseizure medication that is unlike the other antiseizure medications mentioned earlier. It is thought to block sodium and T-type calcium channels, as well as modulating GABAergic and glutamatergic neurotransmission. One advantage is a longer half-life that allows once per day dosing. Zonisamide can cause weight loss similar to topiramate. Zonisamide is useful for both neuropathic pain and migraine prophylaxis.

Antidepressants

Antidepressants, especially tricyclic antidepressants, are useful in treating neuropathic pain. They are less effective than carbamazepine in treating trigeminal neuralgia. Their use includes migraine prophylaxis as listed later. **Tricyclic antidepressants inhibit the reuptake of norepinephrine and serotonin**, both of which appear important in neuropathic pain and pain control.

Adrenocorticosteroids

After nerve injury in which the afferent sensory fibers are crushed or severed, the proximal portion of the nerve is stimulated by nerve growth factor to repair and reestablish a connection with the distal portion. This has been used as a model for neuropathic pain. In this process, the proximal terminal forms a mass of neuronal sprouts known as a **neuroma**. The sprouts generate spontaneous ectopic discharges signaling pain centrally. Application of steroids has been shown to reduce the neuronal activity. The reduction in spontaneous discharge is not caused by a reduction in the number of sprouts, but it probably arises from a stabilization of the neuronal membrane conductivity. A steroid such as dexamethasone may be injected into the area of the neuroma. Often multiple injections with local anesthetic and steroid are needed to stop the spontaneous discharge.

Other Medications

N-methyl-D-aspartate receptor antagonists

It has been shown that 90% of C fibers (unmyelinated, small-diameter, low conduction velocity nerve fibers) contain glutamate and probably release both glutamate and substance P from their peripheral terminals when the stimulus is sufficiently long lasting, at least for several seconds to minutes. Glutamate is an agonist at the *N*-methyl-D-aspartate (NMDA) and α-amino-3-hydroxy-5-methyl-4-isoxazolepropionic acid (AMPA) receptors but cannot activate the NMDA receptor without the presence of the co-agonist glycine. The NMDA receptor has been considered a potential target for modulating chronic pain; however, the current NMDA receptor antagonists have severe side effects, limiting their usefulness. Blocking the glycine site may provide a target without the profound side effects accompanying the currently available NMDA receptor antagonists. Ketamine is a voltage-dependent blocker of the NMDA receptor channels (see Chapter 15). The NMDA receptor is an obvious target for pain intervention because it is known to have a role in long-term potentiation and central sensitization. Ketamine and dextromethorphan are both NMDA channel blockers and are effective in reducing NMDA-mediated responses in the dorsal horn nociceptive system. Recent studies have shown that dextromethorphan and ketamine are able to reduce temporal summation hyperalgesia and spontaneous discharge in neuropathic pain.

These agents are used when other medications have failed to provide adequate relief in centralized neuropathies. Ketamine is a strong NMDA receptor antagonist, but its side effects are disturbing. Dextromethorphan has fewer attendant problems associated with its use but also is only a weak NMDA receptor antagonist with inconsistent benefits. Nevertheless, its antagonistic activity on the NMDA receptor has been reported to be useful for treating chronic pain. Sedation, dizziness, and rash are the most common side effects.

Drugs that act at α-adrenergic receptors

Central neuropathic orofacial pain conditions are often influenced by the sympathetic nervous system. Many of the patients diagnosed with neuropathic pain respond to sympathetic nervous system blockade, relieving their tooth site pain and fulfilling the criteria for a diagnosis of sympathetically maintained pain. Those pain conditions associated with sympathetically maintained pain include reflex sympathetic dystrophy and causalgia. Historically, treatment has involved sympathetic ganglion blockade with local anesthetics or clonidine to stop sympathetic outflow and relieve pain. Phentolamine, an α-adrenergic receptor antagonist, acts on injured nociceptors to reduce sympathetically mediated pain. Continued nociceptor activity is mediated through local sympathetic fiber release of norepinephrine, stimulating the α_1-adrenergic receptors and activating the affected nociceptors. α_2-Adrenergic receptors function as autoreceptors on the peripheral terminals of the postganglionic sympathetic nerve. When these receptors are activated, the release of norepinephrine from the sympathetic fibers is reduced. Tizanidine, like clonidine, is an α_2-adrenergic receptor agonist that decreases sympathetic release of NE. In sympathetically mediated pain states, it is desirable to either block α_1-adrenergic receptor activity to reduce the postjunctional effect of norepinephrine or stimulate α_2-adrenergic receptors to reduce norepinephrine release. These drugs also have utility in decreasing the autonomic-mediated symptoms associated with narcotic withdrawal, such as anxiety, tachycardia, tremor, and sweating.

Other drug targets

Several targets have been identified as potentially important drug development for neuropathic pain. These include calcitonin gene-related peptide (CGRP) receptor antagonists, selective TRVP channel inhibitors, and selective sodium channel subtype inhibitors.

Diagnostic Criteria

Table 37-3 lists the diagnostic criteria for the various neuropathic pain conditions found in the orofacial region. It is crucial to make an accurate diagnosis before instituting treatment. The selection of medications is a complex issue that involves an understanding of the mechanism of the pain. Trigeminal neuralgia and central neuropathic pain conditions are treated by systemic medications. Surgical interventions are often considered if the disorder does not respond to medication. Peripheral neuropathies are often treated by application of agents to

TABLE 37-3 Diagnostic Criteria for Orofacial Neuropathic Pain

Spontaneous chronic peripheral trigeminal neuropathy	• Continuous variable aching pain • No history of trauma or dental treatment in area • No obvious local cause • Pain aggravated by local stimuli (hyperalgesia and allodynia) • Normal radiograph • Positive response to somatic block • Response to thermography not defined • Sympathetic block does not define this disorder
Chronic traumatic trigeminal neuropathy	• Continuous, variable, aching pain • May be punctuated by sharp jolts of pain • History of trauma to area • No obvious local cause • Pain aggravated by local stimuli (hyperalgesia and allodynia) • Equivocal somatic block (may be varying degree of sympathetic involvement) • Normal radiograph • Response to thermography depends on sympathetic involvement • Response to sympathetic block is equivocal
Trigeminal neuralgia I (Classical trigeminal neuralgia)	• Episodic sharp electric-like pain with periods of remission • No obvious local cause • Pain is triggered with minor stimulation • Normal radiograph • Normal thermogram • Positive block • Sympathetic block does not define this disorder.
Trigeminal neuralgia II	• Continuous, variable, diurnal, aching pain • Pain responds to local anesthetic • Pain is not locally triggered.
Sympathetically mediated pain	• Continuous, variable, diurnal aching pain • Responsive to sympathetic block

Continued

TABLE 37-3 Diagnostic Criteria for Orofacial Neuropathic Pain—cont'd

Complex regional pain syndrome	• Pain present longer than 4 months • Pain aggravated by local stimuli (hyperalgesia and allodynia) • No obvious local cause • Normal radiograph • Equivocal response to somatic block • Positive response to sympathetic block (60%) is not a defining characteristic
Sympathetically independent pain	• Continuous, variable, diurnal pain • History of trauma to area • Pain present longer than 4 months • Pain aggravated by local stimuli (hyperalgesia and allodynia) • No obvious local cause • Normal radiograph • Negative response to somatic block • Negative response to sympathetic block, although not a defining characteristic

the site of pain. Systemic medications are often added to the regimen for better pain management.

TREATMENT OF HEADACHE PAIN

Tension-Type Headache

Tension-type headaches and common headaches, such as those caused by viral infections, are routinely treated with an **NSAID** or **acetaminophen.**

Migraine

Migraine comes in different forms, but it is usually characterized by intense headaches. It is associated with elevated serotonin levels, even though the relationship between serotonin and migraine is not well understood.

The sequence of events leading to migraine headaches often begins with a **vasoconstrictor phase** in pia and dura blood vessels. A release of serotonin occurs, and glutamate transmission increases. A **spreading depolarization** of central nerve cells (cortical depression) may also occur, followed by **vasodilation of meningeal vessels and plasma extravasation** with inflammation in the area and excessive stimulation of nociceptive fibers in the trigeminal complex. Serotonin pathways projecting from the pons and midbrain (**raphe nuclei**) to the cortex and limbic system, and other areas of the CNS, are involved as part of the CNS changes (Fig. 37-3). Migraine is therefore composed of **vascular, neuronal, and inflammatory components.**

Drug treatment for migraine is either **abortive** (Table 37-4), given when the acute migraine attack occurs, or **prophylactic** (Table 37-5). Non-opioid analgesic and the triptans are the most commonly used abortive drugs, the latter class selectively targeting serotonin ($5\text{-HT}_{1B/1D}$) receptors. The **triptans** are the mainstay of therapy for moderate to severe migraine (See Table 37-6). Triptans may prevent abnormal dilation of central blood vessels, prevent the release of inflammatory peptides (e.g., CGRP), or other actions (Table 37-4). Nausea is common in the acute attack, and antinausea drugs are used to treat it. Ondansetron, a very effective antiemetic drug, is a 5-HT_3 receptor blocker used to treat nausea occurring with migraine.

Cluster Headaches

Cluster headaches are a rarer form of episodic headaches. Therapy can be similar to that of migraine. In addition, intranasal lidocaine, 100% oxygen, and octreotide can be useful as abortive treatments. Lithium carbonate and occipital nerve blocks may be useful for prophylactic therapy.

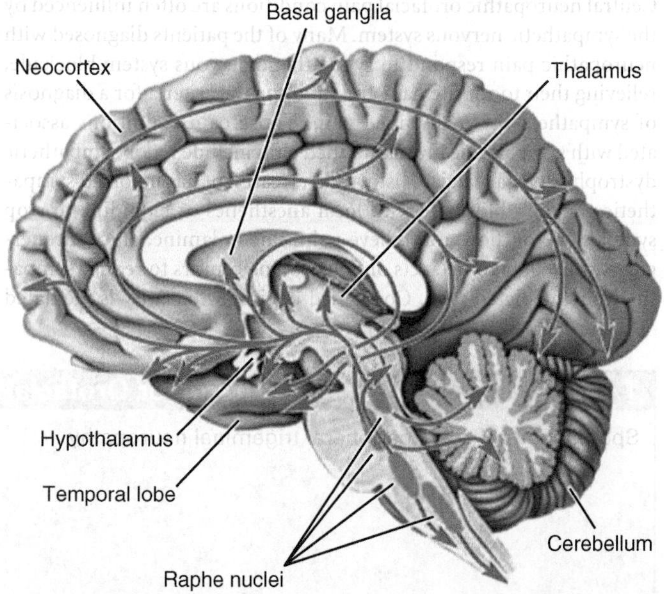

FIG 37-3 The raphe nuclei and their projections. (Modified from Bear MF, Connors WF, Paradiso MA: *Neuroscience: exploring the brain,* ed. 4, 2016, Lippincott, Williams and Wilkins, Philadelphia.)

TOPICAL AGENTS

Topical application of medications to the skin to treat pain has its roots in ancient literature and lore. Compounding pharmacists are able to combine medications in bases such as **pleuronic lecithin organogel (PLO)** for application to the external skin surface or in bases such as **Orabase** for intraoral application. Direct application of topical agents to localized areas of inflammation, irritation, and pain offers several advantages: placement of medications directly over the treatment area potentially decreases side effects, and the direct effect of topical agents on the local receptors may have greater effect than systemic medications.

PLO is a gel base that is able to penetrate the epidermal barrier, carrying the agent through the epidermis to the affected locus. Some systemic absorption occurs, but it is significantly less than would be obtained by systemic administration. The combinations of medications are virtually limitless, but the underlying principle for choosing

TABLE 37-4 Abortive Drugs for the Treatment of Migraine*

Drug	Mechanism	Adverse Effects	Comments
Triptans, e.g., sumatriptan, naratriptan, rizatriptan, zolmitriptan	Agonists at $5\text{-}HT_{1B/1D}$ receptors	Chest tightness, angina, sedation, dizziness, tingling, flushing, GI	Given orally and subcutaneously; sumatriptan and zolmitriptan are also given by nasal spray
Dihydroergotamine	Nonselective 5-HT receptor agonist, vasoconstriction	Similar to triptans, GI, CNS, damage to endothelium	Given IV, intranasally, or subcutaneously
Ergotamine	Nonselective 5-HT receptor agonist	Similar to dihydroergotamine except more severe, including gangrene	Oral absorption is improved with caffeine; ergotamine has largely been replaced by the triptans
NSAIDs	See Chapter 17	See Chapter 17	Ibuprofen, naproxen, aspirin, and diclofenac most commonly used from this group
Acetaminophen	See Chapter 17	See Chapter 17	
Tramadol	See Chapter 16	See Chapter 16	Blocks uptake of catecholamines and serotonin, likely to interact with triptans, ergots, and MAO inhibitors
Adrenocorticosteroids, e.g., prednisone	Antiinflammation, see Chapter 30	See Chapter 30	Used for a short period of time

*Isometheptene is a vasoconstrictor with α- and β-adrenoceptor agonist action. Midrin is a proprietary combination medication that contains isometheptene plus acetaminophen and dichloralphenazone (a mild sedative). This combination is available for treating mild to moderate migraine headache. This combination is less widely used today than in the past.

TABLE 37-5 Prophylactic Drugs in the Management of Migraine

Drug	Mechanism	Adverse Effects	Comments
β-adrenoceptor blockers, e.g., propranolol, metoprolol, atenolol	The mechanism for their effectiveness in migraine is not established	See Chapter 9	
Valproic acid	Blocks calcium and sodium channels; may reduce neuronal activity	GI, dizziness, weakness, dyspepsia, visual changes, tinnitus, drowsiness	May target nociceptive trigeminal vascular inflammatory pathways and reduce cortical nerve spreading depression
Calcium channel blockers, e.g., verapamil	Block "L" type calcium channels; may thereby reduce neuronal and vascular activity	GI, headache, hypotension, edema; see Chapter 19	May prevent relevant vasomotor activity
Topiramate	Several possible mechanisms, reduces spread of cortical stimulation, blocks sodium channels, augments the effects of GABA	Dizziness, weakness, difficulty with concentration, paresthesias, confusion, impotence, GI	May target nociceptive trigeminal vascular pathways and reduce cortical nerve depression
Tricyclic antidepressants, e.g., amitriptyline	Possibly due to inhibition of reuptake of serotonin and norepinephrine	Weight gain, sedation, anti-muscarinic effects, e.g. xerostomia; see Chapter 10	Especially useful in co-morbid depression
Gabapentin	Blocks the $\alpha 2\delta$ subunit of voltage-gated calcium channels	Dizziness, sedation, tremor, ataxia, dry mouth, visual changes	The method of prophylaxis is not established but may resemble that of valproic acid
ACE inhibitors, e.g., lisinopril	Prevents synthesis of angiotensin II	Cough, dizziness, hypotension, hyperkalemia, rarely angioedema	The mechanism of the prophylactic effect may relate to the relaxing effect on blood vessels
Angiotensin II receptor antagonists, e.g., candesartan	Blocks effects of angiotensin II on its receptors	Dizziness, hypotension, hyperkalemia	The mechanism of the prophylactic effect may relate to the relaxing effect on blood vessels
Botulinum toxin type A	Inhibits release of acetylcholine from motor nerves	Hypersensitivity, spread of toxin leading to dysphagia, bronchitis	Given by multiple injections around head and neck, about every 12 weeks

agents to include in the mixture should be based on the assumed pathologic state underlying the painful condition. For example, if the clinician is managing an inflamed temporomandibular joint and the patient is unable or unwilling to take a systemic antiinflammatory drug, an NSAID such as ketoprofen could be included in a PLO base to be applied over the inflamed joint. Presumably, the NSAID would decrease pain and inflammation by inhibiting prostaglandin synthesis locally, avoiding significant systemic effects.

In the past, chronic peripheral trigeminal neuropathy has defied treatment, but recent understanding of the pathophysiologic characteristics of the condition has helped to develop treatment approaches with topical agents that inhibit peripheral sensitizing mechanisms such as C-fiber sensitization. When **capsaicin-responsive vanilloid receptors** were discovered on small-diameter unmyelinated nociceptors (assumed to be C fibers), it was realized that these receptors could be the target for topical intervention. Under new nomenclature, the capsaicin-responsive vanilloid receptors are now described as TRPV1 receptors. Activation causes the affiliated nociceptors to release substance P (SP). Long-term application depletes SP stores and temporarily inhibits the neuron's ability to synthesize more. Persistent application of capsaicin desensitizes chronic peripheral neuropathy, rendering relief from pain. Intraoral application is enhanced by fabricating an acrylic stent to cover the affected area when applying a capsaicin mixture. Capsaicin 0.025% is mixed in Orabase-B paste to give a sticky quality to the paste, helping to hold the stent in place and limiting the dispersion of the agent throughout the mouth. Nevertheless, for conditions such as **trigeminal neuralgia, systemic drugs or surgical procedures** are almost always required.

Topical **ketoprofen** with other agents is useful in applications over inflamed muscles and joints. Ketoprofen 10% to 20% can be mixed in a PLO base and applied three to four times per day after wiping the area with a moist washcloth. In this situation, ketoprofen has a local antiinflammatory effect without gastric irritation. (Other NSAIDs have been used in a similar topical manner.) Patients should be cautioned regarding potential for developing photosensitivity because of the sensitizing properties of the benzophenone moiety of ketoprofen. Ultraviolet light exposure of skin covered with ketoprofen cream promotes the photolysis of erythrocytes. Additionally, the drug is able to induce photoperoxidation of linoleic acid, and ketoprofen may induce DNA damage. There is a concern that repeated use of ketoprofen or other topical agents could lead to sensitization, with the possibility of incurring a greater risk of systemic allergic reactions with oral NSAIDs or other drugs.

The most common neuropathies in the orofacial region include trigeminal neuralgia, traumatic trigeminal neuropathy, postherpetic neuralgia, diabetic neuropathy, cancer-induced neuropathy, and AIDS-induced neuropathy. In general, all these neuropathies have common pain mechanisms and similar treatment protocols. Peripheral nerve damage leads to peripheral sensitization and changes in the CNS. Topical medications are useful for neuropathic pain from peripheral sensitization and may be of some use for centralized neuropathy with peripheral pain trigger zones.

To deliver a drug in the orofacial region by topical application, the agent has to penetrate the natural barriers that the facial skin and oral mucosal tissues provide. The pharmaceutical industry has found different ways to improve the absorption of topical medications, increasing the time and contact between the medications and the target tissues and developing different delivery systems such as creams, gels, dissolvable tablets, chewing gum, adhesive patches, polymeric devices, mouth rinses, and medicated lipsticks. The use of topical drug delivery is quite familiar to the dental profession because the application of creams, gels, and rinses to mucosal sites is a daily activity in dental practice.

The medications often used for oral and perioral neuropathies are topical anesthetics and, recently, capsaicin. Other compounds such as NSAIDs, sympathomimetic agents, and NMDA antagonists are now being used with variable success. Although it is also possible to have other agents such as carbamazepine, baclofen, or amitriptyline compounded for local delivery, their use in peripheral conditions is controversial because their mechanism of action has been described as central, and a peripheral mechanism of action has not been clearly established.

The use of intraoral topical medications is accompanied by some inconveniences. These agents tend to dissolve in saliva and spread throughout the mouth and down the throat. If the topical agent does not have mucosal adhesive properties, it will quickly wash away from the area where it is being applied. Several strategies and delivery systems are being used to counter this problem.

In addition to **capsaicin and NSAIDs, clonidine, ketamine, and eutectic mixtures of local anesthetics** are delivered through the skin by a transdermal carrier or by placing in a material such as Orabase that adheres to the mucous tissue to enhance and maintain tissue/medication contact for longer periods (Table 37-7).

TABLE 37-6 Contraindications, Precautions, and Adverse Reactions of Triptans

Contraindications and Cautions

- Drug allergy
- Prinzmetal (variant) angina
- Pregnancy
- Breastfeeding
- Diabetes
- Hepatic disease
- Uncontrolled hypertension
- Coronary artery disease
- Basilar migraine
- Use of monoamine oxidase (MAO) inhibitor within 14 days
- Hemiplegic migraine
- Peripheral vascular disease
- Cerebrovascular disease
- Impaired liver function
- Use of ergot derivatives or other anti–5-HT medications

Adverse Reactions

Common	Uncommon
• Asthenia	• Anaphylaxis
• Chest pain	• Coronary vasospasm
• Neck tightness	• Acute myocardial infarction
• Jaw tightness	• Cardiac arrest
• Dizziness	• Ventricular tachycardia
• Flushing	• Hypertensive crisis
• Paresthesias	• Stroke

TABLE 37-7 Topical Agents Used for the Treatment of Orofacial Pain

Drug	Mechanism of Action	Dose	Other
Capsaicin	Reduces C-fiber activity	0.025% in an Orabase paste and applied 5-6 times/day	Upon application burning sensation in area of application may last for 10 minutes
Clonidine	α_2-adrenoceptor agonist	0.1-2 mg and applied 3 times/day	Should be compounded by a pharmacist; examination of the painful area may be reported by patient as a cold area
Ketamine	NMDA receptor antagonist	200 mg/mL in transdermal base and applied daily	Presently, a controversial use of ketamine
Local anesthetics	Reduces C-fiber activity	2.5% prilocaine and 2.5% lidocaine mixed in an occlusive dressing and applied daily	If the C-fiber activity can be reduced for a long enough period, normal function will be reestablished

IMPLICATIONS FOR DENTISTRY

This chapter has reviewed the medications used to treat several pain syndromes, including chronic orofacial pain conditions. The medications traditionally used by dentists to treat their patients are generally limited to antibiotics, antiinflammatory agents, opioids, local or general anesthetics, and benzodiazepines. These medications are used to treat acute pain, inflammation, and infections or to anesthetize patients for surgical procedures. With the development of the field of orofacial pain and the increased understanding of painful non–tooth-related conditions that are seen in the orofacial environment, the dental pharmacopoeia has necessarily expanded to include a vast array of medications that have not generally been considered previously. This array will continue to expand as more pharmaceuticals are developed and the understanding of orofacial pain disorders and their mechanisms broadens.

ANTIMIGRAINE DRUGS AND DRUGS FOR NEUROPATHIC AND OTHER PAIN SYNDROMES

Nonproprietary (Generic) Name	Proprietary (Trade) Name
Ergots	
Dihydroergotamine	Migranal, DHE 45
Ergotamine	Ergomar, in Cafergot
Triptans	
Almotriptan	Axert
Eletriptan	Relpax
Frovatriptan	Frova
Naratriptan	Amerge
Rizatriptan	Maxalt
Sumatriptan	Imitrex
Zolmitriptan	Zomig
Antiemetics	
Metoclopramide	Reglan
Prochlorperazine	Compazine
Promethazine	Phenergan
Trimethobenzamide	Tigan
Ondansetron	Zofran
TCAs (see Chapter 10)	
α-Adrenergic Receptor Blockers (see Chapter 9)	
Calcium Channel Blockers (see Chapters 19 and 21)	
Antihistamines (see Chapter 18)	
Centrally Acting Muscle Relaxants	
Baclofen	Lioresal
Carisoprodol	Soma
Cyclobenzaprine	Flexeril
Metaxalone	Skelaxin
Methocarbamol	Robaxin
Tizanidine	Zanaflex
Benzodiazepines (see Chapter 11)	
NSAIDs (see Chapter 17)	
Antiseizure Drugs (see Chapter 12)	
NMDA Antagonists	
Dextromethorphan	Delsym
Ketamine	Ketalar
α-Adrenergic Receptor Agonists	
Clonidine	Catapres
Tizanidine	Zanaflex
Topical Agents*	
Pleuronic lecithin organogel	—
Capsaicin	Zostrix
Others	
Botulinum toxin A	Botox
Botulinum toxin B	Myobloc
Dichloralphenazone	In Midrin
Indomethacin	Indocin
Isometheptene	In Midrin
Sodium hyaluronate	Hyalgan

*See also local anesthetics, Chapter 14; NSAIDs, Chapter 17.

CASE DISCUSSION

The pain experience by this patient is "chronic pain", given its duration. The likelihood is that it is neuropathic pain since there is no observable injury or pathology. The symptoms, i.e. continuous dull aching pain, are not typical of trigeminal neuralgia, which usually presents as episodic, stabbing and electrical type pain. The pain is not provoked by local stimuli, as indicated by the ability to chew on the same side as the pain. These characteristics plus the diurnal variation in the pain strongly suggests trigeminal neuralgia Type II. Topical application or injection of a local anesthetic in the area usually reduces the pain of trigeminal neuralgia Type II significantly. Since local anesthetic relieves the pain, the pain is still being generated peripherally. If the pain did not respond to a local anesthetic, systemic treatment would be required and the diagnosis would be Persistent Idiopathic Facial Pain or Centralized Neuropathic Pain. This case requires referral to a pain specialist for treatment. Drugs used include topical agents, antidepressants, gabapentin, pregabalin, and antiepileptic drugs as indicated for other types of neuropathic pain.

GENERAL REFERENCES

1. Aziz MT, Good BL, Lowe DK: Serotonin-norepinephrine reuptake inhibitors for the management of chemotherapy-induced peripheral neuropathy, *Ann Pharmacother* 48(5):626–632, 2014.
2. Becker WJ: Acute migraine treatment in adults, *Headache* 55:778–793, 2015.
3. Classey JD, Bartsch T, Goadsby PJ: Distribution of 5-HT(1B), 5-HT(1D) and 5-HT(1F) receptor expression in rat trigeminal and dorsal root ganglia neurons: relevance to the selective anti-migraine effect of triptans, *Brain Res* 1361:76–85, 2010.
4. Garnock-Jones KP: Diclofenac potassium powder for oral solution: a review of its use in patients with acute migraine, *CNS Drugs* 28:761–768, 2014.
5. Goadsby PJ, Massiou H, Pascuel J, et al.: Almotriptan and zolmitriptan in the acute treatment of migraine, *Acta Neurol Scand* 115:34–40, 2007.
6. Gobel H, Heinze A: Botulinum toxin type A in the prophylactic treatment of chronic migraine, *Schmerz* 25:563–570, 2011.
7. Lee SE, Kim JH: Involvement of substance P and calcitonin gene-related peptide in development and maintenance of neuropathic pain from spinal nerve injury model of rat, *Neurosci Res* 58:245–249, 2007.

8. Marmura MJ, Silberstein SD, Schwedt TJ: The acute treatment of migraine in adults: the American Headache Society evidence assessment of migraine pharmacotherapies, *Headache* 55:3–20, 2015.
9. Moulin DE, Boulanger A, Clark AJ, et al.: Pharmacological management of chronic neuropathic pain - consensus statement and guidelines from the Canadian Pain Society, *Pain Res Manag* 12:13–21, 2007.
10. Ossipov MH, Dussor GO, Porreca F: Central modulation of pain, *J Clin Invest* 120:3779–3787, 2010.
11. Rapoport AM: The therapeutic future in headache, *Neurol Sci* 33(Suppl 1): S119–S125, 2012.
12. Seena BP, Boros AL, Kumar SKS: Atypical odontalgia – an update, *Calif Dent Assoc J* 40:739–747, 2012.
13. Shamliyan TA, Choi JY, Ramakrishnan R, et al.: Preventive pharmacologic treatments for episodic migraine in adults, *J Gen Intern Med* 28:1225–1237, 2013.
14. Winner P, Linder S, Hershey AD: Consistency of response to sumatriptan/naproxen sodium in a randomized placebo-controlled, cross-over study for the acute treatment of migraine in adolescence, *Headache* 55(4):519–528, 2015.
15. Zakrzewska TH: Trigeminal neuralgia: unilateral episodic facial pain, *J Pain Palliat Care Pharmacother* 29:182–184, 2015.

38

Management of Fear and Anxiety

Daniel A. Haas

KEY INFORMATION

- Fear and anxiety regarding dentistry are common emotions, and their management may require administration of drugs.
- The pillar of safe practice is appropriate training and understanding the differences in the modalities of minimal sedation, moderate sedation, deep sedation, and general anesthesia.
- Nitrous oxide and oxygen can be effective for minimal sedation.
- Administering drugs orally or intravenously can be considered for minimal or moderate sedation.
- Benzodiazepines are the mainstay of sedation by the oral and intravenous routes.

CASE STUDY

A 44-year-old female patient requires general dentistry involving multiple restorative and endodontic procedures. It is estimated that this appointment will take approximately 2 hours. Her anxiety is at a level that she is unable to receive treatment by chairside manner alone. She is classified as an ASA 2 patient, having hypertension controlled by an ACE inhibitor. You are trained to administer minimal and moderate sedation. What are your options for the pharmacologic management of this patient?

BACKGROUND

Fear and anxiety regarding dental procedures are common emotions. The severity ranges widely, with mild apprehension being reported by 75% of the population, and severe anxiety, leading to avoidance of dental treatment, being reported by anywhere from 4% to 21%. Dental anxiety has not diminished but has remained stable over the past 50 years despite advances in the delivery of dentistry. This fear begins in childhood and can persist throughout life, leading to avoidance of dental care. Although mild anxiety may have only a minor effect on oral health, true phobia can lead to avoidance of treatment despite significant symptoms and then result in detrimental consequences for overall health.

Approximately 40% of the population does not receive routine dental care, with apprehension being cited as the most common reason. These patients often require special nonpharmacologic or pharmacologic approaches to allow dental procedures to be done. Pharmacologic approaches involve drugs that produce effects ranging from minimal sedation to general anesthesia.

Behavioral or psychological techniques to manage anxiety in dental patients are the first consideration and are unquestionably important, but their detailed description lies beyond the scope of this chapter. This chapter summarizes the pharmacologic approaches to the management of fear and anxiety in dental patients, with emphasis on the administration of minimal and/or moderate sedation. Complete understanding of this subject requires comprehension of the pharmacologic features of the specific drugs, which are described in other chapters.

GENERAL PRINCIPLES

Indications for Use

The primary indication for pharmacologic methods of patient management is the presence of anxiety, fear, or phobia sufficient to prevent the delivery of needed dental care. Another indication is the presence of motor dysfunction, such as in patients with cerebral palsy or Parkinson disease, whose tremor or uncoordinated movements may be exacerbated by the anxiety of being in the dental office. **Traumatic or extensive dental procedures** are additional potential indications when coupled with anxiety, the need to immobilize the patient, or inability to render the patient pain-free with local anesthesia. Finally, some **patients cannot physiologically tolerate the stress that even a minimal amount of anxiety may induce**; patients with ischemic heart disease, labile hypertension, or stress-induced asthma are included in this group. For these latter groups, minimal or moderate sedation techniques are often successful.

Other potential indications for the use of pharmacologic methods for patient management include **cognitive impairment**, such as in mentally challenged patients or patients with Alzheimer dementia. These patients may be unable to cooperate sufficiently to permit treatment or perhaps even an adequate intraoral examination. Pharmacologic management may also be required for a pediatric patient who may not understand the treatment and is reacting normally for a young child. For these latter two groups, minimal or moderate sedation may be insufficient, and either deep sedation or general anesthesia is often required.

Treatment Planning

To address the needs of fearful or anxious patients, the dentist must first be able to recognize its presence and degree, and this should be determined as part of an appropriate history and patient evaluation.

After identifying an anxious, fearful, or phobic patient, thought should be given to the optimal method of managing the patient. Initially, nonpharmacologic methods of anxiety reduction should be considered. Appropriate chairside manner is often all that is required; this includes use of basic behavioral modification, positive suggestion, and reassurance. This approach is valuable not only when used alone but also when used with pharmacologic approaches.

Despite effective chairside manner, many patients still wish to receive sedation or anesthesia. It has been reported that more than 50% of Americans classified as having high fear or anxiety preferred sedation for their dental care. The same study showed that three times as many subjects reported a preference for parenteral sedation or general anesthesia when undergoing dental treatment than were actually receiving these modalities. This same pattern was seen in a subsequent Canadian study in which patients were asked if they would prefer to have sedation or general anesthesia for each of five procedures. There were large differences in this preference compared with actual prevalence for each procedure—specifically, 3.8-fold difference for cleaning, 2.8-fold difference for restorative dentistry, 9.6-fold difference for endodontics, 15.9-fold difference for periodontal surgery, and 2.2-fold difference for extraction. The low preference/prevalence ratio for extractions suggests that dental patients have better access to sedation/anesthesia services for extractions than for other procedures. Extrapolation of these results suggests that **nearly 25 million American adults are definitely interested in sedation or general anesthesia for dentistry regardless of the cost.**

An absolute requirement basic to the success of patient management is effective local anesthesia. One cannot avoid this necessity in most invasive dental procedures unless complete general anesthesia is being administered. Even then, there may be benefits to the so-called preemptive use of local anesthetic. The dentist should not be misled into thinking that poor local anesthetic technique can be overcome by administering a sedative. Only when the anesthetic failure is strictly caused by anxiety would sedation be fully effective.

The approach to anxiety control should be individualized. It is as faulty to assume that every patient requires general anesthesia for the removal of impacted teeth as it is to assume that no patient requires anxiety control for a simple dental procedure or examination.

The ability to use a particular pharmacologic approach depends on the level of training of the dentist and the applicable laws and regulations. Education for minimal sedation, such as given through inhalation and oral administration, is within the realm of the predoctoral dental curriculum. More advanced forms, such as moderate sedation, given either enterally (orally) or parenterally (intravenously), usually require training at a postdoctoral or continuing education level, although some dental schools have shown that it can be part of a predoctoral program. The most advanced modalities—deep sedation and general anesthesia—require the most formal training. Education for advanced modalities entails a specific postgraduate program devoted to anesthesia (i.e., an accredited residency in dental anesthesiology or an accredited oral and maxillofacial surgery residency, which must include advanced training in anesthesia as part of its curriculum).

Patient Selection

Before choosing pharmacologic adjuncts for patient management, the dentist should carefully review the patient's medical history. In this context, the American Society of Anesthesiologists (ASA) Physical Status Classification System can be helpful (Table 38-1). This assessment tool can be used to estimate the patient's overall ability to tolerate the stress of a planned procedure. It can also help determine the need for further patient evaluation and the degree of monitoring required for the procedure.

ASA I and II patients are usually suitable candidates for sedation or general anesthesia in the outpatient setting. Although outpatient general anesthesia is often inappropriate for ASA III patients, these same patients are at increased risk during stressful procedures when fear and anxiety are not adequately controlled. Techniques to control anxiety involving minimal, moderate, or possibly even deep sedation may be particularly valuable to ASA III patients because they reduce the release of endogenous catecholamines. Patients classified as ASA IV (and higher) are usually not candidates for deep sedation or general anesthesia in the dental office, and minimal or moderate sedation should only be considered by those with advanced training.

TABLE 38-1 American Society of Anesthesiologists Physical Status Classification System

Class	Description
I	Normal, healthy patient
II	Patient with mild systemic disease
III	Patient with severe systemic disease that limits activity, but is not incapacitating
IV	Patient with incapacitating systemic disease that is a constant threat to life
V	Moribund patient not expected to survive 24 hr with or without operation
E	Emergency operation of any type; E is appended to the patient's physical status

PHARMACOLOGIC APPROACHES

Several pharmacologic approaches can be used to manage fear and anxiety in dental patients. These are commonly referred to collectively as the **spectrum of pain and anxiety control**, which incorporates all major routes of administration and levels of central nervous system (CNS) depression. It is important to recognize that the route of administration is not synonymous with the depth of sedation. A spectrum of fear and anxiety control as depicted in Figure 38-1 shows the range of sedation or anesthesia normally sought from the various routes and techniques of administration. In its simplest form, this spectrum is divided into techniques expected to leave the patient awake or to render the patient unconscious. These modalities correspond to sedation and general anesthesia. Definitions of the various levels of sedation have been standardized to include the states of minimal, moderate, and deep sedation. The characteristics of these states and of general anesthesia are defined next and compared in Table 38-2:

Minimal sedation is a minimally depressed level of consciousness, produced by a pharmacologic method, that retains the patient's ability to maintain an airway independently and continuously and to respond normally to tactile stimulation and verbal command. Although cognitive function and coordination may be modestly impaired, ventilatory and cardiovascular functions are unaffected.

Moderate sedation is a drug-induced depression of consciousness during which patients respond purposefully to verbal commands, either alone or accompanied by light tactile stimulation. No interventions are required to maintain a patent airway, and spontaneous ventilation is adequate. Cardiovascular function is usually maintained.

Deep sedation is a drug-induced depression of consciousness during which patients cannot be easily aroused but respond purposefully after repeated or painful stimulation. The ability to maintain ventilatory function independently may be impaired. Patients may require assistance in maintaining a patent airway, and spontaneous ventilation may be inadequate. Cardiovascular function is usually maintained.

General anesthesia is a drug-induced loss of consciousness during which patients are unarousable, even by painful stimulation. The ability to maintain ventilatory function independently is often impaired. Patients often require assistance in maintain-

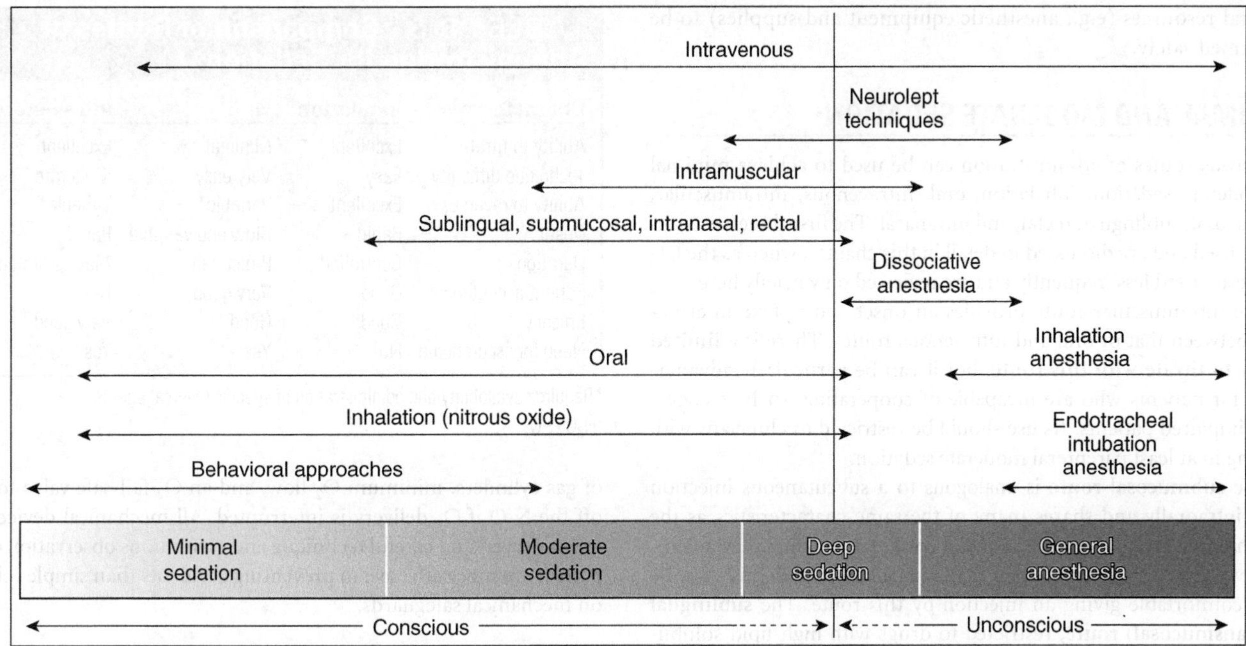

FIG 38-1 The spectrum of fear and anxiety control in dentistry. The range of central nervous system depression normally achieved by various techniques is illustrated by *arrows*. The depth of sedation or anesthesia induced by a given drug primarily depends on the dose administered, route used, and susceptibility of the patient.

TABLE 38-2 Comparison of Minimal Sedation, Moderate Sedation, Deep Sedation, and General Anesthesia

Characteristics	Minimal Sedation	Moderate Sedation	Deep Sedation	General Anesthesia
Consciousness	Maintained	Maintained	Obtunded	Unconscious
Protective reflexes	Intact	Intact	Depressed	Absent
Unassisted airway maintenance	Present	Present	May be absent	Absent
Response to verbal command	Present	May be obtunded	Absent	Absent
Response to tactile stimulation	Present	Present	Absent	Absent
Response to painful stimulation	Present	Present	Reflex withdrawal	Absent
Vital signs	Stable	Usually stable	Usually stable	May be labile
Anxiety	Decreased	Decreased	Absent	Absent
Monitoring required	Basic	Intermediate	Advanced	Advanced
Efficacy	Mild anxiety	Moderate anxiety or fear	Most patients	All patients
Relative risk	Low	Low to intermediate	Intermediate	High
Recovery time	Rapid	Intermediate	Intermediate	May be prolonged
Postoperative sequelae	Uncommon	Uncommon	Uncommon	More common

ing a patent airway, and positive-pressure ventilation may be required because of depressed spontaneous ventilation or drug-induced depression of neuromuscular function. Cardiovascular function may be impaired.

Minimal and moderate forms of sedation are not substitutes for an appropriate chairside manner but are used to reinforce positive suggestion and reassurance in a way that allows dental treatment to be performed with minimal physiologic and psychological stress. These techniques should carry a margin of safety wide enough to render unintended loss of consciousness unlikely. Deep sedation or general anesthesia can be induced by many of the same drugs that induce moderate sedation. The resulting state depends on patient susceptibility, age, medical status, degree of anxiety, and the drug used and dose administered. Either deep sedation or general anesthesia may be indicated when lighter forms of CNS depression are insufficient to permit treatment.

Reliable morbidity and mortality data for the different forms of sedation or general anesthesia are scarce, but several studies have shown that, overall, the techniques used in dentistry should be considered safe. Increased mortality is usually associated with inadequate training or inadequate monitoring of the patient. In a review of adverse events related to sedation in pediatric patients, the use of three or more sedating drugs was more strongly associated with adverse outcomes than was the use of only one or two. If the goal is minimal or moderate sedation, one must avoid administering excessive doses of a sedative to a patient who remains uncooperative while conscious because it could easily lead to a deepening of sedation in which airway patency and protective reflexes may be lost. Any subsequent lack of oxygenation can rapidly lead to a tragic result. Although the progression from moderate to deep sedation can be accomplished easily, it requires a significantly increased degree of practitioner training, patient monitoring, and physical resources (e.g., anesthetic equipment and supplies) to be performed safely.

MINIMAL AND MODERATE SEDATION

Numerous routes of administration can be used to achieve minimal or moderate sedation: inhalation, oral, intravenous, intramuscular, submucosal, sublingual, rectal, and intranasal. The first three are commonly used and are discussed in detail in this chapter, whereas the latter five are used less frequently and are reviewed only briefly here.

The intramuscular route provides an onset and uptake intermediate between that of oral and intravenous routes. There is a **limited ability to titrate with this route**, but it can be particularly advantageous for patients who are incapable of cooperating, such as cognitively impaired patients. Its use should be restricted to clinicians with training in at least parenteral moderate sedation.

The **submucosal route** is analogous to a subcutaneous injection given intraorally and shares many of the same characteristics as the intramuscular route. The submucosal route has no apparent advantage over any of the others, other than the fact that the dentist may be more comfortable giving an injection by this route. The **sublingual (or transmucosal) route**, restricted to drugs with high lipid solubility and available in suitable formulations, is similar to the oral route except that there is a more rapid absorption by the oral mucosa and no first-pass effect. The difference in recommended dosages can be large when comparing oral versus sublingual absorption depending on the extent of first-pass metabolism in the intestine and liver. The onset of effect after sublingual administration may take several minutes for some drugs and considerably longer for others.

The **rectal route** is not often used in dentistry, with the possible exception of pediatric patients. Disadvantages of this route include inability to titrate, inconsistencies in absorption, often poor patient acceptance, and inconvenience.

The **intranasal route** involves the topical application to the nasal mucosa and is characterized by a potentially rapid absorption and onset of action. It has been used as an alternative to intramuscular injection for uncooperative children. Its potential benefits are outweighed, however, by variable absorption, discomfort of mucosal irritation, potential for damage to the nasal mucosa, and, most importantly, the usual need for restraint to achieve administration.

As stated earlier, the route of administration is not synonymous with the depth of sedation. Any route has the potential to induce any degree of sedation or anesthesia. Management of an anxious patient can be discussed according to route of administration, however, because the inhalation and oral techniques are most commonly used for minimal and moderate sedation and are normally the first to be considered. The **intravenous route** is more likely to be selected to induce a greater depth of effect. Table 38-3 compares the routes of administration for sedation.

Inhalation Sedation

Inhalation sedation refers to the administration of nitrous oxide (N_2O), whose pharmacologic features are opioid in nature centrally (involving $GABA_A$ and NMDA receptors), and oxygen (O_2). $N_2O—O_2$ inhalation is a technique of choice for dental procedures that require minimal sedation. The analgesia produced by $N_2O—O_2$ has the potential to ameliorate the incidental discomforts associated with dental treatment. As with other modalities of sedation, however, $N_2O—O_2$ is not a substitute for effective local anesthesia.

Inhalation sedation units must meet stringent safety standards, including color-coding of compressed gas cylinders, a pin-indexed or diameter-indexed safety system to prevent incorrect connection of gas cylinders, minimum O_2 flow, and an O_2 fail-safe valve to shut off the N_2O if O_2 delivery is interrupted. All mechanical devices can fail, however, and careful technique and continuous observation of the patient are more effective in preventing accidents than simple reliance on mechanical safeguards.

TABLE 38-3 Comparison of Routes of Administration for Sedation

Characteristic	Inhalation[†]	Oral	Intravenous
Ability to titrate	Excellent	Minimal	Excellent
Technique difficulty	Easy	Very easy	Moderate
Ability to reverse	Excellent	Variable*	Variable*
Onset	Rapid	Slow and variable	Rapid
Duration	Controlled	Prolonged	May be prolonged
Patient acceptance	Good	Very good	Fair
Efficacy	Good	Good	Very good
Need for escort home	No	Yes	Yes

*Requires availability and administration of specific reversal agents.
[†]$N_2O—O_2$

Advantages

The advantages (and disadvantages) of the inhalation route are summarized in Table 38-3. Because of its relative insolubility in blood, **N_2O has a rapid onset of action**, with clinical effects becoming apparent within a few minutes. This property of **N_2O allows for titration to effect**. In this context, *titration* is defined as the incremental administration of small amounts of a drug until a desired clinical effect is observed. The ability to titrate a drug enables the dentist to control its ultimate effect and eliminates the need to guess the correct dose for a particular patient. This characteristic is a major reason why $N_2O—O_2$ has long been considered a near-ideal technique for minimal or moderate sedation. In the event that a patient inadvertently receives too much drug, the effect can be rapidly decreased by reducing the concentration administered. The inhalation route is the only one in which the actions of a drug can be quickly adjusted in either direction.

Another major advantage of $N_2O—O_2$ inhalation is that **recovery is rapid**. Normally, there is no residual effect on the patient's psychomotor skills and ability to operate a motor vehicle soon after termination of $N_2O—O_2$ inhalation. When it is not combined with any other sedative agent, $N_2O—O_2$ is the only sedation technique in which a patient may be discharged home alone; all other sedation techniques require that the patient be discharged in the care of a responsible adult.

Disadvantages

$N_2O—O_2$ sedation for typical dental procedures has comparatively few disadvantages. There are a few patients for whom this method would be ineffective. Most patients have the desired clinical effect between 20% and 50% N_2O. Another disadvantage is the requirement for patient cooperation. Success with this technique requires the patient to breathe through the nose and to leave a nasal hood in place throughout the procedure. Claustrophobic patients and apprehensive children may be unable to tolerate the nasal hood.

Acute or chronic nasal obstruction precludes the use of $N_2O—O_2$ because the patient is unable to inhale the administered gases. Patients who are mouth breathers for other reasons are also unsuitable candidates. Because of a risk of expansion and rupture of enclosed gas spaces, contraindications include recent vitreoretinal surgery with intraocular gas infusion, pulmonary bullae, pneumothorax, intestinal obstruction, or an obstructed middle ear. Pregnancy may be considered a relative

TABLE 38-4 Steps to Reduce Nitrous Oxide Exposure

Action	Tactic
Facility and equipment preparation	Purchase scavenging nitrous oxide deliver systems with air sweeper capabilities
	Check plumbing for leaks by pressure retention of closed system
	Check all fittings for leaks with disclosing solution or nitrous oxide analyzer
	Ensure exhaust system vents to the outside away from air intake
	Maximize room air circulation
	Consider use of a local exhaust system
Daily use	Adjust vacuum setting to manufacturer's maximum recommended value
	Place hood on nose before administering nitrous oxide
	Adjust flow to patient's minute respiratory volume
	Instruct patient to exhale through nose
	Instruct patient not to talk
	Use rubber dam whenever possible
	Use high-vacuum suction when mouth is open
	Administer 100% oxygen for 3 to 5 minutes before removing hood
Monitoring	Inspect delivery apparatus each day of use, particularly the reservoir bag
	Periodically monitor exposure by passive dosimetry or nitrous oxide analyzer
	Record monitoring results

contraindication because of the usual preference to avoid the administration of any drug during pregnancy. Nevertheless, if drug-induced sedation is to be carried out for a pregnant patient, N_2O—O_2 is preferred over most other sedatives and may be the technique of choice for a short procedure (e.g., <1 hour). Two minor disadvantages are the cost and space needed for the N_2O—O_2 equipment.

There are potential risks for the ability of N_2O to disrupt vitamin B_{12}–dependent biochemical pathways. The primary concern with this is the occupational health hazards from prolonged exposure to trace anesthetic gases. Steps to minimize exposure are summarized in Table 38-4. As well, patients with known mutations causing abnormalities in folate-cycle enzymes may be at risk when administered N_2O.

For two groups of patients, it is not the N_2O that is the concern, but the high inspired O_2. First, patients with severe chronic obstructive pulmonary disease may have chronically elevated carbon dioxide tensions and depend on the hypoxic drive to stimulate breathing. When elevated O_2 concentrations occur, as during N_2O—O_2 administration, the stimulus for involuntary breathing may be removed, leading to respiratory depression and a worsening of respiratory acidosis. Second, patients who have had bleomycin chemotherapy within the past year may be predisposed to pulmonary fibrosis after exposure to high O_2 concentrations.

Clinical application

Administration begins with 100% O_2 at an appropriate flow rate, approximately 6 L/min for most adults. With the reservoir bag filled and O_2 flowing, the mask is placed on the patient. The operator initially adjusts the O_2 flow to meet the patient's minute respiratory volume and then administers a 20% concentration of N_2O to the patient (keeping total gas flow unchanged) and waits 1 to 2 minutes to judge clinical effectiveness. As necessary, the operator increases the N_2O concentration in 5% to 10% increments until the patient exhibits the desired clinical signs and symptoms. In a few patients, doses of 20% or less may be sufficient.

The dentist should advise the patient of the symptoms that may be experienced and that the goal is to feel comfortable. Symptoms occurring during inhalation sedation may include lightheadedness; tingling of the fingers, toes, or lips; warmth; and euphoria. The clinician should not be dogmatic in describing potential symptoms because failure to experience one or more of them may be misinterpreted by the patient as a failure of the technique. When the patient reports being comfortable, the dentist stops increasing the N_2O percentage and begins treatment. Oversedation may be indicated by excessive drowsiness, loss of response to verbal command, inappropriate movement, hearing abnormalities, visual disturbances, sweating, or nausea. Patients should be monitored by clinical assessment of level of consciousness, adequacy of respiration, heart rate, and blood pressure.

Recovery is accomplished by terminating N_2O flow and administering 100% O_2 at the previously established flow rate for approximately 5 minutes (to allow for scavenging of exhaled N_2O) or longer if clinical signs and symptoms warrant. Recovery should be evaluated by visual observation, patient report, and, if necessary, assessment of the postoperative vital signs relative to baseline values.

Enteral (Oral) Sedation

The oral route is the second most frequently used route to accomplish minimal or moderate sedation in dentistry. It has numerous advantages and disadvantages (see Table 38-3).

Advantages

The oral route is commonly used to achieve minimal or moderate sedation because of the ease of administration. Most adults readily accept oral medication; however, young children, the mentally challenged, and those with dementia may not willingly swallow drugs, particularly in tablet or capsule form. Problems such as overdose, idiosyncratic reactions, allergy, and other adverse events may occur whenever drugs are administered, but such reactions are less likely to arise when drugs are given orally, and if they do develop, they are often less intense. Nevertheless, careful administration of any drug by even this route is required because fatal reactions have resulted from oral sedation.

Disadvantages

The major disadvantage of oral sedation is **the inability to titrate reliably**, so the dentist cannot adjust for individual patient response. After a drug is taken orally, it is often impractical to provide an additional dose because of the delay in absorption and onset of action. There can also be a delay in drug equilibration between the plasma and effect site concentrations, which can lead to overdose if additional doses are administered on the basis of patient anxiety. A predetermined dose is best administered while recognizing, on one hand, the risk of an excessive dose leading to prolonged action or inadvertent deep sedation and, on the other hand, the risk of an insufficient dose, in which case the patient would be inadequately sedated to allow dental treatment.

A further disadvantage of oral sedation is the potential for a prolonged duration of action. The patient can remain under the influence of the drug postoperatively and should not leave the dental office unescorted. Specific contraindications to oral sedation depend on the drug used.

Clinical application

The most common indication is the administration of an oral drug for minimal or moderate sedation during the dental procedure. Ideally, a dose used to induce sedation should be administered to the patient in the dental office, taking into account the time required for drug absorption. Although great variability exists, initial clinical effects are often evident approximately 30 minutes after ingestion, with peak effects occurring at about 1 hour. Patients should be monitored by clinical assessment of level of consciousness, adequacy of respiration, heart rate, and blood pressure as necessary. At the end of the case, patients should be discharged to the care of a responsible adult only when they are oriented and ambulatory, have stable vital signs, and show signs of increasing alertness. The patient should be instructed not to drive a vehicle, operate hazardous machinery, or consume alcohol for the remainder of the day.

The oral route may be considered the night before the dental procedure if the patient needs a hypnotic to ensure adequate sleep. Preoperative anxiety reduction before the patient is transported to the dental office may be a second indication for oral premedication. Dosages for these two indications should be kept low enough to minimize the likelihood of oversedation because the dentist is not present to deal with any potential adverse event.

Determinants of dose. The suggested doses for sedation recommended in this chapter apply to a typical 70-kg, healthy adult. Some factors modify these recommendations. The first consideration is the patient's weight. Extremes of age are another consideration. The dosage regimens for pediatric patients may often be determined by body weight or surface area calculations. Geriatric patients may react much more profoundly to CNS depressants with respect to depth and duration of action. As a general recommendation, one should consider an initial dose for an elderly patient of half that usually administered for a typical adult of the same body size.

Medical history and concurrent medication may influence the dose to be used. In particular, drugs affecting the CNS must be assessed, not only regarding interactive potential leading to excessive CNS depression and subsequent respiratory and cardiovascular depression but also regarding the possibility of cross-tolerance and decreased effect of the planned medications. History of the patient's response to mood-altering drugs such as alcohol may indicate an altered dose requirement.

Patients with a substance use disorder require special consideration. Patients who take large amounts of alcohol, opioids, or other mood-altering drugs may require an increased dose of sedative because of tolerance. A patient who is recovering from a substance use disorder should ideally have an oral sedative administered only after consultation with the patient and the health professional treating the dependency.

Finally, **increased anxiety often correlates with increased dose requirement.** Larger doses (although still within the acceptable range) are generally indicated for patients with an increased need for pharmacologic sedation.

Specific drugs

Numerous drugs are available for oral sedation. The following is a summary of the drugs commonly used in dentistry.

Benzodiazepines. Benzodiazepines are typically the drugs of choice for oral sedation and have a wide margin of safety compared with other antianxiety and sedative drugs. They are well absorbed, and most have a rapid onset of action. Relative contraindications to the use of benzodiazepines include myasthenia gravis, obstructive sleep apnea, and acute angle-closure glaucoma. The following benzodiazepines can be considered for use in minimal or moderate sedation in dentistry. Suggested doses for these drugs are listed in Table 38-5.

Triazolam is an effective anxiolytic and amnestic agent; it has a rapid onset of action and a short elimination half-life. This short duration of action is ideally suited to dentistry, allowing for rapid recovery, which is important for outpatient procedures. Triazolam has been shown to be as effective as intravenous diazepam for moderate sedation. Significant adverse reactions of triazolam (e.g., behavioral abnormalities), widely publicized in the lay press, are associated with repeated use of high doses, particularly in elderly patients, and not truly applicable to its use in minimal or moderate sedation for dentistry.

TABLE 38-5 Suggested Adult Dose Regimens for Benzodiazepines for ASA 1 and 2 Patients

Appointment Duration	Minimal Sedation	Moderate Sedation
<2 hr	triazolam 0.125-0.25 mg	triazolam 0.375-0.50 mg
2 to 3 hr	triazolam 0.25 mg	triazolam 0.50 mg
	diazepam 10-15 mg	diazepam 20-30 mg
	temazepam 15 mg	temazepam 30 mg
	oxazepam 10-15 mg	oxazepam 15-30 mg
>3 hr	lorazepam 0.5-1.0 mg	lorazepam 2.0-3.0 mg
	alprazolam 0.25 mg	alprazolam 0.50 mg

Various dose options are given for minimal and moderate sedation. The suggested dose regimens listed in the table are for consideration only and assume that no other sedative is being administered. These doses must be individualized for each patient, taking into account several factors that would include medical history and intended depth of sedation.

A significant interaction can occur with drugs that inhibit the biotransformation pathway of triazolam. Specifically, CYP3A4, which metabolizes triazolam, can be inhibited by numerous drugs, including erythromycin, clarithromycin, azole antifungals (ketoconazole, fluconazole, itraconazole), cimetidine, fluvoxamine, and several antiviral drugs including ritonavir. Concurrent administration of these drugs inhibits triazolam's intestinal and hepatic breakdown, leading to increased and prolonged plasma concentrations; grapefruit juice has the same effect. These drugs may potentiate the magnitude and duration of triazolam's sedative effect.

It is available in 0.125-mg or 0.25-mg tablets.

Diazepam is the prototypic benzodiazepine and has a long history of use in dentistry. It is efficacious, but it has active metabolites and may have a prolonged duration of action. It is available in tablets (2, 5, and 10 mg) and as a syrup (5 mg/5 mL and 25 mg/5 mL).

Lorazepam is another benzodiazepine that has been commonly used. Although it can elicit satisfactory sedation for dental procedures, it has the potential drawbacks of profound anterograde amnesia and an unusually long duration of action. Peak effects may occur 1 to 6 hours after administration, making appropriate scheduling difficult. It may be considered for longer dental appointments (e.g., over 3 hours). It is available as 0.5-, 1-, or 2-mg tablets. Lorazepam is not recommended in pediatric patients.

Midazolam, widely used parenterally, is also available as an oral formulation for use in pediatric patients. It is not normally used orally in adults in the United States or Canada. It has a rapid onset and short duration of action. Similar to triazolam, oral midazolam is contraindicated in patients taking erythromycin or other strong CYP3A4 inhibitors because the resulting interaction can lead to increased plasma concentrations of midazolam with subsequent increased and prolonged sedation. Midazolam's high first-pass effect leads to large differences in the parenteral and oral dosing recommendations. For oral midazolam, the usual dose is 0.5 to 0.6 mg/kg, but doses of 1 mg/kg (to a maximum of 20 mg) have been approved.

Alprazolam may be given for longer procedures as an alternative to lorazepam. Alprazolam (but not lorazepam) is subject to the same

CYP3A4 interactions as triazolam. It is available as 0.25- and 0.5-mg tablets for this purpose.

Temazepam can be considered as an alternative for minimal or moderate sedation if triazolam is unavailable. There is not as much documented use for it in dental anxiety studies, but it does share the properties of other benzodiazepines. It is available as 15- and 30-mg capsules.

Oxazepam, like temazepam, is another benzodiazepine that has less documented use in dental anxiety studies, but it can be considered as an alternative if triazolam is unavailable. It is available as 10-, 15-, and 30-mg tablets.

Zolpidem and zaleplon are sedative-hypnotics related pharmacologically to benzodiazepines because they interact with a subtype of benzodiazepine receptors. They are similar to triazolam (also classified as a sedative-hypnotic) in providing anxiolysis, sedation, and a rapid onset of action, with peak effects occurring in 20 minutes. Prolonged sedation is not a problem because of their short metabolic half-lives and conversion to inactive derivatives. Possible disadvantages are their relative lack of anticonvulsant and muscle relaxant properties. Some question remains regarding whether zolpidem and zaleplon produce specific anxiolytic effects common to the benzodiazepines. The average adult dose is 10 mg; zolpidem and zaleplon are available in 5- and 10-mg tablets (zolpidem) and capsules (zaleplon). Zolpidem is characterized as a category B drug with regard to pregnancy and may be considered an oral sedative of choice for pregnant women. These drugs are contraindicated in patients with liver disease.

Antihistamines. Promethazine is a phenothiazine derivative with antihistaminic properties that has been used for sedation, particularly in pediatric patients, but its use is being superseded by superior drugs, as described here. **Hydroxyzine**, the only antihistamine approved specifically as an antianxiety drug, is similar to promethazine in that it is an antihistamine and induces sedation and has anticholinergic and antiemetic effects. Recommended doses range from 50 to 100 mg for adults, if given alone, and 0.65 to 1 mg/kg for children. If it is combined with another sedative, doses should be reduced. It is available in tablet (10, 25, and 50 mg), capsule (25, 50, and 100 mg), and liquid (10 mg/5 mL syrup and 25 mg/5 mL suspension) formulations.

Other drugs. There are a number of agents that have been used in the past for oral sedation that are no longer recommended, as their risk/benefit balance is inferior to the benzodiazepines and antihistamines. For those trained only in minimal or moderate sedation techniques, agents such as chloral hydrate, opioids, ketamine, and barbiturates are not recommended as oral sedatives.

Parenteral (Intravenous) Sedation

The intravenous route is a very effective method to achieve moderate sedation, as well as deep sedation and general anesthesia. The advantages and disadvantages of this route of administration are summarized in Table 38-3.

Advantages

The intravenous route makes possible the rapid attainment of blood concentrations at which drugs are clinically effective. Intravenous injection leads to a very short latent period, which ranges from 30 seconds—the time it may take to go from the intravenous site to the site of action in the brain—to a few minutes (or longer for drugs of low lipid solubility). **The ability to titrate drugs and minimize the likelihood of overdosage and to enhance drug action rapidly are other advantages.** In clinical practice, the operator requires 2 to 15 minutes to titrate a drug to a desired clinical end point. One more advantage is that a patent intravenous line provides the ideal route for drug administration in the event of an emergency.

Disadvantages

Patients must be cooperative to permit venipuncture. Many children actively resist, and intravenous sedation for children is often undesirable or impossible. Another disadvantage of this route is that the rapid onset of action and the accentuated drug effects likely to be observed tend to magnify problems associated with drug overdose or side effects. As stated earlier, administering intravenous sedation requires advanced training, in part because adverse effects may occur more readily and with more severe consequences.

Clinical applications

For intravenous sedation, monitoring should include, at a minimum, oxyhemoglobin saturation, heart rate, blood pressure, and adequacy of respiration.

Benzodiazepines. As with the oral route, benzodiazepines are the ideal drugs to induce intravenous sedation. **Diazepam** is lipid soluble and water insoluble and is formulated in propylene glycol. This vehicle is often irritating on intravenous administration and may lead to thrombophlebitis. Irritation may be minimized by slow administration into large-caliber veins or by use of a formulation of diazepam dissolved in an injectable emulsion (not currently available in the United States). Diazepam is prepared as a 5-mg/mL solution. The drug must be titrated slowly, with sedative and anxiolytic effects usually beginning at doses of 2 to 10 mg, although great interpatient variability is possible. Appropriate moderate sedation often corresponds with ptosis. By this route, diazepam has a rapid onset of 30 to 60 seconds, with peak effects occurring after approximately 3 minutes. The duration of sedation is dose dependent, but averages approximately 45 to 60 minutes for sedative doses. Overall, diazepam is an effective agent for intravenous sedation, but it has the disadvantages of slow elimination, active metabolites, and the potential for thrombophlebitis.

Midazolam injection is water soluble and, when administered intravenously, does not cause venous irritation. Midazolam is rapidly eliminated and is converted to essentially inactive metabolites. After intravenous administration, it has a rapid onset of 30 to 60 seconds, with peak effects reported to occur after 3 to 5 minutes, which may be slightly slower than with diazepam. The distributional half-life is very short, 6 to 15 minutes, leading to a short duration of action of approximately 45 minutes. The duration of action is dose dependent. It has been suggested that midazolam is approximately three times as potent as diazepam. Moderate sedation is achieved by doses approximating 0.07 mg/kg, titrated slowly in 1-mg increments. Midazolam is provided in strengths of 1 mg/mL and 5 mg/mL. A 1-mg/mL solution is recommended for moderate sedation to facilitate accurate titration.

Opioids. These drugs primarily act centrally to decease pain, fear and anxiety and are not used alone for sedation, but they are commonly given to supplement benzodiazepines or other sedatives either to facilitate moderate sedation or, with increasing doses, to induce deep sedation or general anesthesia. They are useful for painful procedures such as those common in dentistry and oral surgery. Opioids typically provide the advantages of profound analgesia and sedation with minimal cardiovascular effects. The duration of action varies with the drug. Administration of an opioid should be timed so that the peak effect coincides with the most painful part of the procedure.

In general, ASA III patients, such as patients with significant cardiovascular disease, and elderly patients require lower doses of opioids than younger ASA I or II patients. Specific concerns with intravenous opioids include respiratory depression and chest wall rigidity. The latter syndrome is characterized by an increase in muscle tone leading to severe truncal stiffness. It seems to be more prevalent with high doses, with bolus administration of rapidly acting opioids, in elderly patients, and when N_2O is coadministered. Chest wall rigidity is treated with either naloxone or a neuromuscular blocker.

Opioids commonly used for moderate sedation include fentanyl, meperidine, pentazocine, and nalbuphine. **Fentanyl** is particularly suited for procedures of short duration. The dose for sedation is on the order of 1 μg/kg. At this dose, it can be expected to have a duration of action of 30 to 60 minutes. Advantages of fentanyl over other opioids include cardiovascular stability, a relatively short duration of action, and lack of histamine release. Fentanyl is more likely to produce chest wall rigidity.

Meperidine is administered for sedation in doses of 0.5 to 1 mg/kg, usually not exceeding 100 mg. At these doses, meperidine can be expected to have a duration of action of 1 to 2 hours. In addition to its expected effects of analgesia and sedation, meperidine is noted for its antisialagogue effect and potential to induce tachycardia. It is contraindicated in patients taking monoamine oxidase inhibitors or amphetamines and should be used cautiously, or not at all, in patients with asthma because of the potential for histamine release. A more recent concern is its potential to interact with other drugs—serotonin-selective reuptake inhibitors and various other antidepressants—that can increase the activity of endogenous 5-hydroxytryptamine (serotonin).

Pentazocine is a mixed agonist-antagonist, which results in a ceiling effect regarding analgesia and respiratory depression. Adverse reactions include a potential for psychotomimetic effects, such as disorientation, confusion, depression, hallucinations, dysphoria, diaphoresis, and dizziness. In doses approximating 0.5 mg/kg, to a maximum of 30 mg, pentazocine can be expected to have a duration of action of 1 to 2 hours. **Nalbuphine** is also a mixed agonist-antagonist used for sedation. A dose of 0.1 mg/kg, up to a maximum of 10 mg, may be considered.

Propofol, an intravenous general anesthetic, in low doses can be used for moderate sedation or deep sedation by those with training in deep sedation or general anesthesia. Moderate sedation may result in lower doses, such as infusion at a rate of 25 to 100 μg/kg/min.

Dexmedetomidine is a centrally acting α_2-adrenoceptor agonist similar in properties to clonidine. Originally indicated for sedation of intubated patients in the intensive care unit, the drug has been approved for moderate sedation, although not yet widely used. Xerostomia, hypotension, and bradycardia are the most common side effects. An initial evaluation of dexmedetomidine given as a loading dose of 0.1 μg/kg/min for 5 minutes and followed by a continuous infusion of 0.2 μg/kg/hr seemed to be safe and effective for dental patients.

REVERSAL AGENTS

Specific antagonists are available for opioids and benzodiazepines. They should be readily available whenever these agonists are being used for sedation.

Naloxone

Naloxone is a reversal agent for the opioid analgesics. The primary indication is in the treatment of opioid-induced respiratory depression, chest wall rigidity, or overly deep sedation. The drug has a peak effect in 5 to 15 minutes, with a duration of action of 45 minutes. Naloxone should be used with caution. Particular concern is warranted regarding patients with cardiac irritability or opioid dependency. Convulsions, alterations in blood pressure, ventricular tachycardia, and ventricular fibrillation have been reported to occur. Therapeutic doses are best administered by titrating slowly in 0.1-mg increments to effect, often to a final dose of 0.4 to 0.8 mg in cases of true opioid overdosage. The duration of action is short, so there is a danger that the antagonistic effect of naloxone will wear off before the agonistic effect of the opioid, resulting in a return of respiratory difficulties. After the administration of naloxone, the patient should be carefully monitored for 1 hour or more, depending on the opioid being antagonized.

Flumazenil

Flumazenil, a specific benzodiazepine receptor antagonist, exerts little effect by itself. When administered to reverse benzodiazepine-induced CNS depression, however, it causes a rapid reversal of unconsciousness, sedation, amnesia, and psychomotor dysfunction. In the presence of a high dose of agonist, flumazenil first reverses the loss of consciousness and respiratory depression, but drowsiness and amnesia may persist. These latter two signs diminish after higher doses of flumazenil. Onset is rapid, with the peak effect occurring in 1 to 3 minutes. The duration of action is dose dependent, depending on the specific agonist being reversed and how much of it was administered. Incremental doses of 0.1 to 0.2 mg of flumazenil intravenously (up to 3 mg) can be used. Reports indicate that 3 mg may provide 45 to 90 minutes of antagonism.

Flumazenil seems to have few adverse effects other than the important possibility of resedation. The adverse cardiovascular sequelae sometimes seen with naloxone after reversal of opioid overdosage do not occur with flumazenil. Agitation and headache have been reported. Convulsions have occurred in epileptic patients taking benzodiazepines for their condition. Patients taking medications that may cause seizures, such as tricyclic antidepressants, may also be susceptible to convulsions. Flumazenil is indicated whenever rapid reversal of benzodiazepine agonist action is required. As with any reversal agent, the potential for resedation demands that whenever this agent is used to treat an emergency, the patient must be monitored in recovery beyond the potential duration of action of flumazenil.

SUMMARY

Significant progress in the science of dentistry has resulted in important advances in the prevention and treatment of caries and periodontal disease. Many patients fail to benefit from modern dentistry, however, because of fear and anxiety regarding dental treatment. Dentists who are able to use the techniques discussed in this chapter have the capability to carry out dentistry in a compassionate manner for these patients. Patients deserve and expect to be treated as atraumatically as possible, and the administration of judiciously selected drugs can help achieve this goal.

A summary of the drugs to consider for minimal and moderate sedation is listed next.

DRUGS FOR MINIMAL AND MODERATE SEDATION

Drug	Route of Administration
Nitrous oxide	Inhalation
Diazepam	Oral, IV
Midazolam	Oral, IV
Triazolam	Oral
Lorazepam	Oral
Alprazolam	Oral
Temazepam	Oral
Oxazepam	Oral
Hydroxyzine	Oral
Fentanyl	IV
Meperidine	IV
Pentazocine	IV
Nalbuphine	IV
Propofol*	IV infusion
Dexmedetomidine	IV

*The use of propofol is generally restricted in the United States to dentists with formal advanced training in general anesthesia.

CASE DISCUSSION

This patient's history of anxiety shows that there is an indication for the administration of minimal or moderate sedation. The management of her anxiety during the dental procedure is of even greater importance given her history of hypertension. The first choice for inducing minimal sedation is the administration of $N_2O—O_2$. An alternative is to consider the enteral route for minimal sedation. In this latter case, the drug of first choice would be triazolam, at a dose of 0.25mg. If it is determined that moderate sedation is more appropriate, then a dose of 0.5mg would be considered. The patient would be given this drug in the dental office approximately 1 hour prior to the procedure, and then she would be accompanied home after she met the usual discharge criteria.

GENERAL REFERENCES

1. American Academy of Pediatrics and the American Academy of Pediatric Dentistry: Guideline for monitoring and management of pediatric patients during and after sedation for diagnostic and therapeutic procedures, Reaffirmed 2011. Available at: http://www.aapd.org/media/Policies_Guidelines/G_Sedation.pdf. Accessed June 30, 2016.
2. American Dental Association: Guidelines for the use of sedation and general anesthesia by dentists, Adopted 2012. Available at: http://www.ada.org/~/media/ADA/About%20the%20ADA/Files/anesthesia_use_guidelines.ashx.
3. Chanpong B, Haas DA, Locker D: Need and demand for sedation or general anesthesia in dentistry: a national survey of the Canadian population, *Anesth Prog* 52:3–11, 2005.
4. Coté CJ, Karl HW, Notterman DA, et al.: Adverse sedation events in pediatrics: analysis of medications used for sedation, *Pediatrics* 106:633–644, 2000.
5. Coté CJ, Notterman DA, Karl HW, et al.: Adverse sedation events in pediatrics: a critical incident analysis of contributing factors, *Pediatrics* 105:805–814, 2000.
6. Dionne RA, Gordon SM, McCullagh LM, et al.: Assessing the need for anesthesia and sedation in the general population, *J Am Dent Assoc* 129: 167–173, 1998.
7. Dionne RA, Yagiela JA, Coté CJ, et al.: Balancing efficacy and safety for the use of oral sedation in dental outpatients, *J Am Dent Assoc* 137:502–513, 2006.
8. Jackson DL, Milgrom P, Heacox GA, et al.: Pharmacokinetics and clinical effects of multidose sublingual triazolam in healthy volunteers, *J Clin Psychopharmacol* 26:4–8, 2006.
9. Smith TA, Heaton LJ: Fear of dental care: are we making any progress? *J Am Dent Assoc* 134:1101–1108, 2003.

39

Drugs of Abuse

Charles S. Bockman, Peter W. Abel, and Frank J. Dowd

KEY INFORMATION

- Drug abuse is the inappropriate use of a drug for a nonmedical purpose.
- Drugs that are abused cause intense feelings of euphoria or alter perception.
- Categories of abused drugs include opioid analgesics; general depressants of the central nervous system (CNS), e.g., sedative-hypnotics, antianxiety drugs, and alcohol; cocaine, amphetamines, and related psychomotor stimulants; hallucinogens; marijuana; and inhalants.
- Drug addiction refers to compulsive, relapsing drug use despite the negative consequences.
- Drug dependence refers to the physical state produced in response to repeated drug exposure and is defined by a withdrawal syndrome.
- Withdrawal or abstinence syndrome is the drug class–specific group of symptoms that appear when drug administration is discontinued or reduced and is the cardinal sign of dependence.
- Drug tolerance is the reduction in effect in response to repeated drug exposure.
- Ethanol has both acute and chronic effects on several organs, including the brain, liver, heart, and GI tract.
- Ethanol abuse is the most common example of substance abuse, with major impacts on individuals and society.
- Damage to organs from ethanol is due to effects of ethanol, as well as acetaldehyde and nutritional deficiencies.
- Metabolism of ethanol produces acetaldehyde and then acetic acid, displaying zero-order kinetics.

CASE STUDY

Mr. C is a 27-year-old man, who on his first visit to a new dentist complains about recent changes in the appearance of his teeth. He reports losing weight lately, difficulty in sleeping and sometimes having "strange thoughts." Mr. C presents with mild gingivitis and chewed tongue without other signs of soft tissue pathology. He exhibits worn teeth and extensive dental decay, including interproximal surfaces of anterior teeth and buccal surfaces of many maxillary and mandibular teeth. The effects of which drug of abuse are consistent with the signs and symptoms exhibited by Mr. C? Explain the connection between the effects of the abused drug and the oral health of Mr. C.

INTRODUCTION

Drug abuse can be defined as an inappropriate use of a drug for a nonmedical purpose. Drug abuse is considered to cause harm to the individual abuser and to society as a whole. Many variables not directly related to a drug can influence whether a given individual becomes a drug abuser. Many experts argue that cocaine possesses the greatest potential for abuse based on its pharmacologic characteristics alone. For individuals who try nicotine, the risk of developing an addiction is approximately twice that for individuals who try cocaine, however. This statement is not meant to infer that the pharmacologic abuse potential of nicotine is twice that of cocaine; rather, some psychosocial factors are equally important in affecting onset and continuation of drug abuse and addiction. It is beyond the scope of this chapter to discuss these factors related to drug users and their environment; this chapter concentrates solely on the pharmacologic aspects of drugs of abuse.

A wide variety of different types of drugs and other chemical substances are subject to abuse. Anabolic steroids are abused by bodybuilders and other athletes to add muscle mass and enhance athletic performance. The most commonly abused groups of drugs are those that act on the CNS to cause intense feelings of euphoria or alter perception. This chapter focuses on drugs that are abused because they have effects in the CNS that are perceived by some individuals as desirable.

HISTORIC PERSPECTIVE

Natural products such as hemp flowers, opium, and coca leaves have been used for thousands of years for their ability to cause pleasurable sensations or other alterations in consciousness. Other than alcohol, the first major drugs of abuse in the United States were cocaine and opioids. Throughout the nineteenth century, unregulated opium use led to a plethora of patent medicines containing opium derivatives. As a result, many middle-class Americans became dependent on opium because of promiscuous use of such preparations. Nevertheless, social attitudes toward drug abuse remained relaxed until after the Civil War. The widespread use of morphine by injection for dysentery, malaria, and pain resulted in such large numbers of morphine-addicted veterans that morphine dependence became known as "soldier's disease."

The chemical isolation of the alkaloid cocaine in 1859 was followed by a rapid increase in the use of that drug. It was enthusiastically promoted for various disorders, and by the turn of the 20th century, oral abuse of cocaine in the form of patent medicines and tonics was widespread. The manufacturers of Coca-Cola did not stop using cocaine-containing syrup in their soft drink until 1903, after 17 years in production.

In the early 1900s, the mass media developed the myth of cocaine-crazed renegades committing heinous crimes against society. Opioid dependence was still prevalent, and morphine was the major opioid of abuse. During this period, federal laws were enacted to control the widespread drug abuse problem. The introduction of the Pure Food and Drug Act in 1906, the Harrison Narcotic Act in 1914, and the Narcotic Drugs Import and Export Act in 1922, and the enforcement of these acts by law enforcement officials led to the virtual disappearance of cocaine abuse by the 1930s. The increased cost and reduced street availability of cocaine helped lead to the increase of amphetamine as a stimulant drug of abuse. Intravenous (IV) heroin use was also becoming popular, and by 1935, it was as widely abused as morphine. Between World Wars I and II, addiction began to be widely equated with criminality. In the case of marijuana, sensationalized accounts of murders perpetrated by individuals under the influence of the "killer weed" led to the passage of the Marihuana Tax Act of 1937, which effectively banned its production, distribution, and sale.

In the 1960s, drug abuse began to make major inroads into middle-class society. The baby-boom generation began experimenting with lysergic acid diethylamide (LSD) and marijuana. Epidemic amphetamine abuse developed during the 1960s, peaking in 1967 with 32 million legal prescriptions written for amphetamines that suppress appetite and lead to weight loss. To combat the rising tide of drug abuse, the Comprehensive Drug Abuse Prevention and Control Act was enacted in 1970 and replaced previous laws in this area. This act classified drugs into five schedules according to their abuse liability and provided a graded set of penalties for violation of regulations relating to the manufacture, sale, prescription, and record keeping of drugs of abuse. A summary of the abuse potential and examples of drugs falling under this act are provided in Appendix 7. This act is the major regulatory legislation controlling drugs of abuse.

In the early 1970s, cocaine was rediscovered as a recreational drug by the young, upwardly mobile, affluent generation. This second cocaine epidemic necessitated a redefinition of the picture of the typical drug abuser as an unemployed, minority male criminal. For example, the 1993 National Household Survey on Drug Abuse reported that 70% of illicit drug abusers are employed, 80% are white, and 75% live in areas outside of the city. In 1983, a glut in the world market for cocaine combined with the development of a smokable, inexpensive, and very addictive form of the drug called "crack" brought the third cocaine epidemic to the inner cities, where availability of powdered forms of the drug was limited because of its cost. In the 1990s, the preparation of a smokable form of methamphetamine led to the widespread abuse of this stimulant, called "ice" and "crank" on the street. More severe abuse patterns than had ever been seen before emerged with the appearance of these smokable, freebase forms of cocaine and methamphetamine. Smoking these drugs results in a more rapid onset of action and a more intense effect, conferring on them more abuse liability than other forms of these drugs that must be sniffed or taken orally. The abuse potential of these drugs increased so dramatically with this mode of administration that drug seeking became more paramount to this population of abusers than it previously had been. Equally insidious has been the emergence of clandestine laboratories that make "designer drugs," synthetic substances that are inexpensive to produce and difficult to detect. Some examples include the amphetamine analogue 3,4-methylenedioxymethamphetamine (MDMA) (i.e., "ecstasy"), synthetic cathinones (i.e., "bath salts"), and synthetic cannabinoids (i.e., "spice"). In addition, nonmedical use of prescription drugs such as clonazepam (Klonopin), methylphenidate (Ritalin), and oxycodone (OxyContin) has become common.

DRUG ABUSE CHARACTERISTICS AND TERMINOLOGY

The term **addiction** refers to compulsive, relapsing drug use despite the negative consequences. Additional characteristics of addiction, which may or may not be present, are dependence and tolerance. When the administration of a drug is discontinued or, in the case of certain drugs, significantly reduced, **dependence** leads to the appearance of a characteristic and specific group of symptoms, termed a **withdrawal** *or* **abstinence syndrome. Tolerance** exists when administration of the same dose of a drug has progressively less effect. This decreased response to the effects of a drug requires that increasingly larger doses of a drug be given to produce the same pharmacologic actions. The development of tolerance depends on the dose of the drug and the frequency of its administration. Tolerance is caused by compensatory responses that act to decrease the body's response to a drug. The cellular basis for drug tolerance may be related to a decrease in receptors for the drug, a reduction in enzyme activity associated with signal transduction pathways, or other effects. **Cross-tolerance** is the phenomenon whereby chronic use of a drug produces tolerance to that drug's effects and to other drugs that produce the same effect. Cross-tolerance may be observed among drugs of similar or different chemical types. A related but different phenomenon is **cross-dependence**, which refers to an ability of one drug to substitute for another drug, usually in the same class, in a dependent individual without precipitating a withdrawal syndrome.

On the basis of common pharmacologic actions and of cross-tolerance and cross-dependence, the major drugs of abuse can be divided into distinct categories: opioid analgesics; general depressants of the CNS, including sedative-hypnotics, antianxiety drugs, and alcohol; cocaine, amphetamines, and related psychomotor stimulants; hallucinogens; marijuana; and inhalants. Table 39-1 lists the major abuse characteristics of these six drug groups—the abuse potential and degree of dependence and tolerance development commonly associated with the abuse of each drug group. In the following discussion, each drug group is described in terms of three major factors: (1) the pharmacologic effects produced by the drug group; (2) the abuse characteristics of the drug group, including addiction, tolerance, dependence, withdrawal, and other characteristics; and (3) the toxicity caused by the drug group and how it is treated.

ABUSE OF OPIOID ANALGESICS

Opioid analgesics most commonly abused include **heroin, morphine, oxycodone, hydrocodone**, and **fentanyl**. In addition to these agonists, various other synthetic and semisynthetic derivatives are subject to abuse. These agents differ from each other in their abuse characteristics, their onset and duration of action, the intensity of their effects, and, to some extent, the pattern of their abuse. Many of the mechanisms involved in the analgesic response to opioids also produce

TABLE 39-1 Abuse Characteristics of Drug Groups

	Abuse Potential	Dependence	Tolerance
Opioid analgesics	++++	++++	++++
Sedative-hypnotics	+++	++++	+++
Amphetamines	+++	++	++++
Cocaine	++++	++	++
Hallucinogens			
LSD	+	+	++
PCP	+	+	+
Marijuana	++	+	++
Inhalants	+	U	U

++++, Marked; +++, moderate; ++, some; +, slight; *U*, unknown.

euphoria or a perceived state of well-being, and much research has been generated in an attempt to develop efficacious analgesics that are not euphoric and have less abuse potential. Although this research has led to a greater understanding of the physiologic characteristics of pain, at present no opioids or other types of analgesics are superior to morphine. In the following discussion, morphine is considered the prototype for this group, unless another drug is specifically mentioned.

Pharmacologic Effects

In the following discussion, the subjective effects of opioids are the effects observed in individuals who are opioid abusers. Although opioids produce similar pharmacologic effects in most individuals (see Chapter 16), not everyone reports the subjective effects of warmth, contentment, orgasm, and euphoria. In nonabusing individuals, the nausea and vomiting caused by opioids are construed as unpleasant and may obfuscate many of the reinforcing characteristics of these drugs. Many individuals view the mental clouding produced by opioids as an undesirable inability to concentrate, whereas addicts find this quality appealing. Most important, because opioids are the mainstay in the treatment of moderate–severe pain, it is relevant to know that in the therapeutic setting little substantive evidence suggests that effective and controlled pain management with opioids in individuals leads them to develop into opioid abusers.

For individuals who abuse opioids, the IV administration of heroin causes an immediate overwhelming sense of warmth that permeates the abdominal area and that has been described as orgasmic. Nausea, vomiting, and histamine release occur soon after, causing a sense of itching, reddening of the eyes, and a decrease in blood pressure. Feelings of increased energy with talkativeness ("soapboxing") alternate with periods of relaxation or tranquility ("coasting"). This intense euphoria may last several minutes. The depressant effects on the CNS then appear and include mental clouding, decreased visual acuity, and sedation accompanied by a feeling of heaviness in the extremities. The abuser has no motivation to participate in physical activity; the individual appears to be asleep, but only the head and facial muscles are relaxed ("nodding"). This period is followed by episodes of light sleeping accompanied by vivid dreaming. Feelings of anxiety and worry are absent, and a pervasive sense of contentment is present. Taken together, the early euphoric period followed by the sedation and sleeping may last 3 to 5 hours.

Abuse Characteristics

The development of tolerance is a characteristic feature of all opioid agonists. Regardless of whether opioids are administered in a therapeutic setting or are self-administered, repetitive use leads to tolerance or a reduction in response, such that a greater dose of drug is required to achieve the same effect that was produced on initial administration of the drug. Tolerance develops most readily when opioids are given in large doses at short intervals or during constant infusion of the drug; the phenomenon can be observed within days after drug therapy has begun. Tolerance or desensitization to the effects of opioids develops at the cellular level and may be viewed as a homeostatic response by the cell to constant exposure to an agonist. Because the development of tolerance to the effects of opioids is a physiologic phenomenon, it inevitably occurs in patients after repeated drug administration. **The development of tolerance is not a predictor of whether the patient will become an opioid abuser.**

Because most fatalities resulting from opioid overdose are caused by respiratory depression, the prescribing physician must understand that tolerance develops similarly to the respiratory depressant effect and to the analgesic and euphoric effects of opioids. This fact has important ramifications for the clinician, who may be wary about administering 10 times the normal dose of morphine for adequate pain control in a patient who has developed tolerance to the analgesic effects. Out of concern for the respiratory depressant or addictive properties of morphine, the clinician may not provide adequate pain control even though the patient has developed a similar degree of tolerance to the respiratory depressant and euphoric effects of morphine. Because of this use-induced decrease in the ability of opioids to suppress respiration, considerable tolerance to the lethal effects of opioids may develop. Tolerance to the respiratory effect of opioids is rapidly lost during abstinence, however, and death may result if an addict returns to the previously maintained dosage after withdrawal has been completed.

Similar to tolerance, dependence on opioids is also a result of repeated administration of an agonist and occurs for all opioids. Dependence results from cellular adaptation caused by uninterrupted agonist occupation of opioid receptors. Normal function of the individual now requires the presence of an opioid drug at its receptor. When the drug is removed from the receptor during drug withdrawal, an acute withdrawal syndrome ensues. The intensity of the withdrawal syndrome is related to the degree of dependence. As with tolerance, dependence develops most rapidly and to the greatest extent when the opioid receptors are constantly occupied. No outward signs of dependence are observed until the drug is withdrawn. The development of dependence to opioids is a physiologic response seen in all individuals; it does not predict whether they become abusers. In patients who become dependent, the dose of opioid can be decreased by 50% every other day and eventually stopped without overt signs of withdrawal.

Withdrawal symptoms in an opioid-dependent individual include rhinorrhea, lacrimation, vomiting, sweating, yawning, diarrhea, irritability, restlessness, chills, piloerection ("cold turkey"), mydriasis, hyperventilation, tachycardia, hypertension, tremors, and involuntary muscle movements. In general, the appearance and severity of withdrawal signs depend on the duration of action of the opioid being taken. Signs of withdrawal in a heroin-dependent individual appear approximately 6 hours after the last dose, increase in intensity over the next 36 to 72 hours, and subside after about 1 week. In contrast, dependence on a long-acting opioid, such as methadone, results in a mild but protracted withdrawal syndrome with delayed onset. A withdrawal syndrome can also be precipitated in dependent individuals by displacing the opioid from the receptor with an antagonist (naloxone), an agonist-antagonist (pentazocine), or a partial agonist (buprenorphine). Death from opioid withdrawal is rare; however, when it does occur, it is because of cardiovascular collapse from dehydration and acid–base imbalance.

Addiction to opioids is significant, as exemplified by the high relapse rate among addicts after withdrawal. The euphoria, tranquility, and abdominal effects, described as orgasmic, promote abuse of opioids. The rapidity with which opioids penetrate the CNS to cause their psychoactive effects correlates with their ability to cause addiction. Opioid addicts prefer the "rush" sensation produced by the rapid onset of psychoactive effects characteristic of IV administration over the slower onset of effects produced by other routes of administration. Heroin is preferred because its high lipid solubility confers rapid penetration into the brain and an intense effect. Conversely, orally administered methadone for control of chronic pain has much less potential for creating addiction.

Addiction to opioids may occur independently from tolerance and physical dependence and is a result of an addict craving the feelings produced by opioids. This craving may even occur before, or in the absence of, the development of tolerance and dependence. The fact that discontinuance of opioids may precipitate a withdrawal syndrome may provide an incentive to continue their use, however. Because of the short duration of action of heroin, a dependent addict oscillates between feelings of euphoria and sickness related to withdrawal and exhibits drug-seeking behavior. Drug-seeking behavior is manifested by pleas, complaints, demands, and other activities directed toward obtaining the drug to alleviate the discomfort caused by drug withdrawal. However, an individual may become addicted to opioids before developing fear of withdrawal.

Patients in need of pain control should not be denied adequate opioid medication because they show evidence of tolerance or exhibit withdrawal symptoms if the medication is stopped, as these signs do not indicate addiction. In addition, a patient who is in pain and receiving opioids does not respond the same way a psychologically dependent addict responds to opioids. Patients who are able to self-administer their opioid analgesic take the drug solely to reduce the pain, do not increase the dose greatly over time, and stop administration when the pain goes away.

Toxicity

In acute opioid overdose, the classic triad of **coma, respiratory depression**, and **pinpoint pupils** is common to all opioid agonists (except meperidine, in which case the pupils may be dilated in tolerant individuals). Hypoventilation leads to marked hypoxemia and cyanosis, and acute pulmonary edema evidenced by pink, frothy sputum may occur, especially with heroin overdose. Nausea and vomiting may be prominent. Hypotension, as a result of cerebral ischemia, develops gradually and may eventually lead to circulatory shock. Convulsions do not occur with most opioids, although they have been reported in children with codeine overdose, in addicts in response to meperidine, and in cases of propoxyphene poisoning.

The treatment of choice is rapid IV administration of 0.4 mg of **naloxone**, repeated if necessary at 2- to 3-minute intervals. Dramatic improvement occurs within minutes, with enhanced ventilation and dilation of the pinpoint pupils. The patient must be closely monitored because the antagonist's effect lasts only 1 to 4 hours. Monitoring is especially important with methadone overdose because respiratory depression may last 48 hours. If vital signs return to normal, no attempt should be made to arouse the patient with additional naloxone because if the patient is opioid-dependent, large doses of the antagonist may precipitate an acute withdrawal syndrome. Formerly, naloxone was approved for use only in the health care setting. However, in recognition that deaths from opioid overdose, driven largely by prescription abuse, had steadily increased since 2000, naloxone administered by a handheld auto-injector was made available in 2014 by prescription for use by family members or caregivers of opioid drug abusers.

The toxic effects of chronic abuse of opioids are minimal. Other than constipation, addicts with a stable supply of drug, individuals enrolled in a methadone maintenance program, or patients taking opioids long-term for pain control have few difficulties as long as they continue taking the drug. Many addicts share unsterile needles and equipment, however, which increases their risk of contracting acquired immunodeficiency syndrome (AIDS), hepatitis, skin abscesses, deep infections, and endocarditis.

When the supply of an addict's preferred drug is compromised, the addict may substitute substances of unknown content and potency or drugs thought to have a similar effect. Many addicts like the effects caused by IV injection of the agonist-antagonist pentazocine with the antihistamine tripelennamine. The talc contained in the crushed tripelennamine tablet has caused deaths as a result of lung emboli. Overdose leading to death may occur when an addict injects a purer sample than that to which he or she is accustomed or a sample containing a much more potent opioid, such as those seen with China white in the 1980s and fentanyl in the 1990s. Unexpected toxic effects also occurred in the late 1970s and early 1980s, when "bathtub chemists" trying to synthesize potent opioids produced a compound contaminated with 1-methyl-4-phenyl-1,2,3,6-tetrahydropyridine (MPTP), which caused Parkinson-like symptoms in many young abusers (see Chapter 13). Abuse of prescription opioid analgesics has also resulted in unexpected deaths. Beginning in the late 1990s and continuing into the 2000s, deaths from overdosage resulted when individuals crushed tablets of the controlled-release formulation of oxycodone to make the entire dose available for intranasal or IV administration.

Opioid withdrawal or detoxification of heroin addicts or other opioid-dependent individuals can be managed with **methadone** because cross-dependence exists between it and other opioids. Because methadone and all other opioid analgesics act at opioid receptors, methadone can be substituted for the opioid being abused without precipitating a withdrawal syndrome. By substituting longer acting methadone for a short-acting opioid such as heroin, the addict is spared the undesirable effects of withdrawal because the opioid receptor remains occupied. Methadone, with its long duration of action, produces a protracted but tolerable withdrawal syndrome. The dose of methadone is gradually reduced over several weeks until the patient is opioid-free and no longer dependent. Detoxification is effective only if the patient wants to quit abusing opioids and breaks the cycle of relapse and detoxification.

The α_2–adrenergic receptor agonist, **clonidine**, can also be used alone or in combination with methadone to assist in the detoxification of an opioid-dependent individual. Many of the unpleasant effects experienced during opioid withdrawal, such as nausea, vomiting, sweating, tachycardia, cramps, and hypertension, are caused by hyperactivity of the autonomic nervous system. Clonidine, through its stimulation of α_2–adrenergic receptors in the brain, suppresses the outflow of sympathetic nervous system activity, reducing the discomfort of opioid withdrawal.

Although management of acute opioid withdrawal is relatively easy, the recidivism rate (i.e., the number of addicts who return to abusing opioids) is very high. Methadone can also be used in the long-term treatment of opioid abuse, that is, maintenance therapy, when detoxification fails. The pharmacologic basis of methadone maintenance therapy depends on its oral effectiveness in reducing opioid cravings, long duration of action, and the development of cross-tolerance between it and other opioids, particularly heroin. The first step in maintenance therapy is to provide an oral dose of methadone that is not sedating but prevents signs of withdrawal. Maintenance therapy is performed at a government-regulated clinic and is feasible because of the long duration of action of methadone. Patients function normally and do not have the "rush" associated with other routes of administration. If the patient relapses into opioid abuse, the development of cross-tolerance between methadone and heroin or other agents results in a blockade or diminution of the euphoric effect of the abused substance, removing the reinforcing properties of the abused agent. Although the patient is now dependent on a non-intoxicating dose of methadone, he/she can work and participate normally in society.

In 2000, Congress passed the Drug Addiction Treatment Act (DATA), allowing certified physicians to prescribe narcotic medications for the treatment of opioid addiction. DATA produced an important paradigm shift that allowed for the treatment of addiction to opioids such as heroin to occur in physicians' offices, rather than limiting it to highly stigmatized government-regulated methadone clinics. Buprenorphine, an agent now being used under this new legislation, is a long-acting partial agonist that acts on the same receptors as heroin and morphine; it relieves opioid cravings in mildly to moderately addicted individuals and produces less respiratory depression and withdrawal symptoms than the full agonist methadone.

ABUSE OF SEDATIVE-HYPNOTICS

Drugs in the sedative-hypnotic group are general CNS depressants and include sedative-hypnotic and antianxiety drugs (discussed in Chapter 11). Older sedative-hypnotic drugs, including barbiturates, glutethimide, and the widely abused but no longer approved drug methaqualone, have substantial abuse potential. **Benzodiazepines** and related drugs are now the most commonly used sedative-hypnotic and antianxiety drugs. Although these newer drugs have significant abuse potential, they are less frequently abused than the older sedative-hypnotic agents. Sedative-hypnotic drugs are readily available from illicit sources and by prescription abuse when large amounts of the drugs are accumulated by drug abusers visiting different prescribers.

Pharmacologic Effects

The signs of intoxication with sedative-hypnotic and antianxiety drugs are similar to signs produced by alcohol: drowsiness, impairment of motor coordination, ataxia, and slurred speech. Sluggishness, difficulty in reasoning, mood swings, and irritability are also seen. Subjective effects include sensations of well-being, euphoria, and sometimes stimulation. The next day the abuser may experience nervousness, anxiety, tremor, headache, and insomnia. The exact constellation of effects depends on the dose of the drug, the route of drug administration, the frequency of administration, and the user's expectations.

Abuse Characteristics

The degree of addiction with sedative-hypnotic drugs depends on the dose of the drug, the frequency of administration, and the duration of drug use. Sedative-hypnotic drugs differ in onset and duration of action (short-acting and long-acting barbiturates and benzodiazepines are available). Addiction is most commonly associated with abuse of short-acting drugs, such as secobarbital, pentobarbital, oxazepam, and lorazepam. Dependence on longer acting agents, such as phenobarbital and chlordiazepoxide, is less common. Dependence occurs only rarely with intravenously administered ultrashort-acting sedative-hypnotics because they cannot be taken frequently enough to maintain adequate plasma concentrations.

For benzodiazepines, drugs with a higher affinity for the BZ_2 benzodiazepine receptor subtype (e.g., alprazolam) seem to have a greater potential for abuse than drugs with a higher affinity for the BZ_1 benzodiazepine receptor. Initial exposure to sedative-hypnotics may occur when the drug is prescribed to relieve anxiety or insomnia. The dose is slowly increased, and the abuser may become preoccupied with obtaining and using the drug. So-called date rape drugs, such as **γ-hydroxybutyrate**, a metabolite of γ-aminobutyric acid, and the prescription benzodiazepine **flunitrazepam** ("roofies") are also subject to misuse. Both drugs have similar effects as sedative-hypnotics; however, their rapid oral absorption, onset of action, and ability to cause anterograde amnesia have resulted in their surreptitious use as sedatives to facilitate rape of unwitting individuals.

In contrast to opioids, sedative-hypnotics do not induce dependence unless increased doses of drugs are taken over a long period (≥1 month). The onset and severity of the abstinence syndrome also depend, in part, on the dose and the duration of drug use. For instance, some physical dependence is likely to occur with daily doses of secobarbital in excess of 400 mg for about 90 days or more. With chronic use of larger doses, progressively more severe symptoms of withdrawal can be precipitated, even by abruptly reducing the accustomed dose by half. Withdrawal from daily doses of 600 to 800 mg of secobarbital for at least 35 days is sufficient to produce withdrawal seizures. Another important determinant of the onset, severity, and duration of the withdrawal syndrome is the half-life of the specific drug. Drugs with relatively short half-lives (8 to 30 hours) tend to produce a severe withdrawal syndrome that develops quite rapidly. Drugs with longer half-lives (40 to 100 hours) produce a slower onset but less severe withdrawal syndrome of long duration.

The withdrawal syndrome after cessation of sedative-hypnotics resembles that seen after alcohol withdrawal. After a usually symptomless period (8 to 18 hours after the last dose), the individual exhibits increasing symptoms of anxiety, insomnia, agitation, and confusion. Anorexia, nausea and vomiting, sweating, and muscle weakness are also seen. Coarse tremors in the face and hands; dilation of the pupils; and increases in respiratory rate, heart rate, and blood pressure may occur. Orthostatic hypotension and syncope may also occur. These symptoms become more severe during the first 24 to 30 hours of drug withdrawal. By the third or fourth day, major manifestations of abstinence may develop, which include delirium, hallucinations, agitation, hyperthermia, convulsions, and nonspecific symptoms of anxiety. Symptoms associated with benzodiazepine withdrawal also occur; these are persistent tinnitus (≤8 months), muscle twitching, paresthesias, visual disturbances, and confusion and depersonalization. Reports of xerostomia and pain in the jaws and teeth have particular dental significance.

Muscle fasciculations and enhanced deep reflexes may progress to frank seizures. One or more grand mal convulsions lasting less than 3 minutes may occur, with consciousness being regained within 5 minutes. In some cases, status epilepticus may ensue. The prolonged postictal stupor typical of epileptic seizures is not seen, but confusion may persist for 1 or 2 hours. Delirium develops gradually over 2 to 4 days and is heralded by a period of insomnia. Delirium is characterized by confusion, disorientation of time and place, nightmares, and vivid auditory and visual hallucinations. Paranoid delusions with extreme fear and agitation may develop, especially at night ("night terrors"). The symptoms terminate spontaneously after a prolonged period of sleep. This withdrawal psychosis may be caused by rebound rapid eye movement sleep, which, having been suppressed during the period of intoxication, intrudes into the waking state. During the phase of delirium, body temperature is elevated. A continuous marked hyperthermia is a life-threatening problem that, if not immediately and vigorously treated, may (along with agitation) lead to fatal exhaustion and cardiovascular collapse.

After the acute withdrawal syndrome, recovery is gradual but complete after approximately 8 days, although residual weakness may be noted for 6 to 12 weeks. Abrupt withdrawal from large doses of sedative-hypnotics can precipitate a severe, life-threatening withdrawal syndrome that has a significant mortality rate. The withdrawal syndrome from sedative-hypnotics may be more severe than withdrawal caused by opioids.

Tolerance develops to sedative-hypnotic drugs, and partial cross-tolerance also occurs among the various drugs in this class. Tolerance is usually complete to doses of short-acting barbiturates of up to 500 mg/day, but doses of greater than 800 mg/day are associated with signs of intoxication. The onset of tolerance to benzodiazepines in humans develops slowly, beginning in 3 to 5 days, with maximal tolerance in 7 to 10 days. The mechanisms of tolerance to these drugs are unclear. Much of the tolerance to large doses of short-acting barbiturates is associated with hepatic enzyme induction that results in enhanced barbiturate elimination. This metabolic tolerance plays less of a role for benzodiazepines, for which cellular tolerance, a decreased responsiveness of neuronal pathways in the CNS, seems to play a more prominent role.

Toxicity

Ingestion of large doses of sedative-hypnotic drugs may be life-threatening. Coma may develop with progressive deterioration of respiration and blood pressure. The victim exhibits hypoxia, cyanosis, shock, hypothermia, and anuria. Death is usually from cerebral anoxia caused by respiratory failure. Therapy is mainly supportive, consisting of oxygen administered by artificial respiration and fluids or pressor agents (or both) to maintain circulation. For barbiturates, osmotic diuretics with sodium bicarbonate are also used to alkalinize the urine and hasten elimination of the drug. The benzodiazepine receptor antagonist flumazenil has been used specifically to block toxic effects in the treatment of acute benzodiazepine overdose.

Withdrawal from chronic therapeutic abuse of sedative-hypnotic drugs is associated with drug craving, nausea and abdominal cramps, tachycardia, palpitation, and generalized seizures. Panic attacks and disorientation may occur, progressing to paranoid psychosis with aggression, delusions, and visual hallucinations. Coma and respiratory depression cause a significant mortality rate. Treatment includes substitution with a long-acting sedative-hypnotic drug, such as phenobarbital, followed by a modest daily reduction in the maintenance dose. **Seizures** represent a medical emergency and are treated by immediate administration of diazepam, pentobarbital, or carbamazepine. Withdrawal from sedative-hypnotic drugs should be carried out in a hospital setting because life-threatening complications may develop.

ABUSE OF AMPHETAMINES, COCAINE, AND OTHER PSYCHOMOTOR STIMULANTS

Psychomotor stimulants include analogues of phenylethylamine (**D-amphetamine and methamphetamine**), a group of amphetamine derivatives in which the terminal amine nitrogen is part of a heterocyclic group (**methylphenidate**, phendimetrazine) or a diethylated group (diethylpropion), and **cocaine**. The chemical structures of some of these drugs are shown in Figure 39-1. Amphetamines and methylphenidate are generally used for treatment of narcolepsy and attention-deficit/hyperactivity disorder; phendimetrazine and diethylpropion are anorectics. These drugs are available on the street and by prescription. Methamphetamine and cocaine are the most widely abused members of this class. The chemical structure of cocaine is shown in Figure 39-2. Generally, the effects of and abuse patterns associated with the individual drugs in this group are quite similar.

Amphetamine and Related Drugs

Pharmacologic effects

Single oral doses of amphetamine and related drugs produce wakefulness, reduced fatigue and reaction times, and improved performance of psychomotor tasks, especially in sleep-deprived individuals. Feelings of enhanced well-being, moderate exhilaration, and euphoria are common. Judgment may be impaired, and irrational behavior may occur. These drugs can cause signs of increased peripheral adrenergic nerve activity, such as an increase in blood pressure, tachycardia, mydriasis, sweating, and constipation. These effects probably result from the release of norepinephrine from central and peripheral neurons or the blockade of neuronal uptake of norepinephrine at these sites. High oral doses of CNS stimulants induce feelings of cleverness, enhanced abilities, aggressiveness, and fearlessness and may cause a manic "high," paranoid rage, violent diarrhea, and vomiting.

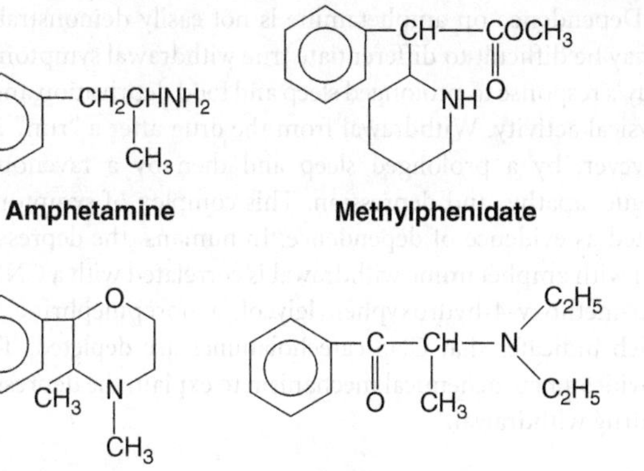

Amphetamine — Methylphenidate — Phendimetrazine — Diethylpropion

FIG 39-1 Structural formulas of amphetamine and related stimulant drugs.

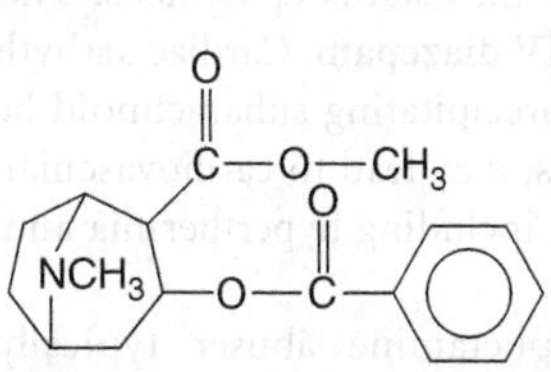

FIG 39-2 Structural formula of cocaine.

Abuse characteristics

Patterns of oral use are usually intermittent and involve lower doses causing milder effects. Oral amphetamines have been abused by students who want to study through the night and by truck drivers who want to stay awake for long hauls. Amphetamine abusers also take these drugs intranasally, intravenously, and by smoking. IV administration of methamphetamine results in a markedly pleasurable rush described as an expanding, flashing, vibration feeling, or a total body orgasm. IV administration of amphetamines is more apt to promote repeated use than oral administration. Because the euphoric effect of IV methamphetamine is long, it can be injected every 3 hours to maintain its euphoric effect.

The standard hydrochloride salt form of methamphetamine can be converted into its freebase, resulting in a form of the drug called "**ice**" or "**crank**" that can be administered by smoking cigarettes laced with the drug. Smoking methamphetamine in its freebase has become the most popular abused form of this drug in recent years. Because smoking the drug is a more acceptable route of administration, the easy availability of this form of the drug has been suggested to be responsible for the more recent increase in its abuse. The onset of effects and the intensity of the euphoria produced by smoking "ice" are reported to be at least as great as those seen when methamphetamine is injected intravenously. Both chemical forms of the drug are usually taken continuously for 2 to 5 days, during which time the abuser does not sleep or eat. This is called a "run" or "binge." The next stage is the "crash," during which the abuser sleeps for 24 to 48 hours. This stage is often followed by hunger, depression, dysphoria, and restlessness.

The degree of addiction and abuse potential is high for all the drugs in this group. Individuals dependent on these drugs have a very strong compulsion to engage in drug-seeking behavior. Marked tolerance to the stimulant effects of amphetamine develops readily. Although the therapeutic dose of amphetamine is 10 to 15 mg, abusers may inject intravenously 2 g/day. The mechanism of tolerance is unknown but has been attributed to the depletion of central catecholamine stores with replacement by *p*-hydroxynorephedrine, a metabolite of amphetamine that may function as a false neurotransmitter in adrenergic nerves.

Dependence on amphetamine is not easily demonstrable because it may be difficult to differentiate true withdrawal symptoms from the body's response to prolonged sleep and food deprivation and enhanced physical activity. Withdrawal from the drug after a "run" is followed, however, by a prolonged sleep and then by a ravenous appetite, fatigue, apathy, and depression. This complex of symptoms is interpreted as evidence of dependence. In humans, the depression associated with amphetamine withdrawal is correlated with a CNS reduction in 3-methoxy-4-hydroxyphenylglycol, a norepinephrine metabolite, which indicates that CNS catecholamines are depleted. This finding provides a neurochemical mechanism to explain the depression caused by drug withdrawal.

Toxicity

Acute severe overdose, although uncommon, is characterized by CNS and cardiovascular stimulation. Coma and convulsions occur, which may develop into status epilepticus. These convulsions may be controlled with **IV diazepam**. Cardiac arrhythmias and hypertension, occasionally precipitating subarachnoid hemorrhage or intracerebral hematomas, may lead to cardiovascular collapse. Enhanced autonomic activity, including hyperthermia and dilated pupils, may also be seen.

A chronic amphetamine abuser typically displays anxiety, akathisia, volatile mood, headaches, and cramps. In addition, the abuser frequently shows signs of mental and physical fatigue, poor personal hygiene, and facial twitching. Of particular interest to dentistry are the **worn teeth and chewed tongue that result from continuous oral movements**. Chronic stimulant abuse leads to stereotypy, psychosis, and overt violence. Stereotypic compulsive behavior is characterized by pleasurable curiosity and fascination with detail. Compulsive, repetitive activity develops, such as cleaning an immaculate home or disassembling and reconstructing mechanical objects. Chronic abuse can cause a drug-induced paranoid psychosis that resembles acute paranoid schizophrenia. Psychosis may develop within 1 to 5 days after beginning drug use and usually lasts 6 to 7 days. The most common symptoms are delusions of persecution; auditory, tactile, and especially visual hallucinations; and hyperactivity. Anxiety, agitation, aggressiveness, and depression are often observed. Paranoia, hallucinations, and terror reactions lead to hostility and difficulty in controlling rage. Amphetamine abusers display a high incidence of unpremeditated, unprovoked, and bizarre acts of violence and assaultive and even homicidal behavior.

After amphetamine use is discontinued, confusion, delusions, and loss of memory may persist for several weeks or months. Treatment of toxicity is based on enhancing the elimination of the drug from the body. Acidification of the urine with ammonium chloride increases the rate of urinary excretion of amphetamine and causes rapid reduction of psychotic symptoms.

Cocaine

The leaves of the coca plant, which contain up to 1.8% of the pure alkaloid, are the primary source of cocaine. The Andean Indians have chewed coca leaves, mixed with an alkaline substance to promote release of cocaine, for many years. Although peak blood concentrations of 95 ng/mL are achieved, little drug-induced euphoria is reported among Andean Indians who chew coca leaves. The leaves are used to make cocaine paste (30% to 90% cocaine), which is converted to pure cocaine hydrochloride, primarily in South America. Many samples of street cocaine apparently contain adulterants such as amphetamines, mannitol, or lidocaine. The local anesthetic procaine shares some characteristics with cocaine and can produce euphoria. Procaine powder is frequently used to cut cocaine and, mixed with mannitol or lactose, is sold as cocaine.

Pharmacologic effects

Cocaine is a local anesthetic that produces adrenergic effects by **blocking neuronal uptake of norepinephrine**. Pharmacologic responses to cocaine are mainly cardiovascular and are similar to those of amphetamine. Cocaine produces a dose-related tachycardia and increase in blood pressure, especially systolic. The onset of action is 2 to 5 minutes by the IV route and approximately 30 minutes by the intranasal route. In both cases the cardiovascular response dissipates over roughly 30 minutes. In IV doses of 32 mg, cocaine promotes a moderate mydriasis and hyperglycemia, but no effects on the electrocardiogram, respiratory rate, or body temperature.

As a recreational drug, cocaine uniformly causes euphoria and signs of CNS stimulation. The subjective effects of cocaine include elation, arousal, and alertness. Garrulousness and enhanced friendliness facilitate social interaction in group settings. Hunger and fatigue are suppressed. The user has a subjective feeling of increased mental agility. As is true of amphetamine, performance may be enhanced in sleep-deprived, but not in rested, subjects. Cocaine can delay ejaculation, which together with heightened sensory awareness and elevated mood, enhances the sexual experience. The orgasmic rush produced by IV cocaine use may become a substitute for coitus. This essentially pleasant high is produced by doses of about 100, 25, and 10 mg of cocaine by the oral, intranasal, and IV routes, respectively.

Negative subjective effects occur in 3% of intoxications in the early stages of abuse, but occur in 82% of compulsive cocaine abusers. The euphoric effects of the drug are followed by restlessness, irritability, and psychomotor agitation. Hyperexcitability and paranoia may occur. Chronic, high-dose cocaine abuse may result in aberrant sexual behavior, such as marathons of promiscuity. Men may have reduced libido, with an inability to maintain an erection or to ejaculate. Women may be unable to achieve orgasm.

Abuse characteristics

Although ingested cocaine can have stimulant effects, it is rarely taken orally. The intranasal route ("snorting") is more commonly used by cocaine abusers. Cocaine hydrochloride usually is inhaled as a "line" of powder containing 20 to 30 mg of the drug. It produces a maximum effect in 15 to 20 minutes and a duration of effect lasting 1 hour or more. Nasal mucosal vasoconstriction and paralysis of membrane cilia prevent complete absorption by this route, and measurable cocaine remains on the nasal mucosa for 3 hours after use. Snorting of cocaine in solution produces effects in 5 to 15 minutes that last 2 to 4 hours. The euphoric effect of cocaine is less intense when the intranasal route is used compared with IV injection or smoking the drug.

When cocaine is injected, the IV route is preferred over the intramuscular or the subcutaneous route because local vasoconstriction delays the onset of action by the latter routes. IV injection produces an intense orgasmic rush in approximately 1 minute that lasts 30 to 40 minutes. Abusers average 16 mg of cocaine per injection in a recreational setting. Cocaine is also used intravenously with heroin. The mixture, referred to as a "speedball," is used to attenuate the excessive stimulation caused by large doses of cocaine.

The smoking of cocaine requires conversion of the hydrochloride salt of the drug to the freebase form. The salt form, when heated, decomposes before the vaporization temperature is reached. The freebase volatilizes at temperatures of approximately 90 °C and is not destroyed by heating. Smokers may manufacture their own freebase by dissolving the salt in an alkaline solution and extracting the alkaloid with a solvent such as ether. Since the mid-1980s, the freebase form has become commonly available as "**crack**," a form of freebase melted down into crystalline balls that can be smoked. Crack may be smoked in cigarettes or by heating with an alcohol flame in a pipe. Because the lung–brain circulation time is only 8 seconds, and the inhalation route bypasses the liver, the effects of smoking cocaine base are just as rapid and intense as IV cocaine and last approximately 20 minutes. Smokers average 100 mg of base with each smoke, increasing to 250 mg with rapid tolerance development. Smoking may be repeated every 5 minutes, with intake in compulsive abusers totaling 1.5 g/day. Smoking freebase cocaine has become the most popular method for administration of this drug, and similar to methamphetamine freebase, the freebase form of cocaine has contributed significantly to the increase in its abuse.

Used intranasally as a low-dose recreational drug, cocaine produces moderate addiction. High-dose IV or inhalation use produces compulsive behavior characterized by loss of control over drug use and an inability to stop the drug despite repeated attempts. Cocaine shares with other addictive drugs a reinforcing property that results in rapid acquisition of self-administration behavior. This reinforcing property may result from activation of a CNS dopaminergic reward system with cell bodies located in the ventral tegmentum projecting to the nucleus accumbens. Cocaine enhances dopaminergic activity at the latter site by blocking dopamine uptake by nerve endings. This endogenous reward system is normally activated by responding to physiologic imperatives such as hunger, thirst, and sex drive. Cocaine directly stimulates this reward circuitry, dominating motivation for essential physiologic needs. Rats given free access to IV cocaine take the drug in preference to food and die of starvation in a few weeks.

Significant tolerance does not develop with occasional cocaine use because of the short half-life of the drug. Frequent use resulting in constant cocaine concentrations in the body does cause tolerance, however. Acute tolerance to subjective and cardiovascular effects is observed within 1 hour after repeated IV doses. Dependence occurs primarily in compulsive, high-dose cocaine abusers. With chronic cocaine use, CNS dopamine depletion may occur, resulting in adverse symptoms during periods of abstinence. Withdrawal results in depression, dysphoria, social withdrawal, craving for the drug, appetite disturbances, tremor, and muscle pain. Such withdrawal phenomena may be severe enough to prevent some abusers from stopping the drug, even though toxic delirium may develop with continued drug use. **Oral diazepam** has been useful in treating withdrawal anxiety; psychotherapy or cautious use of tricyclic antidepressants is recommended for prolonged depression.

Toxicity

Medical complications of cocaine abuse most often involve the CNS and the cardiovascular system. The CNS effects include a toxic psychosis, similar to that caused by amphetamine, which often develops in chronic, heavy abusers of cocaine. The syndrome is characterized by intense anxiety, inability to concentrate, stereotyped compulsive behavior, paranoid delusions, and violent loss of impulse control. Hallucinations may develop that are typically tactile, with sensations of insects burrowing under the skin or snakes crawling over the body. Such psychotic crises are reported in 10% of intoxications in compulsive abusers. Acute depression with suicidal ideation also may develop. Longer term personality changes include a tendency to paranoia with features of depression, reduced frustration threshold, difficulties in impulse regulation, and social maladjustment.

Cardiovascular complications of cocaine include cardiac arrhythmias, with sinus and ventricular tachycardia, ventricular fibrillation, and fatal cardiac arrest. Acute myocardial infarction is a particular hazard among abusers with preexisting coronary artery disease because of the increased systolic blood pressure, heart rate, and myocardial oxygen consumption engendered by cocaine. Abrupt increases in arterial blood pressure, occurring within minutes of intranasal use of cocaine, have resulted in subarachnoid hemorrhage, particularly in individuals with aneurysms of cerebral vessels. One case of fatal rupture of the ascending aorta was reported in an individual with preexisting chronic hypertension who had smoked freebase cocaine. Acute cardiac events may occur even with recreational intranasal use of cocaine in individuals without predisposing cardiac disease.

Hepatotoxicity, with clinical findings of elevated titers of serum transaminases and jaundice, has been reported in chronic cocaine abusers. Such liver damage may occur in plasma cholinesterase–deficient individuals, in whom cocaine metabolism is shunted through hepatic oxidative pathways, resulting in the production of cytolytic superoxides. A significantly increased rate of spontaneous abortion has been noted in pregnant women. Because cocaine can cross the placental barrier, infants born to cocaine abusers may exhibit tremulousness. Frequent intranasal use leads to chronic rhinitis and rhinorrhea, atrophy of the nasal mucosa, loss of sense of smell, and necrosis and perforation of the nasal septum. These changes, occurring as a result of chronic ischemia, should alert the clinician to possible intranasal cocaine abuse. Bruxism and temporomandibular joint disorders are also more frequent in cocaine abusers.

Death from cocaine overdose usually is attributable to generalized convulsions, respiratory failure, or cardiac arrhythmias. Deaths have occurred with each route of cocaine administration and may be so rapid that treatment comes too late. Because cocaine is metabolized by plasma esterases, individuals with low cholinesterase activity are at high risk of cocaine fatality. Treatment of cocaine overdose is symptomatic. CNS stimulation can be treated with IV diazepam, ventricular arrhythmias can be treated with IV lidocaine, and respiratory depression can be treated with oxygen and positive-pressure ventilation.

Other Psychostimulant Drugs

Various other psychostimulant drugs collectively referred to as "**bath salts**" may be classified as synthetic cathinones because they are structurally related to the parent compound cathinone, which is a naturally occurring β-keto amphetamine. Synthetic **cathinones** include methylone, mephedrone, and 3,4-methylenedioxy-N-pryovalerone (MDPV); however, legislation banning the sale, possession, and use of these specific cathinones has promoted the clandestine development of many pharmacologically similar analogues. Synthetic cathinones interact with monoamine transporters on nerve cells analogously to other psychostimulant drugs and thus produce desirable subjective effects similar to those caused by amphetamine or cocaine. At high doses or prolonged use, synthetic cathinones can cause psychosis, tachycardia, hyperthermia, and death.

ABUSE OF HALLUCINOGENS

Hallucinogens are defined as drugs that alter perception, mood, and thought without changes in consciousness or orientation. These drugs are also referred to as **psychotomimetics** because some of their effects mimic naturally occurring psychoses or as **psychedelics** because of their use by some people to induce mystical experiences. These drugs are claimed to provide the abuser with enhanced insight and self-knowledge, leading to new ways of looking at life and new insights into personal relationships.

Psychedelic Hallucinogens

Psychedelic hallucinogens can be divided into different chemical classes. The chemical structures of some psychedelic hallucinogens are shown

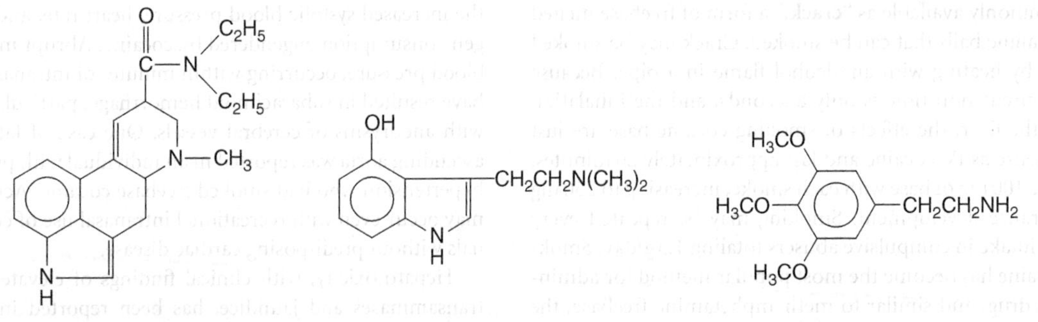

Lysergic acid diethylamide Psilocin Mescaline

FIG 39-3 Structural formulas of representative hallucinogenic drugs.

in Figure 39-3. **Lysergic acid diethylamide (LSD)** is a semisynthetic chemical that does not occur in nature. LSD is a commonly used hallucinogen and has become the standard with which other hallucinogenic substances are compared. Drugs derived from tryptamine include the synthetic compound dimethyltryptamine and its derivative, **psilocin**, and the naturally occurring phosphorylated form of psilocin, psilocybin. The third class of hallucinogens includes amphetamine analogues such as **MDMA** and **mescaline**. Mescaline and psilocybin produce effects that are nearly the same as those produced by LSD. MDMA has stimulant effects similar to those of amphetamine and some psychedelic effects similar to those of LSD. Because MDMA possesses mild psychedelic and stimulant properties, it has become popular in club or dance settings, where it can enhance the light and sound experience and enable users to dance vigorously for extended periods. Under these conditions of prolonged physical exertion, MDMA can cause dangerous levels of dehydration and hyperthermia.

Pharmacologic effects

Symptoms associated with the LSD experience occur sequentially, with somatic symptoms developing first, followed by perceptual and mood changes, and then by psychic or psychedelic phenomena. Within a half hour of ingestion of LSD, a feeling of inner tension develops, accompanied by somatic symptoms of mild sympathetic stimulation and motor alterations. The individual feels dizzy, weak, vaguely numb, and nauseated. Marked mydriasis is accompanied by an increase in blood pressure and pulse rate, tremor, hyperreflexia, and, at high doses, ataxia. These somatic effects are soon submerged by perceptual and psychic effects, which begin approximately 45 minutes after the drug is taken. Some individuals experience euphoria, elation, serenity, or ecstasy, whereas in others the initial tension may progress to anxiety and depression, evoking a panic reaction. A paranoid rage reaction occasionally occurs, although most subjects tend to be passive, quiet, and withdrawn.

Abuse characteristics

The subjective effects of LSD are highly dependent on the psychological makeup of the individual, the environmental influences at the time of the drug experience, the expectations of the individual, and the size of the dose. Distortion of sense perception is the most specific symptom of the LSD experience, affecting all modalities but especially vision. Colors seem unusually bright and vivid, and objects appear distorted and seem to undulate and flow. Fixed objects appear to shift from near to far; fine surface details appear in deep relief; and colorful, dreamlike images occur as vivid streaming filmstrips even with the eyes closed. Frank visual hallucinations are rare, but visual illusions are common, as when a spot on the wall is mistaken for a face. There are distortions of body image, enhanced auditory perception, and, more rarely, alteration of other sensory modalities. Time sense is distorted; it is often described as stopping or going backward. Synesthesias are common, so that music may be experienced visually, or colors may be "heard."

The changes in sensory perception are soon followed by the psychedelic "trip." Subjects may experience depersonalization, and the separation between the self and the environment melts away. The user has a sense of profound insight, revelation, and expanded consciousness. This loss of self is interpreted as a "good trip" by psychedelic drug abusers, but occasionally loss of control and fear of self-disintegration foster panic and even attempts at self-destruction. The individual remains oriented and alert throughout the experience and often remembers all events during the "trip" even months later.

In general, use of these drugs is not associated with marked dependence, and no clear withdrawal syndrome has been reported. If addiction develops at all, it is mild and infrequent. Tolerance to the effects of LSD is not common but has been reported, and cross-tolerance is seen among members of the psychedelic hallucinogens. With repeated use, tolerance to LSD develops within 1 week but lasts only a few days after discontinuance of the drug.

Toxicity

The adult human lethal dose of LSD has been estimated to be 2 mg/kg, although no deaths caused directly by LSD overdosage have been reported. Adverse psychological reactions to hallucinogens are common. Panic reactions or "bad trips" are relatively frequent and are related to an overdose of the drug. Often, companionship and reassurance, or "talking down," is sufficient to control this reaction; if this is insufficient, other treatments include sedation with oral diazepam. Acute depression or psychotic reactions can also occur. Ingestion of 50 mg results in hyperactivity, psychosis, amnesia, upper gastrointestinal tract bleeding, and coma.

Approximately 1 in 20 LSD abusers has "flashbacks," in which episodic visual disturbances resembling previous LSD experiences occur during abstinence from the drug. This alteration is now called **hallucinogen persisting perception disorder**. This disorder may occur months after the previous trip and last a few minutes to a few hours. It is thought to be caused by a drug-induced permanent change in the visual system. This disorder is treated in the same way as panic reactions. In addition, prolonged psychotic states may be precipitated by LSD use, requiring long-term hospitalization and treatment with antipsychotic drugs.

Deliriant Hallucinogens

The ketamine derivative **phencyclidine**, also called PCP or "angel dust," is a synthetic drug that produces a unique state characterized by delirium, hallucinations, insomnia, and agitation. PCP produces what

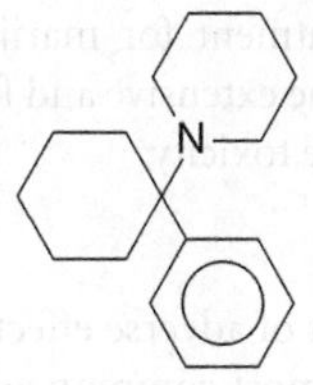

FIG 39-4 Structural formula of phencyclidine.

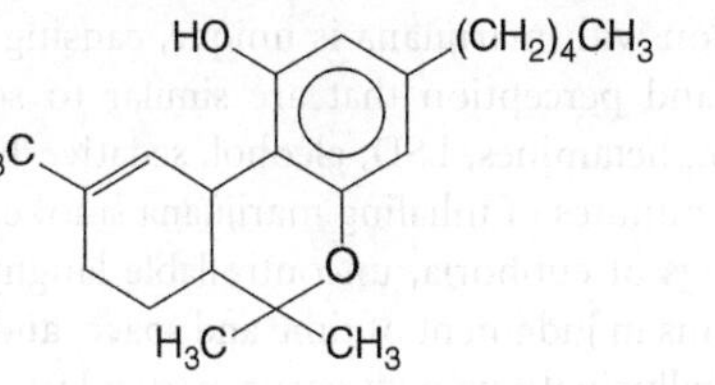

FIG 39-5 Structural formula of Δ-9-tetrahydrocannabinol.

is called a "dissociative state" because it is said to dissociate the mind from the body without loss of consciousness. The drug was investigated in 1958 as an anesthetic in humans, but was subsequently abandoned because of severe postanesthetic dysphoria and hallucinations. Derivatives of PCP, such as thienyl and N-ethyl analogs, are also available on the street. The chemical structure of PCP is shown in Figure 39-4.

Pharmacologic effects

To produce its effects, PCP binds to receptors in the CNS that are associated with the *N*-methyl-D-aspartate acid (NMDA) type of glutamate receptor. NMDA receptors mediate some of the CNS effects of the excitatory amino acid glutamate. The PCP binding site resides within the NMDA-gated Ca^{2+} channel complex, where PCP acts as a noncompetitive antagonist at the NMDA receptor and inhibits some of the CNS effects of glutamate. Receptors that bind PCP have been identified in the CNS in the limbic system and frontal cortex, areas involved in memory, emotion, and behavior. PCP has also been reported to cause dopamine release and to inhibit the active reuptake of dopamine into dopaminergic nerves. This inhibition enhances and prolongs the effects of dopaminergic nerve stimulation.

With lower doses, PCP abusers usually remain alert and oriented, while exhibiting euphoria, agitation, or bizarre behavior. Individuals may be irritable or mute and rigid, stare suspiciously, and exhibit impaired reasoning. They are easily provoked to anger and may exhibit violent behavior. The dissociative state, coupled with effects on limbic-mediated emotional control, may provoke feats of superhuman strength, causing harm to self and others. Inappropriate behavior, such as strolling down a street nude, may occur. Detachment, disorientation, stupor, and coma may also occur, but those are more common at higher doses.

Abuse characteristics

Currently, the most common route of administration of PCP is by smoking, in which the drug is mixed with tobacco or marijuana. At the burning tip of a cigarette, PCP is converted to 1-phenyl-1-cyclohexene (PC), which is largely inactive. In smoking PCP cigarettes, approximately 40% of the dose is received by the smoker as PCP and approximately 30% as PC. Some abusers snort PCP powder or ingest it mixed with alcoholic beverages or in pill form. A small percentage of abusers inject the drug intravenously. Urine and serum concentrations of PCP do not correlate with the state of intoxication. PCP disappears from urine 2 to 4 hours after a single use (largely because of sequestration in fatty tissues), but it may be detected in the urine of chronic abusers for 30 days.

Most PCP use is intermittent rather than chronic. Some PCP abusers develop addiction to the drug, although this is less common than with the drugs of abuse previously discussed. No clearly defined dependence on PCP has been identified, but withdrawal from chronic use has been reported to result in depression, irritability, confusion, and sleep disturbances along with a strong craving for the drug.

Toxicity

Symptoms of acute intoxication appear 15 to 30 minutes after ingestion. Marked analgesia, shivering, salivation, bronchospasm, urinary retention, hypertension, tachycardia, and hyperpyrexia result. Nystagmus is observed in approximately two-thirds of intoxications. Grimacing, localized dystonias, and tremor may progress to grand mal seizures or status epilepticus at doses greater than 70 mg, which also produce deep and prolonged coma with loss of protective reflexes that may last for 1 week or more. Death has been attributed to intracranial hemorrhage, status epilepticus, and respiratory failure. Life-threatening hyperthermia may also develop, sometimes in association with hepatic necrosis. Individuals under the influence of PCP act violently with some regularity, and accidents, including drownings, have been documented in many cases. Acute treatment centers on acidification of the urine to hasten renal excretion of PCP. IV diazepam is used to control seizures and the agitated or excited state caused by the drug. Prolonged psychotic episodes may require treatment with antipsychotic drugs.

ABUSE OF MARIJUANA

Marijuana is ground-up leaves and flowers from the hemp plants, *Cannabis sativa* or *Cannabis indica*, and is one of the most frequently abused drugs in the United States. The cannabinoid **Δ-9-tetrahydrocannabinol (THC)** (Fig. 39-5) is thought to be the main psychoactive ingredient. Preparations of marijuana vary widely in their THC content, depending on the variety and part of the plant used and the environment in which the plant is raised. Stalk fibers from any variety of hemp contain no psychoactive agents, and the type of hemp plant from which stalk fibers are used commercially in the production of rope, twine, cord, and clothing is virtually drug-free because it is grown under conditions that favor high fiber and low THC content. Conversely, more potent samples of marijuana are made from the younger, topmost leaves of hemp varieties that can contain 5% or more THC by weight. Another component of the *Cannabis* plant that is commonly abused is an extract called ***hashish***. In contrast to marijuana, which is ground-up plant material, hashish is an extract containing only the THC-rich resin that is secreted by the hemp plant. Hashish is more potent than marijuana, and it can contain 12% or more THC by weight. Synthetic cannabinoids are also abused. Their chemical structures range from tetrahydrocannabinols and bicyclic cannabinoids to aminoalkylindoles and anandamide analogues. These chemicals are typically sprayed onto plant material and then sold legally as herbal products with names like **"K2"** and **"Spice."** Marijuana, hashish, and synthetic cannabinoids are usually smoked in the form of cigarettes or from a pipe.

Pharmacologic Effects

THC, other phytocannabinoids found in marijuana, and synthetic cannabinoids produce their effects by activating the endocannabinoid system in the brain. The endocannabinoid system consists of CB_1 and CB_2 G protein–coupled receptors, two endogenous ligands (**anandamide and 2-arachidonoyl-glycerol**), and associated metabolic and synthetic enzymes. Although the physiologic significance of the cannabinoid receptors and their ligands remains a matter of much study, evidence suggests a role for the endocannabinoid system in appetite, pain, reward, mental illness, and neurodegenerative disease.

Intoxication with marijuana is unique, causing changes in mood, motivation, and perception that are similar to some of the effects caused by amphetamines, LSD, alcohol, sedative-hypnotics, and opioids. Within minutes of inhaling marijuana smoke, the typical abuser reports feelings of euphoria, uncontrollable laughter, depersonalization, alterations in judgment of time and space, and sharpened vision. Mild visual hallucinations may occur, particularly when the eyes are closed. Similar to LSD, the abuser knows that these visual disturbances are drug-induced. Later, the abuser experiences generalized feelings of well-being, relaxation, and tranquility that may last 2 to 3 hours. The abuser experiences a reduction in attention span, difficulty in thinking and concentrating, and impairment of short-term memory. All these effects are considered desirable by the abuser and are described as "mellowing out." Many abusers report that the feelings of intoxication, dreaminess, and sedation can be more easily suppressed voluntarily than the equivalent effects produced by alcohol. The sedative-hypnotic property of marijuana facilitates the onset of sleep and resembles the effects caused by CNS depressants. This property of marijuana is in sharp contrast to the effects of LSD and other hallucinogens. Although it is generally agreed that a dose-related impairment in psychomotor performance occurs, many experienced abusers exhibit no such decrement in their performance; perhaps this is why no clear correlation has been shown between blood concentrations of THC and an individual's ability to drive a car.

Physiologic effects of smoking marijuana occur within a few minutes, peak in their action in approximately 20 minutes, and wane over 2 to 3 hours. Moderate marijuana use causes reddening of the eyes in association with a euphoric high that is followed by drowsiness. Autonomic effects of marijuana include xerostomia, tachycardia, reduced peripheral resistance, and, in large doses, orthostatic hypotension. These effects may be deleterious in individuals with ischemic heart disease or cardiac failure. Marijuana does not affect respiratory rate, blood glucose concentrations, or pupillary diameter; however, marijuana does reduce intraocular pressure.

Studies of the potential therapeutic uses of **dronabinol**, the nonproprietary name of THC, show it to be effective in treating some conditions. Oral administration of dronabinol has been approved as an antiemetic in cancer patients undergoing chemotherapy and as an appetite stimulant in patients with weight loss resulting from AIDS-related anorexia. Smoking marijuana may also have beneficial effects in the treatment of weight loss in patients with AIDS. Whether smoking marijuana has an advantage over orally administered dronabinol in the treatment of AIDS-related anorexia remains to be determined. Although THC is effective in reducing intraocular pressure in patients with glaucoma, its psychoactive properties make THC less desirable than other forms of drug therapy for this indication.

Abuse Characteristics

In humans, the development of tolerance to marijuana is most apparent among heavy chronic abusers and is evidenced by increases in the amount of drug used over time. Although chronic use of marijuana has a long history, whether dependence on marijuana develops in humans remains controversial. Abrupt withdrawal of marijuana from chronic abusers has been reported to cause sleep disturbances, decreased appetite, nausea, and vomiting. Whether these alterations in normal function are alleviated by the readministration of marijuana has not been shown, and this is necessary to prove that constant exposure to marijuana causes the development of dependence. Although the magnitude of addiction to marijuana is difficult to quantify, marijuana clearly possesses some abuse potential because it is the most commonly used illegal drug in the United States. Perhaps the lack of understanding of the abuse potential of marijuana is related to the fact that few individuals ever seek treatment for marijuana addiction, combined with the knowledge that the extensive and frequent use of this drug has led to few reports of severe toxicity.

Toxicity

Although few reports exist of adverse effects caused by acute administration of marijuana, the most common adverse reaction usually seen in naïve abusers is an acute nonpsychotic panic reaction characterized by anxiety and fear of losing one's mind. Many inexperienced elderly abusers interpret the THC-induced tachycardia combined with the psychological effects of THC as evidence that they are dying. Both of these conditions are best treated with authoritative reassurance or antianxiety agents of the benzodiazepine class. Very high doses of THC may result in self-limiting toxic delirium, acute paranoia, and psychotic episodes. When compared to marijuana, abuse of synthetic cannabinoids is associated with a higher incidence of severe effects such as hypertension, tachycardia, hallucinations, agitation, seizures, and panic attacks that often necessitate medical care.

Chronic use of marijuana seems to cause no functional changes in the CNS; however, heavy smokers may be prone to chronic bronchitis, airway obstruction, poor dentition, and squamous cell metaplasia (similar to smokers of tobacco). Contamination of marijuana with *Aspergillus* or the herbicide paraquat can lead to severe pulmonary damage in abusers. Chronic, intensive use of 5 to 18 marijuana cigarettes weekly is reported to reduce testosterone concentration and cause oligospermia in men. Other studies of shorter exposures to marijuana have not confirmed these findings, although they do show that secondary sexual characteristics in very young abusers can be suppressed by marijuana. Teratogenic effects of THC are known to occur in animals; no such reports exist for humans smoking marijuana. Anecdotal reports suggest marijuana use produces an amotivational syndrome, which is described as an affliction of young abusers of marijuana who drop out of social activities and show little interest in school, work, or other goal-directed activities. Laboratory studies and cross-cultural analyses of marijuana smokers in countries where marijuana use is acceptable do not support the contention that THC use leads to psychosocial deterioration. Others have suggested that the lifestyle and goals of an abuser of any kind of illicit drug may more satisfactorily explain the amotivational syndrome.

ABUSE OF INHALANTS

Modern awareness of the consciousness-altering effects of inhaled compounds began with the discovery of anesthetic agents such as ether, chloroform, and nitrous oxide in the early nineteenth century. Today this list also includes halothane and other halogenated compounds. The use of general anesthetics is discussed in Chapter 15. Although nitrous oxide, halothane, and other volatile anesthetics are usually available only to medical or health care personnel, **nitrous oxide** can also be found in restaurant supply stores as a propellant for making whipped cream and packaged in small metal canisters called **whippets**. Although ether and chloroform are no longer used as anesthetics, they are available through chemical supply houses.

In addition to volatile anesthetics, three other main classes of inhalants are subject to abuse. The first are volatile solvents, which include glue, paint thinners, cleaning fluids, degreasers, and gasoline. The generalized depressant effects on the CNS caused by these solvents are mediated by ingredients such as trichloroethylene, benzene, toluene, naphthalene, hexane, heptaene, and acetone. This class of inhalants is widely abused because of ready availability.

The second class of inhalants includes aerosol propellants such as methanol, ethanol, and isopropanol used in spray paint and cooking sprays. Trichlorofluoromethane and other fluorocarbons used as refrigerants may also be abused. The alcohols are less rewarding than other volatile solvents, and ethanol is more prone to be abused by the oral route of administration.

The third class includes organic nitrites, which include amyl, butyl, and isobutyl nitrite. Amyl nitrite is used as a vasodilator in the treatment of angina pectoris (discussed in Chapter 21) and is packaged in mesh-enclosed glass ampules designed to be crushed between the fingers, allowing for inhalation of the vapors for relief of the pain of angina. **Amyl nitrite ampules** are commonly referred to as "**poppers**" because of the popping sound resulting from their being broken. Amyl nitrite and isobutyl nitrite are perceived to be sexual enhancers, which increases their abuse potential. Although amyl nitrite is available only by prescription, isobutyl nitrite is used as a room deodorizer and can be purchased from shops that sell drug paraphernalia under the names "Locker Room," "Doctor Bananas," and "Rush."

Pharmacologic Effects

With the exception of the organic nitrites, all the abused inhalants have a generalized depressant effect on the CNS similar to that of volatile general anesthetics. Low doses of these agents first produce signs of stimulation followed by depression, unconsciousness, and, with larger doses, death. The desirable effects of these compounds—euphoria, perceptual distortions, ataxia, giddiness, and slurred speech—occur within seconds of inhalation and last 5 to 45 minutes. Undesirable effects may be experienced during use and for variable periods afterward and include coughing, vomiting, rhinitis, photophobia, irritation of the eyes, tinnitus, nausea, and sneezing. The vasodilatory action of the organic nitrites is immediate and produces a feeling of warmth and lightheadedness that is commonly referred to as a "head rush." The "head rush" is brief and is considered desirable; however, it may result in loss of consciousness as a consequence of postural hypotension if the drug is inhaled while standing. Headaches commonly occur after use of organic nitrites and are caused by vasodilation of cerebral blood vessels.

Abuse Characteristics

The euphoria, disinhibition, and general feelings of drunkenness are thought to be the reinforcing characteristics of inhaled CNS depressants; abusers take these agents repeatedly, suggesting addiction to them. Few controlled studies have been performed on the development of tolerance to solvents, aerosols, and nitrites. Because solvents, aerosols, ethanol, barbiturates, and benzodiazepines share many of the same pharmacologic effects, however, considerable interest remains in whether cross-tolerance exists among these agents. There is little evidence that signs of abstinence occur in individuals when inhalants are withdrawn, suggesting that dependence is not part of the experience of these abusers.

Toxicity

Ascribing the toxic effects of an abused inhalant to an individual agent is difficult because the toxic effects of inhaled solvents and aerosols may be caused by more than one substance and because solvents typically contain several volatile compounds or may be tainted with heavy metals such as lead and cadmium. The major health risks associated with acute use of anesthetic gases and volatile liquids are sudden death from asphyxiation, respiratory depression, or arrhythmia-induced cardiopulmonary arrest. Halogenated hydrocarbons, such as trichloroethylene, are particularly likely to cause arrhythmias.

Repeated abuse of inhalation agents may lead to toxic effects caused by chronic exposure. Industrial solvents are known to cause liver and kidney damage, sensory and motor neuropathies, bone marrow suppression, and pulmonary disease. The toxic effects of chloroform on the liver and kidney are so well known that chloroform has not been used as an anesthetic for decades and has been eliminated from commercially available products. Continuous exposure to nitrous oxide can cause megaloblastic anemia, methemoglobinemia, and, rarely, peripheral neuropathy. In industrial settings where chronic exposure to organic nitrites occurs, cases of methemoglobinemia have been reported; however, this is rare in abusers of these compounds.

POLYDRUG ABUSE

Drug abuse problems are often compounded by the practice of taking two or more drugs in combination or in sequence. Polydrug abusers may seek additive or potentiated effects (e.g., the simultaneous use of alcohol and another sedative) or the modulation or termination of effects (e.g., the sequential use of amphetamines and barbiturates). Approximately 20% of chronic alcoholics abuse other drugs, especially barbiturates, antianxiety drugs, and marijuana. Primary heavy abusers of marijuana frequently use amphetamines or psychedelic agents, whereas heroin addicts are particularly apt to abuse amphetamines, cocaine, hallucinogens, and barbiturates. Most patients in methadone maintenance programs apparently are polydrug abusers. When multiple drug dependencies develop, the withdrawal syndrome becomes difficult to treat and is associated with a significantly enhanced mortality rate.

IMPLICATIONS FOR DENTISTRY

Certain signs may alert the dentist to the possible parenteral abuse of drugs. Telltale cutaneous lesions may result from chronic hypodermic administration of drugs of abuse. These lesions include acute septic complications, such as subcutaneous abscesses, cellulitis, and thrombophlebitis, and chronic cutaneous complications, including skin tracks and infected lesions, which occur most commonly in the thigh or antecubital or deltoid regions. Skin tracks result from frequent, multiple injections that produce chronic tissue inflammation. These are typically linear or bifurcated erythematous lesions that become indurated and hyperpigmented. Another sign that may alert the clinician to the problem of drug abuse is the presence of an ill-defined febrile illness. This finding often reflects a low-grade bacteremia resulting from the injection of drugs.

In ascertaining whether a patient is abusing drugs, the dentist cannot depend on being able to identify a particular personality type, recognize cutaneous lesions (which may be concealed under clothing), or diagnose a mild febrile illness. Rather, the dentist must rely on careful and thorough questioning of the patient and on the skillful use of a well-designed **medical history** questionnaire. Drug abuse is a subject of considerable importance to dentists because they are occasionally the unwitting target or victim of drug abusers' need to secure drugs. Also, drug abuse among health professionals has a long history, numerous medical and dental abnormalities are associated with drug abuse, and interactions may occur between drugs that dentists customarily prescribe and drugs the patient is abusing.

Dentists as a Target of Drug Abusers

Inevitably, drug abusers, through pretense and subterfuge, attempt to obtain drugs from dentists. The dentist should be aware of any patient who complains of pain from pulpitis or an abscess and who refuses endodontic or surgical intervention. An opioid abuser may claim to be allergic to codeine or pentazocine in an effort to obtain more positively reinforcing drugs, such as oxycodone, morphine, or hydrocodone. As a general defense against drug abusers, the dentist should never let patients know where such drugs are kept, never leave prescription pads out where they may be taken, and avoid the use of prewritten prescription forms.

Drug Use Among Dentists

Dentists are not immune to the hazards of drug abuse. Similar to physicians, they may be in greater danger of developing drug dependencies than the general population because of the ready accessibility of opioid analgesics and sedative-hypnotic drugs. Opioid addiction among medical personnel is much higher than that of the general population. One form of drug abuse common among dentists and other health professionals is the inhalation of **nitrous oxide.** Evidence suggests that the pleasurable effects of nitrous oxide inhalation can lead to a craving for the drug in some individuals. The abuse potential of nitrous oxide coupled with the ease of availability of the drug contributes to its relatively frequent abuse by dentists.

Medical and Dental Complications of Drug Abuse

The most common and serious medical complications in drug-abusing patients are **AIDS, endocarditis, and hepatitis.** IV drug abusers are at risk of AIDS. Sharing needles for IV injections spreads the AIDS virus. IV drug abusers are responsible for a significant number of AIDS cases among heterosexuals.

Bacterial endocarditis in drug abusers is most commonly caused by *Staphylococcus aureus*, which seems to derive from an increase in endogenous pathogens in the addict rather than from contaminated drugs or drug paraphernalia. In drug-abusing patients, the disease often affects the tricuspid valve, which is unusual in nonabusers. *Pseudomonas* endocarditis, although less common, primarily involves the tricuspid valve and has an overall mortality rate of 50%. *Candida albicans* infects the left-sided valves and is almost invariably fatal. Candidiasis may be disseminated to skin, eyes, bones, or joints.

Viral hepatitis is often seen among drug abusers and is probably transmitted by contaminated needles. The disease is usually mild, but individuals displaying early signs of elevated prothrombin time, fever, elevated leukocyte count, or encephalopathy have a poor prognosis. In 50% to 80% of cases, the acute infection results in chronic inflammatory hepatic disease.

Opioid drugs have been reported to depress the immune system by interacting with opioid receptors on T lymphocytes and leukocytes. Other drugs of abuse have also been suggested either to suppress or to enhance the activity of the immune system. Whether the development of infectious diseases in drug abusers is caused by a direct effect of these drugs on the immune system is unknown.

Specific dental complications of drug use include rampant caries and rapidly progressing periodontal disorders, probably resulting from nutritional deficiencies and neglect of personal hygiene. Xerostomia with an enhanced rate of dental caries has been reported in individuals who abuse opioids, amphetamines, sedative-hypnotic drugs, and marijuana. In other studies, opioid and marijuana use do not seem to reduce the rate of salivary secretion, however. Self-mutilation has occurred among drug abusers; teeth may be deliberately damaged in an effort to obtain drugs. Long-term cocaine and amphetamine abusers may develop facial tics and bruxism, which result in a **traumatized tongue and worn teeth.** These subjects may also chronically rub the tongue along the inside of the lower lip, producing ulcers on the abraded tissues.

Drug Interactions in Drug Abusers

Drug interactions in drug abusers are not unique, but they depend on the drug of abuse. Barbiturates and other sedative-hypnotic drugs induce hepatic cytochrome P450 enzyme activity. Abusers of such substances may be resistant to the therapeutic effects of corticosteroids, oral anticoagulants, and many CNS depressants because the metabolism of these drugs is enhanced by enzyme induction. Opioid abusers generally show tolerance to other opioid analgesics. The dentist should beware of giving pentazocine to such patients because this and other agonist-antagonists may precipitate an acute withdrawal syndrome in opioid-dependent patients. Marijuana may intensify CNS depression produced by barbiturates, general anesthetics, and other CNS depressant drugs. The sympathomimetic effects of cocaine, amphetamine, and marijuana may be enhanced by drugs used in dental practice. Administration of local anesthetics containing epinephrine or gingival retraction cords impregnated with epinephrine may enhance tachycardia and elevations in blood pressure caused by these drugs.

Pain Control and Drug Abusers

Drug abusers may be more anxious and fearful of dental procedures and may have a lower pain tolerance than patients who do not abuse drugs. To counteract these fears, abusers may take their favorite drug of abuse before dental appointments. If the dentist knows that the drug abuser has taken such a drug, the dental procedure should be rescheduled, and the patient should be counseled to avoid drug use before the next visit. Complicating this picture is that tolerance to sedative drugs and local anesthetics has also been reported, particularly in parenteral drug abusers. These patients may need larger amounts of these drugs for pain-free dental treatment. Larger doses of sedatives and local anesthetics carry the risk of enhanced adverse effects caused by these drugs.

Treatment of pain and anxiety in a recovering or reformed substance abuser presents a problem to the dentist. Whether the patient has abused alcohol or other drugs in the past, proper dental care demands a preoperative evaluation of the patient's personal attitude toward drug treatment. Many of these individuals refuse mood-altering drugs, and such wishes must be respected. As a rule, it is best never to administer a drug, or another of its class, that has previously been abused by the patient. In cases in which anxiety is predominantly somatic (e.g., tachycardia, breathlessness, and tremulousness), oral propranolol may be valuable. Intraoperative pain control can be accomplished with local anesthetics, but systemic exposure to **epinephrine** should be minimized in patients being treated with neuronal uptake pump inhibitors such as desipramine for post-dependence depression. Postoperative pain can usually be adequately controlled with nonsteroidal antiinflammatory drugs or acetaminophen.

ETHYL ALCOHOL

The principal medical use of ethyl alcohol (ethanol) is topical disinfection. Although ethanol has limited clinical application, as the most common intoxicant in Western civilization, it is of immense importance because of its potential for abuse and dependence and because it is a major contributing factor to individual and social ills in the United States and other nations.

Ethanol can be obtained as anhydrous alcohol (100% ethanol), as neutral spirits (95% ethanol), and as denatured alcohol. Denatured alcohol, intended primarily for industrial use, is ethanol with a substance added to render it unfit for consumption, such as methanol, benzene, diethyl ether, or kerosene.

The social costs of ethanol abuse are staggering. Ethanol abuse–related costs, including health care costs, criminal damage costs, and workplace costs, are estimated to be several hundreds of billions of U.S. dollars worldwide. Approximately 50% of all fatal

TABLE 39-2 Effects of Ethanol on the CNS and Peripheral Nervous System

Effect	Mechanism	Comments
Encephalopathy* (includes delirium, psychiatric symptoms, dementia)	Ammonia toxicity, thiamine, niacin, and other deficiencies	Hepatic toxicity from alcohol leads to excessive ammonia, and thiamine deficiency
	Direct alcohol effect on glia, neurons, and blood vessels. Alcohol changes proteins, lipids, and DNA	Hypoxia, ischemia, and damage to blood vessels
Increased reward mechanisms	Stimulation of dopaminergic and opioid pathways	Pathways for addiction
Excitement	Disinhibition of inhibitory pathways in the brain	Euphoria, and social uninhibited behavior
Sedation	Increases the effect of GABA	May also involve changes in the NMDA receptor pathway
Aggression	Can deplete serotonin	
Respiratory depression	Depression of medullary respiratory center	Acute toxicity can cause death
Peripheral neuropathy	Thiamine deficiency	Diminished tendon reflexes, sensory loss in feet or legs, muscle atrophy

*Includes Wernicke's encephalopathy and Korsakoff syndrome.
GABA, γ aminobutyric acid; *NMDA*, *N*-methyl-D-aspartate (a glutamate receptor).

traffic accidents are related to the use of ethanol. Drinking aggravates criminal behavior. Ethanol is involved in approximately one-third of suicides and rapes, half of assaults, and one-half to two-thirds of homicides.

Mechanism of Action

It has long been believed that the effects of ethanol on the CNS are mediated by an increase in membrane fluidity, leading to disorder of the membrane lipids and resulting in abnormal activity of ion channels and other proteins. Although there is evidence to support this mechanism, the focus more recently has been on the effect of ethanol on excitatory and inhibitory amino acids in the brain. **Ethanol potentiates the effect of γ-aminobutyric acid (GABA)** at $GABA_A$ receptors. Its mechanism in this respect is similar to that of other sedatives, such as benzodiazepines, which also enhance the effect of GABA at $GABA_A$ receptors and increase Cl^- conductance. In addition, ethanol exerts an inhibitory effect on the CNS by reducing glutamate activation of excitatory ion channels. More specifically, **ethanol inhibits the response of the NMDA receptor** to glutamate. Biochemical mechanisms involved in the CNS effects of ethanol also seem to involve, among others, dopaminergic, adrenergic, serotoninergic, and opioid pathways. Reward mechanisms are enhanced by dopaminergic stimulation and by opioid peptides. Naltrexone, an opioid receptor antagonist, inhibits the desire for alcohol intake, as do dopamine receptor antagonists.

Pharmacologic Effects

Ethanol-induced damage in organs lacking significant ethanol oxidative capacity may result from enzyme-catalyzed esterification of fatty acids with ethanol. Transient accumulation of such fatty acid ethyl esters, or their fatty acid metabolites, seems to inhibit oxidative phosphorylation and may alter plasma membranes, leading to damage in organs such as the heart, pancreas, and brain.

The inflammatory effects of alcohol on the gastrointestinal tract lead to esophagitis and chronic gastritis frequently associated with intense episodes of vomiting, which may lead to gastric laceration and hematemesis. There is a high correlation between heavy drinking and cancer of the mouth and throat. Peptic ulcers and pancreatitis are common among alcoholics.

Effects of alcohol on skeletal muscle may produce acute alcoholic myopathy characterized by muscle cramps, weakness, and swelling, which resolve after a few weeks of alcohol abstinence. In severe cases, extensive muscle degeneration results in myoglobinemia, hyperkalemia, and renal failure. A chronic form of alcoholic myopathy ultimately produces marked muscular atrophy, usually of the pelvic girdle and thighs.

Chronic alcoholism is associated with numerous severe physical complications, including the central and peripheral nervous systems, liver, gastrointestinal tract, and skeletal and cardiac muscle.

Central nervous system

There is a common but mistaken notion that ethanol is a CNS stimulant. To the contrary, **ethanol is a sedative-hypnotic** that depresses the CNS in a dose-dependent fashion. Much of the apparent stimulation resulting from ethanol use results from disinhibition of CNS function because of selective depression of inhibitory pathways at lower concentrations of ethanol. Although mental processes, memory, and concentration are reduced, the individual may feel euphoric, confident, and socially uninhibited. Higher doses (intoxication) lead to overall depression of the CNS. As with other CNS depressants, the major acute toxicity of ethanol is respiratory depression from inhibition of the medullary respiratory center. Effects of ethanol on the brain are shown in Table 39-2.

The concentration of ethanol in alcoholic beverages is often listed as the "proof." The actual concentration of ethanol, in percent by volume, is half the proof number: 80 proof equals 40% ethanol by volume. Because of the variability of absorption of different alcoholic beverages, the effects of ethanol are most commonly correlated with the blood alcohol concentration (BAC), as illustrated in Table 39-3. The effects of ethanol are dose-related and progress through the typical sequence of anxiolysis, sedation, hypnosis, anesthesia, and death. Ethanol is a soporific, increasing the time spent in sleep and decreasing the time it takes to get to sleep.

Liver

A number of effects of ethanol on the liver have been documented (Table 39-4). Acute ingestion of intoxicating amounts of ethanol leads to a reduced liver-metabolizing activity. This effect is reversed when the ethanol is eliminated. In a long-term alcoholic, induction of liver microsomal enzymes is common; if the individual is not intoxicated, drug metabolism may be enhanced. If cirrhosis of the liver occurs, overall metabolism is reduced because of impaired hepatic blood flow and destruction of liver tissue. The use of ethanol has several implications for drug metabolism. Other effects of ethanol on the liver are listed in Table 39-4. The toxic effects on the liver of long-term ethanol abuse are summarized in Figure 39-6.

TABLE 39-3 Correlates of Blood Alcohol Concentration (BAC)

BAC (mg/dL)	Clinical Effects
50	Altered vision, reduced fine motor functions, ataxia, disinhibition, drowsiness, slowed speech, impulsive actions, increased sexual motivation (Drivers younger than 21 are restricted to 20 mg/dL)
80	Legally drunk, lower sexual performance, otherwise heightened effects than those seen at 50 mg/dL
150	Nausea and vomiting, exaggerated action, memory deficits worsened, ataxia, amnesia, rage, nystagmus, analgesia, reduction in the length of rapid eye movement during sleep
300	Dazed, loss of consciousness, hypothermia, hypotension, mydriasis, sweating
400	"Dead drunk" severe medullary paralysis, cardiovascular depression
500	Lethal effect due to medullary paralysis, severe cardiovascular depression

TABLE 39-4 Effects of Ethanol on the Liver

Effect	Mechanism
Toxicity to hepatic cells, increased response to some drugs	Inhibition of liver enzymes with acute high level alcohol intake
Increased liver enzyme activity, reduced effect of some other drugs	Induction of liver microsomal enzymes with chronic alcohol intake during the "sober" period
Altered nutritional status	Lowered levels of vitamins A and D, thiamine, niacin, pyridoxine, and others; acetaldehyde plays a major role
Enhanced lipid peroxidation, membrane damage	Acetaldehyde plays a major role
Damage to liver cells, leading to fatty liver and cirrhosis	Endotoxins from the altered flora of the GI tract stimulate Kupffer cells, leading to inflammatory mediators; recruitment of infiltrating macrophages (see Fig. 39-6)
	Inhibition of insulin-like growth factor

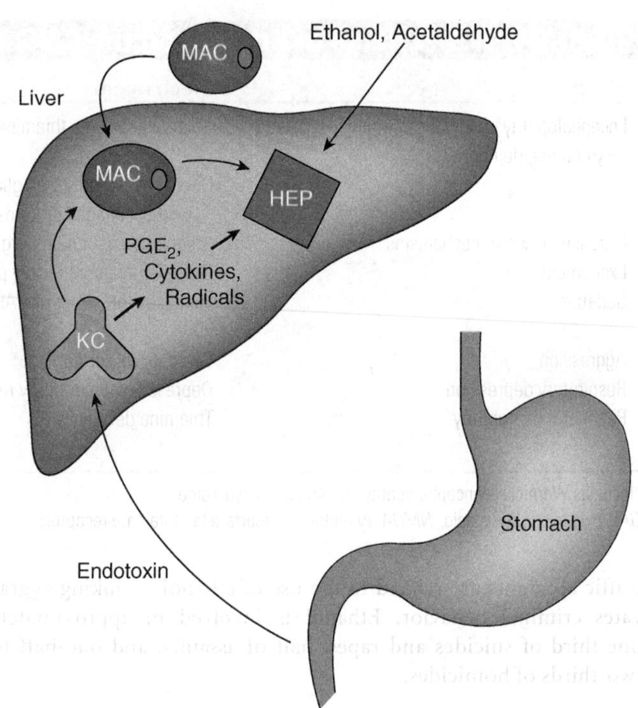

FIG 39-6 Mechanism of liver damage from ethanol. Use of ethanol leads to an increase in certain intestinal gram-negative organisms, resulting in an increase in endotoxins. Damage to the GI tract contributes to the absorption of endotoxins. These stimulate Kupffer cells (*KC*) in the liver to produce mediators, including prostaglandin E_2 (*PGE_2*), cytokines, and free radicals, which damage hepatocytes (*HEP*). Effects on KC lead to the recruitment of infiltrating macrophages (*MAC*), which also release mediators that damage liver cells. Ethanol and acetaldehyde induce cytochrome P450 enzymes (CYP), especially CYP2E1, and damage mitochondria, resulting in production of reactive oxygen species that damage hepatic hepatocytes. Ethanol or acetaldehyde may also act directly on hepatocytes to alter lipid metabolism, damage cell macromolecules, or block the effect of insulin-like growth factor. (Modified from Thurman RG: Mechanisms of hepatic toxicity, II: alcoholic liver injury involves activation of Kupffer cells by endotoxin, *Am J Physiol* 275:G605-G611, 1998; and Wang et al., 2014, in General References.)

Cardiovascular system

Acute alcohol administration results in an elevated catecholamine concentration in blood and urine. Adrenal gland activation results in increased blood concentrations of corticosteroids, epinephrine, and glucose. Adrenal monoamine release is accompanied by compensatory increases in the activity of medullary tyrosine hydroxylase, dopamine β-hydroxylase, and phenylethanolamine-N-methyltransferase. Vascular smooth muscle exhibits hyperreactivity to norepinephrine at low ethanol concentrations and hyporeactivity at high concentrations. The latter effect may be caused by ethanol-induced facilitation of neuronal monoamine uptake.

The direct actions of ethanol on vasomotor tone, coupled with its complex adrenergic effects and centrally mediated influences, produce variable cardiovascular responses. In general, coronary blood flow is slightly enhanced, but there is no concomitant increase in myocardial oxygen uptake. Myocardial contractility is depressed by ethanol. Direct vasoconstriction has been observed in cerebral and renal vascular beds in vitro, but in vivo the effect of ethanol, occurring only at large doses, is an increase in blood flow to the brain and kidneys. Mesenteric blood flow also seems to be increased.

A consistent cardiovascular effect of alcohol ingestion is cutaneous vasodilation. The increased blood flow to the skin provides a feeling of warmth. In cold environments, heat loss may be greatly accentuated, and alcohol generally should be avoided in treating hypothermic individuals. At low ambient temperatures, individuals under the influence of ethanol have a high risk of hypothermia.

The ethanol metabolite acetaldehyde causes catecholamine release and produces tachycardia, increased cardiac output, and increased arterial blood pressure, effects that are abolished by adrenoceptor blockade. The concentrations of acetaldehyde normally resulting from low amounts of ingested ethanol have little acute effect on the cardiovascular system, however. Long-term effects of ethanol differ from its short-term effects. When ingested in excess on a long-term basis, ethanol increases the risk of hypertension and adverse cardiac effects such as stroke. Long-term ethanol abuse can cause a cardiomyopathy characterized by a decreased ventricular ejection fraction and heart failure. Fibrosis of the myocardium may also occur, as well as atrial fibrillation. The "holiday heart syndrome" refers to severe atrial arrhythmias precipitated by bouts of periodic heavy drinking. Hypokalemia and hypomagnesemia are more likely with alcohol abuse.

Kidney

Ethanol has a diuretic effect resulting from inhibition of antidiuretic hormone secretion by the posterior pituitary. Urinary Na^+, K^+, and Cl^- concentrations are reduced, whereas Mg^{++} and norepinephrine are increased.

Sexual function

Ethanol interferes with sexual function in men and women. It can cause temporary impotence even though overall aggressiveness may be enhanced. Long-term alcoholism may lead to more lasting impotence and sterility. Testosterone production may be depressed, and testosterone metabolism may be enhanced, the latter as a result of induction of liver microsomal enzymes. Feminization in men is a possible outcome.

The effects of ethanol on the peripheral vasculature, CNS, antidiuretic hormone secretion, and sexual function are summarized in the following exchange between Macduff and the porter in Shakespeare's *Macbeth*:

> *Macduff: What three things does drink especially provoke?*
> *Porter: Marry, Sir, nose-painting, sleep, and urine. Lechery, sir, it provokes and unprovokes: it provokes the desire but not the performance.*
> ***Shakespeare W: Macbeth. In Wells S, Taylor G, editors:* William Shakespeare, the complete works, *Oxford, 1986, Clarendon Press.***

Blood lipids

A potential salutary effect of moderate consumption of ethanol relates to cholesterol status. Intake on the order of one to two drinks a day increases the ratio of high-density to low-density lipoproteins in the plasma, an effect inversely correlated with the incidence of coronary heart disease and myocardial infarction. Other effects of low to moderate ethanol use, such as reduced platelet aggregation, may also provide some cardioprotective effect.

Alcohol consumption is associated with an increase in serum triglyceride levels. This association may pose a cardiovascular risk, and if the triglyceride levels are high enough, a risk of pancreatitis exists. The overriding issue for the individual and society as a whole is controlling ethanol intake to avoid its many adverse effects.

Gastrointestinal tract

Small oral doses of ethanol temporarily enhance salivary and gastric acid secretion—the increased salivation probably by a conditioned reflex. Large doses of alcohol reduce salivation. Ethanol is a gastric irritant, producing inflammation of the stomach wall in concentrations greater than 15%. Ingestion of solutions of more than 20% ethanol results in increased gastric mucus secretion and in petechial hemorrhage and ulceration. **Ethanol retards intestinal absorption of glucose, amino acids, folic acid, thiamine, and vitamin B_{12}.** Ethanol has also been shown to change the flora in the gastrointestinal tract, favoring the growth of certain gram-negative bacteria. This growth leads to the production of more bacterial endotoxins (lipopolysaccharides). Damage to the gastrointestinal tract leads to greater absorption of toxins. **Endotoxins stimulate liver Kupffer cells,** which produce inflammatory mediators and reactive oxygen species that cause apoptotic changes in hepatic parenchymal cells (see Fig. 39-6). Damage by this mechanism may account partly for short-term and long-term changes.

Absorption, Fate, and Excretion

Ethanol is rapidly absorbed from the stomach and small intestine. After oral ingestion, the rate of absorption largely depends on the gastric emptying time because 75% of a dose is rapidly and completely taken up from the small intestine. Patients with gastrectomy often note enhanced effects of ethanol. The rate of gastric absorption is reduced by the presence of food. Concentrations of ethanol greater than 20% retard absorption by inducing gastric mucosal irritation and pylorospasm.

TABLE 39-5 Equivalents of Alcoholic Beverages

Form of Alcohol	Classification of Drinker: Sex	Classification of Drinker: Age (yr)	Potential Resulting BAC (mg/dL)*
Regular beer (12 oz, 3.5% ethanol)	Male	17-34	22.7
		57-86	25.5
	Female	20-31	27.7
		60-82	30.7
Distilled spirits (1 oz, 40% ethanol)†	Male	17-34	17.1
		57-86	19.3
	Female	20-31	21
		60-82	23.2

*Calculated on the basis of a lean body mass of 153.4 lb (70 kg).
†American proof number is twice the percentage of ethanol by volume.
BAC, Blood alcohol concentration.

Approximately 60% of inspired ethanol vapor is absorbed through the lungs, and intoxication can be achieved by this route. Percutaneous absorption can also occur and has led to death when infants were wrapped in ethanol-soaked cloth to treat hyperthermia.

After oral intake, the arterial BAC exceeds the venous BAC because of rapid tissue uptake of alcohol from capillary blood. Maximum electroencephalogram changes occur approximately 25 minutes before the maximum venous BAC is achieved. The BAC after ingestion of a fixed amount of alcohol is a function of sex, age, and adiposity of the drinker; the nature of the beverage; and the time over which it is ingested. In Table 39-5, which shows the influence of alcoholic beverage, age, and sex on BAC, the BAC has been calculated on the basis of reported age-corrected and sex-corrected values for total body water and blood water content. The tissue alcohol concentration is proportional to lean body weight and tissue water content. Considering the BAC as unity, the relative concentration of ethanol at equilibrium is 1.35 in urine, 1.17 in brain, 1.16 in blood plasma, 1.12 in saliva, 0.05 in alveolar air, and 0.02 in fat.

Under normal circumstances, more than 95% of ingested ethanol is metabolized. High doses of ethanol are associated with lower metabolism (approaching 90% metabolized). Metabolism occurs mostly by a three-phase hepatic oxidation (Fig. 39-7). **Ethanol is initially converted to acetaldehyde** by alcohol dehydrogenase, which requires nicotinamide adenine dinucleotide (NAD) as the hydrogen acceptor:

$$CH_3CH_2OH + NAD^+ \leftrightarrow CH_3CHO + NADH + H^+$$

The binding of substrate and coenzyme to alcohol dehydrogenase involves sites on the enzyme containing zinc and sulfhydryl groups. Human alcohol dehydrogenase also oxidizes methanol, isopropyl alcohol, and ethylene glycol. This dehydrogenase reaction is the rate-limiting step in the metabolism of alcohol except in individuals who have a deficiency in the subsequent enzyme.

The second phase, conversion of acetaldehyde to acetate, occurs in liver and other tissues and is catalyzed by aldehyde dehydrogenase, which has a much greater affinity for acetaldehyde than does alcohol dehydrogenase:

$$CH_3CHO + NAD^+ \leftrightarrow CH_3COOH + NADH + H^+$$

In the third step, acetate, as acetyl coenzyme A, is oxidized further through the Krebs cycle to carbon dioxide and water.

The reductive environment resulting from ethanol oxidation upsets hepatic chemistry and results in reduced gluconeogenesis and enhanced

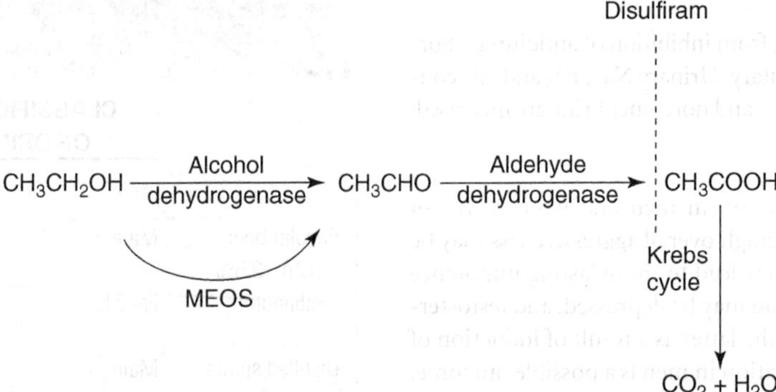

FIG 39-7 Metabolism of ethanol and its blockade by disulfiram. Disulfiram inhibits the mitochondrial and cytoplasmic forms of aldehyde dehydrogenase. *MEOS,* Microsomal enzyme oxidizing system.

triglyceride and lactate formation. Heavy bouts of drinking can cause hypoglycemia, lactic acidosis, and hyperuricemia (because acetate and lactate stimulate the synthesis of uric acid and inhibit its renal excretion), which can precipitate gout, hyperlipidemia, and fatty liver.

An alternate oxidative pathway for alcohol involving the microsomal enzyme oxidation system (MEOS) becomes an important factor in alcohol elimination at high BACs, during which it may account for 10% to 20% of ethanol metabolism. This pathway also yields acetaldehyde. The MEOS pathway is inducible and may account for the higher metabolic inactivation of ethanol seen in individuals who abuse ethanol over the long-term.

Ethanol elimination follows zero-order kinetics even at moderate doses. Thus, metabolism is readily saturated. A 70-kg adult can metabolize approximately 1.0 oz of 80 proof distilled spirits per hour. Approximately 2% to 10% of absorbed alcohol is excreted unchanged, largely through the lungs and kidneys. Minor amounts are detectable in saliva, tears, sweat, and feces. Because ethanol is metabolized to acetate, it can provide calories (a maximum of approximately 1200 kcal/day). It provides no other essential nutrients, however, such as vitamins, amino acids, or fatty acids.

Drug Interactions

Ethanol produces additive effects with all CNS depressants and increases the hypotensive effects of most vasodilators. Long-acting drugs such as diazepam may cause increased depression with ingested alcohol for 24 hours after the drug was given. The benzodiazepine–ethanol combination seems to pose a particular risk. At high BACs, ethanol may inhibit the metabolism of, and potentiate the effects of, benzodiazepines and some other CNS depressants. Short-term alcohol ingestion may also result in exaggerated clinical responses to oral anticoagulants and hypoglycemic agents.

The use of ethanol influences the in vivo absorption of certain drugs. Short-term ethanol ingestion increases, although long-term alcoholism reduces, the oral absorption rate of diazepam. Ethanol also inhibits the absorption and enhances the breakdown of penicillins in the stomach for 3 hours after ethanol intake. Aspirin and other nonsteroidal antiinflammatory drugs (NSAIDs) promote gastric bleeding when combined with ethanol and can cause gastric hemorrhage in alcoholics who have alcoholic gastritis.

In a long-term alcoholic without liver damage, induction of MEOS activity occurs. Increased enzyme activity appears after approximately 3 weeks of heavy drinking and lasts 4 to 9 weeks after the cessation of drinking. A significant reduction in plasma half-life of, and clinical response to, many drugs occurs (e.g., intravenous anesthetics, barbiturates, antianxiety drugs). In long-term alcoholics, the development of hepatic damage offsets the effects of enzyme induction, and drug sensitivity may return to normal. Eventually, cirrhosis leads to significantly reduced drug metabolism. The induction of liver microsomal enzymes with long-term ethanol ingestion is the basis for the enhanced toxicity of acetaminophen in long-term alcohol abusers. Induction of the cytochrome enzymes, CYP2E1 and CYP3A4, favors the production of reactive and hepatotoxic metabolites of acetaminophen (see Chapter 17).

Drugs that inhibit aldehyde dehydrogenase can lead to unpleasant and potentially life-threatening symptoms after ethanol ingestion. These inhibitors include disulfiram (Antabuse), which is given to prevent the use of ethanol by abusers; metronidazole; certain cephalosporins; and oral hypoglycemics. Acutely, acetaldehyde can cause flushing, headache, nausea and vomiting, hypotension, blurred vision, and mental confusion. Because acetaldehyde concentrations vary directly with ethanol intake, high doses of ethanol alone may lead to these symptoms. If aldehyde dehydrogenase is inhibited by drugs such as disulfiram, even low and moderate amounts of ethanol can lead to adverse reactions because of acetaldehyde accumulation. Individuals with a genetic deficiency in aldehyde dehydrogenase, which is common in certain races, also experience the accumulation of acetaldehyde and have alcohol intolerance.

General Therapeutic Uses

Topically applied 70% ethanol is used as a rubefacient, anhidrotic, and antiseptic and as a means to cool the skin in cases of fever. Ethanol is a solvent for the irritating principle of poison ivy, and early ethanol use on affected skin can markedly reduce resulting dermatitis.

Absolute ethanol has been injected to destroy nerves or ganglia in treating intractable pain arising from conditions such as trigeminal neuralgia and inoperable cancer. Other treatment modalities are usually more desirable, however. Ethanol is also used to treat poisoning by methanol, isopropyl alcohol, and ethylene glycol, because ethanol has the highest affinity for alcohol dehydrogenase.

Therapeutic Uses and Implications for Dentistry

Uses of ethanol in dentistry as an antiseptic and disinfectant are discussed in Appendix 3. The dentist can expect to encounter alcoholic patients in everyday practice. **Alcoholics usually exhibit signs of deficient oral hygiene**, such as coated tongue and heavy plaque and calculus deposits. They have twice the rate of tooth loss of the general population, commonly lack mandibular and maxillary first molars, and frequently have severe chronic periodontitis. Chronic asymptomatic enlargement of the parotid, and sometimes submandibular, glands may be observed. The dentist should be aware of the increased incidence of oral leukoplakia in alcoholics and be familiar with its appearance, particularly the erosive form, because 6% of such individuals develop carcinoma, especially of the tongue, within 9 years of diagnosis of the lesion. Postoperative healing time is prolonged in alcoholics; this may be related to a marked increase in collagenase activity, which has been observed in the liver of alcoholics. The potential interactions of ethanol with acetaminophen and NSAIDs should be kept in mind. Large therapeutic doses of acetaminophen should be avoided in moderate to heavy drinkers. Concurrent intake of NSAIDs and ethanol should be avoided.

Alcohol Dependence

Abuse characteristics

Alcoholism is similar to dependence on CNS depressants except that ethanol produces unique direct neurologic, hepatic, and muscular toxicity. Ethanol dependence is characterized by marked psychic and physical dependence, moderate tolerance, and a wide range of pathologic sequelae as well as personal and social problems.

Tolerance develops to ethanol after long-term abuse, but the degree of tolerance, as with other sedative-hypnotics, is much less than that which occurs with opioids. Tolerance to ethanol is partly a result of behavioral adaptation to the effects of ethanol. Adaptive changes by receptor mechanisms and membrane fluidity may also play a role. Induction of MEOS increases the rate of ethanol metabolism. The acute lethal dose of ethanol is not greatly increased, however, over that for nonalcoholics. Cross-tolerance with other sedative-hypnotics also occurs.

Alcohol abstinence syndrome

The severity of acute alcohol abstinence syndrome correlates with the amount and duration of pre-abstinent ethanol intake. The mildest form is the tremulousness and nausea experienced "the morning after," which is readily reversed by "taking a hair of the dog" (i.e., a small amount of ethanol). The most severe abstinence syndrome is delirium tremens. Severe withdrawal symptoms appear 6 to 8 hours after drinking ceases, peak at 48 to 96 hours, and generally resolve in approximately 2 weeks.

Moderate abstinence results in anorexia, nausea, epigastric upset, tremulousness, sweating, apprehension, and insomnia. In more severe abstinence, additional symptoms of diarrhea, vomiting, nightmares, and agitation occur, together with autonomic signs of tachycardia, hyperpnea, and fever. **Delirium tremens**, if it occurs, is manifested by all the preceding symptoms together with possible psychosis, seizures, and hyperthermia. Psychotic manifestations include muttering; delirium; paranoia; delusions; and auditory, visual, and tactile hallucinations of a threatening nature. The individual usually displays agitation, confusion, disorientation, and panic. Neuromuscular hyperexcitability is manifested by gross tremors and grand mal convulsions (with a marked sensitivity to stroboscopically induced seizures), both of which correlate with a rapid urinary excretion of Mg^{++} and a resultant hypomagnesemia during withdrawal. Abstinence may also lead to hyperthermia and circulatory collapse.

Fetal alcohol syndrome

Fetal alcohol syndrome is a cluster of physical and mental defects occurring in children of women who consume ethanol during pregnancy. In more than 90% of cases of fetal alcohol syndrome, there is growth deficiency, microcephaly, and short palpebral fissures. Also common are midfacial hypoplasia, mental retardation, and deficiencies in coordination and fine motor skills. The mental and motor deficiencies may be causally related to the developmental abnormalities of cortical neurons, as observed in rats prenatally exposed to ethanol. The degree of dysmorphogenesis correlates with mental deficiency, with IQs ranging from 55 to 82. Neither the dysmorphic nor the intellectual aspects of fetal alcohol syndrome improve with age. Pregnant patients should be advised to avoid alcoholic beverages and to be aware of the alcoholic content of food and drugs.

Treatment of alcoholism

The treatment of alcoholism involves the detoxification of an acutely inebriated individual, medication to prevent severe symptoms of abstinence, and long-term rehabilitation. The rate of detoxification is determined largely by the rate at which the liver disposes of the ethanol, but the nature of the withdrawal period also depends on the degree of dependence, the environment, and the nutritional status of the patient. The symptoms associated with abstinence are usually treated with a benzodiazepine (e.g., diazepam, if liver function is adequate; oxazepam or lorazepam if liver function is compromised). Supplemental dietary thiamine is given. In addition, three other drugs are approved for treating alcohol dependence: naltrexone, disulfiram, and acamprosate. All modalities of drug treatment for alcoholics are more clinically effective when accompanied by behavioral therapy.

Naltrexone is a long-acting opioid receptor antagonist. Naltrexone reduces the rewarding effects of alcohol by interfering with the activation of dopaminergic reward pathways in the brain. The pharmacology of naltrexone is discussed further in Chapter 16.

Disulfiram is used in avoidance therapy for alcoholics because alcohol intake with disulfiram leads to very unpleasant reactions in patients. Disulfiram is rapidly converted to metabolites such as diethyldithiocarbamate and diethylthiomethylcarbamate. These and possibly other metabolites probably account for the action of the drug (see Fig. 39-7). Disulfiram inhibits aldehyde dehydrogenase through the formation of a covalent disulfide bond between an enzymic thiol group and an active drug metabolite. The enzyme is inhibited irreversibly. Disulfiram also inhibits other enzymes, notably dopamine β-hydroxylase and oxidases of MEOS.

If ethanol is ingested during disulfiram treatment, symptoms of acetaldehyde poisoning develop. Drinking 1.2 oz of 80 proof liquor causes flushing, tachycardia, palpitation, and tachypnea, all lasting approximately 30 minutes. Ingestion of more than 1.6 oz of 80 proof liquor produces intense palpitation, dyspnea, nausea, vomiting, and headache lasting up to 90 minutes. Unconsciousness, hypotensive shock, and sudden myocardial infarction may occur. For this reason, disulfiram must be used only under strict medical supervision.

Acamprosate (calcium acetylhomotaurine) is a GABA analogue that is used to reduce relapse in alcoholics. The drug can reduce nerve excitotoxicity caused by alcohol; this is likely due to its ability to block group 5 metabotropic glutamate receptors (mGluR5) as well as the resulting effects on dopaminergic and other pathways. This action likely promotes abstinence and reduces alcohol withdrawal symptoms.

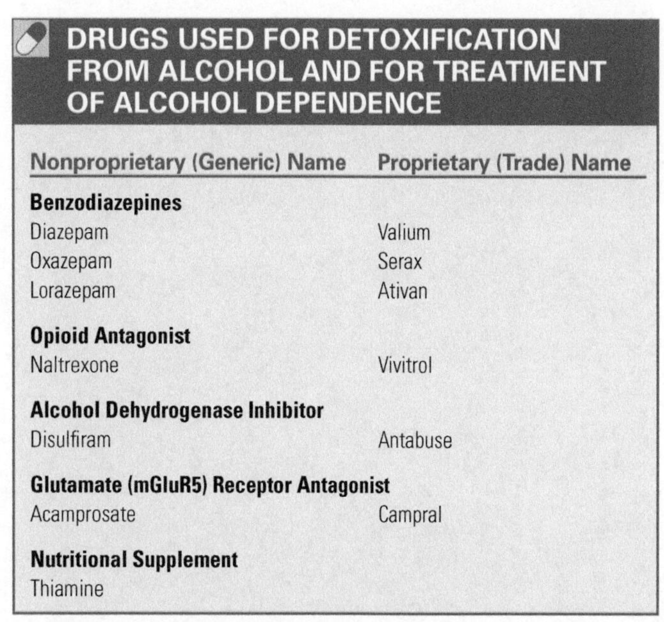

DRUGS USED FOR DETOXIFICATION FROM ALCOHOL AND FOR TREATMENT OF ALCOHOL DEPENDENCE

Nonproprietary (Generic) Name	Proprietary (Trade) Name
Benzodiazepines	
Diazepam	Valium
Oxazepam	Serax
Lorazepam	Ativan
Opioid Antagonist	
Naltrexone	Vivitrol
Alcohol Dehydrogenase Inhibitor	
Disulfiram	Antabuse
Glutamate (mGluR5) Receptor Antagonist	
Acamprosate	Campral
Nutritional Supplement	
Thiamine	

CASE DISCUSSION

Mr. C is abusing methamphetamine, and chronic exposure to it is causing important problems in the oral and overall health of Mr. C. Methamphetamine reduces appetite and salivary flow, and abusers typically have poor nutrition and consume cariogenic carbonated beverages. Together these factors predispose abusers to dental decay. In addition, methamphetamine causes bruxism and continuous oral movements that result in worn teeth and damage to the tongue, respectively. The overall poor condition of the oral cavity and the characteristics of the caries in Mr. C are consistent with chronic methamphetamine abuse. The oral health effects of chronic methamphetamine abuse are sometimes collectively referred to as "Meth Mouth"; however, other stimulants such as amphetamine, cocaine, and MDMA (i.e., "ecstasy") may also produce oral health effects similar to those caused by methamphetamine. The altered sleep pattern and mental changes are also consistent with amphetamine abuse.

Dental treatment for Mr. C should include calculus and plaque removal and polishing of teeth with application of topical fluoride. Mr. C should be encouraged to floss regularly and brush with prescription-strength fluoride toothpaste. Directions should be given to Mr. C on how to improve his diet. For xerostomia, a saliva substitute or cholinergic agonist (pilocarpine or cevimeline) should be considered to stimulate salivary flow. (See Chapter 6.) Mr. C should also be counseled to seek help in treating his substance abuse disorder. Future visits should concentrate on motivating Mr. C to avoid substance abuse, reinforcing preventive practices, and restoring the teeth.

GENERAL REFERENCES

1. Acute reactions to drugs of abuse, *Med Lett Drug Ther* 44:21–24, 2002.
2. Aston R: Drug abuse: its relationship to dental practice, *Dent Clin North Am* 28:595–610, 1984.
3. Baumann MH, Solis E, Watterson LR, Marusich JA, Fantegrossi WE, Wiley JL: Bath salts, spice, and related designer drugs: the science behind the headlines, *J Neurosci* 34:15150–15158, 2014.
4. Cami J, Farre M: Drug addiction, *N Engl J Med* 349:975–986, 2003.
5. De la Monte S, Kril JJ: Human alcohol-related neuropathology, *Acta Neuropathol* 127:71–90, 2014.
6. Karch SB: *Karch's pathology of drug abuse*, ed 3, Boca Raton, FL, 2002, CRC Press.
7. May PA, Baete A, Russo J, Elliot AJ, et al.: Prevalence and characteristics of fetal alcohol spectrum disorders, *Pediatrics* 134:855–866, 2014.
8. O'Brien CP: Drug addiction. In Brunton LL, Chabner B, Knollman B, editors: *Goodman & Gilman's the pharmacological basis of therapeutics*, ed 12, New York, 2011, McGraw-Hill.
9. Rees TD: Oral effects of drug abuse, *Crit Rev Oral Biol Med* 3:163–184, 1992.
10. Stewart A, Maity B, Anderegg SP, Allamargot C, et al.: regulator of G protein signaling 6 is a critical mediator of both reward-related behavioral and pathological responses to alcohol, *Proc Natl Acad Sci* E786–E795, 2015 (online).
11. Wang M, You Q, Lor K, Chen F, et al.: Chronic alcohol ingestion modulates hepatic macrophage populations and functions in mice, *J Leukocyte Biol* 96:657–665, 2014.
12. Winger G, Woods JH, Hofmann FG: *A handbook on drug and alcohol abuse: the biomedical aspects*, ed 3, New York, 2004, Oxford University Press.

40

Toxicology

Harrell E. Hurst and Michael D. Martin

KEY INFORMATION

- Dose is the major determinant that distinguishes therapeutic effects from toxicity with exposure to drugs and chemicals.
- Safety, toxicity, hazard, and risk are terms with specific meanings relevant to toxicology.
- Consideration of cause and effect requires careful assessment of criteria for causal relationships.
- Toxicity varies widely with differences in biologic systems, time-course of exposure, and chemistry of toxicants.
- The dental practitioner has a responsibility to protect both patients and office staff from toxic exposures from environmental and therapeutic sources.
- The dental practitioner should understand and be familiar with principles for managing cases of poisoning.
- Mercury, although an important dental therapeutic agent, is toxic and its use must be managed carefully.
- A great variety of toxic chemical agents, including gases, solvents, pesticides, and natural products, are used in modern society and exposure is virtually inevitable; safety depends on careful use to minimize hazards and reduce risk.

CASE STUDY

Three male dentists, who are within 2 years of each other in age and have been in the same group practice for over 20 years, together attend the American Dental Association annual meeting at which they each have urinary mercury level testing performed. On returning home, they each receive the results. When comparing notes, they are astonished to find that although they each work essentially the same schedule, work in the same environment, and utilize all of the same supplies and techniques, one of the three has a urinary Hg level approximately double that of the others. All three are relatively low, with the two lower at 3.3 and 3.5 μg/L and the higher at 6.1 μg/L. All three are healthy, with no kidney disease or reduced kidney function. Following a discussion of seafood ingestion, a known source of dietary Hg, and a review of their individual practice methods regarding use of mercury amalgam, they cannot determine why one would have such a different urinary Hg level. What might be additional details of a possible cause for this disparity?

Toxicology is a basic science that is concerned with poisonous substances and their toxic actions. This discipline draws on biology, chemistry, and medicine to inform knowledge regarding toxic materials. Toxicology strives to understand key features of biology relevant to adverse interactions of chemicals with living systems. A principal objective is to promote safe use of chemicals, whether encountered as medicines, as food additives or contaminants, as industrial materials, as household products, or in the environment. Topics of interest to toxicologists include management of poisoning, analysis of toxic agents, identification of toxic effects, elucidation of mechanisms of toxicity, characterization of potential chemical risks, forensic and legal applications, and timely application of knowledge to prevent potentially dire consequences of chemical use.

The toxicology of therapeutic agents related to their pharmacologic effects at elevated doses is described in the corresponding chapters of this text. This chapter reviews general principles of toxicology, summarizes key organ systems that are susceptible to toxic effects, and outlines prevention and management of acute poisoning. Toxic materials not described elsewhere in the text are reviewed, and relevant topics related to dental practice are discussed.

GENERAL PRINCIPLES

All chemical substances can cause harm or kill if encountered at sufficiently large concentrations over crucial periods of time. This statement embodies insight articulated by Paracelsus in the 16th century: that dose is the major determinant of toxicity. A subset of substances has relatively specific toxic effects, however. These are considered very harmful based on human experience and are considered poisons or toxins. Beyond this base of experience exists a vast number of uncharacterized, potential toxicants. At this time, there are more than 32 million organic and inorganic substances, over 245,000 inventoried or regulated substances, and some 15 million commercially available chemicals. Because many of these are potentially toxic, this array dictates that toxicologists use some means of triage toward assessment of potential toxicants. At present, selection of chemicals for toxicologic testing is dictated by their potential for use, by funding of basic research on the chemicals, and by evidence of specific adverse effects.

The ultimate aim of toxicologic science in society is to guide safe use of chemicals. The definitions in Box 40-1 can assist in understanding and promoting concise communication in the approach to this objective. **Safety** is a negative entity—that is, the absence of threat of injury. As such, safety cannot be proved directly. Society often simplistically considers chemicals "safe" or "toxic." Such naive characterization can preclude the rational judgment that enables safe uses of

BOX 40-1 Definitions Relevant to Principles of Toxicology

Safety	Condition of being secure from threat of danger, harm, or injury
Toxicity	Property of grave harmfulness or deadliness associated with a chemical that is expressed on biologic exposure
Hazard	Threat of danger directly related to circumstances of use of a chemical
Risk	Expected frequency of occurrence of an adverse effect in a given situation

chemicals. Critical judgment requires understanding of the distinction between the terms **toxicity** and **hazard** to enable assessment of risks (see Box 40-1). Toxicologic studies promote safety by defining hazardous situations of use so that the unsafe use of chemicals can be avoided.

A primary concern of toxicology is evaluation of **risk.** All useful chemicals have some degree of risk associated with their use. Toxicologic science has developed testing paradigms to define toxicity and assess potential risk. Benefits also must be considered relative to the risk of use. A high degree of risk may be acceptable when benefits are great (e.g., use of toxic but potentially life-extending drugs such as chemotherapeutic agents). Otherwise, risk may be unacceptable for less essential uses (e.g., food coloring). In contrast to the science inherent in testing methods, judgment of risk acceptability involves policy. Such judgment invokes economic, social, and ethical values and should consider factors such as needs met by a chemical under consideration, alternative solutions and their risks, anticipated extent of use and public exposure, effects on environmental quality, and conservation of natural resources.

Within such considerations is an issue of major importance to toxicology and to society in general, which is determination of cause-and-effect relationships. This objective of epidemiologic studies is elusive for chronic diseases, such as many types of cancer. Such diseases may involve confounded potential causes, such as chemical or viral exposure and genetic susceptibility factors. Uncritical publication of unscientific observations or incomplete studies lead the public to inappropriate conclusions, which should be characterized more correctly as hypotheses. Adequate processes for determination of causation, as opposed to simple unrelated association or correlation, require scientific discipline and judgment based on considerable experience.

The criteria developed by Sir Austin Bradford Hill (see reference) provide a sound basis for consideration of causal relationships and should be considered a touchstone for expert opinion regarding cause and effect (Box 40-2). None of these criteria should be considered as absolutely essential, and they cannot be considered as proof of causal relationships. Their careful application during evaluation of potential cause-and-effect relationships can assist, however, in organizing knowledge toward a weight-of-evidence judgment and may provide an alternative interpretation for consideration.

Dose–Response Relationships

The relationship between **dose and toxic response** is the fundamental axiom of the science of toxicology. Studies are designed to ascertain dose–response functions associated with specific adverse effects. When simple all-or-nothing criteria, such as death, are used, quantitation of response is simple. More often, objectives require subtler means of assessment that are less readily quantified. Beyond simple indication of the quantity of material required for the toxic effect, dose–response relationships provide strong evidence of the causal relationship between the observed effect and the chemical under study.

BOX 40-2 Hill Criteria for Consideration of Causal Relationships

Criterion	Explanation
Strength of association	Observed magnitude of the association compared with other relevant observations should be considered as a primary indicator in assessment of cause and effect
Consistency	Association of cause and effect can be observed repeatedly by others under appropriate circumstances
Specificity	Particular conditions produce the effect, or a specific group is affected; bounds of causal relationship should be delimited
Temporality	Causation generally occurs before effect, whereas correlational effects can vary in temporality
Biologic gradient	Demonstration of a fundamental dose relationship provides convincing evidence of cause and effect
Plausibility	Some basis in previous knowledge provides a means of common understanding (remember, however, that all phenomena were novel at some point)
Coherence	Care should be taken that interpretation of cause and effect does not unduly conflict with scientifically established facts of biology and medicine
Experiment	Manipulation of accessible variables in the potential cause-and-effect relationship has an effect
Analogy	Previously understood examples provide basis for formulation of testable hypotheses

Data from Hill A: The environment and disease: association or causation? *Proc Roy Soc Med* 58:295, 1965.

Figure 40-1 presents three modes of display of idealized dose–response data to illustrate and describe the dose required for median response in subjects tested. These data are typical of quantal or all-or-nothing responses such as lethality. In this example, the dose axis is logarithmically spaced, and the data describe a log-normal distribution. Responses that arise from mass action, such as reversible occupancy of receptor by drugs, often are most easily interpreted when plotted on a logarithmic axis. Alternatively, effects caused by limited biologic capacity, such as irreversible enzyme inhibition, can exhibit abrupt threshold-like effects and may be more easily analyzed on a linear dose axis. The rule is to plot the data to see what type axis is most informative.

The **lower panel** of Figure 40-1 indicates distribution of responses across the dose axis, with a mean of 10 and standard deviation (SD) of one $\log_{10}$ unit. Response percentages include approximately 68.3% within ±1 SD of the mean, 95.5% within ±2 SD, and 99.7% within ±3 SD of the mean. The distribution indicates hypersusceptibility for individuals at the lowest doses and resistant responders at the highest doses. Such a plot gives a convenient way to visualize the distribution of responses across dose within the test groups.

The **middle panel** of Figure 40-1 plots the cumulative response versus dose across all treated groups. Here the response data are practically linear in the range from −1 to +1 SD for these ideal data. This plot provides a convenient, accurate estimation of dose required for a 50% response, such as the median lethal dose (LD_{50}). Real data are rarely so well behaved, however, as too few data may be available for adequate definition of the sigmoid curve. Another disadvantage is that the sigmoid curve presents difficulty in estimating doses that elicit extremes of response, such as 1% or 99%.

An alternative presented in the **top panel** of Figure 40-1 uses the **probit** transform for the cumulative response. Probit units are derived by conversion of cumulative response percentages to units of SD from the mean. The scale uses normal equivalent deviation units (NED), for which the mean is arbitrarily set to an NED value of 5 to give positive values along the axis. As is evident in the example, the probit transform linearizes the extreme values of the response function, which allows more accurate estimation of doses affecting 1% or 99% of subjects exposed. In addition, the probit transform facilitates determination of the slope, which enables comparison of the dose–response function with other agents or responses.

Such plots are inadequate in dealing with issues of societal risk beyond mean responses, however, as policy often requires estimation of exposure posing a theoretic risk of one in one million, otherwise described as a 10^{-6} risk factor. Practical problems intervene, including the impracticality of experimental studies involving sufficient animals to define adequately the dose–response function at low response levels. A classic toxicologic experiment conducted at the National Center for Toxicological Research illustrates this point. Officially termed the **ED_{01} Study** (See reference, Gaylor, 1980), this experiment examined in detail the response function of mice treated with low doses of the experimental carcinogen 2-acetylaminofluorene. The study, sometimes termed the **megamouse study**, involved more than 24,000 mice to determine, with precision, the dose effective in producing a 1% tumor rate. This work advanced toxicologic understanding of the complexity of genotoxic and proliferative cellular events in chronic cancer bioassays. It also exhibited logistic difficulties in conducting statistical studies of low incidence and illustrated gaps in the evolving understanding of chemically induced cancer.

Factors That Change Dose–Response Relationships

Dose–response relationships can vary with many factors, including differences within and among individuals. Factors responsible for dose–response variations within an individual over time may include age and nutritional status, environmental influences, functional status of organs of excretion, concomitant disease, and various combinations of factors. Changes in pharmacokinetics of toxicants are a frequent basis for altered dose–response relationships. Known influences include increased toxicant **bioactivation** by enzyme induction, such as occurs in certain variants of cytochrome P450 with exposure to phenobarbital or polychlorinated biphenyls. Conversely, inhibition of metabolic clearance is possible with interacting chemicals, increasing the pharmacodynamic action of drugs and chemicals.

The **cytochrome P450 isozyme 3A4** is an important enzyme in human drug metabolism, and its presence in the gut and liver subjects it to inhibition by many drugs and dietary components, such as grapefruit juice. Conversely, substances are often less toxic by the oral route when administered with food as a consequence of less rapid absorption. The time and frequency of administration can be important in altering dose–response relationships through functional changes. Many compounds induce tolerance upon repeated administration, whereas others can become more toxic with closely repeated administration. Receptor densities and sensitivity may vary with time or as a consequence of previous exposure. An example of the latter is the well-known tolerance that develops to long-term administration of opioids.

Responses among individuals differ as a consequence of different genetic traits. Recognition and understanding of relevant aspects of human diversity derived from functional genomic analyses offer potential for therapeutic gains. The rationale is to use appropriate

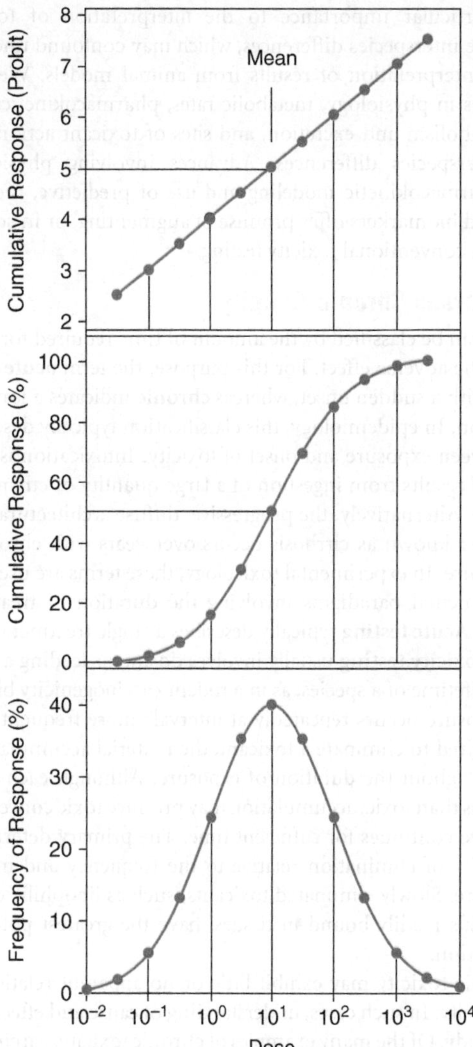

FIG 40-1 Various techniques for graphic display of quantal response versus dose data, including frequency of response (*bottom panel*), cumulative response (*middle panel*), and cumulative response linearized by probit transformation (*top panel*).

drugs in patients best suited to benefit and to reduce use in patients with genetic traits that might result in toxicity. These efforts have spawned new terms, including **pharmacogenetics**, representing characterized genetic differences in drug metabolism and disposition, and **pharmacogenomics**, used to describe the broad spectrum of genes that affect drug response (see Chapter 4). A summary is available that describes progress in determining genetic polymorphisms relevant to drug action and disposition. Known variants linked to altered drug effects in humans include phase I cytochrome P450 enzymes, phase II enzymes such as N-acetyltransferases and glutathione-S-transferases, small molecule transporters, drug and endogenous substrate receptors, and ion channel variants. Similar advances are likely to be applied to understand genetic differences that result in toxic effects aside from those that arise during drug therapy. Approximately 400 million individuals worldwide exhibit a heritable deficiency in the cytoplasmic enzyme glucose-6-phosphate dehydrogenase. Because this enzyme is essential to the cell's capacity to withstand oxidant stress through production of reducing equivalents, sensitive individuals with this enzymatic deficiency have chemically mediated hemolytic anemia when exposed to oxidants.

Of particular importance to the interpretation of toxicologic studies are interspecies differences, which may confound understanding and interpretation of results from animal models. Well-known differences in physiology, metabolic rates, pharmacokinetics of toxicant metabolism and excretion, and sites of toxicant action mediate these interspecies differences. Advances involving physiologically based pharmacokinetic modeling and use of predictive, mechanistically based biomarkers offer promise of augmenting, or in some cases obviating, conventional toxicity testing.

Acute versus Chronic Toxicity

Toxicity can be classified by the amount of time required for development of the adverse effect. For this purpose, the term **acute** describes toxicity with a sudden onset, whereas **chronic** indicates a long latency or duration. In epidemiology, this classification typically describes the time between exposure and onset of toxicity. Intoxication is an acute effect that results from ingestion of a large quantity of ethanol over a brief time. Alternatively, the progressive, diffuse architectural damage to the liver known as cirrhosis occurs over years with chronic ethanol exposure. In experimental toxicology, these terms are used to refer to experimental paradigms involving the duration of treatment or exposure. **Acute testing** typically describes a single treatment, whereas **chronic toxicity testing** usually involves dosing or feeding a chemical over the lifetime of a species, as in a rodent carcinogenicity bioassay.

If exposure occurs repeatedly at intervals more frequent than the time required to eliminate a toxicant, the material accumulates in the body throughout the duration of exposure. Although each exposure may be less than toxic, accumulation may produce toxic concentrations if exposure continues for sufficient time. The primary determinant is the rapidity of elimination relative to the frequency and magnitude of exposure. Slowly eliminated toxicants, such as lipophilic chemicals or materials readily bound in tissues, have the greatest potential for accumulation.

Chronic toxicity may exhibit little or no apparent relationship to acute toxicity. In such cases, understanding of cause and effect requires careful study. Of the many examples of chronic toxicity, carcinogenesis currently is of great concern in society. Precancerous cellular changes occur and develop slowly and may remain undetected over long periods. Periodic dental examinations often play a significant role in detection of cancers of the oral cavity. Knowledge of patient habits with adverse potential health effects, such as the link between tobacco use and occurrence of oral lesions, assists the dental practitioner in being vigilant against such chronic toxicity.

Chemically Related Toxicants

Understanding of chemical toxicity requires knowledge of related chemicals that may be present as impurities because of manufacturing or exist as a result of environmental effects. A classic example is 2,3,7,8-tetrachlorodibenzo-*p*-dioxin (dioxin, or TCDD), which was discovered in the herbicide mixture known as Agent Orange used in the Vietnam War. Although dioxin existed at low part-per-million levels in the herbicide mixture, the extreme toxicity of this contaminant in certain species created grave concern for contaminated areas. This concern led to a ban on the use of the herbicide 2,4,5-trichlorophenoxyacetic acid because TCDD is formed through a condensation reaction involving two molecules of 2,4,5-trichlorophenol. Dioxin also can be formed from other sources, such as combustion of municipal waste, iron ore sintering, and wood pulp and paper mills. The toxic actions of TCDD are mediated through its binding to the aryl hydrocarbon nuclear receptor, which regulates transcription of genes encoding cytochrome P450 enzymes in the CYP1A subfamily and several other genes that regulate cell growth, differentiation, innate immunity, and autoimmune diseases. Despite its extreme toxic potential in some species, epidemiologic studies regarding the effects of low-dose environmental TCDD exposure on humans have been inconclusive to date. High human exposures cause a dermatologic toxicity known as chloracne in some individuals.

The consequences of metabolism of drugs and chemicals after ingestion are extremely important. The following example illustrates the importance of understanding toxic effects relative to drug metabolism. Terfenadine is a nonsedating histamine H_1 receptor antagonist that was widely used for relief of symptoms of seasonal allergy. This drug was removed from the market because studies revealed cardiotoxicity when terfenadine was given with erythromycin. The toxic interaction was traced to the antibiotic's inhibition of the high-affinity oxidative enzyme system CYP3A in human liver and intestinal membranes. This interaction inhibited normal clearance of terfenadine, and the abnormally elevated concentrations produced toxicity in the form of a prolonged cardiac QT interval and the arrhythmia torsades de pointes. This antihistamine has been replaced with its active metabolite, fexofenadine, which apparently does not elicit this toxicity.

Local versus Systemic Effects

Toxic effects can occur at a site of exposure, such as dermal contact, or at some site remote from the point of chemical contact or entry. Local effects dependent on applied concentration are usually diminished by dilution with physiologic fluids and diffusion within tissue away from the site of application. The toxic effect depends on the nature of the interaction at the local site. If the effect is caused by reversible interaction with a receptor, such as that of a local anesthetic, the effect is attenuated by diffusion, and the system is returned to a more normal state as the drug dissociates from receptors. This phenomenon is routinely used in dental practice with the inclusion of epinephrine with local anesthetics, such as lidocaine, to restrict local blood flow and extend duration of local anesthetic action. For toxicants that act through destruction of normal cellular architecture, such as a caustic agent, return to normality requires repair of membranes and cellular structures.

Systemic effects are facilitated by transport within the body fluids and may be influenced by metabolism. Depending on whether biotransformation activates a protoxicant or detoxifies a toxicant, the effects of systemic processing can increase or attenuate toxicity. Compounds may be more or less toxic by the oral route than by other means of systemic exposure, as the first-pass effect of intestine or liver serves to activate or remove toxicants before distribution in the systemic circulation. Alternative systemic exposures, such as inhalation, are not modulated in this manner because systemic exposure occurs directly without first-pass effect.

Target Organ Systems

Most toxic chemicals exhibit specificity in their action on target tissues or organs because these targeted biologic systems reach crucial points in which their physiologic functions are interrupted under the influence of the chemical. This section presents crucial physiologic systems and their characteristics that are important in understanding organ-specific toxicity.

Nervous system

Given the primary importance in control of integrated function, the central nervous system (CNS) is a target of paramount importance for many toxicants. Individual neurons exhibit high metabolic rates and are unable to rely on anaerobic glycolysis. These characteristics make these cells susceptible to toxicants that adversely affect cellular respiration and energy production and lead to neuronal damage when central or peripherally acting toxicants interrupt neuronal metabolism, cerebral circulation, oxygen-carrying capacity of blood, or pulmonary ventilation.

A remarkable cell-selective neurotoxicant is **1-methyl-4-phenyl-1,2,3,6-tetrahydropyridine (MPTP)**, an impurity discovered after attempted illicit synthesis and injection of a meperidine analogue resulted in Parkinson disease-like paralysis. This compound is a protoxicant for **1-methyl-4-phenylpyridinium,** which is formed by monoamine oxidase and concentrated by high-affinity carrier into dopaminergic neurons. The molecular target of 1-methyl-4-phenylpyridinium is reduced nicotinamide adenine dinucleotide dehydrogenase, and the interaction blocks the cellular respiratory exchange of electrons in mitochondria of cells. Its toxic actions result in destruction of **dopaminergic neurons in the substantia nigra**. Death of these cells produces symptoms strikingly similar to Parkinson disease, leading to nonintentional motor actions.

Loss of integrity of neuronal cell metabolism can alter neuronal architecture, particularly the myelin sheath of peripheral neurons. Such effects are common to many forms of toxicity expressed in the nervous system. Various compounds, such as tri-*o*-cresyl phosphate, acrylamide, and metabolites of hexane, cause degeneration of long axons that control neuromuscular activities. Termed **distal axonopathy**, this toxicity involves a "dying back" or retrograde degeneration of distal axons and leads to loss of control of motor functions such as gait. Other effects, such as sensory neuropathy and paresthesia, can result from similar effects of toxicants on small sensory fibers.

Blood and hematopoietic system

Because of the crucial roles of the elements of blood in delivering oxygen and maintaining immune function, toxic effects on blood or the hematopoietic system can be life-threatening. Of these, perhaps no poisoning is more common, preventable, or treatable with timely therapy than the toxic interaction of carbon monoxide (CO) with hemoglobin (Hb). This interaction blocks the vital oxygen-carrying capacity by formation of carboxyhemoglobin (CO-Hb). Characteristics of CO and its toxic effect on various tissues sensitive to anoxia have been concisely reviewed. Details of treatment, which involves displacement of Hb-bound CO with oxygen, are provided in the comprehensive text **Medical Toxicology**. (See reference, Ellenhorn et al., 1997). In mild (CO-Hb < 30%) or moderate (CO-Hb 30% to 40%) cases, therapy includes use of 100% oxygen by nonrebreathing mask until CO-Hb is less than 5%. Severe poisoning can mandate hyperbaric use of oxygen to hasten the exchange.

Another toxic effect that alters the oxygen-carrying capacity of erythrocytes is the formation of methemoglobin. In this toxicity, the heme iron is oxidized from the ferrous (Fe^{++}) to ferric (Fe^{+++}) state by exposure to oxidizing chemicals such as nitrites or aromatic amines. As with CO-Hb, methemoglobin is incapable of carrying molecular oxygen to tissues. Although the effects of resultant anoxia are similar, the treatment differs. Treatment involves use of methylene blue, as a precursor to its metabolite leukomethylene blue, a cofactor that enables erythrocytes to reduce methemoglobin in the presence of reduced nicotinamide adenine dinucleotide phosphate (NADPH). This therapy has complications of potential hemolysis for treatment of infants and individuals with glucose-6-phosphate dehydrogenase deficiency because this enzyme is essential in the production of NADPH.

Other adverse actions affect the blood-forming cells of the bone marrow. Such effects can cause loss of immune functions mediated through leukocytes, as noted with induction of agranulocytosis during treatment with thioamide antithyroid drugs, such as propylthiouracil. Although rare, this adverse effect is devastating because it leaves the patient susceptible to sepsis. Aplastic anemia is a potential complication of therapy with the antiepileptic drugs felbamate and carbamazepine. This condition is very serious because the marrow loses the ability to produce cells. This potential effect requires vigilance for signs of blood dyscrasias and requires laboratory monitoring of blood cell counts during the first months of treatment.

Other adverse effects on the hematopoietic system include overexpression of certain types of cells, such as that noted in the development of acute myelogenous leukemia from benzene. Benzene is a toxicant commonly encountered in petroleum distillates such as gasoline and is considered a causative agent in human leukemia, probably through an active hydroquinone or benzoquinone metabolite. The process of leukemia development seems to involve preferential selection and clonal expansion of stem and progenitor cells through interaction of the toxic benzene metabolites by multiple independent genetic and epigenetic factors.

Respiratory system

The effect of toxicants on the respiratory tract is largely determined by the area of intimate cellular exposure to inhaled chemicals. Such contact is dictated by the structure of the conducting airways and the physical and chemical properties of the toxicant. Larger particles and more water-soluble compounds deposit in the upper regions of the respiratory tract, whereas very fine particles and less soluble gases reach more deeply into the lungs.

Compounds that are rapidly absorbed or highly caustic generally affect the nasal passages. Formaldehyde has a detectable pungent odor at concentrations greater than 0.5 ppm and is highly irritating to the nasal passages. The nasopharyngeal region serves as a filter for particles 10 to 30 μm in diameter. Many of these particles are cleared upward by mucociliary action. Highly water-soluble gases, such as sulfur dioxide, dissolve in moisture present in the upper respiratory membranes and form irritating sulfurous acid. Less soluble compounds, such as oxides of nitrogen and ozone, penetrate more deeply into lung and generally exert effects at membranes in the smallest airways or alveoli. Particles smaller than 5 μm may travel well down into the bronchiolar region, whereas fine particles of 1 μm, nominal size, reach the alveolar region.

Lung toxicity typically involves damage to the delicate architecture vital for efficient gas exchange. Because lung tissues contain many cytokines and immunologic mechanisms for particle clearance and tissue repair, inflammation is a common result of inspired toxic gases such as ozone. With severe acute injury, an exudative phase may progress to pulmonary edema, which alters ventilation, diffusion of oxygen and carbon dioxide, and perfusion. Severity depends on the extent of damage to bronchiolar and alveolar cells and the resolution of inflammation through mitogenic or fibrinogenic processes.

Chronic injury to the lung may result from inhalation of fine particles. Phagocytic mechanisms attempting to remove insoluble particles may produce tissue scarring and interstitial fibrosis, in which collagen fibers replace normal membranes and occupy alveolar interstitial space. This kind of injury is common with inhalation of particles such as asbestos. These actions produce inflexible tissue, diminish surface area, and lead to poor surfaces for gas exchange. Another chronic lung toxicity is emphysema; its major cause is cigarette smoking. This toxic effect produces distended, enlarged air spaces that are poorly compliant but without fibrosis. The pathogenesis of this condition is not fully understood, but an imbalance between proteolytic activities of lung elastase and antiproteases seems to be involved. Lung cancer became a major concern with the increase in popularity of smoking; this health scourge of today was a rare disease a century ago. Smoking is believed to be the most important risk factor for this disease, presenting a tenfold and twentyfold increase in risk for average and heavy smokers.

Organs of excretion

The primary organs of toxicant elimination are the liver and kidneys. The liver provides the major site for metabolic transformation, rendering compounds generally more water-soluble and subject to more efficient excretion in urine by the kidney. The unique physiologic features of each organ provide crucial characteristics that are susceptible to toxic actions and subsequent adverse consequences of impaired function.

The liver possesses remarkable capabilities for regeneration. Hepatotoxicity often results in necrosis and loss of the vital capacities of the liver, however. Essential functions include protein synthesis, nutrient homeostasis, biotransformation, particle filtration, and formation and excretion of bile. Impaired production of proteins such as albumin, clotting factors, and lipoproteins may cause hypoalbuminemia, hemorrhage, and fatty liver. Toxic actions that alter glucose synthesis and storage often lead to hypoglycemia and confusion, whereas effects on cholesterol uptake may produce hypercholesterolemia. Altered biotransformation or biliary excretion of endogenous substrates such as steroid hormones or bilirubin may affect a wide variety of hormonal functions or cause jaundice.

As noted in Chapter 2, various membrane and cytosolic enzymes in the liver provide the essential metabolic functions of oxidation and glucuronide, sulfate, and mercapturate conjugation for removal of toxicants. These reactions usually detoxify compounds, but occasionally metabolic products exhibit enhanced toxicity. Interactions can occur among effects of toxicants within the liver through induction of enzymes or depletion of metabolic resources. Acetaminophen has been widely used as an over-the-counter analgesic without adverse effects on the liver at therapeutic doses. In circumstances of glutathione depletion, however, which occurs with large acetaminophen overdose, malnutrition, or CYP2E1 induction by long-term ethanol use, a reactive electrophilic intermediate forms in sufficient amounts to produce covalent adducts that severely damage the liver.

The kidney plays a vital role in regulating extracellular fluid and excreting soluble wastes through filtration of blood, concentration of wastes, and elimination. To accomplish these vital functions, nephrons are composed of vascular, glomerular, and tubular components. The kidneys possess metabolic and regenerative capabilities, but these resources lead to renal failure when overwhelmed. Nephrotoxicity can be classified as acute or chronic. Acute renal failure can be caused by hypoperfusion from renal vasoconstriction, as elicited by the antifungal amphotericin B, or hypofiltration through glomerular injury resulting from cyclosporine and aminoglycosides. Numerous compounds, including nonsteroidal antiinflammatory drugs, various antibiotics, and heavy metals, cause acute renal failure by nephritis, acute tubular necrosis, or obstruction. Causes of chronic renal failure from many of these toxicants include nephritis from inflammatory and immunologic mechanisms and papillary necrosis through ischemia or cellular injury. Compensatory mechanisms may include hypertrophy and induction of metallothionein synthesis in response to heavy metal exposure.

PREVENTION AND MANAGEMENT OF POISONING

In the practice of dentistry, the practitioner has a responsibility to help protect both office staff as well as patients from accidental poisoning. Steps can be taken by practitioners to limit the possibility of accidental poisoning. Patients should be encouraged to keep all medications out of the reach of children, and drugs should always be kept in child-resistant containers. Medications and toxic agents should be clearly labeled and stored in secure locations. Information on the label of a prescribed drug should be understandable and include the name of the agent and clear directions for use. The prescribing physician or dentist should always indicate the purpose of the medication in the label information on the prescription. The statement of purpose of the medication is known as an "indication." Writing an indication on the prescription helps reduce confusion about drugs in the medicine cabinet and facilitates rapid identification of the drug involved in cases of accidental ingestion. Patients should be instructed to discard unused medication rather than attempt self-medication with drugs remaining from a previous course of therapy.

Diagnosis and treatment of poisoning are the purview of the physician. Principles of therapy for poisoning are summarized in Box 40-3 and apply to the management of any drug overdose. A dentist may be called on to provide emergency treatment of acute poisoning, however, within the practice environment or because of training as a health care professional.

BOX 40-3 First Aid for Poisoning

1. Summon help.
2. Stabilize the patient.
3. Evaluate the cause.
4. Terminate absorption.
5. Consider specific antidotes.
6. Enhance elimination.
7. Provide for supportive care.

Principles of Therapy for Poisoning

Summon help

When acute poisoning is evident, help should be sought through the emergency 911 telephone service if available. For less critical situations, the community poison control center provides an invaluable service. These centers are equipped with extensive files describing the signs and symptoms of poisoning and recommended methods of treatment for most toxic substances distributed within the United States. Poison control centers can be reached by telephone on a 24-hour basis, and phone numbers are usually published inside the cover of telephone directories. If the toxic reaction is serious, expert medical assistance should be sought immediately. In addition, most major medical centers have drug information centers that provide information to practitioners about drugs and drug interactions.

Stabilize the patient

Supportive therapy should be provided. Because hypoxia and shock are two common manifestations of serious toxicity, respiration and circulation must be monitored and assisted if required. For convulsions, physical protective measures may suffice along with the administration of oxygen to help avoid hypoxia. Intravenous diazepam is a drug of choice for pharmacologic control of continuing seizures.

Evaluate the cause

Proper therapy to eliminate exposure to the toxin or reverse its effects depends on identifying the poison. Questioning the victim or the victim's associates, searching for empty containers, or looking for physical signs on the patient (e.g., miosis or needle tracks for opiate or opioid overdose, burn marks in the mouth for ingestion of caustic chemicals) can be important in establishing the cause of poisoning.

Terminate absorption

Any obvious means of contact with the poison should be removed. For dermal exposure to chemicals, removal of contaminated clothing and repeated washing with soap and water are indicated. With ingested compounds other than petroleum products and corrosive substances, induction of vomiting had been suggested, but only in a conscious patient. Vomiting should not be induced for poisoning by petroleum products or agents producing loss of consciousness because of the risk of aspiration. Likewise, corrosive damage to the esophagus and gastric perforations may result from corrosive substances if emesis is induced. Moreover, modern practice is to avoid inducing vomiting because it does not reliably remove ingested poisons. Gastric lavage can be used by qualified personnel if care is taken to avoid aspiration of stomach contents by the victim. Prevention of absorption of many drugs within the gastrointestinal tract can be achieved by activated charcoal (10 to 50 g in water), and cathartics may be used to hasten the exit of drugs from the intestine.

Consider specific antidotes

Specific antidotes are available to treat poisoning by certain classes of compounds. Antidotes may be useful in preventing the absorption of ingested agents (e.g., Ca^{++} salts for F^-), increasing their rate of elimination (e.g., dimercaprol for inorganic mercury), blocking specific receptors (e.g., naloxone for morphine), or blocking other toxic activity (e.g., N-acetyl cysteine for acetaminophen overdose). One specific antidote should be remembered by dentists. For ingestion of toxic amounts of fluoride, which might occur with prescribed tablets or with topical liquids or gels, the local antidote to prevent absorption is Ca^{++} (in milk, calcium lactate, calcium gluconate, or lime water). If necessary, 2 to 10 mL of 10% calcium gluconate may be injected intravenously to bind fluoride and overcome hypocalcemia. Dentists who use benzodiazepines and opioid analgesics for conscious sedation must be familiar with the use of flumazenil and naloxone, respectively, to reverse respiratory depression caused by these drugs.

Enhance elimination

Measures to facilitate elimination of toxicants are in the realm of emergency care physicians; they are mentioned briefly here for completeness. The renal excretion of weak electrolytes can often be accelerated by appropriate modification of urinary pH to promote ionization of the electrolyte. Administration of an osmotic diuretic in conjunction with large volumes of water is helpful in promoting urinary excretion and reducing the renal concentration of nephrotoxic poisons. In limited instances, peritoneal dialysis or hemodialysis may be useful.

Provide for supportive care

Medical assessment of poisoning and continuing treatment, as needed, should be provided by medical staff in an appropriate health care facility.

OCCUPATIONAL SAFETY IN DENTISTRY

Although dentistry is considered to be relatively "occupationally safe," numerous potentially hazardous substances are used in the dental office or laboratory. In addition, dental environments may provide exposure to radiation or to blood-borne pathogens. Since 1988 the **Occupational Safety and Health Administration (OSHA)** has been writing, implementing, and enforcing regulations designed to ensure that employees are informed of hazardous materials in their work environment and given appropriate instruction in the risks and handling of these materials. The primary components of this program include **(1)** labeling of containers for materials, **(2)** on-site maintenance of material safety data sheets for materials used in the workplace that contain hazardous chemicals, and **(3)** employee education and training. For dentistry, OSHA regulations and guidelines include potential exposures to blood-borne pathogens and biologic agents in addition to chemicals. To assist in fulfilling the requirements of OSHA regulations, the American Dental Association has excellent online materials available for study.

To meet OSHA regulations, drugs and chemicals must be labeled with the name of the chemical, appropriate risk warnings regarding the chemical, and name and address of the manufacturer or other responsible party. If a hazardous material is transferred to another container at any time other than for immediate use, an appropriate label must be affixed to the new container.

Material safety data sheets, which provide information on handling, storage, cleanup, disposal, and emergency and first aid procedures, are central to the safety program and are the primary source of risk and hazard information. These sheets are required to be provided by the manufacturer on request and must identify the hazardous substances included in the preparation, the physical and chemical characteristics, the fire and explosion danger, and other health hazard data. These sheets must be present in the workplace and available to employees at all times. Dentists are required to provide appropriate training for employees in the use and management of hazardous substances when they are hired, whenever new hazardous substances are brought into the workplace, and when new information regarding the use of existing substances becomes available.

SPECIFIC TOXICANTS

The toxic effects of several classes of substances are presented. Agents that illustrate general principles presented earlier and that have public health importance or importance in the practice of dentistry are described.

Metals

Metals as a class are toxic primarily because of their ability to bind with biologic structures such as thiol groups in enzymes and other proteins. The major effect in humans is the inhibition of enzyme function. Because of this binding affinity, the effect of metals may be widespread in the organism, but usually a primary or most sensitive system in which clinical manifestations may be detected is evident. Metals as a class are important because of their ubiquitous nature in modern medicine and technology and in nature. Two metals of importance in public health and dental practice are mercury and lead.

Mercury

Mercury is present virtually everywhere in the environment. An estimated 2700 to 6000 tons is released annually from the oceans and the earth's crust into the atmosphere. An additional 2000 to 3000 tons is released through human activities, including the burning of fossil fuels. Mercury exists in three chemical classes: **elemental mercury** (Hg^0), which is a liquid at room temperature and is used as a primary component in dental amalgam; **inorganic mercury salts;** and **organic mercury salts.** Inorganic mercury salts may exist as mercurous (Hg^+) or mercuric (Hg^{++}) forms. Of the many organic forms of mercury, **methylmercury** is the most important toxicologically because of its ability to permeate membranes and the blood–brain barrier, its potency for biologic damage, and its widespread use in human activities.

Mercury toxicity provides an interesting example of several important toxicologic principles. The first is that a single substance may produce differing effects depending on presentation to the organism. Hg^0 is relatively nontoxic when ingested because of poor absorption in the gastrointestinal tract. It may be toxic, however, when injected subcutaneously. In addition, because of its high vapor pressure, it vaporizes readily and is **easily inhaled.** When inhaled, Hg^0 is absorbed readily into the blood, with absorption rates estimated at 74% to nearly 100% of inhaled dose. When in the blood, it is oxidized and is available for binding to enzymes and other proteins, producing toxic effects. Another important principle exhibited by mercury is that when a substance can exist in different chemical forms, the forms may present strikingly different health effects. Organic mercury typically produces signs of toxicity that are neurologic in nature, whereas inorganic salts often produce gastrointestinal destruction and, secondarily, nephritis. These effects are discussed further subsequently.

Inorganic mercury salts are used widely in industry; mercuric chloride is an example of a mercury compound with a wide variety of industrial uses. These compounds, in contrast to organic mercury compounds, are not well absorbed through the gastrointestinal tract and do not readily cross biologic membranes when absorbed. Only approximately 10% of an inorganic mercury dose is absorbed through the gastrointestinal tract compared with more than 90% of an ingested dose of the organic compound methylmercury. Nevertheless, inorganic salts such as mercuric chloride are severely corrosive to tissue and when absorbed produce toxic effects through binding of enzymes. Inorganic mercury compounds have been used medicinally and applied dermally in makeup for hundreds of years until recent times; calomel (a cathartic) and mercurochrome (an antiseptic) are common examples. Virtually all such uses have been discontinued.

Organic mercury compounds represent the most important form of mercury from a toxicologic perspective. This is particularly true of methylmercury because of its widespread use and because it is a by-product of many industrial processes. Organic mercury is known to accumulate in the food chain, and this is particularly evident in seafood, where the pelagic and top-level predators accumulate significant amounts of methylmercury in their flesh.

A number of tragic, inadvertent organic mercury poisonings have occurred in modern times. Two incidents are particularly well documented. From 1932 to 1968, the Chisso Corporation, a company located in Kumamoto, Japan, dumped an estimated 27 tons of mercury compounds into Minamata Bay. Kumamoto is a small town approximately 570 miles southwest of Tokyo. The town consists of mostly farmers and fisherman whose normal diet included fish from the bay. Symptoms of methylmercury poisoning unexpectedly developed in thousands of these people. The illness became known as Minamata disease. Methylmercury has also been widely used to prevent grain spoilage through its antifungal effect. The second major outbreak occurred in the early 1970s when more than 500 people died and many others were made severely ill in Iraq when grain seed treated with methylmercury was inadvertently ground into flour and consumed. In both of these instances, because organic mercury readily crosses the blood–brain and placental barriers, a significant number of fetal deaths and teratogenic results occurred.

Elemental mercury is the form of concern in dentistry because it is a primary component of dental amalgam, constituting approximately 50% by volume of the material. The greatest risk of exposure from Hg^0 is by inhalation of the vapor. Hg^0 vapor is highly lipid-soluble and readily crosses membranes; this gives it ready access to the CNS and other body components, where it is easily oxidized to the mercuric form. Acute, high-level exposure to Hg^0 vapor produces corrosive inflammation of the upper and lower respiratory tract and nephrotoxic and CNS effects. Long-term exposure to low or moderate levels of Hg^0 vapor damages enzymes and structural proteins in the CNS, resulting in blockage of neuromuscular and synaptic transmission. Figure 40-2 shows the currently known range of effects based on urinary mercury concentrations. Urinary mercury concentration is considered a reasonable indicator of recent Hg^0 exposure, but because mercury is

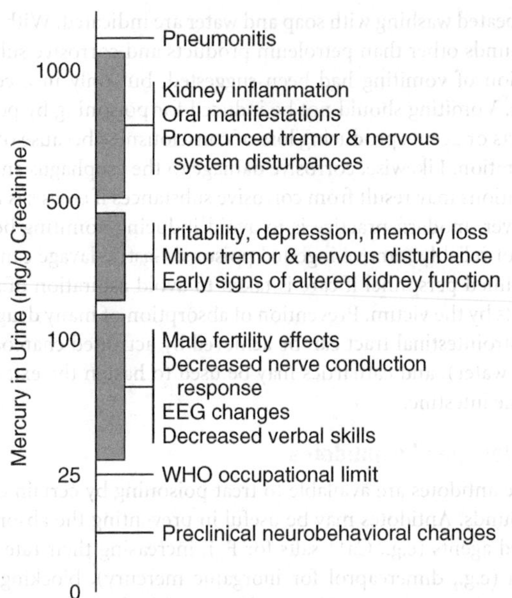

FIG 40-2 Signs and symptoms of mercury toxicity relative to concentrations in urine. Blue areas correspond to the various signs and symptoms seen at that blood level. *EEG*, Electroencephalogram; *WHO*, World Health Organization.

sequestered in organ systems, urinary mercury concentration is not a true indicator of total body burden. Although the three forms of mercury (inorganic, organic, and elemental) produce differing toxicologic effects, the two major target organs of any mercury exposure are the CNS and the kidneys.

Although the earliest indicators of CNS effects of mercury exposure are not always clinically evident, they are measurable with neurobehavioral testing. As exposure increases, behavioral changes may be noticed, such as irritability, memory disturbances, personality changes, drowsiness, or depression. Fine muscle tremors are noted, especially of the fingers, eyelids, and lips, and this loss of neuromuscular control increases as exposure levels increase. Renal damage in the form of tubular necrosis increases in a dose-dependent manner. **Oral manifestations of mercury intoxication include hypersalivation, gingivitis, and gingival discoloration.** Cases of periodontal destruction with tooth loss have been reported at high levels of exposure. Also present at high levels of exposure is a yellow-brown discoloration of the lens of the eye.

Mercury in dentistry

Since the introduction of mercury amalgam into dentistry in the early 19th century, concerns about its safety have been expressed from time to time. Claims of toxic effects cover virtually the entire spectrum of disease, and a vocal "anti-amalgam" contingent currently exists. Much of the confusion regarding the potential health effects of mercury exposure from dental sources is caused by false claims and by flawed studies used to support these claims by anti-amalgam proponents. Two areas of potential concern have been the subject of more recent and ongoing studies. One is the potential occupational risk to dental personnel working with dental amalgam, and the other is to the consumer or patient who has mercury amalgam placed in the teeth as a treatment.

The OSHA and the National Institute for Occupational Safety and Health (NIOSH) have recognized the need to set occupational thresholds over which exposure to mercury must not occur. NIOSH has set a **threshold limit** value of **50 μg of Hg^0 per cubic meter of air**

BOX 40-4 Recommended Guidelines for Minimizing Mercury Exposure in the Dental Environment

1. Use pre-capsulated amalgam preparations only. Reclose disposable capsules after use.
2. Do not use squeeze cloths for expressing mercury from amalgam mix.
3. Monitor office levels of Hg^0 yearly or whenever contamination is suspected.
4. Use exposure badges that sample the air for Hg^0 concentration.
5. Provide periodic urinary mercury concentration testing for personnel.
6. If "free" mercury (rather than pre-capsulated) must be used to mix amalgam, store it away from heat in unbreakable, tightly sealed containers.
7. Store amalgam scrap in a sulfide solution (e.g., used X-ray fixer) or under water.
8. Do not touch amalgam with bare hands.
9. Use a rubber dam for restorative procedures.
10. Use a high-velocity vacuum when manipulating the amalgam and vacuum and water spray when removing old amalgam restorations.
11. In the event of a mercury spill (even a small one), use a mercury spill cleanup kit (commercially available). Do not vacuum the spill because this hastens the volatilization of the mercury into the air.

as a time-weighted average based on a 40-hour workweek, while the legally binding OSHA limit is 100 μg/m³. The World Health Organization has set a more restrictive threshold limit value of **25 μg/m³**. Hg^0, which is readily vaporized, can achieve concentrations of 2000 μg/m³ in a closed room. Studies of ambient air mercury concentrations in dental offices have shown that, under conditions of careless handling of mercury, the occupational threshold levels set by the above organizations can be exceeded. These high concentrations may occur after contamination through accidental spills of Hg^0.

Studies examining occupational exposure among dental personnel show that certain practices in dental offices—now considered outmoded—are the most significant contributors to occupational exposure. These practices include the use of squeeze cloths to express mercury from amalgam; dispensing mercury from a central supply, which leads to accidental spills; and the use of office-prepared capsules. Neurobehavioral changes have been noted in dentists exposed to mercury. Modern dental offices that have good hygiene practices with respect to mercury pose minimal risk to dental personnel, however. **Excellent hygiene remains vital to preventing unnecessary mercury exposure.**

With regard to mercury exposure that patients receive from the placement of amalgams in the course of treatment, anecdotal claims of disease states of every sort attributed to such exposure have been reported. Although rare individuals may be sensitive to very low-level mercury exposure, little or no valid scientific evidence supports such claims in the general population. An important reason for the controversy is the reliance of some individuals on false claims and dubious studies about the dangers of dental amalgams. Two large-scale, randomized, prospective clinical trials have been completed that studied the effect of mercury exposure from dental amalgam in children. These studies each included more than 500 children who were randomly assigned to dental treatment groups that would receive either amalgam or resin composites for necessary restorations in posterior teeth. The subjects were followed annually for five years in the **study by Bellinger and colleagues and seven years in the study by DeRouen and colleagues.** (See references.) Outcome measures included comprehensive batteries of neurobehavioral tests including IQ testing, neurologic examinations including nerve conduction velocities, and renal function tests. Although there were measurable differences in urinary mercury concentrations between the amalgam and non-amalgam treatment groups, there were no significant differences found for any of the outcome measures between groups, indicating that the level of mercury exposure from routine dental treatment with amalgam does not present an important health risk for the measured neurologic or renal outcomes.

A study of 1663 adults participating in the ongoing Air Force Health Study of Vietnam-era veterans to determine possible associations between amalgam exposure and neurologic abnormalities found no association between amalgam exposure and neurologic signs or clinically evident peripheral neuropathy. The body of evidence also indicates no detectable negative effect on general health at the levels of mercury exposure produced by the presence of dental amalgam fillings except in rare cases of allergy to amalgams. (See reference, Dodes.) Following the mercury hygiene guidelines listed in Box 40-4 minimizes any exposure to patients beyond that which results from the amalgam itself.

Lead

Lead has been a toxicologic problem for humans from the earliest times. It was found in early utensils and food storage and preparation vessels. It has been used extensively in plumbing, contaminating drinking water. Occupational exposures to lead occur in miners, smelters, and lead acid battery workers, but the most common chronic exposure is through diet. Perhaps the best recognized sources of lead exposure are from lead-based paint and combustion products of tetraethyl lead antiknock compound added to gasoline before the change to unleaded gasoline. Although Congress produced legislation limiting the lead concentration in paint to 0.06% in the 1970s, many older buildings still contain significant amounts of lead-based paint with very high concentrations of lead. A relatively small chip of this paint may contain 100 mg of lead. When consumed by a child, this amount exceeds the daily allowable intake by a factor of at least 30. Because lead compounds that were included in paint formulas have a sweet taste, young children have frequently consumed these paint chips. (The condition of eating unnatural foods is called **pica.**)

Adults absorb approximately 10% of dietary lead, although children may absorb significantly larger amounts. With normal renal function, absorbed lead is primarily excreted by the kidneys. In the body, lead primarily concentrates in the hard tissues such as bone and teeth. Similar to mercury, lead produces toxic effects primarily by binding with proteins necessary for cellular function. Toxic signs exhibited at various blood levels are illustrated in Figure 40-3. One early effect of lead exposure is inhibition of the **heme biosynthetic pathway.** Intermediary products of heme biosynthesis called **porphyrins** are excreted in the urine in a characteristic pattern indicative of lead poisoning.

Chronic lead poisoning, known as **plumbism**, produces a spectrum of effects depending on the duration and severity of exposure. A microcytic hypochromic anemia may be produced early in exposure and cause lethargy and weakness. Neurologic effects may produce restlessness, irritability, hyperactivity, and impaired intellect. Chronic low-level lead exposure can produce deficits in gross and fine motor

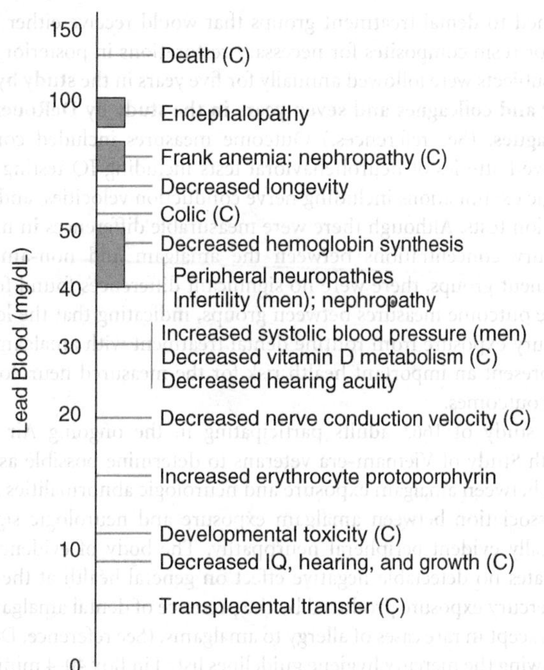

FIG 40-3 Signs and symptoms of lead toxicity relative to concentrations in blood. Children are represented at the more sensitive end of the designated ranges. (C) denotes observations in children. (Adapted from Ellenhorn M, Schonwald S, Ordog G et al: Metals and related compounds: lead. In Cooke D, editor: *Ellenhorn's medical toxicology: diagnosis and treatment of human poisoning*, ed 2, Baltimore, 1997, Williams & Wilkins.)

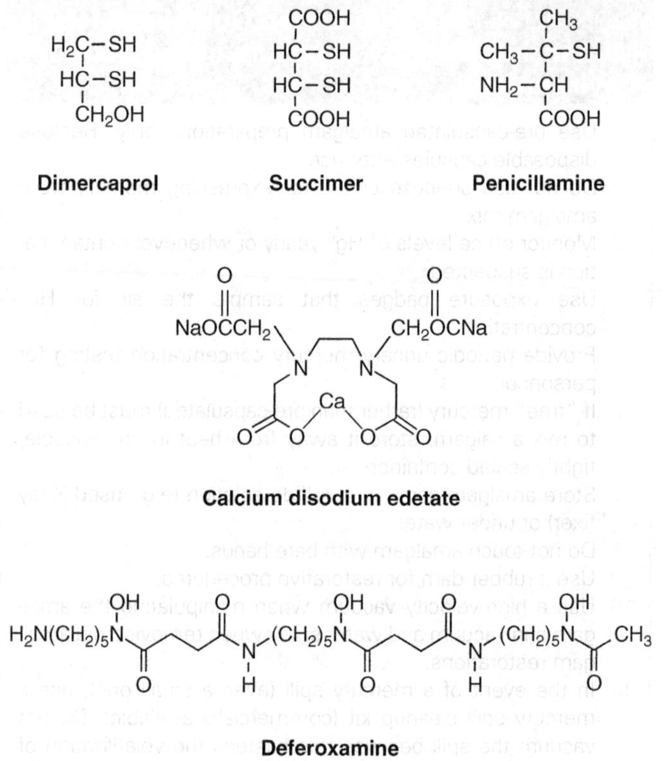

development and in cognitive and intellectual development. Early detection and management of lead exposure is crucial to prevent these permanent effects in children. Peripheral neuropathies may be seen and are manifested as wristdrop, footdrop, and muscular weakness. Gastrointestinal signs such as intestinal spasms may progress to severe abdominal cramping with increased or continued exposure.

The greatest threat from lead poisoning is encephalopathy, which occurs more often in children. Early neurologic signs and symptoms develop as described earlier and progress to delirium, convulsions, and coma. One-fourth of patients with lead encephalopathy do not survive, and 40% of survivors are left with severe neurologic dysfunction. Lead is toxic to the kidney, and reversible tubular damage and irreversible interstitial fibrosis may be seen. Long-term exposure to lead is classically associated with a blue-black line that appears along the gingival margin. This deposit of lead sulfide is known as **Burton lines**, and although associated with lead exposure, it may also be caused by exposures to other metals, such as silver, iron, or mercury.

For treatment, removal of the subject from the source of lead exposure is paramount. Depending on the blood lead levels, chelation therapy is instituted according to protocols for the treatment of lead poisoning recommended by the U.S. Centers for Disease Control and Prevention and the American Academy of Pediatrics. Succimer, calcium disodium edetate, dimercaprol, and penicillamine all are effective, but they differ in advantages of routes of administration and specificities relative to other essential trace metals.

Treatment of poisoning: heavy metal chelators

Chelators are compounds that form complexes with metal ions. The word **chelator** is derived from the Greek word *chele*, meaning "claw." A chelator molecule binds a metal ion by two or more polar functions, such as sulfhydryl, carbonyl, amino, or hydroxyl groups. These form

Dimercaprol | Succimer | Penicillamine

Calcium disodium edetate

Deferoxamine

FIG 40-4 Chemical structures of chelating agents.

bonds similar to the bonds of the protein functional units attacked by metal ions. Through this action, chelators spare endogenous ligands and promote excretion of metals as the chelator-metal complexes. **Dimercaprol, succimer, and penicillamine** are drugs currently marketed to promote the excretion of mercury, lead, and other metals. A few additional agents are available to treat poisoning by metals other than mercury, such as **calcium disodium edetate** for lead and cadmium and **deferoxamine** for iron. Structures of these chelators are shown in Figure 40-4. Selectivity for metal ions varies among chelators. Some, such as edetate, also aggressively remove vital nutrient metals, such as calcium and zinc. Selectivity is important in the choice of the chelator, which should be matched for the heavy metal and circumstances of therapy. Selectivity of chelators for specific heavy metals is presented in Table 40-1.

Dimercaprol (2,3-dimercapto-1-propanol) was developed during World War II as an antidote for the arsenical gas lewisite, and it was formerly known as British Anti-Lewisite (BAL). Subsequently, dimercaprol was found to be an active chelator of various heavy metals. Dimercaprol is prepared as a 10% solution in a peanut oil vehicle (beware of peanut allergy!) and must be injected intramuscularly. It is maximally effective when given shortly after an acute exposure to mercury; however, it is valuable even in chronic mercurialism. Dimercaprol is used with calcium disodium edetate in protocols for treatment of lead poisoning. The drug is usually injected two to three times a day initially, with doses tapering off to once or twice a day over about 10 days. The dimercaprol–mercury complex (actually two dimercaprol molecules to a single mercury atom) is excreted in the urine, which must be kept alkaline to avoid dissociation of the conjugate.

Succimer (meso-2,3-dimercaptosuccinic acid) is structurally similar to dimercaprol. This drug has the advantage of being effective after oral administration and being less toxic than dimercaprol. Succimer is more water-soluble and is the drug of choice for the treatment of lead poisoning because it is more specific for lead chelation than calcium disodium

TABLE 40-1 **Metals and Chelators That Enhance Excretion**

Metal	Chelator	Other Names	Administration
Arsenic	Succimer; dimercaprol	Dimercaptosuccinic acid, DMSA; 2,3-dimercapto-1-propanol, BAL	Oral; IM
Cadmium	$CaNa_2$ EDTA	Calcium disodium edetate	IV infusion
Copper	p-Penicillamine	3-Mercapto-D-valine	Oral
Iron	Deferoxamine		IM
Lead	Succimer; dimercaprol + $CaNa_2$ EDTA; D-penicillamine		Oral; IM + IV infusion; oral
Mercury	Succimer; dimercaprol; penicillamine		Oral; IM; oral

IM, Intramuscular; *IV*, intravenous.

edetate and removes fewer essential minerals such as calcium, copper, iron, and zinc. The dose for lead chelation is 10 mg/kg every 8 hours for 5 days, then 10 mg/kg every 12 hours for 14 days. In animal studies, succimer was more effective than dimercaprol in alleviating acute toxicity and preventing distribution of orally administered mercury from mercuric chloride, particularly to the brain. In addition, oral administration was more efficient than parenteral administration in reducing retention and organ deposition of oral mercuric chloride, probably because of decreased intestinal uptake of the mercuric chloride.

Penicillamine (3-mercapto-D-valine) is a highly effective chelator of **copper** and is of primary importance in the management of **Wilson disease** (hepatolenticular degeneration). Although less effective against other metals, penicillamine is often a useful drug for asymptomatic patients with a moderate body burden of metal because it is orally effective. In general, 1 to 2 g/day is administered as needed for therapy of mercury poisoning. The penicillamine–mercury complex is excreted in the urine.

Calcium disodium edetate complex is a chelator for divalent and trivalent metals that can displace calcium from the molecule. Typically, these metals include lead, zinc, cadmium, manganese, iron, and mercury. Calcium edetate disodium is poorly absorbed from the gastrointestinal tract and is given intramuscularly or intravenously. Calcium disodium edetate must be used carefully according to suppliers' protocols because it can produce nephrotoxicity. Calcium disodium edetate can aggravate symptoms of severe lead poisoning, such as cerebral edema and renal tubular necrosis, and in high doses can lead to severe zinc deficiency.

Deferoxamine is a specific chelating agent for iron. It is available only for parenteral administration. The preferred route is intramuscular; acute iron intoxication treatment involves 1 g as an initial dose, followed by 500 mg every 4 hours for two doses and additional doses of 500 mg every 4 to 12 hours as needed based on clinical response.

Treatment of mercury poisoning

Therapy depends on the type of mercury poisoning. Exposure to elemental or inorganic mercury can be treated with **dimercaprol** (higher mercury levels) or **penicillamine** (lower mercury levels). Hemodialysis may be needed to protect the kidney. **Succimer** is also effective. For short-chain organic mercurials such as methylmercury, chelation therapy is ineffective, and dimercaprol is contraindicated because it concentrates mercury in the brain. Hemodialysis is ineffective. Methylmercury can possibly be bound in the gut with a polythiol resin.

Gases

Perhaps no other toxic pollution issue stirs such universal concern as air pollution because gaseous pollutants are dispersed over broad regions, and inhalation exposure is insidious. Significant regulatory effort is devoted to decreasing air pollutants by the Clean Air Act, and general information on topics important in the control of air pollution is available from the Internet. The U.S. Environmental Protection Agency (EPA) uses six "criteria pollutants" as indicators of air quality and has established a maximum concentration for each to preclude adverse effects on human health. The four gaseous criteria pollutants are discussed subsequently; the remaining two are airborne lead and fine particulate material that is 10 μm or smaller in diameter.

TABLE 40-2 **Carboxyhemoglobin Blood Levels and Symptoms**

CO-Hb Level (%)	Symptoms
0-10	No symptoms
10-20	Mild headache and breathlessness
20-30	Throbbing headache, irritability, emotional instability, impaired judgment and memory, rapid fatigue
30-40	Severe headache, weakness, nausea, vomiting, dizziness, dimmed vision, confusion
40-50	Increasing confusion, severe ataxia, accelerated respiration, possible hallucinations
50-60	Syncope, coma, convulsions, tachycardia with weak pulse
60-70	Increased depth of coma, incontinence
70-80	Profound coma, thread pulse, death
>80	Rapid death

Source: Von Burg R: Carbon monoxide, *J Appl Toxicol* 16:379-386, 1999.

Carbon monoxide

The origin of **carbon monoxide (CO)**, a colorless, odorless gas, is incomplete combustion of carbon. The toxicity of CO results from its combination with hemoglobin (Hb) and exclusion of oxygen from this vital oxygen transfer mechanism. CO exhibits an affinity for Hb 210 to 300 times that of oxygen, and the resultant complex with reduced heme iron, **carboxyhemoglobin (CO-Hb)**, is incapable of combining with oxygen. Moreover, the presence of CO-Hb makes the release of oxygen from Hb in tissues less efficient, which additionally compromises oxygen delivery. Typical symptoms associated with varying CO-Hb levels are presented in Table 40-2. Of the four gaseous criteria pollutants, CO is the most likely to be present in the dental office or home environment, and offices should be equipped with CO detectors.

Ozone

Ozone (O_3) is an odorless, colorless gas composed of three oxygen atoms. Typically, O_3 is not emitted into the air, but it is created at ground level by photochemical reactions among nitrogen oxides and volatile organic compounds in the presence of heat and sunlight. O_3

occurs naturally in the stratosphere (approximately 10 to 20 miles above the earth) and forms a protective barrier that absorbs the sun's harmful ultraviolet rays. In the earth's lower atmosphere and at ground level, O_3 is considered unhealthy because of its oxidative effects. Because of its relative insolubility, inspired O_3 is carried deep into the lung, where it oxidizes membranes in the alveoli. O_3 irritates lung airways and causes inflammation, reduced lung capacity, and increased susceptibility to respiratory illnesses such as pneumonia and bronchitis. Other symptoms include wheezing, coughing, and pain with deep breathing. Oxidation products arising from O_3 reactions with lung proteins or lipids initiate numerous cellular responses, including generation of cytokines and expression of adhesion molecules. These responses promote an influx of **inflammatory cells to the lung** in the absence of a pathogenic challenge, resulting in modification of cellular tight junctions, increased lung permeability, and development of edema. Individuals with preexisting respiratory problems, such as asthma or chronic obstructive pulmonary disease, are most vulnerable. Repeated exposure to O_3 pollution for several months may cause permanent lung damage.

Sulfur dioxide

Sulfur dioxide (SO_2) is a colorless gas with a pungent, irritating odor. SO_2 is used as a preservative of fruits and vegetables, a disinfectant in wineries and breweries, and a bleaching agent in paper and textile industries. It is generated as an air pollutant by industry, such as high-sulfur coal-fired electric power plants, and it is largely responsible for the environmental and public health impact of acid rain. In contrast to the properties and site of impact of O_3, SO_2 is highly soluble in aqueous fluids and affects the upper respiratory tract. On dissolution, it forms sulfurous acid, which is extremely irritating to the nasopharyngeal and respiratory tracts. Acute exposure causes dryness of the nose and throat and a decrease in tidal respiratory volume. Coughing, sneezing, choking, and nasal discharge occur. In dentistry, chronic exposure at SO_2 levels causing these symptoms has been associated with dental caries and gingival and periodontal disorders. Patients have noted rapid dental destruction, loss of restorations, and increased sensitivity of teeth to temperature change.

Nitrogen oxides

Nitrogen dioxide (NO_2) is a brownish, highly reactive gas that is present in all urban atmospheres. The major mechanism for the formation of NO_2 in the atmosphere is the oxidation of the primary air pollutant nitric oxide (NO). Mixtures of nitrogen oxides (NO_x) play a major role, together with volatile organic hydrocarbons, in complex atmospheric reactions that produce O_3 and are important precursors to acid rain. NO_2 is relatively insoluble in aqueous media and decomposes in water to form nitric acid (HNO_3) and NO, a potent vasodilator. When inspired, it reaches deep into the lungs. NO_2 can cause bronchitis, pneumonia, hemorrhagic pulmonary edema, and diffuse alveolar damage. Exposure also seems to reduce resistance to respiratory infections.

Liquids and Vapors

The organic liquid that presents the greatest risks to humans is **ethanol**. The toxicologic profile of this compound is unique among organic liquids and is presented in detail in Chapter 39. Considered in this section are the organic solvents, including hydrocarbons and chlorinated compounds, and methyl methacrylate (because of its common use in dentistry). Figure 40-5 shows structures of some of the compounds discussed below.

Solvents

Although transient exposure to solvents may occur in the home, more significant exposure most commonly occurs in the workplace.

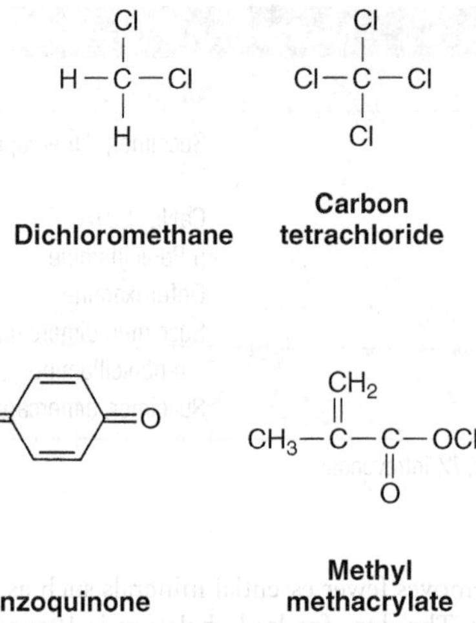

Dichloromethane

Carbon tetrachloride

Benzoquinone

Methyl methacrylate

FIG 40-5 Chemical structures of chlorinated solvents, the benzene metabolite benzoquinone, and the acrylic plastic monomer methyl methacrylate.

Exposure most often occurs through inhalation; absorption through the skin is also a common route of exposure. Absorption from the gastrointestinal tract is variable. Compounds that are well absorbed, such as benzene or toluene, can produce significant systemic toxicity. Others, such as naphtha or gasoline, are not as well absorbed. A major risk from ingestion is the potential for pneumonitis as a result of emesis and aspiration.

Regardless of the site of absorption, the great lipid solubility of this group of compounds allows them to cross the blood–brain barrier readily. Individuals exposed to high concentrations of organic solvents usually exhibit profound CNS depression. Chronic exposure to lower concentrations of these chemicals produces toxic effects characteristic of the individual compounds.

Chlorinated solvents

Dichloromethane, otherwise known as **methylene chloride**, is a common solvent in paint remover and is used for liquid–liquid extraction in laboratories. Acute toxicity is caused by **CNS depression**, and fatalities have resulted from exposure. Symptoms include mental confusion, fatigue, lethargy, headache, and chest pain. Dichloromethane is metabolized to carbon monoxide. Evidence of its carcinogenicity, obtained in mice, seems to be related to toxic metabolites formed by glutathione-S-transferase and may be specific to the very high activity and localization of this enzyme in this species.

Carbon tetrachloride is metabolized in the liver to a highly reactive free radical metabolite that, in the presence of oxygen, reacts with proteins and lipids. The resulting **hepatotoxicity** may take days to develop and is accompanied by severe renal toxicity. Compounds that increase the rate of carbon tetrachloride biotransformation, such as cytochrome P450 enzyme inducers, increase the danger of toxicity. Substances that inhibit its metabolism are protective.

In a similar manner, **perchloroethylene** (also known as tetrachloroethylene) has been found to produce reactive metabolites that are thought to produce renal toxicity. This compound has also been associated with an increased risk of oral, laryngeal, and esophageal cancer in workers occupationally exposed to dry-cleaning processes that use perchloroethylene. Its use has declined due to these adverse effects.

Benzene

Benzene is another widely used industrial solvent commonly encountered in petroleum distillates such as gasoline. Benzene is considered a causative agent in human leukemia, probably through active hydroquinone or benzoquinone metabolites formed at oxidation.

Methyl methacrylate

Methyl methacrylate is widely used in dentistry for the production of prosthetic devices and in orthopedic medicine as a luting agent. Although properly cured polymers from methyl methacrylate seem to be biologically inert, numerous adverse effects have been associated with the monomer. Exposure to the monomer can lead to toxicity and allergic reactions. A slight, transient decrease in blood pressure has occasionally been reported when methyl methacrylate was used to cement orthopedic devices. The assumption in these cases was that the effects were caused by absorption of the monomer into the patient's vasculature. Adverse effects have also been reported by personnel in operating rooms, where, because of improper mixing, concentrations of more than 200 ppm have been measured. Surgeons have developed contact dermatitis and paresthesias, and nurses have reported dizziness, nausea, and vomiting.

A survey of dental laboratories suggests exposure to more moderate concentrations (≤5 ppm) of the monomer, although peak concentrations can be double that amount. Although the concentrations to which dental technicians are exposed are moderate, a study of dental technicians suggested that cutaneous absorption of the monomer, a result of dipping the fingers in the liquid to smooth and improve the finish of the polymer surface, caused a localized slowing of nerve conduction. Other studies have found more generalized neuropathies attributed to methyl methacrylate exposure in dental technicians. In addition, cutaneous reactions have been reported from monomer and "cured" methacrylate polymer.

Numerous studies have confirmed more recently that dental resins and composites release methacrylates and many similar components that are known to have the potential for endocrine-disrupting effects. The term **endocrine-disrupting** refers to alterations in the natural biosynthesis, metabolism, or receptor occupancy of hormones such as estrogen and testosterone. Many of these endocrine-disrupting compounds found in dental filling materials are uncured monomers, such as **bisphenol A (BPA) and bisphenol A glycidylmethacrylate (Bis-GMA),** and chemically related compounds such as phthalates. BPA, which is present in many food-use containers, is also present in many dental sealants and restorative materials, and it has been shown to be detectable from these sources in children.

Although little is definitively known about the effects of low-dose exposure of these components of dental composites and sealants, some evidence exists of the potential for detectable effects on human metabolic systems. Much of this evidence is from animal model and human in vitro studies, and little or no research has been reported that uses in vivo studies to examine these potential effects. Potential systemic effects on the organism of endocrine disruption are wide-ranging and biologically important. These may include developmental defects, behavioral effects, fertility problems, and tumorigenic effects. There have been no safety studies or randomized clinical trials in humans to examine the potential effects of low-dose exposures to these substances, such as one might get from dental sources, but available data suggest that such exposures produce minimal effects, if any. Two additional **precautions can be used with sealants and composites** in dentistry: removal of residual monomer during sealant/composite placement, and minimizing elective use of these materials during pregnancy. (See www.ada.org.)

Pesticides

Pesticides play a unique societal role as these products are designed and produced for their toxic effects. Much research has been devoted to develop the concept of selective toxicity, in which products have toxic actions on pests, while affording advantage of less toxicity to other species. Selective toxicity can be derived from differential metabolism between target and nontarget species or can be due to entirely different physiologic receptors that mediate toxicity in target organisms. The diversity of target receptors is detailed in an excellent comprehensive, short review detailing primary mechanisms of toxic actions of pesticides including insecticides, herbicides, and fungicides. (See reference, Casida, 2009.)

In the United States, pesticides are regulated by the EPA under auspices of the Federal Insecticide, Fungicide, and Rodenticide Act (FIFRA). Before a pesticide can be legally used, it must be registered with the EPA Office of Pesticide Programs (OPP). Pesticide registration typically extends for 15 years. By this process the EPA examines the ingredients of a pesticide; the site or crop on which it is to be used; the amount, timing, and frequency of its use; and storage and disposal practices. The EPA OPP evaluates each pesticide to ensure no adverse effects on humans, nontarget species, or the environment under specified use before initial registration. Older, previously registered pesticides undergo re-registration to assess health effects as new information becomes available.

Depending on the toxicity of the marketed product, pesticides are registered for general public use or are restricted for use only by or under the direct supervision of a certified pesticide applicator. Pesticides are restricted from residential or institutional use if the product, as diluted for use, has an oral LD_{50} of 1.5 g/kg or less and restricted for other uses if the product, as diluted for use, has an oral LD_{50} of 50 mg/kg or less.

Certain pesticides have been banned or severely restricted for export or import through the auspices of the United Nations Environment Programme and the Food and Agriculture Organization, which developed international guidelines for exchange of information on banned or severely restricted industrial chemicals and pesticides. These guidelines eventually evolved into the United Nations Rotterdam Convention on the Prior Informed Consent Procedure, which lists banned and restricted pesticides.

The Food Quality Protection Act of 1996 amended FIFRA to require evaluation of pesticide safety with consideration of potential aggregate exposures from nondietary and dietary routes. From this mandate, pesticide registrations are being revised. The current status of pesticides is available electronically via a Website that the EPA OPP maintains with extensive information regarding pesticide use, regulation, data sources, consumer alerts, and educational materials. The EPA OPP also has supported production of a manual, Recognition and Management of Pesticide Poisonings, available electronically, that is designed to provide health professionals with current information regarding health hazards of pesticides. (See reference, Roberts and Reigart, 2015.)

Insecticides

Most insecticides in common use by the public today fall into three classes based on their mode of toxic action: **neonicotinoids**, which act as **ligands** for the insect **nicotinic** receptors; **anticholinesterases,** characterized by their inhibitory action on acetylcholinesterase; and **pyrethroid** insecticides, so named after their origin as pyrethrum extract from flowers of the genus *Chrysanthemum*. Organochlorine insecticides, such as DDT, were widely used from 1945 to 1969, but they have been banned for use in the United States because of their adverse effects, including their biologic and environmental persistence, biomagnification through diet in lipid tissues of higher organisms, demonstrated interaction with estrogen receptors, and enzyme-inducing properties.

Neonicotinoids, the newest class insecticides developed during the past 25 years, (structure presented in Figure 40-6). Of these, imidacloprid is most widely used at present. These compounds exhibit selective

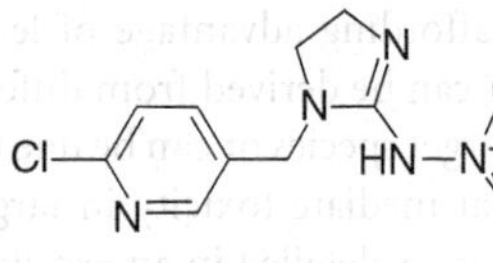

FIG 40-6 Chemical structures of the neonicotinoid insecticides.

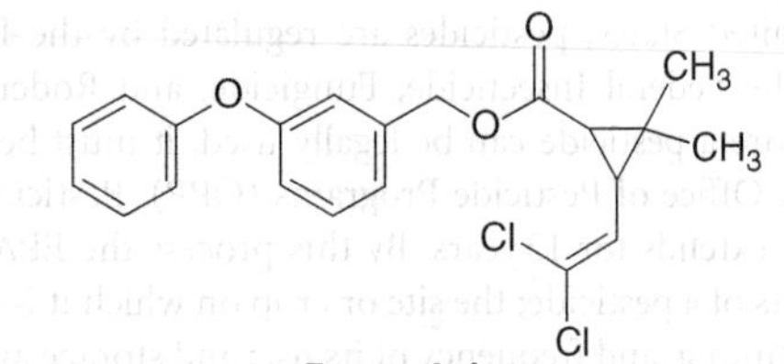

toxicity through greater affinity for insect nicotinic receptors than those of mammals. Neonicotinoid insecticides have been described as partial agonists, super-agonists, or antagonists at nicotinic receptors, depending on the compound. As a result, they disrupt receptor function and cause paralysis and death. Although these compounds offer selectivity through differential affinity, this is not absolute, and mammalian toxicity ensues at higher concentrations.

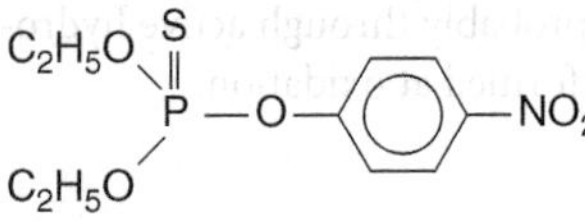

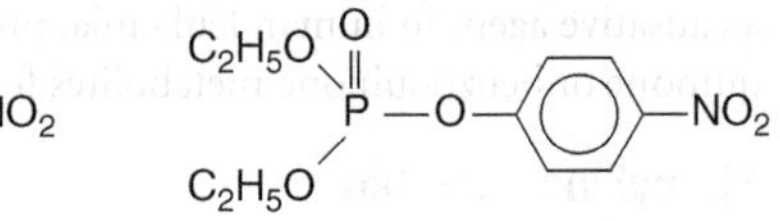

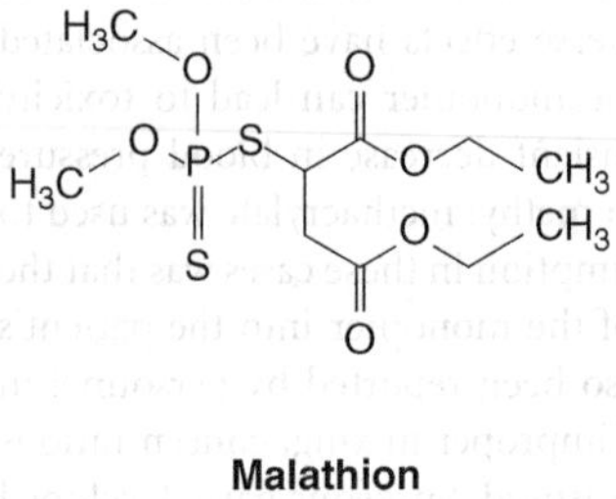

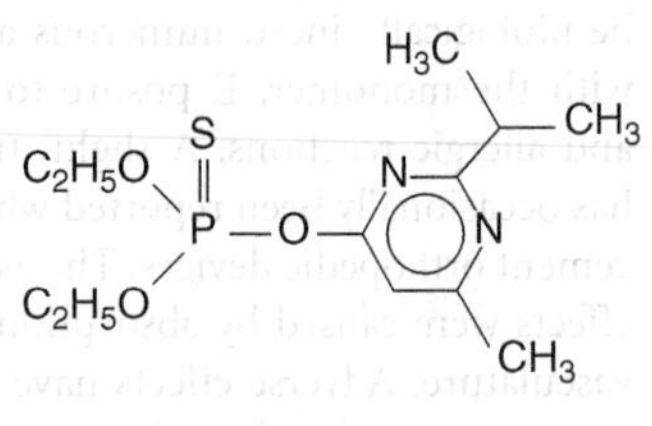

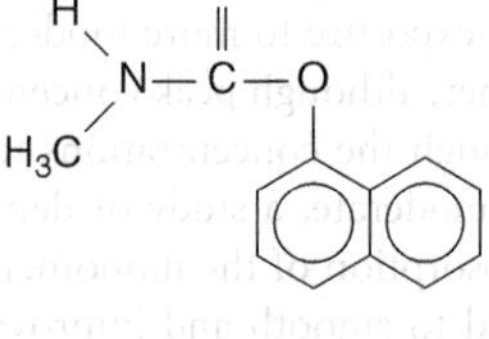

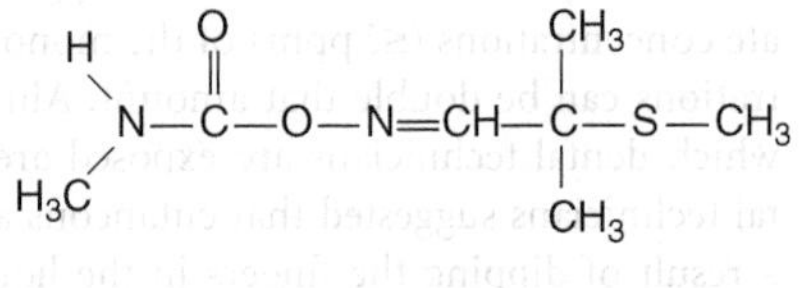

Acute human poisonings with neonicotinoids are increasing with increased use of this class of insecticides. The majority of case reports of neonicotinoid poisoning to date indicate oral ingestion in suicidal attempts, rather than inhalation or dermal exposure, as normal protective garments prevent applicator exposure. Syndromes of poisoning are typical of hyper-cholinergic stimulation at nicotinic receptors. CNS effects include dizziness, disorientation, and coma. Initially the autonomic nervous system is stimulated, and diaphoresis, tachycardia, and elevation of blood pressure occur. As the nervous system fails with exhaustive overstimulation, dyspnea or apnea, mydriasis, bradycardia, hypotension, and coma occur in severe poisoning cases.

Neonicotinoids currently are under increasing regulatory scrutiny due to their toxicity to pollinating insects such as honey bees. Although the role of neonicotinoids in recent bee colony collapse syndrome is not yet clear, it is apparent that these insecticides are extremely toxic to these beneficial insects and must be carefully applied to prevent adverse environmental impact.

The **anticholinesterase** insecticides are organophosphate or methylcarbamate esters. Representative structures are shown in Figure 40-7. The mechanism of action of anticholinesterase drugs is described in greater detail in Chapter 6. These compounds inhibit the hydrolytic action of the neurologically essential enzyme system, acetylcholinesterase, which is transiently acetylated during normal hydrolysis of acetylcholine. Anticholinesterases interact with the enzyme in a manner similar to the endogenous substrate, but with hydrolytic turnover numbers several orders of magnitude smaller than those of the natural substrate, acetylcholine. This interaction leaves the enzyme phosphorylated or carbamylated and incapable of physiologic function. Poisoning causes an overwhelming abundance of acetylcholine at cholinergic receptors in synapses of autonomic nerves, neuromuscular junctions, in the adrenal medulla, and in the CNS. As hydrolysis of acetylcholine is the controlling step in termination of synaptic cholinergic transmission, inactivation of acetylcholine is neurotoxic particularly in the autonomic nervous system of the CNS and the neuromuscular junctions of the somatic nervous system.

FIG 40-7 Chemical structures of organophosphate and methylcarbamate anticholinesterase insecticides.

As many as 100 organophosphate-class insecticides have been used in the United States. Many are analogues of phosphorothioic acid and are relatively poor anticholinesterases. These are activated preferentially in insects to phosphate homologues by oxidative mechanisms. A classic example of differences in toxicity of thio versus oxo organophosphate homologues is exhibited by **parathion versus paraoxon.** Substitution of the sulfur atom with oxygen results in a tenfold increase in mammalian toxicity. The venerable insecticide **malathion** has been used widely for nonagricultural applications, and it is the active ingredient in Ovide lotion used topically to treat head lice. Other organophosphates such as chlorpyrifos, diazinon, and terbufos are now restricted to use only by certified applicators.

Of some 20 methylcarbamates in use, **carbaryl** has been used most widely in home and garden applications. It is relatively nontoxic to mammals but is highly toxic to honeybees. In contrast, aldicarb, a methylcarbamate designed with molecular dimensions based on acetylcholine, is some 200 times more toxic to mammals. Aldicarb is available only to certified applicators; it is applied to the soil and taken up for systemic action in plants.

Treatment of acute **anticholinesterase poisoning** by either organophosphates or methylcarbamates involves liberal use of **anticholinergic drugs**, particularly atropine, to antagonize muscarinic cholinergic signs. **Pralidoxime** has been used successfully to reverse cholinesterase inhibition when used early in treatment of cases of **organophosphate poisoning**, but it may aggravate poisoning with methylcarbamate insecticides.

The **pyrethroids** consist of a group of natural or synthetic compounds that modify properties of ion channels in nerves. Pyrethroids maintain Na^+ channels in the open state for prolonged periods, leading to **hyperexcitation of the nervous system.** These compounds elicit repetitive activity, particularly in sensory nerves, along with membrane depolarization, enhanced neurotransmitter release, and eventual block of excitation. These actions occur as a consequence of prolongation of

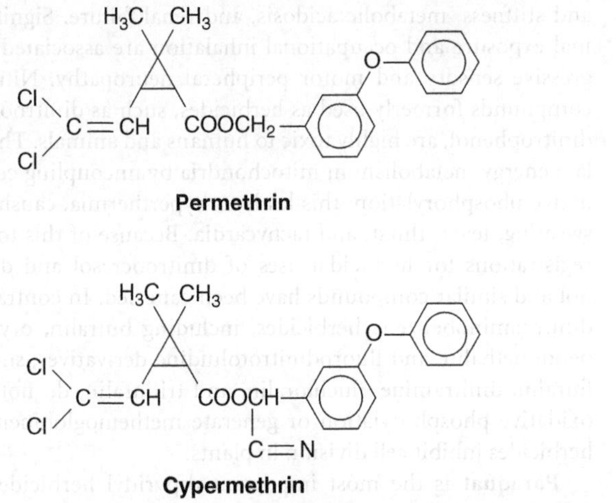

FIG 40-8 Chemical structures of several synthetic pyrethroid insecticides.

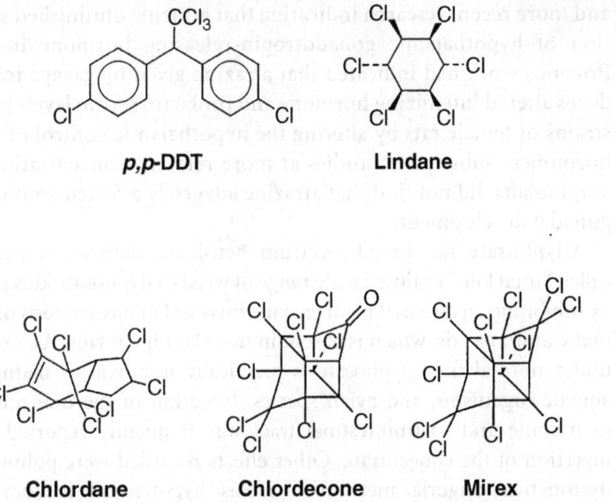

FIG 40-9 Chemical structures of several organochlorine insecticides.

Na^+ ion current in voltage-dependent Na^+ channels. The pyrethroids have remarkably selective toxicity for insects relative to mammals. They are largely contact insecticides with rapid "knock-down" properties.

Natural pyrethroids (pyrethrin I, pyrethrin II) are short-lived as a consequence of rapid oxidation and photodegradation in the environment and are rapidly hydrolyzed or oxidized when taken orally. These properties have resulted in rapid acceptance with minimal risk from use, but disadvantages are short duration of action and expense of natural product isolation. Synthetic pyrethroids have been designed to be more persistent. These include two types, determined by the presence or absence of a cyano function; two examples are shown in Figure 40-8. Of these, permethrin is stable to light and has low toxicity in adult mammals, but it is more toxic to neonates with undeveloped hydrolytic and oxidative mechanisms. Other synthetic analogues substituted with a cyano group are more toxic. Occupational exposure to pyrethroid insecticides leads to temporary paresthesia and respiratory irritation. Treatment is generally supportive.

Organochlorine insecticides, previously used extensively, are now only of historic importance in the United States, but some are still used in other regions of the world because of their low cost, stability, and efficacy. Figure 40-9 shows structures of some of these organochlorine insecticides. The Nobel Prize for Physiology and Medicine in 1948 was awarded to Paul Mueller, who discovered the insecticidal properties of DDT, the organochlorine prototype. DDT is a member of the dichlorodiphenylethane subclass of organochlorine insecticides, but it is now restricted under the UN PIC (Prior Informed Consent) procedure. The chlorinated cyclodiene structure subclass includes **chlordane**, dieldrin, and heptachlor, which also are restricted under the UN PIC procedure. Chlordecone and mirex represent another unique subgroup of cage-like, highly-chlorinated C10 structures that are restricted from use. The hexachlorocyclohexane-type compounds include **lindane,** a specific insecticidal isomer that is still used in lindane lotion as an ectoparasiticide and ovicide for crab and head lice.

The toxic actions of organochlorines, similar to pyrethroids, **alter conduction in the ion channels of nerves.** DDT alters Na^+ and K^+ ion permeability, Na^+, K^+-ATPase and Ca^{++}-dependent ATPase functions, and inhibition of calmodulin in nerves. These actions reduce the rate of nerve membrane repolarization and increase sensitivity to small stimuli. The chlorinated cyclodienes are different because their actions seem to be more localized within the CNS. These compounds inhibit Na^+, K^+-ATPase and Ca^{++}-dependent ATPase and act as γ-aminobutyric acid antagonists, eliciting uncontrolled neurotoxic excitation.

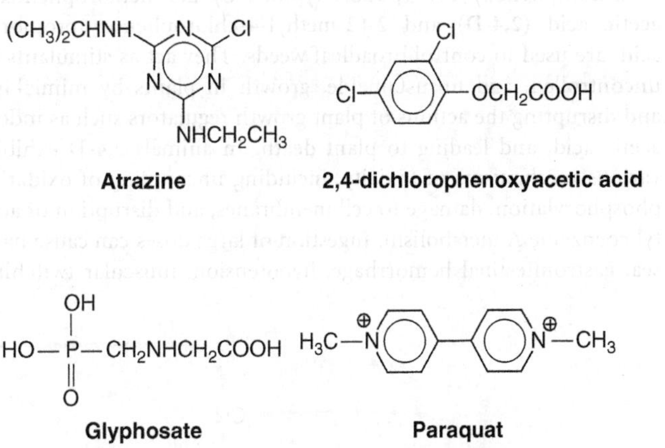

FIG 40-10 Chemical structures of various herbicides.

Herbicides

Herbicides are the most widely used type of pesticides. Given the broad use of these pesticides with apparently low relative risk in normal use, some herbicides in common use are presented, with selection based on high usage or significant toxicity where evident. Research efforts by crop scientists in recent decades have produced diverse structures, many of which offer selective toxicity against weeds, while sparing economic crops. An example is the use of herbicides in "no-till" production of grains, in which fields are sprayed to kill grasses, and seeds are planted without the need for plowing fields. Structures of some herbicides are illustrated in Figure 40-10.

Atrazine is a member of the class of chemically similar compounds known as the triazine herbicides that block photosynthesis in plants. Atrazine is one of the most widely used agricultural pesticides in the United States, as approximately 80 million pounds of the atrazine active ingredient are applied annually to control broadleaf weeds in field corn and sorghum, in lawns and turf, and after production of wheat. Epidemiologic studies of workers exposed in chemical plants and farming populations have not shown a significant incidence of disease related to atrazine use, and little acute toxicity is evident in suicide attempts with atrazine. Atrazine is undergoing review, however, for re-registration by the EPA Health Effects Division. This decision for re-review was based on the high volume of use, persistence of atrazine in surface and ground water, and more recent research indicating that atrazine diminished secretion of hypothalamic gonadotropin-releasing hormone in rats. Previous work had indicated that atrazine given by gavage in high doses altered luteinizing hormone and prolactin serum levels in two strains of female rats by altering the hypothalamic control of these hormones. Subsequent studies at more relevant concentrations in amphibians did not find that atrazine adversely affected amphibian gonadal development.

Glyphosate has broad-spectrum herbicidal activity, sometimes called "total kill," against a wide range of weeds. Glyphosate kills plants by inhibiting an essential plant enzyme involved in biosynthesis of aromatic amino acids, which is absent in nonplant life forms. As a result, under normal use, glyphosate is practically nontoxic to mammals, aquatic organisms, and avian species. Irritation of the oral mucous membrane and gastrointestinal tract was frequently reported with ingestion of the concentrate. Other effects recorded were pulmonary dysfunction, oliguria, metabolic acidosis, hypotension, leukocytosis, and fever. Various reviews, which indicated absence of toxicity in long-term animal studies of glyphosate, have been summarized.

Chlorophenoxy compounds, typified by 2,4-dichlorophenoxyacetic acid **(2,4-D)** and 2-(2-methyl-4-chlorophenoxy)propionic acid, are used to control broadleaf weeds. They act as stimulants of uncontrolled, and unsustainable, growth in plants by mimicking and disrupting the actions of plant growth regulators such as indole acetic acid, and leading to plant death. In animals 2,4-D exhibits various mechanisms of toxicity, including uncoupling of oxidative phosphorylation, damage to cell membranes, and disruption of acetyl coenzyme A metabolism. Ingestion of large doses can cause nausea, gastrointestinal hemorrhage, hypotension, muscular twitching and stiffness, metabolic acidosis, and renal failure. Significant dermal exposure and occupational inhalation are associated with progressive sensory and motor peripheral neuropathy. Nitrophenolic compounds formerly used as herbicides, such as dinitroocresol and dinitrophenol, are highly toxic to humans and animals. These stimulate energy metabolism in mitochondria by uncoupling cellular oxidative phosphorylation; this leads to hyperthermia, causing profuse sweating, fever, thirst, and tachycardia. Because of this toxicity, the registrations for herbicidal uses of dinitroocresol and dinitrophenol and similar compounds have been canceled. In contrast, certain dinitroaminobenzene herbicides, including butralin, oryzalin, and pendimethalin, and fluorodinitrotoluidine derivatives, such as benfluralin, dinitramine, fluchloralin, and trifluralin, do not uncouple oxidative phosphorylation or generate methemoglobinemia. These herbicides inhibit cell division in plants.

Paraquat is the most important dipyridyl herbicide for toxicologic consideration because it has delayed, severe, and specific pulmonary toxicity. Paraquat exhibits its particular and unique toxicity in part because of its selective accumulation in lung tissue by a diamine transport system located in the alveolar epithelium. In addition, paraquat is involved in a single-electron cyclic reduction–oxidation reaction that attacks unsaturated lipids in membranes to form lipid peroxides. The oxidative destruction and subsequent fibrotic lesions developed during reparative processes lead to severely diminished lung function, anoxia, and death days after ingestion of paraquat. The comprehensive treatise by Ellenhorn and associates (**See references**) presents pharmacokinetic plots indicating likely survival or death based on blood concentrations versus time after ingestion of paraquat.

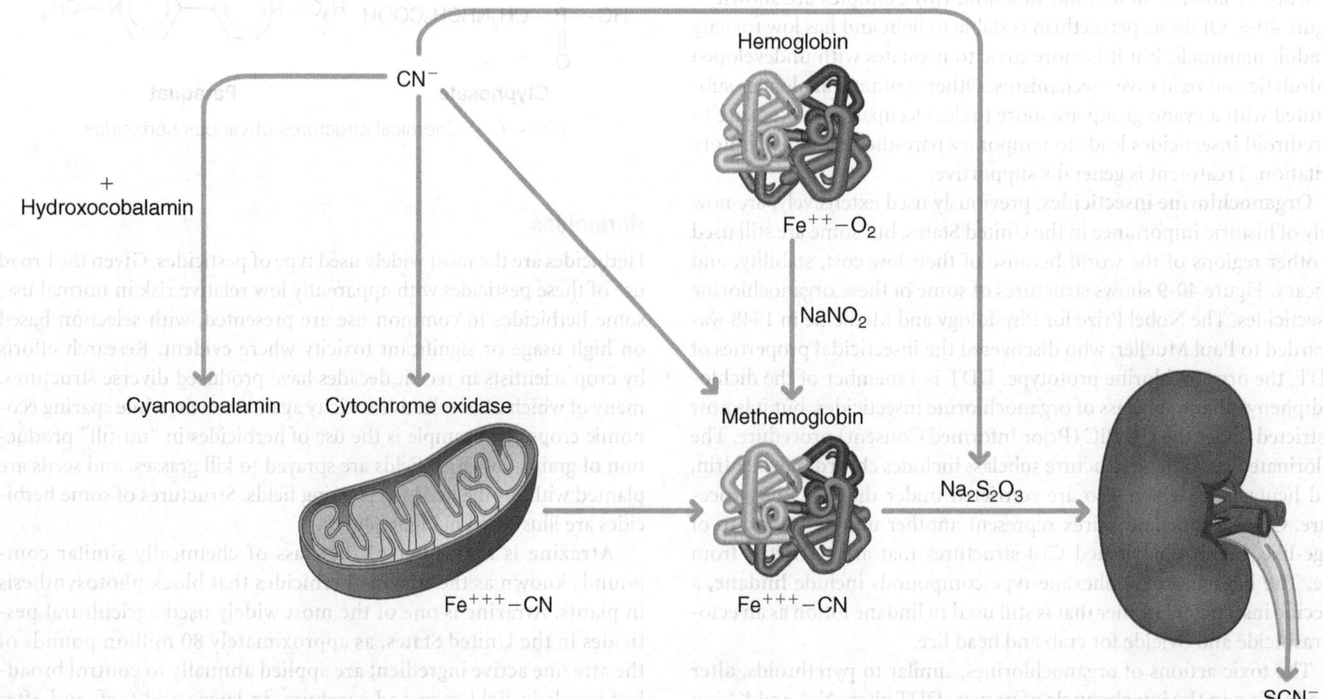

FIG 40-11 Treatment of cyanide poisoning. Cyanide (CN^-), whether inhaled or ingested, combines with ferric ions (Fe^{+++}) in cytochrome oxidase to inhibit cellular respiration. Therapy is aimed at eliminating cyanide from the cells by a two-step process: (1) sodium nitrite ($NaNO_2$) is administered intravenously to oxidize the iron in hemoglobin from the ferrous (Fe^{++}) to the ferric state; the methemoglobin that is formed competes for cyanide, freeing cytochrome oxidase from attack by cyanide. (2) Cyanide is inactivated by the administration of sodium thiosulfate ($Na_2S_2O_3$) to yield thiocyanate (SCN^-), which is readily excreted in the urine. Cyanide can also be removed by the use of hydroxocobalamin as shown. Experimentally, these steps reduce the lethal potency of cyanide by 80%.

Cyanide

Sodium cyanide, which liberates hydrogen cyanide, is occasionally used against predatory animals. this is the only current registered use for sodium cyanide as a pesticide. This use is controversial. Because of its extreme toxicity, sodium cyanide is restricted to use only by trained applicators. Cyanide inactivates cellular oxidative phosphorylation by binding to the Fe^{+++} in the cytochrome oxidase. The inability of cells to use oxygen, particularly in the brain and heart, is rapidly lethal to warm-blooded animals. Therapy for poisoning involves treatment with 100% oxygen and rapid provision of an alternative, less critical source of Fe^{+++} for cyanide binding. This is accomplished through induction of methemoglobinemia by administering amyl nitrite or sodium nitrite. Treatment with sodium thiosulfate solution follows to assist conversion of cyanide to thiocyanate by the mitochondrial enzyme rhodanese (Fig. 40-11). A newer treatment of cyanide poisoning involves the use of hydroxocobalamin to form cyanocobalamin and reduce cyanide complexed with the cytochrome complex. The cyanocobolamin is excreted in the urine.

Rodenticides

Various compounds have been used to attack rodents. Some are quite toxic to rodents, humans, and wildlife through acute exposure, whereas others require multiple doses to elicit significant toxicity. Most of these act as anticoagulants, and their structures are shown in Figure 40-12.

Warfarin

Diphacinone

Brodifacoum

Bromadiolone

FIG 40-12 Chemical structures of anticoagulant rodenticides.

The oldest, **warfarin,** is a coumarin derivative that has been used as a rodenticide since 1950. Warfarin derives its action through antagonism of vitamin K action as a cofactor in synthesis of coagulation factors (see Chapter 26).

Resistant strains of rodents have emerged, which has led to development of new hydroxycoumarin derivatives (so-called "superwarfarins") that are much more potent and do not require repeated doses to kill. Brodifacoum and bromadiolone are characterized as single dose in use. Necropsies after poisonings support the diagnosis of coagulopathy with findings of hemoperitoneum, hemothorax, and pulmonary hemorrhage. Because of the increased potency and increased duration of action in some of these newer rodenticides, poisoning has occurred in pets, wildlife, and exposed humans. Treatment is based on assessment of prothrombin time, which should be monitored at 24 and 48 hours after ingestion. If prothrombin time is elevated at these times, treatment with phytonadione (phylloquinone, vitamin K_1) should be instituted with continued assessment of prothrombin time over 4 to 5 days.

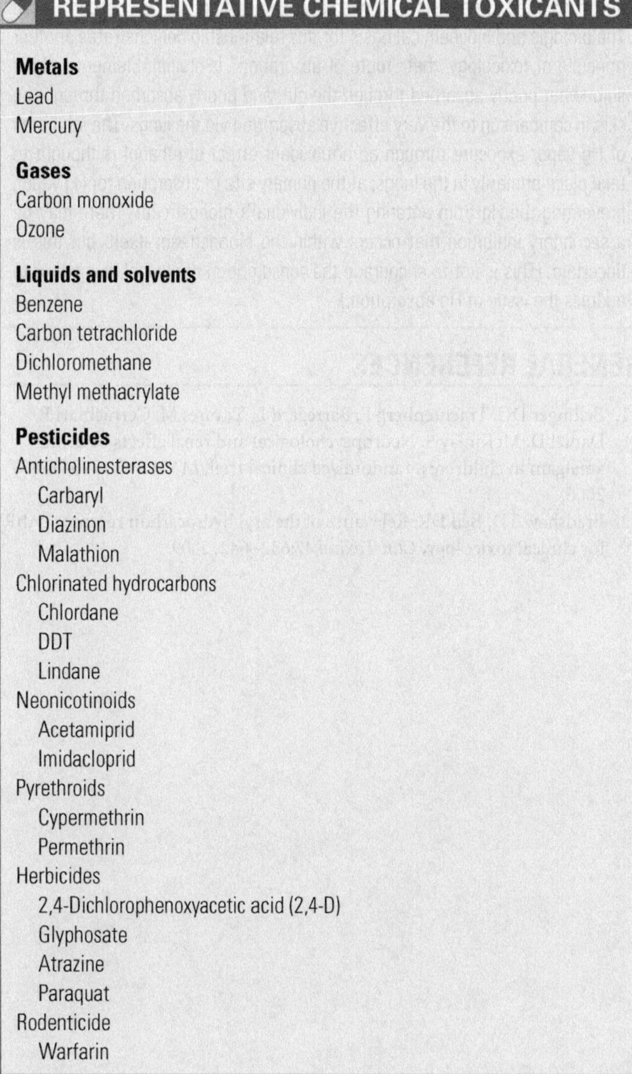

REPRESENTATIVE CHEMICAL TOXICANTS

Metals

Lead
Mercury

Gases

Carbon monoxide
Ozone

Liquids and solvents

Benzene
Carbon tetrachloride
Dichloromethane
Methyl methacrylate

Pesticides

- Anticholinesterases
  - Carbaryl
  - Diazinon
  - Malathion
- Chlorinated hydrocarbons
  - Chlordane
  - DDT
  - Lindane
- Neonicotinoids
  - Acetamiprid
  - Imidacloprid
- Pyrethroids
  - Cypermethrin
  - Permethrin
- Herbicides
  - 2,4-Dichlorophenoxyacetic acid (2,4-D)
  - Glyphosate
  - Atrazine
  - Paraquat
- Rodenticide
  - Warfarin

CASE DISCUSSION

This case of three dentists of the same age, gender, health status, and occupational exposure to Hg allows several principles of toxicology to be examined. One is that of exposures. The primary source of Hg exposure in a dental office is via absorption through the lungs. Elemental Hg, which is the form used in dental offices, whether pre-capsulated or mixed on-site, produces Hg vapor which is readily absorbed through the lungs. All three dentists in this case use approximately the same amount of amalgam in their practice, all use the same pre-capsulated brand, and all are exposed to the same ambient levels of Hg vapor since they all work the same number of hours. The degree to which each dentist scavenged mercury vapor during operative procedures was presumed to be similar although this is another relevant variable.

Because elemental Hg is absorbed so readily through the lungs, control of Hg vapor in the dental environment is important. A second toxicologic principle is that of consideration of multiple exposures and how one exposure might influence another. In this case, one of the dentists, abstains from alcohol. The other two each have, on average, two drinks of alcohol per day.

As demonstrated in a study (Martin and Naleway, 2004), the amount of ethanol consumed by dentists was inversely related to urinary Hg concentrations. The biologic and biochemical basis for this relationship demonstrates another principle of toxicology, that "route of absorption" is crucial. Elemental Hg is somewhat poorly absorbed through the gut, and poorly absorbed through the skin in comparison to the very effective absorption via the lungs. The inhibition of Hg vapor exposure through an antioxidant effect of ethanol is thought to take place primarily in the lungs, at the primary site of absorption for Hg vapor, preventing the Hg from entering the individual's bloodstream. There may be a secondary inhibition that occurs within the bloodstream itself, but this is uncertain. (This is not to encourage the consumption of alcohol, but rather to address the issue of Hg absorption.)

GENERAL REFERENCES

1. Bellinger DC, Trachtenberg F, Barregard L, Tavares M, Cernichiari E, Daniel D, McKinlay S: Neuropsychological and renal effects of dental amalgam in children: a randomized clinical trial, *JAMA* 295:1775–1783, 2006.
2. Bradshaw TD, Bell DR: Relevance of the aryl hydrocarbon receptor (AhR) for clinical toxicology, *Clin Toxicol* 47:632–642, 2009.
3. Casida JE: Pest Toxicology: the primary mechanisms of pesticide action, *Chemical Research in Toxicology* 22:609–619, 2009.
4. Danielson PB: The cytochrome P450 superfamily: biochemistry, evolution and drug metabolism in humans, *Current Drug Metabolism* 3:561–597, 2002.
5. DeRouen TA, Martin MD, Leroux BG, Townes BD, Woods JS, Leitao J, Castro-Caldas A, Luis H, Bernardo M, Rosenbaum G, Martins IP: Neurobehavioral effects of dental amalgam in children: a randomized clinical trial, *JAMA* 295:1784–1792, 2006.
6. Dodes JE: The amalgam controversy. An evidence-based analysis, *Journal of the American Dental Association* 132:348–356, 2001.
7. Dresser GK, Spence JD, Bailey DG: Pharmacokinetic-pharmacodynamic consequences and clinical relevance of cytochrome P450 3A4 inhibition, *Clinical Pharmacokinetics* 38:41–57, 2000.
8. Ellenhorn MJ, Schonwald S, Ordog G, Wasserberger J, editors: *Ellenhorn's Medical Toxicology; Diagnosis and Treatment of Human Poisoning*, ed 2, Baltimore, 1997, Williams & Wilkins.
9. Gaylor DW: The ED01 study: summary and conclusions, *Journal of Environmental Pathology and Toxicology* 3:179–183, 1980.
10. Hanieh H: Toward understanding the role of aryl hydrocarbon receptor in the immune system: current progress and future trends, *BioMed Research International* 2014, 520763.
11. Hill AB: The environment and disease: association or causation? *Proceedings of the Royal Society of Medicine* 58:295–300, 1965.
12. Kingman A, Albers JW, Arezzo JC, Garabrant DH, Michalek JE: Amalgam exposure and neurological function, *Neurotoxicology* 26:241–255, 2005.
13. Langston JW, Ballard P, Tetrud JW, Irwin I: Chronic Parkinsonism in humans due to a product of meperidine-analog synthesis, *Science* 219:979–980, 1983.
14. Martin MD, Naleway C: The inhibition of mercury absorption by dietary ethanol in humans: cross-sectional and case-control studies, *Occupational and Environmental Medicine* 61:e8, 2004.
15. McKinney C, Rue T, Sathyanarayana S, Martin M, Seminario AL, DeRouen T: Dental sealants and restorations and urinary bisphenol A concentrations in children in the 2003-2004 National Health and Nutrition Examination Survey, *Journal of the American Dental Association* 145:745–750, 2014.
16. Roberts JR, Reigart JR: *Recognition and Management of Pesticide Poisonings*, ed 6, www2.epa.gov, 2015.

41

Drugs for Medical Emergencies

Morton B. Rosenberg and James C. Phero

KEY INFORMATION

- Both minor and major medical emergencies can occur during dental treatment.
- Dental offices must have critical emergency management drugs readily available.
- Dentist and chairside personnel must be current and competent in basic life support (BLS) for health care providers.
- Supplemental oxygen must be available, as well as the ability to deliver it under positive pressure.
- Advanced cardiac life support (ACLS) is required in certain dental settings. Training and competence in ACLS requires an in-depth knowledge of the pharmacology of the recommended management drugs.

CASE STUDY

Ms. BR, your 45-year-old patient, is a severe dental phobic. Her medical history includes a history of asthma treated with fluticasone propionate and salmeterol xinafoate. She occasionally uses an albuterol inhaler for acute episodes and has brought it with her. On arrival into the dental operatory, her vital signs on your automated vital signs monitor are the following: blood pressure (BP) 145/87, heart rate 90 bpm, respiratory rate 12 rpm, and oxygen saturation 96%. During your injection of local anesthesia containing 2% lidocaine with 1:100,000 epinephrine, she begins to complain of tightness in her chest and inability to catch her breath. You immediately stop the procedure and give her the albuterol inhaler to use. After two inhalations, she has no relief of symptoms. She is diaphoretic, tachypneic, and wheezing. You record her vital signs again, and her BP is 165/82, heart rate 102 bpm, and oxygen saturation 88%. What is your next course of action?

Every dentist should expect to be involved in the diagnosis and treatment of medical emergencies during the course of his or her clinical practice. These emergencies vary in their cause and nature of occurrence. They may be directly related to dental therapy, or they may simply occur by chance in the dental environment. In studies surveying the incidence and type of medical emergencies in dental practice, many of the respondents reported medical emergencies. Although most of the reported emergencies were minor (e.g., syncopal episodes that resolved uneventfully), life-threatening or major emergencies were also reported. **Many medical emergencies occur during the administration of local anesthesia and during painful procedures** such as extractions and pulp extirpation where local anesthesia may be inadequate. The potential need for acute medical intervention during dental treatment may be increased for practitioners treating a high percentage of medically compromised, elderly patients or patients with special needs. Additionally, practitioners using minimal, moderate, or deep sedation and general anesthesia have unique considerations that may influence the incidence and severity of medical emergencies in the office.

It has been postulated that the incidence of medical emergencies in dentistry is increasing. This increase may be attributed to the following factors:

1. **Increasing age of the general population.** As the number of elderly individuals in the general population increases, the likelihood of encountering a medical emergency as a result of the physiologic and pathologic changes associated with aging also increases. In addition to the normal deterioration of major organ systems that occurs with age, elderly patients are more likely to exhibit chronic clinical manifestations of organ deterioration (e.g., angina pectoris, congestive heart failure, chronic obstructive lung disease) that may become acute emergencies from patient-perceived stress during the dental visit requiring intervention. **Elderly patients take more prescription and over-the-counter drugs than young patients**, and the effects of these compounds can be significantly different from the effects seen in younger patients. The pharmacokinetics of many drugs are altered by aging; pharmacodynamic and physiologic changes also may result in greater sensitivity to many drugs, especially central nervous system (CNS) depressants.
2. **Effect of medical and dental advances.** Advances in the diagnosis and treatment of many medical conditions have permitted an increasing population of medically compromised and complex patients to survive and seek comprehensive dental treatment. Medical advances in such diverse areas as cancer, cardiovascular disease, and psychiatric illness are of concern. Surgical advances such as organ transplants, cardiac valve replacements, coronary artery revascularization, pacemakers, and automatic implantable cardioverter-defibrillators are of concern. They can be directly related to the occurrence of acute medical problems in the dental office. In general, **the growing number of medically stabilized yet chronically ill patients seeking dental treatment is paralleled by a concomitant increase in the incidence of medical emergencies during dental treatment**. Dental advances such as intraosseous implants and comprehensive periodontal and restorative treatment leading to “lifelong dentistry” are attracting older, less healthy patients into the dental environment.
3. **Pharmacologic therapies. Therapeutic choices for dentists are constantly increasing** with the introduction of new generations of

antibiotics, analgesics, local anesthetics, and sedative drugs. Each new drug has its own inherent indications, contraindications, and possible side effects. These drugs also have the capacity to interact with each other and with other drugs the patient may be taking for medical conditions. Such drug interactions have the potential to elicit acute adverse reactions during the dental appointment. The growing popularity of herbal supplements, over-the-counter preparations, and other alternative medical therapies has implications that are being recognized and studied. Many of the side effects of these alternative medical therapies, such as antihemostatic, hypotensive, and hypoglycemic properties, can directly affect dental treatment.

4. **Drug abuse.** Substance abuse is a fact of life in modern society. Many dental patients "premedicate" themselves with prescribed or illicit CNS depressants before dental therapy. These drugs may present acute problems by themselves or interact with drugs administered or prescribed by the dentist.

EMERGENCY PREPARATION

Many chronic medical conditions, such as asthma, congestive heart failure, coronary artery disease, and cerebrovascular disease, may become acute medical emergencies when exacerbated by the stress of the dental appointment. Stress, anxiety, fear, and phobia may cause other minor stress-related emergencies, such as syncopal and hyperventilation episodes. A thorough **preoperative evaluation**, meticulous detail to achieving profound local anesthesia in a safe manner, consideration of nonpharmacologic stress reduction protocols, and the use of pharmacologic sedative techniques to minimize pain, fear, and anxiety help reduce this risk.

Preoperative evaluation includes the use of a medical history questionnaire, oral history, review of systems, physical examination, vital signs, and appropriate laboratory tests and consultations. This evaluation should determine the risk/benefit ratio of the contemplated procedure, what drugs should be used or avoided, the potential for a medical emergency, and the type of monitoring best suited for the particular patient.

EMERGENCY PREPAREDNESS

Almost any medical emergency can occur during the course of dental treatment or by other individuals in the dental office, which means that **dental personnel must be prepared to provide effective basic life support for health care providers (BLS-HCP) and seek emergency medical services in a timely manner.** Dentists must be able to diagnose and treat common medical problems (e.g., syncope or hyperventilation syndrome) definitively and respond effectively to certain less common (or even rare) but potentially life-threatening emergencies, especially emergencies that may arise as a result of dental treatment (e.g., anaphylactic reaction to an administered drug). These emergencies are listed in Table 41-1.

Many factors determine the degree of preparedness for medical emergencies needed in a specific dental practice, but all dental offices must be ready at some basic level. The use of local anesthesia is an indication for the dentist to be prepared to handle medical emergencies, as evidenced by the following language in product literature approved by the U.S. Food and Drug Administration: "Dental practitioners who employ local anesthetic agents should be well versed in diagnosis and management of emergencies that may arise from their use. Resuscitative equipment, oxygen, and other emergency drugs should be immediately available for immediate use." An overall emergency preparedness plan, as outlined in Table 41-2, is essential for every

TABLE 41-1 Potential Medical Emergencies in the Dental Office That May Require Drug Therapy

Medical Emergency Category	Medical Emergency
Psychogenic	Syncope Hyperventilation syndrome
Respiratory	Asthma Pulmonary edema
Cardiovascular	Angina pectoris Myocardial infarction Hypertension Hypotension Tachycardia Bradycardia Acute heart failure
Central nervous system	Cerebrovascular accident Seizure
Endocrine	Hypoglycemia Hyperglycemia Adrenal insufficiency
Drug related	Allergic reactions Sedative/anesthetic

TABLE 41-2 Emergency Preparedness Checklist

Completed	Duties
________	All staff members have specific assigned duties
________	Alternative plans have been made in case of a missing staff member
________	All clinical staff are current in basic life support for health care providers (BLS-HCP) and have proper training in the diagnosis and treatment of medical emergencies
________	The dental office is appropriately equipped with emergency equipment and supplies
________	Periodic unannounced emergency drills are conducted routinely
________	Appropriate emergency phone numbers are placed prominently by each phone
________	Oxygen tanks and oxygen delivery systems are checked regularly
________	All emergency equipment is in good working order and located in an appropriate location based on the emergency plan
________	Monthly checks are made for all emergency medications and replacement of expired drugs
________	All emergency supplies are restocked immediately after use
________	A specific individual has been assigned to ensure that these items have been completed and to document this checklist review
________	Cognitive aids to assist correct algorithms are reviewed and immediately available

(Modified from: Fast TB, Martin MD, Ellis TM: Emergency preparedness: a survey of dental practitioners, *J Am Dent Assoc* 112:449-501, 1986.)

dental practice. Implicit in Table 41-2 is the necessity to develop a team approach in preparing for and responding to medical emergencies in the dental office, with each staff member (receptionist, dental auxiliary, dental hygienist, and dentist) responsible for a specific role.

Preparedness must be individually tailored according to the type of patient treated (e.g., young, healthy patients in an orthodontic practice versus medically compromised patients in a periodontal practice), location (e.g., an urban setting where emergency medical service personnel [EMS] are readily available versus a rural location where there may be a significant delay until EMS arrives), and training (i.e., whether the dentist and staff are competent to perform advanced emergency procedures and protocols). Although a comprehensive guide to the pathophysiologic characteristics, prevention, diagnosis, and management of specific medical emergencies is beyond the scope of this chapter, several sources for this purpose are listed in the general references. In practices where sedation or general anesthesia is administered, advanced emergency training and equipment are required and regulated by state dental practice acts.

EMERGENCY DRUGS

Although many medical emergencies may be properly treated without the use of drugs, every dental office must have a **medical emergency management kit** with drugs, equipment, and supplies appropriate to the training of the individual dentist, the patient being treated, and the type of procedures being performed. However, no drug can take the place of a properly trained health professional and support staff in diagnosing and treating emergencies. Nevertheless, the design and purchase of an appropriate emergency kit often play an integral role in dictating the course and outcome of emergency treatment.

Besides determining which drugs should be included in an emergency kit, **the dentist must understand that he or she must maintain the knowledge base and skills to use them**. In the midst of a medical emergency, with the patient by definition in an acutely abnormal or even critical situation, there is no time to begin reading labels, leafing through emergency texts, or administering drugs as suggested by a brochure in the emergency kit. In addition, there is a significant difference between the theoretic knowledge of how to treat an emergency and being able to put such cognitive skills to practical use. Constant review and training keeps the dental team sharp. Regular continuing education in medical emergencies, review of new advances in pharmacology, certification and recertification in BLS-HCP and ACLS, and emergency drills are all good in preparing for emergencies.

Many states mandate certification in BLS for dental licensure. Plus, in offices that use deep sedation/general anesthesia, additional training in ACLS is the standard of care. Without prompt attention to the CABDs (circulation, airway, breathing, defibrillation) of cardiopulmonary resuscitation (CPR), drug therapy is of little value. The advent of automatic external defibrillators has made early defibrillation an integral part of the BLS "chain of survival" for the treatment of cardiac arrest. Since January 1998, health care provider CPR courses conducted by the American Heart Association have include a mandated module on automatic external defibrillator application and use. Some states mandate the presence of an automatic external defibrillator in dental offices.

The correct approach to **the use of drugs in any dental office medical office should be conservative and supportive.** If any consequence of dental treatment is foreseeable and results in harm, liability may be imposed. Emergency drugs are potent, rapidly acting agents that require insight and training for proper administration and patient management.

TABLE 41-3 Suggested Basic Emergency Equipment for the General Dental Office

General Equipment	Portable E tank of oxygen with regulator and key	Regulator includes pressure gauge and flow meter providing 15 L/minute
	Supplement "passive" oxygen delivery systems:	Nasal cannula Face mask nonrebreathing
	Oropharyngeal airways (Guedel type: 80, 90, 100 mm)	
	Magill forceps for foreign body removal	
	Yankauer tip suction handle, suction tubing, operatory high volume system adapter	
Monitoring Devices	Stethoscope and sphygmomanometer and/or automated vital signs monitor	Pediatric, small, medium, large, and extra large cuff as appropriate for each patient
	Wall clock with second hand	
	Automated external defibrillator adhering to AHA 2015 guidelines	

Emergency drug kits may either be organized by the individual practitioner or purchased commercially. In the past, many dentists were uncomfortable choosing and purchasing individual drugs for their emergency kits without having trusted information and recommendations as a resource, so the purchase of high-quality, commercially available emergency drug kits modified for dentistry provided recommended drugs with consistent drug potency through automatic drug updating. The Anesthesia Research Foundation of the American Dental Society of Anesthesiology has been actively addressing the importance for dentists to respond effectively to medical emergencies. Their "Ten Minutes Saves a Life!" program integrates emergency equipment and drugs into a comprehensive response kit as a professional courtesy to the profession.

There is a general tendency to over equip basic dental emergency kits with equipment and drugs that are beyond the expertise of many dentists not trained and experienced in intravenous drug administration. An office emergency kit should include equipment (Table 41-3) and the drugs that may be needed for dental office medical emergencies, and these items must be familiar to the dentist. Many authors, state boards of dental registration, commercial vendors, and professional groups have suggested the composition of dental medical emergency kits. The composition of these kits varies greatly and depends on the training and philosophy of emergency care of the creator, whether the kit is dental specific, and whether sedation or anesthesia is used. The definitive pharmacologic features of these drugs are discussed in other chapters.

Basic Emergency Drugs

All dentists must keep unexpired drugs readily available in the office in fresh supply for immediate administration (Table 41-4). Dentists must know immediately when, how, and in what doses to give these specific agents for acutely life-threatening situations, and this can only be accomplished by ongoing dentist and office team training that incorporates the use of checklists and algorithms.

TABLE 41-4 Basic Medical Emergency Drugs for the General Dental Office

Drug	Indications	Mode of Action	Preparations
Oxygen	For use in all medical emergencies in which hypoxemia may be present	Elevates arterial oxygen tension	Cylinders (green); E tanks, 690 L
Epinephrine	Acute allergic reactions, severe acute asthma (not responding to adrenergic inhaler)	α and β receptor agonist	Adult 1:1000, 0.3 mg Pediatric 1:1000, 0.15 mg
Nitroglycerin	Angina pectoris, acute myocardial infarction	Vasodilator	Sublingual tablets 0.4 mg Aerosol/spray, 0.4 mg/actuation
Albuterol	Mild to moderate bronchospasm	Selective β2 receptor agonist	Aerosol, 90 μg/actuation
Glucose	Hypoglycemia	Anti-hypoglycemic	Only if conscious: oral/transmucosal preparations (orange juice, cake icing, cola)
Aspirin	Evolving myocardial infarction	Reduces platelet aggregation	Chewable aspirin, 325 mg
Diphenhydramine	Mild to moderate allergic reactions	Antihistamine	Oral or IM, 25-50 mg
Aromatic ammonia	Syncope	General arousal agent	Vaporole crushed and held 4-6 inches under nose

Oxygen

Oxygen is a fundamental if not the primary, emergency drug indicated in any medical emergency where hypoxemia may be present. These emergencies include, but are not limited, to acute disturbances involving the cardiovascular system, respiratory system, and the CNS. In a hypoxemic patient, breathing-enriched oxygen elevates the arterial oxygen tension, which improves oxygenation of peripheral tissues. Due to the steep properties of the oxyhemoglobin dissociation curve, a modest increase in oxygen tension can significantly alter hemoglobin saturation in a hypoxemic individual. Hypoxemia leads to anaerobic metabolism and metabolic acidosis, which often adversely affect the efficacy of emergency pharmacologic interventions.

Clinically, hypoxemia in the spontaneously breathing patient is frequently seen as agitation. Oxygen can be delivered to a spontaneously breathing patient by full face mask, nasal cannula, or nasal hood. Additionally, the office must have a portable system of oxygen delivery to cover problems outside the operatory. Dental offices must also have the capacity to deliver oxygen via positive-pressure ventilation. This may be accomplished with the use of a bag-valve-mask device (consisting of a mask, self-inflating bag, and nonrebreathing valve) or with a manually triggered oxygen-powered breathing device (consisting of a mask connected by a valve activated by a lever and high-pressure tubing to the oxygen supply). Each method of providing positive-pressure ventilation requires training for effective use. Practice is necessary in learning how to provide a mask seal around the nose and mouth and learning the correct pressure, volume, and rate for ventilation when squeezing the bag. The oxygen-powered device may appear to be easier to use, but frequently the pressurized flow of oxygen inflates the stomach, pressurizing the gastric contents and leading to aspiration. Both techniques are preferred, however, over mouth-to-mouth, mouth-to-nose, or mouth-to-mask techniques. Airway adjuncts such as oropharyngeal and nasopharyngeal airways and advanced airway rescue aids such as endotracheal equipment, laryngeal mask airways, and the means of establishing an emergency airway by cricothyrotomy and transtracheal ventilation can be useful or even lifesaving in the hands of a trained and experienced health professional. Without appropriate training, however, their use may prove deleterious in an acute emergency.

Although oxygen toxicity may occur after prolonged therapy with high concentrations of oxygen, it is not an issue during clinical urgent/emergency oxygenation and/or ventilation. This statement is true even for the rare patient whose respiratory drive depends on hypoxemia because of chronically elevated carbon dioxide concentrations. If clinically indicated, oxygen should never be withheld during any medical emergency. Inspired oxygen concentrations depend on the delivery system used. The ability to understand the oxygen concentrations that can be delivered to spontaneously breathing or apneic patients is important in determining the best airway oxygenation/ventilation device (Table 41-5).

TABLE 41-5 Inspired Oxygen Concentration with Different Delivery Systems

Delivery System Liters/Minute (LPM)	Liters/Minute (LPM)	Inspired Oxygen Concentration (Percentage)
Spontaneous Breathing		
Nasal cannula/nasal hood	1-6	25-45
Resuscitation face mask	6-15	40-60
Nonrebreather mask	10-15	60-90
Positive-Pressure Ventilation		
Mouth-to-mouth		17
Mouth-to-mask	10-15	80
Bag-valve-mask	15-25	75-95
Manually triggered, oxygen-powered breathing device		75-95

Epinephrine

Epinephrine is the most important injectable drug in the dental emergency kit. Epinephrine is an endogenous catecholamine with α-adrenergic receptor–stimulating and β-adrenergic receptor–stimulating activity. It is the drug of choice for the management of the cardiovascular and respiratory manifestations of acute allergic reactions. The beneficial pharmacologic actions of epinephrine when used in resuscitative dosages include bronchodilation, increased systemic vascular resistance, increased arterial BP, increased heart rate, increased myocardial contractility, and increased myocardial and cerebral blood flow.

For the effective treatment of acute anaphylactic or anaphylactoid reactions, epinephrine must be administered immediately as the condition is diagnosed. The drug dose of 0.3 to 0.5 mg can be injected intramuscularly as 0.3 to 0.5 mL of a 1:1000 solution. Epinephrine should be available for immediate use as an auto-injector or vial plus 1-mL syringe with IM needle. The intravenous route using 1:10,000

TABLE 41-6 Important Emergency Support Drugs

Drug	Indications	Mode of Action	Route of Administration
Diazepam	Prolonged seizures	Anticonvulsant	Intravenous
Hydrocortisone	Adjunctive drug for major allergic reactions	Corticosteroid	Intravenous
Atropine	Bradycardia	Anticholinergic	Intravenous

is reserved for an overwhelming reaction, but its use may induce or exacerbate ventricular ectopy, and it should be administered with great caution.

Because of its profound bronchodilating effects, epinephrine is also indicated for the treatment of acute asthmatic attacks unrelieved by sprays or aerosols of β_2-adrenergic receptor agonists. Epinephrine is one of the major vasoactive compounds indicated for use during cardiac arrest because of its ability to elevate coronary perfusion pressure.

Nitroglycerin

Although nitroglycerin is available in many preparations—long-acting oral and transmucosal preparations, transcutaneous patches, and intravenous solutions—**the appropriate forms for the dental office are the sublingual tablet or translingual spray**. Nitroglycerin is the treatment of choice for acute angina pectoris. It acts primarily by relaxing vascular smooth muscle, dilating systemic venous and arterial vascular beds, and reducing venous return and systemic vascular resistance. These actions all combine to reduce myocardial oxygen consumption. One tablet or spray (0.4 mg) should be given initially. This dose may be repeated twice at 5-minute intervals to a total dose of three administrations provided the patient does not become bradycardic or hypotensive. Relief should occur within 1 to 2 minutes; if the discomfort is not relieved, the diagnosis of evolving myocardial infarction must be considered for first-time chest pain patients or patients with a history of angina that is not relieved with nitroglycerin.

Contraindications to the administration of nitroglycerin include patients who are hypotensive and patients who have recently taken sildenafil (Viagra) or another phosphodiesterase type 5 inhibitor. The combination of nitroglycerin and sildenafil, or like drug, can lead to profound hypotension and unconsciousness.

Bronchodilator

Inhalation of a β_2-adrenergic receptor agonist, such as metaproterenol, terbutaline, or albuterol, is used in the treatment of acute bronchospasm encountered during asthma and anaphylaxis. The use of a bronchodilating agent results in bronchial smooth muscle relaxation and the inhibition of chemical mediators released during hypersensitivity reactions. Albuterol or levalbuterol is an excellent choice because both have fewer cardiovascular side effects than other bronchodilators.

Glucose

Glucose preparations are used to treat hypoglycemia that results either from fasting or insulin/carbohydrate imbalance in a patient with diabetes mellitus. If the patient is conscious, carbohydrates may be administered orally. Treatment may include commercially available oral glucose that can be placed in the buccal fold or other sources such as orange juice, a chocolate bar, cake icing, or carbonated glucose-containing soft drinks, which act rapidly to restore circulating blood glucose. If the patient is unconscious and acute hypoglycemia is suspected, intravenous administration of 50% dextrose solution or intravenous or intramuscular administration of glucagon (which increases blood glucose by its effects on liver glycogen) is the treatment of choice. The treatment of hyperglycemia using insulin in not indicated in the dental office.

Aspirin

The antiplatelet properties of aspirin have been shown to decrease myocardial ischemia dramatically when administered to patients during an evolving myocardial infarction; aspirin has no substitute for this indication. Contraindications to aspirin use include patients with aspirin intolerance and patients with severe bleeding disorders.

Antihistamine

Antihistamines such as diphenhydramine are useful in the treatment of minor or delayed allergic reactions and as adjuncts in the management of an acute allergic or anaphylactoid reaction. Adverse effects of antihistamines include CNS depression resulting in sedation, thickening of tracheobronchial secretions, and decreased BP.

Respiratory stimulant

Aromatic ammonia is a pungent, noxious irritant to the mucous membranes and stimulates the respiratory and vasomotor centers of the medulla. It is used as a general arousal agent during syncope where the patient is still breathing.

Primary Support Drugs

Primary support drugs are helpful for treating medical emergencies that are usually not acutely life-threatening (Table 41-6). Although dentists do not have to include these drugs in the emergency kit, they are useful, particularly for situations in which the dentist is familiar with their use and where EMS may not be immediately available.

Anticonvulsant

Seizures that may require acute medical intervention may be associated with epilepsy, hyperventilation episodes, cerebrovascular accidents, hypoglycemic reactions, or vasodepressor syncope. Local anesthetic overdoses or accidental intravascular injection may also require the administration of an anticonvulsant. Current management of a seizure that interferes with ventilation or persists for longer than 5 minutes includes intravenous or intramuscular administration of benzodiazepines such as midazolam or diazepam.

Corticosteroid

Corticosteroids are used in the definitive management of acute allergic reactions and acute adrenal insufficiency. Even though the onset of even an intravenous corticosteroid, such as hydrocortisone sodium, is delayed, the drug can be useful in halting the progression of a major allergic or anaphylactoid reaction. The dentist may encounter what initially appears to be a syncopal episode but is actually the more serious problem of acute adrenal insufficiency in a patient taking long-term systemic corticosteroids to treat a chronic medical condition or a patient with primary adrenal insufficiency (i.e., Addison disease). For this life-threatening emergency, prompt diagnosis, BLS techniques, and infusion of corticosteroids are needed.

Anticholinergic

For the treatment of bradycardia, atropine is the first drug to consider. As an anticholinergic drug, it stimulates heart rate by blocking the action of the vagus nerve, thereby increasing firing of the SA node. In patients with myocardial ischemia and hypoxia, atropine should be used carefully because it increases oxygen demand of the heart and can worsen ischemia. The intravenous dosing for atropine is 0.5 mg every 3 to 5 minutes as needed, with a maximal total dosage of 3 mg (6 dosages).

Drugs for Advanced Cardiac Life Support

ACLS is the standard of care for comprehensive patient resuscitation by health care providers with advanced skills and training. Cardiac arrest and sudden cardiac death are major causes of mortality. Pharmacotherapy plays an important role in the ACLS management of these patients. Guidelines for ACLS provide recommendations for specific drug therapies. These guidelines are constantly reviewed and updated and are now subdivided into ACLS and pediatric advanced life support. Included in this training is the use of many antiarrhythmic and vasoactive drugs (Table 41-7). Training in ACLS is necessary for dentists administering deep sedation or general anesthesia and is often required by state law for providers of moderate sedation. State regulations should be consulted to determine which of the drugs described here must be available in locations where sedation or anesthesia is administered. Newer ACLS guidelines have reduced the emphasis on multiple medications, rhythm checks, and maneuvers that interrupt chest compressions for more than 10 seconds. Additionally, there is increased emphasis on searching for and addressing the cause of the cardiac arrest.

Pulseless arrest rhythms are divided into shockable and non-shockable rhythms (Fig. 41-1). Shockable rhythms are ventricular fibrillation (VF) or ventricular tachycardia (VT). In VT/VF, definitive therapy consists of BLS CPR with defibrillation. Drug therapy may be administered via intravenous, intraosseous, and endotracheal routes. If VT/VF persists, vasoactive drugs such as epinephrine or vasopressin or both are recommended to facilitate defibrillation. The antiarrhythmic, amiodarone, may also be indicated. Non-shockable pulseless arrest rhythms include asystole and pulseless electrical activity. These rhythms require drug therapy including epinephrine and vasopressin.

Symptomatic bradycardia is defined as a heart rate less than 60 beats/min combined with symptoms such as hypotension, altered mental status, chest pain, syncope, or other signs of shock. Besides basic CPR, atropine doses or epinephrine, dobutamine, or dopamine infusions may be indicated depending on the degree of atrioventricular (AV) block, followed by transcutaneous pacing if these medications are ineffective.

Symptomatic tachycardia is defined as a heart rate greater than 100 beats/min combined with symptoms of shock. Treatment can range from immediate synchronized cardioversion to drug therapy. Treatment for stable patients is based on the classification of the rhythm into narrow-complex or wide-complex tachycardia. Vagal maneuvers, administration of adenosine, or administration of second-line drugs such as calcium channel blockers or β blockers may be considered. These drugs should not be used for Wolff-Parkinson-White syndrome.

Regular, **wide-complex tachycardias** (QRS >0.12 second) include VT, supraventricular tachycardia with aberrancy, and tachycardias associated with or mediated by accessory pathways. Immediate synchronized cardioversion is performed for unstable supraventricular tachycardia owing to reentry, unstable atrial fibrillation, unstable flutter, and unstable monomorphic VT. Adenosine is recommended for wide-complex tachycardias that are believed to be supraventricular tachycardia. If the tachycardia is VT and the patient is stable, an antiarrhythmic drug, such as amiodarone or procainamide, may be given.

TABLE 41-7 Advanced Cardiac Life Support Drugs

Drug	Indication
Antiarrhythmics	
Lidocaine	Ventricular tachycardia, pulseless ventricular tachycardia, or ventricular fibrillation
Amiodarone	Pulseless ventricular tachycardia or ventricular fibrillation, supraventricular tachycardia (most forms)
Procainamide	Intermittent/recurrent ventricular tachycardia
Verapamil, diltiazem	Atrial flutter or atrial fibrillation, supraventricular tachycardia
Adenosine	Supraventricular tachycardia
Atropine	Bradycardia, asystole, certain types of atrioventricular block
Magnesium sulfate	Torsades de pointes, ventricular fibrillation (if hypomagnesemia is present)
β Blockers (e.g., propranolol)	Atrial flutter or atrial fibrillation, supraventricular tachycardia, refractory ventricular tachycardia
Inotropes	
Epinephrine	Anaphylactic shock, asystole, pulseless electrical activity, pulseless ventricular tachycardia or ventricular fibrillation, bradycardia
Vasopressin	Pulseless ventricular tachycardia or ventricular fibrillation
Norepinephrine	Refractory hypotension
Dopamine	Bradycardia, hypotension
Dobutamine	Congestive heart failure
Isoproterenol	Refractory symptomatic bradycardia, long QT syndrome
Digoxin	Atrial flutter, fibrillation, heart failure
Inamrinone	Refractory congestive heart failure
Milrinone	Refractory congestive heart failure
Vasodilators/Antihypertensives	
Nitroprusside	Hypertension, acute heart failure
Nitroglycerin	Hypertension, acute heart failure, angina pain
Others	
Sodium bicarbonate	Hyperkalemia, metabolic acidosis with bicarbonate loss, hypoxic lactic acidosis
Morphine	Acute pulmonary edema, pain, and anxiety
Furosemide	Acute pulmonary edema
Thrombolytic agents (e.g., alteplase, streptokinase)	Acute thrombosis

Antiarrhythmic agents

Beyond defibrillation, which is the only proven intervention to achieve return of spontaneous circulation in patients experiencing VF, antiarrhythmic drugs have been advocated as adjunctive treatments potentially to normalize abnormally depolarizing and conducting myocardial cells. Amiodarone is recommended for the treatment of VF or pulseless VT unresponsive to other measures. Amiodarone is a complex drug that acts on Na^+, K^+, and Ca^{++} channels and has α-adrenergic–blocking and β-adrenergic–blocking properties. In the emergency setting, it is administered as an intravenous bolus of 150 mg over 10 minutes followed by an initial maintenance infusion of 1 mg/min. The patient should be monitored carefully for hypotension and bradycardia.

Lidocaine, a class IB antiarrhythmic, acts by inhibiting the ion flux via Na^+ channels and has been used for years for pulseless VT/VF. It

Adult Cardiac Arrest Circular Algorithm–2015 Update

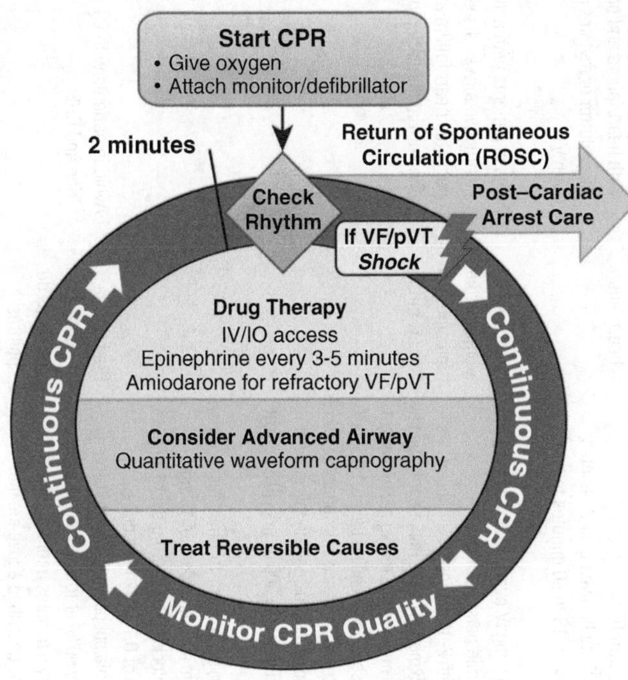

CPR Quality

- Push hard (at least 2 inches [5 cm]) and fast (100-120/min) and allow complete chest recoil.
- Minimize interruptions in compressions.
- Avoid excessive ventilation.
- Rotate compressor every 2 minutes, or sooner if fatigued.
- If no advanced airway, 30:2 compression-ventilation ratio.
- Quantitative waveform capnography
  – If P_{ETCO_2} <10 mm Hg, attempt to improve CPR quality
- Intra-arterial pressure.
  – If relaxation phase (diastolic) pressure <20 mm Hg, attempt to improve CPR quality.

Shock Energy for Defibrillation

- **Biphasic:** Manufacturer recommendation (eg, initial dose of 120-200 J); if unknown, use maximum available. Second and subsequent doses should be equivalent, and higher doses may be considered.
- **Monophasic:** 360 J

Drug Therapy

- **Epinephrine IV/IO dose:** 1 mg every 3-5 minutes
- **Amiodarone IV/IO dose:** First dose: 300 mg bolus. Second dose: 150 mg.

Advanced Airway

- Endotracheal intubation or supraglottic advanced airway
- Waveform capnography or capnometry to confirm and monitor ET tube placement
- Once advanced airway in place, give 1 breath every 6 seconds (10 breaths/min) with continuous chest compressions

Return of Spontaneous Circulation (ROSC)

- Pulse and blood pressure
- Abrupt sustained increase in P_{ETCO_2} (typically ≥40 mm Hg)
- Spontaneous arterial pressure waves with intra-arterial monitoring

Reversible Causes

- **H**ypovolemia
- **H**ypoxia
- **H**ydrogen ion (acidosis)
- **H**ypo-/hyperkalemia
- **H**ypothermia
- **T**ension pneumothorax
- **T**amponade, cardiac
- **T**oxins
- **T**hrombosis, pulmonary
- **T**hrombosis, coronary

FIG 41-1 Adult cardiac arrest treatment. *IO*, Interosseous; *J*, Joule; *PETCO₂*, partial pressure of end tidal CO_2; *VF*, ventricular fibrillation; *VT*, ventricular tachycardia. See American Heart Association Guidelines 2015, Web-based Integrated 2010 & 2015 American Heart Association Guidelines for Cardiopulmonary Resuscitation and Emergency Cardiovascular Care, Part 7: Adult Advanced Cardiovascular Life Support https://eccguidelines.heart.org/wp-content/themes/eccstaging/dompdf-master/pdffiles/part-7-adult-advanced-cardiovascular-life-support.pdf (accessed July 14, 2016).

has been relegated more recently to an alternative drug for the treatment of VF and pulseless VT, but it still has utility as an alternative to amiodarone when amiodarone is unavailable.

Verapamil and diltiazem are nondihydropyridine Ca^{++} channel blockers that inhibit extracellular Ca^{++} influx through slow Ca^{++} channels, inhibiting automaticity in the sinoatrial node and conduction via the AV node. Verapamil is used to terminate reentrant tachyarrhythmias that require AV nodal conduction for their continuation and to control the ventricular rate in patients with atrial fibrillation or flutter or multifocal atrial tachycardia. Diltiazem is used for the same indications, but it seems to produce less myocardial depression than verapamil. Because of its narrow safety margin, digitalis has been largely superseded by Ca^{++} channel blockers and β blockers to manage acute atrial fibrillation.

Adenosine is an endogenous purine nucleoside that acts by temporarily depressing AV and sinus node activity. It is an important drug for controlling AV nodal reentrant tachycardia and junctional tachycardias. Bolus administration is indicated for paroxysmal supraventricular tachycardia.

Atropine inhibits cholinergic responses that decrease heart rate and systemic vascular resistance and is used to increase heart rate during periods of symptomatic sinus bradycardia resulting from excessive parasympathetic nervous system activity. Because atropine can increase myocardial oxygen demand, precipitate tachyarrhythmias, and expand the zone of infarction, it must be used carefully in patients with presumptive myocardial infarction.

Hypotensive patients may require a continuous infusion of a powerful inotrope or vasopressor for hemodynamic support. Typical infusions include epinephrine, dopamine, dobutamine, phenylephrine, norepinephrine, or vasopressin.

Mg^{++} replacement is advocated when hypomagnesemia is present. Hypomagnesemia can precipitate polymorphic VT (torsades de pointes) and VF.

β-Adrenergic blockers, such as atenolol, metoprolol, propranolol, and esmolol, may enhance the benefits of thrombolytic agents in patients receiving these agents and have been shown to reduce the incidence of VF in post–myocardial infarction patients not receiving thrombolytic agents. These drugs are also used to control the ventricular rate in the presence of atrial tachyarrhythmias. Adverse effects of β-adrenergic blockers relate to their actions on the cardiac conduction system and exacerbation of bronchospasm in patients with preexisting lung disease.

Summaries of core antiarrhythmic agents used for ACLS in situations of tachycardia, are found in Table 41-8.

TABLE 41-8 IV Drugs Used for Tachycardia

Drug	Characteristics	Indication(s)	Dosing	Side Effects	Precautions or Special Considerations
Intravenous Drugs Used to Treat Supraventricular Tachyarrhythmias					
Adenosine	Endogenous purine nucleoside; briefly depresses sinus node rate and AV node conduction; vasodilator	• Stable, narrow-complex regular tachycardias • Unstable narrow-complex regular tachycardias while preparations are made for electrical cardioversion • Stable, regular, monomorphic, wide complex tachycardia as a therapeutic and diagnostic maneuver	6 mg IV as a rapid IV push followed by a 20 mL saline flush; repeat if required as 12 mg IV push	Hypotension, bronchospasm, chest discomfort	Contraindicated in patients with asthma; may precipitate atrial fibrillation, which may be very rapid in patients with WPW; thus a defibrillator should be readily available; reduce dose in post–cardiac transplant patients, those taking dipyridamole or carbamazepine and when administered via a central vein
Diltiazem, Verapamil	Non-dihydropyridine calcium channel blockers; slow AV node conduction and increase AV node refractoriness; vasodilators, negative inotropes	• Stable, narrow-complex tachycardias if rhythm remains uncontrolled or unconverted by adenosine or vagal maneuvers or if SVT is recurrent • Control ventricular rate in patients with atrial fibrillation or atrial flutter	Diltiazem: Initial dose 15 to 20 mg (0.25 mg/kg) IV over 2 minutes; additional 20 to 25 mg (0.35 mg/kg) IV in 15 minutes if needed; 5 to 15 mg/h IV maintenance infusion (titrated to AF heart rate if given for rate control) Verapamil: Initial dose 2.5 to 5 mg IV given over 2 minutes; may repeat as 5 to 10 mg every 15 to 30 minutes to total dose of 20 to 30 mg	Hypotension, bradycardia, precipitation of heart failure	Should only be given to patients with narrow-complex tachycardias (regular or irregular). Avoid in patients with heart failure and pre-excited AF or flutter or rhythms consistent with VT
Atenolol, Esmolol, Metoprolol, Propranolol	β-Blockers; reduce effects of circulating catecholamines; reduce heart rate, AV node conduction and blood pressure; negative inotropes	• Stable, narrow-complex tachycardias if rhythm remains uncontrolled or unconverted by adenosine or vagal maneuvers or if SVT is recurrent • Control ventricular rate in patients with atrial fibrillation or atrial flutter • Certain forms of polymorphic VT (associated with acute ischemia, familial LQTS, catecholaminergic)	Atenolol (β1 specific blocker) 5 mg IV over 5 minutes; repeat 5 mg in 10 minutes if arrhythmia persists or recurs Esmolol (β1 specific blocker with 2- to 9-minute half-life) IV loading dose 500 mcg/kg (0.5 mg/kg) over 1 minute, followed by an infusion of 50 mcg/kg per minute (0.05 mg/kg per minute); if response is inadequate, infuse second loading bolus of 0.5 mg/kg over 1 minute and increase maintenance infusion to 100 mcg/kg (0.1 mg/kg) per minute; increment; increase in this manner if required to maximum infusion rate of 300 mcg/kg [0.3 mg/kg] per minute Metoprolol (β1 specific blocker) 5 mg over 1 to 2 minutes repeated as required every 5 minutes to maximum dose of 15 mg Propranolol (nonselective β-blocker) 0.5 to 1 mg over 1 minute, repeated up to a total dose of 0.1 mg/kg if required	Hypotension, bradycardia, precipitation of heart failure	Avoid in patients with asthma, obstructive airway disease, decompensated heart failure and pre-excited artrial fibrillation or flutter
Procainamide	Sodium and potassium channel blocker	• Pre-excited atrial fibrillation	20 to 50 mg/min until arrhythmia suppressed, hypotension ensues, or QRS prolonged by 50%, or total cumulative dose of 17 mg/kg; or 100 mg every 5 minutes until arrhythmia is controlled or other conditions described above are met	Bradycardia, hypotension, torsades de pointes	Avoid in patients with QT prolongation and CHF

Amiodarone	Multichannel blocker (sodium, potassium, calcium channel, and noncompetitive α/β-blocker)	• Stable irregular narrow complex tachycardia (atrial fibrillation) • Stable regular narrow-complex tachycardia • To control rapid ventricular rate due to accessory pathway conduction in pre-excited atrial arrhythmias	150 mg given over 10 minutes and repeated if necessary, followed by a 1 mg/min infusion for 6 hours, followed by 0.5 mg/min. Total dose over 24 hours should not exceed 2.2 g.	Bradycardia, hypotension, phlebitis	
Digoxin	Cardiac glycoside with positive inotropic effects; slows AV node conduction by enhancing parasympathetic tone; slow onset of action	• Stable, narrow-complex regular tachycardias if rhythm remains uncontrolled or unconverted by adenosine or vagal maneuvers or if SVT is recurrent • Control ventricular rate in patients with atrial fibrillation or atrial flutter	8 to 12 mcg/kg total loading dose, half of which is administered initially over 5 minutes, and remaining portion as 25% fractions at 4- to 8- hour intervals	Bradycardia	Slow onset of action and relative low potency renders it less useful for treatment of acute arrhythmias
Intravenous Drugs Used to Treat Ventricular Tachyarrhythmias					
Procainamide	Sodium and potassium channel blocker	• Hemodynamically stable monomorphic VT	20 to 50 mg/min until arrhythmia suppressed, hypotension ensues, or QRS prolonged by 50%, or total cumulative dose of 17 mg/kg; or 100 mg every 5 minutes until arrhythmia is controlled or other conditions described above are met	Bradycardia, hypotension, torsades de pointes	Avoid in patients with QT prolongation and CHF
Amiodarone	Multichannel blocker (sodium, potassium, calcium channel, and noncompetitive α/β-blocker)	• Hemodynamically stable monomorphic VT • Polymorphic VT with normal QT interval	150 mg given over 10 minutes and repeated if necessary, followed by a 1 mg/min infusion for 6 hours, followed by 0.5 mg/min. Total dose over 24 hours should not exceed 2.2 g.	Bradycardia, hypotension, phlebitis	
Sotalol	Potassium channel blocker and nonselective β-blocker	• Hemodynamically stable monomorphic VT	In clinical studies 1.5 mg/kg infused over 5 minutes; however, US package labeling recommends any dose of the drug should be infused slowly over a period of 5 hours	Bradycardia, hypotension, torsades de pointes	Avoid in patients with QT prolongation and CHF
Lidocaine	Relatively weak sodium channel blocker	• Hemodynamically stable monomorphic VT	Initial dose range from 1 to 1.5 mg/kg IV; repeated if required at 0.5 to 0.75 mg/kg IV every 5 to 10 minutes up to maximum cumulative dose of 3 mg/kg; 1 to 4 mg/min (30 to 50 mcg/kg per minute) maintenance infusion	Slurred speech, altered consciousness, seizures, bradycardia	
Magnesium	Cofactor in variety of cell processes including control of sodium and potassium transport	• Polymorphic VT associated with QT prolongation (torsades de pointes)	1 to 2 g IV over 15 minutes	Hypotension, CNS toxicity, respiratory depression	Follow magnesium levels if frequent or prolonged dosing required, particularly in patients with impaired renal function

AF, Atrial fibrillation; *CHS*, congestive heart failure; *IV*, intravenous; *LQTS*, long QT syndrome; *SVT*, supraventricular tachycardia; *VF*, ventricular fibrillation; *VT*, ventricular tachycardia; *WPW*, Wolff-Parkinson-White Syndrome.

Note: Amiodarone, lidocaine and magnesium can be administered by intraosseous administration in certain circumstances.

See American Heart Association Guidelines 2015, Web-based Integrated 2010 & 2015 American Heart Association Guidelines for Cardiopulmonary Resuscitation and Emergency Cardiovascular Care, Part 7: Adult Advanced Cardiovascular Life Support https://eccguidelines.heart.org/wp-content/themes/eccstaging/dompdf-master/pdffiles/part-7-adult-advanced-cardiovascular-life-support.pdf (accessed July 14, 2016).

Vasoactive drugs

In the absence of adequate circulation, **vasoconstricting drugs such as catecholamines or vasopressin may enhance organ perfusion by increasing arterial and aortic pressures**, resulting in desirable increases in cerebral and coronary perfusion pressures, while reducing blood flow to visceral and muscle tissues. Indications for their use include ischemic heart disease, acute heart failure, cardiogenic shock, and cardiac arrest.

Epinephrine is currently the preferred initial catecholamine recommended in ACLS for pulseless VT/VF, asystole, and pulseless electrical activity arrest (Table 41-9). The benefits of epinephrine in this application are its ability to cause vasoconstriction, to act as a cardiotonic, and to facilitate cardiac perfusion during CPR, thus increasing the success of defibrillation.

Vasopressin causes peripheral vasoconstriction by stimulation of vasopressin receptors located in skin and skeletal muscle and vasopressin receptors located in the mesenteric circulation, resulting in shunting of blood to vital organs. In addition, vasopressin potentiates the effects of catecholamines, enhancing vasoconstriction and resulting in greater coronary perfusion, which leads to more effective CPR and greater survival.

Hypotensive patients may require a continuous infusion of a powerful inotrope or vasopressor for hemodynamic support. Typical infusions include epinephrine, dopamine, dobutamine, phenylephrine, norepinephrine, or vasopressin.

Norepinephrine is indicated in patients with low peripheral resistance and severe hypotension. Under these conditions, the drug is a potent vasoconstrictor and inotropic agent. Sloughing and necrosis of tissues may occur if extravasation occurs during administration. Dopamine is a chemical precursor of norepinephrine and has α_1-adrenergic–stimulating and β_1-adrenergic–stimulating properties. Specific dopaminergic receptors also contribute to the drug's cardiovascular pharmacologic characteristics. Indications for dopamine include certain types of shock, such as that associated with heart failure. Dobutamine is a synthetic catecholamine and potent inotrope used in the treatment of heart failure when signs and symptoms of shock are absent. Inamrinone and milrinone are nonadrenergic cardiotonic agents that also cause vasodilation with hemodynamic effects similar to dobutamine. They increase cardiac function and induce peripheral vasodilation. Calcium chloride was initially thought to be beneficial during resuscitation by increasing myocardial contractility, but studies have shown that high concentrations of Ca^{++} may be detrimental.

Vasodilators

Intravenous nitroglycerin permits controlled titration in relaxing vascular smooth muscle. This drug may cause severe hypotension when administered to a hypovolemic patient. Sodium nitroprusside is an extremely potent, rapidly acting, direct peripheral vasodilator. It is used for the treatment of acute heart failure and hypertensive emergencies.

Sodium bicarbonate

Sodium bicarbonate is administered intravenously to correct metabolic acidosis occurring during protracted resuscitative efforts. The use of this drug should be guided by blood gas analysis if possible.

Diuretics

Diuretics such as furosemide are used intravenously for their venodilating and diuretic effects for the treatment of acute pulmonary edema and cerebral edema after cardiac arrest.

Morphine

Morphine is the opioid of choice to manage ischemic chest pain and acute pulmonary edema. The drug is titrated in small intravenous or intramuscular doses to avoid respiratory depression.

Thrombolytic agents

Thrombolytic therapy is often instituted early in evolving myocardial infarction to promote fibrin digestion and clot dissolution. Many studies are being conducted with streptokinase, urokinase, anistreplase, and alteplase to determine their respective roles in the early treatment of myocardial infarction.

Emergency Drugs Specific to Sedation and Anesthesia

Supplementary drugs are additional emergency drugs that must be available when certain sedative or anesthetic drugs are administered. They include drugs that are used to reverse untoward effects of anesthetics and others that are used to treat specific medical conditions that may occur during anesthesia (Table 41-10).

Naloxone is a specific opioid antagonist that reverses opioid-induced respiratory depression. It is mandatory in practices where parenteral opioids are administered. Flumazenil is a specific benzodiazepine antagonist that reverses sedation and respiratory depression resulting from benzodiazepine administration. Succinylcholine is used to overcome laryngospasm during deep sedation/general anesthesia by

TABLE 41-9 Use of Epinephrine in Advanced Cardiac Life Support

Characteristics	Indications	Dosing	Side Effects	Precautions
Non-selective α- and β-adrenergic receptor agonist	Pulseless VT of VF	1 mg IV or IO, repeat every 3-5 minutes	Excessive increase in heart rate and blood pressure. Increased myocardial oxygen demand	Use with caution in cases of myocardial infarction
	Symptomatic bradycardia	2-10 mcg/min in a continuous infusion		
	Asystole	1 mg IV or IO, repeat every 3-5 minutes		

IO, Intraosseous; *IV*, intravenous; *VF*, ventricular fibrillation; *VT*, ventricular tachycardia.

TABLE 41-10 Drugs for Reversal of Sedation and Anesthesia Agents

Drug	Indication	Mode of Action	Route of Administration
Naloxone	Respiratory depression; oversedation	Opioid antagonist	Intravenous or intramuscular
Flumazenil	Respiratory depression; oversedation	Benzodiazepine antagonist	Intravenous
Succinylcholine	Laryngospasm	Skeletal muscle relaxant	Intravenous or intramuscular
Dantrolene sodium	Malignant hyperthermia	Prevents Ca^{++} release in muscle cell	Intravenous

relaxing skeletal muscle controlling the vocal cords. Succinylcholine is also used to treat fentanyl-induced chest wall rigidity. It should be used only by practitioners with advanced anesthesia training. Dantrolene arrests the development of malignant hyperthermia syndrome, a genetically transmitted disorder of excessive Ca^{++} release in skeletal muscle occurring during general anesthesia in which succinylcholine or volatile inhalation anesthetics are routinely administered.

The use of parenteral vasopressors to treat hypotension may be indicated during anesthesia. Some vasopressors, such as methoxamine and phenylephrine, increase BP by causing peripheral vasoconstriction selectively, whereas ephedrine acts by a combination of peripheral vasoconstriction and cardiac stimulation.

CASE STUDY DISCUSSION

This is a major medical emergency and an immediate call for help should be instituted. The patient should be placed in a semi-sitting position to allow for better utilization of the accessory muscles of respiratory. Oxygen should be administered via a nonrebreathing mask. Epinephrine, 0.3 mg of a 1:1000 solution, should be injected intramuscularly via an auto-injector or with a 1-ml tuberculin syringe with an intramuscular needle after drawing up from the vial. Vital signs should be continuously monitored until help has arrived.

GENERAL REFERENCES

1. Web-based Integrated 2010 & 2015 American Heart Association Guidelines for Cardiopulmonary Resuscitation and Emergency Cardiovascular Care, Part 7: Adult Advanced Cardiovascular Life Support https://eccguidelines.heart.org/wp-content/themes/eccstaging/dompdf-master/pdffiles/part-7-adult-advanced-cardiovascular-life-support.pdf (accessed July 14, 2016).
2. DeAngelis AF, Barrowman RA, Harrod R, Nastri AL: Review article: maxillofacial emergencies: oral pain and odontogenic infections, *Emerg Med Australas* 26(4):336–342, August 2014, http://dx.doi.org/10.1111/1742-6723.12266.
3. Gesek Jr DJ: Respiratory anesthetic emergencies in oral and maxillofacial surgery, *Oral Maxillofac Surg Clin North Am* 25(3):479–486, August 2013.
4. Haas DA: Emergency drugs, *Dent Clin North Am* 46(4):815–830, October 2002.
5. Josell SD, Abrams RG: Managing common dental problems and emergencies, *Pediatr Clin North Am* 38(5):1325–1342, October 1991.
6. Maher NG, de Looze J, Hoffman GR: Anaphylaxis: an update for dental practitioners, *Aust Dent J* 59(2):142–148, June 2014.

42

Clinical Rationale for and Significance of Prescription Writing

Vahn A. Lewis

KEY INFORMATION

- A prescription is an order transmitted from the prescriber to a qualified supplier of a treatment for the benefit of a patient.
- A drug prescription for a patient requires thoughtful crafting to provide safe and effective treatment and to avoid unnecessary adverse actions or drug interactions.
- The prescription is a legal document; it is regulated by medical and legal considerations.
- The requirements for prescribing change with time, and it is the practitioner's duty to keep current with these requirements.
- Electronic databases and prescribing systems are part of current practice and available to facilitate and assist with the challenges in prescribing.
- The process of prescribing has many stakeholders; prescribing can be restricted by the needs of these various parties.

CASE STUDY

JP Dentist is treating Ms. S., his dental patient who has cellulitis and fever due to abscessed tooth #1. He notes that the patient is 35 years old and weighs 130 lbs. He notes that the patient is taking omeprazole, to treat a bleeding gastric ulcer. The patient has pain and fever. He knows from practice that a facial cellulitis can be dangerous.

JP considers the case and decides to treat this infection with an antibiotic and also wants to treat the patient for moderate pain while the infection is resolving. He prescribes amoxicillin, 500 mg every 8 hours to be taken for the next 7 days to treat the infection. He calculates that he will need to supply the patient with 21 tablets to complete the therapy. In addition, the patient may experience moderate pain that may last a few days while the antibiotic treatment is being given. He decides to treat the patient with acetaminophen/codeine (Tylenol #3), one tablet every 4 hours for 3 days. He calculates that it will take 18 tablets to complete this course of therapy for 3 days. He writes his prescriptions, following the laws that regulate prescribing controlled substances. After writing the prescriptions, what should JP Dentist discuss with Ms. S.?

PRESCRIPTION

A **prescription** is a written, verbal, or electronic order for medication to be used for the diagnosis, prevention, or treatment of a specific patient's disease by a licensed physician, dentist, podiatrist, or veterinarian. In some states, a prescription may also be written by appropriately trained persons from other medical professions. A prescription is a legal document for which the prescriber and the pharmacist are responsible. Prescriptions are subject to state, federal, and local regulations, with multiple stakeholders at each level.

The writing of a prescription is one step in many that must be properly performed to initiate a course of therapy (Fig. 42-1). This process starts with establishing a proper prescriber–patient relationship, which includes patient identification, proper diagnostic procedures, presentation and discussion of a treatment plan to the patient, availability of counseling, and follow-up care. Prescribing outside the proper prescriber–patient relationship is unprofessional conduct. These fundamental concepts have been reasserted recently with respect to prescribing for patients on the Internet who are unknown to the practitioner (thus there is no prescriber–patient relationship). A prescription is **prima facie** evidence in court that such a relationship exists.

Selection of therapy requires a multitude of factors to be considered: factors related to the patient (e.g., has difficulty swallowing tablets, age, gender) and the therapeutic goal (cure or symptom control); evaluation of drug interactions; recognition of the various relationships among the patient, prescriber, and insurance companies and governmental bodies (that may establish guidelines or limits on payment for medications); and the medication costs and whether the patient can afford to buy it. There are increasing concerns about drug availability or purity of medications. Prescribing should be done in a thoughtful and deliberate way, and the conditions for error-free prescribing must be ensured. In 1999, The **Institute of Medicine** report "To Err is Human" documented a concern about medical errors. The report analyzed the nature of errors and categorized them into slips, lapses, and mistakes. Slips and lapses occur when the prescriber knows the correct procedure but fails to perform it properly. Mistakes result from incorrect understanding of the correct course of action.

Slips and lapses can be influenced by the conditions under which the prescribing is done, interruptions during the writing of the prescription, or writing an incorrect drug name from memory, although the intended drug choice was sound. In this regard, several suggestions were made, including standardizing prescribing rules, using automated prescriber drug order entry systems and pharmaceutical software, having necessary patient information available at the point of care, and improving the patient's knowledge about his or her treatment. Some areas in which errors often occur include poor handwriting, incorrect calculation of pediatric drug doses, look-alike drug name mix-ups, prescriptions for drugs to which the patient is allergic or intolerant, inappropriate dosage forms, and failure to appreciate toxicity of each drug in drug combinations. There is a relationship between increased

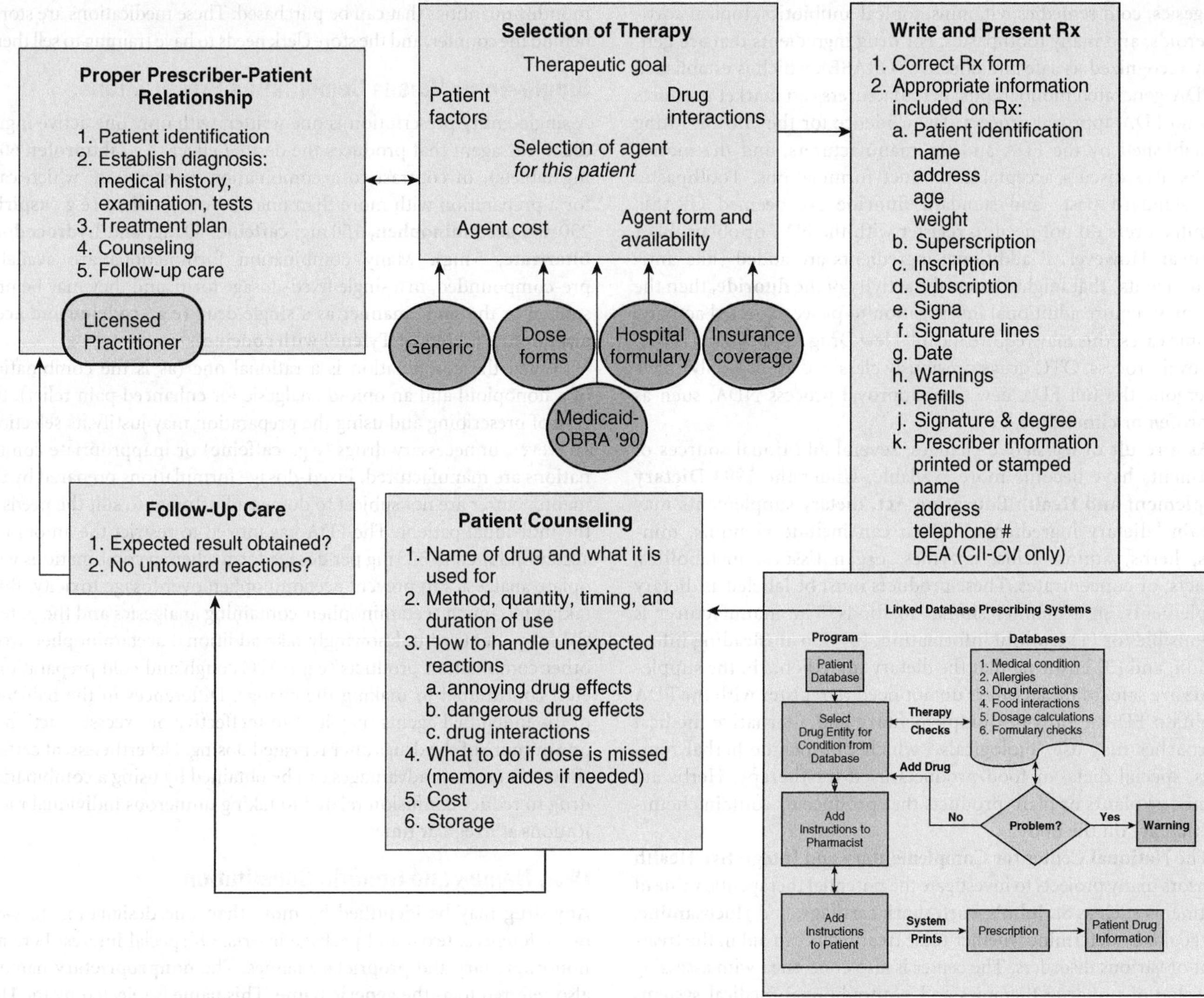

FIG 42-1 Steps involved in proper prescribing. After selecting the correct therapy, the prescriber must fill out the various components of the prescription to meet professional and legal requirements established by state, federal, and professional organizations. The next step is to present the prescription to the patient and provide the name of the drug and what it is being prescribed for, how to take it, what kinds of untoward effects the patient might expect, and what the patient should do about them if they occur. Some discussion of storage and cost of the medication may be included when indicated. After the presentation of the prescription, it is still important to monitor the progress of the patient. If the therapeutic goals are not being achieved, the process may need to be started over. *OBRA,* Omnibus Budget Reconciliation Act.

admissions (practitioner overloading) and increased errors. New errors also occur as new therapeutic entities and/or dosage forms are introduced. Surveys of prescriptions find errors not only within single prescriptions but also between multiple prescriptions for the same patient in the form of drug interactions or incompatibilities.

Legal Categories of Drugs

Drugs may be categorized according to legal restrictions governing their use as **over-the-counter** (**OTC**), prescription (synonyms: **legend, dangerous, Rx only**), or **controlled drugs**. As determined by the **U.S. Food and Drug Administration** (**FDA**), a prescription drug (now designated "**Rx only**") is one that requires a prescription to be dispensed by a pharmacist, whereas an OTC drug can be purchased without a prescription. Several state laws refer to prescription drugs as "legend" or "dangerous" drugs, meaning that they are unsafe for use except under the supervision of a licensed practitioner and available only by prescription. The legend that is on the dispensed agent reads: "Caution: Federal law prohibits dispensing without prescription." Drugs such as antibiotics, local anesthetics, and systemic corticosteroids are examples of prescription drugs.

Drugs with an abuse potential, called **controlled substances**, have additional restrictions placed on their use. The **Drug Enforcement Administration** of the Department of Justice is responsible for identifying and regulating such drugs. Controlled substances may be OTC, prescription, or unavailable for medical use. Examples of controlled drugs include opioids, such as **codeine** or **morphine**, that are characterized as having medical use, or **heroin**, characterized as having no accepted medical use in the United States. Most controlled substances have their principal site of action in the central nervous system. The widely abused anabolic steroids are an important exception to this rule and are controlled substances.

OTC agents are deemed to be safe and effective without professional guidance when used according to their labeled instructions. Examples of OTC (nonprescription drugs) include some nonopioid analgesics, cold remedies, vitamins, topical antibiotics, topical corticosteroids, and many toothpastes. For drug ingredients that are generally recognized as safe and effective (**GRASE**), which is established by FDA-generated monographs, manufacturers can market products with no FDA approval process. The evidence for the GRASE rating is established by the FDA and the manufacturers, and the monographs also discuss acceptable product formulations. Toothpastes with standard paste and standard **fluoride** are deemed GRASE. Manufacturers do not need to register with the FDA or obtain FDA approval. However, if additional ingredients are added (like antiplaque agents) that might change the activity of the **fluoride**, then the FDA may require additional investigation to prove expected activity. In some cases, this may require the full New Drug Application (NDA) approval process. OTC drugs previously classified as "RX only" have undergone the full FDA new drug approval process NDA, such as **ibuprofen** or **cimetidine**.

As a result of legislative changes, several additional sources of treatments have become more available. Under the 1994 **Dietary Supplement and Health Education Act**, dietary supplements may contain "dietary ingredients," which can include vitamins, minerals, herbs, amino acids, enzymes, organ tissues, metabolites, extracts, or concentrates. These products must be labeled as dietary supplements, in a manner similar to foods. The manufacturer is responsible for (1) truthful information, (2) non-misleading information, and (3) ensuring that the dietary ingredients in the supplements are safe. Manufacturers do not need to register with the FDA or obtain FDA approval. Complementary and alternative medical approaches may use "biologicals," which can include herbal remedies, special diets, or food products used for therapy. Herbs are defined as plants or plant products that produce or contain chemicals that act on the body.

The **National Center for Complementary and Integrative Health** sponsors many projects to investigate the potential therapeutic value of treatments such as **St. John's wort, shark cartilage**, and **glucosamine**. The goal is to determine whether these treatments can aid in the treatment of various disorders. The center is also concerned with assessing the value of nondrug therapies and nontraditional medical systems such as acupuncture, Eastern medicine, and homeopathic medicine. The FDA can provide guidelines for the therapeutic claims made for these various products through the Center for Food Safety and Applied Nutrition, whose role is primarily educational.

The **United States Pharmacopeia (USP)** has developed a **Dietary Supplement Verification** (DSV) Program. For a dietary supplement to bear the **USP-DSV** seal, it must include its ingredients on the label, indicate the strength and amounts of ingredients, prove that the product is shown to be absorbable when taken, document that it has been screened for heavy metals, microbes, and pesticides, and confirm that it has been manufactured in safe, sanitary, and controlled conditions. The need for verification has been emphasized in 2015 by New York State's issuing Cease and Desist orders for the sale of several dietary supplements that failed to contain any DNA fingerprint evidence that they contained the labeled drug. Also, the FDA issued a warning to health care professionals on the dangers of using probiotic dietary supplements in hospitals after a premature infant died after receiving a dietary supplement probiotic tainted with *Rhizopus oryzae* fungus. Dietary supplements are sometimes contaminated with various unlabeled prescription drugs (and thus mislabeled); an example is an herbal promoted for "male enhancement" containing **sildenafil,** an "Rx only" drug.

A new class of drugs has been created by the **Combat Methamphetamine Epidemic Act** of 2005, which created restrictions for the sale of ephedrines and phenylpropanolamine from retail stores. These products require the buyer to present identification and limit the monthly quantities that can be purchased. These medications are stored behind the counter, and the store clerk needs to have training to sell them.

Single-Entity Versus Combination Prescriptions

A single-entity prescription is one written with only one active ingredient, the agent that produces the desired effect (e.g., **ibuprofen** 600-mg tablets), in contrast to a combination prescription, which calls for a preparation with more than one active ingredient (e.g., **aspirin,** 230 mg; **acetaminophen**, 150 mg; **caffeine**, 30 mg; and **hydrocodone bitartrate**, 5 mg). Many combination formulations are available pre-compounded, in a single fixed-dosage form, and they may be prescribed in the same manner as a single drug (e.g., **codeine and acetaminophen tablets** or **Tylenol with codeine**).

When the combination is a rational one (as is the combination of a nonopioid and an opioid analgesic for enhanced pain relief), the ease of prescribing and using the preparation may justify its selection. However, unnecessary drugs (e.g., **caffeine**) or inappropriate combinations are manufactured. Fixed-dosage formulations prepared by the manufacturer are not subject to dosage adjustment to suit the needs of the individual patient. The FDA has moved to restrict the amount of acetaminophen to 325 mg per dosage form when in combinations with opiate analgesics to prevent acetaminophen overdosage toxicity. Both taking too much acetaminophen-containing analgesics and the potential for patients to unknowingly take additional acetaminophen from other combination products (e.g., OTC cough and cold preparations, etc.) contributed to making the change. Differences in the half-lives of the individual agents may lead to ineffective or excessive action of one or more of the drugs after repeated dosing. Nevertheless, at certain times, therapeutic advantages can be obtained by using a combination drug to reduce confusion related to taking numerous individual medications at irregular times.

Drug Names and Generic Substitution

Any drug may be identified by more than one designation in various references, texts, and package inserts. Of special interest here are nonproprietary and proprietary names. The **nonproprietary** name is also referred to as the **generic name.** This name is selected by the **U.S. Adopted Names Council**, a body hosted by the American Medical Association. The steady increase in the number of new drugs and the marketing of existing drugs by different manufacturers are making similarities between different drug names an increasing challenge. The practitioner must be vigilant in prescribing the correct agent and spelling drug names correctly. Because, with few exceptions, individual drugs have only one nonproprietary name, it is this name by which the drug is primarily identified. Nonproprietary names may differ among countries (e.g., **the United States uses acetaminophen, whereas England uses paracetamol**). The same agent may also have many **proprietary** or **trade names**, which are given to it by the various manufacturers or marketers to identify their brand of the drug. In advertisements and labeling with the trade name, the nonproprietary name of the drug must also be prominently identified.

In recent years, governmental regulatory agencies have had a strong tendency to encourage or mandate the prescription and dispensation of drugs by nonproprietary name. The principal motivation for these regulations is to control rapidly increasing drug costs. Currently, all states and the District of Columbia have repealed their existing anti-substitution laws and replaced them with drug substitution laws permitting or, in some states, requiring the pharmacist to dispense lower cost generic drugs (preparations containing the same active chemicals in identical amounts but sold under the common nonproprietary name), unless specifically prohibited by the prescriber. Also, the federal government has instituted "maximum allowable cost" programs in an effort to contain the cost of prescription drugs to the consumer by limiting prescription by proprietary name. These programs require the prescriber to certify the necessity of prescribing a specific brand of drug by hand writing "**Brand necessary**" or "**Brand medically necessary**" rather than its nonproprietary counterpart. According to the FDA, the savings may range from 30% to 80%. Recently, some low-cost generics have undergone very large increases in price, from hundreds to thousands of percent. Patients, pharmacists, and lawmakers are questioning the appropriateness of such large increases. Some of the causes of these increases include drug shortages, policies of the FDA adopted to meet such shortages, and aggressive private equity firms.

Equivalence: Chemical, Pharmaceutical, Biologic, and Therapeutic

If two brands of the same drug are to be considered for substitution, the basis for identifying them as equivalent must be carefully defined. Drug products that contain the same amounts of the same active ingredients in the same dosage forms and meet current official compendium standards are considered chemical equivalents. **Pharmaceutical equivalents** are drug products that contain the same amounts of the same therapeutic or active ingredients in the same dosage form and meet standards based on the best currently available technology. This description means that pharmaceutical equivalents are formulated identically and must pass certain laboratory tests for equivalent activity, including dissolution tests when appropriate, by standards set for various classes of drugs.

Bioavailability refers to the extent and rate of absorption of a dosage form as reflected by the time–concentration curve of the administered drug in the systemic circulation. **Bioequivalent** drugs are drugs that, when administered to the same individual in the same dosage regimen, result in comparable bioavailability. Insofar as the extent of absorption is concerned, pharmaceutical equivalence is a proxy for biologic equivalence.

Therapeutic equivalents are chemical or pharmaceutical equivalents that, when administered to the same individual in the same dosage regimen, provide essentially the same efficacy (and toxicity). Therapeutic equivalency can be shown only by controlled human clinical trials, which are expensive and time-consuming. In the absence of contradictory clinical evidence, drugs that are bioequivalent are assumed to be therapeutically equivalent.

Chemically equivalent drugs may not share comparable bioavailability. Problems of bioequivalence can arise from many areas. First, although the amounts of the therapeutic ingredients may be the same in two dosage forms, the preparations may contain different binders, diluents, stabilizers, preservatives, and various other pharmacologically inactive excipients to give them their physical form. Second, the pressure used to compress the mixture into the tablet or capsule dosage form may vary and alter the dissolution rate. For suspensions or solutions, the methods used to dissolve, disperse, or suspend the drug in a liquid formulation may differ. Third, the quality control, age, purity, and physical consistency of any of the chemical constituents contained in different formulations of chemically equivalent products can differ. All these various and sometimes poorly controlled factors can influence the rate at which the product disintegrates or dissolves in the gastrointestinal tract, affecting absorption of the active ingredients.

Variations in bioavailability have been shown to be responsible for some treatment failures with certain categories of drugs. Approximately 5% of drug products pose challenges to generic drug manufacturers. Drugs with poor bioavailability, high lipid solubility, nonlinear pharmacokinetics, or narrow therapeutic ranges cause difficulty; examples include steroids, digitalis glycosides, and anticoagulants. Advanced or complex dosage forms with coatings or layers are also difficult to match. Drugs with potential bioavailability problems that are likely to be used by dentists include the various dosage forms of erythromycin, diazepam, and ibuprofen.

To facilitate the wider use of generic drugs, the FDA has published a list of all FDA-approved drugs that it regards as therapeutically equivalent, entitled ***Approved Drug Products with Therapeutic Equivalence Evaluations*** (also known as the **Orange Book**). This source can be used as a guide to identifying generic alternatives that pharmacists can substitute for a brand-name product designated the "**reference-listed drug**" or as the innovator drug. This list indicates drugs that are considered therapeutically equivalent (termed a **positive formulary**), designated with a rating beginning with the letter *A*; drugs that may not be therapeutically equivalent (termed a **negative formulary**), designated with a starting letter *B*; and drugs about which the agency has not yet made a determination (blanks). The FDA's policy is to consider pharmaceutically equivalent drugs as therapeutically equivalent unless scientific evidence to the contrary exists. In the **Orange Book** (available on the Internet), the reference-listed drug, therapeutically equivalent rating, and generic drug rating are provided in tabular form. If a generic oral dosage form preparation is considered therapeutically equivalent, it is given the designation of *AB* (the second letter, *B* in this case, refers to the class of dose form). At the time of this writing, 100% of **ibuprofen, diazepam, and erythromycin ethyl succinate suspensions** were considered *AB*.

Although FDA recalls of generic drugs greatly outnumber recalls of brand-name drugs, most American pharmaceutical firms follow **Good Manufacturing Practice** regulations and are inspected periodically by the FDA for compliance with quality control standards. However, FDA has estimated that 40% of finished dosage forms and 80% of drug ingredients are now being imported. This creates a challenging situation for the FDA as only in some cases is the FDA allowed to inspect foreign drug manufacturing. The **Generic Drug User Fee Act** of 2012 has established a voluntary program of review of foreign manufacturers, which will be funded by user fees. It is left to the practitioner to know the properties of the drugs used and to decide whether to prescribe by trade or nonproprietary name. If the condition being treated is not serious or life-threatening and if the therapeutic index of the drug category being prescribed is not critical, a generic drug can save the patient a substantial amount of money, and the drug should be prescribed by its nonproprietary name.

The development of potent biologic-based treatments, such as therapeutic antibodies, is a rapidly growing area of medicine. In some diseases, these agents have remarkable therapeutic efficacy. Several biologic antibodies have been developed to attack various components of the inflammatory process seen in arthritis. Some of these agents have been referred to as **DMARDS (i.e., disease modifying anti-rheumatic drugs)**. As these agents lose their patent protection, drugs called "**biosimilars**," "**follow-on biologic**," or "**subsequent entry biologic**" may be marketed or manufactured by a different company, to be similar to the innovator product. Hopefully, this would lead to reductions in cost for these agents, which frequently cost thousands of dollars for a month's supply.

Issues related to prescription writing

Off-label prescribing. When an NDA is approved, it indicates for which conditions the use of the drug has been approved, based on the scientific evidence submitted to the FDA, and these are indicated in the package insert (labeling) for the drug. However, if clinical evidence develops that the drug is useful for other conditions, it can be prescribed legally for those conditions. There should be adequate literature to support these other uses, and indeed, for use of many drugs in dentistry, such uses are often **off-label** but supported by literature that justifies their use. However, the practitioner should realize that if a problem develops with the off-label use of the drug, then the use may need to be justified in a court of law. A second practice has developed with respect to off-labeled drug use where the motivation for use is encouragement by the drug industry, through salesmen or through providing of favorable literature that encourages use for off-label indications. However, since many of the studies have been sponsored by the drug company themselves, the potential for bias and marketing forces rather than scientific evidence justifying the off-label use exists. There have been several attempts to regulate this kind of activity, but the history in this area has been varied. Practitioners using drugs for off-labeled indications should be aware that they are doing so and should be sufficiently educated in the literature and general practice standards that they would be able to justify the use in court.

Decision support. Several sources of drug information should be available during selection of drug therapy. Good sources for identifying the drug, dosage form, and dose include **The Physicians' Desk Reference, Facts and Comparisons**, and **ePocrates Rx**. In addition, it is valuable to have a compilation of drug interactions available to screen for possible adverse interactions. A book such as **Drugs in Pregnancy and Lactation** is helpful when a course of therapy is being planned for women of childbearing potential and for pregnant or nursing women. The American Pharmacists Association's **Handbook of Nonprescription Drugs** may be useful if the practitioner is uncertain whether an OTC, herbal, or complementary drug might affect his therapy.

Additional sources of drug information are available as computer software programs, compact disks, and personal digital assistant programs and on the Internet. Electronic resources can have advantages if the text is accompanied by a sophisticated search engine. An innovation in prescribing is the concept of "linked database prescribing" (Fig. 42-2). This type of system has the potential to reduce several sources of prescribing errors, such as poor handwriting, selection of the wrong drug name (selection is based on therapeutic classification), nonexistent product strengths and dosage forms, orders for drugs to which patients are allergic, and therapeutic duplication or incompatibilities. Other errors such as dosing and patient instruction errors could also be reduced by appropriately designed systems. A development in this area is the integration of the information from resources in the previous paragraphs into a single database. A good database will include Rx, OTC drugs, herbals, drug interaction checkers, advice for use in pregnancy and lactation, etc. Although integrating the drug database with a patient databases seems to have a bright future, implementation would be challenging for professional, technical, and legal reasons. If patient data are entered into such a system, the system would need to comply with the **Health Insurance Portability and Accountability Act** of 1996. Specialties such as dentistry may use drugs in a different way than the drugs are generally used in medicine; this can lead to false rejections or warnings for valid prescriptions. Who would be responsible for programming and maintaining the quality of the databases? Who would pay for the use of such a system?

An example of a linked database prescribing system is Elsevier/Gold Standard **Clinical Pharmacology**. Some of what this database covers are the following: Rx only; OTC; dietary supplements; Beer's list (drugs to avoid in the elderly); high-alert medications; narrow therapeutic index drugs; confused drug names, do not crush, and black box warnings from the FDA labeling; and drug information for patients, as well as drug interaction and therapeutic duplication reports. **Lexicomp Online for Dentistry** is another database system that may have some dental-related guidance included.

Filling Prescriptions

Increasingly, prescriptions are being filled at sites remote from where the patient lives. Prescriptions may be mailed or in some cases submitted by the telephone or Internet to a pharmacy. Remote pharmacies

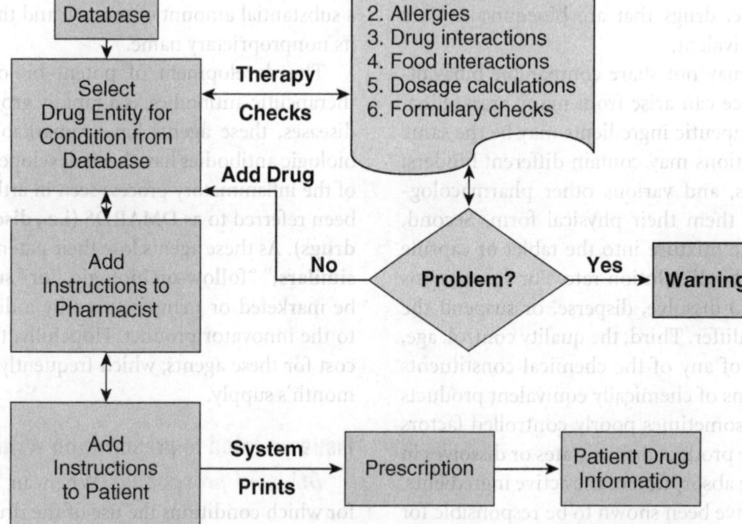

FIG 42-2 The complex process of prescribing can be facilitated by a linked database prescribing system. These systems can assist the prescriber by putting patient, drug, drug interaction, and formulary information at the prescriber's fingertips. The systems can provide warnings when problems are discovered. Current systems leave the instructions to the pharmacist and patient up to the prescriber. Written drug information for the patient is frequently generated automatically.

may be used to obtain medications at a better price or may be required by insurance carriers. In some cases, these pharmacies may not be in the United States.

The FDA is charged with regulating the production of prescription drugs from development to distribution. It has set standards that require compliance during drug development (e.g., **NDA**), **labeling** (package inserts), drug manufacturing (i.e., **Good Manufacturing Practices**), and drug distribution and postmarketing surveillance (e.g., **MedWatch**). The FDA is challenged, however, by limited funding (**Prescription Drug User Fee Act**), changes in international agreements (the **North American Free Trade Agreement** and the **General Agreement on Tariffs and Trade**), changes in public attitudes toward regulation of medications (1994 **Dietary Supplements and Health Education Act**), increased availability of drugs or dietary supplements manufactured outside the United States, increased threats to drug and food safety (bioterrorism, "mad cow disease"), increased production of counterfeit or substandard copies of therapeutic agents, and the use of the Internet to market drugs.

Mail-Order Pharmacies

For long-term medications for which the cost is covered by an insurance company, patients may be directed to submit the prescription to a central pharmacy if the company is to cover the cost. The medication is shipped to the patient by domestic mail, and if the shipment crosses state or national borders, the pharmacy must comply with FDA requirements.

Internet Prescriptions

The development of Internet drug distribution has added an additional area of challenge for the control of the drug supply. Many of the solicitations for drug sales over the Internet are illegal in the United States, and the FDA has moved to close such practices. The **National Association of Boards of Pharmacy** has reviewed the quality of Internet pharmacies over 7 years and found that 96.3% of the sites reviewed operate out of compliance with the U.S. Pharmacy laws and practice standards. These sites may come and go, sometimes before the FDA can act. The medications sold may be of unknown quality and may come from distant sources. Cursory Internet health histories may not properly reflect the patient's health status or may not be reviewed by qualified personnel. In addition, if a patient has an adverse reaction to a drug obtained from a distant source, recognizing and treating adverse reactions may be difficult. There is also a potential financial risk to the patient when using the Internet because the seller may be unknown to the buyer. ***Caveat Emptor*** ("let the buyer beware") is very much the operating principle for these transactions. To help reduce some of the risks associated with the use of Internet pharmacies, the NAPB has developed a voluntary certification program called **Verified Internet Pharmacy Practices Site (VIPPS)**. A VIPPS seal of approval indicates that the pharmacy complies with state licensing and additional requirements, including the patient's right to privacy.

Re-Importation of Drugs

Technically, no unapproved drugs may be imported into the United States. Travelers and immigrants may feel more comfortable, however, taking medications they are familiar with from their home countries. The FDA and U.S. Customs Service regulate drug importation for personal use by guidance documents used for interpreting the various laws administered by the FDA. Small quantities of medications unavailable in the United States, intended to continue a course of treatment begun in a foreign country, may be allowed to enter. The FDA narrows the scope of such drug importations to small amounts (generally less than a 3-month supply) for personal use. If the product's use is properly identified, it is not for a serious condition, and it is deemed not a health risk, it can be approved. If it is an unapproved product for treatment of a serious illness for which treatment is unavailable domestically, not for commercial sale, and not deemed to pose an unreasonable risk, and the patient can document that a physician is responsible for the patient's care, it may be approvable. These provisions were prompted by the concerns for patients with acquired immunodeficiency syndrome who were willing to assume the greater risk of non-FDA-approved drugs to treat their often fatal condition.

There are examples of seized drugs that were previously banned from the United States for safety concerns being illegally imported into the United States. In some cases, labeling for the imported drugs fails to mention offending agents contained in the container. Drugs that are outright counterfeits have been discovered. Control over the manufacturing of imported products may be unknown, and they are sometimes contaminated with bacteria, fungi, or other "filth." In some cases, drugs that are older than their expiration date are received, resulting in subtherapeutic blood concentrations or, in worst cases, toxicity from a degraded drug.

The cost savings of using drugs from foreign sources can be substantial, however. A prescription that may cost more than $100 to fill in the United States may be available from Canada for less than half that amount and may be available from India for pennies per dose. Mexico is also a source for low-cost medicines. In many cases, these foreign drugs are just as effective as the more expensive versions available in the United States. For patients taking lifesaving medications who have no insurance or have a fixed or low income, their choice may be between no medication or cheaper imported drugs. Programs have been developed for physicians licensed to practice in the United States and Canada to write prescriptions for busloads of patients who get their prescriptions filled in Canada and then return to the United States. The variations in the value of the dollar affect some of these savings; nevertheless, there are still considerable savings in buying outside the United States. In other cases, "storefront" pharmacies have opened that receive prescriptions in various cities in the United States, fax them to Canadian pharmacies for filling, and then deliver the medications to the patients by mail. The FDA has judged the latter operations to be illegal commercial importers and has moved to shut them down.

The **Food and Drug Administration Safety and Innovation Act** (**FDASIA**-2012) addresses some of these problems for domestic and foreign drug manufacturers. The act permits the charging of fees to support the activities of registering and reviewing drug manufacturing facilities, both domestic and foreign. This program is still under development and includes drugs, medical devices, biologicals, and biosimilars. In addition, the penalties for intentionally adulterated or counterfeit drug trafficking have been increased.

Noncompliance

A subject of current interest regarding directions on prescriptions is patient compliance or, more accurately, noncompliance. Twenty-five percent to 60% of all patients fail to take medications as intended by their physicians. Noncompliance includes such practices as improper or inappropriate timing of doses or premature discontinuation of the medication. The many possible reasons for patient noncompliance may involve a lack of knowledge or understanding of the drug or the purpose for which it was prescribed, misinformation from nonmedical sources, negative patient attitudes toward illness or "taking drugs," development of an adverse effect, economic factors, or inadequate communication (instruction and emphasis) by the practitioner.

Failure to take medications correctly has been linked to readmission in 20% of Medicare patients released from the hospital. The **Affordable Care Act** required a Readmission Reduction Program for several serious disorders. Although post-dental treatment failures are unlikely to be this dramatic, patient education about the drugs you prescribe is likely to improve therapy and reduce recalls.

Patient compliance is probably improved when the prescriber explains the condition for which the patient is being treated, what the alternative treatment regimens are, and the anticipated benefits of the selected drug treatment. After the drug therapy is selected, patients should be informed of the name of the drug and, in layman's terms, its therapeutic purpose. This information helps the patient recognize the importance of each prescription. Specific instructions on drug use should include how and when to take the medication, how much to take, and when to expect the benefits. The patient should also be made aware of possible adverse reactions and side effects. Some side effects such as drowsiness may be disturbing and interfere to an extent with daily living, but they do not require discontinuation of therapy. Other adverse reactions, such as acute allergic reactions, require immediate discontinuation of therapy. Finally, drug and food interactions should be mentioned. The patient should be given an opportunity to ask questions or clarify the instructions.

For patients on a strict budget, a discussion of drug costs may be important. Little is accomplished by prescribing a drug that the patient is unable or unwilling to buy. The patient should also be informed of what to do if a dose is missed and whether the drug should be taken immediately or at the next dosing interval. It is also useful to tell the patient about any special storage requirements, such as the need for keeping the drug refrigerated (emulsions) or at room temperature (syrups). Practitioners need to familiarize themselves with the instructions for use and storage of the medications they prescribe because these instructions can vary among dosage forms and preparations of the same drug entity.

Patient information sheets for numerous drugs, especially newly approved agents, are available online from the FDA. These sheets may be downloaded and given to patients to help address many of the informational issues that can influence compliance. The practitioner should read these before they are provided to the patient as the dental use of the drug may not match the medical use and require different instructions.

The prescription enhances the physician–patient relationship and contributes to patient compliance if care is used in presenting it. Writing a prescription in English and the instructions in a language the patient understands and in the patient's presence and then explaining it, in addition to improving compliance, may equip the patient to detect any errors that may occur in prescribing or filling the prescription.

Because few patients are able to recall oral instructions accurately, the labeled directions should be specific. Failure to be specific can provide the basis for malpractice lawsuits. If the patient has many prescriptions or has a special difficulty with oral instructions, a written reminder should accompany the prescription.

Patient compliance may also be improved by selecting drugs that need to be taken only once or twice daily instead of agents that have to be administered more frequently. When multiple drug therapy is necessary, combination products, when appropriate, are helpful in reducing the "confusion over pill profusion," as is prescribing drugs with distinctive physical characteristics (e.g., a red tablet, a white tablet, and a capsule instead of three white tablets).

Dosage Calculations (Posology)

The dosage of a prescribed drug may vary according to several factors: the degree or severity of the condition for which it is being prescribed; the age, weight, sex, or temperament of the patient; the route, frequency, or timing of administration; concurrent medication; patient suggestibility (placebo effect), habits, sensitivities, or previous medication history (hyperreaction or hyporeaction); and the systemic health of the patient. Important changes in clearance or volume of distribution can produce changes in expected half-lives of drugs. Because drug metabolism and elimination are primarily accomplished by the liver and kidneys, any significant change in the function of these organs may necessitate a change in dosing. For the fluoride prescription, the age of the patient and the amount of fluoride in the water supply are the primary determinants of the dosage.

The manufacturer's package insert, pharmacology texts, and the compendial sources mentioned earlier in this chapter and in Chapter 3 list the official, average, or usual 150-lb adult male dose for a drug. A listed dose or dosage range is a guide for prescription purposes, and although it does not carry the weight of a regulation, it does have medicolegal implications if an adverse effect occurs. Practitioners are well advised to stay within the recommended dosage range unless they have a sound reason to vary from it (see later).

For many drugs intended for pediatric use, the packaging may suggest dosing for children of various weight brackets or may suggest doses based on a mg-per-kilogram basis. These are useful unless the child has an extreme body type.

No uniform format is used in references to express dosing information. For most drugs, the dose is reported as the amount of drug to be given at a single dose, which is repeated at a stated interval each day. Alternatively, the manufacturer may indicate the total amount of drug to be administered "in divided doses" per day. The practitioner is expected to know what dosage forms are available and how often to give them on the basis of the pharmacokinetics of the drug and the nature of the patient (these can be found in an appropriate reference or drug databases). For dosage determination, an "adult" is usually interpreted to mean an individual 18 years old or older and weighing approximately 70 kg (150 lb).

Children and many underweight, diseased, or elderly patients require a dosage that is lower than that suggested for a nominal adult. Very large or obese patients may require dosage adjustment, but this adjustment can depend on the characteristics of each drug; with some drugs (e.g., gentamicin), the increased dosage can increase the risk of toxicity. Patient pharmacogenomics can also be a factor, such as a patient who is a CYP2D6 poor or ultra-metabolizer.

When no package label dosing adjustments are available, several general rules have been proposed for computing the dosage of a drug for children, as follows:

1. Clark's rule:

   Child's weight (lb [or kg])/150 lb (or 70 kg) × adult dose = child's dose

   This determines the dose suitable for a child based on the typical adult weight of 150 lb (or 70 kg).

2. Young's rule:

   Child's age (yr)/child's age + 12 (yr) × adult dose = child's dose

   This calculates the dose for the child based on age, with a 12-year-old child receiving half the adult dose.

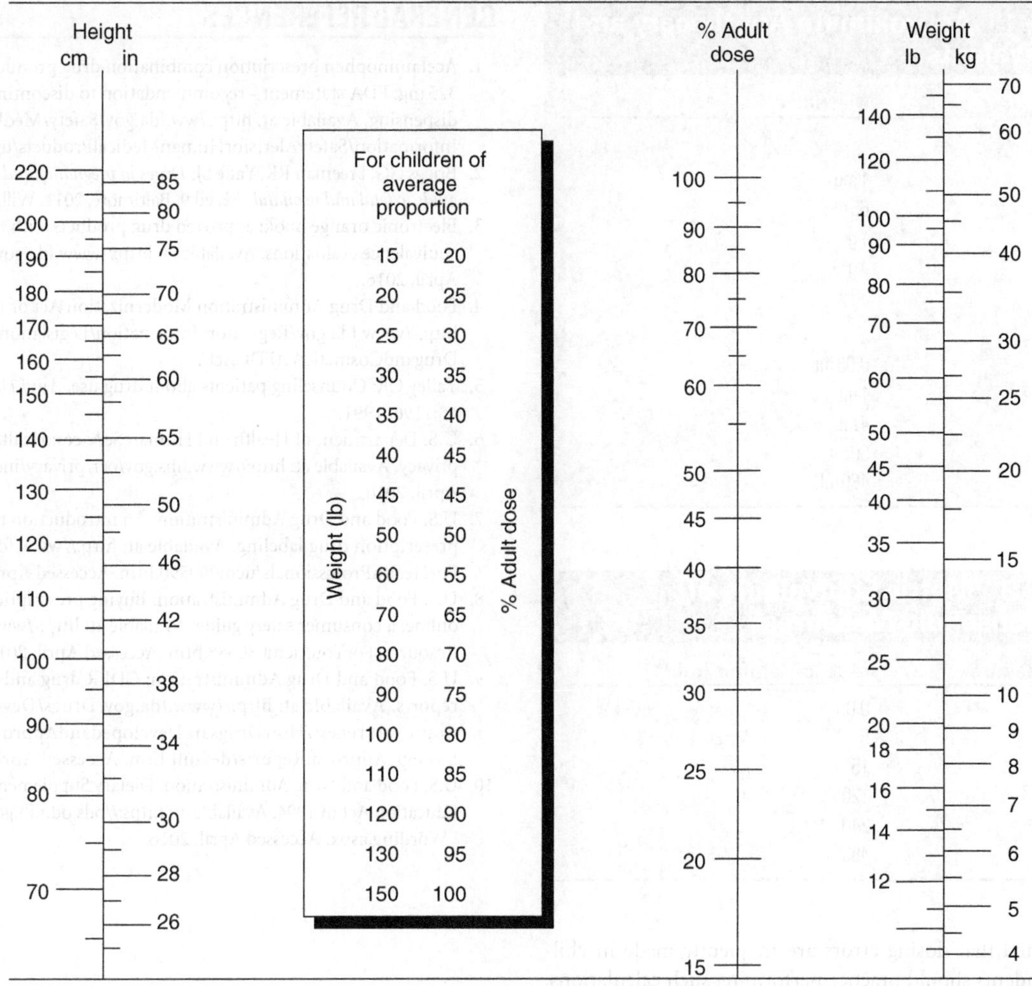

FIG 42-3 Nomogram for estimating dose based on surface area. A value of 1.73 m^2 is used as the adult surface area standard. The intersection of a *straight line* connecting the patient's height and weight with the dosage column indicates the correct percentage of the adult dose. A simplified table for children of normal height and weight is also provided.

3. Surface area:

   This is extrapolated from the patient's height and weight, and it is divided by the average adult surface area to determine the fraction of the adult dose. This method is seldom used in dentistry. Dosage tables or graphs (Fig. 42-3) are available, which obviate time-consuming and error-prone calculations.

Of all these methods, Clark's rule is the most widely used, and Young's rule is the most subject to error. Because physiologic functions dealing with drug disposition are generally proportional to body surface area, the surface area method is probably the most accurate of the three. This distinction is dubious, however, because drug responses in children, especially very young children, are modified by factors other than body size. When dosage information is unavailable, and one of these methods has to be used to estimate the child dose, it is important to monitor the patient carefully to ensure that therapeutic effects are obtained and toxic reactions are minimized.

Weights and Measures

Two systems of designating weights and measures of drugs and preparations are the apothecary and the metric systems. Although the older apothecary measures may still be used by some clinicians for some drugs, the metric system is now standard. Approximate equivalents between the two systems are given in Table 42-1. Apothecary measures are not equivalent to measures used for commercial purposes in the United States or the Troy measures used for precious metals.

Household measures are commonly encountered when liquid preparations are prescribed. If the directions call for the patient to take a certain volume of drug solution, the pharmacist converts the metric value given into its household equivalent, as indicated in Table 42-2. Utensils likely to be used by patients may yield different volumes of medicine than were initially intended. To circumvent this problem, calibrated measuring devices can be purchased to administer liquid medicines; patients should be encouraged to use these when taking their medications.

Calculating the appropriate patient dose, calculating the amount of drug product needed to achieve this dose, expressing the dose in a household measure, and calculating the total amount of the drug to be dispensed by the pharmacist for the full course of treatment are common calculations performed in the practice of dentistry. Such calculations are required when prescribing an antibiotic suspension for a child. Although the mathematics is simple, teaching experience indicates that 40% of students are unable to perform calculations correctly on examination. The 1999 Institute of Medicine report on

TABLE 42-1 Approximate Apothecary and Metric Equivalents

Apothecary	Metric
Weight	
1/65 grain	1 mg
1 grain	65 mg
15 grains	1 g
1 dram	4 g
1 ounce	30 g
Volume	
1 minim	0.06 mL
16 minims	1 mL
1 fluid dram	4 mL
1 fluid ounce	30 mL
1 pint	480 mL

TABLE 42-2 Metric Equivalents of Common Household Measures

Household Measure	Metric Volume (mL)
1 USP drop	0.05
1 teaspoon	5
1 tablespoon	15
1 teacup	120
1 glass	240
1 pint	480

medical error noted that dosing errors are frequently made in children's dosing. Students should practice performing such calculations, and any time drug doses are calculated for a patient, they should be double-checked for accuracy.

CASE DISCUSSION

After writing his prescriptions, JP Dentist should talk to Ms. S. and explains what the drugs do, how they should be taken, and for how long. Antibiotics should be taken for the full course of therapy, and he may want to make sure that she is not allergic to the penicillins and warn her about what to do if she experiences signs of an allergy. The dentist should describe the common adverse actions and tell her which are benign and which would signal that she should stop the therapy. He should tell the patient that she should start to feel better in a few days (penicillins often produce rapid improvement in infections). For Tylenol #3, (acetaminophen 300 mg plus codeine 30 mg) he should warn about possible drowsiness, not to drive while taking it, that she should not take it with alcohol, and she should take it as prescribed to reduce the risk of adverse effects. It is advisable to tell her that she may not need to take the prescribed medication for 3 days , substituting with acetaminophen if this is sufficient. One extra pain tablet may be taken at initial dosing intervals if needed, but not to exceed 10 tablets per day to limit the acetaminophen dose. He should tell her what to do if it causes nausea or vomiting. Also, she should not give or sell it to anyone else. He may wish to tell her about what the prescriptions cost and ask if she would have a problem paying for them. In this case the prescriptions should be relatively inexpensive. Finally, he should ask if she has any other questions about the medications he has prescribed. He reschedules the patient for a dental extraction in one week. A prescription for pain may be needed at that time as well.

GENERAL REFERENCES

1. Acetaminophen prescription combination drug products with more than 325 mg: FDA statement - recommendation to discontinue prescribing and dispensing. Available at: http://ww.fda.gov/Safety/MedWatch/SafetyInformation/SafetyAlertsforHumanMedicalProducts/ucm381650.htm.
2. Briggs GG, Freeman RK, Yaffe SJ: *Drugs in pregnancy and lactation: a reference guide to fetal and neonatal risk*, ed 9, Baltimore, 2011, Williams & Wilkins.
3. Electronic orange book: approved drug products with therapeutic equivalence evaluations. Available at: http://www.fda.gov/cder/ob. Accessed April, 2016.
4. Food and Drug Administration Modernization Act of 1997. Available at: http://www.fda.gov/RegulatoryInformation/Legislation/FederalFoodDrugandCosmeticActFDCAct/.
5. Talley CR: Counseling patients about drug use, *Am J Hosp Pharm* 48:1196, 1991.
6. U.S. Department of Health and Human Services: Health information privacy. Available at: http://www.hhs.gov/ocr/privacy/index.html. Accessed April, 2016.
7. U.S. Food and Drug Administration: An introduction to improved FDA prescription drug labeling. Available at: http://www.fda.gov/Training/ForHealthProfessionals/ucm090590.htm. Accessed April, 2016.
8. U.S. Food and Drug Administration: Buying prescription medicine online: a consumer safety guide. Available at: http://www.fda.gov/Drugs/ResourcesForYou/ucm080588.htm. Accessed April, 2016.
9. U.S. Food and Drug Administration: CDER drug and biologic approval reports. Available at: http://www.fda.gov/Drugs/DevelopmentApprovalProcess/HowDrugsareDevelopedandApproved/DrugandBiologicApprovalReports/default.htm. Accessed April, 2016.
10. U.S. Food and Drug Administration: Dietary Supplement Health and Education Act of 1994. Available at: https://ods.od.nih.gov/About/DSHEA_Wording.aspx. Accessed April, 2016.

APPENDIX 1

Protein Biopharmaceuticals

Frank J. Dowd

Representatives of protein-based drugs are used to treat disorders such as immune diseases, inflammatory reactions, blood lipid disorders, or infections. Most are monoclonal antibodies or fusion proteins containing an antibody component. Similar drugs used in cancer chemotherapy are listed in Chapters 35 and 36. Immune-related drugs are discussed in Chapter 35.

Name (Proprietary Name)	Composition	Mechanism	Indication(s)
Abatacept (Orencia)	Fusion of IgG fragment and T-cell antigen	Binds to CD80 and CD86, blocks T cells	RA, JA
Abciximab (ReoPro)	MAB versus glycoprotein IIb/IIIa receptor on platelets	Inhibits platelet aggregation	Unstable angina, used during percutaneous coronary intervention
Adalimumab (Humira)	MAB versus TNF-α	Prevents interaction of TNF-α with p55 and p75 receptors	RA, JA, AS, CD, PA, PP
Alirocumab (Praluent)	MAB versus PCSK9	Prevents PCSK9 from binding to the LDL receptor and thus prevents LDL receptor degradation	Hypercholesterolemia
Anakinra (Kineret)	Recombinant protein antagonist of IL-1 receptor	Blocks IL-1 from binding to receptor	RA, CAPS
Basiliximab (Simulect)	MAB versus IL-2 receptor α on T lymphocytes	Prevents T-cell-mediated rejection	Prevent organ rejection
Belimumab (Benlysta)	MAB versus B lymphocyte stimulator protein	Blocks binding of B-cell survival protein, BLγS, to its receptor	SLE
Certolizumab (Cimzia)	MAB versus TNF-α	Blocks effect of TNF-α	RA, CD, PA
Eculizumab (Soliris)	MAB versus complement protein, C5	Prevents generation of terminal complement complexes	PNH, AHUS
Etanercept (Enbrel)	Fusion of IgG fragment and p75 TNF receptor	Blocks effect of TNF-α and TNF-β	RA, JA, PA, PP, AS
Golimumab (Simponi)	MAB versus TNF-α	Blocks effect of TNF-α	RA, PA, UC, AS
Infliximab (Remicade)	MAB versus TNF-α	Blocks effect of TNF-α	RA, PA, UC, PP, AS, CD
Natalizumab (Tysabri)	MAB versus α4-integrin	Inhibits α4-integrin and cell adhesion	CD, MS
Omalizumab (Xolair)	MAB versus IgE	Blocks binding of IgE to IgE receptors on mast cells and basophils	Asthma, chronic idiopathic urticaria
Palivizumab (Synagis)	MAB versus specific site of gp120/gp41 protein of respiratory syncytial virus (RSV)	Blocks fusion of membrane of RSV with host cell	Respiratory syncytial virus
Rilonacept (Arcalyst)	Fusion of IgG fragment and IL-1 receptor component	Blocks IL-1 receptor signaling	CAPS
Rituximab (Rituxan)	MAB versus CD20	Blocks B cells	RA
Tocilizumab (Actemra)	MAB versus IL-6	Reduces inflammation	RA, JA
Ustekinumab (Stelara)	MAB against p40 subunit of IL-12 and IL-23	Blocks IL-12 and IL-23 signaling	PA, PP

AHUS, Atypical hemolytic uremic syndrome; *AS*, ankylosing spondylitis; *CAPS*, Cryopyrin-associated periodic syndromes; *CD*, Crohn's disease; *IL*, interleukin; *JA*, juvenile arthritis; *MAB*, monoclonal antibody; *MS*, multiple sclerosis; *PA*, psoriatic arthritis; *PCSK9*, proprotein convertase subtilisin/kexin type 9; *PNH*, paroxysmal nocturnal hemoglobinuria; *PP*, plaque psoriasis; *RA*, rheumatoid arthritis; *SLE*, systemic lupus erythematosus; *TNF*, tumor necrosis factor; *UC*, ulcerative colitis.

2 APPENDIX

Use of Herbs and Herbal Dietary Supplements in Dentistry*

Angelo J. Mariotti

Alternative (integrative, complementary, natural, holistic) medicine is composed of a broad range of treatments that are often preventive in nature and commonly directed at treating the whole person rather than a specific disease. Substances used in alternative therapies are most often derived from natural sources. Many of these—particularly herbal medicines—have been used for more than 2000 years and are relied on by approximately 80% of the world's population in developing countries. Most people who use alternative care modalities do so because they are following traditions handed down from one generation to the next. What Western culture calls **alternative treatments** are in most cultures often the only available options for health care. Most such treatments have lacked rigorous scientific evidence of efficacy; however, there is a growing body of clinical research documenting the activity and utility of some of these regimens. The National Institutes of Health have designated such therapies as **complementary and alternative medicine** (**CAM**). In contrast, Western medicine (sometimes referred to as **allopathic**) includes a diverse array of scientific, mostly evidence-based pharmacologic and surgical technologies, which, although described as "mainstream," "conventional," "orthodox," or "traditional," have been practiced for little more than a century. These treatments focus almost exclusively on eliminating disease.

The term **alternative medicine** is used in this chapter to indicate "interventions neither taught widely in medical schools nor generally available in hospitals." This selection is not meant to exclude other terms. The increasingly popular term **integrative medicine** may be preferable because it stresses that these treatment protocols often can be effectively integrated with conventional medicine to optimize the health of the patient.

For decades in the United States and in some European countries, alternative medicine—and alternative (or holistic) dentistry—has implied care at the "fringe" of accepted medical (or dental) practice. There is an increasing trend now to incorporate many of these forms of care into the mainstream and include them as covered benefits in health insurance plans. Alternative medical therapies, depending on how they are defined (e.g., whether prayer is included as a CAM therapy), are used by an estimated 25% to 42% of the U.S. population. About 20% use natural products, including vitamins, minerals, herbs, and other dietary supplements. Table A2.1 lists the reasons why patients pursue CAM therapies. CAM therapies have become popular considering that visits to alternative care practitioners exceed visits to allopathic primary care physicians by more than 200 million annually, and Americans spend an estimated $30 billion a year on these services plus $18.8 billion on dietary supplements; most of these expenses are not reimbursed. In response to these trends, most medical and some dental schools in the United States now provide at least introductory coursework in CAM.

This appendix focuses on natural pharmacologic and therapeutic agents—principally botanical (herbal) remedies—that constitute one of the alternative or integrative means of health maintenance and disease treatment.

REGULATIONS AND QUALITY CONTROL

The growth of alternative therapies in the United States was spurred by the passage of the **Dietary Supplement Health and Education Act (DSHEA) of 1994**. This act greatly boosted the market for dietary supplements, including vitamins, minerals, and botanical remedies. Under DSHEA (Table A2.2), manufacturers could promote herbal products for the maintenance of health by using "structure/function" claims, such as the product "enhances the immune system" and "improves memory." It also permits, but does not require, manufacturers to list product safety precautions. Clarification of DSHEA in 1998 allowed herbal product manufacturers and distributors to make some additional claims, primarily to suggest their use for modifying natural life events, including menopause, pregnancy, and aging.

Under DSHEA, **dietary supplements**, including herbal products, are legally **classified as foods**. They are exempted from the normal review process the U.S. Food and Drug Administration (FDA) requires for drugs. DSHEA also requires that manufacturers must be able to substantiate, when challenged, all claims made either on the container or in the literature that accompanies the dietary supplement product. Such challenges can come from the FDA or from self-regulatory mechanisms, such as the industry-funded program of the National Advertising Division of the Better Business Bureau, wherein ad claims are being reviewed for accuracy, resulting in the revision of such claims where evidence may be lacking or, if the manufacturer does not comply, referral to the Federal Trade Commission for possible action.

TABLE A2.1 Reasons for Using Complementary and Alternative Medicine Therapies*

Reason	%
Thought CAM combined with conventional medicine would help	54.9%
Thought CAM would be interesting to try	50.1%
Thought conventional medicine would not help	27.7%
Conventional medicine professional suggested CAM	25.8%
Conventional medicine too expensive	13.2%

*Based on survey of 31,044 adults ≥18 years old from the U.S. civilian noninstitutionalized population.

CAM, Complementary and alternative medicine.

* The author wishes to acknowledge Drs. Richard P. Cohan and Mark Blumenthal for authoring the chapter, "Use of Herbs and Herbal Dietary Supplements in Dentistry", in the previous edition.

TABLE A2.2 Important Components of the Dietary Supplement Health and Education Act (DSHEA)

Definition of Dietary Supplement	
A product (other than tobacco) that:	Contains one or more vitamins, minerals, herbs, amino acids Is formulated in capsules, tablets, liquids, powders, soft gels Is not a conventional food or sole item of a meal or diet Is labeled as a dietary supplement
Safety of Dietary Supplements	
FDA has burden of proof that the supplement is dangerous or constitutes a risk to public health. New dietary ingredients introduced into the market after October 15, 1994, must have safety data submitted to FDA for premarket acceptance.	
Supplement Claims and Labeling	
Manufacturers can make nutrient content claims and claims on how dietary supplement affects structure or function of body. Manufacturer must have reasonable evidence/research supporting claims but is normally not required to disclose it. FDA has burden of proof that claim is inadequately substantiated.	
Statement of Nutritional Support (on Label or in Advertising)	
Permitted if a classic nutrient-deficiency benefit is claimed. Permitted if role of supplement is to affect structure or function of body. Can include documented mechanism of action. Can describe general well-being from consuming the ingredients. Must prominently display disclaimer that statements have not been evaluated by FDA and that product is not intended to treat, mitigate, cure, or prevent a disease.	
Supplement Ingredient Labeling and Nutrition Information	
Must include the following (or would be considered misbranded and removed):	Commonly accepted name of each ingredient Quantity of each ingredient Total weight of ingredients Part(s) of the plant from which ingredient(s) is (are) derived The term: dietary supplement

Adapted from Israelsen LD: *Summary of the Dietary Supplement Health and Education Act of 1994. Quarterly review of natural medicine*, Seattle, WA, Spring 1995, Natural Product Research Consultants.

TYPES OF HERBAL DIETARY SUPPLEMENTS AND RELATED BOTANICAL PRODUCTS

Natural products of plants are marketed in unmodified forms (such as the whole leaf, bark, berry, or root), as powders in capsules and tablets, as herbal teas, and in various extracts and other derivatives. The recorded use of natural preparations for their pharmacologic effects dates from at least 2735 BCE, when a Chinese emperor recommended the use of ephedra (*Ephedra sinica*, which contains ephedrine and at least five other sympathomimetic agents) for a respiratory condition. Approximately 25% to 30% of prescription medications commonly used to treat diseases today are derived from natural sources. Examples include digoxin from the foxglove plant (*Digitalis purpurea* and *Digitalis lanata*, used to treat congestive heart failure) and quinidine from the cinchona plant (*Cinchona* species, used as an antiarrhythmic drug). Tables A2.3 summarizes some common herbal remedies; their possible uses and indications; and their potential liabilities, including potential adverse drug interactions.

Most therapeutic products used as alternative therapies are the natural herb material or extracts of the herb. Water-based extracts include infusions (teas) and decoctions, whereas alcohol extracts are usually marketed as tinctures or other forms of extracts. An increasing number of products are combinations of herbs or mixtures of herbs and so-called nutraceuticals. **Nutraceuticals** are nutritional compounds—usually food extracts or their derivatives (e.g., the carotenoid lycopene derived from tomato)—promoted for use in a therapeutic way to treat or prevent specific problems or diseases.

INTEGRATED HEALTH CARE AND DENTISTRY

Patient Evaluation

An important part of the health history is the solicitation of the patient's medication usage. Although some patients provide this information unsolicited under the "medication" question usually asked in health questionnaires, other patients do not for various reasons. One reason is that they may not believe or understand that their alternative therapy products are considered medications. They also may not feel comfortable telling a conventional health care provider that they are using alternative therapies for fear of disapproval. In either case, there is a much greater probability that they would provide the information if it is specifically solicited, such as by a question requesting the patient to list "natural remedies" being taken. Therefore, if a patient is taking any alternative product, the dentist should inquire about its identity and doses and whether the product is being used preventively or to treat specific problems.

Modifications of Dental Treatment

Sometimes the use of alternative medicines by a dental patient requires modification of the treatment plan. Most commonly, before surgical procedures, modification involves stopping **herbal remedies that inhibit hemostasis.** As listed in Tables A2.3 and A2.4, numerous alternative products may potentially exert antiplatelet or anticoagulant activity, but chief among them are **garlic and ginger.** A second consideration regarding these herbal medicines is the possibility of postoperative bleeding if the dentist prescribes a nonsteroidal antiinflammatory drug for postoperative pain relief (see Table A2.4). There is a potential for added risk of bleeding if a nonsteroidal antiinflammatory drug, especially aspirin, is administered to a patient taking supplemental garlic or **ginkgo.** The use of acetaminophen, opioids, or the cyclooxygenase-2–selective analgesic celecoxib may avoid this potential drug interaction.

Orthostatic hypotension may be more likely to occur in patients taking herbal products capable of decreasing arterial blood pressure. Such products include astragalus, dong quai, and sage. Patients taking these remedies—especially elderly patients, patients with cardiovascular disease, and patients fasting for sedation or anesthesia—should be monitored for hypotension. In addition, changes in body position (as in moving from the supine to the standing position) should be made slowly and with careful patient observation.

Several herbal agents, including kava and valerian, can cause sedation. Their combination with standard doses of prescribed anxiolytics and sedative-hypnotics may result in severe central nervous system depression. Conversely, long-term use of these agents may decrease responsiveness to benzodiazepines and related drugs. Meperidine and tramadol probably should be avoided in patients taking **St. John's wort** because of the agents' shared potential for increasing 5-hydroxytryptamine activity in the brain, possibly resulting in a serotonergic syndrome of restlessness, motor hyperactivity, and coma.

TABLE A2.3 **Pharmacologic Profiles of Common Herbal Products**

Herbal Product*	Uses/Effects	Precautions/Adverse Effects	Drug Interactions
Aloe vera: *Aloe vera* (and related species); aloe, Zanzibar	Topical anesthetic (gel); soothes wounds and burns; accelerates wound healing; latex form is a laxative	Topical use to abraded skin may cause burning sensation; ingestion of latex derivative causes powerful catharsis by irritating the large intestine; may cause GI cramps and congenital malformation	Cathartic effect of latex form often hastens passage of oral medications, often inhibiting their absorption and may potentiate anticoagulant therapy by reducing intestinal absorption of vitamin K
Asian ginseng: *Panax ginseng*; Chinese ginseng	Adaptogen and immunomodulator; fights fatigue; improves concentration and performance; enhances healing; generally increases ability to tolerate stress and recuperate; principal male adaptogen in Chinese medicine	Inhibited blood clotting from effects on platelet adhesion and blood coagulation; may reduce blood glucose concentrations; a "ginseng abuse syndrome," with diarrhea, hypertension, and nervousness has been described, which may be linked to concomitant intake of caffeine and large doses of unknown "ginseng" preparations	May increase effect of hypoglycemic drugs but promote diuretic resistance when combined with loop diuretics; may potentiate headache, tremors, and mania with MAO inhibitors and increase responses to caffeine; may potentiate bleeding with antiplatelet agents and anticoagulants (but may decrease effect of warfarin)
Astragalus: *Astragalus membranaceus*; milk vetch, huang chi	Adaptogen and immunostimulant; speeds metabolism	Subject to bacterial degradation when used as a component of denture adhesive; mutagenic by the Ames test	May decrease effectiveness of immunosuppressants
Bilberry fruit: *Vaccinium myrtillus*; huckleberry, European blueberry	Mild antiinflammatory of mucous membranes; slows cataracts, diabetic retinopathy; leaf used as a tea to treat diarrhea	Mild antiplatelet effects; may cause diarrhea in some individuals and should be discontinued if it persists for >3 days; bilberry leaf is toxic and can cause hypoglycemia	Potentiation of antiplatelet and anticoagulant drugs; effects may be inhibited by phenobarbital; leaf may increase effect of hypoglycemic drugs
Cascara sagrada: *Rhamnus purshiana*; buckthorn, sacred bark	Laxative/cathartic	K^+ may be lost, causing weakness and coagulation deficits	Cathartic-induced hypokalemia may potentiate or increase toxicity of muscle relaxants, antiarrhythmics, cardiac glycosides, and K^+-depleting diuretics
Dong quai: *Angelica sinensis*; Chinese angelica	Manage pain from injury, arthritis; improve circulation, treat allergic reactions; principal female remedy in Chinese medicine for overcoming fatigue and treating gynecologic/menopausal symptoms	Excessive doses may cause hypotension and interfere with platelet activity	Increased hypotensive effects with antihypertensives and opioids; potentiation of antiplatelet and anticoagulant drugs
Echinacea: *Echinacea purpurea* (and related species); purple cone flower	Immunomodulator; boost immunity and treat symptoms of upper respiratory infections	Possible allergic reactions in individuals with ragweed and related allergies; potential aggravation of autoimmune illness (e.g., lupus) and progressive diseases (HIV, tuberculosis)	Antiinflammatory activity of herb can be inhibited by phenobarbital and other microsomal enzyme inducers; potential adverse interactions with immunosuppressants (e.g., corticosteroids, cyclosporine)
Feverfew: *Tanacetum parthenium*	Antipyretic antiinflammatory; used for prophylaxis of migraine headache and to treat arthritis, premenstrual and menstrual discomfort, and fevers	Chewing fresh leaves or seeds may cause mouth irritation (swelling, ulcers), dysgeusia, nausea, vomiting, insomnia, and diarrhea; discontinuation may cause post-feverfew syndrome of nervousness, tension headaches, insomnia, and joint discomfort; may cause abortion during pregnancy and interfere with platelet aggregation	Possible increased bleeding with concurrent use of antiplatelet and anticoagulant drugs
Garlic: *Allium sativum*; allium, stinking rose	Used as digestive aid and to treat hypertension and as broad-spectrum topical antibiotic; may decrease LDL cholesterol and triglycerides and increase HDL cholesterol	Possible bleeding from inhibition of platelet aggregation and antithrombotic effects; allergic reactions possible; ingestion of large dose may cause burning sensation in mouth and throat; theoretic risk of increased autoimmune reactions and organ transplant rejection	Possible increased bleeding with concurrent use of antiplatelet and anticoagulant drugs; possible increased hypoglycemia in patients taking insulin

TABLE A2.3 Pharmacologic Profiles of Common Herbal Products—cont'd

Herbal Product*	Uses/Effects	Precautions/Adverse Effects	Drug Interactions
Ginger: *Zingiber officinale*; black ginger, zingiberis rhizome	Antibiotic, antioxidant, antiinflammatory, and antiemetic; used principally for prophylaxis of motion sickness and to treat digestive disorders, nausea, and vomiting (via local action on stomach receptors)	Possible bleeding from inhibition of platelet aggregation	Possible increased bleeding with concurrent use of antiplatelet and anticoagulant drugs
Ginkgo: *Ginkgo biloba*; maidenhair tree	Leaf extract is used to improve cerebral and peripheral circulation, for enhanced concentration, memory, and hearing; amelioration of dementia; and relief of peripheral vascular disease	Possible bleeding from inhibition of platelet aggregation; mild GI upset and headache, occasional nausea and vomiting	Possible increased bleeding with concurrent use of antiplatelet and anticoagulant drugs
Goldenseal: *Hydrastis canadensis*; yellow root, orange root, Indian turmeric	Antiinflammatory and broad-spectrum antimicrobial; treats digestive and respiratory infections; promotes wound healing	Fresh plant or high doses may cause irritation to oral mucosa and GI distress	None documented
Kava–kava: *Piper methysticum*; kava–kava	Anxiolytic, sedative-hypnotic; used to treat anxiety, insomnia, and muscle tension	Local anesthetic action causes temporary mouth numbness; may rarely cause hepatotoxicity and liver failure; high doses may cause inebriation, with incoordination, ataxia, and drowsiness; long-term use may cause reversible scaly skin rash	Summation of effects with benzodiazepines and other CNS depressants; high doses may increase dystonic reactions with antipsychotics and levodopa
Red yeast rice: *Monascus purpureus*; ZhiTai	Antihypercholesterolemic; blocks cholesterol synthesis and decreases total plasma cholesterol, LDL cholesterol, and triglycerides	Rarely causes hepatic and skeletal muscle damage; allergic reactions in individuals sensitive to yeast or rice	Inhibitors of CYP3A4 (e.g., erythromycin, itraconazole) potentiate hepatic and skeletal muscle toxicity; risk is also increased with coadministration of other lipid-lowering drugs (statins, fibrates, gemfibrozil, niacin); oral anticoagulant effects are potentiated
Saw palmetto: *Serenoa repens*; sabal	Treats benign prostatic hypertrophy; may inhibit dihydrotestosterone; may have antiestrogenic effects	May occasionally cause GI disturbances	Possible interaction with sex steroids
St. John's wort: *Hypericum perforatum*; Klamath weed	Treats mild-moderate depression and anxiety; antiinflammatory in GI and respiratory tracts; eases menstrual cramps; antiviral in large doses against enveloped viruses in vitro; topical use as an antibacterial and antiinflammatory analgesic for minor wounds and infections	Photosensitivity in rare cases, such as with high doses, prolonged treatment, and excessive sun exposure; induces CYP3A4, CYP1A2, and several CYP2 enzymes in liver and GI tract; may cause drowsiness	Increased phototoxic/photoallergic reactions with tetracyclines, sulfonamides, and proton pump inhibitors; summation effects with benzodiazepines, opioids, and other CNS depressants; serotonergic crisis possible with meperidine, MAO inhibitors, and other antidepressants; decreases plasma concentrations of protease inhibitors, cyclosporine, digoxin, and warfarin
Valerian: *Valeriana officinalis*	Sedative-hypnotic; used to reduce anxiety, alleviate motor activity and muscle spasms, and promote sleep	Drowsiness	Summation of effects with benzodiazepines, sedative-hypnotics, and other CNS depressants

CNS, Central nervous system; *GI*, gastrointestinal; *HDL*, high-density lipoprotein; *HIV*, human immunodeficiency virus; *LDL*, low-density lipoprotein; *MAO*, monoamine oxidase.
*Listed in order are the principal **common name**, scientific name, and other common names. Some of the uses described in this table have not been validated by well-controlled clinical studies; likewise, many of the adverse effects and drug interactions listed are either speculative or of potential concern but not proved to be clinically significant.

Finally, the potential for interactions between herbal supplements and conventional medications used in dentistry has been an increasing concern among practitioners as more consumers use more herbal products along with conventional medications. Although there is a documented growth in the use of the herbal products with conventional medications, there has not been a significant increase in reports of adverse herbal–drug interactions (HDIs) associated with the growing herb use. Nonetheless, four most common classes of prescription medications with a **potential for interaction (antithrombotic medications, sedatives, antidepressants, and antidiabetic agents)** should be considered for potential clinically significant interactions.

Herbal Therapies for Oral Conditions

An important area of interest for dentists, hygienists, and patients is the use of alternative remedies to manage dental and other oral problems. Agents listed in Table A2.3 that have antimicrobial,

TABLE A2.4 Potential Herbal and Other Dietary Supplement Drug Interactions in Dentistry*

Dental Drug	Herbal/Nutraceutical Product	Effect	Recommendation
NSAIDs	Bilberry fruit, bromelain, cat's claw, coleus, cordyceps, devil's claw, evening primrose, feverfew, fish oils, garlic, ginger, ginkgo, ginseng, grape seed, green tea, guggul, horse chestnut, licorice, prickly ash, red clover, reishi, S-adenosylmethionine, turmeric, vitamin E	Antihemostatic effects (primarily antiplatelet actions) may result in increased bleeding after surgical procedures for which NSAIDs are prescribed	Avoid aspirin; use other NSAIDs cautiously after procedures likely to cause postoperative bleeding
	Deglycyrrhizinated licorice	May reduce or prevent GI bleeding	Dissolve deglycyrrhizinated licorice sublingually 20-30 minutes before consuming NSAID†
Meperidine, tramadol	5-hydroxytryptophan, L-tryptophan, S-adenosylmethionine, St. John's wort	Theoretic concern of serotonin syndrome	Avoid combined use
Benzodiazepines, barbiturates, opioids, other CNS depressants	Kava, melatonin, St. John's wort, valerian, astragalus, coleus, hawthorn, dong quai, garlic, parsley, sage	Increased CNS depression Postural hypotension more likely	Avoid combined use Protect patient against postural hypotension: change position slowly; avoid dehydration
Penicillin VK	Guar gum	Penicillin absorption inhibited	Avoid concurrent administration
Sulfamethoxazole-trimethoprim	*p*-Aminobenzoic acid	Competitive inhibition of antimicrobial effect	Avoid combination
Sulfamethoxazole-trimethoprim, tetracyclines	Dong quai (related species), St. John's wort	Phototoxic/photoallergic reactions more likely	Avoid combination
Tetracyclines	Calcium, iron, magnesium, zinc salts	Decreased tetracycline absorption	Avoid concurrent administration
Antibiotics	Probiotic supplements‡	Possible decreased GI adverse effects	Administer probiotic 20-30 minutes before or 2-3 hours after antibiotic

CNS, Central nervous system; *GI*, gastrointestinal; *NSAIDs*, nonsteroidal antiinflammatory drugs.

*Many of the interactions noted in this table are speculative and theoretic and are lacking adequate clinical evidence in humans. For an evidence-based assessment of hundreds of herbs and their potential or actual interactions with conventional pharmaceutical medications, see Brinker F: *Herb contraindications and drug interactions*, ed 3, Sandy, OR, 2001, Eclectic Medical Publications. Electronic updates with new information not included in the book are available at http://www.eclecticherb.com/emp. Accessed April 18, 2016.

†Some of the proposed interactions noted in this table are beneficial (e.g., the effect of sublingual licorice on reducing potential gastric irritation caused by oral administration of NSAIDs).

‡Preparations of normal gut flora used to help restore the normal microbial ecology disrupted by the antibiotic.

TABLE A2.5 Herbal Ingredients in Oral Health Care Products

Herbal Ingredient	Products	Possible Uses and Effects
Aloe vera (*Aloe vera*)	Mouth rinse, toothpaste, lubricating gel, antiseptic gel	Antiinflammatory, antiseptic, promotes healing of canker sores and wounds
Anise (*Pimpinella anisum*)	Mouth rinse, toothpaste	Breath freshener; may increase bleeding
Bloodroot (*Sanguinaria canadensis*)	Mouth rinse, toothpaste	Inhibits oral bacteria, used for gingivitis/periodontitis; may cause leukoplakia
Calendula (*Calendula officinalis*)	Mouth rinse, toothpaste	Antiinflammatory, promotes wound healing
Carrageenan (from red seaweed)	Toothpaste, tooth gel	Stabilizer, thickener
Cinnamon (*Cinnamomum verum* and related species)	Mouth rinse, toothpaste	Breath freshener
Clove (*Eugenia caryophyllata*)*	Toothache balm, mouth rinse, toothpaste, temporary filling material	Antiinflammatory, analgesic, antifungal; may cause increased bleeding
Eucalyptus (*Eucalyptus globulus*)	Mouth rinse, toothpaste	Antiseptic
Ginkgo (*Ginkgo biloba*)	Toothpaste	No use reported
Goldenseal (*Hydrastis canadensis*)	Mouth rinse, toothpaste, antiseptic gel, tooth gel	Immunostimulant, antibiotic, used for cold sores
Green tea (*Camellia sinensis*)	Toothpaste	Antiviral, cariostatic, antineoplastic, used for gingivitis/periodontitis; if swallowed may decrease absorption of basic drugs
Lemon balm (*Melissa officinalis*)	Antiseptic gel, lip balm	Antiherpetic; used to treat cold sores, nerve pain; may increase intraocular pressure
Licorice (*Glycyrrhiza glabra*)	Toothpaste, topical gel	Flavoring, antiherpetic, used to treat cold sores, canker sores
Myrrh (*Commiphora molmol*)	Mouth rinse, floss, tincture	Antiinflammatory, anticandidal, breath freshener, astringent; used to promote healing and for gingivitis
Neem (*Azadirachta indica*)	Toothpaste	Antimicrobial, mild abrasive, plaque inhibitor

TABLE A2.5 Herbal Ingredients in Oral Health Care Products—cont'd

Herbal Ingredient	Products	Possible Uses and Effects
Peelu (*Salvadora persica*)	Toothpaste, natural toothbrush	Mild abrasive, antibacterial, hemostatic, breath freshener
Peppermint (*Mentha piperita*)[†]	Mouth rinse, oral gel, dental gum, breath freshener, antiseptic gel, temporary filling material	Antibacterial, breath freshener, used for gingivitis/periodontitis and externally for myalgia and neuralgia; peppermint oil can cause burning sensation; possible tongue spasm; respiratory arrest contraindicates use in young children
Prickly ash (*Zanthoxylum americanum*)	Mouth rinse	None reported (proposed to be analgesic and to promote healing)
Propolis (*Propolis balsam*)	Toothpaste, flossing ribbon, in lysine gel	Analgesic, antibacterial, antifungal, mild antiinflammatory, promotes healing
Spearmint (*Mentha spicata*)[‡]	Toothpaste	Breath freshener
Stevia (*Stevia rebaudiana*)	Dental gel, mouth rinse	Cariostatic sweetener, weak antimicrobial
Tea tree oil (*Melaleuca alternifolia*)	Mouth rinse, breath freshener, antiseptic (in lozenges, toothpicks)	Antibacterial, antifungal, antiviral; may cause irritation in sensitive individuals
Thyme (*Thymus vulgaris*)	Mouth rinse	Antiseptic, breath freshener
Vegetable glycerin (glycerol)	Toothpaste, antiseptic gel	Lubricant, soother, sweetener
Witch hazel (*Hamamelis virginiana*)	Mouth rinse (alcoholic extract)	Antiinflammatory, soothing astringent (from alcoholic content), promotes wound healing; may cause stomach irritation if accidentally ingested
Xylitol (from birch tree bark)	Toothpaste, chewing gum	Cariostatic sweetener[§]

*Derivatives used in dentistry: eugenol, clove oil.
[†]Derivatives used in dentistry: menthol, peppermint oil.
‡Distillate used in dentistry: spearmint oil.
[§]Bacteria cannot metabolize xylitol, which is converted to glucose in the liver.

immunostimulant, and antiinflammatory actions may be used systemically for various oral conditions. In addition, there is a growing range of natural and **herbal products formulated for topical oral use**, including numerous mouth rinses, toothpastes, and irrigating solutions. Herbal dental products typically include agents that may be classified as astringents, antimicrobials, antiinflammatories, immunostimulants, circulation enhancers, tissue healers and soothers, and breath fresheners. The efficacy of therapeutic benefits of many of these agents has not been substantiated. Some of these natural agents are listed in Table A2.5.

WEB-BASED SOURCES OF INFORMATION ON HERBAL MEDICINE AND HERBAL DIETARY SUPPLEMENTS

www.consumerlab.com (ConsumerLab)
Free quality ratings of herbal and nutraceutical products. Subscription includes access to Natural Products Encyclopedia.

www.factsandcomparisons.com (Facts and Comparisons)
Access for subscription to Review of Natural Products and Drug Interaction Facts: Herbal Supplements and Food and for purchase of printed versions.

www.herbalgram.org (American Botanical Council)
Membership access to various information sources, including HerbClip, a biweekly abstract service; Herbalgram, a bimonthly journal; HerbMedPro, an evidence-based herbal database; and the German Commission E monographs.

www.herbmed.org (Alternative Medicine Foundation)
Subscription access to HerbMedPro and free access to Herbmed (75 herbal products) and Resource Guides on alternative medicine modalities, including herbal medicine.

www.naturaldatabase.com (Therapeutic Research Center)
Subscription access to the Natural Medicines Comprehensive Database and purchase access to printed and handheld computer versions.

www.naturalstandard.com (Natural Standard)
Free and expanded subscription access to the Natural Standard databases, which provide evidence-based information about alternative therapies, including herbal supplements.

www.nccam.nih.gov (National Center for Complementary and Alternative Medicine)
General information on complementary and alternative medicines, listing of alerts and advisories, and research results.

GENERAL REFERENCES

1. Hotwani K, Baliga S, Sharma K: Phytodentistry: use of medicinal plants, *J Complement Integr Med* 11:233–251, 2014.
2. Taheri JB, Azimi S, Rafieian N, Zanjani HA: Herbs in dentistry, *Int Dent J* 61:287–296, 2011.
3. Zheng LW, Hua H, Cheung LK: Traditional Chinese medicine and oral diseases: today and tomorrow, *Oral Dis* 17:7–12, 2011.

3 APPENDIX

Antiseptics and Disinfectants

Angelo J. Mariotti

It is important to understand the differences between the terms **sterilization, disinfection, and antisepsis. Sterilization** is the ultimate goal of any infection control protocol because it is the killing of all forms of microorganisms. To eradicate resistant viruses and bacterial endospores effectively requires the application of high heat or chemicals or both for a sufficient time. The most widely used means of attaining this objective in a dental office are dry heat, steam, and chemical vapor sterilization units. **Disinfection** is the application of chemicals to destroy most pathogenic organisms on inanimate surfaces. Although some chemicals used for disinfection are capable of achieving sterilization given sufficient time of exposure, their use to effect sterilization is discouraged because of the number of conditions that can lead to failure in this application. **Antisepsis** is the use of chemicals to destroy or inhibit pathogenic organisms on skin or living tissue. The difference between disinfection and antisepsis may seem small, but it leads to a wide divergence in the products used and the regulation of the products. Disinfectants fall under the regulatory authority of the U.S. Environmental Protection Agency and are subject to that agency's rules for demonstration of effectiveness and use in the workplace. Antiseptics, because they are intended for application on living tissue, fall under the regulations of the U.S. Food and Drug Administration regarding effectiveness and clinical use.

The table lists representative classes of compounds used as disinfectants or antiseptics with their dental uses. The aldehyde and certain halogen-based and oxidizing compounds have the broadest range of effectiveness. These agents also tend to be the most toxic to human tissue. Consequently, their use has been primarily limited to disinfection. The other chemical classes are less effective antimicrobial agents, but they also tend to be less harmful to human tissue and find use as disinfectants and antiseptics.

Commonly Used Disinfectants in Dentistry

Class	Agents	Mechanism of Action	Uses in Dentistry
Alcohols	Isopropanol, ethanol, n-propanol	Denaturation of bacterial proteins	Alcohol-based hand sanitizers in gel or rub delivery systems have been shown to be an effective alternative to washing unsoiled hands with soap and water or antimicrobial soap.
Aldehydes	Glutaraldehyde	Alkylation of sulfhydryl, hydroxyl, carboxyl, and amino groups of microorganisms, which alters RNA, DNA, and protein synthesis	Glutaraldehyde is used to disinfect equipment that cannot be steam sterilized. Currently, glutaraldehyde is the most common active ingredient for cold sterilization. However, cold sterilization is not extensively used because of the introduction of heat-resistant materials available for steam sterilization as well as the requirement for prolonged immersion in (6-10 hours) and thorough removal of glutaraldehyde from equipment.
Halogens	Chorine, iodines	Free chlorine acts in a number of ways including oxidization of sulfhydryl groups on enzymes and amino acids, amino acid ring chlorination, decreased uptake of nutrients, inhibition of protein synthesis, destruction of DNA, and/or decreased oxygen uptake	These are some of the most effective antimicrobial compounds used for disinfection but are not extensively used in dentistry due to their corrosiveness. Dilute concentrations of chlorine (5% sodium hypochlorite) have been used to disinfect and debride root canals, while more concentrated formulations (50 ppm chlorine dioxide) have been recently used to disinfect dental unit waterlines. Iodine and iodophors were used in dentistry to identify plaque and to disinfect wounds, but currently they have very limited use in dentistry.
Heavy metals	Tin	Disruption of bacterial enzymatic processes, binds to sulfhydryl groups	Tin, the stannous ion, is an effective antimicrobial. Stannous fluoride has become a popular fluoride source in dentifrices, particularly in dentifrices marketed for their effect on gingival health. The ability of tin to inhibit bacterial growth and biofilms has supported the use in dentifrices. However, there are problems with stability, taste, and staining.
Oxidizing compounds	Hydrogen peroxide	Destructive hydroxyl free radicals attack membrane lipids, DNA, and other essential cell components	Hydrogen peroxide is the most common of numerous oxidizing compounds that have been used primarily as antiseptics in health care. Oxygenating agents release oxygen as an active intermediate, loosening debris in inaccessible areas. The germicidal activity of these agents in the oral cavity is negligible.

Commonly Used Disinfectants in Dentistry—cont'd

Class	Agents	Mechanism of Action	Uses in Dentistry
Phenolic compounds	Eugenol, chlorhexidine, triclosan	Denaturation of proteins and inactivation of essential bacterial enzyme systems and leakage of essential metabolites from the cell wall	Phenolic compounds are used extensively in dentistry. Eugenol (2-methoxy-4-allylphenol) has weak antimicrobial activity but is useful for rapid analgesic properties. Eugenol remains a common component in many sedative pastes. Chlorhexidine (1,1′-hexamethylene bis(5-(*p*-chlorophenyl) biguanide)) is a common antiseptic used as an oral rinse to reduce dental biofilms. As a result of the binding of chlorhexidine to oral structures, the drug exhibits substantivity in the mouth. Triclosan (2,4,4′-trichloro-2′-hydroxydiphenyl ether) is a nonionic bisphenol with broad antimicrobial activity as well as a direct antiinflammatory effect. When combined with a copolymer, triclosan in a dentifrice has significant substantivity.
Surface-active agents	Sodium dodecyl sulfate, quarternary ammonium compounds	Inactivation of energy-producing enzymes, denaturation of essential cell proteins, and disruption of the cell membrane	Surface-active agents are not used to disinfect equipment in the dental office; rather, these agents are used in toothpastes and mouth rinses to reduce dental biofilms. Detergents such as sodium dodecyl sulfate are effective primarily as a result of their cleaning and emulsifying ability. Quaternary ammonium compounds, such as cetylpyridinium chloride, have broad but modest antimicrobial activity and are used in mouth rinses.

GENERAL REFERENCES

Best Practices for the Safe Use of Glutaraldehye in Health Care, Occupational Safety and Health Administration, https://www.osha.gov/Publications/glutaraldehyde.pdf.

Guidelines for Disinfection and Sterilization in Healthcare Facilities, 2008, http://www.cdc.gov/hicpac/Disinfection_Sterilization/13_0Sterilization.html.

Harte JA: Standard and transmission-based precautions: an update for dentistry, *J Am Dent Assoc.* 141:572–581, 2010.

Kumar S, Atray D, Paiwal D, Balasubramanyam G, Duraiswamy P, Kulkarni S: Dental unit waterlines: source of contamination and cross-infection, *J Hosp Infect* 74:99–111, 2010.

4 APPENDIX

Drug Interactions in Clinical Dentistry

Angelo J. Mariotti

Numerous studies have documented that drugs are rarely taken in isolation. For example, adults in contemporary society may take an average of four to five drugs daily, and hospitalized patients may receive from 9 to 13 different agents every 24 hours, depending on the institution, the patient's status, and the intercommunication among attending physicians. As the number of administered drugs increases arithmetically, the risk of an adverse drug reaction increases geometrically. Although some of this increase undoubtedly reflects a greater severity of disease and reduced physiologic reserve in patients requiring multidrug therapy, it also underscores the fact that drugs may interact with each other in producing toxicologic effects. Drug interactions, in fact, account for 5% to 10% of all adverse reactions to drugs and may be responsible for extending the hospital stay of approximately 15% of admitted patients. However, not all drug interactions are clinically significant or undesired, and some are actively sought in pharmacotherapeutics to increase drug effectiveness, decrease toxicity, or both. This section reviews the basic principles and general mechanisms of drug interactions and illustrates these interactions with selected examples. Some interactions are not included here, for example, medication interference with laboratory tests and metabolic interactions with environmental chemicals, such as pesticides that alter in vivo enzyme activity. Interactions involving herbal products are described in Appendix 2. Finally, it is generally assumed, in this appendix, for the sake of simplicity that only two agents are interacting concurrently, and that the drugs are given systemically.

The sources of drugs that may be involved in drug interactions are varied. They may be prescribed or administered by a single physician or dentist or by several practitioners. Patients may also medicate themselves with over-the-counter preparations, with drugs provided by relatives or friends, or with medication remaining from a previous prescription. Finally, certain substances in foods and in cigarette smoke may interact with administered drugs. Potential interactions between concurrently administered drugs are both dose and duration dependent; nevertheless, the degree or severity of an adverse interaction is seldom predictable. In the discussion that follows, drug interactions are reviewed according to type and mechanism, and examples of each are included for illustration.

CLASSIFICATION OF DRUG INTERACTIONS

Drug interactions are expressed in a bewildering diversity of altered responses. Quantitative changes in reactions to one or more drugs can occur, and complex systems of nomenclature and mathematic description have been developed to characterize the combined effects of drugs. Although such approaches are of theoretic and experimental value, they are less useful in the clinical setting and fail to take into account some qualitative changes in drug effect that can occur.

The simplest clinical classification scheme recognizes three basic types of drug interactions: **antagonism**, **potentiation**, and **unexpected drug effect** (Table A4.1). Implicit in this classification is a primary or "object" drug whose effects are modified (i.e., reduced, increased, or transformed) and an interacting or "precipitant" drug responsible for altering the effects of the object drug. Omitted from Table A4.3 (see later in this appendix), however, are drugs that produce identical or similar actions, yielding a **summation** of drug effects when the drugs are administered together. Inasmuch as summation is commonly exploited in therapeutics and is often responsible for adverse drug reactions, its description is included in Table A4.1. A last category, **synergism**, is used to identify agonist combinations that yield a magnitude of effect beyond that obtainable with a single agonist regardless of dose (Table A4.1).

MECHANISMS OF DRUG INTERACTIONS

Drug interactions can occur at any point along the pharmacologic pathway of the agonist, from even before the drug is administered to a patient, to the period when it is in contact with its site of action, to the point at which it is eliminated. The various mechanisms involved in drug interactions can be grouped taxonomically into three broad categories: **pharmaceutical, pharmacokinetic, and pharmacodynamic interactions** (Table A4.2).

FACTORS INFLUENCING DRUG INTERACTIONS

Several variables can affect the occurrence and intensity of potential drug interactions. Prime among these are variations in the handling of and reaction to administered drugs, including the genetic-based differences described in Chapter 4. Drug interactions and drug effects are both dose dependent and duration dependent; thus an interaction may not be clinically discernible each time interacting drugs are administered. The higher the dosage and the longer the administration, the greater is the chance that an interaction may occur. Previous exposure affecting drug transport, metabolism, or responsiveness may alter the potential for interaction. In addition, many drugs have a long biologic half-life, and effective concentrations may be present in the blood or tissue for many days after the cessation of therapy; interactions may occur, therefore, days and occasionally weeks after discontinuation of therapy with one of the interacting drugs.

DRUG INTERACTIONS USED IN PHARMACOTHERAPEUTICS

Combinations of drugs are used in therapy to provide enhanced effects and to prevent adverse reactions. Purposeful drug interactions are especially common in the treatment of certain diseases, such as essential hypertension, tuberculosis, and cancer, in which the concurrent administration of two or more drugs is routine. Drugs may also be given sequentially so the second agent abruptly terminates the action of the first. Thus edrophonium, a cholinesterase inhibitor, is administered to reverse the neuromuscular blockade of vecuronium, and leucovorin (folinic acid) is administered to "rescue" patients given potentially lethal doses of methotrexate, a folic acid analogue used in cancer chemotherapy. Agents useful as specific antidotes in accidental drug overdosage include protamine for heparin, naloxone for opioid analgesics, and atropine for anticholinesterases.

Particular mention should be made of fixed-dose combination products. Such preparations make up a significant fraction of all drugs sold in the United States, from over-the-counter remedies to prescription items to agents administered by practitioners. The fixed combination of a local anesthetic with epinephrine to provide more effective and more prolonged anesthesia is a notable example. In general, drug mixtures include a principal ingredient for the main therapeutic effect; adjuvants that summate with, potentiate, or otherwise complement the first drug; and correctives that antagonize or minimize undesired side effects.

The major criticisms of fixed-dose combinations are (1) the inability to adjust the dosages of the individual ingredients to the needs of a particular patient; (2) discrepancies in half-lives of individual agents, leading to the accumulation of some, but not other, constituents during repeated administration; (3) the likelihood of taking unnecessary drugs; (4) the possibility of increased toxicity or allergenicity without correspondingly increased therapeutic efficacy; and (5) the possibility of a higher cost from the manufacturer. However, fixed-dose combinations have certain potential advantages. Certain mixtures offer therapeutic gains in effectiveness or safety (e.g., acetaminophen with hydrocodone combinations, local anesthetic-vasoconstrictor solutions, and hydrochlorothiazide with triamterene). In addition, drug combinations may improve patient compliance by reducing the number of medications the patient must take. Finally, the reduced number of individual prescriptions can be less expensive to the patient. Although certain fixed-dose combinations are useful, such preparations should be avoided as a general rule, and only those

TABLE A4.1 The Effects of Different Types of Drug Interactions

Drug Interaction Classification	Definition	Possible Mechanisms
Antagonism	The biologic or clinical response to a drug is reduced by administering a second agent.	A substance produces a physical or chemical change in the agonist, reducing or abolishing its activity. One drug modifies the disposition of a second agent. Competition exists between drugs for the same receptor site, diminishing or even abolishing the effectiveness of the active drug. Antagonism of receptor activation exists that is of a noncompetitive nature. Drugs having opposing actions at different receptor sites partially or completely antagonize the effects of either or both drugs.
Potentiation	Occurs when a combination of two drugs that do not share similar pharmacologic activities results in an effect of one of the drugs that is greater than expected that can lead to toxicity.	Not active in producing the effect by itself, the precipitant or potentiating drug sensitizes the person to the active object drug. Interaction occurs when the precipitant drug elevates the free concentration of the active drug by increasing its absorption, altering its distribution, or inhibiting its elimination.
Unexpected drug effect	The combination of two or more drugs resulting in a response typically not observed when any of the drugs is given singly, even in overdose.	A novel drug effect involves perturbation of the metabolism of one drug by another, leading to the formation of a highly active metabolite.
Summation	The combined activities of two or more drugs that elicit identical or related pharmacologic effects.	If the drugs act at the same site and produce simple arithmetic summation of effects, they are said to be **additive.**
Synergism	The combination of two or more agonists produces an effect that is greater quantitatively than what can be achieved by maximally effective doses of any one drug given alone.	More than one mechanism is involved in a synergistic response.

TABLE A4.2 Mechanisms of Drug Interactions

Mechanism	Definition	Effects
Pharmaceutical	**Pharmaceutical interactions** represent drug incompatibilities of a physical or chemical nature.	In general, pharmaceutical interactions can be anticipated between organic acids and bases, resulting in precipitation of one or both drugs. Chemical reactions between drugs may also occur, but these are less common.
Pharmacokinetic	**Pharmacokinetic interactions** derive from the influence of one drug on the absorption, distribution, biotransformation, or excretion of another drug.	**Absorption**. Many times an interaction affects the rate or extent of effective absorption of a drug into the systemic circulation, causing a decrease or increase in that drug's effect. Factors influencing absorption include the pH of lumen fluids, enzyme activity, and intestinal motility. **Distribution**. After a drug is absorbed, an interaction may modify its distribution or the rate of transfer of the drug from one location to another. Drug distribution can be affected by plasma protein binding as well as distribution across cellular membranes.

Continued

TABLE A4.2 Mechanisms of Drug Interactions—cont'd

Mechanism	Definition	Effects
		Metabolism. The degree and duration of activity of a drug are often functions of its metabolism; therefore an interacting drug can modify the effect of an agonist by altering its rate of biotransformation. Most drugs used therapeutically are metabolized in the liver by the microsomal enzyme system and drugs that alter these enzymes can affect drug concentrations.
		Excretion. Increasing or decreasing the rate of excretion, or renal or biliary clearance, of a drug also alters its elimination rate constant and therefore the amount of drug available in the circulating plasma, thus affecting the duration and the degree of activity of the drug. Renal excretion is influenced by urinary pH and tubular reabsorption, as well as inhibition of active tubular transport.
Pharmacodynamic	**Pharmacodynamic interactions** represent modifications in the pharmacologic effects of a drug independent of any change in the quantitative disposition of that drug.	Such interactions may increase, diminish, or qualitatively alter the therapeutic effect. Many interactions take place at or near receptor sites. The mechanisms involved can include competition for the receptor or alterations of either the receptor or its natural ligand, whereas, interacting drugs may also exert their effects at sites of action in different locations.

TABLE A4.3 Examples of Interactions of Drugs Commonly Used in Dentistry

Drug	Interacting Drug	Effect and Recommendation
Antibiotics		
Penicillins, cephalosporins	Bacteriostatic antibiotics (e.g., macrolides, tetracyclines, clindamycin)	Bacteriostatic antibiotics (second group) may interfere with the action of bactericidal antibiotics (first group). Consult with informed sources for optimal therapy
Penicillins, cephalosporins, tetracyclines, ciprofloxacin	Oral contraceptives	There is a **low risk** that these antibiotics may stimulate estrogen elimination and may decrease effectiveness of contraceptive agent. Advise patient accordingly
Penicillins, cephalosporins	Probenecid	Urinary excretion of antibiotic is retarded. Consult with prescribing physician for appropriate dosage schedule
Penicillins	Enoxaparin, heparin	High-dose penicillins can increase bleeding time. Use cautiously
	Methotrexate	Urinary excretion of methotrexate may be inhibited. Use cautiously
Ampicillin, amoxicillin	Allopurinol	High incidence of skin rash has been reported
	Atenolol	Atenolol concentrations may be reduced. Use cautiously
Cephalosporins	Drugs that cause nephrotoxicity or ototoxicity (e.g., aminoglycosides, aspirin, amphotericin B, cisplatin, cephalosporins, colistimethate)	Additive toxicity may occur. Cephalexin and cefoxitin are apparently safe
Clindamycin, macrolides, tetracyclines	Bactericidal antibiotics (e.g., penicillins, cephalosporins)	Action of bactericidal antibiotics may be inhibited. Avoid concurrent use, or consult with informed sources
Clindamycin	Erythromycin, clarithromycin, azithromycin	Antagonism can occur between these drugs. Avoid concurrent use. Do not use one agent for prophylaxis of endocarditis after recent use of other agent
	Kaolin	Absorption of clindamycin is delayed. Avoid concurrent use of clindamycin
Macrolides	Chloramphenicol, clindamycin	Erythromycin and other macrolides may interfere with the antibacterial effects of the other agents. Avoid concurrent use. Do not give clarithromycin or azithromycin for prophylaxis of endocarditis after recent use of one of these drugs
Macrolides, tetracyclines	Digoxin	Absorption of digoxin preparations may be increased. Advise patient accordingly
Erythromycin, clarithromycin	Alfentanil, bromocriptine, caffeine, calcium channel blockers, carbamazepine, corticosteroids, cyclosporine, disopyramide, ergot drugs, felodipine, midazolam, theophylline drugs, triazolam, valproic acid, warfarin	Erythromycin and clarithromycin may interfere with metabolism of these drugs. Use intravenous agents cautiously. Administration of clarithromycin prophylaxis of endocarditis is probably of little consequence, but a full course of macrolide therapy requires consultation with physician, especially regarding carbamazepine, cyclosporine, and warfarin
	HMG-CoA reductase inhibitors (statins)	Erythromycin and clarithromycin interfere with metabolism of these agents, possibly causing rhabdomyolysis. Avoid concurrent use

TABLE A4.3 Examples of Interactions of Drugs Commonly Used in Dentistry—cont'd

Drug	Interacting Drug	Effect and Recommendation
Erythromycin	Drugs that cause ototoxicity or especially hepatotoxicity (e.g., furosemide, fluorouracil)	Use of erythromycin for prophylaxis of endocarditis is probably not a problem. Increased risk of ototoxicity or hepatotoxicity may warrant consultation with prescribing physician
Tetracyclines	Antacids, bismuth, Ca^{++}, iron, Mg^{++}, or zinc salts, H_2 antihistamines, colestipol	Absorption of tetracycline is impaired. Space administration schedules to avoid simultaneous ingestion. Occasionally, increased dosage necessary
	Li^+ salts	Plasma Li^+ concentrations may be increased. Advise patient accordingly
	Anisindione, warfarin	In patients with poor dietary vitamin K, tetracyclines may increase effect of oral anticoagulants. Use cautiously
Doxycycline	Barbiturates, alcohol (chronic use), carbamazepine, phenytoin	Hepatic clearance of doxycycline is increased. Adjust dosage upward, or use alternative tetracycline
Oxytetracycline	Insulin	Hypoglycemic action of oxytetracycline reduces insulin requirements. Substitute with another antibiotic
Metronidazole	Alcohol	Alcohol metabolism is altered, leading to buildup of acetaldehyde. Avoid concurrent use
	Cimetidine	Hepatic clearance of metronidazole is decreased. Use cautiously
	Chloroquine, disulfiram	Psychotomimetic reactions possible. Avoid concurrent use
	Barbiturates, phenytoin	Hepatic clearance of metronidazole is increased. Consider increasing dose if therapy proves to be suboptimal. Metronidazole may decrease phenytoin, however, which may warrant consultation with prescribing physician
	Li^+ salts	Renal toxicity of Li^+ may occur. Avoid concurrent use
	Warfarin	Hepatic clearance of warfarin is decreased. Full course of therapy requires consultation with prescribing physician
Azole antifungal drugs	Antivirals, benzodiazepines, carbamazepine, calcium channel blockers, digoxin, colchicine, lovastatin, simvastatin. atorvastatin, oxycodone, quinidine, phenytoin, sirolimus, tacrolimus	The levels of these drugs may be increased due to inhibition of cytochrome enzymes and other effects of the azole antifungal drugs
Azole antifungal drugs	Barbiturates, rifampin	Increased metabolism of itraconazole
Azole antifungal drugs	H_2 histamine receptor blockers, proton pump inhibitors	Decreased absorption of the azoles
Analgesics		
Aspirin and other NSAIDs	NSAIDs	Ulcerogenic and platelet-inhibiting effects of these agents are increased, but not the analgesia. Aspirin may decrease effectiveness of some NSAIDs. Avoid concurrent use, but ensure optimal NSAID therapy
	Drugs that cause nephrotoxicity and ototoxicity (e.g., aminoglycosides, cyclosporine, furosemide, vancomycin)	Short courses for pain relief are probably of little concern, but avoid or minimize concurrent use
	Antidiabetic sulfonylurea drugs	Hypoglycemic effects are enhanced. Substitute with acetaminophen
	Baclofen, methotrexate, Li^+ salts, phenytoin, Ca^{++} channel blockers	Plasma concentrations of these agents are increased by aspirin-like drugs. Substitute with acetaminophen
	Probenecid, sulfinpyrazone	Probenecid interferes with renal and biliary excretion of NSAIDs. Aspirin may block uricosuric effects of probenecid and sulfinpyrazone. Substitute with acetaminophen
	Alcohol, corticosteroids	Combination may result in gastrointestinal ulceration and bleeding. Corticosteroid may also increase salicylate clearance. Avoid concurrent use
	ACE inhibitors, β blockers, diuretics	Hypotensive effect of ACE inhibitors, β blockers, and diuretics may be reduced. Advise patient accordingly
Aspirin, other NSAIDs, and acetaminophen	Anticoagulants and thrombolytics, extended-spectrum β-lactam antibiotics (e.g., ticarcillin)	Combination may result in increased bleeding, especially with aspirin. Cautious use of acetaminophen acceptable (<2 g/day)
Aspirin	Valproic acid	Increased plasma concentrations of valproic acid and additive antiplatelet effects may increase bleeding tendencies. Use cautiously
	Carbonic anhydrase inhibitors	Increased central nervous system (CNS) toxicity from aspirin or carbonic anhydrase inhibitor may result. Use cautiously
	Antacids, griseofulvin	Salicylate concentrations reduced. Use alternative NSAID

TABLE A4.3 Examples of Interactions of Drugs Commonly Used in Dentistry—cont'd

Drug	Interacting Drug	Effect and Recommendation
	Ibuprofen and other NSAIDs	Ibuprofen and other NSAIDs can interfere with the antiplatelet effect of aspirin. Avoid concurrent use if used together for longer than a few days. Alternatively, administer the non-aspirin NSAID after the daily aspirin has been absorbed
Ibuprofen	Digoxin	Ibuprofen decreases clearance of digoxin. Substitute acetaminophen to avoid possibility of increased toxicity
Acetaminophen	Alcohol	Acetaminophen hepatotoxicity is more likely in chronic alcoholics. Use cautiously
	Cholestyramine	Concurrent ingestion inhibits acetaminophen absorption. Administer acetaminophen at least 1 h before cholestyramine
	β Blockers, barbiturates, isoniazid, phenytoin, sulfinpyrazone	Alteration of acetaminophen metabolism may increase risk of hepatotoxicity. Use cautiously
Opioid analgesics and opioid agonist-antagonists	Alcohol, CNS depressants, local anesthetics, antidepressants, antipsychotics, centrally acting antihypertensives, antihistamines, cimetidine, $MgSO_4$ (parenteral)	Increased CNS and respiratory depression may occur. Use cautiously, perhaps in reduced dosage
	Antimuscarinics, antidiarrheals, antihypertensives	Opioids increase effects of these drugs. Use cautiously
	Naltrexone, opioid agonist-antagonists	These drugs block the analgesic effects of opioids. Substitute with ibuprofen or similar NSAID for pain relief
	Monoamine oxidase inhibitors, furazolidone, procarbazine	Meperidine results in marked toxicity and is absolutely contraindicated. Use other opioids cautiously
	Aprepitant, diltiazem, HIV protease inhibitors, verapamil	These drugs may increase the plasma concentrations and effects of the opioids. Avoid concurrent use if possible
Codeine, hydrocodone	Amiodarone, celecoxib, diphenhydramine, duloxetine, fluoxetine, paroxetine, quinidine, ritonavir, sertraline,	Conversion to analgesic metabolites may be impaired. Avoid use of codeine; may need increased doses of hydrocodone
Alfentanil	Erythromycin	Erythromycin may interfere with metabolism of alfentanil. Use cautiously
Opioid agonist/antagonist	Opioid analgesics	Antagonism of opioid analgesic effect may lead to withdrawal symptoms in dependent patients. Avoid concurrent use
Local Anesthetic Preparations		
Local anesthetics	Alcohol, CNS depressants, opioids, antidepressants, antipsychotics, centrally acting antihypertensives, antihistamines, $MgSO_4$ (parenteral)	Increased CNS and respiratory depression may occur. Use cautiously
	Antiarrhythmic drugs	Increased cardiac depression may occur. Use cautiously
	Anticholinesterases	Local anesthetics may antagonize effects of anticholinesterases on muscle contractility. Treat myasthenic patients in consultation with physician
Amides	Amiodarone, β blockers, cimetidine	Metabolism of amides in liver is reduced. Use cautiously
Esters	Anticholinesterases	Metabolism of esters is reduced. Use cautiously
	Sulfonamides	Inhibition of sulfonamide action may occur. Avoid concurrent use
Adrenergic vasoconstrictors	Inhalation anesthetics	Increased possibility of cardiac arrhythmias exists with some agents. Consult with anesthesiologist
	Methyldopa, tricyclic antidepressants	Sympathomimetic effects may be enhanced. Use epinephrine cautiously. Avoid levonordefrin and norepinephrine
	β Blockers, adrenergic neuron blockers, entacapone, tolcapone	Hypertensive and cardiac reactions are more likely. Use cautiously
	Antipsychotics	Vasoconstrictor action is inhibited, which may lead to hypotensive responses to epinephrine. Use cautiously
Antianxiety-Sedative Agents		
Barbiturates, benzodiazepines, chloral hydrate, hydroxyzine, propofol	Alcohol, CNS depressants, opioids, local anesthetics, antidepressants, antipsychotics, centrally acting antihypertensives, antihistamines, $MgSO_4$ (parenteral)	Increased CNS and respiratory depression may occur. Use cautiously, perhaps in reduced dosage
Barbiturates, benzodiazepines, propofol	Antihypertensives, antipsychotics, intravenous opioids, Li^+ salts	Intravenous administration in patients receiving these medications can lead to hypotension. Use cautiously

TABLE A4.3 Examples of Interactions of Drugs Commonly Used in Dentistry—cont'd

Drug	Interacting Drug	Effect and Recommendation
Barbiturates	Acetaminophen, anticoagulants (oral), β blockers (except renally excreted congeners), carbamazepine, chloramphenicol, cimetidine, corticosteroids, corticotropin, cyclophosphamide, cyclosporine, dacarbazine, delavirdine, disopyramide, doxorubicin, doxycycline, estrogen and estrogen-containing contraceptives, fenoprofen, griseofulvin, guanfacine, haloperidol, hydantoin anticonvulsants, levothyroxine, methadone, metronidazole, mexiletine, phenothiazines, quinidine, protease inhibitors, theophylline-containing preparations, tricyclic antidepressants, valproic acid, verapamil	Barbiturates stimulate metabolism of many drugs. Avoid multidose use. Single administration of short-acting drug (e.g., pentobarbital) is not known to be a problem
	Antipsychotics	Increased tendency for hypothermia. Evaluate temperature as needed
	Chloramphenicol, methylphenidate, valproic acid	Metabolism of barbiturate decreased. Avoid multidose use. Advise patient of possibility of post-sedation drowsiness
	Methsuximide	Metabolism of the barbiturate is decreased. Avoid multidose use. Advise patient of possibility of post-sedation drowsiness
Thiopental, methohexital	Probenecid, sulfonamides	Decreased binding of barbiturate to plasma proteins can potentiate anesthetic effect. Use cautiously
Benzodiazepines	H_2 antihistamines	Delayed absorption of benzodiazepine. Advise patient accordingly
	Carbamazepine	Increased metabolism of both agents. Avoid multidose use
	Cimetidine, disulfiram, fluconazole, fluoxetine, isoniazid, itraconazole, metoprolol, omeprazole, oral contraceptives, posaconazole, propranolol, probenecid, valproic acid	Metabolism of benzodiazepine may be decreased. Lorazepam and oxazepam least likely to be affected; avoid multidose use of other agents. Advise patient of possibility of post-sedation drowsiness
	Levodopa	Decreased therapeutic effect of levodopa. Advise patient accordingly
	Amiodarone	Increased cardiovascular toxicity. Avoid concurrent use
	Digoxin	Digoxin elimination rate may be decreased. Substitute with short-acting benzodiazepine (e.g., triazolam), and avoid multidose use
	Disulfiram	May increase the half-life of benzodiazepines, except lorazepam, oxazepam and temazepam
Lorazepam	Alcohol, scopolamine	Increased anxiety with alcohol and irrational behavior with scopolamine. Avoid concurrent use
Midazolam, triazolam	Diltiazem, cimetidine, erythromycin, fluconazole, fluoxetine, fluvoxamine, itraconazole, quinupristin/dalfopristin, nefazodone, verapamil	Metabolism of midazolam and triazolam impaired. Avoid concurrent oral use; otherwise use cautiously
	Clozapine, HIV protease inhibitors	Serious CNS adverse effects may occur. Avoid concurrent use
Chloral hydrate	Anisindione, warfarin	Oral anticoagulants are displaced from protein binding sites, which may lead to bleeding. Avoid concurrent use
	Alcohol	Combination causes increased cardiovascular toxicity and CNS depression. Avoid concurrent use

mixtures that have been demonstrated to be therapeutically advantageous to the patient should be used.

This appendix lists important interactions that may occur between drugs a patient is taking for non-dental conditions and common antimicrobial, analgesic, local anesthetic, and antianxiety-sedative preparations prescribed or used in clinical practice. It is assumed that all prescriptions are for short-term therapy (i.e., ≤1 week) and that all drugs are in conventional dosages. Antimicrobial drugs include oral forms of penicillins (e.g., penicillin V, amoxicillin), cephalosporins (e.g., cephalexin, cefaclor), macrolides (including the various salt forms of erythromycin), tetracyclines (e.g., tetracycline, doxycycline), clindamycin, and metronidazole. Analgesics covered consist of NSAIDs, acetaminophen and opioid analgesics, opioid agonist-antagonists, and their combinations. Local anesthetics include all formulations currently available for dental use in the United States. Antianxiety-sedative drugs listed include short-acting and ultrashort-acting barbiturates, propofol, benzodiazepines, chloral hydrate, and hydroxyzine. The term **use cautiously** indicates that the interaction is rare or not usually dangerous (or both) and that careful administration within recommended dosage limits and increased surveillance of drug effects should suffice to avoid serious toxicity.

5 APPENDIX

Drugs Used in the Treatment of Glaucoma

Frank J. Dowd

Class	Drugs	Mechanism	Chapter
Muscarinic receptor agonists	Carbachol, pilocarpine	Constrict pupils and ciliary muscle leading to exit of aqueous fluid via canal of Schlemm and trabecular network as well as uveoscleral pathway	6
Anticholinesterases			
Short-acting	Physostigmine		
Long-acting	demecarium, echothiophate		
Adrenergic receptor agonists		Reduce production of aqueous humor and increase outflow, vasoconstriction	8
α and β agonist	Epinephrine		
Prodrug	Dipivefrin		
α_2 Agonist	Apraclonidine, brimonidine	Decrease aqueous humor production	
β-Adrenergic receptor antagonists		Decrease aqueous humor production	9
Nonselective	Carteolol, levobunolol, metipranolol, timolol		
β_1 Selective	Betaxolol		
Prostaglandin $F_{2\alpha}$ analogues	Bimatoprost, latanoprost, travoprost, unoprostone	Increase outflow of aqueous humor through the uveoscleral and trabecular meshwork pathways	
Carbonic anhydrase inhibitors	Acetazolamide, brinzolamide, dorzolamide	Reduce aqueous humor secretion	22
Osmotic agents	Glycerine, isosorbide, mannitol	Osmotic removal of aqueous humor	22

Glaucoma results in an increase in intraocular pressure that can damage the retina. There are two basic types of glaucoma: open angle and closed or narrow angle. These refer to the angle between the iris and the exit channels for aqueous humor, primarily the canal of Schlemm and the trabecular meshwork. Open-angle glaucoma is the more common type, but closed-angle glaucoma can present an acute emergency. Open-angle glaucoma is treated pharmacologically. The definitive treatment for closed-angle glaucoma is surgical correction of the occluded exit channels. Drug therapy is useful as a temporary adjunct to surgery for closed-angle glaucoma. Drugs that cause mydriasis pose a high risk in patients with closed-angle glaucoma. Drugs are given as eye drops except for some carbonic anhydrase inhibitors and some osmotic agents.

APPENDIX 6

Prescription Writing

Vahn A. Lewis

COMPONENT PARTS OF THE PRESCRIPTION

A complete, ideal prescription comprises several parts, each of which provides specific information about the prescriber, the patient, and the drug. The patient's **full name**, **age**, and **address** are required on prescriptions for DEA-controlled substances. Including the patient's age and/or weight is especially desirable on prescriptions for children younger than 12 years or elderly patients needing dosage adjustment, permitting the pharmacist to confirm the dosage. The **name and full address** of the prescriber are necessary. The **telephone** number may be required and is usually included as a convenience to the pharmacist. The **date** on which the prescription is written and signed is always desirable and is required on prescriptions for DEA-controlled substances or in states in which prescriptions expire.

The symbol **Rx**, known as the **superscription**, is generally understood to be an abbreviation of the Latin *recipe*, meaning "take thou," but it was probably derived from the ancient Roman symbol for Jupiter and used in the physician's prayer for the survival of the patient.

The **inscription** provides specific information about the drug preparation: (1) the name of the drug, which can be either the nonproprietary or the proprietary name, or possibly both, with the proprietary name following the nonproprietary name in parentheses, as with **pentazocine (Talwin)**, and (2) the unit dosage or amount of the drug in milligrams (e.g., **penicillin VK 500 mg**) or other appropriate unit of measure (e.g., **penicillin G 250,000 U**) and the dosage form (e.g., **tablets, suspension, sprinkles**). If the prescription is for a liquid preparation, the individual unit of dosage is usually contained in a **teaspoonful** or 5 mL (e.g., **amoxicillin 125 mg/5 mL**). The inscription should provide an unambiguous identification of the drug and any other ingredients that the pharmacist must assemble to fill the prescription order. Drug products are available in unique strengths and dosage forms. When prescribing, a product, strength, and dosage form that is available to the pharmacist should be designated. The inscription should be written just below and to the right of the superscription.

The next part of the prescription is the **subscription**. The subscription is the prescriber's directions to the pharmacist regarding fulfilling the inscription. Because almost all drugs used by dentists are available in manufactured dosage forms, the subscription is usually brief, including the following:

1. The quantity (and dosage form) of the drug to be dispensed; that is, the number of tablets or capsules or the volume of a liquid preparation needed for a course of therapy (e.g., "dispense 28 tablets").
   a. This direction is written, preferably in Arabic numerals, for an appropriate amount of the drug to supply the patient for the full course of the intended therapy. The prescriber also considers the toxicity and abuse potential of the drug and the cost to the patient. For DEA-controlled drugs, the quantity must be written in numbers and spelled out (in English, not Latin) to avoid alteration. (Without this precaution, 15 is easily changed to 45, 75, or 150.) Alternatively, the prescription may have a check-off box for the range of doses that includes the amount to be dispensed. In any prescription, no greater quantity of drug than is needed should be ordered. In the case of electronic prescriptions, sent directly to the pharmacy, only the numerical designation of the quantity is required as the patient does not handle the prescription. In some cases, the amount prescribed should be limited to prevent obscuring symptoms, such as prescribing analgesics for 3 or 4 days rather than the 7 to 10 days as is common for antibiotics. If multiple appointments are anticipated, it may be more cost-effective to write the amount to reflect several appointments. The subscription should be on the line below the last line of the inscription. Directions to the pharmacist to list the name of the medication will be on the container label and this is indicated by writing "label." The current trend in most states is to require the pharmacist to identify medications on the label unless such identification is not considered to be in the patient's best interest and is specifically prohibited by the prescriber. Identifying the drug can help the patient identify which medication he or she is taking, and it can prevent allergic reactions or adverse interactions with other medications and misuse of the unused portion of the prescription. It may be especially helpful in directing the management of victims of drug poisoning. When present, this information is often physically located below the transcription on the prescription.
2. Instruction to the pharmacist if the prescription can be refilled without the prescriber writing a new prescription.
   a. The number and its time limitation are specified for DEA-controlled drugs, but they are otherwise left to the discretion of the practitioner. Some state laws dictate, however, that prescriptions expire at the end of each year. If refill directions are not authorized by the prescriber, no refills may be dispensed. With controlled substances, care should be taken to devise a refill authorization system that is not easily altered, such as crossing out all except the desired number in a series (e.g., 0, 1, 2, etc.). The refill instructions are usually physically located below the transcription.
3. Dispensing characteristics of the drug.
   a. To save patients money, some states allow dispensing up to three refills (for a 90-day supply of drug) at the same time unless the practitioner notes that the "**refill schedule is medically necessary**" on the prescription. This exception is not made for controlled substances or psychotropics. In the case of fluoride prescriptions, it would be wise to specify "refill schedule is medically necessary."

The **transcription**, or **signature**—from the Latin ***signa***, meaning "label" or "let it be labeled" and indicated on the prescription by "**Label:**"

TABLE A6.1 Some Latin Abbreviations Used in Prescription Writing

Abbreviation	Latin	English
ad lib.	ad libitum	at pleasure
a.c.	ante cibum	before meals
aq.	aqua	Water
b.i.d.	bis in die	twice a day
caps.	capsula	Capsule
disp.	dispensa	Dispense
gtt.	guttae	Drops
h.	hora	Hour
h.s.	hora somni	at bedtime
non rep.	non repetatur	do not repeat (or refill)
p.c.	post cibum	after meals
p.r.n.	pro re nata	as needed
q.h.	quaque hora	every hour
q.4h.	quaque quarta hora	every 4 hours
q.i.d.	quater in die	four times a day
Sig.	signa	let it be labeled, label
stat.	statim	immediately
tab.	tabella	Tablet
t.i.d.	ter in die	three times a day

Label: Take two tablets immediately. Take one or two tablets every 4 hours as needed for relief of pain. (much preferred form)

Sig: Tab 2 stat. Tab 1 or 2 q.4h. p.r.n. for relief of pain.

FIG. A6.1 Sample of the same transcription or signature (instructions to the patient) written in English and with Latin abbreviations.

or "**Sig:**"—is the prescriber's directions to the patient that appear on the medicine container. At one time, such directions were uniformly written in Latin, but modern practice is to use English. Latin abbreviations are still used by many clinicians in prescriptions and progress notes to save time (Table A6.1); however, such gains are minor in general dental practice and may contribute to prescription errors (e.g., "q4h" instead of "qid" represents a 50% dosage increase). Fig. A6.1 depicts the same signature for an analgesic medication, one written entirely in English and the other written in Latin abbreviations. Items written in the transcription are transferred onto the prescription bottle label by the pharmacist, so they should be complete but concise. The use of Latin in writing prescriptions is outmoded and can be confusing. Its use in prescriptions is highly discouraged.

The phrase "use as directed" should not be used. Rather, the transcription should be explicit and include (1) the route and method (e.g., take, instill, or insert); (2) the number of dose forms to be taken each time (e.g., take two tablets); (3) how frequently to administer the medication (e.g., every 6 hours or at bedtime); (4) for what length of therapy (e.g., for 7 days or until all taken); (5) for what purpose (now required by law in some states; e.g., for an analgesic, "to relieve pain" or "for pain"); and (6) any special instructions (e.g., shake well before using or refrigerate). The instructions to the patient should be consistent with the patient characteristics, drug, and dosage form. Prescriptions written for children should use the verb **give** instead of **take** to indicate that the parent or guardian is to administer the drug. Enteric-coated drugs should be "swallowed whole" to ensure that the coating is still intact when the drug reaches the stomach. Directions for suspensions should include the phrase "shake well then take ..." to ensure administration of a uniform dose. The transcription should be located on the next line after the subscription. (The arrangement of information on the prescription is by custom, but by observing this order the practitioner is less likely to omit an essential part of the instructions.)

The handwritten **signature** and **professional degree** of the prescriber convey the authority of the prescriber to order the medication and of the pharmacist to fill the prescription. Although all prescriptions should be signed, a signature is required by law only for certain controlled substances (Schedule II drugs); other prescriptions may be telephoned to a pharmacy, where the pharmacist writes them down. When it appears, the dentist's signature is followed by the prescriber's professional degree rather than preceded by "Dr." as the abbreviation for "Doctor." If several dentists work in a clinic that use the same prescription form, several states require that the prescriber's name be mechanically printed or stamped on the prescription on an extra line under the signature line. Most state dental practice acts specify that prescriptions may be written only for patients under active care. Many state laws stipulate that only the classes of drugs directly involved with dental treatment may be prescribed by the dentist. Another form of identifier needed on some prescriptions is the National Provider Identifier (NPI), which was established by HIPAA. The NPI serves as a unique provider identifier for all electronic prescribing and billing.

Finally, the prescriber's DEA registration number must appear on any prescription for a controlled or scheduled drug in compliance with the Controlled Substances Act of 1970. This number should not be routinely entered on prescriptions that do not require it, to prevent its use by potential drug abusers or inappropriate use for insurance prescriber identification.

Many states have their own acts related to controlled substances. If state, federal, or local regulations governing any drug or procedure differ, the most stringent of the regulations applies. The state and federal certificates of registration must be renewed periodically. DEA registration is not required of practitioners in the military or the Public Health Service or of recent graduates in internship or residency programs; in the latter case, the institutional DEA registration number may be used but with addition of a suffix to identify the unique practitioner in training (PIT). Practitioners in a hospital or institutional setting may also use the hospital DEA with a unique practitioner identifier code that is issued and recorded by the hospital.

After the prescribing of the drug, but before the prescription is filled, the pharmacist evaluates the prescription again. The pharmacist has responsibility to the patient and the practitioner to check the prescription for possible errors in drug selection, dosage form and dosage, and patient instructions and therapeutic appropriateness (e.g., prescribing excess quantities of controlled substances).

PRESCRIPTION FORMAT AND PAD FORMS

Increasingly, prescriptions are being written using certified digital systems that securely transmit an electronic prescription to the pharmacy of the patient's choice. These systems offer some advantages for drugs that may be abused or are covered under Medicaid. Because the patient never has possession of the prescription, there is no need for tamper-proof prescription forms or the need to write drug quantity in numbers and letters, as is required for paper prescriptions. These exceptions do not apply to faxed prescriptions.

Handwritten prescriptions should be written concisely, accurately, and legibly. Ink, indelible pencil, or typing is required for prescriptions

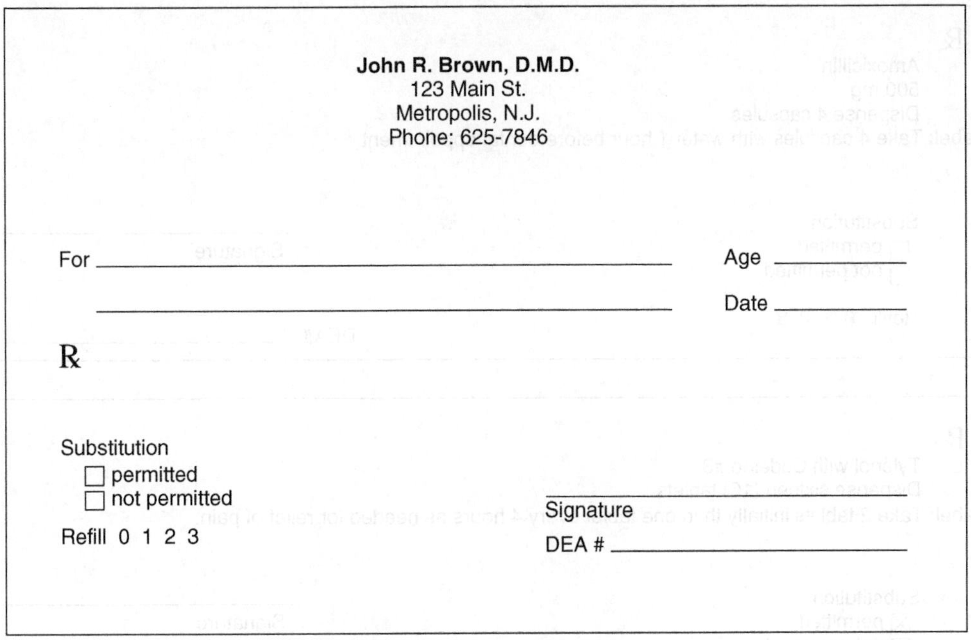

John R. Brown, D.M.D.
123 Main St.
Metropolis, N.J.
Phone: 625-7846

For ______________________________ Age ________

______________________________ Date ________

℞

Substitution
☐ permitted
☐ not permitted

Refill 0 1 2 3

____
Signature

DEA # ______________

FIG. A6.2 Typical prescription form.

for Schedule II drugs and is preferable for all prescriptions. Use of "gel" pens to write prescriptions to prevent washing away of the original prescription information is recommended because gel pen ink is absorbed into a paper's fibers and resists its removal by chemical solvents. These pens are widely available. With the advent of safe and effective drugs, consumer education, and the concept of informed consent, the need for therapeutic mysticism of an illegible prescription written in a foreign language (e.g., medical Latin) no longer exists. Similarity between the names of some highly active and potentially toxic drugs makes illegibility all the more indefensible. Typed electronic prescriptions help in this regard.

Prescription pads should also be kept secured in a locked drawer or under similar cover when not in use to avoid loss or theft. Inventories of prescription pads and drug stocks should be performed regularly to detect theft and diversion of prescription forms and drugs. Sequentially numbered prescription blanks make detection of diversion easier. If theft of a prescription pad is suspected, such loss should be reported to the local pharmacies or state board or drug control agency. In addition, for good dental practice and for medicolegal reasons, a duplicate of each prescription or a record thereof should be kept in the patient's chart or record.

Blank printed prescription pads should not have the name of a pharmacy or pharmaceutical company imprinted anywhere on the form because such an implicit endorsement may direct the patient to a particular pharmacy or manufacturer's product. Similarly, phone, fax, or electronic prescriptions should be sent to the pharmacy of the patient's choice, not the practitioner's.

The **U.S. Troop Readiness, Veterans' Care, Katrina Recovery, and Iraq Accountability Appropriations Act** of 2007 requires the use of tamper-resistant prescription forms for prescriptions for Medicaid patients. To be considered tamper-resistant, a prescription pad must contain industry-recognized features designed to prevent the following: (1) unauthorized copying, (2) erasure or modification, and (3) counterfeiting of a completed or blank prescription form. The prescription should include a statement alerting the pharmacist of the tamper-resistant features and how the pharmacist can verify authenticity. The rule applies to all written and computer-generated prescriptions (OTC, Rx, and controlled) delivered to patients for which Medicaid reimbursement is expected.

Exceptions to the rules include (1) prescriptions phoned, faxed, or emailed from the prescriber to the pharmacy; (2) emergency fills on a noncompliant prescription form, for which a prescriber provides the pharmacy with a verbal, faxed, electronic, or compliant written prescription within 72 hours after the date on which the prescription was filled; and (3) prescriptions for certain specified institutions and clinical settings. The need for tamper-resistant prescription forms for non-Medicaid prescriptions varies on a state-by-state basis and needs to be determined for the dentist's area of practice.

Fig. A6.2 presents a typical preprinted prescription form used, with minor variations, by most practitioners. Because of state laws permitting or, in some instances, mandating the substitution of a generic preparation for a proprietary drug, state laws permitting accelerated refills may have a feature on the prescription form to indicate whether a substitution is permitted or an accelerated refill. Because no physical prescription is written for telephone orders, the practitioner must indicate verbally to the pharmacist whether substitution is permitted or refills can be accelerated. In some hospitals, prescriptions are generated by the patient information system and sent directly to the pharmacy.

Fig. A6.3 presents three sample prescriptions. The first, for antibiotic prophylaxis before dental therapy, is written by nonproprietary name; the second, for postoperative pain relief, is written by proprietary name for the sake of convenience. In the latter case, the dosage is implicit in the particular formulation selected (e.g., **Tylenol with Codeine No. 3: acetaminophen [Tylenol] 300 mg and codeine 30 mg**, with the notation three indicating the 30-mg strength of codeine). The third prescription, for **fluoride** supplementation in a child (2 years old) living in a low-fluoride area, is one of the few instances in which long-term drug use and the use of refills is appropriate in clinical dentistry.

℞
Amoxicillin
500 mg
Dispense 4 capsules
Label: Take 4 capsules with water 1 hour before dental appointment.

Substitution
☐ permitted
☐ not permitted

Signature

Refill ~~0~~ ~~1~~ 2 ~~3~~

DEA#

℞
Tylenol with Codeine #3
Dispense sixteen (16) tablets
Label: Take 2 tablets initially then one tablet every 4 hours as needed for relief of pain.

Substitution
☒ permitted
☐ not permitted

Signature

Refill 0 ~~1~~ ~~2~~ ~~3~~

DEA# AB1234567

℞
Sodium fluoride oral solution 0.5 mg fluoride/1 ml
Dispense 50 mL
Label: Give one-half dropperful (0.5 ml) once daily.

Substitution
☐ permitted
☐ not permitted

Signature

Label ☒ Refill ~~0~~ ~~1~~ ~~2~~ 3

DEA#

FIG. A6.3 Sample prescriptions. The top and bottom prescriptions are by nonproprietary name. The middle prescription, for a combination product, is written by trade name for convenience (generic substitution is permitted).

Controlled Substance Laws and Drug Schedules

Vahn A. Lewis

In addition to laws regulating drugs in general, special legislation has been enacted pertaining to drugs of abuse. A historical perspective of this legislation is given in Appendix 8. Control of the distribution of commonly abused drugs (e.g., **opioids, barbiturates, and amphetamines**) by the **Drug Enforcement Administration (DEA) is regulated by the Controlled Substances Act.** This act divides drugs of abuse into five schedules based on the drugs' potential for abuse, their medical usefulness, and the degree to which they may lead to physical or psychological dependence. The criteria for inclusion within the five schedules are presented in Table A7.1.

To prescribe controlled substances, the licensed practitioner must register with the DEA. Many of these regulations are administered by the DEA **Office of Diversion Control**. The registration must be renewed periodically, and the certificate of registration must be retained and displayed by the practitioner. When registered, the practitioner assumes several responsibilities, including keeping records of all controlled substances obtained, administered, dispensed, prescribed, lost, (including by theft) (DEA Form 106) destroyed (DEA Form 106), or surrendered to a reverse distributor, form 41) and the secure storage of the drugs and prescription pads. To purchase Schedule II drugs, the practitioner must use the **DEA 222C** order form or enroll in CSOS to order CII drugs electronically.. Although Schedules III, IV, and V drugs may be obtained without special forms, a biennial inventory of all controlled substances on hand must be performed. Office supplies of CIII-V drugs are not ordered using a prescription form but on the dentist's office stationary. Inventory of all controlled substances on hand must be kept for inspection and copying by officers for at least 2 years.

TABLE A7.1 Classification of Controlled Substances

Schedule	Criteria for Inclusion	Examples of Drugs
I	High abuse potential, no currently accepted medical use, may lead to severe dependence	Research use only: heroin, lysergic acid diethylamide, marijuana*, mescaline, methaqualone, peyote, psilocybin
II	High abuse potential, accepted medical use, may lead to severe dependence	Amphetamines, cocaine, codeine, dronabinol, meperidine, methadone, methylphenidate, morphine, oxycodone, pentobarbital, secobarbital all hydrocodone products
III	Abuse potential less than drugs in Schedules I or II, accepted medical use, moderate to low physical dependence liability, possibly high psychological dependence	Benzphetamine, butabarbital, methyprylon, mixtures of codeine with aspirin or acetaminophen, stanozolol
IV	Abuse potential less than drugs in Schedule III, accepted medical use, low dependence liability	Chloral hydrate, diazepam, meprobamate, phenobarbital, propoxyphene, triazolam
V	Abuse potential less than drugs in Schedule IV, accepted medical use, limited dependence liability	Cough preparations containing codeine or similar opioid derivatives, pseudoephedrine-containing decongestants

*Marijuana was placed in Schedule I by Congress with the intent that its proper schedule would be determine by study. The Shafer commission found that marijuana of the day was relatively harmless when used intermittently and did not need to be scheduled. This finding was unacceptable to President Richard Nixon. Marijuana has remained in Schedule I since that time.

Schedule I drugs may not be prescribed. **Schedule II** drug prescriptions may not be refilled. Emergency, partially filled prescriptions must be completely filled within 72 hours. For patients in long-term care facilities or for patients with terminal illnesses, partial filling of Schedule II drugs may be permitted for 60 days after the date on the prescription. Multiple sequentially dated prescriptions for Schedule II drugs can be written for legitimate medical purposes to extend treatment to 90 days from the initial prescription's inception. In dentistry, there is very little need for pain control prescriptions supplying more than 3 or 4 days of analgesics. In many states, special prescription forms or restrictions are applied to Schedule II drugs.

Controlled substances in **Schedules III, IV, and V** can be refilled five times within 6 months, assuming that the prescriber authorizes these refills. After the final permitted refill, a new prescription for the product must be obtained. Drugs in **Schedule V**, which consist of preparations containing limited quantities of certain opioid agents as well as pseudoephedrine-containing decongestants, may be sold without a prescription (if permitted by the state), assuming that the drug is dispensed by a pharmacist to a purchaser who is at least 18 years old and that a record of the transaction is kept by the pharmacist.

A pharmacist is permitted to fill oral prescriptions for any prescription drug except Schedule II products, provided that they are subsequently committed to writing and filed by the pharmacist. The law allows for the dispensing of verbal prescriptions for opioid and other Schedule II drugs in emergency situations, but the quantity must be limited to the amount needed for the emergency, the prescription must be put in writing by the pharmacist, and the prescriber must furnish the pharmacist with a signed, written prescription within 72 hours. Labeling on prescription bottles for all controlled substances must contain the warning "**Caution: Federal law prohibits the transfer of this drug to any person other than the patient for whom it was prescribed.**"

PRESCRIPTION DRUG MONITORING PROGRAMS

A prescription drug monitoring program uses information collected by state drug enforcement agencies to monitor the controlled substance prescription use and potential abuse of controlled substances. Information is sent from pharmacies to the enforcement agency who monitors use and suggests the need for review in situations where the prescribing appears excessive. These programs have been effective at reducing abuse. A more recent innovation has been to make this information available by online database to doctors and pharmacists who can review patients for excessive use (from patients visiting numerous practitioners to obtain additional controlled substances, i.e., **"doctor shopping"**) at the time of writing the prescription.

Small amounts of controlled substances in Schedules II through V may be imported or exported by U.S. citizens for their personal use if the following conditions are met: (1) the controlled substance is in its original container dispensed to the individual and (2) the prescription is declared to Customs Service stating that (a) the controlled substance is for his or her personal use or for an animal traveling with him or her and (b) the trade name and schedule symbol are on the label or the name and address of the dispenser and the prescription number are on the label. In addition, the total of controlled substance dosage units cannot exceed 50.

Information and applications for registration may be obtained from the DEA, Office of Diversion Control, Registration Unit, PO Box 28083, Central Station, Washington, DC 20005; online at http://www.deadiversion.usdoj.gov/online_forms_apps.html or from the DEA Regional Office in the area in which the applicant practices. The DEA has created a Website that provides current information on registration and contacts and laws dealing with controlled substances. It is now possible to submit registration documents electronically to this Website or to print out forms that can be mailed to the DEA for registration.

Regulations and Drug Prescribing

Vahn A. Lewis

Various federal, state, and local laws have been enacted to control the manufacture, sale, and dispensing of drugs. To comply with these regulations, the clinician should be aware that the most stringent of these laws takes precedence, whether it is federal, state, or local. A summary of federal laws that affect dental prescribing is provided in Table A8.1.

HISTORICAL DEVELOPMENT OF DRUG LEGISLATION

A major concern of nations has always been the establishment of criteria for drug identity and purity; to this end, the development of pharmacopeias has proved invaluable. A pharmacopeia is a written description of the source, identification, and preparation of medicinal agents. The first pharmacopeia to gain legal status was one adopted by the city-state of Nuremberg in the early sixteenth century. Today the trend is for the development of **international pharmacopeial standards** (referred to as **harmonization** of standards).

The first USP was published in 1820 by a group of physicians, pharmacists, and chemists. This first **United States Pharmacopeial Convention** established certain policies, notably that only drugs of proven merit would be included in the USP and that regular revisions of the document would be issued. The USP published in 2015 is the thirty-eighth edition. Drugs with combinations of drugs were excluded from the USP; in 1888, the American Pharmaceutical Association began to publish the **National Formulary of Unofficial Preparations.** In 1975, the National Formulary was joined into the USP-NF, and it is in its thirty-third edition. Around the turn of the twentieth century, a growing public clamor over the quality, purity, and safety of food and drug products led to the passage of the **Federal Food and Drugs Act of 1906**, also known as the Pure Food and Drug Act. In this legislation, the USP and National Formulary were given quasi-legal status regarding defining the purity and quality of drugs. Standards were also established for the labeling of medicinal products. In the years that followed, these standards were extended by court decisions and congressional actions to cover promotional materials in addition to the products themselves (see Table A8.1).

Before 1937, the testing of drugs and ingredients used in medications was not required before marketing. In 1937, a relatively new solvent, diethylene glycol, was used in an "elixir of sulfonamide." This agent caused the death of many children and was responsible for the swift passage of the **Federal Food, Drug, and Cosmetic Act** of 1938. This act required manufacturers to provide the FDA with evidence of drug safety in the form of a **New Drug Application (NDA)** before distributing the agent. The Act of 1938 also introduced the principle of separating drugs into prescription and nonprescription categories by requiring companies selling over-the-counter (OTC) drugs to furnish purchasers with the information necessary for their safe and effective use. Questions concerning which drugs could be sold OTC and which had to be reserved for prescription use were not resolved, however, until passage of the **Durham-Humphrey Amendment in 1951**.

In response to the thalidomide tragedy in Europe, Congress passed the **Kefauver-Harris Amendments of 1962.** These amendments required manufacturers of new drugs to follow set standards of animal and human pharmacologic and toxicologic testing, with the data from each step to be reviewed by the FDA. Requirements for evaluating safety and studying chronic and fetal toxicity and efficacy (omissions of the 1938 Act) were included in this legislation.

Two federal laws controlling prescription drugs are the **Durham-Humphrey Amendment (Section 503B)** of 1951 to the Food, Drug, and Cosmetic Act of 1938 and the **Comprehensive Drug Abuse Prevention and Control Act (Controlled Substances Act)** of 1970. The Durham-Humphrey law prohibited the dispensing of certain kinds of drugs (e.g., systemic antibiotics and corticosteroids and other agents whose unsupervised use may be unsafe) except on the prescription order of a licensed practitioner. Under this law, a prescription for these drugs may not be refilled unless authorized by the prescriber.

The FDA has the responsibility for determining how a drug may be dispensed. The FDA is also responsible for reviewing the labeling and advertising of the use of prescription and OTC drugs. It is not illegal to use a drug for indications not initially intended. However, casual use of drugs for unlisted indications can lead to excess use and increased toxicity that was not evaluated during initial testing.

In 2006, the FDA incorporated new conventions in the formatting of the drug labeling for the "package insert" information. The labeling now includes a half-page summary of major points at the beginning of the labeling. The new labeling also makes provisions for electronic hot links between the summary and full discussion in the label. "**Black box**" warnings indicate adverse effects with particularly serious consequences that are featured prominently at the top of the drug labeling.

In the 1980s, the high cost of drugs became the subject of congressional legislation. Substantive changes in drug substitution laws, simplified approval of generic drugs (using **abbreviated NDA** applications, **ANDA**), and Medicaid drug reimbursement controls were introduced in attempts to curtail explosive drug costs. One component of the increased cost stems from the development of new drug entities. Because of the complexity of the approval process, much of the patent protection for a drug can expire before a drug is ever marketed. To recover their investments, manufacturers charge high prices for new drugs, contributing to the upsurge in medical costs. To blunt this trend, the **Drug Price Competition and Patent Term Restoration Act** of 1984 (**Waxman-Hatch Act**) was passed. It extended marketing protection for **innovator** drugs. An innovator product is an original, newly developed drug that requires an approved NDA for marketing; a synonym is **New Molecular Entity**.

Under the Waxman-Hatch Act, innovator drugs may be given extensions on their patent protection. The law also simplified the process of obtaining an ANDA for approval to market generic drugs to help reduce overall drug costs of known agents. In conjunction with the **Orphan Drug Amendment** of 1983, this law also made provisions for the development of "orphan drugs" (i.e., drugs used for rare

TABLE A8.1 Federal Laws Regulating Drugs and Prescribing

Law	Effect
Pure Food and Drug Act 1906 (Wiley Act)	Prohibited mislabelling and adulteration of drugs Triggered by decades of problems with impure, misbranded, and unwholesome practices in the food and drug industries
Opium Exclusion Act of 1909	Prohibited importation of opium. A bill passed to appease the mainland Chinese who were opposed to the opium trade of the British but also to restrict the use of smoked opium used principally by Chinese emigrants in California
Amendment (1912) to the Pure Food and Drug Act	Prohibited false or fraudulent advertising claims or labeling made about medications
Harrison Narcotic Act of 1914	Established regulations for use of opium, opiates, and cocaine (marijuana added in 1937)
Food, Drug, and Cosmetic Act of 1938	Triggered by "Elixer of Death" tragedy, required evidence that new drugs be safe and pure by data submitted in a New Drug Application (NDA) (but did not require proof of efficacy); enforcement by FDA established prescription and over-the-counter classifications
Durham-Humphrey Amendment of 1951	Vested in the FDA the power to determine which products were dangerous and should be provided only with a prescription from a trained practitioner and which drugs could be used safely by reading the labeling on the package (and therefore could be sold "over-the-counter"). Also allowed verbal prescriptions and refills
Kefauver-Harris Amendments (1962) to the Food, Drug, and Cosmetic Act	Required proof of efficacy and safety for new drugs and for drugs released since 1938; established guidelines for reporting information about adverse reactions, clinical testing, and advertising of new drugs
Radiation Control for Health and Safety Act, 1968	Established standards for ionizing and non-ionizing radiation including sonic radiation. (X-ray machines, ultra-sonic cleaners, TVs, phones, etc.)
Drug Efficacy Study Implementation 1966–1969	Required proof of efficacy and safety of legacy drugs not included in the Kefauver-Harris amendments. Led to the development of Abbreviated New Drug Application (ANDA) for generic drugs
Comprehensive Drug Abuse Prevention and Control Act (1970), Controlled Substances Act, as amended	Outlined strict controls in the manufacture, distribution, and prescribing of habit-forming drugs; established programs to prevent and treat drug addiction
1972 FDA over-the-counter review process	OTC ingredients generally recognized as safe and effective when following FDA monograph guidelines may be sold without further safety and efficacy studies. Drugs not meeting this criteria generally follow the NDA process
Orphan Drug Amendments of 1983	Amended Food, Drug, and Cosmetic Act of 1938, providing incentives for the development of drugs to treat conditions suffered by <200,000 patients in the United States
Drug Price Competition and Patent Restoration Act of 1984 (Waxman-Hatch Act)	Abbreviated NDA for generic drugs; required bioequivalence data; patent life extended by amount of time delayed by FDA review process; cannot exceed 5 extra yr or extend >14-yr post-NDA approval; authorized abbreviated NDA
Omnibus Budget Reconciliation Act of 1990	Deepened governmental involvement in prescription writing through legislation relating to best discount prices, rebates, formularies, and pharmacy reimbursements; placed restrictions on payment for prescriptions for barbiturates and benzodiazepines
Generic Drug Debarment Act of 1991 and the Food, Drug, Cosmetic, and Device Enforcement Amendment of 1991	Increased penalties for abuses of generic drug regulations
1992 Expedited Drug Approval Act	Allowed accelerated FDA approval for drugs of high medical need; required detailed postmarketing patient surveillance
1992 Prescription Drug User Fee Act	Required manufacturers to pay user fees for certain NDAs, Prescription Drug User Fee Act (PUDFA I); FDA states review time for new chemical entities has decreased from 30 mos in 1992 to 20 mos in 1994
1994 Dietary Supplements and Health Education Act	Required dietary supplement manufacturers to ensure that a dietary supplement is safe before it is marketed; FDA is responsible for taking action against any unsafe dietary supplement product after it reaches the market; generally, manufacturers do not need to register with FDA or get FDA approval before producing or selling dietary supplements; manufacturers must ensure that product label information is truthful and not misleading
North American Free Trade Act (1994) and General Agreement on Tariffs and Trade (1948, revised 1994), World Trade Organization (1995)	Necessitated harmonization of pharmacopeias and drug regulations between trading partners. Changed patent procedures for pharmaceutical companies worldwide. Established the World Trade Organization with international legal reach
1996 Health Insurance Portability Accountability Act (HIPAA)	Standardized third-party payment for medical treatment and increased confidentiality and privacy for patient information maintained in medical databases; impacts electronic prescribing
1997 FDA Modernization Act	Replaced "legend" with label "Rx only"; allowed manufacturer to provide literature on off-label uses of drugs with practitioners if requested by the practitioner; revised accelerated track approval for drugs that treat life-threatening disorders; made provisions for pediatric drug research; revised interaction of agency with individuals doing clinical trials Reauthorized PDUFA II

TABLE A8.1 **Federal Laws Regulating Drugs and Prescribing—cont'd**

Law	Effect
Medication Equity and Drug Safety Act of 2002	Would permit re-importation of drugs manufactured in the United States but exported to a second country to help overcome the premium price Americans pay for their medications if authorized by Secretary of the Health and Human Services Department; no HHS secretary has given authorization
Best Pharmaceuticals for Children (2002), Pediatric Research Equity Act 2003	Provides for testing of drugs in pregnant women and children to improve the science basis for making therapeutic decisions in these understudied populations
2002 Public Health and Bioterrorism Preparedness Act	Provided procedures for use of certain drugs under emergency conditions; reauthorized PDUFA III
2005 Combat Methamphetamine Epidemic Act	Establishes new regulations for the sale of ephedrine, pseudoephedrine, and phenylpropanolamine that differ from the Control Substance V regulations by not requiring sale in a pharmacy
U.S. Troop Readiness, Veterans Care, Katrina Recovery, and Iraq Accountability Appropriations Act of 2007	Established requirement for the use of tamper-resistant written prescriptions for Medicaid prescription reimbursement; prescriptions must have three tamper-resistant features
FDAAA-2007 Food and Drug Administrative Amendments Act 2007	Reauthorized PDUFA (IV), reuse controls for medical devices; best pharmaceuticals for children; pediatric research equity; modernization of certain practices; clinical trials reporting on clinical trials.gov, outsourcing of evaluations for medical devices to third parties (MDUFMA).
Family Smoking Prevention and Tobacco Control and Federal Retirement Reform (2009)	FDA given certain authority to regulate tobacco products
Affordable Care Act (ACA) of 2010: Title VII: Subtitle A Biologics Price Competition and Innovation Act	Authorizes biosimilar medications Zarxio (filgrastim-sndz) is biosimilar to Neupogen (filgrastim Amgen) recombinant colony-stimulating factor; this is the first biosimilar approved in the United States http://www.medscape.com/viewarticle/841021
Affordable Care Act 2010: Prescription Drug Coverage	Health coverage obtained under ACA needs to cover prescription drugs
Generic Drug User Fee Amendments of 2012	User fees will be collected to defray the expense of regulating generic drugs; this legislation has an international scope
FDA Food Safety Modernization Act 2011	Shifts focus from responding to food contamination to a focus on preventing food contamination
FDA Safety and Innovation Act of 2012	Reauthorizes and extends users' fees (PDUFA-V) promotes innovation; increases stakeholder's involvement; enhances the safety of the drug supply chain
Pandemic and All-Hazards Preparedness Reauthorization of 2013	Medical continuity in disasters; FDA emergency use authorization; many regulations for drug expiration dates or good manufacturing procedures may be suspended during an emergency
Drug Quality and Security Act 2013	Fills legal gaps caused by a supreme court decisions* that limited the role of the FDA for overseeing "pharmacy compounded" drug distribution
Designer Anabolic Steroids Control Act of 2014	Concerned with updating anabolic steroid target drugs

NDA, New Drug Application.
*Thompson versus Western State Medical Center, 2002.

diseases). In general, it is not economically feasible to produce these drugs for the small groups of patients (often <200,000) who need them. Exclusive rights can be granted under this law for production and marketing of a drug or for specific labeling to permit the use of a drug in a rare disease. No price restrictions are placed on drugs developed under the Orphan Drug Act, and these treatments can be expensive. Recent orphan developments have led to numerous "biological," nuclear, and medical device treatments. This led to the renaming of this group to **Orphan Products**.

Drug companies have taken an interest in "discovering" new uses of known drugs in small population groups. The drug **thalidomide**, which was withdrawn from the market when it produced the severe birth defect phocomelia, has been rereleased for use in treating multiple myeloma, leprosy and aphthous ulcers seen in human immunodeficiency virus and Behçet disease based on data indicating that it inhibits tumor necrosis factor-α production.

Because of advances in understanding of the human genome and the development of diagnostic gene chips, more small population disorders are expected to fit within the Orphan Drug Act. There were 27 orphan drugs designated in 1984 when the program started. New developments and a desire by pharmaceutical companies to exploit the benefits of this category have increased the interest. There were 283 orphan agents designated in 2014 for a total of 2861 **Orphan Product Designations** at the time of this writing. Although relatively few novel new drugs are approved, there are numerous changes in the labeling for existing entities (changes include new indications, dosage forms, or new warnings). Some well-known treatments such as **Botox (botulinum toxin**-onabotulinum toxin A) were developed under orphan legislation. **Botox** is now widely used beyond the original expected population. This "popularization" of orphan drugs appears to be a new drug development strategy.

The 1984 **Waxman-Hatch Act** led to a surge of ANDAs by generic manufacturers, and FDA personnel became overloaded with work. In an attempt to speed up the processing of their applications, several generic drug manufacturers pressured FDA officials for quick approval, and others submitted samples of the innovator drug as examples of their own product. Other problems that have occurred included the selling of counterfeit drugs and physician drug samples to pharmacists at below-market prices. Their use may lead to therapeutic failure. To discourage these practices, the **Generic Drug Debarment Act** of 1991 and the **Food, Drug, Cosmetic, and Device Enforcement Amendment** of 1991 were passed to increase substantially the penalties for such activities. In 2014 the **Safety and Innovation Act** authorized the collection of review fees from the medical industry, for both generic (**Generic Drug User Fee Amendments**) and biosimilar (**Biosimilar Drug User Fee Agreement**) drugs to facilitate the review of these therapies.

The 1990s represented a revolutionary period for drug regulation. Lawsuits and legal challenges of FDA actions led to substantial changes in the regulation of dietary supplements, natural product drugs, and complementary and alternative medications. In 1994, the U.S. Congress passed the **Dietary Supplements and Health Education Act**, which allows numerous agents with pharmaceutical activity to be identified as dietary supplements. In addition, international trade agreements such as **NAFTA** and **GATT** necessitated the development of harmonization agreements between member countries by the **International Conference on Harmonization**. Harmonization seeks to unify pharmacopeias and laws related to the international pharmaceutical trade. Outside these agreements, there are additional trade agreements, such as those associated with normalization of relations between the United States and China.

These changes have led to increased availability of natural products from domestic and foreign sources. Natural products can have therapeutic potential, but they can also complicate therapy by inducing unexpected toxic effects and drug interactions. One example is **St. John's wort,** which has been found to produce an antidepressant effect. It can also induce hepatic drug metabolism, which could decrease blood concentrations of other drugs, such as antiviral protease inhibitors. In addition, imported natural products are occasionally found to be adulterated with conventional drugs such as **phenylbutazone**, **sildenafil**, or **chlordiazepoxide**. These findings underscore the need for complete patient medical histories, including questions on prescription drugs, OTC drugs, dietary supplements, alternative medicines, and drugs of abuse.

The 1992 **Prescription Drug User Fee Act** (**PDUFA I**) authorized the FDA to charge pharmaceutical companies who are having their NDAs evaluated by the agency. This financial resource has enabled the FDA to double the rate of approval of new drug entities. An increased number of postmarketing withdrawals of new drugs has also occurred. The 1997 **FDA Modernization Act** has modified the role of the FDA further. For dentists, a key provision allows manufacturers to disseminate information about non-labeled or unapproved uses of drugs and medical devices. This provision may increase drug company interest in promoting "off-label dental" uses of medical drugs and promoting dosing of agents that were not studied in the original application.

HIPAA also affects dental prescribers (see Table A8.1). This legislation is concerned with standardizing the process of third-party payment for medical treatment (requiring each practitioner to obtain an individual National Provider Identifier (NPI) number for use in insurance forms), but it has also substantially tightened the standards for confidentiality and privacy of patient information maintained in medical databases. As an unintended outcome, it has occasionally become more difficult for dentists to obtain medical information necessary to evaluate their patients for prescribing purposes. The fines for violating these new rules can be substantial.

Although the federal government has set no standards concerning which prescription drugs a dentist may use clinically, many state laws regulating the practice of dentistry restrict drugs used to those associated with orofacial or dental treatment. A typical law of this kind states that dentists can "diagnose, treat, operate, or prescribe for any disease, pain, injury, deficiency, deformity, or physical condition of the human teeth, alveolar process, gums, or jaws." Thus, a dentist can prescribe smoking cessation aides "to prevent oral cancer."

The dispensing of drugs by physicians and dentists is a more recent development in the United States. The **Federal Trade Commission** has agreed to allow the sale of drugs by practitioners to their patients, and almost all states have recognized physician/dentist dispensing under strict regulatory requirements regarding storage, labeling, and record keeping. The ethical implications of this practice have been questioned on numerous grounds, including conflict of interest, lack of training and facilities for appropriate drug handling, and loss of the traditional practitioner–pharmacist double-checking of prescriptions. There has been a serious problem of **"pill mill pain clinics"** dispensing large quantities of opiate drugs to poorly qualified patients.

APPENDIX 9

Glossary of Abbreviations*

Frank J. Dowd and Angelo J. Mariotti

1,25[OH]D	1,25-Dihydroxycholecalciferol, calcitriol
25[OH]D	Calcifediol
5-FdUTP	5-Fluorodeoxyuridine triphosphate
5-FU	Fluorouracil
5-FUdR	Floxuridine
5-HIAA	5-Hydroxyindoleacetic acid
5-HT	5-Hydroxytryptamine (serotonin)
5-HTT	5-Hydroxytryptamine transporter
6-APA	6-β-Aminopenicillanic acid
6-MNA	6-Methoxy-2-naphthylacetic acid
ā	Before
Å	Angstrom
a.c.	Before meals (ante cibum)
A/G ratio	Albumin/globulin ratio
A_1, A_2, A_3	Adenosine receptors
AAOS	American Academy of Orthopaedic Surgeons
ABC	ATP-binding cassette
ABCD	Airway, breathing, circulation, defibrillation
ABO	Antigenic determinants
ABVD	Adriamycin (doxorubicin), bleomycin, vinblastine, dacarbazine (regimen)
ABX	Antibiotics
AC	Adenylyl (or adenylate) cyclase
ACE	Angiotensin-converting enzyme
ACh	Acetylcholine
AChE	Acetylcholinesterase
AChR	Acetylcholine receptor
ACLS	Advanced cardiac life support
ACTH	Adrenocorticotropic hormone
ACVD	Acute cardiovascular disease
ad lib	As much as desired
ADA	Adenosine deaminase
ADA	American Dental Association
ADH	Antidiuretic hormone
ADHD	Attention-deficit/hyperactivity disorder
ADP	Adenosine 5′-diphosphate
ADT	Accepted Dental Therapeutics
AED	Automatic external defibrillator
AEDs	Anti-epileptic drugs
AF (A. fib)	Atrial fibrillation
AFB	Acid-fast bacillus
AFHS DI	American Hospital Formulary Service Drug Information
$AgNO_3$	Silver nitrate
AHA	American Heart Association
AHPA	American Herbal Products Association
AIDS	Acquired immunodeficiency syndrome
AIMs	Abnormal involuntary movements
AIP	Acute intermittent porphyria
Al^{+++}	Aluminum ion
ALA	δ-Aminolevulinic acid
ALL	Acute lymphocytic leukemia
ALS	Amyotrophic lateral sclerosis
ALS	Antilymphocytic serum
ALT	Alanine aminotransferase (formerly SGPT)
AMA	American Medical Association
AML	Acute monocytic leukemia
AMP	Adenosine 5′-monophosphate
amp	Ampule
AMPA	α-Amino-3-hydroxy-5-methyl-4-isoxazole propionate
AMPK	Adenosine-activated protein kinase
AMPT	α-Methyl-para-tyrosine
amt	Amount
ANA	Antinuclear antibody
ANS	Autonomic nervous system
ANUG	Acute necrotizing ulcerative gingivitis
AODM	Adult-onset diabetes mellitus
AP	Antiplasmin
AP-1	Activating protein-1
AP5	2-Amino-5-phosphonovaleric acid
AP7	2-Amino-7-phosphonoheptanoic acid
APAP	Acetaminophen
APC	Aspirin-phenacetin-caffeine
aPC	Activated protein C
APD	Action potential duration
APF	Acidulated phosphate fluoride
APSAC	Anisoylated plasminogen-SK activator complex
aPTT	Activated partial thromboplastin time
AR	Adrenergic receptor
Ara-A	Vidarabine, adenosine arabinoside
ARA-C	Cytosine arabinoside (cytarabine)
ara-g	9-beta-D-arabinofuranosylguanine

*This list includes abbreviations used in medicine in addition to those used in the book. For a complete list of receptors and their nomenclature, refer to the website of the International Union of Basic and Clinical Pharmacology (IUPHAR) http://www.guidetopharmacology.org/nomenclature.jsp

ARAS	Ascending reticular activating system
ARBs	Angiotensin II receptor blockers
ARC	AIDS-related complex
ARDS	Acute respiratory distress syndrome
ARONJ	Antiresorptive-agent-induced osteonecrosis of the jaw
ASA	American Society of Anesthesiologists
ASA	Aspirin
ASAP	As soon as possible
ASHD	Atherosclerotic heart disease
AST	Aspartate aminotransferase (formerly SGOT)
ATIII	Antithrombin III
ATM	Atmosphere
ATN	Acute tubular necrosis
ATP	Adenosine 5′-triphosphate
ATPase	Adenosine triphosphatase
AV	Atrioventricular/arteriovenous
AZT	Zidovudine (azidothymidine)
Ba	Barium
BAC	Blood alcohol concentration
BBB	Blood–brain barrier
BBB	Bundle branch block
BCG	Bacillus Calmette-Guerin
BCL-ABL	Breakpoint cluster region-Abelson
BCNU	Carmustine
BCR	β-Cell antigen receptor
bcr	Breakpoint cluster region
BDP	Beclomethasone dipropionate
β-arr	β-Arrestin
BE	Bacterial endocarditis
bFGF	Basic fibroblastic growth factor
bid	Twice a day (bis in die)
Bis-GMA	Bisphenol A glycidyl methacylate
BMD	Beclomethasone dipropionate
BMP	Beclomethasone monopropionate
BMR	Basal metabolic rate
BoNT-A	Botulinum toxin type A
BoNT-B	Botulinum toxin type B
BP	Blood pressure
BPA	Bisphenol A
BPH	Benign prostatic hypertrophy
BSA	Body surface area
BSAC	British Society for Antimicrobial Chemotherapy
BuChE	Butyrocholinesterase
BUN	Blood urea nitrogen
BZ_1, BZ_2	Benzodiazepine receptors
C	Centigrade
C&S	Culture and sensitivity
C_1, C_2, ...	First cervical vertebra, second cervical vertebra, ...
C6	Hexamethonium
CA	Cancer/carcinoma
Ca^{++}, Ca^{2+}	Calcium ion
CABG	Coronary artery bypass graft
CAD	Coronary artery disease
CAM	Complementary and alternative medicine
cAMP	Cyclic adenosine 3′,5′-monophosphate
Cap	Capsule
CBC	Complete blood count
cc	Cubic centimeter

CCB	Calcium channel blocker
CCNU	Lomustine
CCR5	Cysteine–cysteine chemokine receptor 5
CCU	Cardiac care unit
CD	Cluster of differentiation
CD40L	CD40 ligand
CDAC	*Clostridium difficile*-associated colitis
CDAD	*Clostridium difficile*-associated diarrhea
CDC	Centers for Disease Control and Prevention
CDK	Cyclin-dependent kinase
Cdk5	Cyclin-dependent kinase 5
cDNA	Complementary DNA
CDR	Complementarity-defining region
CETP	Cholesteryl ester transfer protein
CF	Cystic fibrosis
CG	Chorionic gonadotropin
cGMP	Cyclic guanosine 3′,5′-monophosphate
CGRP	Calcitonin gene-related peptide
ChAc	Choline acetylase
CHD	Congenital or coronary heart disease
CHF	Congestive heart failure
CHG	Chlorhexidine gluconate
CI	Cardiac index
CIWA	Clinical Institute Withdrawal Assessment (alcohol/drug toxicology screen tool)
CL	Clearance
Cl^-	Chloride ion
cl liq	Clear liquid
CLL	Chronic lymphatic/lymphocytic leukemia
cm	Centimeter
CMI	Cell-mediated immunity
CML	Chronic myelogenous/myelocytic leukemia
CMV	Cytomegalovirus
CNS	Central nervous system
CO	Cardiac output
CO	Carbon monoxide
CO_2	Carbon dioxide
CoA	Coenzyme A
CO-Hb	Carboxyhemoglobin
COMT	Catechol-O-methyltransferase
CoNS	Coagulase-negative staphylococci
COPD	Chronic obstructive pulmonary disease
cor	Heart
COX	Cyclooxygenase
CP	Cerebral palsy
CPK	Creatine phosphokinase
CPR	Cardiopulmonary resuscitation
CRF	Chronic renal failure
CRH	Corticotropin-releasing hormone
CRP	C-reactive protein
CSF	Cerebrospinal fluid
CT	Computed tomography
CTLA-4	Cytotoxic T-lymphocyte-associated antigen-4
CTZ	Chemoreceptor trigger zone
CV	Cardiovascular
CVA	Cerebrovascular accident
CXCR4	β-Chemokine receptor 4
CYP	Cytochrome P450
Cys	Cysteinyl
cysLTs	Cysteinyl leukotrienes
D	Dopamine (receptor)

d	Dalton
DAT	Dopamine transporter
DATA	Drug Addiction Treatment Act
D_5LR	Dextrose 5% in lactated Ringer's
D_5W	Dextrose 5% in water
DAG	Diacylglycerol
DDAVP	Desmopressin
DDT	Dichlorodiphenyltrichloroethane
DEA	Drug Enforcement Administration
DES	Diethylstilbestrol
DFP	Isoflurophate (formerly diisopropylfluorophosphate)
DHFR	Dihydrofolate reductase
DHT	Dihydrotachysterol
DIC	Disseminated intravascular coagulation/coagulopathy
DIT	Diiodotyrosine
DKA	Diabetic ketoacidosis
DM	Diabetes mellitus
DMARD	Disease-modifying antirheumatic drug
DMFT	Decayed, missing, and filled teeth
DMPP	Dimethylphenylpiperazinium
DMSO	Dimethyl sulfoxide
DMT	Dimethyltryptamine
DNA	Deoxyribonucleic acid
DOA	Dead on arrival
DOB	Date of birth
Dopa (DOPA)	Dihydroxyphenylalanine
DPP-4	Dipeptidyl peptidase 4
DPT	Diphtheria, pertussis, tetanus vaccine
DSHEA	Dietary Supplement Health and Education Act of 1994
DSM-V-R	*Diagnostic and Statistical Manual of Mental Disorders*, Ed 5
DSV	Dietary Supplement Verification Program
DT	Delirium tremens
DTH	Dihydrotachysterol
DTIC	Dacarbazine
DVT	Deep vein thrombosis
Dx	Diagnosis
E	Epinephrine
e.g.	For example
ea	Each
EACA	ε-Aminocaproic acid
EATT	Excitatory amino acid transporter
EBV	Epstein-Barr virus
EC_{50}	Concentration that yields a half-maximal response
ECG	Electrocardiogram
ECHO	Echocardiogram
ECL	Enterochromaffin-like cell
ECT	Electroconvulsive therapy
ED_{50}	Median effective dose
ED_{99}	Dose effective in 99% of the population
EDRF	Endothelium-derived relaxing factor
EDTA	Ethylenediamine tetraacetic acid
EEG	Electroencephalogram/electroencephalography
EENT	Eye, ear, nose, and throat
EGFR	Epidermal growth factor receptor
EGFR-TK	Epidermal growth factor receptor-tyrosine kinase
eIF-2	Eukaryotic initiation factor
EKG	Electrocardiogram
elix	Elixir
EMG	Electromyogram
EMLA	Eutectic mixture of local anesthetics
ENT	Ear, nose, and throat
EPA	Environmental Protection Agency
EPO	Erythropoietin
EPP	End plate potential
EPS	Extrapyramidal symptoms
EPSP	Excitatory postsynaptic potential
ER	Emergency room
ER/PR	Estrogen receptor/progesterone receptor
erm	Erythromycin-resistant methylase
ERP	Effective refractory period
ESBL	Extended-spectrum β-lactamase
ESR	Erythrocyte sedimentation rate
ETOH	Ethyl alcohol
F-	Fluoride ion
Fc	Crystallizable fragment (region) of antibody
FDA	U.S. Food and Drug Administration
Fe^{++}	Ferrous ion
Fe^{+++}	Ferric ion
FEV_1	Forced expiratory volume in 1 s
fib	Fibrillation
FIFRA	Federal Insecticide, Fungicide, and Rodenticide Act
FKBP	Tacrolimus-binding protein
fl	Fluid
FMO	Flavine monooxygenase
FRAP	FKBP-rapamycin-associated protein
FSH	Follicle-stimulating hormone
FUTP	Fluorouridine 5′-triphosphate
FVC	Forced vital capacity
G protein	Guanine nucleotide-binding regulatory protein
GABA	γ-aminobutyric acid
GAT	GABA transporter
G-CSF	Granulocyte colony-stimulating factor (filgrastim)
GDP	Guanosine diphosphate
GERD	Gastroesophageal reflux disease
GH	Growth hormone
GHRF	Growth hormone-releasing factor
GI	Gastrointestinal
GILZ	Glucocorticoid-induced leucine zipper protein
GIP	Glucose-dependent insulinotropic polypeptide
Gla	γ-carboxyglutamic acid
GLP-1	Glucagon-like peptide 1
GLSA	Glycopeptide *Staphylococcus aureus*
Glut 4	Glucose transporter 4
GlyT	Glycine transporter
gm	Gram
GM-CSF	Granulocyte-macrophage colony-stimulating factor (sargramostim)
GMP	Good Manufacturing Practices
GnRH	Gonadotropin-releasing hormone
GP	Glycoprotein
GPCR	G protein–coupled receptor
gr	Grain

GRE Glucocorticoid response element
GRIP-1 Glucocorticoid receptor interacting protein-1
GRK G protein–coupled receptor kinase
GSK-3β Glycogen synthase kinase-3β
GTP Guanosine 5′-triphosphate
GU Genitourinary
GVHD Graft-versus-host disease
GYN/Gyn Gynecology
H&P History and physical
H^+ Hydrogen ion
H_1, H_2, H_3 Histamine receptors
H_2O Water
H_2O_2 Hydrogen peroxide
HAART Highly active antiretroviral therapy
HACEK (group) *Haemophilus influenzae, Aggregatibacter actinomycetemcomitans, Cardiobacterium hominis, Eikenella corrodens, Kingella kingae*
HAV Hepatitis A virus
Hb, Hgb Hemoglobin
HbA_{1c} Hemoglobin A_{1c}
HBV Hepatitis B virus
HCG Human chorionic gonadotropin
HCN Hyperpolarization-activated cyclic nucleotide-gated K^+ channels
HCl Hydrochloric acid
HCT Hematopoietic cell transplantation
Hct Hematocrit
HCV Hepatitis C virus
HCVD Hypertensive cardiovascular disease
HDAC Histone deacetylase
HDL High-density lipoprotein
HEENT Head, eyes, ears, nose, throat
hERG Human ether-a-go-go-related gene (K^+ channel)
HETE Hydroxyeicosatetraenoic acid
Hg^+ Mercurous
Hg^{++} Mercuric
Hg^0 Elemental mercury (in dental amalgam)
Hgb Hemoglobin
HGT Horizontal gene transfer
HIO Hypoiodous acid
HIPAA Health Insurance Portability and Accountability Act (of 1996)
HIT Heparin-induced thrombocytopenia
HIV Human immunodeficiency virus
HLA Human leukocyte antigen
HMG-CoA 3-Hydroxy-3-methylglutaryl coenzyme A
HMWK High-molecular-weight kininogen
HPV Human papillomavirus
hr Hour
HR Heart rate
hs At bedtime (hora somni)
HSCT Hematopoietic stem cell transplant
HSV Herpes simplex virus
Ht Height
HTN Hypertension
HVD Hypertensive vascular disease
Hx History
Hz Hertz
HZV Herpes zoster virus
I^- Iodide ion
i.e. That is
IADHS Inappropriate antidiuretic hormone syndrome
IAP Inhibitor of apoptosis protein
IBS Irritable bowel syndrome
ICD Implanted cardiac defibrillator
ICU Intensive care unit
ID Infectious disease
IDDM Insulin-dependent diabetes mellitus
IDL Intermediate-density lipoprotein
IE Infective endocarditis
IFIS Inoperable floppy iris syndrome
IFN Interferon
IFN-γ Interferon-γ
Ig Immunoglobulin
IgA Gamma A immunoglobulin
IgD Gamma D immunoglobulin
IgE Gamma E immunoglobulin
IGF, IGF-I Insulin-like growth factor I
IgG Gamma G immunoglobulin
IgM Gamma M immunoglobulin
IHD Ischemic heart disease
IHSS Idiopathic hypertrophic subaortic stenosis
I_K Potassium current
IL Interleukin
IL-1 Interleukin-1
IL-1R Interleukin-1 receptor
IL-1RA Interleukin-1 receptor antagonist
IL-2 Interleukin-2
IL-3 Interleukin-3
IM Intramuscular
IMF Intermaxillary fixation
IND Notice of Claimed Investigational Exemption for a New Drug
INH Isonicotinic hydrazide
iNOS Inducible nitric oxide synthetase (or synthase)
INR International Normalized Ratio
int Internal
IOP Intraocular pressure
IP Inositol phosphate
IP International Pharmacopoeia
IP_2 Inositol bisphosphate
IP_3 Inositol 1,4,5-trisphosphate
IPG Inositol phosphoglycan
IPSP Inhibitory postsynaptic potential
IQ Intelligence quotient
ISA Intrinsic sympathomimetic activity
ITP Idiopathic thrombocytopenia purpura
IUD Intrauterine device
IV Intravenous
IVC Inferior vena cava
IVP Intravenous pyelogram
K^+ Potassium ion
KNCQ Neuronal potassium channels
K_D Dissociation constant
kDa Kilodalton
Kg, kg Kilogram
KGD Lysine-glycine-aspartic acid sequence
Kir Inwardly rectifying K^+ channels
L Liter

L	Long-lasting current
L_1, L_2, ...	First lumbar vertebrae, second lumbar vertebrae
LAD	Left anterior descending (coronary artery)
LAK	Lymphokine-activated killer (cell)
LAP	Laparotomy
LAP	Left atrial pressure
LAP	Leucine amino peptidase
LAP	Leukocyte alkaline phosphatase
lat	Lateral
lb	Pound
LBBB	Left bundle branch block
LC	Locus coeruleus
LD_{50}	Median lethal dose
LDH	Lactic dehydrogenase
LDL	Low-density lipoprotein
L-dopa	Levodopa
LFA-1	Leukocyte function antigen-1
LGV	Lymphogranuloma venereum
LH	Luteinizing hormone
LHRH	Luteinizing hormone-releasing hormone
Li^+	Lithium ion
liq	Aqueous solution
LJP	Localized juvenile periodontitis
LMWH	Low-molecular-weight heparin
LNAT	Large neutral amino acid transporter
LPH	Lipotropic pituitary hormone
LR	Lactated Ringer's solution
LRRK2	Leucine-rich repeat kinase 2
LSD	Lysergic acid diethylamide
LT	Leukotriene
LTB4	Leukotriene B4
LV	Left ventricle
LVAD	Left ventricular assist device
LVH	Left ventricular hypertrophy
M	Muscarinic receptor (protein)
m	meter
Mab	Monoclonal antibody
MAC	Minimum alveolar concentration
MAO	Monoamine oxidase
MAOI	Monoamine oxidase inhibitor
MAP	Mean arterial blood pressure
MAPK or MAP kinase	Mitogen-activated protein kinase
mcg, µg	Microgram
MCH	Mean corpuscular hemoglobin
MCHC	Mean corpuscular hemoglobin concentration
mChR	Muscarinic cholinergic receptor
MCP-1	Monocyte chemoattractive protein-1
m-CPP	*m*-Chlorophenylpiperazine
M-CSF	Monocyte/macrophage colony-stimulating factor
MCV	Mean corpuscular volume
MD	Muscular dystrophy
MDD	Major depressive disorder
MDMA	3,4-Methylenedioxymethamphetamine
MDP	Maximum diastolic potential
MDR	Multidrug resistant protein
MDR-1	Multidrug resistance protein-1
MDS	Myelodysplastic syndrome
MEA	Multiple endocrine adenoma syndrome
meds	Medications/medicine
MEOS	Microsomal enzyme oxidation system
MEPP	Miniature end plate potential
mEq	Milliequivalent
MFP	Sodium monofluorophosphate
MG	Myasthenia gravis
mg	Milligram
Mg^{++}	Magnesium ion
MGluR	Metabotropic glutamate receptor
MH	Malignant hyperthermia
MHC	Major histocompatibility gene complex
MHPG	3-Methoxy-4-hydroxyphenylglycol
MI	Myocardial infarction
MIC	Minimum inhibitory concentration
MIT	Monoiodotyrosine
MKP-1	Mitogen-activated protein kinase phosphatase-1
µL	Microliter
mL	Milliliter
MLC	Minimum lethal concentration
MLCK	Myosin light-chain kinase
MLKS (resistance)	Macrolide, lincosamide, ketolide, streptogramin
MLS_B	Macrolide-lincosamide-streptogramin B (aggregate gene)
mm	Millimeter
MMPI	Matrix metalloprotease inhibitor
MOPP	Mechlorethamine, Oncovin (vincristine), procarbazine, prednisone (regimen)
MPP^+	1-Methyl-4-phenylpyridinium
MPTP	1-Methyl-4-phenyl-1,2,3,6-tetrahydropyridine
MRCoNS	Methicillin-resistant coagulase-negative staphylococci
MRD	Maximum recommended dose
MRI	Magnetic resonance imaging
MRP	Multidrug resistance-associated protein
MRSA	Methicillin-resistant *Staphylococcus aureus*
MS	Morphine sulfate
MS	Multiple sclerosis
MSSA	Methicillin-sensitive *Staphylococcus aureus*
MTIC	Monomethyl 5-triazinoimidazole carboxamide
MTTP	Microsomal triglyceride transfer protein
MW	Molecular weight
N	Nicotinic
N&V	Nausea and vomiting
N/A	Not applicable
N_2O	Nitrous oxide
Na^+	Sodium ion
Na^+,K^+-ATPase	Na^+,K^+-activated adenosine triphosphatase
NAD (NADH)	Nicotinamide adenine dinucleotide
NADPH	Nicotinamide adenine dinucleotide phosphate
NAM	N-acetylmuramic acid
NAPA	N-acetylprocainamide
NAPQI	N-acetyl-*p*-benzoquinoneimine

NCCAM	National Center for Complementary and Alternative Medicine
NCCLS	National Committee for Clinical Laboratory Standards
NCEP	National Cholesterol Education Program
NCX	Na^+-Ca^{++} exchanger
NDA	New Drug Application
NE	Norepinephrine
NED	Normal equivalent deviation units
neg	Negative
NET	Nasoendotracheal
NET	Norepinephrine transporter
NF	National Formulary
NF-ATc	Cytoplasmic component of nuclear factor of activated T cells
NF-ATn	Nuclear component of nuclear factor of activated T cells
NF-κB	Nuclear factor (κB)
NHANES	National Health and Nutrition Examination Survey
NHL	Non-Hodgkin lymphoma
NHLBI	National Heart, Lung, and Blood Institute
NIDDM	Non-insulin-dependent diabetes mellitus
NK	Natural killer (cell)
NK	Neurokinin
N_M	Nicotinic receptor on neuromuscular junction
NMDA	N-methyl-D-aspartate
NME	New molecular entity
NMR	Nuclear magnetic resonance
NMS	Neuroleptic malignant syndrome
N_N	Nicotinic (receptor), nerve type
NNT	Number needed to treat
NO	Nitric oxide
noc	Night
NOS	Nitric acid synthetase (or synthase)
NPH (insulin)	Neutral protamine Hagedorn
NPI	National Provider Identifier
NPN	Nonprotein nitrogen
NPO	Nothing by mouth
NPT-1	Na^+/phosphate transporter-1
NPY	Neuropeptide Y
NRM	Nucleus raphe magnus
NSAID	Nonsteroidal antiinflammatory drug
NSCLC	Non-small cell lung cancer
NSILA	Nonsuppressible insulin-like activity
NTG	Nitroglycerin
NTS	Nucleus tractus solitarius
NVDC	Nausea, vomiting, diarrhea, constipation
NYHA	New York Heart Association
O_2	Oxygen
O_3	Ozone
OA	Osteoarthritis
OAT	Organic anion transporter
OATP	Organic anion-transporting polypeptide
OB	Obstetrics
OBRA	Omnibus Budget Reconciliation Act
OCT	Organic cation transporter
OD	Overdose
oint	Ointment
OM	Otitis media
OmpF	Outer membrane protein F (*E. coli*)
ONJ	Osteonecrosis of the jaw
OR	Operating room
ORL	Opioid receptor-like
ORN	Osteoradionecrosis
OSHA	Occupational Safety and Health Administration
OT	Occupational therapy
OTC	Over-the-counter
p	Para
PABA	*p*-Aminobenzoic acid
PAC	Premature atrial contraction
$PaCO_2$	Partial pressure of carbon dioxide in arterial blood
PAE	Post-antibiotic effect
PAF	Platelet-activating factor
PAG	Periaqueductal gray matter
PAI-1	Plasminogen activator inhibitor type 1
PALC	Post-antibiotic leukocyte effect
PALS	Pediatric advance life support
PaO_2	Partial pressure of oxygen in arterial blood
PAR	Protease-activated receptor
PAS	*p*-Aminosalicylic acid
PAT	Paroxysmal atrial tachycardia (now usually said SVT)
PBI	Protein-bound iodine
PBP	Penicillin-binding protein
pc	After meals (post cibum)
PCA	Patient-controlled analgesia
PCP	Phencyclidine
PCP	*Pneumocystis carinii* (now *jiroveci*) pneumonia
PCSK9	Proprotein convertase subtilisin/kexin type 9 (important in LDL receptor disposition)
PDGF	Platelet-derived growth factor
PDR	*Physician's Desk Reference*
PDUFA	Prescription Drug User Fee Act
PEG	Polyethylene glycol
PEG-MGDF	Pegylated megakaryocyte growth and development factor
per	By/through
PET	Positron emission tomography
P-F	Phosphofluoride linkage
PF-3	Platelet factor 3
PFC	Perfluorocarbon
PG	Prostaglandin
PGG_2, PGH_2	Prostaglandin endoperoxides
PGI_2	Prostacyclin
pH	Negative log of the hydrogen ion concentration
PI	Principal investigator
PID	Pelvic inflammatory disease
PIGR	Polymeric immunoglobulin receptor
PIP_2	Phosphatidylinositol 4-5-bisphosphate
pK_a	Negative log of the ionization constant of an acid
PKU	Phenylketonuria
PLC	Phospholipase C
PLO	Pleuronic lecithin organogel
PMC	Pseudomembranous colitis
PMN	Polymorphonuclear (leukocyte)

PNMT	Phenylethanolamine-N-methyltransferase
po	By mouth (per os)
PO/IM	Oral/intramuscular potency ratio
PPARs	Peroxisomal proliferators-activated receptors
PPI	Proton pump inhibitor
ppm	Parts per million
PRH	Prolactin-releasing hormone
prn	Pro re nata (as needed)
PRON	Postradiation osteonecrosis
PSI, psi	Pounds per square inch
PT	Prothrombin time
PT	Physical therapy
pt	Patient
PTH	Parathyroid hormone
PTT	Partial thromboplastin time
PUD	Peptic ulcer disease
PUFA	Polyunsaturated fatty acids
ω-3 PUFA	Omega-3 polyunsaturated fatty acid
pulv	Powder
PUVA	Psoralen plus ultraviolet A
q	Every (quaque)
q.s.	Quantity sufficient
q2 (3, 4, …) d.	Every 2 (3, 4, …) days
q2 (3, 4, …) h.	Every 2 (3, 4, …) hours
RA	Rheumatoid arthritis
RAI	Radioactive iodine
RANK	Receptor activator of nuclear factor Kappa-B
RANKL	RANK ligand
RAR	Retinoid acid receptor
RBC	Red blood count
RDS	Respiratory distress syndrome
reg	Regular
REM	Rapid eye movement (sleep)
RF	Rheumatic fever
RGD	Arginine-glycine-aspartic acid sequence
RH	Releasing hormone
Rh	Rhesus factor
RHD	Rheumatic heart disease
RNA	Ribonucleic acid
RNP	Ribonucleoprotein
ROC	Receptor-operated channel
ROS	Reactive oxygen species
RSV	Respiratory syncytial virus
RVM	Rostroventral medulla
R_x (or Rx)	Prescription
RXR	Retinoid X receptor
RyR	Ryanodine receptor
S	Svedberg unit
S_1, S_2, S_3	First, second, and third sacral vertebrae
S_1, S_2, S_3, S_4	Systolic heart sounds
SA	Sinoatrial (node)
SaO_2	Saturation of oxygen in arterial blood
SAR	Structure–activity relationship
SBE	Subacute bacterial endocarditis
SC	Subcutaneous
SCF	Stem cell factor
SD	Standard deviation
SEM	Standard error of the mean, or scanning electron microscope
SERCA	Sarcoplasmic endoplasmic reticulum Ca^{++}-ATPase
SERM	Selective estrogen receptor modulator
SERT	Serotonin transporter
SGLT2	Sodium-glucose co-transporter 2
SGOT	Serum glutamic-oxaloacetic transaminase (now AST)
SGPT	Serum glutamic-pyruvic transaminase (now ALT)
SIADH	Syndrome of inappropriate antidiuretic hormone secretion
SIF	Small, intensely fluorescent (cell)
Sig	Let it be labeled
SK	Streptokinase
SKF 525A	Proadifen
SLC	Solute carrier
SLE	Systemic lupus erythematosus
SLUD	Salivation, lacrimation, urination, defecation
SNARE (complex)	Synaptobrevin, syntaxin, SNAP-25
SNC	Substantia nigra pars compacta
SNP	Single nucleotide polymorphism
SNRI	Serotonin norepinephrine reuptake inhibitor
SNS	Sympathetic nervous system
SO_2	Sulfur dioxide
sol	Solution
SP	Substance P
sp gr	Specific gravity
SQ (or SC)	Subcutaneous
SR	Sarcoplasmic reticulum
SRC-1	Steroid receptor coactivator-1
SRS-A	Slow-reacting substance of anaphylaxis (leukotrienes)
SSRI	Selective serotonin reuptake inhibitor
STAT	Signal transducers and activators of transcription
STAT	Immediately (statum)/at once
STD	Sexually transmitted disease
STD	Standard
supp	Suppository
SV2	Synaptic plasma membrane protein
SVT	Supraventricular tachycardia
syr	Syrup
T	Temperature
T&A	Tonsillectomy and adenoidectomy
T_1, $T_{2, \ldots}$	Thoracic vertebrae first, second, …
$T_{½}$	Half-life, half-time
T_3	Triiodothyronine, liothyronine
T_4	Tetraiodothyronine/thyroxine/levothyroxine
tab	Tablet
TALH	Thick ascending limb of the loop of Henle
TB	Tuberculosis
TBG	Thyroid-binding globulin
TCA	Tricyclic antidepressant
TCDD	Dioxin
TCR	T-cell antigen receptor
TD_{50}	Median toxic dose
TEA	Tetraethylammonium
TF	Tissue factor
TFPI	Tissue factor pathway inhibitor
TGF-γ	Transforming growth factor-γ
THC	Tetrahydrocannabinol
THO	Activated T cells that have yet to differentiate

TI Therapeutic index
TIA Transient ischemic attack
TIBC Total iron-binding capacity
tid Three times a day
TM Transmembrane domain
TM Tympanic membrane
TM1 Transmembrane domain 1
TMD Temporomandibular disorder
TMD Transmembrane domain
TMJ Temporomandibular joint
TNF Tumor necrosis factor
TNF-α Tumor necrosis factor-α
TO Telephone order
TOA Tubo-ovarian abscess
TOF Tetralogy of Fallot
t-PA Tissue-type plasminogen activator
TPMT Thiopurine S-methyltransferase
TPN Total parenteral nutrition
TPO Thrombopoietin
TPR Total peripheral resistance
tr Tincture
TRH Thyrotropin-releasing hormone
TRP Transient receptor potential (channels)
TRPV1 Transient receptor potential vanilloid receptor 1
tRNA Transfer RNA
trt Treatment
TSH Thyroid-stimulating hormone; thyrotropin
TT Thrombin time
Tx Treatment, therapy
TXA_2 Thromboxane A_2
U Uptake
UA Urinalysis
UC Uterine contraction
UCHD, UCD Usual childhood diseases
UE Upper extremity
UGI Upper gastrointestinal
UGT Uridine diphosphate glucuronosyltransferase
Unit (formerly IU) International unit
u-PA Urokinase plasminogen activator
UPDRS Unified Parkinson Disease Rating Scale
USAN United States Adopted Name
USANC United States Adopted Name Council
USP United States Pharmacopeia
USPDI United States Pharmacopeia Dispensing Information
UTI Urinary tract infection
UV Ultraviolet
V Fib Ventricular fibrillation
V_d Volume of distribution
VD Venereal disease
V_D/V_T Physiologic dead space in percent of tidal volume
VEGF Vascular endothelial growth factor
VF Ventricular fibrillation
VGS Viridans group streptococci
VIP Vasoactive intestinal peptide
VIPPS Verified Internet Pharmacy Practices Site
VISA Vancomycin-intermediate-resistant *Staphylococcus aureus*
viz Namely
VKOR Vitamin K epoxide reductase
VLDL Very low-density lipoprotein
VMA Vanillylmandelic acid
vol Volume
VRE Vancomycin-resistant enterococci
VRG Vessel-rich group
vs Versus
VT Ventricular fibrillation
vWD von Willebrand disease
vWf von Willebrand factor
VZV Varicella-zoster virus
WBC White blood cell, leukocyte count
WHO World Health Organization
wt Weight
y/o, yo, yrs Years old

INDEX

Note: Page numbers followed by *f* indicate figures, *t* indicate tables and *b* indicate boxes.

G

M